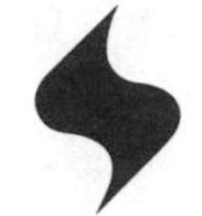

Stedman's

RADIOLOGY WORDS

THIRD EDITION

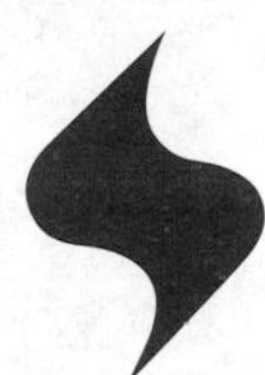

Stedman's RADIOLOGY WORDS

THIRD EDITION

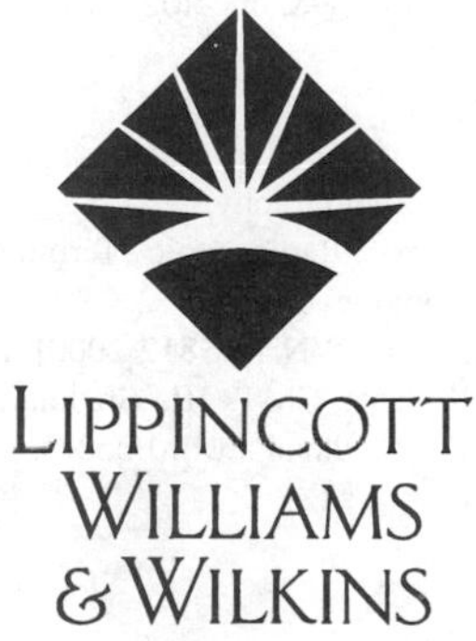

LIPPINCOTT WILLIAMS & WILKINS

Series Editor: Beverly J. Wolpert
Associate Managing Editor: William A. Howard
Art Direction: Jonathan Dimes
Art Coordinator: Jennifer Clements
Production Manager: Tricia Smith
Typesetter: Peirce Graphic Services, Inc.
Printer & Binder: Victor Graphics

351 West Camden Street
Baltimore, MD 21201-2436

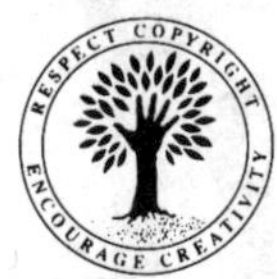

Printed in the United States of America

Third Edition, 2000

Library of Congress Cataloging-in-Publication Data

01 02 03
3 4 5 6 7 8 9 10

Library of Congress Cataloging-in-Publication Data

Stedman's radiology words.--3rd ed.
p. ; cm. -- (Stedman's word book series)
Editor: Kathryn Mason.
Rev. ed. of part of: Stedman's radiology & oncology words. 2nd ed. c1995.
Includes bibliographical references.
ISBN 0-7817-2653-0
1. Radiology--Terminology. 2. Radiography, Medical--Terminology. 3. Diagnosis, Radioscopic--Terminology. [DNLM: 1. Radiology--Terminology--English. 2. Radiography--Terminology--English. WN 15 S812 2000] I. Title: Radiology words. II. Mason, Kathryn, CMT. III. Stedman's radiology & oncology words. IV. Stedman's word books.
RC78.A3 S74 2000
616.07'57'014--dc21

00-064001

Contents

Acknowledgments

An important part of our editorial process is the involvement of medical transcriptionists—as advisors, reviewers and/or editors.

We extend special thanks to Kathryn Mason, CMT, for editing the contents of this new edition and to Martha Richards, RRA, for reviewing, researching, and resolving many difficult content questions. We also extend special thanks to Patricia L. White, CMT, and to Sandi Alvarez for performing final prepublication reviews.

Thanks as well to to our MT Editorial Advisory Board members, including Cheryl Bennett, CMT; Mary Kathryn Murphy; Peg Nelson, CMT; Diana Rezac, CMT; Suzanne Taubert, CMT; and Jenifer Walker, MA. These medical transcriptionists and medical language specialists served as important contributors, editors, and advisors.

Other important contributors to this edition include Kay Deering, who focused on the appendix sections, and Jeanne Bock; Marty Cantu; Janice Deal; Shemah Fletcher; Kathy Hess; Darcy Johnson; Robin Koza; Helen Littrell; and Déborah Wiggins.

Barb Ferretti played an integral role in the process by reviewing the content files for format, updating the database, and providing a final quality check.

As with all our *Stedman's* word references, this resource incorporates the suggestions and expertise of our many contacts in the medical transcriptionist community. Thanks to all of our advisory board participants, reviewers, and editors; AAMT meeting attendees; and others who have written us with requests and comments—keep talking, and we'll keep listening.

Acknowledgments

Editor's Preface

Radiology encompasses not only diagnostic but also therapeutic techniques, crossing over a wide range of specialties. We transcribe radiologic terms on every imaginable occasion, not just for the radiologist. From the emergency room physician to the neurologist to the family practitioner, doctors routinely dictate results of imaging studies. Almost every specialty relies on radiologic imaging. A current reference covering terms from simple anatomy to complex equipment and the bewildering array of vascular, nuclear, and ultrasonographic techniques in between is a necessary and fundamental resource in every medical transcriptionist's library.

In this edition, you will find that radiology has been separated from oncology and the other specialties included in the last edition. When we began compiling the third edition, we started with the database of terms from the second edition and added new terms culled from a wide variety of clinical texts, journals, CD-ROM references, and websites. We also knew we wanted to include more comprehensive anatomic illustrations.

We ended up with such a large database of terms that it was necessary to break radiology and oncology into separate volumes. Careful pruning of obsolete or irrelevant terms and redundancies, meticulous research to rectify style discrepancies, and numerous editorial passes left us with the most accurate and relevant radiology reference we could create. This edition includes diagnostic and interventional radiology; abdominal, chest, gastrointestinal, genitourinary and skeletal imaging; and mammography, CT, MRI, neuroradiology, nuclear medicine, and ultrasonographic terms, all thoroughly cross-referenced in one exhaustive volume.

Throughout my association with Stedman's, I have been continually impressed not only that they are willing to listen, but that they actually seek out the opinions and suggestions of the medical transcriptionists who use their references. I can attest to the fact that at the core of each of their references are the ideas, vision, and research of countless MTs. It is truly a team effort to put together a reference such as this, and I am privileged to be a part of it.

Kathryn Mason, CMT

Publisher's Preface

Stedman's Radiology Words, Third Edition offers an authoritative assurance of quality and exactness to the wordsmiths of the healthcare professions—medical transcriptionists, medical editors and copyeditors, health information management personnel, court reporters, and the many other users and producers of medical documentation.

We received many requests for updates to *Stedman's Radiology & Oncology Words, Second Edition*. As the requests continued to accumulate, we realized that medical language professionals needed a current, comprehensive reference for radiology. We also realized that the terminology had expanded to the point that the terms for both radiology and oncology would no longer fit within the same binding; therefore, we developed separate new editions for each.

In *Stedman's Radiology Words, Third Edition,* users will find thousands of words encompassing diagnostic, therapeutic, and interventional radiology; abdominal, chest, gastrointestinal, genitourinary and skeletal imaging; mammography, CT, MRI, neuroradiology, nuclear medicine, and ultrasonographic terms; and related drugs. Users will also find terms for protocols, diagnostic and therapeutic procedures, new techniques, and lab tests, as well as equipment names, and abbreviations with their expansions. The appendix sections provide anatomical illustrations with useful captions and labels, contrast media, sample reports, and common terms by procedure.

This compilation of more than 70,000 entries, fully cross-indexed for quick access, was built from a base vocabulary of approximately 50,000 medical words, phrases, abbreviations and acronyms. The extensive A-Z list was developed from the database of *Stedman's Medical Dictionary, 27th Edition,* and supplemented by terminology found in current medical literature (please see list of References on page xvi).

We at Lippincott Williams & Wilkins strive to provide you with the most up-to-date and accurate word references available. Your use of this word book will prompt new editions, which we will publish as often as updates and revisions justify. We welcome your suggestions for improvements, changes, corrections, and additions—whatever will make this *Stedman's* product more useful to you. Please complete the postpaid card at the back of this book, and send your recommendations care of "Stedman's" at Lippincott Williams & Wilkins.

Explanatory Notes

Medical transcription is an art as well as a science. Both approaches are needed to correctly interpret the dictation of a physician, whose language is a product of education, training, and experience. This variety in medical language means that there are several acceptable ways to express certain terms, including jargon. *Stedman's Radiology Words, Third Edition,* provides variant spellings and phrasings for many terms. These elements, in addition to complete cross-indexing, make *Stedman's Radiology Words, Third Edition,* a valuable resource for determining the validity of terms as they are encountered.

Alphabetical Organization

Alphabetization of main entries is letter by letter as spelled, ignoring punctuation, spaces, prefixed numbers, Greek letters, or other characters. For example:

γ-aminobutyric acid (GABA)
aminocaproic acid
ε-aminocaproic acid (EACA)
aminoglycoside
aminophylline
4-aminoquinoline

In subentry alphabetization, the abbreviated singular form or the spelled-out plural form of the noun main entry word is ignored.

Format and Style

All main entries are in **boldface** to expedite locating a sought-after term, to enhance distinction between main entries and subentries, and to relieve the textual density of the pages.

Irregular plurals and variant spellings are shown on the same line as the singular or preferred form of the word. For example:

incus, pl. incudes

hygroma, hydroma

Hyphenation

As a rule of style, multiple eponyms (e.g., Mears-Rubash approach) are hyphenated. Also, hyphens have been added between a manufacturer and one or more eponyms (e.g., Vital-Metzenbaum dissecting scissors). Please note that in many cases, hyphenation is a question of style, not of accuracy, and thus is a matter of choice.

Possessives

Possessive forms have been dropped in this reference for the sake of consistency and conformance with the guidelines of the American Association for Medical Transcription (AAMT) and other groups. Please note, however, that in many cases, retaining the possessive, like hyphenating, is a question of style, not of accuracy, and thus is a matter of choice. To form the possessive of a word, simply add the apostrophe or apostrophe "s" to the end of the word.

Cross-indexing

The word list is in an index-like main entry-subentry format that contains two combined alphabetical listings:

(1) A *noun* main entry-subentry organization, which is typical of the A-Z section of medical dictionaries like *Stedman's:*

plaque
 arterial p.
 p. cleaving

tabes
 burned-out t.
 t. dorsalis

(2) An *adjective* main entry-subentry organization, which lists words and phrases as you hear them. The main entries are the adjectives or modifiers in a multi-word term. The subentries are the nouns around which the terms are constructed and to which the adjectives or modifiers pertain:

direct
 d. ray
 d. visualization

tagged
 t. atom
 radioactively t.

This format provides the user with more than one way to locate and identify a multi-word term. For example:

duct	**main**
main pancreatic d.	m. pancreatic duct
palate	**high**
high arched p.	h. arched palate

It also allows the user to see together all terms that contain a particular descriptor, as well as all types, kinds, or variations of a noun entity. For example:

intussusception	**line**
appendiceal i.	absence of innominate l.
i. target sign	gaussian l.
i. of vein	l. shadow

Wherever possible, abbreviations are separately defined and cross-referenced. For example:

MALT
mucosa-associated lymphoid tissue

mucosa-associated
m.-a. lymphoid tissue (MALT)

tissue
mucosa-associated lymphoid t. (MALT)

References

In addition to the manufacturers' literature we gather at various medical meetings, scientific reports from hospitals, and the lists of our MT Editorial Advisory Board members (from their daily transcription work), we used the following sources for new terms in *Stedman's Radiology Words, Third Edition:*

Books

Billups NF, Billups SM. The American Drug Index 1999, 43rd Edition. St. Louis: Facts & Comparisons, 1999.

Chew FS, Maldjian C, Leffler SG. Musculoskeletal Imaging: A Teaching File. Baltimore: Lippincott Williams & Wilkins, 1999.

Dahnert WF. Dahnert's Radiology Review Manual, Fourth Edition. Baltimore: Lippincott Williams & Wilkins, 1999.

Lance LL. 2000 Quick Look Drug Book. Baltimore: Lippincott Williams & Wilkins, 2000.

The Merck Manual, 16th Edition. Rahway, NJ: Merck Research Laboratories, 1992.

Perez CA, Brady LW, eds. Principles and Practice of Radiation Oncology, Third Edition. Philadelphia: Lippincott-Raven, 1997.

Pittman SC. Radiology Imaging Words and Phrases. Modesto: Health Professions Institute, 1997.

Pyle V. Current Medical Terminology, 7th Edition. Modesto: Health Professions Institute, 1998.

Sloane SB. A Word Book in Radiology: With Anatomic Plates and Tables. Philadelphia: Saunders, 1988.

Stedman's Medical Dictionary, 27th Edition. Baltimore: Lippincott Williams & Wilkins, 2000.

Tessier C. The AAMT Book of Style. Modesto: AAMT, 1995.

Journals

Applied Radiology. Ocean, NJ: Anderson Publishing, 1998–1999.

Diagnostic Imaging. San Francisco: Miller Freeman, 1996–1999.

Emergency Radiology. Berlin: Springer-Verlag, 1996–1999.

Internal Medicine. Montvale, NJ: Medical Economics, 1995–1999.

Journal of Magnetic Resonance Imaging. Baltimore: Lippincott Williams & Wilkins/ International Society for Magnetic Resonance in Medicine, 1998.

The Latest Word. Philadelphia: Saunders, 1996–1999.

Magnetic Resonance in Medicine. Wiley: New York. 1997.

MT Monthly. Gladstone, MO: Computer Systems Management, 1996–1999.

Perspectives on the Medical Transcription Profession. Modesto: Health Professions Institute, 1993–1999.

RadioGraphics. Oak Brook, IL: Radiological Society of North America, 1998–1999.

Radiologic Technology. Albuquerque: American Society of Radiologic Technologists. 1996–999.

The Radiologist. Baltimore: Lippincott Williams & Wilkins, 1998–1999.

Radiology. Oak Brook, IL: Radiological Society of North America, 1998–1999.

CDs

Atlas SW, ed. MRI of the Brain and Spine on CD-ROM, Second Edition. Philadelphia: Lippincott Williams & Wilkins, 1997.

Baum S, ed. Abrams' Angiography, Fourth Edition, on CD-ROM. Philadelphia: Lippincott Williams & Wilkins, 1998.

Bradley Jr. WG, Crues III JV, eds. MRI of the Central Nervous System, Mastering MRI: An Educational and Reference Series on CD-ROM. Baltimore: Lippincott Williams & Wilkins, 1996.

Clinical Reference Library on CD-ROM, Version 1999.4. Hudson, OH: Lexi-Comp, 1999.

Hricak H, Lipson S. Abdominal Imaging: Genitourinary Radiology. Baltimore: Lippincott Williams & Wilkins, 1997.

Jeffrey Jr. RB, ed. Abdominal and Pelvic Ultrasound on CD-ROM with CT and MR Correlation. Baltimore: Lippincott Williams & Wilkins, 1995.

Johnson KA, Becker JA. The Whole Brain Atlas CD-ROM. Baltimore: Lippincott Williams & Wilkins, 1999.

Kopans DB. Breast Imaging, Second Edition on CD-ROM. Baltimore: Lippincott Williams & Wilkins, 1998.

Lee JKT, Sagel SS, Stanley RJ, Heiken JP, eds. Computed Body Tomography with MRI Correlation. Baltimore: Lippincott Williams & Wilkins, 1998.

McGahan JP, Goldberg BB. Diagnostic Ultrasound: A Logical Approach. Baltimore: Lippincott Williams & Wilkins, 1997.

Steinbach LS. Musculoskeletal Imaging, CD-ROM. Baltimore: Lippincott Williams & Wilkins, 1999.

Stoller DW. Magnetic Resonance Imaging in Orthopaedics & Sports Medicine. Baltimore: Lippincott Williams & Wilkins, 1997.

Webb WR, ed. High-Resolution Lung CT. Baltimore: Lippincott Williams & Wilkins, 2000.

Websites

http://hpisum.com

http://mtdaily.com

http://www.mtdesk.com

A
A. phenomenon
A. point
A. ring of esophagus
A1-A5 segments of anterior cerebral artery
AA
ascending aorta
AAA
abdominal aortic aneurysm
AAI
atrial inhibited
AAI mode
AAI rate-responsive mode
AAOS acetabular abnormalities classification
Aaron sign
abandonment
mode a.
abapical pole
Abbott artery
Abbreviated Injury Scale
ABC
aneurysmal bone cyst
aortic-brachiocephalic
abdomen
distended a.
flat plate of a.
gasless a.
scaphoid a.
abdominal
a. abscess
a. adenopathy
a. adhesion
a. air collection
a. aorta
a. aorta crescent sign
a. aorta thrombosis
a. aortic aneurysm (AAA)
a. aortic aneurysm rupture
a. aortic artery
a. aortic coarctation
a. aortic plexus
a. aortography
a. apron
a. blunt trauma
a. canal
a. carcinosis
a. cascade
a. cavity
a. collection of fluid
a. contents
a. cystic fetal mass
a. diffuse calcification
a. distention
a. ectopic pregnancy
a. fat
a. fat pad
a. fibromatosis
a. fissure
a. fistula
a. fluid wave
a. football sign
a. gas
a. gas collection
a. girth
a. great vessel
a. heart
a. hemorrhage
a. heterotaxia
a. hysterectomy
a. inflammation
a. irradiation
a. kidney
a. left ventricular assist device (ALVAD)
a. lymph node
a. pain
a. paracentesis
a. pseudotumor
a. raphe
a. ring
a. roentgenography
a. sac
a. series
a. situs inversus
a. situs solitus
a. sonography
a. space
a. splenosis
a. stoma
a. string-of-beads sign
a. strip radiotherapy
a. triangular ligament
a. ultrasound
a. vascular accident
a. vascular calcification
a. view
a. viscera
a. wall calcification
a. wall defect
a. wall desmoid tumor
a. wall hernia
abdominis
rectus a.
abdominopelvic
a. actinomycosis
a. cavity
a. mass
a. viscera

abducens
abducted and externally rotated (ABER)
abduction
a. fracture
a. stress test
abduction-external rotation fracture
abductor
a. digiti quinti (ADQ)
a. digiti quinti muscle
a. hallucis muscle
a. pollicis brevis (APB)
a. pollicis brevis muscle
abductovalgus
hallux a.
abductus
pes a.
ABER
abducted and externally rotated
Abernethy sarcoma
aberrant
a. artery
a. bundle
a. ganglion
a. intrahepatic bile duct
a. pancreas
a. papilla
a. right subclavian artery
a. spleen
a. tissue
a. umbilical stomach
a. vascular channel
a. venous drainage
aberration
intersegmental a.
intraventricular a.
ventricular a.
ABGd imaging agent
ABI
ankle-brachial index
ability
cardiac pumping a.
ablation
percutaneous radiofrequency a.
radiofrequency a. (RFA)
radiofrequency catheter a. (RFCA)
radiopharmaceutical a.
saline-enhanced RF tissue a.
stereotactic a.
total a.
transaortic radiofrequency a.
transapical endocardial a.
transcatheter a.
transseptal radiofrequency a.
ultrasound-guided percutaneous interstitial laser a.
ablative laser therapy
abnormal
a. adherence of placenta
a. bright signal
a. cisterna magna
a. dimensions of cardiac chamber
a. ejection fraction response
a. esophageal fold
a. esophageal peristalsis
a. fold esophagus
a. heart chamber dimension
a. lung pattern
a. ossification
a. peristalsis esophagus
a. placental size
a. position of foot
a. small bowel fold
a. tissue
a. tracer accumulation
a. tracking
a. tubular function
a. umbilical cord attachment
abnormality
accumulation a.
acral a.
akinetic segmental wall motion a.
arch of aorta a.
bony a.
bronchocentric a.
bulbar a.
caliceal a.
cardiopulmonary a.
congenital a.
cytoarchitectonic a.
D'Antonio classification of acetabular a.
definitive a.
dyskinetic segmental wall motion a.
ectopic wall motion a.
facial a.
fetal a.
figure-of-eight a.
focal limb a.
focal wall motion a.
focal white matter signal a.
frontal plane growth a.
functional a.
gestational sac a.
global wall motion a.
gray matter a.
high-signal a.
hyperkinetic segmental wall motion a.
hypokinetic segmental wall motion a.
ileocecal valve a.
intracranial vascular a.
labeling a.

left ventricular regional wall motion a.
limb reduction a.
migrational a.
mucosal a.
nonpalpable a.
obstructive a.
osseous a.
paraspinal a.
perfusion a.
restrictive a.
rostrocaudal extent signal a.
screening-detected a.
segmental bronchus perfusion a.
snowman a.
soft tissue a.
spinal cord injury without radiographic a. (SCIWORA)
subsegmental perfusion a.
torsional a.
tracer a.
ultrastructural a.
urachal a.
vascular a.
vertebral border a.
vertebral endplate a.
vessel wall a.
wall motion a. (WMA)
white matter a.

abnormally thin skull

aboral direction

abortion
complete a.
missed a.
a. in progress
spontaneous a.

abortive
a. appendicitis
a. neurofibromatosis

abortus

above
a. diaphragm (AD)
a. selected threshold (AST)

above-elbow (AE)

above-elbow amputation

above-knee amputation (AKA)

ABPA
allergic bronchopulmonary aspergillosis

ABR
American Board of Radiology

Abrahams sign

Abrams biopsy needle

abrasion
cortical a.
subperiosteal cortical a.

Abrikosov tumor

abruptio
placenta a.
a. placentae

abruption
placental a.

abrupt vessel closure

abscess
abdominal a.
actinomycotic brain a.
anaerobic lung a.
anchovy paste a.
annular a.
aortic annulus a.
appendiceal a.
arthrifluent a.
Aspergillus cerebral a.
bone a.
brain a.
breast a.
Brodie metaphyseal a.
cerebral a.
chocolate sauce a.
chronic breast a.
cold breast a.
cold spine a.
collar-button a.
cuff a.
daughter a.
deep interloop a.
deep pelvic a.
diverticular a.
encapsulated brain a.
enteroperitoneal a.
epidural a.
extradural a.
frontal a.
gallbladder wall a.
granulomatous brain a.
growth plate a.
hepatic a.
horseshoe a.
iliac fossa a.
interloop a.
intermesenteric a.
intersphincteric a.
intraabdominal a.
intradural a.
intrahepatic a.

NOTES

abscess *(continued)*
intramesenteric a.
intraosseous a.
intraperitoneal a.
intrascrotal a.
ischiorectal a.
kidney a.
lacunar a.
left upper quadrant a.
liver a.
lung a.
mediastinal a.
metaphyseal a.
metastatic a.
midpalmar a.
orbital a.
ovarian a.
Paget a.
pancreatic a.
paracolic a.
parapharyngeal a.
pararectal a.
pararenal a.
paraspinal a.
parotid a.
partial pericardial a.
pelvic a.
perianal a.
periappendiceal a.
pericecal a.
pericholecystic a.
pericolic a.
pericolonic a.
perinephric a.
perirenal a.
pharyngeal a.
phoenix a.
Pott a.
premasseteric space a.
prostate a.
psoas a.
pulmonary a.
pyogenic brain a.
pyogenic liver a.
renal a.
retropharyngeal a.
scrotal a.
soft tissue a.
space of Retzius a.
spinal epidural a. (SEA)
splenic a.
sternal a.
subaponeurotic a.
subdiaphragmatic a.
subdural a.
subgaleal a.
subhepatic a.
subperiosteal a.
subphrenic a.
subungual a.
testicular a.
thecal a.
thenar space a.
thyroid a.
tuboovarian a.
ventral epidural a.

abscessogram

abscission needle

abscopal
a. effect

abscopalt

absence
congenital pericardial a.
a. of innominate line
limb a.
a. of outer end of clavicle
partial pericardial a.
psoas a.
a. seizure
a. of spleen
a. of uptake

absent
a. aortic knob
a. bronchial cartilage
a. diaphragm sign
a. greater sphenoid wing
a. kidney
a. kidney outline
a. kidney sign
a. peripheral vein
a. peristalsis
a. runoff
a. sphenoid wing
a. valve
a. ventricle

absolute
a. artery dimension
a. blood flow
a. curative resection
a. dose intensity (ADI)
a. emission probability
a. ethanol
a. linearity
a. noncurative resection

absolute-peak
a.-p. efficiency
a.-p. efficiency calibration

absorbed
a. dose (AD)
a. dose range

absorbent gland

absorptiometer
single-energy x-ray a. (SXA)

absorptiometry
dual-energy x-ray a. (DEXA, DXA)

dual-photon a. (DPA)
single-photon a. (SPA)

absorption
a. atelectasis
bone a.
bone radiation a.
a. cavity
a. coefficient
electromagnetic a.
laser energy a.
a. line
photoelectric a.
radiofrequency a.
radioiron oral a.
a. of radionuclide
a. unsharpness
a. x-ray spectrum

abut

abutment

abutting

AC
aortic closure

ACA
anterior cerebral artery

Acacia
Skiodan A.

ACAD
atherosclerotic carotid artery disease

acalculia

acalculous cholecystitis

acanthiomeatal line

acanthopelvis

acanthosis nigricans

acardia

ACAT
automated computed axial tomography

ACBE
air-contrast barium enema

accelerated
a. acute kidney rejection
a. atherosclerosis
a. fractionation
a. hyperfractionated radiation therapy
a. interstitial pneumonia
a. particle
a. peristalsis
a. phase
a. phase gain

acceleration
fetal growth a.
growth a.
a. map
a. time

accelerator
alpha particle a.
Bevatron a.
dual-energy linear a.
electron linear a.
a. factor
heavy ion medical a. in Chiba (HIMAC)
high-energy bent-beam linear a.
linear a. (LINAC)
a. mass spectrometry (AMS)
Mevatron 74 linear a.
microtron a.
particle a.
Philips linear a.
racetrack microtron a.
Siemens Mevatron 74 linear a.
University of Florida linear a.
Varian a.

accentuation
a. of markings
paramagnetic enhancement a.

accessory
a. adhesion molecule
a. atlantoaxial ligament
a. blood supply
a. breast
a. canal
a. cephalic vein
a. cusp
a. diaphragm
a. digit
a. duct of Santorini
a. fissure
a. hemiazygos vein
a. hemidiaphragm
a. hepatic duct
a. hepatic vein
a. lobe
a. lymph node
a. middle cerebral artery
a. multangular bone
a. muscle
a. nasal cartilage
a. navicular bone
a. nerve
a. organ
a. ossicle
a. ossification center
a. pancreas

NOTES

accessory *(continued)*
a. pancreatic duct
a. placenta
a. process
a. renal artery
a. saphenous vein
a. sesamoid bone
a. sign colon
a. sinus
a. spleen
a. thyroid gland
a. tubercle
a. ureteral bud
a. vertebral vein
accident
abdominal vascular a.
cardiovascular a. (CVA)
cerebrovascular a. (CVA)
vascular a.
accidental correction
accompanying vein
accordion
a. fold
a. vertebra
accreta
placenta a.
Accucore II biopsy needle
accuDEXA
a. bone densitometer
a. bone mineral density assessment device
accumulation
a. abnormality
abnormal tracer a.
dependent extracellular fluid a.
fluid a.
a. of gas
nonspecific a.
parenchymal tracer a.
residual urine a.
Thorotrast a.
tracer a.
accumulative phase
AccuProbe
accuracy calibrator
ACD
annihilation coincidence detection
ACE
angiotensin-converting enzyme
ACE inhibition renography
ACE inhibition scintigraphy
Ace-Colles half ring
acervuloma
ace of spades sign
acetabula (*pl. of* acetabulum)
acetabular
a. angle
a. bone
a. cavity
a. cup
a. depth to femoral head diameter (AD/FHD)
a. fossa
a. fracture
a. index
a. labrum
a. notch
a. posterior wall fracture
a. protrusion
a. reconstruction plate
a. residual dysplasia
a. rim fracture
a. roof
a. shell
acetabular-prosthetic interface
acetabuli
protrusio a.
acetabulum, pl. **acetabula**
cartilaginous a.
deep-shelled a.
os a.
weightbearing dome of a.
Y-shaped a.
acetanilidoiminodiacetic acid
acetate
^{11}C a.
manganese a.
medroxyprogesterone a.
octreotide a.
acetazolamide-enhanced SPECT
acetrizoate
meglumine a.
a. sodium
acetrizoic acid
acetylsalicylic acid
ACF
anterior cervical fusion
ACG
apexcardiogram
achalasia
cricopharyngeal a.
a. of esophagus
megaesophagus of a.
primary a.
secondary a.
ureteral a.
vigorous a.
acheiria
achievable
as low as reasonably a. (ALARA)
Achiever balloon dilatation catheter
Achilles
A. bulge sign
A. bursa
A. tendon

A. tendon rupture
A. tendon shortening

Achilles densitometer

Achillis

tendo A.

acholangic biliary cirrhosis

achondrogenesis

achondroplasia

achondroplastic dwarfism

achoresis

acid

acetanilidoiminodiacetic a.
acetrizoic a.
acetylsalicylic a.
ametriodinic a.
amidotrizoic a.
a. aspiration pneumonitis
benzoic a.
beta-oxybutyric a. (BOBA)
butyl iminodiacetic a. (BIDA)
chenodeoxycholic a. (CDCA)
^{11}C-labeled fatty a.
deoxyribonucleic a.
diatrizoic a.
diethylenetriamine pentaacetic a.
diethyl iminodiacetic a. (DIDA)
diisopropyl iminodiacetic a. (DISIDA)
dimethyl iminodiacetic a. (DIDA)
dimethylsuccinic a. (DMSA)
ethylenediaminetetraacetic a. (EDTA)
ethylenediamine tetramethylene phosphoric a. (EDTMP)
flavone acetic a.
fluoro-6-thia-heptadecanoic a.
free fatty a. (FFA)
gadolinium cyclohexanediaminetetraacetic a. (Gd-CDTA)
gadolinium-diethylenetriamine pentaacetic a.
gadolinium ethylenediaminetetraacetic a. (Gd-EDTA)
gadolinium tetraazacyclododecanetetraacetic a. (Gd-DOTA)
gadopentetic a.
glucoheptanoic a. (GHA)
hepatic 2,6-dimethyliminodiacetic a. (HIDA)
hepatoiminodiacetic a. (HIDA)
homovanillic a.
hydroxyindole acetic a.
^{123}I heptadecanoic a.
iminodiacetic a. (IDA)
iobenzamic a.
iobutoic a.
iocarmic a.
iocetamic a.
iodamic a.
iodoalphionic a.
iodopanoic a.
iodoxamic a.
ioglicic a.
ioglycamic a.
iopanoic a.
iophenoxic a.
ioprocemic a.
iopronic a.
iosefamic a.
ioseric a.
iosumetic a.
ioteric a.
iothalamic a.
iotroxic a.
ioxaglic a.
ioxithalamic a.
iozomic a.
ipodic a.
long-chain fatty a.
low-dose folic a.
meclofenamic a.
mefenamic a.
metrizoic a.
nitriloacetic a.
nonesterified fatty a. (NEFA)
okadaic a.
ophenoxic a.
paraaminobenzoic a. (PABA)
paraaminosalicylic a. (PAS)
paraisopropyliminodiacetic a. (PIPIDA)
pentetic a.
a. peptic ulcer
phenoxyacetic a.
polylactic a.
a. reflux
technetium-99m acetanilide iminodiacetic a.
technetium-99m diethylenetriamine penta-acetic a.

NOTES

acid *(continued)*
technetium-99m dimercaptosuccinic a.
a. test
tetraazacyclododecanetetraacetic a.
triiodobenzoic a.
tyropanoic a.
ursodeoxycholic a.
acidophilic
a. adenoma
a. pituitary tumor
acinar
a. adenocarcinoma
a. nodule
a. pancreatic cell carcinoma
a. pattern
a. rosette
a. sarcoidosis
a. tuberculosis
acinarization
acini (*pl. of* acinus)
acinic
a. cell adenocarcinoma
a. cell carcinoma
a. cell tumor
acinous
a. adenoma
a. cell carcinoma
acinus, pl. **acini**
Ackerman criteria for osteomyelitis
Ackrad balloon-bearing catheter
ACL
anterior cruciate ligament
aclasis
diaphyseal a.
tarsoepiphyseal a.
ACM
automated cardiac flow measurement
ACM ultrasound
ACMI ulcer measuring device
ACoA
anterior communicating artery
Acoma scanner
acoprosis
acoprous
acoustic
a. artifact
a. canal
a. crest
a. cyst
a. enhancement
a. gel
a. imaging
a. impedance
a. interface
a. lens
a. meatus
a. nerve
a. nerve sheath tumor
a. neuroma
a. noise
a. papilla
a. pressure
a. pressure amplitude
a. quantification
a. response technology (ART)
a. schwannoma
a. shadowing
a. trauma
a. tubercle
a. velocity
a. vesicle
a. wave
a. window
acousticofacial
a. crest
a. ganglion
AC-PC
anterior commissure-posterior commissure
AC-PC line
AC-PC plane
ACPL
antibody-conjugated paramagnetic liposome
AcQsim CT simulator
acquired
a. acroosteolysis
a. aortic valve stenosis
a. atelectasis
a. bronchiectasis
a. cystic disease of uremia
a. cystic kidney disease
a. epidermoid
a. hepatic cyst
a. hepatocerebral degeneration
a. hydrocephalus
a. ichthyosis
a. immunodeficiency syndrome (AIDS)
a. intestinal lymphangiectasis
a. left ventricle aneurysm
a. megacolon
a. mitral stenosis
a. porencephaly
a. renal cystic disease
a. spinal stenosis
a. tracheobronchomalacia
a. unilateral hyperlucent lung
a. urethral divertculum
acquisition
continuous volumetric a.
data a.
double-helix a.
gradient a.
image a.

interleaved a.
long axis a.
a. matrix
multiple gated a. (MUGA)
multiple overlapping thin-slab a. (MOTSA)
multiple slice a.
multisection multirepetition a.
multislice a.
polarity-altered spectral-selective a. (PASTA)
primary digital a.
reduced a.
segmented k-space a.
sequential image a.
short-axis a.
signal a.
spirometric a.
spoiled gradient-recalled a.
a. technique
a. time
volume a.
a. window

ACR
American College of Radiology
ACR rate
ACR teleradiology standard

acral
a. abnormality

acrania

Acrel ganglion

acridine orange

acridinyl anisidide

acrocephalosyndactyly, acrocephalosyndactylia
Pfeiffer a.
Saethre-Chotzen a.

acrodermatitis enteropathica

acrodysostosis

acrofacial

acrokeratosis

acromegaly

acromelia

acromelic
a. dwarfism
a. dysplasia

acromial
a. angle
a. articular surface
a. bone
a. spur

acromiale
os a.

acromicria

acromioclavicular
a. articulation
a. injury classification
a. joint
a. joint disk
a. joint separation
a. ligament
a. space

acromiocoracoid ligament

acromiohumeral
a. distance
a. interval (AHI)

acromion
hooked a.
a. process

acromutilation

acroosteolysis
acquired a.
familial idiopathic a.

acroosteosclerosis

acropachy
thyroid a.

acropectorovertebral dysplasia

acrosomal vesicle

acrosyndactyly

acrylic microsphere

ACS balloon catheter

Act
Mammography Quality Standards A.

ACTH-producing tumor

actinic
a. granuloma
a. ray
a. reticuloid

actinium
a. emanation

actinomycetes
thermophilic a.

actinomycosis
abdominopelvic a.
retroperitoneal a.

actinomycotic brain abscess

action
phase-specific a.

activate

activated
a. atom
a. partial thromboplastin time

NOTES

activation
a. analysis
a. factor
activation-sequence mapping
active
a. biplanar MR imaging guidance
a. congestion
a. duodenal ulcer
a. emptying fraction
a. hyperemia
a. infiltrate
a. mode
a. osteomyelitis
a. parenchymal disease
a. precordium
activity
a. assessment
bilary excretion bowel a.
blood pool a.
body background a.
bone morphogenetic a.
brain a.
colonic a.
cortical a.
crossover of a.
decreased a.
dihydropyrimidine dehydrogenase a.
electrical a.
increased a.
lung/heart ratio of thallium 201 a.
mast cell-enhancing a.
osteoblastic a.
peak parenchymal a.
peristaltic a.
physiologic high a.
problematic abdominal a.
radiotracer a.
reflux a.
retained cortical a. (RCA)
specific a.
time to peak a.
tracer a.
ventricular ectopic a. (VEA)
ACTR
American Club of Therapeutic Radiologists
acuminata
condyloma urethra a.
papilloma a.
Acuson
A. computed sonography
A. 128EP imager
A. 128EP scanner
A. linear array transducer
A. 5-MHz linear array
A. transvaginal sonography
A. ultrasound
A. ultrasound scanner
A. 128XP ultrasound system
acute
a. abdominal obstruction
a. abdominal series
a. allergic extrinsic alveolitis
a. alveolar hypoperfusion
a. alveolar infiltrate
a. appendicitis
a. atelectasis
a. avulsion fracture
a. central cord syndrome
a. cerebellar hemispheric lesion
a. cerebral infarct imaging
a. cerebrovascular insufficiency
a. cholecystitis
a. compartment syndrome
a. compression triad
a. coronary insufficiency
a. cortical necrosis
a. diffuse bacterial nephritis
a. diffuse interstitial fibrosis
a. disseminated encephalomyelitis (ADEM)
a. diverticulitis
a. eosinophilic pneumonia
a. erosive gastritis (AEG)
a. esophagitis
a. extrinsic allergic alveolitis
a. flank pain
a. focal bacterial nephritis
a. gastroenteritis (AGE)
a. glomerulonephritis
a. heart failure
a. hematogenous osteomyelitis (AHO)
a. hemodynamic overload
a. hemorrhagic leukoencephalitis
a. hepatitis
a. hydrocephalus
a. hydronephrosis
a. interstitial lung disease sign
a. interstitial lung edema
a. interstitial nephritis (AIN)
a. interstitial pneumonia (AIP)
a. interstitial pneumonitis
a. intramural hematoma
a. ischemic brain infarct
a. juvenile cirrhosis
a. laryngotracheobronchitis
a. lethal carditis
a. lymphoblastic lymphoma
a. marginal branch
a. mediastinal widening
a. mesenteric ischemia
a. myelofibrosis
a. myocardial infarct
a. native kidney tubular necrosis

a. neuropathy
a. nonsuppurative ascending cholangitis
a. obstructive cholangitis
a. pancreatitis
a. peptic ulcer
a. phase of inflammation
a. pleurisy
a. pulmonary edema
a. radiation bone marrow syndrome
a. radiation pneumonitis
a. radiation syndrome
a. renal failure (ARF)
a. renal infarct
a. renal transplant rejection
a. renal transplant tubular necrosis
a. renal vein thrombosis
a. respiratory distress syndrome (ARDS)
a. respiratory failure (ARF)
a. retroviral syndrome
a. sclerosing hyaline necrosis (ASHN)
a. sinusitis
a. splenic tumor
a. sprain
a. stretch injury
a. subdural hematoma
a. suppurative ascending cholangitis
a. suppurative pyelonephritis
a. suppurative sialadenitis
a. suppurative thyroiditis
a. testicular torsion
a. thromboembolic pulmonary arterial hypertension
a. traumatic aortic injury (ATAI)
a. tubular necrosis (ATN)
a. vertebra collapse

AcuTect
A. imaging agent

acutely symptomatic scrotum

AD
above diaphragm
absorbed dose
Alzheimer disease
aortic diameter

ADAC gamma camera

adactyly, adactylia

adamantinoma

adamantinomatous craniopharyngioma

Adamkiewicz
arteries of A.
A. artery

Adams-Stokes syndrome

adapted standard mammography unit

adaptive
a. correction
a. hyperplasia
a. hypertrophy

Addison
A. disease
A. plane
A. point
A. syndrome

addressed
regional lymph node cannot be a. (NX)

adducta
coxa a.

adducted thumb

adduction
a. fracture
a. frame
a. to neutral
a. stress

adductor
a. canal
a. hallucis
a. hiatus
a. longus
a. magnus
a. magnus muscle
a. muscle strain
a. pollicis
a. sweep of thumb
a. tubercle

adductus
Bleck classification of metatarsus a.
metatarsus a.
pes a.
true metatarsus a. (TMA)

ADEM
acute disseminated encephalomyelitis

adenectomy

adenitis
mesenteric a.
sclerosing a.

adenocanthoma
endometrial a.

adenocarcinoma
acinar a.

NOTES

adenocarcinoma *(continued)*
acinic cell a.
ampullary a.
bronchiolar a.
cervical a.
colloid a.
cystic a.
distal rectal a. (DRA)
ductal pancreatic a.
duct cell a.
duodenal a.
endometrial secretory a.
exophytic a.
gastrointestinal tract a.
giant cell a.
hepatoid a.
infiltrating a.
intraluminal a.
kidney a.
lung a.
medullary-type a. (MTA)
metastatic a.
a. of Moll
mucinous a.
mucin-producing a.
nonmucinous a.
pancreatic ductal a.
papillary serous a.
poorly differentiated a. (PDA)
renal a.
scirrhous infiltrating a.
secretory a.
serous a.
a. in situ
small bowel a.
stomach a.
ulcerating a.
urinary bladder a.
a. of uterus
vulvar adenoid cystic a.
adenocystic carcinoma
adenofibroma
adenofibromyoma
adenohypophysial
adenohypophysis
adenoid
a. cystic carcinoma parotis
a. cystic lung carcinoma
a. squamous cell carcinoma
a. tumor
adenoleiomyofibroma
adenolipoma
adenoma
acidophilic a.
acinous a.
adnexal a.
adrenal a.
adrenocortical a.
apocrine a.
autonomous thyroid a.
basal cell a.
basophilic brain a.
benign oxyphilic a.
bile duct a. (BDA)
a. of breast
bronchial a.
bronchoalveolar cell a.
Brunner gland a.
carcinoma ex pleomorphic a.
carotid sheath a.
colloid a.
colonic a.
colorectal a.
cortical a.
cutaneous a.
cystic kidney a.
cystic pituitary a.
ductal a.
ectopic parathyroid a.
embryonal a.
eosinophilic brain a.
a. familial polyposis
fetal a.
fibroid a.
a. fibrosum
follicular thyroid a.
Fuchs a.
functioning pituitary a.
gallbladder a.
giant villous a.
glycoprotein-secreting a.
gonadotroph cell a.
gonadotropin-secreting a.
growth hormone-producing a.
hepatic a.
hepatocellular a.
Hürthle cell a.
intraspinal a.
kidney a.
Leydig cell a.
liver cell a.
macrocystic a.
malignant pleomorphic a.
a. malignum
mediastinal a.
microcystic a.
moderately differentiated a.
mucinous a.
nephrogenic bladder a.
a. of nipple
nonfunctioning pituitary a.
nonhyperfunctioning adrenal a.
oncocytic thyroid a.
oxyphilic kidney a.
oxyphilic thyroid a.
pancreatic macrocystic a.

pancreatic microcystic a.
papillary cystic a.
parathyroid a.
parotid pleomorphic a.
Pick tubular a.
pituitary a.
pleomorphic lung a.
polypoid a.
poorly differentiated a.
prostatic a.
proximal tubular a.
renal cortical a.
retrotracheal a.
sebaceous a.
a. sebaceum
sessile a.
small bowel a.
suprasellar a.
sweat duct a.
testicular tubular a.
thyroid a.
thyrotroph cell a.
toxic a.
tubulovillous colon a.
villotubular a.
villous colon a.
villous duodenal a.
villous esophageal a.
well-differentiated a.

adenomatoid
a. malformation
a. odontogenic tumor

adenomatosis

adenomatous
a. colonic polyp
a. goiter
a. hyperplasia
a. polyp (AP)
a. polyposis syndrome

adenomyoma

adenomyomatosis

adenomyosarcoma

adenomyosis
diffuse a.
ureteral a.
uterine a.

adenopapillomatosis
gastric a.

adenopathy
abdominal a.
axillary a.
bilateral hilar a.
cervical a.
hilar a.
mediastinal a.
mesenteric a.
metastatic a.
paratracheal a.
postinflammatory a.
pulmonary a.
reticulation with hilar a.
retrocrural a.
retroperitoneal a.
sandwich configuration a.
secondary axillary a.
thoracic a.
tuberculous mediastinal a.

adenosarcoma
breast a.

Adenoscan
A. contrast medium
A. imaging
A. imaging agent

adenosine
echocardiogram a.
a. echocardiography imaging
a. triphosphate

adenosis
breast a.
microglandular a.
sclerosing a.

adenovirus pneumonia

adequate
a. cardiac output
a. coronary perfusion
a. stroke volume

AD/FHD
acetabular depth to femoral head diameter

ADH
atypical ductal hyperplasia

adherence

adherent
a. pericardium
a. placenta
a. thrombus

adhesed

adhesion
abdominal a.
attic a.
bandlike a.
fibrous pleural a.
inflammatory a.
intraarticular a.

NOTES

adhesion *(continued)*
a. molecule
pericardial diaphragmatic a.
peritendinous a.
pleuropericardial a.
pleuropulmonary a.
subacromial bursal a.
subdeltoid bursal a.
adhesive
a. arachnoiditis
a. atelectasis
a. capsulitis
a. ileus
a. inflammation
a. platelets
ADI
absolute dose intensity
atlantodens interval
adiabatic
a. demagnetization
a. fast passage
a. fast scanning technique
a. off-resonance spin locking
a. slice-selective radiofrequency pulse
adiadochokinesia
adipiodone
adipose
a. fold
a. fossa
a. ligament
a. tissue
a. tumor
adiposogenital dystrophy
adiposum
cor a.
aditus
a. ad antrum
a. ad pelvem
a. laryngis
a. orbitae
a. pelvis
a. vaginae
adjacent
a. field x-ray dosimetry
a. voxels
adjunctive therapy
adjuvant
a. analgesic
a. analgesic drug
a. chemoradiation
a. chemotherapy
a. chronotherapy
a. irradiation
a. radiation
a. therapy
adjuvanticity
admaxillary gland
administration
competitive iron a.
contrast a.
drug a.
Food and Drug A. (FDA)
intralymphatic radioactivity a.
intraperitoneal drug a.
vasodilator a.
Administration of Radioactive Substances Advisory Committee (ARSAC)
Administrators
American Hospital Radiology A. (AHRA)
admixture
a. lesion
a. lesion of heart
adnexa
transposed a.
adnexal
a. adenoma
a. carcinoma
a. cyst
a. embryo
a. mass
a. metastasis
a. torsion
adnexectomy
adolescent
a. hallux valgus
a. idiopathic scoliosis (AIS)
ADQ
abductor digiti quinti
adrenal
a. adenoma
a. angiography
a. artery
bilateral large a.
a. calcification
a. capsule
a. carcinoma
a. chemodectoma
a. cortex
a. cyst
a. cystic mass
a. failure
a. feminizing syndrome
a. ganglioneuroma
a. gland
a. gland cancer
a. hematoma
a. hemorrhage
a. hyperplasia
a. imaging
a. imaging metaiodobenzylguanidine
a. imaging MIBG
a. incidentaloma
a. insufficiency

a. lesion
a. medulla
a. medullary disease
a. metastasis
a. myelolipoma
a. neuroblastoma
a. paraganglioma
a. pheochromocytoma
a. pseudocyst
a. scintigraphy
a. tuberculosis
a. tumor
a. vein
a. venography
a. virilizing syndrome

adrenalectomy

adrenal-to-spleen ratio (ASR)

adrenarche
premature isolated a.

adrenocortical
a. adenoma
a. carcinoma
a. disease
a. hyperfunction
a. hyperplasia
a. macrocyst
a. neoplasm
a. rest cell tumor
a. secretion

adrenocorticotropin microadenoma

adrenogenital syndrome

adrenoleukodystrophy

adrenoleukodystrophy-adrenomyeloneuropathy (ALD-AMN)

adrenomyeloneuropathy

Adrian-Crooks type cassette

ADR Ultramark 4 ultrasound

Adson
A. maneuver
A. sign

adsorption
competitive a.

adult
a. dose
a. polycystic kidney disease
a. progeria
a. respiratory distress syndrome (ARDS)
a. T-cell lymphoma

adult-type coarctation of aorta

advanced
A. Breast Biopsy Instrument
a. cortical disease
a. life support (ALS)
a. multiple-beam equalization radiography (AMBER)
A. NMR Systems scanner

advancement
frontoorbital a.
vastus medialis a. (VMA)

adventitia
tunica a.

adventitial
a. fibroplasia
a. tissue

adventitious bursa

adverse
a. effect
a. event

adynamic
a. ileus
a. intestinal obstruction

adynamic/paralytic ileus

AE
above-elbow

AE amputation

Aeby muscle

AEC
automatic exposure control
Automic Energy Commission

AEG
acute erosive gastritis

AEGIS sonography management system

AER
apical ectodermal ridge

aerated tissue

aeration

AeroChamber

aerodigestive
a. cancer
a. tract

aerophagia

aerosol
radioactive a.
technetium-99m DTPA a.
a. ventilation scan
a. ventilation study

aerosolized
a. Tc-PYP
a. technetium Tc DTPA imaging agent

AF
aortic flow
arcuate fasciculus

NOTES

A-FAIR
arrhythmia-insensitive flow-sensitive alternating inversion recovery
A-FAIR imaging
afferent
a. digital nerve
a. loop
a. loop syndrome
a. lymph vessel
a. nerve lesion
a. view
African
A. Burkitt lymphoma
A. Kaposi sarcoma
afterload
increased ventricular a.
left ventricular a.
afterloader
Fletcher a.
Henschke a.
^{192}I high-dose-rate remote a.
Nucletron MicroSelectron/LDR remote a.
afterloading
high-dose-rate remote a.
a. radiation
a. tandem and ovoids
a. technique
AG
angular gyrus
aganglionic
a. bowel
a. megacolon
a. segment
aganglionosis
skip a.
AGC
anatomically graduated component
AGE
acute gastroenteritis
angle of greatest extension
age
biologic a.
bone a.
chronologic a.
delayed bone a.
fetal a.
gestational a.
indeterminate a.
large for gestational a. (LGA)
menstrual a.
age-indeterminate infarct
Agency
International Atomic Energy A. (IAEA)
agenesis
Bayne classification of radial a.
corpus callosum a.
gallbladder a.
liver a.
lumbosacral a.
lung a.
partial corpus callosum a.
pulmonary artery a.
renal a.
sacral a.
thymic a.
unilateral pulmonary a.
uterine a.
vaginal a.
vermian a.
agenetic
a. fracture
a. porencephaly
agent (*See* contrast, material, medium)
^{18}F estradiol imaging a.
^{18}F fludeoxyglucose imaging a.
^{18}F fluorodeoxyglucose imaging a.
^{18}F fluoro-DOPA imaging a.
^{18}F fluoroisonidazole imaging a.
^{18}F fluorotamoxifen imaging a.
^{18}F L-DOPA imaging a.
^{18}F N-methylspiperone imaging a.
^{18}F spiperone imaging a.
ABGd imaging a.
AcuTect imaging a.
Adenoscan imaging a.
aerosolized technetium Tc DTPA imaging a.
aggregated albumin with technetium imaging a.
aggregated iodinated I-131 serum albumin imaging a.
air imaging a.
Albunex ultrasound heart imaging a.
aminopolycarboxylic acid imaging a.
Amipaque imaging a.
Angio-Conray imaging a.
Angiocontrast imaging a.
Angiografin imaging a.
AngioMARK contrast a.
Angiovist 282, 292, 370 imaging a.
antifibrin-MoAb antibody imaging a.
antimony imaging a.
antimyosin monoclonal antibody imaging a.
antitoxoplasmosis a.
baby formula with ferrous sulfate imaging a.
Baricon imaging a.
barium sulfate imaging a.
Baro-CAT imaging a.

Baroflave imaging a.
Barosperse 110 imaging a.
B-19026 chelate imaging a.
benzamide imaging a.
Biligrafin imaging a.
Biliscopin imaging a.
Bilivist imaging a.
Bilopaque imaging a.
Biloptic imaging a.
bioreductive a.
bis-Gd-mesoporphyrin imaging a.
bone marrow a.
bromodeoxyuridine imaging a.
bromophenol blue imaging a.
bromospirone imaging a.
bunamiodyl imaging a.
^{45}Ca imaging a.
calcium-47 imaging a.
CA15-3 antigen radioimmunoassay imaging a.
^{11}C acetate imaging a.
calcium-45 imaging a.
carbogen radiosensitizer imaging a.
carbonated saline solution imaging a.
carbon imaging a.
Cardiografin sodium imaging a.
Cardio-Green imaging a.
Cardiolite imaging a.
cardioselective a.
Cardiotec imaging a.
^{11}C butanol imaging a.
^{11}C carbon monoxide imaging a.
^{11}C carfentanil imaging a.
^{11}C deoxyglucose imaging a.
CEAker imaging a.
CentoRx imaging a.
Ceretec radioisotope imaging a.
cerium silicate imaging a.
cesium chloride imaging a.
^{11}C flumazenil imaging a.
Cholebrine imaging a.
Cholografin meglumine imaging a.
chromated ^{51}Cr serum albumin imaging a.
chromium imaging a.
^{11}C imaging a.
^{11}C-labeled cocaine imaging a.
^{11}C-labeled fatty acids imaging a.
^{11}C L-159 imaging a.
^{11}C L-884 imaging a.
^{11}C L-methylmethionine imaging a.
^{11}C methoxystaurosporine imaging a.
^{11}C N-methylspiperone imaging a.
^{11}C N-methylspiroperidol imaging a.
^{11}C nomifensine imaging a.
CO_2-negative imaging a.
Conray 30, 43, 60, 280, 325, 400 imaging a.
contrast a.
copper (Cu) imaging a.
copper-zinc superoxide dismutase imaging a. (Cu/Zn-SOD imaging agent)
corn oil and ferric ammonium citrate imaging a.
^{11}C palmitate imaging a.
^{11}C palmitic acid radioactive imaging a.
^{11}C raclopride imaging a.
Cr-HIDA chelate imaging a.
^{11}C thymidine imaging a.
^{67}Cu imaging a.
^{62}Cu PTSM imaging a.
^{62}Cu pyruvaldehyde-bis-(4N-thiosemicarbazone) imaging a.
Cu/Zn-SOD imaging a.
   copper-zinc superoxide dismutase imaging agent
cyanocobalamin imaging a.
Cysto-Conray II imaging a.
Cystografin imaging a.
Cystokon imaging a.
DDFP imaging a.
   dodecafluoropentane imaging agent
degassed tap water imaging a.
denatured technetium Tc RBC imaging a.
deuterium imaging a.
dextrose 5% in water imaging a.
d,1-HMPAO imaging a.
diatrizoate-60 imaging a.
diatrizoate meglumine imaging a.
diatrizoate sodium imaging a.
diazepam imaging a.
diethylenetriaminepentaacetic acid imaging a. (DTPA imaging agent)
dihydroxyphenalalanine imaging a. (DOPA imaging agent)
Diodrast imaging a.
Dionosil imaging a.
diprotrizoate imaging a.
dispersing a.

NOTES

agent *(continued)*
dodecafluoropentane imaging a. (DDFP imaging agent)
DOPA imaging a.
dihydroxyphenalalanine imaging agent
DTPA imaging a.
diethylenetriaminepentaacetic acid imaging agent
Duografin imaging a.
Dy-DTPA-BMA imaging a.
dysprosium HP-DO3A imaging a.
Eaton a.
EchoGen ultrasound imaging a.
Echovist imaging a.
EDTMP imaging a.
effervescent a.
etanidazole imaging a.
Ethiodol imaging a.
Ethodian imaging a.
Evans blue imaging a.
exametazime imaging a.
FCR 9501HQ high-resolution storage phosphor imaging a.
Feridex MRI contrast a.
ferumoxsil imaging a.
^{18}F-labeled HFA-134a imaging a.
^{18}F-labeled polyfluorinated ethyl imaging a.
fluid embolic a.
fluid vascular occluding a.
fluorine imaging a.
fluorocarbon-based ultrasound contrast a.
fluorodeoxyglucose imaging a.
furosemide imaging a.
gadobenate dimeglumine imaging a.
gadobenic acid imaging a.
gadobutrol imaging a.
gadodiamide imaging a.
gadolinium oxide imaging a.
gadoteridol imaging a.
gadoversetamide imaging a.
gallium imaging a.
Gastrografin imaging a.
GastroMARK oral imaging a.
Gastrovist imaging a.
Gd-BOPTA/Dimeg imaging a.
Gd-DTPA/Dimeg imaging a.
Gd-enhanced imaging a.
Gd-EOB-DTPA imaging a.
Gd-HP-DO3A imaging a.
Gd-153 imaging a.
glomerular filtration a.
glucagon imaging a.
Glucarate imaging a.
GSA imaging a.
halistatin-1 imaging a. (H1 imaging agent)
hand-agitated imaging a.
H-benzapine imaging a.
Hedspa imaging a.
hepatobiliary contrast a.
Hexabrix imaging a.
high-density barium imaging a.
high-osmolar contrast a. (HOCA)
H1 imaging a.
halistatin-1 imaging agent
Hippuran imaging a.
Hipputope imaging a.
holmium imaging a.
human serum-ABGd imaging a.
human serum-albumin imaging a.
hybrid MRI imaging a.
hydrogen peroxide imaging a.
hyoscine butylbromide imaging a.
Hypaque-Cysto imaging a.
Hypaque-50 imaging a.
Hypaque-76 imaging a.
Hypaque Meglumine imaging a.
Hypaque-M imaging a.
Hypaque Sodium imaging a.
hyperpolarized He-3 imaging a.
hyperpolarized ^{129}Xe imaging a.
Imagent GI imaging a.
Imagopaque imaging a.
imidoacetic acid radioactive a.
ImmuRAID antibody imaging a.
Immurait imaging a.
imodoacetic acid imaging a.
Indiclor imaging a.
indium imaging a.
indocyanine green imaging a.
inhaled oxygen imaging a.
intercalating a.
intratumoral a.
Intropaque imaging a.
iobenzamic acid imaging a.
iobitridol imaging a.
iocarmic acid imaging a.
iocetamic acid imaging a.
iodamine meglumine imaging a.
iodinated imaging a.
iodipamide meglumine imaging a.
iodized oil imaging a.
5-iodoacetamidofluorescein imaging a.
5-iodo-2-deoxyuridine imaging a.
Iodo-gen imaging a.
iodohippurate sodium imaging a.
iodomethamate sodium imaging a.
iodophthalein sodium imaging a.
iodophylated chelates imaging a.
Iodotope imaging a.
iodoxamate meglumine imaging a.

iodoxamic acid imaging a.
iohexol imaging a.
ionic paramagnetic imaging a.
iopamidol imaging a.
Iopamiron 310, 370 imaging a.
iopanoic acid imaging a.
iopentol nonionic imaging a.
iophendylate imaging a.
iopydol imaging a.
iopydone imaging a.
iosefamic acid imaging a.
iotetric acid imaging a.
iothalamate meglumine imaging a.
iothalamate sodium imaging a.
iothalmic acid imaging a.
iotrol imaging a.
iotroxic acid imaging a.
ioversol imaging a.
ioxaglate meglumine imaging a.
ioxaglate sodium imaging a.
ioxilan with iohexol imaging a.
ipodate calcium imaging a.
ipodate sodium imaging a.
iridium imaging a.
isoflurane imaging a.
Isopaque imaging a.
Isovue-128 imaging a.
Isovue-250 imaging a.
Isovue-300 imaging a.
Isovue-370 imaging a.
Isovue-M 200, 300 imaging a.
Isovue nonionic imaging a.
K4-81 imaging a.
kinase C antiglioma monoclonal antibody imaging a.
Kinevac imaging a.
Kontrast U imaging a.
krypton-81m radioactive imaging a.
LeukaScan imaging a.
Levovist imaging a.
ligand a.
lighter-than-bile contrast a.
lipiodol myelographic imaging a.
lipophilic imaging a.
Liquipake imaging a.
long-scale imaging a.
low-osmolality contrast a. (LOCA)
low-osmolar contrast a. (LOCA)
L-tyrosine imaging a.
lymphangiographic imaging a.
Lymphazurin imaging a.
macroaggregated albumin imaging a.
macromolecular imaging a.
Macrotec imaging a.
magnetic resonance receptor a.
magnetite albumin imaging a.
Magnevist imaging a.
Mallinckrodt imaging a.
mangafodipir trisodium imaging a.
manganese imaging a.
mannitol and saline imaging a.
MD-Gastroview imaging a.
meglumine iodipamide imaging a.
meglumine iotroxate imaging a.
Metastron imaging a.
methiodal sodium imaging a.
methyl methacrylate imaging a.
metrizamide imaging a.
metrizoate sodium imaging a.
metrizoic acid imaging a.
microbubble contrast imaging a.
mineral oil imaging a.
monoclonal antibody imaging a.
MS-325 contrast a.
myelographic imaging a.
Myoscint imaging a.
Myoview imaging a.
naloxone imaging a.
nanoparticulate imaging a.
negative contrast imaging a.
nephrotropic MR imaging a.
Neurolite imaging a.
neurotropic imaging a.
nicotinamide imaging a.
nimodipine imaging a.
Niopam imaging a.
nitrogen-13 ammonia imaging a.
nitrous oxide imaging a.
no-carrier-added ^{18}F imaging a.
nonionic paramagnetic contrast imaging a.
nonsteroidal antiphlogistics imaging a.
normal human serum albumin imaging a.
novel a.
Novopaque imaging a.
Nycomed imaging a.
OctreoScan imaging a.
Octreotide imaging a.
oil emulsion imaging a.
olsalazine imaging a.

NOTES

agent *(continued)*
Omnipaque imaging a.
Omniscan imaging a.
OncoScint breast imaging a.
OncoSpect imaging a.
OncoTrac imaging a.
Optiray 320 imaging a.
Optison ultrasound contrast a.
Orabilex sodium imaging a.
Oragrafin Calcium imaging a.
Oragrafin Sodium imaging a.
oral bile desaturating a.
oral contrast imaging a.
Oralex ultrasound imaging a.
Oravue imaging a.
Oxilan imaging a.
oxygen imaging a.
palladium imaging a.
Pantopaque imaging a.
paramagnetic imaging a.
pentagastrin imaging a.
pentavalent DMSA imaging a.
pentetreotide imaging a.
peppermint oil imaging a.
peptide imaging a.
perflubron imaging a.
perfluorocarbon imaging a.
perfusion a.
pertechnetate sodium imaging a.
phenobarbital imaging a.
Phentetiothalein imaging a.
phosphoric acid imaging a.
phosphorus imaging a.
polygelin colloid imaging a.
potassium imaging a.
Priodax imaging a.
ProHance imaging a.
propyliodone imaging a.
ProstaScint monoclonal antibody imaging a.
Racobalamin-57 radioactive imaging a.
radioactive cancer-specific targeting a.
radioactive isotope imaging a.
radiolabeled MoAb imaging a.
radiopaque imaging a.
radioprotective a.
radiotherapeutic a.
renal cortical isotope scanning a.
Renografin-60 imaging a.
Renografin-76 microbubbles imaging a.
Reno-M-Dip imaging a.
Reno-M-30 imaging a.
Reno-M-60 imaging a.
Renotec imaging a.
Renovist II imaging a.
Renovist imaging a.
Renovue-Dip imaging a.
Renovue-65 imaging a.
residual imaging a.
reticuloendothelial imaging a.
rhenium imaging a.
RIGScan CR49 imaging a.
Robengatope radioactive imaging a.
rose bengal sodium ^{131}I radioactive biliary a.
rubidium chloride imaging a.
Rubratope-57 imaging a.
Salpix imaging a.
samarium imaging a.
satumomab pendetide imaging a.
sclerosing a.
selenium imaging a.
^{75}Se selenomethionine radioactive a.
sestamibi imaging a.
Sethotope radioactive imaging a.
Sinografin imaging a.
Skiodan imaging a.
SmartPrep imaging a.
sodium bicarbonate solution imaging a.
sodium chloride imaging a.
sodium diatrizoate imaging a.
sodium diatrizoate with Menoquinon imaging a.
sodium iodide ring imaging a.
sodium iodipamide imaging a.
sodium iodohippurate imaging a.
sodium iodomethamate imaging a.
sodium iothalamate imaging a.
sodium ipodate imaging a.
sodium methiodal imaging a.
sodium pertechnetate imaging a.
sodium thorium tartrate imaging a.
sodium tyropanoate imaging a.
Solu-Biloptin imaging a.
Somatostatin imaging a.
sonicated meglumine sodium imaging a.
sonicated Renografin-76 imaging a.
sorbitol 70% imaging a.
SPIO imaging a.
superparamagnetic iron oxide imaging agent
sprodiamide imaging a.
Sterling imaging a.
stool-tagging a.
strontium imaging a.
sucrose polyester imaging a.
sulfobromophthalein imaging a.
sulfur colloid imaging a.
superparamagnetic iron oxide imaging a. (SPIO imaging agent)
tantalum imaging a.

^{99m}Tc albumin aggregated imaging a.
^{99m}Tc albumin colloid imaging a.
^{99m}Tc albumin microaggregated imaging a.
^{99m}Tc albumin microspheres imaging a.
^{99m}Tc biciromab imaging a.
^{99m}Tc bicisate imaging a.
^{99m}Tc colloid imaging a.
^{99m}Tc dimercaptosuccinic acid imaging a.
^{99m}Tc disofenin imaging a.
^{99m}Tc etidronate imaging a.
^{99m}Tc exametazime imaging a.
^{99m}Tc ferpentetate imaging a.
^{99m}Tc furifosmin imaging a.
^{99m}Tc Glucarate hot spot imaging a.
^{99m}Tc gluceptate imaging a.
^{99m}Tc human serum albumin imaging a.
^{99m}Tc lidofenin imaging a.
^{99m}Tc mebrofenin imaging a.
^{99m}Tc medronate disodium imaging a.
^{99m}Tc mertiatide imaging a.
^{99m}Tc oxidronate imaging a.
^{99m}Tc pentetate calcium trisodium imaging a.
^{99m}Tc pentetate sodium imaging a.
^{99m}Tc pentetic acid imaging a.
^{99m}Tc polyphosphate imaging a.
^{99m}Tc riisocyanide imaging a.
^{99m}Tc rimetaphosphates imaging a.
^{99m}Tc sestamibi imaging a.
^{99m}Tc siboroxime imaging a.
^{99m}Tc sodium gluceptate imaging a.
^{99m}Tc sodium pertechnetate imaging a.
^{99m}Tc succimer imaging a.
^{99m}Tc sulfur colloid imaging a.
^{99m}Tc sulfur microcolloid imaging a.
^{99m}Tc teboroxime imaging a.
^{99m}Tc tetrofosmin imaging a.
teboroxime imaging a.
Techneplex imaging a.
TechneScan MAG3 imaging a.
TechneScan Q-12 imaging a.
technetated aggregated human albumin imaging a.
technetium imaging a.
Telepaque imaging a.
teratogenicity of contrast a.
Tesuloid imaging a.
thallium imaging a.
thallous chloride imaging a.
TheraSeed imaging a.
Thixokon imaging a.
thorium dioxide imaging a.
Thorotrast imaging a.
ThromboScan imaging a.
tissue imaging a.
Tomocat imaging a.
triiodinated imaging a.
triisocyanide ^{99m}Tc imaging a.
Tru-Scint imaging a.
tumorostatic a.
tyropanoate sodium imaging a.
Tyropaque imaging a.
ultrasmall-particle superparamagnetic iron oxide imaging a. (USPIO imaging agent)
Ultravist imaging a.
uniphasic imaging a.
uranium imaging a.
Urografin 290 imaging a.
urokinase imaging a.
Urovist Cysto imaging a.
Urovist Meglumine imaging a.
Urovist Sodium imaging a.
USPIO imaging a.
    ultrasmall-particle superparamagnetic iron oxide imaging agent
Vascoray imaging a.
vasodilating a.
visualization of imaging a.
water-soluble iodinated imaging a.
water-soluble nonionic positive imaging a.
xenon imaging a.
xylenol orange imaging a.

AGF
    angle of greatest flexion

Agfa
    A. CR system
    A. Medical scanner
    A. PACS system

agglutinin

aggregated
    a. albumin with technetium imaging agent

NOTES

aggregated *(continued)*
a. iodinated I-131 serum albumin imaging agent
a. lymphatic follicle
aggregometer
aggressive
a. infantile fibromatosis
a. interstitial infiltrate
a. malignancy
a. perivascular infiltrate
aggressiveness
bone tumor a.
aging gut
AGL
anterior glenoid labrum
agnogenic
a. myeloid metaphysis
a. myeloid metaplasia
agonal clot
agranulocytosis
agretope
agyria
a. pachygria complex
ahaustral
AHC
apical hypertrophy
AHI
acromiohumeral interval
apnea-hypopnea index
AHO
acute hematogenous osteomyelitis
AHRA
American Hospital Radiology Administrators
AI
A. 5200 diagnostic ultrasound
A. 5200 diagnostic ultrasound system
AICA
anterior-inferior cerebellar artery
anterior-inferior cerebral artery
anterior-inferior communicating artery
Aicardi syndrome
AICD
automatic implantable cardioverter-defibrillator
AICS
artery of inferior cavernous sinus
AIDS
acquired immunodeficiency syndrome
AIDS cholangitis
AIDS cryptococcosis
AIDS cystitis
AIDS-related
A.-r. cholangiopathy
A.-r. esophagitis
A.-r. gastritis
A.-r. lymphoma
AIN
acute interstitial nephritis
AIOD
aortoiliac obstructive disease
AIP
acute interstitial pneumonia
American Institute of Physics
air
ambient a.
a. block
a. bolus
bowel loop a.
a. bronchogram
a. cavity
a. cisternography
a. collection
colonic a.
a. conditioner lung
a. crescent
a. cyst
a. cystogram
a. density
a. dose
a. embolus
a. encephalography
a. enema fluoroscopic imaging
a. esophagogram
a. exchange
extraalveolar a. (EAA)
extraluminal a.
flail a.
free a.
free intraperitoneal a.
a. gap
a. hunger
a. imaging agent
a. inflation
a. injection
inspired a.
a. insufflation
a. interface
intracranial a.
intraluminal a.
intramural colonic a.
intraorbital a.
intraperitoneal a.
a. leak
a. luminogram
mediastinal a.
a. myelography
a. plasma spray hydroxyapatite
a. plethysmography
a. pocket
retrocrural a.
a. sac
a. space
subcutaneous a.
transradiant a.

a. trapping
a. vesicle
air/bone/tissue boundary
airborne transmission
air-containing
a.-c. mass of neck
a.-c. neck mass
air-contrast
a.-c. barium enema (ACBE)
a.-c. enema
a.-c. imaging
a.-c. view
air-core magnet
air-crescent lung sign
air-driven artificial heart
air-filled
a.-f. loop
a.-f. lung
air-filtration system
air-fluid
a.-f. level
a.-f. line
air-gap
a.-g. radiography
a.-g. technique
Airis II MRI system
air-kerma
integrated reference a.-k. (IRAK)
a.-k. rate constant
a.-k. strength
total reference a.-k. (TRAK)
airless
a. lung
a. mass
air–soft tissue interface
airspace
air-space
a.-s. consolidation
a.-s. disease
a.-s. edema
a.-s. enlargement
a.-s. metastasis
a.-s. nodule
a.-s. opacity
airspace-filling pattern
airway
a. anatomy
asthmatic a.
a. constriction
embryology of a.
a. embryology
esophageal obturator a.
a. fluoroscopy
a. fluoroscopy imaging
hypertonic a.
increased a.
large a.
mucoid plugging of a.
a. narrowing
a. obstruction
oropharyngeal a.
a. pattern
a. pressure
a. pressure peak
a. pressure release ventilation
a. resistance
resistance a. (RAW)
a. responsiveness
small a.
a. tree
airways tuberculosis
AIS
adolescent idiopathic scoliosis
Aitken
A. acromioclavicular injury classification
A. classification of epiphyseal fractures
A. femoral deficiency
AIUM
American Institute of Ultrasound in Medicine
AIVV
anterior internal vertebral vein
Ajmalin liver injury
AKA
above-knee amputation
Akerlund deformity
AK-Fluor injection
akinesis
inferior wall a.
akinetic
a. left ventricle
a. segment
a. segmental wall motion
a. segmental wall motion abnormality
AL
anterolateral
ala, pl. **alae**
sacral a.
a. of sacrum
Alagille syndrome

NOTES

alakalinity
Engel a.
alanine-silicone pellet
Alanson amputation
alar
a. bone
a. cartilage
a. chest
a. dysgenesis
a. fold
a. ligament
a. plate
a. process
a. spine
ALARA
as low as reasonably achievable
alba
linea a.
phlegmasia dolens a.
Albarran gland
Albers-Schönberg
Albers-Schönberg position
A.-S. bone
A.-S. marble bone
Albert position
Albini nodule
Albinus muscle
Albrecht bone
Albright
A. hereditary osteodystrophy
A. syndrome
Albright-McCune-Sternberg syndrome
albuginea
tunica a.
albumin
Gd-DTPA-labeled a.
human serum a.
I-labeled macroaggregated a.
iodinated I-131 aggregated a.
iodinated I-131 serum a.
iodinated ^{125}I serum a.
^{131}I serum a.
macroaggregated a. (MAA)
neogalactosyl a.
radioiodinated serum a. (RISA)
^{99m}Tc macroaggregated a.
technetium-99m human serum a.
technetium-99m macroaggregated a.
technetium-99m mini-microaggregated a. (^{99m}Tc MMAA)
Albunex
A. ultrasound contrast medium
A. ultrasound heart imaging agent
ALCL
anaplastic large-cell lymphoma
Alcock canal
alcoholic
a. cardiomegaly
a. cirrhosis
a. dilated cardiomyopathy
a. fatty liver
a. fibrosis
a. gastritis
a. heart
a. liver disease (ALD)
a. pneumonia
ALD
alcoholic liver disease
ALD-AMN
adrenoleukodystrophy-adrenomyeloneuropathy
Alderson anthropomorphic phantom
aldosterone-producing carcinoma
aldosterone-secreting carcinoma
Aldrich syndrome
aleukemic
a. presentation
aleukocytosis
Alexander
A. disease
A. view
algebraic reconstruction technique (ART)
algorithm
annealing a.
bioeffects a.
bone a.
Clarkson scatter-summation a.
clustering a.
cone-beam reconstruction a.
contour-following a.
Cookey-Tukey a.
correlation a. (CR)
decryption a.
defuzzification a.
3D elastic subtraction a.
digital imaging processing a. (DIP algorithm)
DIP a.
digital imaging processing algorithm
document-recognition a.
DRC a.
dynamic range control algorithm
dual-lookup table a.
dynamic range control a. (DRC algorithm)
edge-enhanced error diffusion a.
elastic subtraction a.
encryption a.
Feldkamp a.
fringe thinning a.
geometric optimization a.
high-spatial-frequency reconstruction a.
histogram equalization a.

image restoration a.
interpolation a.
iterative a.
K-means clustering a.
least-squares a.
lossy a.
mapping a.
maximum intensity projection a.
maximum likelihood a.
memory-intensive a.
mensuration a.
neural evaluation a.
pixel-oriented a.
quantizer-design a.
radix-two a.
Ramesh and Pramod a.
reconstruction a.
restoration a.
shaded-surface display a. (SSD algorithm)
Shinnar-LeRoux a.
SSD a.
shaded-surface display algorithm
Z-interpolation a.

aliased flow

aliasing
a. artifact
a image
a. phenomenon
temporal a.

Alibert-Bazin form of mycosis fungoides

alignment
anatomic a.
angular a.
bony a.
field a.
a. of fracture fragment
a. and registration of 3D image
rotational a.
torsional a.
transverse plane a.
vertebral body a.
a. of vertebral body

alimentary
a. canal
a. tract
a. tract calcification

alimentation
enteral a.

Alken-Marberger nephroscope

allantoic
a. circulation
a. cyst
a. vesicle

Allen sign

allergic
a. bronchopulmonary aspergillosis (ABPA)
a. disease
a. granulomatosis
a. granulomatous angitis
a. pneumonia
a. reaction
a. sinusitis

allergy
iodine a.

Allis sign

Allman classification of acromioclavicular injury

allocation
bit-rate a.
a. of treatment

allocortex

allodynia

alloesthesia

allogeneic, allogenic
a. bone marrow transplant
a. disease
a. peripheral cell transplant
a. stem-cell transplantation (SCT)

allograft
aortic a.
bone a.
bone-chip a.
a. rejection
renal a.

allograft-mediated

alloimmune disease

allowed beta transition

alloxan-Schiff reaction

All-Tronics scanner

ALN
axillary lymph node

alobar holoprosencephaly

Aloka
A. color Doppler real-time 2D blood flow imaging with Cine Memory
A. imaging
A. linear ultrasound
A. sector ultrasound
A. SSD ultrasound system
A. ultrasound linear scanner
A. ultrasound sector scanner

NOTES

Alouette amputation
Alpers disease
alpha (α)
a. cradle
a. frequency band
a. particle
a. particle accelerator
a. particle bombardment
a. radiation
a. ray
a. sigmoid loop
thyrotropin a.
a. tocopherol
alpha-actinin protein
alpha-particle emitter
Alpine hunter's cap deformity
ALPSA
anterior labroligamentous periosteal sleeve avulsion
ALPSA lesion
ALS
advanced life support
amyotrophic lateral sclerosis
alta
patella a.
alteration
bilateral a.
hemodynamic a.
altered blood flow
alternans
pulsus a.
alternating
a. hemifield stimulation
a. sinus
alternator
film a.
altitudinal hemianopsia
Altman classification
ALT ultrasound system
altus
calcaneus a.
aluminum
a. ion breakthrough test
a. pneumoconiosis
ALVAD
abdonimal left ventricular assist device
alveodental ridge
alveolar
a. atrophy
a. basal cell carcinoma
a. bone fracture
a. border
a. border of mandible
a. bronchiole
a. canal
a. clouding
a. consolidation
a. consolidative process
a. crest
a. dead space
a. dilatation
a. disease
a. disease sign
a. duct
a. duct emphysema
a. echinococcosis
a. ectasia
a. epithelial hyperplasia
a. foramen
a. gland
a. hemorrhage
a. hydatid
a. hypersensitivity
a. infiltrate
a. macrophage
a. microlithiasis
a. mucosal carcinoma
a. overdistention
a. overventilation
a. pattern
a. pneumonia
a. point
a. pressure
a. pulmonary edema
a. rhabdomyosarcoma
a. ridge
a. sac
a. sarcoidosis
a. septal inflammation
a. septal necrosis
a. septum
a. soft part sarcoma
a. supporting bone
a. ventilation (VA)
a. volume
alveolar-capillary block
alveolarization
alveoli (*pl.* of alveolus)
alveolingual groove
alveolitis
acute allergic extrinsic a.
acute extrinsic allergic a.
chronic diffuse sclerosing a.
chronic extrinsic allergic a.
chronic fibrosing a.
cryptogenic fibrosing a.
desquamative fibrosing a.
diffuse sclerosing a.
extrinsic allergic a.
fibrosing a.
fibrosing cryptogenic a.
mural fibrosing a.
subacute extrinsic allergic a.
alveolobuccal groove
alveolodental canal
alveologram

alveololabial groove
alveolus, pl. **alveoli**
pulmonary a.
alvine calculus
alymphocytosis
alymphoplasia
Alzheimer disease (AD)
AM
arterial malformation
Am
americium
^{241}Am
americium-241
AMA
American Medical Association
AMA-Fab scintigraphy
amastia
amastrozole
amaurosis
central a.
cerebral a.
uremic a.
amazia
AMBER
advanced multiple-beam equalization radiography
ambient
a. air
a. wing of the quadrigeminal cistern
ambiguous
a. genitalia
ambilevosity
ambilevous
amblyaphia
AMBRI
atraumatic, multidirectional, bilateral radial instability
AMBRI syndrome
ambulatory
a. equilibrium angiocardiography
a. equilibrium angiography
a. Holter echocardiography
amelanotic tumor
ameloblast
ameloblastic
a. adenomatoid tumor
a. carcinoma
a. fibroma
a. fibrosarcoma
a. sarcoma
ameloblastoma
a. of the jaw
amentia
Americaine
American
A. Board of Radiology (ABR)
A. Club of Therapeutic Radiologists (ACTR)
A. College of Radiology (ACR)
A. Hospital Radiology Administrators (AHRA)
A. Institute of Physics (AIP)
A. Institute of Ultrasound in Medicine (AIUM)
A. Medical Association (AMA)
A. Medical Association Ligament Injury Classification System
A. Registry of Diagnostic Medical Sonographers (ARDMS)
A. Registry of Radiologic Technologists
A. Rheumatism Association (ARA)
A. Roentgen Ray Society
A. Shared-CuraCare scanner
A. Society of Neuroradiology
A. Society of Radiologic Technologists (ASRT)
A. Society of Registered Technologists (ASRT)
A. Society for Therapeutic Radiology and Oncology (ASTRO)
A. Spinal Cord Injury Association (ASCIA)
A. Spinal Cord Injury Association classification
A. Standards Association (ASA)
A. Urological Association (AUA)
americium (Am)
a.-241 (^{241}Am)
a. radioactive source
ameroid occluder
Ames test
ametriodinic acid
AMI
anterior myocardial infarct
AMI 121 contrast medium
AMI 227 contrast medium
amidotrizoic acid
aminopolycarboxylic acid imaging agent

NOTES

amiodarone
a. liver
a. lung
Amipaque
A. contrast medium
A. imaging agent
Ammon
A. horn
A. horn sclerosis
ammonia
anhydrous a. (NH_3)
ammonium excretion
amniocentesis
therapeutic a.
amniography
amnioinfusion
amnion
a. ring
a. rupture
a. rupture sequence
amnionic, amniotic
a. band
a. band syndrome
a. cavity
a. duct
a. fluid
a. fluid embolus
a. fluid index
a. fluid volume
a. fold
a. inclusion cyst
a. membrane
a. raphe
a. sac
a. sheet
amnionicity
A-mode
A.-m. display
A.-m. echocardiography
A.-m. encephalography
A.-m. ultrasound
amorphous
a. fetus
a. high signal intensity
a. selenium plate
a. silicon
Amoss sign
amphiarthrodial
amphiarthrosis
amphoric echo
Amplatz
A. angiography needle
A. dilator set
A. radiolucent handle
amplifier
buffer a.
gradient a.
image a.
linear a.
log a.
nuclear pulse a.
Servox a.
amplitude
acoustic pressure a.
a. asymmetry
gradient a.
a. imaging
a. modulation
output a.
pressure a.
septal a.
ampulla, pl. **ampullae**
phrenic a.
a. of semicircular canal
a. tumor
a. of Vater
a. of Vater anatomy
a. of Vater cyst
ampullar
a. pregnancy
ampullary
a. adenocarcinoma
a. aneurysm
a. carcinoma
a. crest
a. stenosis
amputated-foot view
amputation
above-elbow a.
above-knee a. (AKA)
AE a.
Alanson a.
Alouette a.
Beclard a.
below-knee a. (BKA)
Berger interscapular a.
Bier a.
Boyd ankle a.
Bunge a.
Burgess below-knee a.
button toe a.
Callander a.
Carden a.
chop a.
Chopart hindfoot a.
circular supracondylar a.
closed flap a.
congenital a.
digital a.
femoral head a.
fetal a.
fingertip a.
fishmouth a.
forearm a.
Hey a.
interscapulothoracic a.

Jaboulay a.
Kirk distal thigh a.
Le Fort a.
Lisfranc a.
midthigh a.
nonreplantable a.
one-stage a.
Pirogoff a.
ray a.
replantable a.
a. sign
supramalleolar open a.
Syme ankle disarticulation a.
Teale a.
transcarpal a.
transcondylar a.
translumbar a.
transmetatarsal a. (TMA)
traumatic a.
two-stage a.
Vladimiroff-Mikulicz a.

AMS
accelerator mass spectrometry

Amsterdam dwarfism

Amstutz classification

AMT-25-enhanced
A.-e. MR image
A.-e. MR imaging

amu
atomic mass unit

amygdala
a. of cerebellum

amygdalofugal pathway

amygdaloid
a. area
a. fossa
a. nuclear complex
a. tubercle

amyl nitrite

amyloid
a. deposit
a. oral cavity disease
a. tumor

amyloidoma

amyloidosis
chronic renal failure a.
CNS a.
GI tract a.
heart a.
hereditary a.
idiopathic a.
kidney a.
lung a.
a. of multiple myeloma
primary a.
secondary a.
senile a.
skeletal a.

amyloidotic cardiomyopathy

amyotonia congenita

amyotrophic lateral sclerosis (ALS)

amyotrophy
Aran-Duchenne a.

anacrotic notch

anaerobic lung abscess

anal
a. atresia
a. bulge
a. canal
a. cleft
a. column
a. crypt
a. disk
a. fascia
a. fissure
a fistula
a. intermuscular septum
a. intersphincteric groove
a. manometry
a. orifice
a. pit
a. plate
a. protrusion
a. stenosis
a. stricture
a. vein
a. verge

analeptic enema

analgesic
adjuvant a.
a. nephropathy

analog, analogue
dysprosium a.
halogenated thymidine a.
pyrimidine a.
radiolabeled estrogen a.
a. scan converter
technetium-labeled phosphate a.
technetium-99m IDA a.

analogous

analog-to-digital converter

analogue (*var. of* analog)

analysis, pl. **analyses**
activation a.

NOTES

analysis *(continued)*
basic volume image a.
5-bromodeoxyuridine a.
cephalometric a.
Cerenkov scintillation a.
clinicopathological a.
Collett a.
cue-based image a.
deconvolutional a.
diagnostic efficacy a.
digital frequency a.
direct immunofluorescence a.
discriminant a.
Doppler spectral a.
Doppler waveform a.
duplex ultrasound a.
eigenvector a.
electrooculographic a.
fast Fourier spectral a.
field-fitting a.
fission track a.
folding potential a.
footprint a.
Fourier a.
fractal a.
frequency a.
gamma spectrometric a.
high-definition three-dimensional a.
image display and a. (IDA)
Khan scatter a.
kinetic parameter a.
late effect a.
liquid scintillation a.
multielemental neutron activation a.
multivariant regressional a.
neutron activation a.
nuclide a.
phase a.
planar thallium with quantitative a.
pole figure texture a.
power spectral a. (PSA)
prospective a.
pulse height spectral a.
quantitative a.
range-gated Doppler spectral flow a.
rate a.
recursive partitioning a.
residual stress a.
roentgen stereophotogrammetric a. (RSA)
Sassouni a.
sensitivity a.
signal sonographic feature a.
slope blot a.
sonographic feature a.
spectral a.
S-phase a.
Steel-Dwaas a.
stepwise regression a.
thin film a.
volumetric a.
x-ray diffraction a.

analytic
a. reconstruction
subjective, objective, management, and a. (SOMA, SOMA scale)

analyzer
automated cerebral blood flow a.
Dow hollow fiber a.
Medigraphics a.
multichannel a. (MCA)
pulse height a.

anaphylactic reaction

anaplasia
cerebellar a.

anaplastic
a. astrocytoma
a. cerebral glioma
a. ependymoma
a. large-cell lymphoma (ALCL)
a. mixed oligoastrocytoma
a. plasmacytoma
a. thyroid carcinoma

anastomosis, pl. **anastomoses**
arterial brain a.
Baffe a.
bidirectional cavopulmonary a.
biliary-enteric a.
Billroth I, II a.
cobra-head a.
coiling of a.
colocolic a.
colorectal a.
Damus-Kaye-Stancel a. (DKS anastomosis)
DKS a.
Damus-Kaye-Stancel anastomosis
embryonic a.
extradural a.
Glenn a.
hepatojejunal a.
heterocladic a.
Hofmeister a.
Horsley a.
ileal pouch-anal a.
ileorectal a. (IRA)
ileotransverse colon a.
intercavernous a.
J-shaped a.
Kocher a.
Kugel a.
laser-assisted microvascular a.
left internal mammary artery (LIMA) a.
splenorenal a.

stenotic esophagogastric a.
Sucquet-Hoyer a.
tracheal a.
ureteroureteral a.

anastomotic
a. aneurysm
a. arterial circle
a. disruption
a. hemorrhage
a. leakage
a. pseudoaneurysm
a. site
a. stenosis
a. stoma
a. stricture
a. ulcer
a. vein

anatomic
a. alignment
a. axis
a. barrier
a. bile duct variant
a. brain classification
a. dead space
a. distribution
a. fracture
a. landmark
a. moment erratum
a. neck
a. plane
a. position
a. reduction
a. root
a. shunt flow
a. snuffbox
a. variability

anatomically
a. dominant
a. graduated component (AGC)

anatomy
airway a.
ampulla of Vater a.
anomalous a.
basal ganglia a.
breast a.
bronchopulmonary lung segment a.
bulbourethral gland a.
carpal bone a.
cochlear a.
coronary vessel a.
coronory artery a.
craniovertebral junction a.
cross-sectional lung segment a.
Daseler-Anson classification of plantaris muscle a.
distorted a.
endometrial a.
facial nerve a.
hepatic artery a.
inner ear a.
internal auditory canal a.
kidney a.
left-dominant coronary a.
liver segment a.
lobar breast a.
Lowsley lobar a.
maxillary nerve a.
medullary venous a.
normal planar MR a.
ovarian a.
pituitary gland a.
plantar compartmental a.
prostate a.
radiologic a.
renal a.
renal vascular a.
right dominant coronary a.
Saltzman a.
scrotal a.
sectional segmental a.
segmental liver a.
small bowel fold a.
stapedial nerve a.
superior orbital fissure a.
teardrop pelvic a.
temporal bone a.
thoracic spine a.
trigeminal nerve a.
umbilical cord a.
uterine a.
vascular kidney a.
vascular renal a.
zonal prostate a.
zonal uterine a.

anchoring villus

anchovy paste abscess

anconeal, anconal
a. fossa

anconeus muscle

anconoid

ancyroid, ankyroid
a. cavity

Anderson-D'Alonzo odontoid fracture classification

NOTES

Anderson-Hutchins tibial fracture
Andren method
androblastoma
androgen-independent prostate cancer
androgen-producing tumor
android pelvis
anechoic
a. area
a. center
a. fluid
a. fluid collection
a. lesion
a. mantle
a. mass
a. thrombus
anembryonic pregnancy
anemia
radiation a.
refractory a.
anemic infarct
anencephaly
aneriosus
ductus a.
aneroid manometry
aneuploid cell line
aneurysm
abdominal aortic a. (AAA)
acquired left ventricle a.
ampullary a.
anastomotic a.
aortic a.
aortic arch a.
aortic sinus a.
aortoiliac a.
arterial a.
arteriosclerotic intracranial a.
arteriosclerotic thoracoabdominal aortic a.
arteriovenous pulmonary a.
ascending aortic a.
aspergillotic a.
atherosclerotic aortic a.
atrial septal a.
axillary a.
bacterial a.
basilar artery a.
berry intracranial a.
bifurcation a.
bland aortic a.
brachiocephalic arterial a.
brain a.
bulging a.
calcified wall of a.
cardiac ventricle a.
carotid artery a.
carotid-ophthalmic a.
cavernous sinus a.
cavity of a.
celiac artery a.
cerebral a.
circle of Willis a.
circumscript a.
cirsoid a.
clinoid a.
clip ligation of a.
clipping of a.
coating of a.
coiling of a.
communicating artery a.
compound a.
congenital aortic sinus a.
congenital arteriosclerotic a.
congenital cerebral a.
congenital intracranial a.
congenital left ventricular a.
congenital pulmonary artery a.
congenital renal a.
contained leak of aortic a.
coronary artery a.
coronary vessel a.
cranial a.
cylindroid a.
degenerative aortic a.
de novo a.
dilatation of a.
dissecting abdominal a.
dissecting aortic a.
dissecting basilar artery a.
dissecting intracranial a.
distal aortic arch a.
dome of a.
Dorendorf sign of aortic arch a.
Drummond sign of aortic a.
ductal a.
ductus arteriosus a.
ectatic a.
eggshell border of a.
embolic a.
extracerebral a.
extracranial a.
false a.
feeding artery of a.
fenestration of dissecting a.
fundus of a.
fusiform a.
Galen vein a.
giant brain a.
great cerebral vein of Galen a.
hematoma of a.
hemorrhage of a.
hepatic artery a.
hernial a.
hunterian ligation of a.
Hunt-Kosnik classification of a.
iliac artery a.
imperforate a.

induced thrombosis of aortic a.
infected a.
inflammatory aortic a.
infrarenal abdominal aortic a.
innominate a.
internal carotid artery a.
a. of internal carotid artery
intracavernous carotid a.
intracerebral a.
intracranial a. (ICA)
intracranial berry a.
intramural coronary artery a.
isthmus a.
juxtarenal aortic a.
kidney a.
late false a.
lateral a.
leaking abdominal aortic a.
left ventricular a.
lower basilar a.
luetic aortic a.
malignant bone a.
miliary a.
mirror image a.
mixed a.
M1 segment a.
mural a.
mycotic a.
mycotic aortic a.
mycotic brain a.
mycotic intracranial a.
neck of a.
neoplastic a.
nodular a.
orbital a.
pararenal aortic a.
pelvic a.
perforating a.
phthisis of a.
popliteal artery a.
portal vein a.
a. of posterior communicating artery
posterior communicating artery a.
posterior-inferior cerebellar artery a.
postinfarction ventricular a.
Pott a.
precursor sign to rupture of a.
prerenal aortic a.
prerupture of a.
pulmonary arteriovenous a.
pulmonary artery a.
pulmonary artery compression ascending aortic a.
racemose a.
Rasmussen mycotic a.
rebleeding of a.
renal artery a.
rerupture of a.
ruptured a.
ruptured intracranial a.
sac of a.
sacciform a.
saccular a.
sacral a.
serpentine a.
Shekelton a.
sinus of Valsalva a.
spindle-shaped a.
splanchnic a.
splenic artery a.
spontaneous infantile ductal a.
spurious a.
subclavian a.
subvalvular a.
supraclinoid carotid a.
suprarenal aortic a.
suprarenal extension of a.
suprasellar a.
syphilitic aortic a.
thoracic aortic a.
thoracoabdominal aortic a.
thrombosed giant vertebral artery a.
thrombotic a.
trapping of a.
traumatic intracranial a. (TICA)
true aortic a.
true heart a.
true ventricular a.
tubular a.
uterine cirsoid a.
varicose a.
varix of a.
vein of Galen a.
venous a.
ventricular septal a.
verminous a.
wall of a.
windsock a.
worm a.

aneurysmal
a. bone cyst (ABC)
a. bone cyst doughnut sign
a. clip

NOTES

aneurysmal *(continued)*
a. coil
a. dissection
a. fundus
a. hematoma
a. hemorrhage
a. neck
a. phthisis
a. proportion
a. rupture
a. sac
a. vein
a. wall
a. wall calcification
a. wall gas
a. widening of aorta
aneurysmectomy
aneurysmogram
aneurysmography
AngeLase combined mapping-laser probe
angel-wing sign
Anger
A. camera
A. scintillation camera
Anghelescu sign
angiitis (*var. of* angitis)
angiitis-granulomatosis disorder
angioblastic lymphadenopathy
angioblastoma
bone a.
cord a.
malignant a.
angiocardiography
ambulatory equilibrium a.
biplane a.
equilibrium radionuclide a.
exercise radionuclide a.
first-pass radionuclide exercise a.
gated radionuclide a.
radionuclide a.
transseptal a.
angiocentric
a. immunoproliferative disorder
a. immunoproliferative lesion
a. lymphoproliferative lesion
a. T-cell lymphoma
Angio-Conray
A.-C. contrast medium
A.-C. imaging agent
Angiocontrast imaging agent
angio-CT
superselective a.-C.
angiodynagraphy
angiodysgenetic
angiodysplasia
a. of colon
angioedema
angioendotheliomatosis
reactive proliferating a.
angioendotheliosis
angiofibroblastic
a. hyperplasia
a. proliferation
a. tendinosis
angiofibroma
juvenile nasopharyngeal a. (JNPA)
angiofollicular
a. hyperplasia lymph node
a. lymph node hyperplasia
a. and plasmacytic polyadenopathy
angiogenesis
Angiografin
A. imaging agent
angiogram (*See* angiography)
balloon occlusion pulmonary a.
biplane left ventricular a.
digital subtraction pulmonary a.
percutaneous transluminal coronary a., PTCA a.
projection a.
radionuclide a. (RNA)
small-angle double-incidence a. (SADIA)
spinal a.
visceral a.
angiographic
a. corkscrew artery
a. finding
a. guide wire
a. muscle mass index
a. occlusion
a. target
a. targeting
a. Teflon dilator
angiographically
a. occult intracranial vascular malformation (AOIVM)
a. occult vascular malformation (AOVM)
a. occult vessel
a. visualized vascular malformation (AVVM)
angiography
adrenal a.
ambulatory equilibrium a.
aortic arch a.
axial a.
basilar a.
biplane a.
black blood magnetic resonance a.
blood pool radionuclide a.
blush of dye on a.
brain capillary a.
breath-hold contrast-enhanced three-dimensional MR a.

bronchial a.
Brown-Dodge method for a.
cardiac gated MR a.
carotid a.
cavernous brain a.
celiac a.
cerebral a.
CO_2 a.
computed tomographic a. (CTA)
computerized tomographic hepatic a. (CTHA)
contrast a.
coronary a.
cut-film a.
cystic duct a.
2DFT time-of-flight MR a.
3D gadolinium-enhanced magnetic resonance a.
diagnostic a.
digital celiac trunk a.
digital rotational a. (DRA)
digital subtraction a. (DSA)
digital subtraction rotational a.
3D inflow MR a.
directional color a. (DCA)
dobutamine thallium a.
3D phase-contrast magnetic resonance a.
dynamic tagging magnetic resonance a.
ECG-synchronized digital subtraction a.
edge-detection a.
elastic subtraction spiral CT a.
electrocardiogram-synchronized digital subtraction a.
Epistar subtraction a.
equilibrium radionuclide a.
femoral runoff a.
femorocerebral catheter a.
first-pass radionuclide a.
fluorescein a.
FluoroPlus a.
four-vessel cerebral a.
frameless stereotactic digital subtraction a.
functional magnetic resonance a. (fMRA)
gated blood pool a.
gated equilibrium radionuclide a.
gated nuclear a.
helical computed tomographic a. (HCTA)
hepatic a.
a. imaging
indocyanine green a.
innominate a.
intercostal artery a.
internal carotid a.
interventional a.
intraarterial digital subtraction a. (IADSA)
intraarterial stereotactic digital subtraction a.
intracranial MR a.
intraoperative digital subtraction a. (IDIS, IDSA)
intravenous digital subtraction a. (IVDSA)
intravenous fluorescein a. (IVFA)
intravenous stereotactic digital subtraction a.
left coronary a. (LCA)
left ventricular a.
low field MR a.
magnetic resonance a. (MRA)
magnification a.
mesenteric a.
multislab magnetic resonance a.
noncardiac a.
nonselective a.
nontriggered phase-contrast MR a.
nuclear a.
occlusion a.
orthogonal view on a.
pancreatic a.
phase-contrast a.
phase-contrast MR a.
postangioplasty a.
postembolization a.
postoperative a.
posttourniquet occlusion a.
preoperative a.
PTCA coronary a.
pulmonary artery wedge a.
pulmonary vein wedge a.
renal a.
resistive index a.
rest and exercise gated nuclear a.
right coronary a. (RCA)
scintigraphic a.
segmented k-space time-of-flight MR a.

NOTES

angiography *(continued)*
Seldinger a.
selective a.
selective arterial magnetic resonance a.
selective presaturation MR a.
selective venous magnetic resonance a.
shaded-surface display CT a.
single-plane a.
sitting-up view a.
spiral CT a. (SCTA)
stereotactic cerebral a.
a. suite
superselective a.
Tagarno 3SD cine projector for a.
therapeutic a.
thoracic a.
three-compartment wrist a.
three-dimensional gadolinium-enhanced MR a.
three-dimensional helical CT a.
three-dimensional inflow MR a.
three-dimensional phase-contrast MR a.
time-of-flight magnetic resonance a.
transseptal a.
transvenous digital subtraction a.
tumor blush on a.
velocity encoding on brain MR a.
venous brain a.
vertebral a.
angioimmunoblastic
a. lymphadenopathy
a. lymphadenopathy-like T-cell lymphoma
angioinfarction
angioleiomyoma
angiolipofibroma
angiolipoma
epidural a.
angiolithic
a. degeneration
a. sarcoma
angiolymphoid hyperplasia
angioma, pl. **angiomata**
arterial a.
arteriovenous interhemispheric a.
capillary a.
cavernous a.
cutaneous a.
encephalic a.
extracerebral cavernous a.
intracranial cavernous a.
intradermal a.
a. lymphaticum
pulmonary a.
a. serpiginosum
spider a.
superficial a.
telangiectatic a.
a. venosum racemosum
venous a.
AngioMARK contrast agent
Angiomat 6000 contrast delivery system
angiomatoid
a. malignant fibrous histiocytoma
a. tumor
angiomatosis
cystic bone a.
encephalotrigeminal a.
epithelioid a.
meningofacial a.
a. of retina
retinal a.
retinocerebellar a.
visceral a.
angiomatous
a. disease
a. lymphoid hamartoma
a. nasal polyp
a. syndrome
angiomyofibroma
angiomyolipoma
hepatic a.
kidney a.
renal a.
angiomyoma
angiomyosarcoma
angiomyxoma
umbilical cord a.
angioneuromyoma
angioneurotic edema
angioosteohypertrophy syndrome
angiopathy
cerebral amyloid a.
angioplastic meningioma
angioplasty sheath
angiopneumography
AngioRad radiation system
angioreticuloendothelioma of heart
angioreticuloma
spine a.
angiosarcoma
bone a.
breast a.
cavernous a.
a. of heart
hepatic a.
liver a.
spleen a.
angioscopic guidance
Angio-Seal
angiotensin
a. II
angiotensin-converting enzyme (ACE)

angiotherapy
vasoocclusive a. (VAT)
angiotomomyelography
angiotropic large cell lymphoma
Angiovist
A. contrast medium
A. 282, 292, 370 imaging agent
AngioVista angiographic system
angitis, angiitis
allergic granulomatous a.
cutaneous leukocytoclastic a.
necrotizing a.
angle
acetabular a.
acromial a.
anorectal a.
antegonial a.
anterior angulation a.
anterior talocalcaneal a.
a. of anteversion
arch a.
basal a.
Baumann a.
Beatson combined ankle a.
bimalleolar a.
blunting of costophrenic a.
blunting of costovertebral a.
blurring of costophrenic a.
Böhler a.
Boogaard a.
Bowman a.
Bragg a.
brain tumor at cerebellopontine a.
C a.
calcaneal inclination a.
calcaneal pitch a.
calcaneoplantar a.
capital epiphysis a.
capitolunate a.
cardiodiaphragmatic a.
cardiohepatic a.
cardiophrenic a.
carinal a.
carpal wrist a.
carrying a.
CCD a.
central collodiaphyseal a.
cephalic a.
cephalometric a.
cerebellopontine a. (CPA)
Citelli a.
Clarke arch a.
clivus-canal a.
Cobb scoliosis a.
Codman a.
condylar a.
congruence a.
costal a.
costolumbar a.
costophrenic a.
costosternal a.
costovertebral a. (CVA)
craniofacial a.
craniovertebral a.
a. of declination of metatarsal
distal articular set a. (DASA)
Doppler a.
dorsiflexion a. (DFA)
dorsoplantar talometatarsal a.
dorsoplantar talonavicular a.
Drennan metaphyseal-epiphyseal a.
duodenojejunal a.
Ebstein a.
epigastric a.
exposure a.
fan a.
femoral torsion V a.
femorotibial a. (FTA)
Ferguson a.
first-fifth intermetatarsal a.
first metatarsal a.
first-second intermetatarsal a.
flip a.
focal spot-to-film a.
foot-progression a. (FPA)
Frankfort mandibular incisor a.
Garden a.
gastroesophageal a.
Gissane a.
gonial a.
a. of greatest extension (AGE)
a. of greatest flexion (AGF)
hallux dorsiflexion a. (DFA)
hallux interphalangeus a.
hallux valgus a. (HVA)
hallux valgus interphalangeus a.
hepatic a.
hepatorenal a.
Hibbs metatarsocalcaneal a.
Hilgenreiner a.
His a.
a. of His
incident a.
a. of inclination of urethra

NOTES

angle *(continued)*
a. of incongruity
increased carrying a.
infrasternal a.
a. of insonation
intermetatarsal a. (IMA)
kite a.
Konstram a.
lateral patellofemoral a.
lateral plantar metatarsal a.
lateral talocalcaneal a.
lateral talometatarsal a.
lateral tarsometatarsal a.
Laurin a.
Lewis a.
Louis a.
Ludovici a.
Ludwig a.
lumbosacral joint a.
magnetization precession a.
a. of mandible
mandibular a.
Meary metatarsotalar a.
medial a.
mediolateral radiocarpal a.
Merchant a.
metaphyseal-epiphyseal a.
metatarsocalcaneal a.
metatarsotalar a.
metatarsus adductus a.
metatarsus primus a.
Mikulicz a.
navicular to first metatarsal a.
neck shaft a.
nidus a.
nutation a.
obliterated costophrenic a.
occipitocervical a.
a. of orientation
Pauwel a.
pelvic femoral a.
phase a.
phrenopericardial a.
Pirogoff a.
plantar metatarsal a.
pontine a.
posterior urethrovesical a.
precession a.
proximal articular set a. (PASA)
psoas shadow a.
pulse flip a.
Q a.
radiocarpal a.
Ranke a.
resting forefoot supination a.
a. of rib
Rolando a.
sacrohorizontal a.
sacrovertebral a.
scapular a.
set a.
slip a.
sphenoid a.
spinographic a.
splenic a.
splenorenal a.
sternal a.
sternoclavicular a.
subcarinal a.
substernal a.
subtalar a.
sulcus a.
surgical a.
talar tilt a.
talocalcaneal a.
talocrural a.
talometatarsal a.
talonavicular a.
tarsometatarsal a.
thigh-foot a. (TFA)
tibiofemoral a. (TFA)
tibiotalar a.
tip a.
tracheal bifurcation a.
transmalleolar axis-thigh a.
transmetatarsal-thigh a.
unsharpness of the costophrenic a.'s
urethrovesical a. (UVA)
valgus carrying a.
a. variation resolution
varus a.
varus metatarsophalangeal a.
venous a.
venous brain a.
venous neck a.
vertebrophrenic a.
vesicourethral a.
wedge isodose a.
Welcher basal a.
Wiberg a.
Wiltze a.
xiphoid a.

angled
a. pleural tube
a. slice

angles of trigone

Angström unit

angular
a. alignment
a. artery
a. curvature
a. deformity
a. deviation
a. frequency
a. gyrus (AG)

a. momentum
a. notch
a. process of orbit
a. sampling
a. vein
a. velocity

angularis
a. body
incisura a.
a. sulcus

angulated
a. catheter
a. fracture
a. lesion
a. segment

angulation
anterior a.
caudal-cranial a.
cephalic a.
coronal a.
cranial a.
forefoot a.
gantry a.
kyphotic a.
palmar a.
posttraumatic a.
spinal a.
a. of spine
valgus a.
varus a.
volar a.

angulus of stomach

anhaustral colonic gas pattern

anhydrous ammonia (NH_3)

ani (*gen. and pl. of* anus)

aniline cancer

aniridia

anisidide
acridinyl a.

anisoleukocytosis

anisopoikilocytosis

anisotrophy

anisotropic
a. 3D imaging
a. resolution
a. rotation
a. tissue
a. volume study

anisotropically
a. rotational diffusion (ARD)
a. rotational diffusion imaging

anisotropy
curvature a.
a. factor
magnetic a.

anisura

ankle
a. bone
disk of a.
eccentric axis of rotation of the a.
eversion of a.
footballer's a.
fused a.
a. fusion
a. instability
inversion injury of a.
a. joint
a. joint complex
laciniate ligament of a.
a. mortise
a. mortise axis
a. mortise fracture
a. mortise widening
neuropathic a.
sprained a.
a. swelling
syndesmosis sprain of a.
synthetic graft bypass to a.
a. systolic pressure
tailor's a.
transmalleolar a.
twisted a.

ankle-arm
a.-a. index
a.-a. pressure

ankle-brachial
a.-b. index (ABI)
a.-b. pressure measurement
a.-b. pressure ratio

ankylosing
a. hyperostosis
a. spondylitis

ankylosis
bony a.
extracapsular a.
false a.
fibrous a.
intracapsular a.
joint a.
ligamentous a.
shoulder a.
spurious a.
vertebral a.

NOTES

ankyroid (*var. of* ancyroid)
anlage, pl. **anlagen**
cartilaginous a.
pancreatic dorsal a.
ventral pancreatic a.
ANMR Insta-scan MR scanner
Ann Arbor classification
annealing
a. algorithm
simulated a.
annectant gyrus
annihilation
a. coincidence detection (ACD)
a. radiation
a. reaction
anniversary phenomenon
annotated imaging
annular
a. abscess
a. array
a. calcification
a. cartilage
a. constricting lesion
a. detector
a. dilatation
a. disk bulge
a. disruption
a. epiphysis
a. esophageal stricture
a. fiber
a. fibrosis
a. foreshortening
a. fracture
a. hypoplasia
a. ligament
a. ligament of trachea
a. pancreas
a. phased-array hyperthermia
a. placement
a. placenta
a. ring
annularis
digitus a.
annuli (*pl. of* annulus)
annuloaortic ectasia
annulospiral organ
annulus, anulus, pl. **annuli**
aortic valve a.
atrioventricular a.
bulging a.
calcified a.
a. fibrosus
a. fibrosus tear
fissure of a.
friable a.
mitral valve of a.
a. ovalis
pulmonary valve a.
redundant scallop of posterior a.
septal tricuspid a.
tricuspid valve a.
a. umbilicalis
valve a.
a. of Vieussens
Vieussens a.
ano
fissure in a.
fistula in a.
anococcygeal
a. ligament
a. raphe
anodal block
anode
molybdenum a.
a. ray
rhodium a.
rotating a.
a. tube
a. tube reloading
tungsten a.
anogenital
a. band
a. raphe
anomalad
Robin a.
anomalous
a. anatomy
a. branching
a. bronchus
a. craniovertebral junction
a. distribution
a. drainage
a. innominate artery compression syndrome
a. insertion
a. left coronary artery
a. left pulmonary artery
a. origin
a. origin of artery
a. pathway
a. pulmonary venous connection
a. pulmonary venous return
a. serum chemistry
a. vein of scimitar syndrome
a. vessel
anomaly, pl. **anomalies**
anorectal a.
aortic arch a.
atlas a.
atrioventricular junction a.
axis a.
back-angle a.
bell-clapper a. (BCA)
cardiac a.
cardiovascular a.
cloacal a.

congenital cardiac a.
congenital conotruncal a.
congenital gallbladder a.
congenital pancreatic a.
conjoined nerve root a.
conotruncal congenital a.
cranial a.
craniofacial a.
craniovertebral a.
Cruveilhier-Baumgarten a.
cutaneous vascular a.
developmental renal a.
double-inlet ventricle a.
duplication a.
Ebstein a.
extracardiac a.
fast-flow vascular a.
fetal cardiac a.
fetal chest a.
fetal CNS a.
fetal gastrointestinal a.
fetal heart a.
fetal neck a.
fetal urinary tract a.
Freund a.
gastrointestinal fetal a.
genitourinary a.
heart a.
jugular bulb a.
kidney a.
limb reduction a.
May-Hegglin a.
Michel a.
migrational a.
Mondini a.
müllerian duct a.
multiple congenital anomalies (MCA)
numerary renal a.
occipitoatlantoaxial a.
presacral a.
radial ray a.
segmentation a.
Shone a.
slow-flow vascular a.
structural a.
Taussig-Bing a.
tricuspid valve a.
Uhl a.
Undritz a.
urachal a.
urinary tract a.
uterine a.
in utero detection of cardiac a.
vascular a.
vena cava a.
venous a.
vertebral segmentation a.
Zahn a.

anonymous vein

anorectal
a. angle
a. anomaly
a. atresia
a. dysgenesis
a. fistula
a. junction
a. line
a. lymph node
a. malformation
a. manometry
a. melanoma
a. ring
a. tuberculosis

anorectum

anovular ovarian follicle

anoxia
brain a.
cerebral a.
perinatal a.

anoxic
a. encephalopathy
a. ischemia

Anrep effect

ansa, pl. **ansae**
a. of Vieussens

anserine
a. bursa
a. bursitis

anserinus
pes a.

antebrachial
a. fascia
a. vein

antebrachium

antecedent sign

antecolic

antecubital
a. fossa
a. space
a. vein

ante fenestram fissula

anteflexed uterus

anteflexion

NOTES

antegonial
a. angle
a. notch
antegrade
a. aortography
a. bile flow
a. blood flow
a. catheterization
a. cystography
a. diastolic flow
a. fast pathway
a. filling of vessels
a. perfusion
a. perfusion pressure measurement (APPM)
a. puncture
a. pyelography
a. pyelography imaging
a. refractory period
a. urography
a. venography
antepartum hemorrhage
anteprostatic gland
anterior
a. abdominal wall
a. angulation
a. angulation angle
a. aspect
a. atlas arch
a. atrial myocardial bundle
a. band
a. band of colon
a. basal bronchus
a. border
a. border of heart
a. bowing of sternum
a. bowing tibia
a. capsular shift
a. cardiac vein
a. cerebellar artery syndrome
a. cerebral artery (ACA)
a. cervical fusion (ACF)
a. choroidal artery
a. clear space
a. colliculus
a. column fracture
a. column of spine
a. commissure
a. commissure-posterior commissure (AC-PC)
a. communicating artery (ACoA)
a. communicating artery complex
a. communicating artery distribution infarct
a. compartment syndrome
a. condylar canal
a. condyloid foramen
a. cord syndrome
a. coronary plexus
a. corpus
a. corticospinal tract
a. cruciate deficit of knee
a. cruciate ligament (ACL)
a. cruciate ligament injury
a. current (AC) generator
a. curvature
a. cusp
a. cutaneous branch
a. descending artery
a. dislocation
a. drawer sign
a. epidural fat
a. exenteration
a. fascicular block
a. feet view
a. fibular ligament
a. fontanelle
a. fornix of vagina
a. glenoid labrum (AGL)
a. gray column
a. gray column of cord
a. horn
a. horn cell disease
a. horns of spinal cord
a. humeral line
a. hypothalamus
a. iliac crest
a. inferior tibiofibular ligament
a. intercostal artery
a. interhemispheric cistern
a. interhemispheric fissure
a. internal vertebral vein (AIVV)
a. internodal pathway
a. internodal tract of Bachmann
a. interventricular groove
a. jugular vein
a. junction line
a. labral avulsion
a. labral disruption
a. labroligamentous periosteal sleeve avulsion (ALPSA)
a. labroligamentous periosteal sleeve avulsion lesion
a. labrum periosteal sleeve avulsion lesion
a. leaflet prolapse
a. lobe
a. maxillary spine
a. median fissure
a. mediastinal compartment
a. mediastinal mass
a. mediastinum
a. meningeal artery
a. metatarsal arch
a. mitral valve leaflet

a. motion of posterior mitral valve leaflet
a. myocardial infarct (AMI)
a. oblique position
a. osteophyte
a. palatine foramen
a. papillary muscle (APM)
a. pararenal space (APS)
a. parietal lesion
a. pillar of fauces
a. planar image
a. planar imaging
a. precordium
a. predominance
a. projection
a. pulmonary plexus
a. recess of ischiorectal fossa
a. rectus fascia
a. rectus sheath
a. sacral foramen
a. sacral meningocele
a. sagittal diameter (ASD)
scalenus a.
a. scalloping of vertebra
a. semicircular canal
a. semilunar valve
a. septal myocardial infarct
serratus a. (SA)
a. spinal artery
a. spinal artery syndrome
a. spinal ligament calcification
a. spinocerebellar tract
a. spinothalamic tract
a. spur
a. surface of pancreas
a. talar dome
a. talocalcaneal angle
a. talofibular ligament (ATF)
a. temporal branch of posterior cerebral artery
a. terminal vein (ATV)
a. tibial artery
a. tibial bowing
a. tibial compartment
tibialis a.
a. tibial sign
a. tibial subluxation
a. tibial tendon
a. tibiofibular ligament
a. tip of temporal lobe
a. tracking
a. tricuspid leaflet (ATL)
a. tricuspid valve leaflet
a. urethra
a. urethral injury
a. wall antral ulcer
a. wall motion
a. wall myocardial infarct

anterior-inferior
a.-i. cerebellar artery (AICA)
a.-i. cerebral artery (AICA)
a.-i. communicating artery (AICA)
a.-i. iliac spine

anterior/posterior

anterior-posterior flow direction

anterior-superior iliac spine (ASIS)

anterior-to-posterior sagittal canal diameter

anteroapical
a. defect
a. trabecular septum

anterobasal segment

anterochiasmatic lesion

anterofundal placenta

anterograde
a. block
a. peristalsis

anteroinferior
a. dislocation
a myocardial infarct
a. triangular fragment

anterolateral (AL)
a. abdominal wall
a. aspect
a. compression fracture
a. fontanelle
a. groove
a. impingement
a. myocardial infarct
a. rotary knee instability
a. segment
a. surface
a. system
a. white matter of cord

anterolisthesis

anteromedial
a. superior humeral head impaction
a. surface

anteromedian groove

anteroposterior (AP)
a. (AP) film
a. (AP) projection
a. aspect
a. diameter

NOTES

anteroposterior *(continued)*
a. iliac spine
superior labral a.
a. talocalcaneal (APTC)
a. view
anteroseptal
a. commissure
a. myocardial infarct
antetorsion
femoral a.
anteversion
angle of a.
femoral a.
Magilligan technique for measuring neutral a.
anteverted uterus
anthracosilicosis
anthracosis
anthracotic material
anthrax pneumonia
anthrocotic tuberculosis
anthropoid pelvis
anthropologic baseline
anthropometric imaging
anthropometry
3D surface a.
anthropomorphic baseline
antialiasing technique
antibody
a. half-life
a. labeling
antibody-conjugated paramagnetic liposome (ACPL)
antibody-labeled circulating granulocyte
anticoagulation
anticoincidence circuit
antiestrogen radiologic therapy
antiferritin
iodine-131 a.
antiferromagnetism
antifibrin
a. antibody imaging
a. scintigraphy
antifibrin-MoAb antibody imaging agent
antigravity muscle
anti-idiotypic affinity chromatography
antimesenteric
a. border
a. border of distal ileum
a. fat pad
antimesocolic side of cecum
antimony
a. antimotility drug
a. imaging agent
antimyosin
a. antibody-Fab scintigraphy (AMA-Fab scintigraphy)
a. monoclonal antibody imaging agent
antitoxoplasmosis agent
antitragohelicine fissure
antitubercular therapy
antler sign
Anton syndrome
antra (*pl. of* antrum)
antral
a. beaking
a. edema
a. gastritis
a. G-cell hyperplasia
a. mucosal diaphragm
a. mucosal thickening
a. nipple sign
a. padding
a. polyp
a. pouch
a. sphincter
a. stasis
a. stenosis
a. stomach narrowing
a. stricture
a. ulcer
a. web
antritis
antrochoanal polyp
antroduodenal motility
antropyloric canal
antrum, pl. **antra**
aditus ad a.
cardiac a.
a. cardiacum of Highmore
gastric a.
Highmore a.
Malacarne a.
mastoid a.
maxillary a.
prepyloric a.
pyloric a.
retained gastric a.
a. of stomach
a. of Willis
Willis a.
anulus (*var. of* annulus)
anuria
anus, gen. and pl. **ani**
ectopic a.
imperforate a.
levator ani
anvil
a. bone
a. sign
AO, Ao
aorta
aortic opening
AO ankle fracture classification

AO classification of ankle fracture
AO tension band
AO:AC ratio
AO-Danis-Weber ankle fracture classification
AOIVM
angiographically occult intracranial vascular malformation
aorta, pl. **aortae (AO, Ao)**
abdominal a.
adult-type coarctation of a.
aneurysmal widening of a.
arch of a.
ascending a. (AA)
ascending hypoplasia of a.
bifurcation of a.
biventricular origin of a.
biventricular transposed a.
brachiocephalic trunk of a.
calcified a.
central a.
cervical a.
coarctation of a.
descending thoracic a.
dextropositioned a.
D-malposition of a.
double arch a.
double-barrel a.
draped a.
dynamic a.
ectasia of a.
elongated a.
feminine a.
Hodgson aneurysmal dilatation of the a.
infantile coarctation of a.
infrarenal abdominal a.
intramural hematoma of a.
juxtaductal coarctation of a.
kinked a.
L-malposition of a.
native a.
overriding a.
pericardial a.
porcelain a.
postductal coarctation of a.
preductal coarctation of a.
pseudocoarctation of a.
recoarctation of a.
reconstruction of a.
retroesophageal a.
reversed coarctation of a.
root of a.
sclerosis of a.
small feminine a.
stenosis of a.
supraceliac a.
supradiaphragmatic a.
symptomatic coarctation of a.
terminal a.
thoracic a.
thoracoabdominal a.
tortuous a.
transposed a.
tulip bulb a.
unwinding of a.
ventral a.
widening of a.
wide tortuous a.
aorta-left ventricular fistula
aorta-right ventricular fistula
aortic
a. allograft
a. aneurysm
a. annulus abscess
a. aperture
a. arch
a. arch aneurysm
a. arch aneurysm sign
a. arch angiography
a. arch anomaly
a. arch atresia
a. arch calcification
a. arch hypoplasia syndrome
a. arch interruption
a. arch lesion
a. arch malformation
a. arch obstruction
a. atherosclerosis
a. atresia
a. attenuation
a. bifurcation
a. body tumor
a. bulb
a. button
a. calcification sign
a. cannulation
a. cartilage
a. closure (AC)
a. coarctation
a. cuff
a. cusp
a. cusp separation
a. deviation

NOTES

aortic *(continued)*
a. diameter (AD)
a. dissection
a. distensibility
a. elongation
a. enlargement
a. flow (AF)
a. flow volume
a. foramen
a. gland
a. graft
a. graft infection
a. hiatus
a. idiopathic necrosis
a. impedance
a. incisura
a. inflow
a. insult
a. isthmus
a. kinking
a. knob
a. knuckle
a. lumen
a. lymph node
a. motion artifact
a. nipple
a. nipple sign
a. nitrogen-nipple sign
a. node metastasis
a. notch
a. opening (AO, Ao)
a. opening of heart
a. orifice
a. ostium
a. outflow gradient
a. outflow obstruction
a. override
a. oxygen saturation
a. paravalvular leak
a. penetrating ulcer
a. plexus
a. prominence
a. pseudoaneurysm
a. pullback
a. reconstruction
a. regurgitation (AR)
a. root
a. root cineangiography
a. root diameter
a. root dilatation
a. root dimension
a. root echocardiography
a. root homograft
a. root pressure
a. root ratio
a. root replacement
a. runoff
a. rupture
a. sac
a. sclerosis
a. segment
a. septal defect
a. septum
a. shag
a. sinotubular junction
a. sinus aneurysm
a. sinus fistula
a. sinus to right ventricle fistula
a. spindle
a. stenosis (AS)
a. stiffness
a. stump blowout
a. subvalvular ring
a. thromboembolism
a. thrombosis
a. tract complex hypoplasia
a. transsection
a. tube graft
a. valve (AoV)
a. valve annulus
a. valve area (AVA)
a. valve atresia
a. valve calcification
a. valve deformity
a. valve echocardiography
a. valve endocarditis
a. valve gradient (AVG)
a. valve leaflet prolapse
a. valve lesion
a. valve nodule
a. valve obstruction
a. valve opening
a. valve opening to aortic valve closing ratio (AO:AC ratio)
a. valve peak instantaneous gradient
a. valve pressure gradient
a. valve replacement (AVR)
a. valve sinus
a. valve thickening
a. valvular disease (AVD)
a. valvular incompetence
a. valvular insufficiency
a. vasa vasorum
a. vent suction line
a. vestibule of ventricle
a. wall thickening
a. window
a. window node
a. wrap

aortic-brachiocephalic (ABC)
a.-b. (ABC) injury

aortic-left ventricular tunnel

aorticopulmonary (*var. of* aortopulmonary)

aorticorenal
a. ganglion
a. graft
aortitis
bacterial a.
infectious a.
luetic a.
noninfectious a.
a. syndrome
syphilitic a.
Takayasu a.
aortoarteritis
aortocaval fistula
aortocoronary valve
aortoduodenal fistula
aortoenteric fistula
aortoesophageal
a. fistula
aortofemoral
a. arteriography
a. bypass graft
a. runoff
aortofemorofemoral
descending thoracic a. (DTAF)
aortogastric
aortogram
aortography
abdominal a.
antegrade a.
arch a.
ascending a.
balloon occlusive a.
biplanar a.
contrast a.
countercurrent a.
digital subtraction a.
flush a.
a. imaging
postangioplasty a.
retrograde a.
retrograde femoral a.
retrograde transaxillary a.
retrograde transfemoral a.
retrograde translumbar a.
selective visceral a.
supravalvular a.
thoracic arch a.
translumbar a. (TLA)
ultrasonic a.
aortoiliac
a. aneurysm
a. bypass graft
a. inflow assessment
a. inflow system
a. obstruction
a. obstructive disease (AIOD)
a. stenosis
a. thrombosis
aortoiliofemoral artery
aortomegaly
diffuse a.
aortopathy
idiopathic medial a.
aortoplasty
balloon a.
patch-graft a.
posterior patch a.
subclavian flap a.
a. with patch graft
aortopulmonary, aorticopulmonary
a. fenestration
a. fistula
a. septal defect
a. septum
a. trunk
a. window
a. window mass
aortosclerosis
aortoseptal continuity
aortosigmoid fistula
aortovelography
transcutaneous a. (TAV)
aortoventriculoplasty
AoV
aortic valve
AOVM
angiographically occult vascular malformation
AP
adenomatous polyp
anteroposterior
AP inversion stress vagina view
AP malleolar bisection
AP supine portable view
apallic syndrome
APB
abductor pollicis brevis
APC-3 collimator
APC-4 collimator
ape hand of syringomyelia
apelike hand
aperiodic
a. complex

NOTES

aperiodic *(continued)*
a. functional MR imaging
a. wave
aperistalsis
aperistaltic
a. distal ureteral segment
a. esophagus
aperta
spina bifida a.
aperture
aortic a.
a. diaphragm
superior thoracic a.
APEX
A. 409, 415 camera
apex, pl. **apices**
a. beat
a. of bladder
cardiac a.
a. cordis
displaced left ventricular a.
duodenal bulb a.
a. of external ring
external ring a.
a. of femur
a. of fibula
F point of cardiac a.
a. of head of patella
a. of the heart
Koch triangle a.
a. of Koch triangle
a. of left ventricle
left ventricular a.
lung a.
orbital a.
petrous a.
a. of petrous portion of temporal bone
a. of prostate
right ventricular a. (RVA)
sternal a.
systolic retraction of a.
uptilted cardiac a.
ventricular a.
apexcardiogram (ACG)
aphagia
aphalangia
aphtha, pl. **aphthae**
aphthous
a. stomach ulcer
apical
a. air space
a. aspect
a. atelectasis
a. bronchus
a. canaliculus
a. cap
a. capping
a. cap sign
a. complex
a. corn
a. distribution lung disease
a. duodenal ulcer
a. ectodermal ridge (AER)
a. fenestration
a. five-chamber view echocardiography
a. foramen
a. gland
a. granuloma
a. hypertrophy (AHC)
a. hypokinesis
a. hypoperfusion
a. impulse
a. infiltrate
a. lesion
a. ligament
a. lordotic projection
a. lordotic view
a. lymph node
a. myocardial infarct
a. notch
a. petrositis
a. pleural thickening
a. pneumonia
a. posterior artery
a. process
a. scarring
a. segment
a. short-axis slice
a. and subcostal four-chambered view
a. surface of heart
a. suture
a. thinning
a. tissue
a. two-chamber view
a. two-chamber view echocardiography
a. wall
a. wall motion
a. window
apical-lateral wall myocardial infarct
apically directed chest tube
apices (*pl. of* apex)
apicitis
petrous a.
apicoposterior
a. bronchus
a. segment
apiculate waveform
aplasia
bone marrow a.
cerebellar a.
cochlea a.
a. of deep vein

deep venous a.
lung a.
Michel a.
pulmonary a.
radial a.
uterine a.
aplastic uterus
Apley sign
APM
anterior papillary muscle
apnea
apnea/bradycardia ratio
apnea-hypopnea index (AHI)
apocrine
a. adenoma
a. carcinoma
a. cyst
a. sweat gland
Apogee
A. CX 200 echo system
A. RX400
A. ultrasound device
Apollo DXA bone densitometry system
aponeurosis
bicipital a.
digital a.
epicranial a.
external oblique a.
flexor carpi ulnaris a.
internal oblique a.
palmar a.
plantar a.
tendon a.
aponeurotic
a. band
a. fibroma
a. portion of diaphragm
a. triangle
a. troika
aponeurotica
galea a.
apophyseal, apophysial
a. fracture
a. injury
a. joint
a. lesion
a. point
a. pouch
apophysis, pl. **apophyses**
bone lesion a.
fragmentation of a.
a. of Rau
rim a.
ring a.
apophysitis
calcaneal a.
iliac a.
apoplexy
Broadbent a.
cerebellar a.
delayed pineal a.
mesenteric a.
pineal a.
postpartum pituitary a.
pulmonary artery a.
pulmonary vein a.
aporic gland
apotentiality
cerebral a.
APP
average pixel projection
apparatus, pl. **apparatus, apparatuses**
extensor a.
Hilal embolization a.
juxtaglomerular a. (JGA)
mitral a.
oculomotor a.
valvular a.
vestibular a.
zero time of the x-ray a.
apparent
a. diffusion coefficient
a. paramagnetism
appearance
apple-core a.
apple-peel a.
applesauce a.
ball-in-hand a.
banding a.
batwing a.
beaded a.
beaked a.
beaten brass a.
beaten silver a.
beavertail a.
bilaminar a.
birdlike a.
blade-of-grass a.
bone-within-bone a.
bubble-like a.
bull-neck a.
bull's eye a.
bunch of grapes a.
catheter tip hockey-stick a.

NOTES

appearance *(continued)*
cauliflower a.
Christmas tree a.
cobblestone a.
cobra-head a.
cobweb a.
cockscomb a.
coffee-bean a.
coiled-spring a.
collar-button a.
colonic lead-pipe a.
corkscrew a.
cottage loaf a.
cotton-ball a.
cotton-wool a.
crabmeat-like a.
cushingoid a.
cystic a.
double-bubble a.
double-bulb a.
double-halo a.
drooping lily a.
duodenal teardrop a.
feathery a.
fine-speckled a.
fish-flesh a.
flame a.
frayed string a.
froglike a.
frondlike a.
hair-standing-on-end a.
hammered brass a.
hammered silver a.
heterogeneous a.
hole-within-hole a.
homogeneous a.
Honda sign a.
honeycombed a.
horseshoe a.
hot-cross-bun a.
inverse comma a.
inverted-T a.
isodense a.
jail-bars a.
jelly-belly a.
kernel of popcorn a.
lacelike a.
leafless tree a.
light bulb a.
lobulated saccular a.
lollipop tree a.
meconium ileus soap-bubble a.
moth-eaten a.
mottled a.
multiseptate a.
mushroom a.
Neptune trident a.
onion peel a.
onionskin a.
owl's eye a.
pancake a.
panda a.
picket fence a.
picture frame a.
popcornlike a.
pruned-tree a.
pseudo-post Billroth I a.
punched-out a.
railroad track a.
reticulogranular a.
rugger jersey a.
saber-shin a.
sandwich a.
sawtooth a.
scalloped a.
scottie dog a.
serrated a.
shell-of-bone a.
sign of the burnuous a.
signet ring a.
snake's head a.
spadelike a.
spiderweb a.
spiral a.
spongy a.
stacked-coin a.
stepladder a.
stippled a.
string-of-beads a.
string-of-pearls a.
sunburst a.
Swiss Alps a.
Swiss cheese a.
tam-o-shanter a.
target a.
teardrop a.
tree-in-winter bile duct a.
trefoil a.
trilaminar a.
trilayer a.
twisted small bowel ribbon a.
ventricle batwing a.
walking-stick a.
waterfall a.
weblike a.
whorled a.
windsock a.
wineglass a.
wormy a.

appendage
atrial a.
cecal a.
coccygeal a.
epiploic a.
juxtaposition of atrial a.
left atrial a. (LAA)

left auricular a. (LAA)
right atrial a. (RAA)
testicular torsion a.
torsed a.
truncated atrial a.
vermicular a.
wide-based, blunt-ended right-sided atrial a.

appendectomy

appendiceal
a. abscess
a. cancer
a. intussusception
a. mass
a. stump

appendices (*pl. of* appendix)

appendicitis
abortive a.
acute a.
epiploic a.
target sign a.

appendicolith (*var. of* appendolith)

appendicolithiasis (*var. of* appendolithiasis)

appendicular
a. lymph node
a. skeleton
a. vein

appendix, pl. **appendices**
cecal a.
double a.
ensiform a.
a. of epididymis
epiploic a.
filiform a.
a. of Morgagni
Morgagni a.
a. mucocele
paracecal a.
perforated gangrenous a.
retrocecal a.
retroileal a.
a. rupture
subcecal a.
a. testis
a. of ventricle of larynx
vermicular a.
vermiform a.
vesiculosa a.
xiphoid a.

appendolith, appendicolith

appendolithiasis, appendicolithiasis

apperceptive mass

apple-core
a.-c. appearance
a.-c. carcinoma
a.-c. tumor

apple-green birefringence

apple-peel
a.-p. appearance
a.-p. appearance of the GI tract
a.-p. bowel

applesauce
a. appearance
a. sign

application
interstitial radioelement a.
intracavitary radioelement a.
ribbon a.
surface-dose a.
surface radioelement a.

application-specific integrated circuit (ASIC)

applicator
beta-ray a.
Blocdorn a.
Burnett a.
colpostat a.
Henschke seed a.
intracavitary afterloading a.
Mick seed a.
MIRALVA a.
Nucletron a.
^{90}Sr-loaded eye a.
Syed-Puthawala-Hedger esophageal a.
tandem a.
Wang a.

APPM
antegrade perfusion pressure measurement

apposing articular surface

apposition
bone-to-bone a.
bony a.
close a.
fracture in close a.
a. of leaflets
margin of a.

approach
axillofemoral a.
brachial artery a.
femoral artery a.
femoral venous a.

NOTES

approach *(continued)*
mask-based a.
pencil-beam a.
retrograde femoral arterial a.
approximation
Born a.
apron
abdominal a.
lead a.
quadriceps a.
a. shield
APS
anterior pararenal space
APT
automatic peak tracking
APT intrathecal
APTC
anteroposterior talocalcaneal
AquaSens
A. FMS 1000 fluid monitoring system
aqueduct
cerebral a.
cochlear a.
a. compression
forking of sylvian a.
gliosis of sylvian a.
mesencephalon a.
midbrain a.
Monro a.
sylvian a.
a. of Sylvius
ventricular a.
vestibular a.
aqueductal
a. CSF stroke volume
a. forking
a. obstruction
a. occlusion
a. stenosis
aqueous
a. solution
a. vein
Aquilion CT scanner
AR
aortic regurgitation
atrial rate
ARA
American Rheumatism Association
arabinsylguanosine triphosphate
arachnodactilia
arachnodactyly
a. bone
a. CHD
arachnoid
a. brain cyst
a. canal
a. diverticulum
a. fibrosis
a. granulation
a. granulation calcification
a. loculation of the spine
pia a.
a. retrocerebellar pouch
a. space
a. spine cyst
a. of uncus
a. villi obstruction
a. villus
arachnoidal foramen
arachnoiditis
adhesive a.
cystic a.
fibrosing a.
Aran-Duchenne amyotrophy
Arantius
A. canal
A. ligament
A. nodule
nodulus A.
A. ventricle
arborescens
lipoma a.
arborescent
arborization
a. block
a. of ducts
arborize
arc
pulmonary a.
reflex a.
a. ring
a. therapy
a. welder's lung
arcade
collateral a.
a. of Frohse
Frohse ligamentous a.
gastroepiploic a.
mitral a.
septal a.
Struthers a.
subpleural pulmonary a.
superficialis a.
Arcelin view
arch
a. angle
anterior atlas a.
anterior metatarsal a.
a. of aorta
a. of aorta abnormality
aortic a.
a. aortography
articular a.
atlas a.
a. of atlas

a. of bone
carpal a.
cervical aortic a.
chimney-shaped aortic a.
chimney-shaped high aortic a.
circumflex retroesophageal a.
congenital interruption of aortic a.
coracoacromial a.
cortical kidney a.
deep a.
distal aortic a.
double aortic a.
ductal a.
embryonic aortic a.
embryonic branchial a.
a. of fauces
first branchial a.
flattened a.
a. of foot
fourth branchial a.
a. fracture
Hapad metatarsal a.
hemal a.
high a.
Hillock a.
hyoid a.
hypochordal a.
hypoplastic aortic a.
interruption of aortic a.
keystone of calcar a.
a. length index
longitudinal a.
lung a.
medial a.
midaortic a.
mural a.
neural vertebral a.
osseocartilaginous a.
osseoligamentous a.
palmar arterial a.
plantar arterial a.
posterior metatarsal a.
pubic a.
retroesophageal a.
right aortic a.
right-sided a.
a. of Riolan
Riolan a.
a. rupture
second branchial a.
subpubic a.
superciliary a.
superficial palmar arterial a.
target a.
tarsal a.
third branchial a.
tortuous aortic a.
transverse aortic a.
a. of vertebra
vertebral a.
Zimmerman a.
zygomatic a.

arched crest

archenteric canal

Archer syndrome

archicortex

arching

a. of back
a. of mitral valve leaflet

architectural

a. alterations of bone
a. disturbance
a. effacement

architecture

bone a.
bony a.
brain a.
a. of brain
ductal a.
foot a.
hepatic a.
intestinal villous a.
intranodal a.
lobular a.
lung a.
mural a.

archive

digital a.

arciform vein

Arcitumomab diagnostic imaging system

Arco classification

arcuate

a. artery
a. artery of foot
a. complex
a. crest
a. eminence
a. fasciculus (AF)
a. fiber involvement
a. ligament
a. ligament of diaphragm
a. movement
a. nucleus
a. uterus

NOTES

arcuate *(continued)*
a. vein
a. vessel
arcuatus
arcuate uterus
pes a.
talipes a.
uterus a.
ARD
anisotropically rotational diffusion
ARDMS
American Registry of Diagnostic Medical Sonographers
ARDS
acute respiratory distress syndrome
adult respiratory distress syndrome
area
a. of abnormal density
amygdaloid a.
anechoic a.
aortic valve a. (AVA)
arrhythmogenic a.
Bamberger a.
bare a.
body surface a. (BSA)
Broca a.
Brodmann a.
callosal a.
cardiac frontal a.
cortical motor a.
cross-sectional a. (CSA)
denervated a.
a. of denudation
echo-free a.
effective balloon-dilated a. (EBDA)
Erb a.
fat-density a.
fluid-filled a.
fractional a.
a. gastrica
gastrohepatic bare a.
Gorlin formula for aortic valve a.
Gorlin formula for mitral valve a.
Haeckerman a.
Hatle method to calculate mitral valve a.
hilar a.
hot a.
hyperechoic a.
hypodense a.
hypoechoic a.
hypometabolic a.
a. of increased radiolabeling
infraclavicular a.
infrahilar a.
ischemic a.
jet a. (JA)
language a.
lenticular a.
luminal a.
lytic a.
midsternal a.
mitral regurgitant signal a.
mitral valve a. (MVA)
motor a.
olfactory a.
parietal association a.
parietooccipital a.
parietotemporal a.
peak a.
periaortic a.
perihilar a.
periportal a.
peroneal a.
pharyngeal a.
photopenic a.
postcricoid a.
premotor a.
proliferation a.
puboischial a.
pulmonic a.
punched-out a.
radiodensity a.
radiolucent a.
rarefied a.
regurgitant orifice a. (ROA)
retrocardiac a.
retroperitoneal a.
retrosternal a.
Rolando a.
sclerotic a.
scrotal a.
septal a.
skip a.
sonolucent a.
speech a.
stenosis a.
subglottic a.
subhepatic a.
suprapubic a.
tricuspid a.
a. under the (concentration-time) curve (AUC)
valve a.
water density a.
watershed a.
Wernicke a.
xiphopubic a.
zygomaticomalar a.
area/hemidiameter variation
area-length method for ejection fraction
areflexia
detrusor a.
Arelin method

arena
simulation of treatment a.
areola, pl. **areolae**
areolaa of bone
areolar
a. connective tissue
a. plane
ARF
acute renal failure
acute respiratory failure
argentaffinoma
argon-pumped dye laser
arhinencephaly
arm
Leyla a.
linebacker's a.
outrigger a.
Popeye a.
Armanni-Ebstein lesion
armored heart
Arnoff external fixation device
Arnold
A. canal
A. convolution
Arnold-Chiari
A.-C. deformity
A.-C. malformation
A.-C. syndrome
arrangement
string-of-pearls nuclear a.
array
Acuson 5-MHz linear a.
annular a.
cartesian reference coordinate voxel a.
convex linear a.
detector a.
electrode a.
gate a.
high-density linear a.
linear electrode a.
linear phased a.
NMR quadrature detection a.
parallel a.'s
silicon diode a.
symmetric phased a.
thin-film transistor a.
voxel a.
arrest
circulatory a.
electrical circulatory a.
epiphyseal a.
flow a.
growth plate a.
intermittent sinus a.
profound hypothermic circulatory a. (PHCA)
a. reaction
sinus a.
transient sinus a.
arrested circulation
arrhenoblastoma
arrhinencephaly
arrhythmia circuit
arrhythmia-insensitive
a.-i. flow-sensitive alternating inversion recovery (A-FAIR)
a.-i. flow-sensitive alternating IR
arrhythmic myocardial infarct
arrhythmogenic
a. area
a. border zone
a. right ventricular cardiomyopathy
a. right ventricular dysplasia syndrome
ArrowFlex sheath
arrowhead-shaped
ARSAC
Administration of Radioactive Substances Advisory Committee
ART
acoustic response technology
algebraic reconstruction technique
ART transducer
artefact (*var. of* artifact)
arteria
a. lusoria
a. radicularis anterior magna
arterial
a. aneurysm
a. angioma
a. avulsion
a. blockage
a. brachiocephalic trunk
a. brain anastomosis
a. brain displacement
a. branch
a. bulb
a. bypass graft
a. calcification
a. canal
a. cannulation
a. capillary
a. circle

NOTES

arterial *(continued)*
a. circle of Willis
a. cone
a. cutoff
a. deficiency pattern
a. degenerative disease
a. dilatation
a. dilatation and rupture
a. dimension
a. duct
a. embolus
a. endothelium
a. flow-phase image
a. flow phase imaging
a. gland
a. groove
a. hemorrhage
a. hyperemia
a. hypertension
a. hypotension
a. insufficiency
a. intima
a. invasion
a. kinking
a. ligament
a. linear density
a. lumen
a. lung malformation
a. malformation (AM)
a. narrowing
a. nephrosclerosis
a. obstruction
a. occlusion
a. oxygen saturation
a. patency
a. peak systolic pressure
a. phase
a. plaque
a. portography
a. pulsatility
a. pulsation artifact
a. return
a. runoff
a. sclerosis
a. scrotum supply
a. segment
a. sheath
a. spasm
a. steal
a. stenosis
a. supply
a. thrombosis
a. tonus
a. topography
a. tree
a. varix
a. vein
a. wall
a. wall dissection
a. wall thickness
a. waveform
arterial-arterial fistula
arterialization
hypervascular a.
a. of venous blood
arterial-portal fistula
arteries of Adamkiewicz
arteriobiliary fistula
arteriocapillary sclerosis
arteriococcygeal gland
arteriogenic impotence
arteriogram
arteriography
aortofemoral a.
balloon occlusion a.
bilateral carotid a.
biplane pelvic a.
biplane quantitative coronary a.
brachial a.
brachiocephalic a.
bronchial a.
carotid cerebral a.
celiac a.
cerebral a.
contrast a.
coronary a.
cortical kidney a.
CT a.
delayed phase of a.
digital subtraction a. (DSA)
documentary a.
elective a.
femoral runoff a.
four-vessel a.
hepatic a.
infrahepatic a.
intraoperative a.
ipsilateral antegrade a.
Judkins coronary a.
longitudinal a.
lumbar a.
mesenteric a.
pelvic a.
percutaneous femoral a.
peripheral a.
postdilatation a.
pruned-tree a.
pulmonary a.
quantitative coronary a. (QCA)
renal a.
retrograde a.
ring blush on cerebral a.
runoff a.
selective cerebral a.
selective coronary a.
selective visceral a.

Sones selective coronary a.
spiral computed tomography a. (SCTA)
splenic a.
subclavian a.
superior mesenteric a.
transfemoral a.
vertebral a.
visceral a.
wedge a.
x-ray a. (XRA)

arteriohepatic dysplasia

arteriolar
a. ischemic ulcer
a. narrowing
a. necrosis
a. resistance
a. sclerosis

arteriole
reactive a.

arteriolovenular bridge

arteriomyomatosis

arteriopathy
plexogenic pulmonary a.

arterioportobiliary
a. fistula

arteriorenal

arteriosclerosis
calcific a.
cerebral a.
coronary a.
generalized a.
hyaline a.
hypertensive a.
idiopathic pulmonary a. (IPA)
infantile a.
intimal a.
kidney a.
medial a.
Mönckeberg a., Moenckeberg arteriosclerosis
a. obliterans (ASO)
obliterative a.
obscuration a.
obstructing embolus a.
peripheral a.
presenile a.
pulmonary a.
renal a.
senile a.

arteriosclerotic
a. cardiovascular disease (ASCVD)
a. deposit
a. heart disease (ASHD)
a. intracranial aneurysm
a. kidney
a. occlusive disease
a. peripheral vascular disease
a. plaque
a. renal disease
a. thoracoabdominal aortic aneurysm

arteriosinusoidal
a. fistula
a. penile fistula

arteriostenosis

arteriosum
cor a.
ligamentum a.

arteriosus
calcified ductus a.
ductus a.
embryonic truncus a.
patent ductus a. (PDA)
persistent ductus a.
persistent truncus a. (PTA)
premature closure of ductus a.
pseudotruncus a.
railroad track ductus a.
reversed ductus a.
silent patent ductus a.
truncus a.

arteriovascular calcification

arteriovenous (A-V)
a. brain malformation
a. colon malformation
a. cord malformation
a. fistula
a. fistula bone
a. fistula transplant
a. hemangioma
a. interhemispheric angioma
a. intraosseous malformation
a. kidney malformation
a. malformation (AVM)
a. pressure gradient
a. pulmonary aneurysm
a. shunt imaging
a. varix

arteritis, pl. **arteritides**
carotid artery a.
cranial granulomatous a.
luetic a.

NOTES

arteritis *(continued)*
Takayasu a.
temporal granulomatous a.
artery
A1-A5 segments of anterior cerebral a.
Abbott a.
abdominal aortic a.
aberrant a.
aberrant right subclavian a.
accessory middle cerebral a.
accessory renal a.
Adamkiewicz a.
adrenal a.
aneurysm of internal carotid a.
aneurysm of posterior communicating a.
angiographic corkscrew a.
angular a.
anomalous left coronary a.
anomalous left pulmonary a.
anomalous origin of a.
anterior cerebral a. (ACA)
anterior choroidal a.
anterior communicating a. (ACoA)
anterior descending a.
anterior-inferior cerebellar a. (AICA)
anterior-inferior cerebral a. (AICA)
anterior-inferior communicating a. (AICA)
anterior intercostal a.
anterior meningeal a.
anterior spinal a.
anterior temporal branch of posterior cerebral a.
anterior tibial a.
aortoiliofemoral a.
apical posterior a.
arcuate a.
ascending frontoparietal a.
ascending pharyngeal a.
atrial circumflex a.
atrioventricular node a. (AVNA)
auricular a.
axillary a.
azygos anterior cerebral a.
basal cerebral a.
basal perforating a.
basilar a.
beading of a.
bifurcation of anterior communicating a.
bifurcation of common carotid a.
bifurcation of internal carotid a.
bifurcation of middle cerebral a.
blocked a.
brachial a.
brachiocephalic a.
branch of a.
bronchial a.
buckled innominate a.
bulbourethral a.
calcarine a.
calcific a.
callosomarginal a.
candelabra a.
cannulated a.
caroticotympanic a.
carotid a.
cavernous internal carotid a.
C1-C5 segments of internal carotid a.
celiac a.
central a.
cerebellar a.
cerebellolabyrinthine a.
cerebral a.
cervical a.
CF a.
circumflex artery
choroidal pericallosal a.
circumflex a. (CF artery, CX artery)
circumflex coronary a.
circumflex groove a.
colic a.
collateral circulation in compression of a.
common carotid a. (CCA)
common femoral a.
common hepatic a.
common iliac a.
common peroneal a.
communicating a.
complete transposition of great a.'s
congenital absence of pulmonary a.
congenital aneurysm of pulmonary a.
conus a.
a. of the conus medullaris
corduroy a.
corkscrew appearance of hepatic a.
coronary a.
corrected transposition of great a.'s
cortical a.
costocervical a.
course of a.
cremasteric a.
CX a.
circumflex artery
cystic a.
deep a.
deferential a.
deltoid branch of posterior tibial a.
descending septal a.
dextrotransposition of great a.'s

diagonal branch of a.
a. diameter
dilated pulmonary a.
dissection of a.
distal circumflex marginal a.
dominant left coronary a.
dominant right coronary a.
dorsal a.
Drummond marginal a.
ductus deferens a.
duodenal a.
duplex ultrasound carotid a.
dural a.
dynamic entrapment of vertebral a.
eccentric coronary a.
ectatic carotid a.
elastic recoil of a.
en passage feeder a.
a. entrapment
epicardial coronary a.
ethmoidal a.
external carotid a. (ECA)
external iliac a.
extracranial vertebral a.
extradural a.
facial a.
falx a.
familial fibromuscular dysplasia of a.
feeder a.
feeding branch of a.
femoral a.
femoropopliteal a.
first diagonal branch a.
first obtuse marginal a.
FP a.
  frontopolar artery
friable a.
frontal a.
frontopolar a. (FP artery)
fusiform narrowing of a.'s
gastric a.
gastroduodenal a.
gastroepiploic a.
gonadal a.
helicine a.
hepatic a.
Heubner a.
high left main diagonal a.
hilar a.
hyaloid a.
hypogastric a.
idiopathic dilated pulmonary a.
ileocolic a.
iliac a.
iliofemoral a.
a. of inferior cavernous sinus (AICS)
inferior epigastric a.
inferior mesenteric a. (IMA)
infragastric infragenicular popliteal a.
infrageniculate popliteal a.
innominate a.
intercostal a.
interlobar a.
intermediate coronary a.
internal aberrant carotid a.
internal carotid a. (ICA)
internal iliac a.
internal mammary a. (IMA)
internal pudendal a.
internal thoracic a. (ITA)
interruption of pulmonary a.
intraacinar pulmonary a.
intracavernous internal carotid a.
intracranial vertebral a.
invisible main pulmonary a.
ipsilateral downstream a.
kinking of carotid a.
Kugel a.
a. of labyrinth
labyrinthine a.
lacrimal a.
left anterior descending a.
left atrioventricular groove a.
left circumflex coronary a.
left common carotid a.
left common femoral a.
left coronary a. (LCA)
left internal mammary a. (LIMA)
left main coronary a. (LMCA)
left pulmonary a. (LPA)
lenticulostriate a.
leptomeningeal a.
lingual a.
lingular a.
lumbar a.
main pulmonary a. (MPA)
mainstem coronary a.
major aorticopulmonary collateral a.'s
mammary a.

NOTES

artery *(continued)*
marginal branch of left circumflex coronary a.
marginal branch of right coronary a.
marginal circumflex a.
maxillary a.
medial plantar a.
median sacral a.
medullary a.
meningeal a.
meningohypophyseal a.
mesencephalic a.
mesenteric a.
middle cerebral a.
middle meningeal a.
midmarginal branch of a.
M1-M5 segments of middle cerebral a.
musculophrenic a.
narrowing of a.
native coronary a.
nodular induration of temporal a.
obtuse marginal coronary a.
occipital a.
occlusion of a.
OM a.
operculofrontal a.
ophthalmic a.
origin of a.
a. ostium
ovarian a.
overriding great a.
pancreaticoduodenal a.
paracentral a.
paramalleolar a.
paramedian thalamic a.
paramedian thalamopeduncular a.
paricallosal a.
parietal middle cerebral a.
parietooccipital branch of posterior cerebellar a.
partial transposition of great a.'s
patency of a.
peduncular segment of superior cerebellar a.
pelvic a.
penile a.
a. of Percheron
perforating a.
pericallosal a.
perimedial renal fibroplasia a.
periosteal a.
peripancreatic a.
peroneal a.
persistent primitive trigeminal a.
persistent sciatic a.
petrous segment of carotid a.
pharyngeal a.
phrenic a.
pipestem a.
plantar metatarsal a.
plaque-containing a.
pontine a.
popliteal a.
posterior aorta transposition of great a.'s
posterior cerebral a. (PCA)
posterior choroidal a.
posterior circumflex humeral a.
posterior communicating a. (PCA, PCoA)
posterior descending a. (PDA)
posterior-inferior cerebellar a. (PICA)
posterior-inferior communicating a. (PICA)
posterior intercostal a.
posterior parietal a.
posterior spinal a.
posterior temporal a.
posterior tibial a.
posterolateral spinal a. (PLSA)
posttemporal middle cerebral a.
P1-P4 segments of posterior cerebral a.
precentral a.
precommunicating segment of anterior cerebral a.
prefrontal a.
premammillary a.
primitive acoustic a.
primitive hypoglossal a.
primitive trigeminal a. (PTA)
profunda femoris a.
proximal anterior descending a.
proximal anterior tibial a.
proximal circumflex a.
proximal digital a.
proximal left anterior descending a.
proximal popliteal a.
pterygoid a.
pulmonary a. (PA)
radial digital a.
radicular a.
radiculomedullary a.
radiculospinal a.
radiomedullary a.
ramus intermedius a.
ramus medialis a.
recanalized a.
reconstitution of blood flow in a.
reconstitution via profunda a.
redundant carotid a.
renal a.
reperfused a.

resilient a.
retinal a.
retroesophageal right subclavian a.
right coronary a. (RCA)
right descending pulmonary a. (RDPA)
right femoral a.
right inferior epigastric a.
right internal iliac a.
right internal jugular a.
right pulmonary a. (RPA)
right ventricular branch of right coronary a.
Riolan a.
rolandic a.
scalp branch of external carotid a.
sclerotic coronary a.
segmental branch of a.
septal perforator a.
shared coronary a.
side-by-side transposition of great a.'s
single umbilical a.
sinoatrial node a. (SANA)
sinus nodal a.
spermatic a.
spinal a.
splenial branch of posterior cerebral a.
splenic a. (SA)
stapedial a.
stenotic coronary a.
subclavian a.
subcostal a.
subscapular a.
sudden blockage of coronary a.
superdominant left anterior descending a.
superficial external pudendal a.
superficial femoral a. (SFA)
superficial temporal a.
superior cerebellar a. (SCA)
superior epigastric a.
superior genicular a.
superior intercostal a.
superior mesenteric a.
superior pulmonary a.
superior thyroid a.
supernormal a.
supraclinoid carotid a.
supraorbital a.
supratrochlear a.
takeoff of a.
telencephalic ventriculofugal a.
temporal a.
temporooccipital a.
testicular a.
thalamocaudate a.
thalamogeniculate a.
thalamoperforating a.
thoracoacromial a.
thoracodorsal a.
thrombotic pulmonary a. (TPA)
thyrocervical trunk of subclavian a.
thyroid a.
tibial a.
translocation of coronary a.
transposition of great a.'s (TGA)
trifurcation of a.
truncal a.
twig of a.
ulnar digital a.
umbilical a.
uterine a.
ventriculofugal a.
vertebral a.
vertebrobasilar a.
vidian a.
visceral a.
weakened a.
a. of Willis

artery/aortic velocity ratio
artery-vein-nerve bundle
arthrempyesis
arthrifluent abscess
arthritic talonavicular changes
arthritis, pl. **arthritides**
Bekhterev a.
Cedell-Magnusson classification of a.
collagen disease a.
cystic rheumatoid a.
degenerative a.
destructive brucellar a.
facet joint a.
gouty a.
hamate a.
hand/wrist a.
inflammatory bowel disease a.
juvenile rheumatoid a.
Kellgren a.
metatarsophalangeal joint a.
mixed rheumatoid and degenerative a.

NOTES

arthritis *(continued)*
a. mutilans
pancarpal destructive a.
psoriatic a.
Reiter syndrome a.
rheumatoid a.
septic a.
a. syphilitica deformans (ASD)
traumatic a.
tuberculous a.
arthrodesed digit
arthrodial cartilage
arthrogram
arthrography
Brostrom-Gordon a.
coronal computed tomographic a. (CCTA)
CT a.
double-contrast a.
Gordon-Brostrom single-contrast a.
a. imaging
indirect MR a.
joint a.
magnetic resonance a.
saline-enhanced MR a.
single-contrast a.
temporomandibular joint a.
three-compartment a.
vacuum a.
arthrogryposis
a. multiplex congenita
arthropathy
Charcot a.
facet a.
gouty a.
neuropathic a.
rotator cuff a.
arthrophyte
arthroplasty
Girdlestone a.
total hip a.
arthropneumoradiography
arthropyosis
arthroscintigraphy
arthroscopic
a. decompression
arthroscopy
arthrosis
crystal-induced a.
a. deformans
degenerative a.
spiral a.
arthrosteitis
pustulotic a.
arthrotomography
contrast computed a.
a. of shoulder

articular
a. arch
a. calculus
a. capsule
a. cartilage
a. cartilage attenuation
a. cartilage degeneration
a. cartilage violation
a. cartilage volume
a. cortex
a. crest
a. disk
a. disorders wrist
a. eminence
a. erosion
a. facet
a. fluid
a. fossa
a. fragment
a. gout
a. hand disorder
a. instability
intercarpal a.
a. labrum
a. lamella
a. lamella of bone
a. mass separation fracture
a. meniscus
a. network
a. pillar fracture
a. pit
a. process
a. process of vertebra
a. rheumatism
a. surface
a. tubercle
a. tubercle of temporal bone
a. vascular circle
a. wrist disorder
articularis
meniscus a.
articulated skeleton
articulating surface
articulation
acromioclavicular a.
atlantoaxial a.
body contour orbit a.
calcaneocuboid a.
carpometacarpal a.
carporadial a.
cartilage a.
condylar a.
congruent a.
costovertebral a.
DIP a.
distal interphalangeal joint a.
disturbance of a.
femoral a.

fixation a.
humeroradial a.
humeroulnar a.
intercarpal a.
intermetacarpal a.
interphalangeal a.
interval a.
joint a.
metacarpophalangeal a.
occipitocervical a.
patellofemoral a.
PIP a.
pisotriquetral a.
posterior membrane a.
proximal interphalangeal joint a.
radiocapitellar a.
radiocarpal a.
radiohumeral a.
radiolunate a.
radioscaphoid a.
radioulnar a.
sacroiliac a.
scapuloclavicular a.
subluxation a.
subtalar a.
talocalcaneal a.
talocalcaneonavicular a.
talonavicular a.
tarsometatarsal a.
thorax a.
tibiofibular a.
triquetropisiform a.
zygapophyseal a.

artifact, artefact
acoustic a.
aliasing a.
aortic motion a.
arterial pulsation a.
asymmetric a.
attenuation a.
barium a.
baseline a.
beam-hardening a.
black boundary a.
black comets a.
blooming a.
bone-hardening a.
bounce-point a.
bowel gas a.
braces a.
breast a.
breathing a.
broadband noise detection error a.
bulk susceptibility a.
calibration failure a.
catheter impact a.
catheter tip motion a.
catheter tip position a.
catheter whip a.
center line a.
central point a.
chemical shift a.
chemical shift phenomena a.
clothing a.
coin a.
comet-tail a.
computer-generated a.
construction a.
corduroy a.
crescent a.
crinkle a.
crosstalk effect a.
crown a.
crush a.
data-clipping detection error a.
data spike detection error a.
DC offset a.
developer a.
direct current offset a.
distortion of limitations of image reconstruction algorithm a.
double-exposure drift a.
eddy current a.
eddy ringing a.
edge-boundary a.
edge misalignment a.
edge ringing a.
a. effect
effusion a.
end-pressure a.
entry slice phenomenon a.
equipment a.
external a.
faulty radiofrequency shielding a.
ferromagnetic a.
flow effect a.
flow-induced a.
flow-related enhancement a.
fluid-flow a.
fog a.
foreign material a.
gaseous oxygen a.
geophagia a.
ghosting a.

NOTES

artifact *(continued)*
Gibbs phenomenon a.
glass eye a.
glove phenomenon a.
half-moon a.
hot spot a.
a. image
image postprocessing error a.
imbalance of gain a.
imbalance of phase a.
intensifying screen a.
iron overload a.
kink a.
kissing a.
lettering a.
linear a.
low-attenuation pulsation a.
low signal intensity a.
magic angle effect a.
magnetic susceptibility a.
main magnetic field inhomogeneity a.
mercury a.
metallic a.
micrometallic a.
mirror-image a.
misregistration a.
mitral regurgitation a.
moiré fringes a.
mosaic a.
motion a.
movement a.
muscle a.
noise spike a.
orbit a.
out-of-slice a.
overlying attenuation a.
pacemaker a.
pacing a.
paramagnetic a.
partial volume effect a.
patient motion a.
pellet a.
phase cancellation intensity a.
phase discontinuity a.
phase-encoding motion a.
phase-shift a.
pica a.
popliteal artery pulsation a.
propagation speed a.
pseudofracture a.
pulsation a.
quadrature phase detector a.
radiofrequency overflow a.
radiofrequency spatial distribution problem reconstruction a.
reconstruction a.
respiratory motion a.
reticulation a.
reverberation a.
ring-down a.
scintigraphy a.
screen craze a.
shading a.
side lobe a.
signal drop-out a.
simulated echo a.
skin crease a.
skin fold a.
skin lesion a.
slice overlap a.
slice profile a.
spatial misregistration a.
spatial offset image a.
split image a.
stairstep a.
star a.
subcutaneous injection of contrast a.
summation shadow a.
superimposition a.
surgical a.
susceptibility a.
swallowing a.
swamp-static a.
T a.
temporal instability a.
tree a.
truncation band a.
twinkling a.
venetian blind a.
view insufficiency a.
voluming a.
wheelchair a.
white noise a.
wraparound ghosting a.
wrinkle a.
zebra stripe a.
zero-fill a.
zipper a.

artifactual

artificial
a. cardiac valve
a. fracture
a. heart
a. left ventricular assist device
a. lung
a. neural network
a. pneumothorax
a. radioactivity

Artma Virtual Patient

Artoscan
A. M
A. MRI imaging
A. MRI scanner
A. MRI system

Arvidsson dimension-length method for ventricular volume
aryepiglottic
a. cyst
a. fold
a. fold carcinoma
a. fold neurofibroma
arytenoid
a. cartilage
a. sparing
arytenoidal articular surface
AS
aortic stenosis
ASA
American Standards Association
asbestos
a. bodies
a. exposure
a. fibers
a. pleural plaque
asbestos-induced pleural fibrosis
asbestosis
pulmonary a.
asbestos-related
a.-r. lung cancer
a.-r. mesothelioma
a.-r. pleural disease
A-scan
A.-s. imaging
A.-s. ultrasound
ascariasis
binary a.
bowel a.
liver a.
ascendant follicle
ascending
a. aorta (AA)
a. aorta dilatation
a. aorta hypoplasia
a. aortic aneurysm
a. aortography
a. cholangitis
a. colon
a. contrast MR phlebogram
a. contrast phlebography
a. contrast phlebography imaging
a. frontal convolution
a. frontoparietal (ASFP)
a. frontoparietal artery
a. hypoplasia of aorta
a. lumbar vein
a. medullary vein thrombosis
a. parietal convolution
a. parietal gyrus
a. pharyngeal artery
a. process
a. ramus of ischium
a. tract
Aschner phenomenon
Aschoff
A. node
A. nodule
Aschoff-Tawara node
ASCIA
American Spinal Cord Injury Association
ascites
chylous a.
fetal a.
gelatinous a.
massive a.
neonatal a.
pancreatic a.
urine a.
ascitic fluid
ASCVD
arteriosclerotic cardiovascular disease
atherosclerotic cardiovascular disease
ASD
anterior sagittal diameter
arthritis syphilitica deformans
atrial septal defect
Aselli pancreas
aseptic necrosis
ASFP
ascending frontoparietal
ASH
asymmetric septal hypertrophy
ASHD
arteriosclerotic heart disease
Asherman syndrome
Asherson syndrome
Ashhurst
A. fracture classification system
A. sign
Ashhurst-Bromer classification of ankle fractures
ash leaf patch
Ashman
A. index
A. phenomenon
ASHN
acute sclerosing hyaline necrosis

NOTES

ASIC
application-specific integrated circuit
ASIC circuit
ASIS
anterior-superior iliac spine
Ask-Upmark kidney
as low as reasonably achievable (ALARA)
ASO
arteriosclerosis obliterans
atherosclerosis obliterans
asoma
aspect
anterior a.
anterolateral a.
anteroposterior a.
apical a.
axial a.
dorsal a.
dorsolateral a.
dorsoplantar a.
inferior a.
infrapatellar a.
lateral a.
lordotic a.
medial a.
mediolateral a.
mesial a.
plantar a.
posterior a.
posterolateral a.
proximal a.
superior a.
superolateral a.
ventral a.
Aspect computer
Aspen
A. digital ultrasound
A. digital ultrasound system
aspergillosis
allergic bronchopulmonary a. (ABPA)
bronchopulmonary a.
chronic necrotizing a.
invasive pulmonary a.
noninvasive a.
primary a.
saprophytic a.
semiinvasive a.
aspergillotic aneurysm
Aspergillus
Aspergillus bronchiolitis
Aspergillus cerebral abscess
asphyxia
fetal a.
perinatal a.
asphyxiating thoracic dysplasia
aspiration
barium a.
a. biopsy
bone marrow a.
breast cyst a.
CT-guided needle a.
a. cytology
fine-needle a.
meconium a.
a. of ova
pleural fluid a.
a. pneumonia
a. pneumonitis
pulmonary a.
tracheal a.
transbronchial needle a. (TBNA)
transtracheal a.
ultrasound-guided transthoracic needle a.
aspirator
Sonocut ultrasonic a.
Aspire
A. continuous imaging
A. continuous imaging system
asplenia
asplenia syndrome R
ASPVD
atherosclerotic pulmonary vascular disease
ASR
adrenal-to-spleen ratio
ASRT
American Society of Radiologic Technologists
American Society of Registered Technologists
assembly
linear array-hydrophone a.
assessment
activity a.
aortoiliac inflow a.
BFM arm impairment a., Brunnstrom-Fugl-Meyer arm impairment a.
Diagnostic and Therapeutic Technology A. (DATTA)
Doppler a.
hemodynamic a.
invasive a.
in vivo stereologic a.
myocardial function a.
noninvasive a.
Office of Health Technology A.
preoperative a.
quantitative Doppler a.
real-time a.
regional wall motion a.
sonographic a.

ultrasonic a.
vascular a.
assimilation
atlantooccipital a.
a. pelvis
assist
intraaortic balloon a.
assistance
fluoroscopic a.
Assmann focus
associated sequestrum
association
American Medical A. (AMA)
American Rheumatism A. (ARA)
American Spinal Cord Injury A. (ASCIA)
American Standards A. (ASA)
American Urological A. (AUA)
a. cortex of parietal lobe
a. fiber
A. of University Radiologic Technicians (AURT)
A. of University Radiologists (AUR)
New York Heart A. (NYHA)
a. tract
VATER a.
AST
above selected threshold
astatine (At)
asterixis
asteroid body
asthmatic
a. airway
a. bronchitis
a. pneumonia
astragalar bone
astragalocalcanean
a. bone
astragalocrural
a. bone
astragaloscaphoid
a. bone
astragalotibial
a. bone
astragalus
aviator's a.
a. bone
fracture of a.
ASTRO
American Society for Therapeutic Radiology and Oncology
astroblastoma
astrocytic
a. gliosis
a. hamartoma
a. tumor
astrocytoma
anaplastic a.
calcified a.
cerebellar a.
cerebral a.
chiasmatic-hypothalamic pilocytic a.
CNS juvenile pilocytic a.
cord a.
a. cord
cystic pilocytic a.
desmoplastic infantile a.
gemistocytic a.
giant cell a.
infiltrative a.
juvenile orbital pilocytic a.
juvenile pilocytic a. (JPA)
low-grade a. (LGA)
macrocystic pilocytic cerebellar a.
microcystic pilocytic cerebellar a.
multifocal anaplastic a.
orbital juvenile pilocytic a.
pilocytic a.
piloid a.
protoplasmic a.
retinal a.
solid pilocytic a.
subependymal giant cell a.
supratentorial a.
temporoinsular a.
well-differentiated a.
astroglial tumor
asymmetric
a. appearance time
a. artifact
a. bile duct
a. breast density
a. closure of cusp
a. data sampling
a. echo
a. intrauterine growth retardation
a. IUGR
a. pulmonary congestion
a. septal hypertrophy (ASH)
a. thorax

NOTES

asymmetry
amplitude a.
congestive a.
facial a.
focal a.
hypertrophic a.
interhemispheric a.
left-right a.
limb-length a.
narrowing a.
septal a.
skull a.
thoracic a.
asymptomatic
a. coarctation
a. gallstone
a. hydrocephalus
a. hypertrophy
asynchronous transfer mode (ATM)
asynchrony
heart a.
asyndetic communication
asyneresis
asynergic myocardium
asynergy
infarct-localized a.
left ventricular a.
regional a.
segmental a.
asystolic pause
At
astatine
ATAI
acute traumatic aortic injury
atavistic epiphysis
ataxia
infantile-onset spinocerebellar a.
spinocerebellar a.
a. telangiectasia
ataxia-hemiparesis syndrome
ataxia-telangiectasia
CNS a.-t.
atelectasis
absorption a.
acquired a.
acute a.
adhesive a.
apical a.
basilar a.
bibasilar discoid a.
bronchopulmonary a.
chronic a.
compressive a.
confluent areas of a.
congenital a.
congestive a.
dependent a.
discoid a.
disklike a.
initial a.
lobar a.
lobular a.
lower pulmonary lobe a.
massive a.
middle pulmonary lobe a.
nonobstructive a.
obstructive a.
passive a.
patchy a.
peripheral parenchymal a.
platelike a.
platterlike a.
primary a.
reabsorption a.
relaxation a.
resorptive a.
rounded a.
secondary a.
segmental a.
slowly developing a.
streaks of a.
subsegmental a.
subsegmental bibasilar a.
subsegmental lower lobe a.
upper pulmonary lobe a.
atelectatic
a. asbestos pseudotumor
a. lung
atelosteogenesis
ATF
anterior talofibular ligament
atherectomized vessel
atherectomy
directional coronary a. (DCA)
extraction catheter a.
percutaneous coronary rotational a. (PCRA)
retrograde a.
rotational coronary a. (RCA)
Simpson a.
transcutaneous extraction catheter a.
transluminal a.
AtheroCath
DVI Simpson A.
Simpson A.
atheroembolic renal disease
atheroembolism
atherogenesis
atherolysis
ultrasonic a.
atherolytic
atheroma
carotid bifurcation a.
coral reef a.
a. molding
protruding a.

atheromatous
a. debris
a. degeneration
a. embolus
a. lesion
a. material
a. plaque
a. stenosis
a. ulcer
atheroocclusive disease
atherosclerosis
accelerated a.
aortic a.
carotid a.
coronary a.
extracranial carotid artery a.
fatty streak a.
fibrous plaque a.
intimal a.
intracranial carotid artery a.
juxtarenal aortic a.
native a.
a. obliterans (ASO)
pararenal aortic a.
premature a.
virulent a.
atherosclerotic
a. aortic aneurysm
a. aortic ulcer
a. cardiovascular disease (ASCVD)
a. carotid artery disease (ACAD)
a. change
a. debris
a. fatty streak
a. lesion
a. narrowing
a. occlusive syndrome
a. plaque
a. pulmonary vascular disease (ASPVD)
a. stenosis
atherostenosis
atherothrombotic brain infarct
athlete's
a. heart
a. pseudonephritis
Atkin epiphyseal fracture
ATL
anterior tricuspid leaflet
ATL HDI 3000 ultrasound system
ATL Mark 600 real-time sector scanner
ATL Neurosector real-time scanner
ATL real-time Neurosector scan imaging
ATL real-time ultrasound
atlantal ligament
atlantoaxial
a. articulation
a. instability
a. interval
a. joint
a. rotary displacement
a. rotary fixation
a. separation
a. subluxation
atlantodens interval (ADI)
atlantodental
atlantomastoid
atlantooccipital
a. assimilation
a. dislocation
a. fusion
a. junction
a. membrane
a. separation
atlantoodontoid
atlas
a. anomaly
a. arch
arch of a.
a. articular sinus
burst fracture of a.
compression fracture of a.
A. 2.0 diagnostic ultrasound system
a. facet
a. fracture
Greulich and Pyle a.
a. matching
a. occipitalization
occipitalization of a.
rachischisis of a.
split a.
transverse ligaments of a.
ATL Ultramark 8, 9
ATM
asynchronous transfer mode
ATM mode
atmospheric pressure
ATN
acute tubular necrosis
atom
activated a.

NOTES

atom *(continued)*
Bohr a.
excited a.'s
ionized a.
labeled a.
nuclear a.
radioactive a.
recoil a.
stripped a.
tagged a.
atomic
a. absorption spectrophotometry
a. absorption spectroscopy
a. mass
a. mass unit (amu)
atonic
a. esophagus
a. ureter
a. urinary bladder
atony, atonia
chronic gastric a.
collecting system a.
gastric a.
intestinal a.
renal collecting system a.
sphincter a.
stomach a.
urinary bladder a.
atopic
atopy
atraumatic, multidirectional, bilateral radial instability (AMBRI)
atraumatic occlusion of vessels
atresia
anal a.
anorectal a.
aortic a.
aortic arch a.
aortic valve a.
biliary a.
bronchial a.
choanal a.
congenital biliary a.
congenital intestinal a.
congenital laryngeal a.
duodenal a.
esophageal a.
external auditory canal a.
extrahepatic biliary a. (EBA)
familial a.
ileal a.
infundibular a.
inner ear a.
intestinal congenital a.
intrahepatic a. (IHA)
laryngeal a.
mitral valve a.
nasopharyngeal a.
phenobarbital biliary a.
prepyloric a.
Pulec and Freedman classification of congenital aural a.
pulmonary artery a.
pulmonary valve a.
pulmonary vein a.
pulmonic a.
small bowel a.
tricuspid valve a.
urethral a.
valvular a.
ventricular a.
atresic
atretic
a. ovarian follicle
a. segment
atria (*pl. of* atrium)
atrial
a. activation time
a. appendage
a. appendage juxtaposition
a. bigeminal rhythm
a. canal
a. cannulation
a. circumflex artery
a. complex
a. cuff
a. disk
a. diverticulum of brain
a. dome
a. echo
a. ectopic automatic tachycardia
a. emptying volume
a. fetal flutter
a. fibrillation
a. focus
a. infarct
a. inhibited (AAI)
a. irritability
a. isomerism
a. kick
a. mesenchymoma
a. myxoma
a. ostium primum defect
a. partition
a. rate (AR)
a. ring
a. septal aneurysm
a. septal defect (ASD)
a. septal defect occlusion
a. septal resection
a. septostomy
a. septum
a. situs
a. situs solitus
a. standstill
a. systole

a. thrombosis
a. transposition

atrialized ventricle

atrial-phase volumetric function

atriocaval junction

atriofascicular tract

atriography
contrast left a.
negative contrast left a.

atrio-His, atriohisian
a.-H. bypass tract
a.-H. fiber
a.-H. pathway

atrioventricular (AV, A-V)
a. annulus
a. band
a. block
a. bundle
a. canal
a. canal defect
a. connection
a. gradient
a. groove
a. groove branch
a. junction
a. junction anomaly
a. nodal bypass tract
a. nodal node mesothelioma
a. nodal orifice
a. nodal ostium
a. nodal rhythm
a. nodal ring
a. nodal septal defect
a. nodal septum
a. nodal valve
a. node
a. node artery (AVNA)
a. node of His
a. opening of His
a. septal defect
a. sulcus
a. time
a. trunk
a. valve

atrium, pl. **atria**
common a.
a. dextrum cordis
giant left a.
high right a. (HRA)
left a. (LA)
low right a. (LRA)
low septal right a.
maximal volume of left a.
nontrabeculated a.
oblique vein of left a.
a. pulmonale
pulmonary a.
respiratory a.
right a. (RA)
shunt with normal left a.
single a.
a. sinistrum
a. sinistrum cordis
stenosing ring of left a.
thin-walled a.
trabeculated a.
a. of ventricle
ventricular a.

atrophic
a. brain lesion
a. breast
a. cirrhosis
a. degeneration
a. emphysema
a. fracture
a. gastritis
a. inflammation
a. kidney
a. lesion of brain
a. nonunion
a. pyelonephritis
a. thrombosis

atrophied ovary

atrophy
alveolar a.
bone a.
a. of bone
brachial a.
brain a.
brown a.
cerebellar a.
cerebral surface a.
compensatory a.
compression a.
cord a.
cortical a.
degenerative a.
denervation a.
dentatorubral-pallidoluysian a.
disuse a.
divopontocerebellar a.
a. of dorsum sella
dorsum sellae a.
eccentric a.

NOTES

atrophy *(continued)*
focal a.
frontotemporal a.
gastric a.
hemisphere a.
hippocampal a.
Hoffmann a.
interstitial a.
kidney a.
Kugelberg-Welander juvenile spinal muscle a.
lesser a.
lobar lung a.
lobular lung a.
localized muscular a.
multiple system a. (MSA)
muscle a.
neurogenic a.
olivopontocerebellar a.
pancreatic a.
parenchymatous a.
peroneal muscular a.
physiologic a.
postinflammatory renal a.
postmenopausal uterine a.
postneuritic a.
postobstructive renal a.
primary optic a.
progressive neuropathic muscle a.
progressive postpolio muscle a. (PPPMA)
quadriceps a.
reflux a.
renal reflux a.
scapuloperoneal muscular a.
seminal vesicle a.
small bowel folds a.
spinal cord a.
spinal muscular a. (SMA)
subacute denervation a.
subcortical Sudeck osteoporotic a.
Sudeck a.
sulcal a.
temporal horn a.
testicular a.
vascular villous a.
villous a.

attachment
abnormal umbilical cord a.
biopsy-guided a.
capsular a.
central rhomboid a.
cerebellar a.
commissural a.
dural a.
epicardial a.
fibroosseous a.
fibrous a.
Hudson a.
intimate a.
lateral pterygoid tendinous a.
ligamentous a.
meniscocapsular a.
meniscofemoral a.
meniscotibial a.
mesenteric a.
Pearson a.
peritoneal a.
tendinous a.
tentorium cerebelli a. (TCA)
vascular pterygoid a.

attack
heart a.
transient hemispheric a.
transient ischemic a. (TIA)

attention
raptus of a.

attenuate

attenuated
a. cortical surface
a. dura
a. image
a. intercarpal articular cartilage
a. ligament
a. lumen

attenuating

attenuation
aortic a.
articular cartilage a.
a. artifact
beam a.
breast a.
a. coefficient
a. compensation
a. correction
decreased a.
diaphragmatic a.
digital beam a.
a. effect
expiratory a.
focal a.
gamma ray a.
ground-glass a.
hemidiaphragm a.
a. by hemidiaphragm
a. imaging
increased a.
a. level
linear a.
liver a.
a. measurement
nonuniform a.
photon a.
a. scan
signal a.
tendon a.

theophylline a.
a. threshold
ultrasonic a.
a. value
valve a.
x-ray a.
attenuator
attic
a. adhesion
a. cholesteatoma
a. recess
a. temporal bone
attritional tear
attrition rupture of tendon
ATV
anterior terminal vein
atypical
a. aortic valve stenosis
a. benign fibrous histiocytoma
a. brain teratoma
a. bronchial pneumonia
a. carcinoid
a. chest pain
a. ductal hyperplasia (ADH)
a. epithelium
a. interstitial pneumonia
a. lobular breast hyperplasia
a. measles pneumonia
a. meningioma
a. primary pneumonia
a. regenerative hyperplasia
a. renal cyst
a. subisthmic coarctation
a. tuberculosis
a. verrucous endocarditis
a. vessel colposcopic pattern
^{198}Au
gold-198
^{198}Au colloid
AUA
American Urological Association
AUC
area under the (concentration-time) curve
auditory
a. canal
a. capsule
a. cartilage
a. cortex
a. ganglion
a. pit
a. plate
a. process
a. tube
a. vein
a. vesicle
Auenbrugger sign
Auerbach
A. mesenteric plexus
myenteric plexus of A.
Auger
A. effect
A. electrons
Auger-electron emitter
augmentation
bladder a.
breast a.
a. mammoplasty
mechanical a.
reverse a.
thiol a.
augmented
a. breast
a. cardiac output
a. filling
a. filling of right ventricle
a. stroke volume
AUR
Association of University Radiologists
aura
uncinate a.
aureus
methicillin-resistant
Staphylococcus a.
auricle
left a.
right a.
auricular
a. artery
a. canaliculus
a. cartilage
a. complex
a. fissure
a. ganglion
a. ligament
a. lymph node
a. muscle
a. notch
a. point
a. surface
a. triangle
a. tubercle
a. vein
auriculoinfraorbital plane
auriculoventricular groove

NOTES

Aurora
A. dedicated breast MRI system
A. MR breast imaging
A. MR breast imaging system scanner
AURT
Association of University Radiologic Technicians
auscultatory finding
Aussies-Isseis unstable scoliosis
Austin Flint phenomenon
autoamputation
terminal tuft a.
autocancellation
Autocorrelator
autofluorescence
autofluoroscope
autofusion
autogenous
a. bone
a. vein
a. vein bypass graft
autograft
bridge a.
double a.
autoimmune
a. leukopenia
a. phenomenon
a. response
a. sialadenitis
auto injector
autologous
a. blood clot
a. bone marrow rescue
a. bone marrow support
a. bone marrow transplant
a. labeled leukocytes
a. patch graft
a. pericardium
a. stem-cell transplantation
a. vein graft
automated
a. airway tree segmentation method
a. angle-encoder system
a. border detection by echocardiography
a. cardiac flow measurement (ACM)
a. cardiac flow measurement ultrasound (ACM ultrasound)
a. cardiac flow measurement ultrasound technology
a. cerebral blood flow analyzer
a. computed axial tomography (ACAT)
a. large-core breast biopsy
a. quantification
a. synthesis
automatic
a. bladder
a. exposure control (AEC)
a. extraction
a. implantable cardioverter-defibrillator (AICD)
a. lumen edge segmentation
a. motion correction
a. peak tracking (APT)
automaticity
sinus node a.
Automic Energy Commission (AEC)
automotility factor
autonephrectomy
autonomic
a. denervation
a. hyperventilation
a. insufficiency
a. nerve block
a. nervous system
a. plexus
autonomous
a. nodule
a. thyroid adenoma
autoparenchymatous metaphysis
autoprescanning
autoradiogram
autoradiograph
autoradiographic localization
autoradiography
quantitative track etch a.
autoregressive moving average
autoregulation of cerebral blood flow
AutoSPECT
autosplenectomy
autostereoscopic
autotopagnosia
auxiliary ventricle
AV, A-V
atrioventricular
AV block
AV node
AV Wenckebach heart block
AVA
aortic valve area
avalanche
Townsend a.
avascular
a. bone necrosis
a. brain mass
a. cortical infarction necrosis
a. femoral head necrosis
a. fibrocartilage
a. kidney mass
a. necrosis (AVN)
a. necrosis lunate
a. renal mass

a. tarsal scaphoid necrosis
a. vertebral body necrosis
avascularity
AVD
aortic valvular disease
Avellis syndrome
average
autoregressive moving a.
a. gradient number
a. pixel projection (APP)
a. positron energy
a. radiation dose
signal a.
spatial average-pulse a. (SAPA)
spatial average-temporal a. (SATA)
spatial peak-temporal a. (SPTA)
averaging
motional a.
partial volume a.
spike a.
volume a.
AVG
aortic valve gradient
aviator's astragalus
avis
calcar a.
Aviva mammography system
AVM
arteriovenous malformation
intradural spinal AVM
AVM radiotherapy
AVN
avascular necrosis
AVNA
atrioventricular node artery
Avogadro number (Λ)
AVR
aortic valve replacement
AVSD
avulse
avulsed
a. fracture fragment
a. ligament
a. retinaculum
avulsion
anterior labral a.
anterior labroligamentous periosteal sleeve a. (ALPSA)
arterial a.
bony humeral a.
a. chip fracture
coracoid tip a.
epiphysis a.
iatrogenic a.
ligament a.
lumbar root a.
nail plate a.
peroneus longus muscle a.
spinal nerve root a.
spinous process a.
a. stress fracture
testicular artery a.
traumatic a.
venous a.
avulsive cortical irregularity
AVVM
angiographically visualized vascular malformation
A-wave pressure
axes (*pl. of* axis)
axial
a. angiography
a. aspect
a. carpal dislocation
a. cineangiography
a. compression fracture
a. compression injury
a. dimension
a. grade echo imaging
a. gradient echo image
a. hiatal hernia
horizontal long a. (HLA imaging, HLA)
a. joint dissection
a. left anterior oblique ventriculogram
a. localizer
a. manual traction test
multiecho a.
a. musculature
a. neuritis
a. plane
a. plane imaging
a. plate
a. projection
a. radiograph
a. resolution
a. scan
a. section
a. sesamoid view
a. skeleton
a. slice
a. spinal system
a. spin density

NOTES

axial *(continued)*
a. surface
a. transabdominal image
a. transabdominal imaging
a. view
a. wall
a. weight loading
axilla, pl. **axillae**
axillary
a. adenopathy
a. aneurysm
a. artery
a. cavity
a. fascia
a. fossa
a. hematoma
a. irradiation
a. line
a. lymphadenopathy
a. lymph node (ALN)
a. muscle
a. node involvement
a. node metastasis
a. plexus
a. pouch
a. sheath
a. space
a. sweat gland
a. tail
a. tail of Spence
a. tail view
a. triangle
a. tumor downstaging
a. ultrasonography
a. vein
a. vein traumatic thrombosis
a. vessel
axillary-axillary bypass graft
axillary-brachial bypass graft
axillary-femoral bypass graft
axillary-femorofemoral bypass graft
axillobifemoral bypass graft
axillofemoral approach
axillosubclavian vein thrombosis
axiolabiolingual plane
axiomesiodistal plane
axis, pl. **axes**
anatomic a.
ankle mortise a.
a. anomaly
basibregmatic a.
basicranial a.
bimalleolar foot a.
a. body
bowel a.
celiac a.
coordinate a.
cortical hinge a.
craniospinal a.
distal reference a. (DRA)
enteroinsular a.
femoral shaft a.
a. fracture
a. of heart
HPA a.
hypothalamic-pituitary a.
hypothalamic-pituitary-adrenal a.
hypothalamic-pituitary-gonadal a.
hypothalamoneurohypophysial a., hypothalamoneurohypophyseal
leg a.
a. ligament
long a.
longitudinal a.
mechanical a.
metatarsal a.
proximal reference a. (PRA)
renal a.
single a.
spinal a.
subtalar a.
transcondylar a. (TCA)
transporionic a.
vertical a.
weightbearing a.
X a.
Y a.
Z a.
axonal shearing
axonopathic neurogenic thoracic outlet syndrome
Ayerza disease
azotemic osteodystrophy
azozurine
azygoesophageal
a. line
a. recess
azygogram
azygography
azygos
a. anterior cerebral artery
a. artery of vagina
a. blood flow
a. continuation
a. continuation of inferior vena cava
a. fissure
a. hematoma cap
a. lobe
a. lobe of lung
a. lymph node
nodus arcus venae a.
a. vein
a. vein distention
a. vein enlargement
Azzopardi tumor

B-19026 chelate imaging agent
B-19036 chelate
B6 bronchus sign
Baart de las Faille sign
baby
b. formula with ferrous sulfate contrast
b. formula with ferrous sulfate imaging agent
Baccelli
B. sign
B. sign of pleural effusion
Bachman
Bachmann
anterior internodal tract of B.
B. bundle
bacillary embolus
***Bacillus anthracis* pneumonia**
back
arching of b.
b. crease
b. projection
b. stroke volume
back-angle anomaly
backbleeding
backfire fracture
backflow
b. of blood
pyelolymphatic b.
pyelorenal b.
pyelotubular b.
pyelotumoral b.
pyelovenous b.
venous b.
backflux
background (BKG)
b. equivalent radiation time
b. radiation
b. subtraction technique
back-knee deformity
backprojection
back-projection
filtered b.-p. (FBP)
backrush of blood into left ventricle
backscatter
b. of blood
b. electrons
back-to-back configuration
backup of blood
backward
b. curvature
b. flow
b. heart failure
backwash ileitis
bacteremia
catheter-associated b.
bacterial
b. aneurysm
b. aortitis
b. endocarditis
b. ependymitis
b. epiglottitis
b. nephritis
b. osteomyelitis
b. pneumonia
b. pneumonitis
b. sinusitis
b. toxin
badge
ring b.
Baehr-Lohlein lesion
Baeyer-Villiger oxidation
Baffe anastomosis
baffled tunnel
baffle leak
bag
b. of bagassosis
bile b.
ostomy b.
stomal b.
Tedlar b.
bagassosis
bag of b.
bagpipe sign
Baillarger stripe
Baillinger
inner stripe of B.
bail-lock knee joint
baja
patella b.
BAK-1 interbody fusion system
baked-brain phenomenon
Baker cyst
baker's leg
balance
mass b.
B. sign
balanced
b. circulation
b. hemivertebra
b. ischemia
b. pneumoperitoneum
balancing subdural hematoma
bald gastric fundus
Balint syndrome
Balkan
B. fracture frame
B. nephritis
B. nephropathy

B

Balke protocol for cardiac exercise stress testing
Balke-Ware treadmill exercise stress testing protocol
ball
b. catcher view
b. of foot
fungus b.
keratin urinary tract b.
kidney fungus b.
lung fungus b.
myelin b.
renal fungus b.
sludge b.
ball-and-seat valve
ball-and-socket
b.-a.-s. ankle mortise
b.-a.-s. epiphysis
b.-a.-s. joint
ball-bearing eye sign
ballerina-foot pattern
ball-in-hand appearance
ballism
ballismus
ballistic
b. injury
b. material
ballistocardiography
ball-occluder valve
balloon
b. aortoplasty
b. atrial septostomy
barium enema retention b.
b. bronchoplasty
b. catheter fenestration
b. cholangiogram
b. counterpulsation
b. dilatation
b. dilator
b. epiphysis
b. expulsion imaging
b. inflation
b. occlusion arteriography
b. occlusion pulmonary angiogram
b. occlusive aortography
PET b.
positron emission tomography balloon
positron emission tomography b. (PET balloon)
b. proctogram
b. pump
rectal b.
scintigraphic b.
b. tamponade
b. test occlusion
b. test occlusion imaging
b. topography
b. tuboplasty
USCI PET b.
waist in b.
ballooned
b. floor of ventricle
b. sella
ballooning
b. degeneration
disk b.
b. mitral valve prolapse syndrome
b. of vertebral interspace
balloon-occluded arterial infusion
balloon-shaped heart
balloon-tipped angiographic catheter
ball-type valve
ball-valve
b.-v. obstruction
b.-v. thrombus
b.-v. tumor
Baló concentric sclerosis
BALT
bronchus-associated lymphoid tissue
Bamberger
B. area
B. sign
Bamberger-Marie disease
bamboo spine
banana-shaped uterine cavity
Bancaud phenomenon
Bancroft sign
band
alpha frequency b.
amnionic b.
anogenital b.
anterior b.
AO tension b.
aponeurotic b.
atrioventricular b.
b. of Broca
Broca diagonal b.
calf b.
Clado b.
constriction b.
coronary b.
dense metaphyseal b.
b. of density
b. of deossification
external b.
fascial b.
fibroelastic b.
fibromuscular b.
fibrous b.
free band of colon b.
Gennari b.
b. of Gennari
H b.
Harris b.
His b.

Hunter-Schreger b.
hypoechoic b.
iliotibial b.
intercaval b.
internal b.
intratesticular b.
IT b.
Ladd b.
Lane b.
lateral b.
longitudinal b.
low-signal-intensity fibrous b.
low-signal-intensity peripheral b.
lucent b.
Mach b.
Maissiat b.
Marlex b.
Meckel b.
mesocolic b.
metaphyseal lucent b.
moderator b.
omental b.
parenchymal fibrous b.
parenchymal lung b.
Parham-Martin b.
parietal b.
peritoneal b.
pretendinous b.
radiofrequency saturation b.
Reil b.
scar b.
septal b.
septomarginal b.
septum b.
serpiginous b.
silicone elastomer b.
Simonart b.
tendinous b.
b. tenodesis
transverse b.
walking saturation b.
Z b.

bandbox resonance
banding
b. appearance
halftone b.
bandlike
b. adhesion
b. shadow
bandpass filter
Bankart
B. dislocation
B. fracture
B. lesion
Bannayan-Riley-Ruvalcaba syndrome
Bannister angioedema disease
Banti
B. disease
B. syndrome
BAP
brightness area product
bar
Bill b.
bony b.
cartilaginous b.
cecal b.
congenital b.
coracoclavicular b.
cricopharyngeal b.
b. defect
fibrous b.
hyoid b.
median b.
parallel-line equal spacing b.
Passavant b.
physeal b.
PLES b.
pterygoalar b. (PTAB)
unsegmented vertebral b.
barber
b. chair position
b. pole sign
barber's
b. chair sign
b. pilonidal sinus
Barclay niche
Bard
B. CPS system
B. percutaneous cardiopulmonary support system
B. rotary atherectomy system (BRAS)
Bardeen primitive disk
Bardinet ligament
bare
b. area
b. area of liver
b. lymphocyte syndrome
Baricon
B. contrast medium
B. imaging agent
baritosis
barium
b. artifact

NOTES

barium *(continued)*
b. aspiration
b. bolus
double tracking of b.
b. enema (BE)
b. enema imaging
b. enema retention balloon
b. enema through colostomy
b. enema with air contrast
b. esophagogram
b. examination
flocculation of b.
b. fluorochloride
fragmentation of b.
high-density b.
holdup in flow of b.
hydrophilic nonflocculating b.
b. injection
b. injection through colostomy
b. lead sulfate
b. meal
b. mixture
b. platinocyanoide
b. pneumoconiosis
pocketing of b.
reflux of b.
residual b.
retained b.
retention of b.
b. segmentation
b. snake-head sign
b. strontium sulfate
b. study
b. sulfate ($BaSO_4$)
b. sulfate contrast medium
b. sulfate imaging agent
b. suspension
b. swallow
b. swallow imaging
b. vaginography
barium-filled colon
barium-impregnated poppet
barium-sulfate impregnated shunt
barium-water esophagogram
barked injury
Barkow ligament
barlike
Barlow
B. disease
B. hip instability test
B. sign
B. syndrome
Baro-CAT
B.-C. contrast medium
B.-C. imaging agent
Baroflave
B. contrast medium
B. imaging agent
baroreceptor
b. bulb
carotid bulb b.
Barosperse
B. contrast medium
B. 110 imaging agent
Baros space
barotrauma
intrapulmonary b.
pulmonary b.
barrel chest
Barré-Lieou syndrome
barrel-shaped
b.-s. lesion
b.-s. stone
Barrett
B. disease
B. epithelium
B. esophagus
B. ulcer
barrier
anatomic b.
b. beam
Bart abdominoperipheral angiography unit
Barth hernia
Bartholin
B. duct
B. gland
B. gland carcinoma
B. gland cyst
Barton fracture
Barton-Smith fracture
Bartter syndrome
basal
b. angle
b. arachnoid cistern
b. bone
b. cell adenoma
b. cell carcinoma
b. cell nevus syndrome
b. cell papilloma
b. cerebral artery
b. chorda
b. descent
b. extension
b. ganglia anatomy
b. ganglia calcification
b. ganglia of cerebellum
b. ganglia echogenic focus
b. ganglia hematoma
b. ganglia infarct
b. ganglion
b. hypodense ganglia lesion
b. joint
b. joint of thumb
b. lamella
b. layer

b. neck fracture
b. nucleus
b. perforating artery
b. placenta vein
b. plate
b. ridge
b. segmental bronchus
b. short-axis slice
b. skull fracture
b. sphincter
b. surface
b. tuberculosis
b. vein of Rosenthal (BVR)
b. zone

bascule
cecal b.

base
b. of bladder
b. of brain
broad b.
cranial b.
b. deficit
b. density
Dycal b.
b. of finger
b. fog
b. of heart
invagination skull b.
lung b.
b. of lung
b. of metacarpal
orbital b.
b. of phalanx
b. projection
respiratory disturbance of acid b.
skull b.
b. of skull (BOS)
b. of skull foramen
b. of thumb
b. of toe
ulcer b.
b. view

baseball
b. bat shape
b. finger
b. finger fracture
b. pitcher's elbow
b. shoulder

Basedow goiter

baseline
anthropologic b.
anthropomorphic b.
b. artifact
b. of bulb
b. chest x-ray
b. mammography
radiographic b. (RBL)
Reid b. (RBL)
reproducible b.
return to b.
b. tenting
b. view

basibregmatic axis

basic
b. cycle length (BCL)
b. drive cycle length (BDCL)
b. volume image analysis

basicranial axis

basilar
b. angiography
b. artery
b. artery aneurysm
b. artery bifurcation
b. artery ectasia
b. artery insufficiency
b. artery syndrome
b. atelectasis
b. bone
b. cartilage
b. cistern
b. crest
b. distribution lung disease
b. femoral neck fracture
b. fibrosis
b. groove
b. impression
b. intracerebral hemorrhage
b. invagination
b. line
b. occlusion
b. pleural scarring
b. plexus
b. pneumonitis
b. pneumothorax
b. process
b. sinus
b. skull fracture
b. sulcus
b. suture
b. vertebra
b. zone infiltrate

basilar-vertebral artery disease

basilic vein

basioccipital bone

NOTES

basiocciput
b. hypoplasia
b. tumor
basion
basion-axial interval
basion-dens interval
basipharyngeal canal
basisphenoid bone
basivertebral vein
basket guide wire
basketlike calcification
$BaSO_4$
barium sulfate
basocervical fracture
basophilic brain adenoma
batch
b. reading
b. reading of x-rays
Batson
B. plexus
B. vertebral brain system
bat's wing shadow
Batten disease
battered child syndrome
battledore placenta
Battle sign
batwing
b. appearance
b. configuration
b. configuration of ventricle
b. formation
b. lung consolidation
Baudelocque diameter
Bauer Temno biopsy needle
Bauhin valve
Baumann angle
bauxite
b. fibrosis of lung
b. pneumoconiosis
Bayer Immuno 1 Dpd assay automated bone-resorption test
bayesian
b. calculation
b. formula
b. image estimation (BIE)
b. technique
Bayes theorem
Bayler-Pinneau method
Bayliss effect
Baylor total artificial heart
Bayne
B. classification of radial agenesis
B. radial agenesis classification
bayonet
b. deformity
b. dislocation
b. fracture position
b. leg
b. position of fracture
b. sign
Bazin disease
BBBB
bilateral bundle-branch block
BBC
biceps, brachialis, coracobrachialis
BBC muscles
BBD
benign breast disease
BBOT
2,5-bis(5-t-butylbenzoxazol-2-yl)thiophene
BBR
bundle-branch reentry
BBs
both bones
BCA
bell-clapper anomaly
B-cell
B.-c. monocytoid lymphoma
B.-c. tumor
BCL
basic cycle length
BD
below diaphragm
BDA
bile duct adenoma
B-D bone marrow biopsy needle
BDCL
basic drive cycle length
BDM
border detection method
BE
barium enema
beachchair position
bead
b. chain cystogram
Dynal M450 magnetic b.'s
immunomagnetic b.'s
methyl methacrylate b.'s
packed b.'s
Sephadex b.'s
targeting b.'s
beaded
b. appearance
b. bile duct
b. bronchus
b. ductal dilatation
b. hepatic duct
b. pancreatic duct
b. rib
b. thickening
b. ureter
beading
b. of artery
rosary b.
b. sign

beak
dorsal talar b.
b. fracture
b. ligament
b. sign
beaked
b. appearance
b. cervicomedullary junction
b. pelvis
beaking
antral b.
b. of head of talus
talar b.
talonavicular b.
tectal b.
beaklike
b. configuration
b. osteophyte formation
beak-shaped nose
BEAM
beam
b. attenuation
barrier b.
blended b.
cobalt-60 b.
cone b.
coplanar b.
b. current
b. diffraction
electron b.
b. energy
fan b.
b. filtration
gaussian mode profile laser b.
b. hardening
helium ion b.
b. intensity
intensity-modulated photon b.
laser b.
lateral opposed b.
b. limitation
lucite b.
megavoltage treatment b.
b. monitor
multifield b.
noncoplanar therapy b.
open b.
parallel-opposed b.'s
b. pattern
pencil electron b.
primary b.
b. quality comparison
radiation b.
b. restrictor
b. shaper
sound b.
b. splitter
b. steering
b. therapy
wedged-pair b.
x-ray b.
beam-hardening
b.-h. artifact
b.-h. effect
beam-modifying device
beam's eye view (BEV)
beam's-eye view dosimetry
beam-splitting mirror
bear
b. claw ulcer
b. paw sign
bear's paw hand
beat
apex b.
ectopic b.
escape b.
inferolateral displacement of apical b.
ventricular capture b. (VCB)
ventricular ectopic b. (VEB)
ventricular premature b. (VPB)
ventricular pseudoperfusion b.
beaten
b. brass appearance
b. brass skull
b. silver appearance
b. silver appearance of skull
Beath view
beat-knee syndrome
Beatson
B. combined ankle angle
B. combined ankle length
beat-to-beat variability
Beau disease
Beauvais disease
beavertail appearance
Beckenbaugh technique
Becker
B. nevus
B. sign
Beck triad
Beckwith-Wiedemann syndrome

NOTES

Beclard
B. amputation
B. hernia
Beclere
B. method
B. position
becquerel (Bq)
Becton Dickinson FAC scan
BED
bioeffect dose
biologically equivalent dose
bed
bladder b.
gallbladder b.
hepatic b.
liver b.
portal vascular b.
primary tumor b.
prostatic b.
pulmonary vascular b.
b. of rib
skeletal b.
stomach b.
tumor b.
vascular b.
Bednar tumor
bedroom fracture
bedside
b. chest radiography
b. radiography
Beemer disease
beep-o-gram
beer
b. drinker's beriberi cardiomyopathy
b. heart
B. law
Beevor sign
Behçet
B. chest syndrome
B. GI tract
Behr syndrome
BEI
butanol-extractable iodine
Bekhterev
B. arthritis
B. layer
B. tract
Bell
B. brachydactyly
B. palsy
B. phenomenon
bell-and-clapper deformity
bell-clapper anomaly (BCA)
Bell-Dally cervical dislocation
belli
Bellini
duct of B.
B. ligament
papillary duct of B.
bellomedullary
belly
bubble of the b.
b. of muscle
below diaphragm (BD)
below-knee amputation (BKA)
Benassi
B. method
B. position
bend
hand-shaped b.
knee-like b.
bending fracture
Bends asbestos pleurisy
benediction posture
Benedict-Talbot body surface area method
beneficial atrial septal defect
bengal
I-labeled rose b.
benign
b. asbestos-related pleural disease
b. Bergman ossicle
b. biliary stricture
b. bone lesion
b. breast calcification
b. breast disease (BBD)
b. cerebellar ectopia
b. chondroblastoma
b. conal cyst
b. congential Wilms tumor
b. cortical defect
b. duct ectasia
b. duodenal tumor
b. fetal hamartoma
b. fibrous bone lesion
b. fibrous bone tumor
b. fibrous histiocytoma
b. gastric ulcer
b. infiltrate
b. intracranial hypertension
b. juvenile melanoma
b. lung tumor
b. lymphadenopathy
b. lymphoepithelial lesion
b. lymphoepithelial parotid tumor
b. lymphoma of rectum
b. lymphoproliferative lesion
b. mass
b. meningeal fibrosis
b. mesenchymoma
b. mesothelioma
b. mixed tumor parotis
b. neoplasm
b. nephrosclerosis
b. nevus

b. ovarian tumor
b. oxyphilic adenoma
b. papillary stenosis
b. pleural fibroma
b. polyp
b. prostatic hyperplasia (BPH)
b. prostatic hypertrophy (BPH)
b. sclerosing ductal proliferation
b. small bowel tumor
b. subdural effusion
b. teratoid mediastinum tumor
b. thymoma
b. urethral tumor
b. vascular lesion

benignity
benignum
Benink tarsal index
Bennett
B. comminuted fracture
B. dislocation
B. lesion

Benoist penetrometer
bent-knee pelvic tilt
benzalkonium chloride
benzamide
b. imaging agent
substituted b.

benzocaine
benzoic acid
Berger
B. interscapular amputation
B. space

Bergman sign
Bergqvist triad
beriberi heart
berkelium
Berman angiographic catheter
Bernard canal
Bernard-Horner syndrome
Berndt-Harty
B.-H. talar lesion staging
B.-H. talar lesion staging classification

berry
B. aneurysm rupture
b. intracranial aneurysm
B. ligament

Berteil projection
Bertel
B. method
B. position

Bertillon cephalometer
Bertin
B. bone
large column of B.
B. ligament
septum of B.

berylliosis
beryllium granuloma
BES
British engineering system

beta (β)
b. decay
b. particle
b. radiation
b. ray
b. transition

beta-methyl-p-iodophenyl-pentadecanoic acid SPECT scan imaging
beta-oxybutyric acid (BOBA)
beta-ray
b.-r. applicator
b.-r. ophthalmic plaque therapy
b.-r. spectrometer

beta-spectra shapefactor coefficient
betatron
Bethea sign
Bethesda bone
Beuren syndrome
BEV
beam's eye view
billion electron volts

Bevalac system
Bevatron accelerator
beveled
b. edge sign
b. electron beam cone

beveling
bezoar
B_0 field variation
BFM
Brunnstrom-Fugl-Meyer
BFM arm impairment assessment

Biad
B. camera
B. SPECT imaging
B. SPECT imaging system

Bianchi nodule
bias
lead-time b.
length-time b.
overdiagnostic b.
selection b.

NOTES

bias *(continued)*
self-selection b.
time-to-treatment b.
biatrial
b. hypertrophy
b. myxoma
BIB
biliointestinal bypass
bibasilar
b. bronchopneumonia
b. discoid atelectasis
bibasilarly
bicameral uterus
bicanalicular sphincter
BICAP unit
bicaval cannulation
biceps
b., brachialis, coracobrachialis (BBC)
b. brachii
b. brachii tendon
b. femoris
b. femoris muscle
long head of b. (LHB)
short head of b.
biceps-labral complex
bicerebral infarct
Bichat
B. canal
B. fat pad
B. foramen
B. ligament
B. membrane
bicipital
b. aponeurosis
b. bursitis
b. fascia
b. groove
b. rib
b. ridge
b. synovial sheath
b. tendon sheath
b. tuberosity
bicipitoradial bursa
bicisate
technetium-99m b.
Bickel ring
bicollis
bicornis b.
bicommissural aortic valve
biconcave
b. deformity
b. disk
biconcavity
bicondylar
b. T-shaped fracture
b. Y-shaped fracture
biconvex
bicornate uterus
bicornis
b. bicollis
uterus b., bicornate uterus
b. uterus
bicornuate
b. uterus
bicoronal synostosis
bicortical
b. iliac bone
b. screw
bicuspid
b. aortic valve
b. atrioventricular valve
b. valvular aortic stenosis
bicycle
b. ergometer
b. exercise radionuclide ventriculogram
b. spoke fracture
BIDA
butyl iminodiacetic acid
Bid-Gd mesoporphyrine
bidirectional
b. cavopulmonary anastomosis
b. interface
b. shunt
BIE
bayesian image estimation
Biello criteria
Bielschowsky-Jansky disease
Bier amputation
Biermer sign
bifascicular bundle branch block
bifemoral graft
bifid
b. aortic branch
b. biceps tendon
b. clitoris
b. pelvis
b. precordial impulse
b. rib
b. thumb deformity
bifida
spina b.
bifidum
cranium b.
bifocal manipulation with distraction
biforate uterus
bifrontal
b. index
b. oligodendroglioma
bifurcate
bifurcated ligament
bifurcating branch
bifurcation
b. aneurysm
b. of anterior communicating artery

b. of aorta
aortic b.
basilar artery b.
carotid artery b.
common bile duct b.
b. of common carotid artery
common carotid artery b.
b. graft
hepatic duct b.
iliac b.
b. of internal carotid artery
b. lesion
b. lymph node
b. of middle cerebral artery
middle cerebral artery b.
patent b.
pulmonary artery b.
pulmonary trunk b.
tracheal b.
b. of trunk
ureteral bud b.

Bigelow
B. ligament
ligament of B.

bigeminal
b. pattern
b. pregnancy

Bigliani classification

bihemispheral insult

biischial diameter

bilaminar
b. appearance
b. zone

bilary excretion bowel activity

bilateral
b. alteration
b. anterior chest bulge
b. arachnoid cyst
b. bronchogram
b. bundle-branch block (BBBB)
b. carotid arteriography
b. carotid stenosis
b. choroid plexus cyst
b. consolidation
b. cortical necrosis
b. diaphragmatic elevation
b. diffuse increased uptake
b. ductal ectasia
b. fetal chest mass
b. hallux valgus
b. hilar adenopathy
b. hydrocephalus
b. hyperlucent lung
b. iliac crest
b. incomplete ureteral injury
b. infarct
b. interstitial pulmonary infiltrate
b. intrafacetal dislocation
b. large adrenal
b. large kidney
b. left-sidedness
b. lesion
b. locked facets
b. lower lobe pneumonia
b. lymphadenectomy
b. myocutaneous graft
b. narrowing of urinary bladder
b. obstruction
b. occlusion
b. orbital frontal cortex
b. pleural tube
b. pyramidal sign
b. renal mass
b. right-sidedness
b. salpingo-oophorectomy
b. small kidney
b. superior vena cava
b. upper lobe cavitary infiltrate
b. vagotomy effect

bilaterally symmetric

bile
b. bag
b. capillary
concentrated b.
b. concretion
b. duct
b. duct adenoma (BDA)
b. duct carcinoma
b. duct cystadenoma
b. duct dilatation
b. duct dyskinesia
b. duct filling defect
b. duct gas
b. duct infundibulum
b. duct lumen
b. duct multiple hamartoma
b. duct narrowing
b. duct pressure
b. duct proliferation
b. duct scan
b. duct scan imaging
b. duct stone
b. duct stricture
b. encrustation

NOTES

bile *(continued)*
b. extravasation
b. flow
b. flow obstruction
gastric reflux of b.
high-density b.
b. lake
b. leakage
lithogenic b.
b. papilla
b. plug
b. pulmonary embolus
b. reflux
b. reflux gastritis
b. stasis
bileaflet valve
bilharzial
b. carcinoma
b. granuloma
bilharziasis
cardiopulmonary b.
protopulmonary b.
biliary
b. atresia
b. calculus
b. canal
b. cirrhosis
b. cirrhotic liver
b. colic
b. cystadenoma
b. decompression
b. dilatation
b. drainage
b. duct
b. dyskinesia
b. dyssynergia
b. endoprosthesis
b. fistula
b. lithotripsy
b. manometry
b. mud
b. obstruction syndrome
b. passage
b. piecemeal necrosis
b. plexus
b. saturation index
b. sludge
b. stent
b. stricture
b. structure
b. system
b. tract
b. tract cancer
b. tract CT scan imaging
b. tract disease
b. tract obstruction
b. tract stone
b. tree
b. tree gas
b. tree obstruction
biliary-cutaneous fistula
biliary-duodenal
b.-d. fistula
b.-d. pressure gradient
biliary-enteric
b.-e. anastomosis
b.-e. anastomosis operation
b.-e. fistula
biliary-to-bowel transit
Biligrafin
B. imaging agent
Biligram
Biliodyl
bilioenteric
b. bypass
b. fistula
biliointestinal bypass (BIB)
biliopancreatic
b. bypass (BPB)
b. diversion
b. shunt
bilious bronchial pneumonia
bilirubinate stone
Biliscopin
B. contrast medium
B. imaging agent
Bilivist
B. contrast medium
B. imaging agent
Bilivistan
Bill bar
billion electron volts (BEV)
billowing
b. mitral valve
b. mitral valve prolapse
Billroth
B. I, II anastomosis
B. I, II gastroduodenostomy
B. I, II gastrojejunostomy
bilobate placenta
bilobed
b. configuration
b. gallbladder
b. mass
b. polypoid lesion
bilocular
b. stomach
b. uterus
biloculare
cor b.
biloma
intrahepatic b.
subphrenic b.
Bilopaque
B. imaging agent
Biloptic imaging agent

Biloptin
bimalleolar
b. angle
b. ankle fracture
b. foot axis
bimastoid line
binary
b. ascariasis
b. digit
b. image
b. imaging
bind
^{99m}Tc Ceretec b.
technetium-99m Ceretec bind
binding
b. energy
ionic b.
receptor b.
b. site
Bing-Horton syndrome
binning
projection b.
binocular stereoscope
Binswanger
B. disease
B. encephalopathy
biodegradable
b. implant
b. magnetic microcluster
b. stent
biodistribution
bioeffect
b. dose (BED)
thermal b.
bioeffects algorithm
Biograft
Dardik B.
biologic
b. age
b. half-life
b. window
biological
b. osteosynthesis
b. tissue valve
biologically equivalent dose (BED)
biology
radiation b.
biomagnetometer
Magnes b.
biomechanical
b. imbalance
b. stress
biomechanics of limb length discrepancy
biometry
longitudinal ultrasonic b.
biomodulator
biophysical profile score (BPS)
biopotential
induced b.
bioprosthesis
biopsy
aspiration b.
automated large-core breast b.
bone marrow b.
breast b.
computerized tomography-guided needle b.
core needle b.
CT-directed b.
CT-guided needle b.
CT-guided percutaneous b.
CT-guided transsternal core b.
fetal liver b.
fetal skin b.
guided b.
interactive MR-guided b.
intramedullary tumor b.
MRI-guided breast b.
b. needle
needle b.
percutaneous transhepatic liver b.
placenta b.
point-in-space stereotactic b.
skeletal b.
stereotactic percutaneous needle b.
systematic ultrasound-guided b.
b. transducer
transthoracic needle aspiration b. (TTNAB)
ultrasound-guided stereotactic b.
vacuum needle b.
ventricular endomyocardial b.
biopsy-guided attachment
Biopsys mammotome
bioptome
Kawai b.
bioreductive agent
Biosound AU (Advanced Ultrasonography) system
Biospec
B. MR imaging system
B. MR imaging system scanner
biosynthesis

NOTES

Biot sign
biparietal
b. bossing
b. diameter (BPD)
b. lesion
b. suture
biparietotemporal hypometabolism
bipartite
b. fracture
b. sesamoid
b. sesamoid bone
b. uterus
bipartition
facial b.
bipedal lymphangiography
bipennate muscle
bipenniform muscles of hand
biphasic
b. CT
b. curve
b. helical CT scan
b. system
biplanar
b. aortography
b. MR imaging guidance
biplane
b. angiocardiography
b. angiography
b. axial film
b. cineangiography
b. cinefluorography
b. fluoroscopy
b. left ventricular angiogram
b. orthogonal view
b. pelvic arteriography
b. pelvic oblique study
b. quantitative coronary arteriography
b. sector probe
b. sector scanner
b. transesophageal echocardiography
b. ventriculogram
bipolar
b. gradient
b. hip replacement
b. lead
b. pacemaker
BIRADS
Breast Imaging Reporting and Data System
bird
b. beak esophagus
b. breeder's lung
b. fancier's lung
b. handler's lung
bird-beak
b.-b. configuration or narrowing
b.-b. taper at esophagogastric junction
birdcage
b. head coil
b. resonator
b. splint
bird-headed dwarfism
birdlike appearance
bird's
b. eye view
b. nest filter
b. nest lesion
Bird sign
birefringence
apple-green b.
biricodar
birth canal
bisacodyl tannex
bisagittal ridge
bisection
AP malleolar b.
bisferious pulse rhythm
bis-gadolinium-mesoporphyrine (bis-Gd-MP)
bis-Gd-mesoporphyrin imaging agent
bis-Gd-MP
bis-gadolinium-mesoporphyrine
bismuth
B. classification of benign bile duct stricture
b. germanate-68
1,4-bis(5-phenyloxazol-2-yl)benzene
bispinous diameter
2,5-bis(5-t-butylbenzoxazol-2-yl)thiophene (BBOT)
bit
b. CT
parity b.
bite
b. plane
b. sign
bitewing
b. film
b. radiograph
b. x-ray
bit-rate allocation
bituberous diameter
bivalve
biventricular
b. assist device (BVAD)
b. configuration
b. enlargement
b. hypertrophy
b. origin of aorta
b. support system (BVS)
b. transposed aorta
biventricularly
Bjork-Shiley heart valve

BKA
below-knee amputation
BKG
background
black
b. blood magnetic resonance angiography
b. blood T2-weighted inversion-recovery MR imaging
b. boundary artifact
b. comets artifact
b. echo writing
b. epidermoid
b. faceted stone
b. lung
b. lung disease
b. pleura sign
b. star breast lesion
black-dot heel
Blackett-Healy
B.-H. method
B.-H. position
Blackfan-Diamond syndrome
bladder
apex of b.
atonic urinary b.
b. augmentation
automatic b.
base of b.
b. bed
bilateral narrowing of urinary b.
b. cancer
b. capacity
b. carcinoma
centrally uninhibited b.
contracted b.
b. contractility study
b. contusion trauma
b. distention
b. diverticulitis
b. diverticulum
b. dome
dome of urinary b.
b. dysfunction
b. endometriosis
b. exstrophy
exstrophy of b.
b. flap hematoma
flat-top b.
b. floor
b. fundus
b. hemorrhage
hourglass b.
hypertrophic b.
b. hypertrophy
hypotonic b.
b. incontinence
intraperitoneal rupture of b.
kidneys, ureters, b. (KUB)
b. laceration
b. map
motor paralytic neurogenic b.
neck of b.
b. neck contracture
neurogenic urinary b.
neuropathic b.
nonneurogenic b.
b. outlet obstruction
papilloma of b.
pear-shaped urinary b.
b. perforation
b. pheochromocytoma
refluxing spastic neurogenic b.
b. rupture
b. rupture trauma
sensitive b.
sensory neurogenic b.
sensory paralytic b.
shrunken b.
spastic urinary b.
squamous urinary b.
b. stasis
b. stone
teardrop b.
thickened b.
transurethral resection of b.
trigone of b.
b. tumor
uninhibited b.
unstable b.
urinary b.
urinary bladder within a b.
urinary blunt trauma b.
uvula of b.
b. wall
b. wall calcification
b. wall thickening
b. wall thickness
BladderManager
B. ultrasound
B. ultrasound device
bladder-prostate rhabdomyosarcoma
BladderScan ultrasound
bladder-within-bladder sign

NOTES

blade
b. bone
b. plate
blade-of-grass
b.-o.-g. appearance
b.-o.-g. osteolysis
Blalock shunt
Blalock-Taussig shunt
bland
b. aortic aneurysm
b. embolus
b. infarct
blast
b. chest
extrafollicular b.
blastic
b. lesion
b. metastasis
b. phase
b. transformation
b. variant
blastocyst
blastocytoma
blastoma
parenchymal b.
pleuropulmonary b.
blastomycosis
nasopharyngeal b.
North American b.
bleb
emphysematous b.
ruptured emphysematous b.
subpleural b.
Bleck
B. classification of metatarsus adductus
B. metatarsus adductus classification
bleed
gastrointestinal b. (GI bleed)
herald b.
technetium-99m pertechnetate GI b.
technetium-99m sulfur colloid GI b.
bleeding
first-trimester b.
gastrointestinal b.
b. into brain parenchyma
intrapericardial b.
b. lesion
b. point
b. polyp
postmenopausal b.
postmenopausal uterine b.
b. site
splenic b.
b. time
b. ulcer
b. uterus
blended
b. beam
b. beam technique
blennorrhagic swelling
blennothorax
bleomycin lung
Blessig cyst
blind
b. dimple
b. enema
b. foramen
b. gut
b. intestine
b. loop syndrome
b. percutaneous puncture of subclavian vein
b. pouch syndrome
b. segment
b. tibial outflow tract
b. upper esophageal pouch
Blineau projection
blink mode
blister
b. of bone
fracture b.
BLL
Burkitt-like lymphoma
bloc
en b.
block
air b.
alveolar-capillary b.
anodal b.
anterior fascicular b.
anterograde b.
arborization b.
atrioventricular b.
autonomic nerve b.
AV b.
AV Wenckebach heart b.
bifascicular bundle branch b.
bilateral bundle-branch b. (BBBB)
bone b.
bundle-branch heart b.
celiac b.
celiac ganglion b.
Cerrobend b.
complete atrioventricular b. (CAVB)
complete congenital heart b.
complete fetal heart b.
complete heart b. (CHB)
conduction b.
congenital complete heart b.
congenital heart b.
congenital symptomatic AV b.
custom shielding b.
deceleration-dependent b.
divisional b.

donor heart-lung b.
entrance b.
exit b.
false bundle-branch b.
familial heart b.
fascicular b.
filler b.
first-degree AV b.
first-degree heart b.
fixed third-degree AV b.
fluoroscopy-guided subarachnoid phenol b.
heart b.
high-grade AV b.
incomplete atrioventricular b. (IAVB)
incomplete heart b.
incomplete left bundle-branch b. (ILBBB)
incomplete right bundle-branch b. (IRBBB)
inflammatory heart b.
infra-His b.
intermittent third-degree AV b.
interventricular b.
intraatrial b.
intra-His b.
intranodal b.
intravenous b.
intraventricular b. (IVB)
intraventricular conduction b.
intraventricular heart b.
inverted-Y b.
ipsilateral bundle-branch b.
irregular b.
left anterior fascicular b. (LAFB)
left anterior hemiblock b.
left bundle-branch b. (LBBB)
mantle b.
midline mucosa-sparing b.
Mobitz I or II heart b.
mucosa-sparing b.
multiple b.'s
paroxysmal AV b.
partial heart b.
periinfarction b. (PIB)
peripheral nerve b.
pixel b.
posterior fascicular b.
pseudo-AV b.
regional neurolytic b.
retrograde b.
right bundle-branch b. (RBBB)
second-degree AV b.
second-degree heart b.
shielding b.
shock b.
simple b.
sinoatrial b. (SAB)
sinoatrial exit b.
sinus node exit b.
subarachnoid nerve b.
subarachnoid phenol b.
suprahisian b.
sympathetic b.
third-degree AV b.
third-degree heart b.
transient AV b.
transmission b.
trifascicular b.
unidirectional b.
unifascicular b.
ventricular b.
ventriculoatrial b.
b. vertebra
vesicular b.
Wenckebach AV b.
Wilson b.
8 x 8-pixel b.

blockade
coil b.

blockage
arterial b.
bronchus b.
pulmonary artery b.
ventricular catheter b.

blocked
b. artery
b. bronchus
b. pleurisy
b. shunt tube
b. vertex field

blocker's exostosis

blocking factor

Bloedorn applicator

Blom-Singer tracheoesophageal fistula

blood
arterialization of venous b.
backflow of b.
backscatter of b.
backup of b.
b. channel
b. clearance half-time
b. clot

NOTES

blood *(continued)*
deoxygenated b.
disseminated intravascular coagulation of b.
egress of b.
epidural b.
extravasated b.
b. extravasation
b. flow
b. flow extraction fraction
b. flow imaging
b. flow measurement
b. flowmetry
b. flow pattern
b. flow redistribution
b. flow reserve
b. flow response
b. flow study
b. flow velocity
hydrostatic pressure of b.
b. inflow
intracerebral b.
intraparenchymal b.
intraventricular b.
b. leak
left-to-right shunting of b.
marked shunting of b.
mixed venous b.
occult b.
b. oxygenation level-dependent
b. oxygenation level-dependent contrast
b. oxygenation level-dependent effect
b. oxygenation level-dependent imaging
parenchymal b.
b. patch
b. perfusion
b. perfusion monitor (BPM)
peripheral b.
periportal tracking of b.
b. plate thrombus
b. pool
b. pool activity
b. pool imaging
b. pool phase image
b. pool phase imaging
b. pool radionuclide angiography
b. pool radionuclide cardioangiography
b. pool radionuclide echocardiography
b. pool radionuclide scan
b. pool scintigraphy
b. pressure
b. pressure response
right-to-left shunting of b.
shunted b.
b. sludge
sluggishly flowing b.
b. speckle
splanchnic b.
subdural b.
upstream b.
vascular b.
venous b.
b. vessel
b. vessel invasion
b. vessel kinking
b. vessel thermography
b. vessel tumor
b. viscosity reduction
b. volume
b. volume per minute

blood-clotting mechanism

blood-filled bone sponge

bloodless
b. fluid
b. zone of necrosis

blood-tumor-barrier leakage

blooming
b. artifact
b. focal spot
signal b.

Bloom syndrome

Blount
B. disease
B. tibia vara

blow-in fracture

blowing pneumothorax

blowout
aortic stump b.
b. bone lesion
bone lesion b.
b. fracture
b. lesion of posterior vertebral element

blue
bromophenol b.
cresyl b.
isosulfan b.
b. rubber-bleb nevus syndrome
toluidine b. (TB)

blueberry muffin syndrome

blue-digit syndrome

blue-toe syndrome

Blumberg sign

Blumenbach clivus

Blumensaat line

Blumenthal lesion

Blumer rectal shelf

blunt
b. border of lung
b. chest trauma
b. gastrointestinal trauma

b. injury
b. pancreatic trauma
b. trauma gallbladder
b. trauma kidney

blunted
b. ejection fraction
b. posterior sulcus

blunt-end sialogram needle

blunting
caliceal b.
b. of costophrenic angle
costophrenic angle b.
b. of costovertebral angle
haustral b.
b. of valve

blur
focal spot b.
geometric b.
motion b.
object-plane b.

blurred-image tomogram

blurring
b. of aortic knob
b. of costophrenic angle
b. of disk margins
radiographic b.

blush
choroid plexus b.
cortical b.
b. of dye on angiography
kidney papillary b.
myocardial b.
renal parenchymal b.
tumor b.
vascular b.

BMC
bone mineral content

BMD
bone mineral density

BMI
body mass index

BMIPP SPECT scan imaging

B mode
longitudinal B. m.
pseudocolor B. m.

B-mode
B.-m. display
B.-m. echocardiography
B.-m. echography
B.-m. imaging
B.-m. ultrasonography

BMP
bone marrow pressure

Board
National Radiological Protection B. (NRPB)

boat-shaped heart

BOBA
beta-oxybutyric acid

Bochdalek
foramen of B.
B. foramen
B. gap
B. hernia
B. muscle

body
alignment of vertebral b.
angularis b.
asbestos b.'s
asteroid b.
axis b.
b. background activity
b. box plethysmography
b. burden
calcific round b.
calcified pineal b.
carotid b.
caudate b.
b. cavity
coccygeal b.
b. coil
b. coil imaging
compressed b.
b. contour orbit
b. contour orbit articulation
enlargement of vertebral b.
b. of epididymis
esophageal b.
b. of femur
ferruginous b.
foreign b. (FB)
free b.
b. of gallbladder
Gamna-Gandy b.
geniculate b.
glenoid labral ovoid b.
b. glomus
b. habitus
height of vertebral b.
Howell-Jolly b.
H-shaped vertebral b.
b. interface
intraarticular loose b.

NOTES

body *(continued)*
intraluminal foreign b.
intraocular foreign b.
intravascular foreign b.
juxtarestiform b.
Langerhans b.
lateral geniculate b.
loose intraarticular b.
Luys b.
malpighian b.
mamillary b.
b. mass index (BMI)
Masson b.
medial geniculate b.
metallic foreign b.
Michaelis-Gutmann b.
multilaminar b.'s
navicular b.
b. nitrogen
nonradiopaque foreign b.
ossified b.
osteochondral loose b.
osteochondrotic loose b.
pacchionian b.'s
pacchionian b.
b. of the pancreas
Pappenheimer b.
pharmacoradiologic disimpaction of esophageal foreign b.
Pick b.
picture frame pattern of vertebral b.'s
pineal b.
pleura fibrin b.
Prowazek b.
Prowazek-Greeff b.
psammoma b.
radiopaque foreign b.
Reilly b.
restiform b.
retained foreign b.
rhinencephalic mamillary b.
rice joint b.
Ross b.
Russell b.
scalloping of margin of vertebral b.
b. scanning
b. of scapula
scapular b.
Schaumann b.
Schiller-Duval b.
b. section radiography
b. section radiography imaging
Seidelin b.
small vertebral b.
squared vertebral b.
b. stalk
b. of the stomach
b. surface area (BSA)
b. surface area calculation
b. surface potential mapping
thyroid psammoma b.
tracheobronchial foreign b.
trapezoid b.
b. of the uterus
b. of vertebra
vertebral b.
vesalianum of vertebral b.
b. wall
Weibel-Palade b.
Zuckerkandl b.'s

Boeck lung sarcoid

Boehler (*var. of* Böhler)

Boerhaave syndrome

Boettcher canal

boggy
b. synovitis
b. synovium

Bogros space

Böhler, Boehler
B. angle
B. calcaneal view
B. view

Bohr
B. atom
B. effect
B. equation
B. magneton
B. radius
B. theory

BOLD
BOLD effect

bolster finger

Bolton-Hunter technique

bolus
air b.
barium b.
b. challenge imaging
b. challenge test
b. chase
contrast b.
b. contrast enhancement
b. dose
dynamic b.
electron b.
food b.
intravenous b.
b. intravenous injection
radioactive b.
simple b.
special b.
b. tagging
tracer b.
b. tracking

b. transit
water b.
bombard
bombardment
alpha particle b.
end of saturated b. (EOSB)
neutron b.
bond
Tc b.
technetium bond
technetium b. (Tc bond)
valence b.
wedge b.
bone
b. abscess
b. absorption
accessory multangular b.
accessory navicular b.
accessory sesamoid b.
acetabular b.
acromial b.
b. age
b. age imaging
b. age ratio
alar b.
Albers-Schönberg bone
Albers-Schönberg marble b.
Albrecht b.
b. algorithm
b. allograft
alveolar supporting b.
b. angioblastoma
b. angiosarcoma
ankle b.
anvil b.
apex of petrous portion of temporal b.
arachnodactyly b.
arch of b.
architectural alterations of b.
b. architecture
areolae of b.
arteriovenous fistula b.
articular lamella of b.
articular tubercle of temporal b.
astragalar b.
astragalocalcanean b.
astragalocrural b.
astragaloscaphoid b.
astragalotibial b.
astragalus b.
atrophy of b.
b. atrophy
attic temporal b.
autogenous b.
basal b.
basilar b.
basioccipital b.
basisphenoid b.
Bertin b.
Bethesda b.
bicortical iliac b.
bipartite sesamoid b.
blade b.
blister of b.
b. block
Bonfiglio b.
both b.'s (BBs)
bowed long b.
breast b.
bregmatic b.
Breschet b.
brittle b.
b. bruise
brush border margin of b.
bundle b.
calcaneal b.
Calcitite b.
calvarial b.
b. canaliculus
cancellated b.
b. cancer
candle-wax appearance of b.
cannon b.
b. capillary hemangioma
capitate b.
carpal navicular b.
cartilage b.
cavalry b.
b. cement
b. center
central b.
chalky b.
cheek b.
chevron b.
b. chip
b. chloroma
b. coccidioidomycosis
coccygeal b.
coccyx b.
coffin b.
collar b.
compact b.
cone-and-socket b.

NOTES

bone *(continued)*
continuity of b.
convoluted b.
b. core
coronary b.
b. cortex
cortical b.
corticocancellous b.
costal b.
coxal b.
cranial b.
cribriform b.
cubital b.
cuboid b.
cuneiform b.
dancer's b.
dead b.
b. debris
b. demineralization
dense structure of b.
b. densitometer
b. density imaging
b. density measurement
b. density study
depression of nasal b.
dermal b.
devitalized portion of b.
diastasis of cranial b.
dimple of b.
displaced fragment of b.
dorsal talonavicular b.
b. dysplasia
b. dystrophy
eburnated b.
b. echinococcosis
b. end
endochondral b.
entrapped plantar sesamoid b.
epactal b.
epihyal b.
epihyoid b.
epiphysis b.
epipteric b.
episternal b.
erosion of epiphyseal b.
ethmoid b.
exoccipital b.
facial b.
femoral b.
fencer's b.
b. fibrosarcoma
fibular sesamoid b.
first cuneiform b.
b. fixation device
flank b.
b. flap
b. flap fixation plate
flat b.
Flower b.
b. formation
b. formation cloaca
fourth turbinated b.
b. fracture
fracture running length of b.
fragile b.
b. fragment
fragment of b.
frontal b.
gallium imaging in b.
Goethe b.
gracile b.
b. graft
greater multangular b.
great toe sesamoid b.
growth center of b.
b. growth stimulator
hallux sesamoid b.
hamate b.
b. hardening
Hardy-Clapham classification of sesamoid b.
haunch b.
heel b.
hemangioendothelial b.
heterotopic b.
highest turbinated b.
hip b.
hollow b.
hooked b.
humeral b.
hyoid b.
hyperplastic b.
b. hypertrophy
b. hypothyroidism
iliac cancellous b.
immature b.
b. implant
b. implantation cyst
incarial b.
incisive b.
incomplete fracture of b.
incus b.
b. infarct
infected b.
b. infection
inferior turbinated b.
inflammation of b.
b. ingrowth
b. injury radiation
^{111}In-labeled leukocyte b.
innominate b.
intermaxillary b.
intermediate cuneiform b.
interparietal b.
b. interstice
intracartilaginous b.

intrachondral b.
intramembranous b.
irregular b.
ischial b.
b. island
isolated dislocation of semilunar b.
ivory b.
jaw b.
knuckle b.
lacrimal b.
b. lacuna
lamellar b.
lamellated b.
lateral sesamoid b.
b. length imaging
b. length study
lenticular b.
lentiform b.
b. lesion
b. lesion apophysis
b. lesion blowout
b. lesion epiphysis
b. lesion of the rib
lesser multangular b.
lingual b.
b. lipoma
long b.
long axis of b.
lunate b.
lunocapitate b.
luxated b.
b. lymphoma
malar b.
malignant fibrous histiocytoma
of b. (MFH-B)
malleolus b.
marble b.
b. marrow
b. marrow agent
b. marrow aplasia
b. marrow aspiration
b. marrow biopsy
b. marrow boundary
b. marrow depression
b. marrow dose
b. marrow edema
b. marrow embolus
b. marrow fibrosis
b. marrow hypoplasia
b. marrow infiltrate
b. marrow lesion
b. marrow lymphoid hyperplasia
b. marrow microenvironment
b. marrow myeloid precursor
b. marrow pressure (BMP)
b. marrow purging
b. marrow relapse
b. marrow rescue
b. marrow scintigraphy
b. marrow stroma
b. marrow suppression
b. marrow toxicity
b. marrow transplant
b. marrow transplantation
b. mastocytosis
mastoid b.
b. matrix
b. maturation
mature b.
maxillary b.
maxilloturbinal b.
medial cuneiform b.
medial sesamoid b.
medullary b.
membrane of b.
mesocuneiform b.
metacarpal b.
b. metastasis
metatarsal b.
middle cuneiform b.
middle turbinate b.
b. mineral content (BMC)
b. mineral content imaging
b. mineral content study
b. mineral density (BMD)
b. mineralization
morcellized b.
b. morphogenetic activity
mortise of b.
multangular b.
nasal b.
navicular b.
b. neck
necrotic b.
b. neoplasm
newly woven b.
Nicoll b.
occipital b.
odontoid b.
omovertebral b.
orbicular b.
orbital b.
orbitosphenoidal b.
os calcis b.

NOTES

B

bone *(continued)*
ossifying fibroma of long b.
osteonal b.
osteopenic b.
osteoporosis of b.
osteoporotic b.
os trapezium b.
os trapezoideum b.
b. overdevelopment
b. oxalosis
pagetoid b.
b. pain
palatine b.
parietal b.
b. particle
pedal b.
pelvic b.
pencil b.
perichondral b.
perilesional b.
periosteal b.
periotic b.
peroneal b.
petrosal b.
petrous temporal b.
phalangeal b.
phantom b.
b. phase image
b. phase imaging
b. pinhole
Pirie b.
pisiform b.
b. plug
pneumatic b.
pole of scaphoid b.
porous b.
postsphenoid b.
posttraumatic atrophy of b.
postulnar b.
b. powder
preinterparietal b.
premaxillary b.
presphenoid b.
primitive b.
proliferation of b.
prominence of b.
pterygoid b.
pubic b.
pyramidal b.
quadrilateral b.
quadripartite sesamoid b.
b. quantitative CT (BQCT)
radial b.
b. radiation absorption
reactive woven b.
Recklinghausen disease of b.
refractured b.
b. remodeling
replacement b.
b. resorption
resurrection b.
reticulated b.
rider's b.
Riolan b.
rudimentary b.
sacral b.
sandbagging fracture of long b.
b. sarcoidosis
b. scan
scaphoid b.
scapular b.
b. scintigraphy
b. scintiscan imaging
sclerosed temporal b.
scorings on b.
b. screw
scroll b.
second cuneiform b.
semilunar b.
septal b.
sesamoid b.
b. shaft
shank b.
shin b.
short b.
sieve b.
b. sliver
solid b.
sphenoid b.
sphenoidal turbinated b.
splintered b.
spoke b.
spongy b.
b. spur
squamooccipital b.
squamous b.
stirrup b.
b. strut
subchondral b.
subperiosteal new b.
b. substance
b. substitute
substitution b.
superior turbinated b.
supernumerary sesamoid b.
supracollicular spike of cortical b.
suprainterparietal b.
supraoccipital b.
suprapharyngeal b.
suprasternal b.
supreme turbinate b.
b. surface
b. survey
sutural b.
b. syphilis
tail b.

talus b.
target b.
tarsal b.
telephone handle b.
temporal b.
thick b.
thigh b.
thoracic b.
three-cornered b.
tibia b.
tibial sesamoid b.
tongue and trough b.
trabecular b.
trabeculated b.
trapezium b.
trapezoid b.
trapezoid of Henle b.
triangular b.
tripartite sesamoid b.
triquetral b.
trumpet b.
b. tuberculosis
tuberculous b.
tubular b.
b. tumor
b. tumor aggressiveness
tumor-bearing b.
b. tumor matrix
turbinate b.
tympanic b.
tympanohyal b.
ulnar b.
ulnar sesamoid b.
unciform b.
upper jaw b.
vascular b.
vertebral body subchondral b.
vesalian b.
Vesalius b.
vomer b.
waist of scaphoid b.
weightbearing b.
whettle b.
b. window
wing of sphenoid b.
wormian b.
woven b.
wrist triquetrum b.
b. xanthogranuloma
xanthomatosis of long b.
xiphoid b.
yoke b.
zygomatic b.

bone-air interface
bone-chip allograft
bone-forming
b.-f. bone tumor
b.-f. sarcoma
bone-hardening artifact
bone-implant interface
bonelet
bone-on-bone contact
bone-tendon-bone graft
bone-tendon exposure
bone-to-bone apposition
bone-within-bone
b.-w.-b. appearance
b.-w.-b. vertebra
Bonfiglio bone
bonnet
gluteal b.
bony
b. abnormality
b. alignment
b. ankylosis
b. apposition
b. architecture
b. bar
b. bridge
b. callus
b. callus formation
b. change
b. coalition
b. contusion
b. decompression
b. defect
b. deformity
b. degeneration
b. deposit
b. destruction
b. disruption
b. eburnation
b. encroachment
b. enlargement
b. erosion
b. excrescence
b. exostosis
b. fossa
b. fusion
b. glenoid marrow fat
b. glenoid rim
b. healing
b. heart

NOTES

bony *(continued)*
b. humeral avulsion
b. hyperostosis
b. island
b. labyrinth
b. lysis
b. necrosis
b. nonunion
b. orbit
b. osteophyte
b. overgrowth
b. palate
b. pelvis
b. plate
b. process
b. projection from vertebra
b. proliferation
b. prominence
b. protuberance
b. rarefaction
b. reabsorption
b. ridge
b. sclerosis
b. semicircular canal
b. sequestrum
b. skeleton
b. skull landmark
b. spicule
b. spurring
b. stability
b. structure
b. thoracic cage
b. thorax
b. tissue
b. trabecular injury
b. trabecular pattern
b. tuft of finger
b. union
b. vertebra projection

Boogaard angle

book cassette

boomerang
b. configuration of brain
b. tendon

BOOP
bronchiolitis obliterans with organizing pneumonia

Boorman classification of gastric cancer

boost
brachytherapy b.
b. dose
electron beam b.
interstitial b.
b. therapy

booster
b. heart
b. phenomenon

boot-shaped heart

boot-top fracture

border
alveolar b.
anterior b.
antimesenteric b.
cardiac b.
ciliated b.
corticated b.
crescentic b.
b. detection method (BDM)
diaphragmatic b.
echocardiographic automated b.
heart b.
inferior b.
interosseous b.
irregular b.
lateral b.
left sternal b. (LSB)
lobulated b.
lower left sternal b.
lower sternal b. (LSB)
medial b.
mediastinal b.
mesenteric b.
midleft sternal b.
periventricular b.
posterior b.
rounded convex b.
scapulovertebral b.
serpiginous low signal intensity b.
shagging of cardiac b.
shaggy heart b.
smooth b.
sternal b.
sternocleidomastoid muscle b.
straight anterior vertebral b.
straightening of anterior vertebral b.
superior b.
thin b.
upper sternal b.
b. zone

borderline
b. cardiomegaly
b. heart size
b. malignancy
b. normal
b. severe rejection

Borg scale of treadmill exertion

Born
B. approximation
B. method

Bornholm disease

boron
b. counter
b. neutron capture

BOS
base of skull

Bosniak classification
boss
  carpal b.
  parietal b.
bossa
  parietal b.
bosselated
  b. stone
  b. surface
bosselation
bossing
  biparietal b.
  frontal b.
  occipital b.
Bosworth
  B. bone peg insertion
  B. fracture
Botallo
  B. duct
  B. foramen
  ligament of B.
  B. ligament
both-bone fracture
both bones (BBs)
both-column fracture
Böttcher canal
bottle sign
bottoming out of prosthetic component
Bouchard disease
bouche de tapir
bougie
bougienage
  b. technique
Bouillaud
  B. disease
  B. sign
bounce-point artifact
bouncing
  ligamentous b.
bound
  Cramer-Rao minimum variance b. (CR-MVB)
  b. electrons
boundary
  air/bone/tissue b.
  bone marrow b.
  b. edge
  horizontal b.
  b. layer
  tumor b.
bouquet
  fixed shaped coplanar or nonplanar radiation beam b.
Bourgery ligament
Bourneville disease
Bourneville-Pringle disease
boutonnière
  b. deformity
  b. dislocation
Bouveret
  B. disease
  B. syndrome
Bouveret-Hoffmann syndrome
Bovero muscle
bovine
  b. heart
  b. heart xenograft
bovinum
  cor b.
Bowditch
  B. effect
  B. staircase phenomenon
bowed
  b. legs
  b. long bone
  b. micromelia
bowel
  aganglionic b.
  apple-peel b.
  b. ascariasis
  b. axis
  b. and bladder dysfunction
  b. cancer
  b. containing opaque material
  b. contents
  b. continuity
  corkscrew appearance of small b.
  dead b.
  dilated dry small b.
  dilated fetal b.
  dilated loops of b.
  dilated wet small b.
  distal small b.
  b. distention
  echogenic fetal b.
  fixed segment of b.
  fluid-filled loop of b.
  b. gas
  b. gas artifact
  b. gas pattern
  herniated b.
  hoop-shaped loops of b.

NOTES

bowel *(continued)*
b. incontinence
b. infarct
infarcted b.
intussuscepted b.
b. intussusception
irritable b.
ischemic b.
kinked b.
b. kinking
large b.
loop of b.
b. loop
b. loop air
b. loop dilatation
b. lumen
b. motion
b. movement
multiple loops of small b.
multiple stenotic lesions of small b.
b. necrosis
normal-caliber b.
b. obstruction
peristalsing b.
b. peristalsis
pleating of small b.
b. preparation
proximal small b.
b. pseudoobstruction
ribbon b.
b. secretion
shock b.
b. shock
small b.
b. sounds
b. spasm
b. stenosis
b. stoma
strangulated b.
b. wall
b. wall hematoma
b. wall penetration
bowing
anterior tibial b.
b. deformity
b. fracture
b. of mitral valve leaflet
b. of tendon
bowleg
bowler's thumb
Bowman
B. angle
B. capsule
B. disk
B. muscle
B. space
bowstring
b. sign
b. tear
bowstringing
bow-tie
b.-t. morphology
b.-t. sign
bowtie filter
box
carpal b.
ligamentous b.
mammographic view b.
shadow b.
view b.
boxer's
b. elbow
b. punch fracture
boxlike cardiomegaly
Boyce sign
Boyd
B. ankle amputation
B. formula
B. perforating vein
B. type II fracture
Boyden
B. sphincter
B. test meal
Boyd-Griffin trochanteric fracture classification
Bozzolo sign
BP
bronchopleural
bronchopulmonary
bypass
BP fistula
Imagent BP
BPB
biliopancreatic bypass
BPD
biparietal diameter
bronchopulmonary dysplasia
BPH
benign prostatic hyperplasia
benign prostatic hypertrophy
BPM
blood perfusion monitor
BPS
biophysical profile score
fetal BPS
BPS spinal angiographic catheter
Bq
becquerel
BQCT
bone quantitative CT
Br-76 bromospiperone
Bracco
B. system

brace
Milwaukee b.
bracelet
^{89}Sr (strontium) b.
braces artifact
brachia (*pl. of* brachium)
brachial
b. arteriography
b. artery
b. artery approach
b. artery compression
b. artery cuff pressure
b. artery end-diastolic pressure
b. artery peak systolic pressure
b. artery pulse pressure
b. atrophy
b. bypass
b. fascia
b. lymph node
b. plexus
b. plexus birth injury
b. plexus compression
b. plexus infiltrate
b. plexus neuritis
b. vein
brachial-basilar insufficiency
brachialis
brachicephaly
brachii
biceps b.
triceps b.
brachiocephalic
b. arterial aneurysm
b. arteriography
b. artery
b. branch
b. ischemia
b. lymph node
b. trunk
b. trunk of aorta
b. vein
b. vessel
brachiocubital
brachioproctic eroticism
brachioradialis muscle
brachium, pl. **brachia**
b. of colliculus
b. conjunctivum
b. pontis
Bracht-Wachter lesion
brachycephalic head shape
brachycephaly
brachydactyly
Bell b.
Christian b.
Mohn-Wriedt b.
brachymelia
rhizomelic b.
brachymetatarsia
brachypellic pelvis
brachytherapy boost
bracing
fracture b.
Bradbury-Eggleston
B.-E. syndrome
B.-E. triad
bradycardia
fetal b.
bradyphemic
bradyphrenia
Braescia-Cimino
Bragard sign
Bragg
B. angle
B. curve
B. equation
B. ionization peak
B. law
B. peak photon-beam therapy
B. peak radiosurgery
B. spectrometer
Bragg-Gray cavity
braided diagnostic catheter
brain
b. abscess
b. activity
b. anatomy classification
b. aneurysm
b. aneurysm target sign
b. anoxia
architecture of b.
b. architecture
atrial diverticulum of b.
atrophic lesion of b.
b. atrophy
base of b.
boomerang configuration of b.
b. bridging vein
Broca motor speech area of b.
buckling cortical b.
b. calcification hemangioma
b. cancer
b. candle drippings
b. capillary angiography

NOTES

brain *(continued)*
b. cavernoma
b. concussion
b. contusion
b. cord sign
b. cyst
b. death
b. degeneration
b. disease
dura mater of b.
b. dysfunction
b. dysgerminoma
b. edema
edematous b.
b. electrical activity mapping
eloquent areas of b.
b. empyema
b. ependymoma
b. fissure
b. function
b. geography
b. hematoma
b. homeostasis
horseshoe configuration of b.
b. incidentaloma
b. infarct
inflammation of b.
insular region of b.
b. ischemia
b. laceration
b. lesion
b. lesion ring
b. lipoma
b. lymphoma
b. mantle
b. mass
b. mass in jugular foramen
meninges of b.
b. metastasis
b. paragonimiasis
b. parenchyma
b. perfusion
b. perfusion reserve
b. perfusion scintigraphy
b. perfusion SPECT
b. plasticity
puff-of-smoke b.
b. region vesicle
b. scan
b. scan imaging
silent area of b.
smooth b.
softening of b.
split b.
b. stenosis hemorrhage
b. substance
b. surface matching technique
b. swelling
b. tissue herniation
b. tuber
b. tuberculoma
b. tumor
b. tumor at cerebellopontine angle
b. tumor classification
unicameral b.
Virchow-Robin space of b.
b. water contents
water on the b.
wet b.
b. window

brain-core gradient

brainstem
b. compression
b. demyelination
b. disease
b. displacement
b. edema
b. encephalitis
b. ependymoma
b. glioma
b. hemorrhage
b. infarct
b. ischemia
ischemic b.
b. lesion
b. pyramidal tract
b. reticular formation
reticular formation of the b.
b. sign
tegmentum of b.

brain-to-background ratio

braking radiation

branch
acute marginal b.
anterior cutaneous b.
arterial b.
b. of artery
atrioventricular groove b.
bifid aortic b.
bifurcating b.
brachiocephalic b.
bronchial b.
b. bronchus
cardiac b.
caudal b.
circumflex b.
collateral b.
cortical b.
cutaneous lateral b.
diagonal b.
diagonal b. #1 (D1)
digital b.
distal b.
dorsal b.
feeding b.
first major diagonal b.

first septal perforator b.
geniculate b.
inferior cardiac b.
inferior wall b.
intrahepatic portal vein b.
large obtuse marginal b.
left bundle b.
marginal b.
midmarginal b.
motor b.
muscular b.
musculophrenic b.
nonlingular b.
obtuse marginal b. (OMB)
paired parietal b.
paired visceral b.
pancreatic duct b.
perforating b.
phalangeal b.
b. point
posterior descending b.
posterior intercostal b.
posterior ventricular b.
proper digital nerve b.
pruning of pancreatic duct b.
pudendal b.
b. pulmonary artery stenosis
ramus intermedius artery b.
ramus medialis artery b.
right bundle b.
second diagonal b.
segmental b.
septal perforating b.
side b.
sinoatrial b.
subcostal b.
superior phrenic b.
unpaired parietal b.
unpaired visceral b.
ventral b.
ventricular b.

branched
b. calculus
b. chain
b. decay

branches of vein

branchial
b. cartilage
b. cleft
b. cleft development
b. duct
b. efferent column
b. fistula
b. pouch
b. sinus

branching
anomalous b.
b. calcification
b. line
b. linear structure
mirror-image brachiocephalic b.
b. pattern
right aortic arch with mirror image b.
b. tubular structure

BRAS
Bard rotary atherectomy system

Brasdor method

Braun
B. canal
B. tumor

Braune muscle

Braunwald sign

bread-and-butter
b.-a.-b. heart
b.-a.-b. pericarditis
b.-a.-b. pericardium

bread-loaf technique

breakthrough
normal perfusion pressure b.
b. vasodilation
b. visualization

breast
b. abscess
accessory b.
adenoma of b.
b. adenosarcoma
b. adenosis
b. anatomy
b. angiosarcoma
b. artifact
atrophic b.
b. attenuation
b. augmentation
augmented b.
b. biopsy
b. bone
b. cancer
b. cancer risk factor
b. cancer screening
b. carcinoma
central solitary papilloma b.
b. coil
b. comedocarcinoma

NOTES

breast *(continued)*
compression of b.
b. core biopsy specimen
b. cyst
b. cyst aspiration
cystic disease of b.
b. degeneration
b. disease
b. edema
b. embryology
fascia of b.
b. fibroadenolipoma
b. fibroadenoma
fibroadenoma of b.
b. fibroadenomatosis
fibrocystic b.
b. fibrosis
b. hamartoma
b. hematoma
b. hyperplasia
B. Imaging Reporting and Data System (BIRADS)
b. irradiation
lactating b.
b. lesion
b. lipofibroadenoma
b. lipoma
lobule b.
b. localizer
b. lymph node
b. lymphoma
b. mammographic technique
b. metastasis
b. microcalcification
milky way b.
b. mucocele
nonlactating b.
papilloma b.
b. papilloma
b. parenchyma
b. phyllode tumor
b. pneumocystography
b. popcorn calcification
b. preservation
b. prosthesis rupture
b. pseudolymphoma
b. reconstruction
b. sarcoma
b. shadow
shoemaker's b.
b. skin thickening
b. sonography
tail of b.
b. thrombophlebitis
b. tissue
b. traction
b. trigger point
b. ultrasound
variocele tumor of b.

breastbone

breaststroker's knee

breath-hold
b.-h. cine-MR
b.-h., contrast-enhanced 3D MR angiography scan imaging
b.-h. contrast-enhanced three-dimensional MR angiography
b.-h. gradient-recalled echo (GRE) sequence
b.-h. T1-weighted MP-GRE MR imaging
b.-h. ungated imaging
b.-h. velocity-encoded cine MR imaging

breathing
b. artifact
b. feedback

breath pentane measurement

breech
b. presentation

bregma

bregmatic
b. bone
b. fontanelle

bregmatomastoid
b. suture

bremsstrahlung scan

Brenner tumor

Breschet
B. bone
B. canal
B. sinus

Brescia-Cimino
B.-C. fistula
B.-C. graft

Brett
B. sun
B. syndrome

Breuerton
B. view
B. x-ray view of hand

breve
vinculum b.

brevis
abductor pollicis b. (APB)
coxa b.
extensor carpi radialis b. (ECRB)
extensor digitorum b. (EDB)
extensor pollicis b. (EPB)
flexor digiti minimi b.
flexor digiti quinti b. (FDQB)
flexor digitorum b.
flexor hallucis b. (FHB)
flexor pollicis b.
palmaris b.

BRH
Bureau of Radiological Health
bridegroom's palsy
bridge
arteriolovenular b.
b. autograft
bony b.
b. circuit
interthalamic b.
intraductal b.
loop ostomy b.
mucosal b.
muscular b.
myocardial b.
nasal b.
osseous b.
osteophytic b.
portal-to-portal b.
skin b.
transphyseal bone b.
ventral b.
Wheatstone b.
bridged loop-gap resonator
bridging
b. callus
b. defect
b. necrosis
b. osteophyte
bright
b. contrast enhancement
b. echo
b. layer
b. pixel value
b. signal
bright-field imaging
brightly increased renal parenchymal echogenicity
brightness
b. area product (BAP)
b. gain
b. mode
b. modulation
brightness-time curve
bright-signal-intensity tumor
brim
pelvic b.
b. of the pelvis
quadrilateral b.
b. sign
brimstone liver
B ring of esophagus
Brinton disease
brisement therapy
brisk wall motion
Brissaud syndrome
Bristol-Myers system
British
B. engineering system (BES)
B. thermal unit (BTU)
brittle
b. bone
b. bone failure
broad
b. band of pleural fluid
b. base
b. fascia
b. ligament
b. ligament hernia
b. ligament pregnancy
b. maxillary ridge
b. thumb syndrome
broadband
b. noise detection error artifact
b. transducer
broad-based polyp
Broadbent
B. apoplexy
B. inverted sign
broadening
dipolar b.
quadripolar signal b.
spectral b.
Broca
B. area
band of B.
B. convolution
B. diagonal band
B. gyrus
B. index
B. motor speech area of brain
B. pudendal pouch
Brockenbrough-Braunwald sign
Brock meddle lobe syndrome
Broden
B. position
B. view
Broders tumor index classification
Brodie
B. bursa
B. disease
B. knee
B. ligament
B. metaphyseal abscess

NOTES

Brodmann
B. area
B. cytoarchitectonic field
broken bough pattern
bromide
ethidium b.
perfluorooctyl b. (PFOB)
potassium b.
silver b.
bromine-76 bromospirone
brominized oil
bromodeoxyuridine
b. imaging agent
b. labeling index
5-bromodeoxyuridine
-b. analysis
bromophenol
b. blue
b. blue imaging agent
bromospiperone
Br-76 b.
bromospirone
bromine-76 b.
b. imaging agent
bromsulphalein (BSP)
bronchi (*pl. of* bronchus)
bronchial
b. adenoma
b. angiography
b. annular cartilage
b. arteriography
b. artery
b. atresia
b. branch
b. bud
b. calculus
b. caliber
b. carcinoid tumor
b. carcinoma
b. cleft cyst
b. collateral circulation
b. cuff sign
b. dehiscence
b. diameter
b. dilatation
b. distortion
b. erosion
b. fracture
b. groove
b. inflammation
b. kinking
b. lumen
b. mucocele
b. mucosa
b. mucosal edema
b. obstruction
b. polyp
b. provocation imaging
b. provocation testing
b. reactivity
b. rupture
b. septum
b. sinus
b. smooth muscle spasm
b. spur
b. stenosis
b. stricture
b. tract
b. tree
b. tube
b. type B disease
b. vein
b. vessel
b. wall thickening
bronchiectasis
acquired b.
capillary b.
congenital b.
cylindrical b.
cystic b.
dry b.
follicular b.
fusiform b.
Polynesian b.
postinfectious b.
recurrent b.
reversible b.
saccular b.
b. traction
tuberculous b.
tubular b.
varicose b.
bronchiectasis-bronchomalacia syndrome
bronchiectasis-ethmoid sinusitis
bronchiectatic pattern
bronchiolar
b. adenocarcinoma
b. carcinoma
b. dilatation
b. disease
b. edema
b. emphysema
b. narrowing
b. obstruction
bronchiole
alveolar b.
conducting b.
irreversible narrowing of b.'s
lobular b.
membranous b.
respiratory b.
terminal b.
tree-in-bud b.
bronchiolitis
Aspergillus b.
constrictive b.

exudative b.
b. fibrosa obliterans
follicular b.
b. obliterans
b. obliterans with organizing pneumonia (BOOP)
obliterative b.
proliferative b.
respiratory b.
smoker's b.
vesicular b.

bronchiolus, pl. **bronchioli**

bronchitis
asthmatic b.
follicular b.

bronchoadenitis

bronchoalveolar
b. carcinoma
b. cell adenoma

bronchoarterial bundle

bronchobiliary fistula

bronchocavernous

bronchocavitary fistula

bronchocele

bronchocentric
b. abnormality
b. granulomatosis
b. inflammatory infiltrate

bronchoconstriction
exercise-induced b.
isocapnic hyperventilation-induced b.

bronchoconstrictor

bronchocutaneous fistula

bronchodilation, bronchodilatation

bronchodilator effect

bronchoesophageal fistula

bronchogenic
b. carcinoma
b. cyst

bronchogram
air b.
bilateral b.
Cope method b.
fiberoptic b.
fluid-filled b.
b. imaging
mucous b.
scattered air b.
Swiss cheese air b.
tantalum b.
unilateral b.

bronchography

broncholith

broncholithiasis

bronchomalacia

bronchomediastinal lymph trunk

bronchomotor effect

bronchoplasty
balloon b.

bronchoplegia

bronchopleural (BP)
b. fistula

bronchopleuropneumonia

bronchopneumonia
bibasilar b.
hemorrhagic b.
hypostatic b.
inhalation b.
subacute b.
tuberculous b.

bronchopneumonitis

bronchopulmonary (BP)
b. aspergillosis
b. atelectasis
b. dysplasia (BPD)
b. fistula
b. foregut
b. foregut malformation
b. lung segment anatomy
b. lymph node
b. neoplasm
b. segment
b. sequestration

bronchoradiography

bronchorrhea

bronchosinusitis

bronchospasm
paradoxical b.
uncontrolled b.

bronchospastic effect

bronchostaxis

bronchostenosis

bronchotracheal

bronchovascular
b. anatomy cross-section
b. bundle
b. markings
b. pattern

bronchovesicular markings

bronchus, pl. **bronchi**
anomalous b.
anterior basal b.
apical b.
apicoposterior b.

NOTES

bronchus *(continued)*
basal segmental b.
beaded b.
b. blockage
blocked b.
branch b.
cardiac segmental b.
contracted b.
depression of left mainstem b.
dilated b.
ectatic b.
edematous b.
epiarterial b.
extrapulmonary b.
fractured b.
granulomatous inflammation of b.
hyparterial b.
inferior lobe b.
inflamed b.
inflamed edematous b.
intermediate b.
b. intermedius
intrapulmonary b.
inverted-T appearance mainstem b.
lateral basal segmental b.
left main stem b.
left primary b.
lingular b.
lobar b.
mainstem b.
major b.
medial basal segmental b.
medium-sized b.
middle lobe b.
mucoid impaction of b.
nonlingular branches of upper lobe b.
normal-appearing b.
posterior basal segmental b.
primary left b.
primary right b.
principal b.
right lobe b.
right mainstem b.
right primary b.
secondary b.
secretion-filled b.
segmental b.
b. sign
b. stem
subapical b.
subsegmental b.
superior lobe b.
superior segmental b.
tracheal b.
bronchus-associated lymphoid tissue (BALT)
bronchus-pulmonary artery ratio
bronzed sclerosing encephalitis
bronze liver
Brooker
B. classification of heterotopic ossification
B. periarticular heterotopic ossification classification
Brooke tumor
Brostrom-Gordon arthrography
brow-down skull view
brown
b. atrophy
b. cell cyst
b. edema
b. induration of lung
b. tumor
Brown-Bovari machine
Brown-Dodge method for angiography
brownian water motion
Brown-Roberts-Wells
B.-R.-W. frame
B.-R.-W. technique
Brown-Séquard
B.-S. lesion
B.-S. syndrome
brow presentation
brow-up skull view
Bruce
B. and Muir tract
B. protocol
brucellar
b. myositis
b. osteomyelitis
b. synovitis
Bruck disease
Brücke muscle
Brudzinski sign
Bruel-Kjaer
B.-K. ultrasound
B.-K. ultrasound scanner
bruise
bone b.
Bruker
B. AMX 300 NMR spectrometer
B. console
B. CSI MR system
B. PC-10 relaxometer
B. scanner
B. TC-10 relaxometer
Brunner
B. gland
B. gland adenoma
B. gland hyperplasia
B. gland hypertrophy
Brunnstrom-Fugl-Meyer (BFM)
B.-F.-M. arm impairment assessment

brush
 b. border margin of bone
 Castaneda thrombolytic b.
 Cragg thrombolytic b.
Bryant sign
BSA
 body surface area
B-scan imaging
BSP
 bromsulphalein
BTU
 British thermal unit
bubble
 b. of the belly
 encapsulated gas b.
 free gas b.
 Garren-Edwards gastric b. (GEG bubble)
 gas b.
 gastric air b.
 GEG b.
  Garren-Edwards gastric bubble
 intragastric b.
 b. sign
 stomach b.
 b. ventriculogram
bubble-like appearance
bubbly
 b. bone lesion
 b. bulb
 b. lung
 b. lung syndrome
 b. opacity
bucca, pl. **buccae**
buccal
 b. cavity
 b. groove
 b. lymph node
 b. mucosa
 b. mucosal cancer
 b. shelf
 b. space
 b. space infection
 b. surface
buccinator
 b. crest
 b. lymph node
buccocervical ridge
buccogingival ridge
buccolingual plane
bucconeural duct
buccopharyngeal fascia
Buck
 B. extension
 B. fascia
bucket-handle
 b.-h. meniscus tear
 b.-h. pelvic fracture
buckle
 b. fracture
 wire-fixation b.
buckled
 b. innominate artery
 b. innominate artery syndrome
buckling
 b. cortical brain
 innominate artery b.
Bucky
 B. diaphragm
 B. digital x-ray device
 B. tomogram
 B. view
 B. view tray
bud
 accessory ureteral b.
 bronchial b.
 capillary b.
 dorsal pancreatic b.
 end b.
 limb b.
 ureteral b.
 vascular b.
 ventral pancreatic b.
Budd
 B. cirrhosis
 B. syndrome
Budd-Chiari syndrome
budding plate
Budge
 ciliospinal center of B.
budgerigar fancier's lung
Budin-Chandler anteversion determination
Budin joint
Budlinger-Ludlof-Laewen disease
Buerger thromboangiitis obliterans disease
buffalo hump
buffer
 b. amplifier
 Spli-Prest b.
Buford complex
Buhl desquamative pneumonia

NOTES

bulb
aortic b.
arterial b.
baroreceptor b.
baseline of b.
bubbly b.
carotid b.
dehiscent jugular b.
dental b.
duodenal b.
end b.
b. of heart
heart b.
high jugular b. (HJB)
inferior jugular vein b.
internal jugular b.
b. of occipital horn of lateral ventricle
olfactory b.
b. of penis
b. of posterior horn of lateral ventricle
sinovaginal b.
superior jugular vein b.
b. of vein
bulbar
b. abnormality
b. intracerebral hemorrhage
b. peptic ulcer
b. ridge
b. septum
b. tract
bulbocavernosus muscle
bulbocavernous gland
bulbosity
bulbospongiosus muscle of penis
bulbourethral
b. artery
b. gland
b. gland anatomy
b. gland lesion
bulbous
b. costochondral junction
b. enlargement
b. stump
b. urethra
bulge
anal b.
annular disk b.
bilateral anterior chest b.
disk b.
epiphrenic b.
inguinal b.
late systolic b.
palpable presystolic b.
parasternal b.
precordial b.
suprasternal b.
bulging
b. aneurysm
b. annulus
b. disk
b. dura
b. fontanelle
b. lung fissure
b. precordium
bulk
b. laxative
b. magnetization vector
mediastinal b.
muscle b.
b. susceptibility artifact
bulky tumor
bulla, pl. **bullae**
emphysematous b.
b. ethmoid
ethmoidal b.
b. formation
bullet
hollow-point b.
metallic track of b.
stabilizing b.
tri-point b.
bullet-shaped vertebra
bull-neck appearance
bullosa
concha b.
junctional epidermolysis b.
bullous
b. disorder
b. edema
b. edema of bladder wall
b. emphysema
b. emphysema of intestine
b. lung disease
bull's
b. eye appearance
b. eye deformity
b. eye image
b. eye imaging
b. eye polar map
b. eye sign
b. eye stomach lesion
b. eye technique
bump
hip b.
inion b.
runner's b.
splenic b.
bumper fracture
bunamiodyl
b. imaging agent
bunch
b. of flowers in kidney
b. of grapes appearance

bundle
aberrant b.
anterior atrial myocardial b.
artery-vein-nerve b.
atrioventricular b.
Bachmann b.
b. bone
bronchoarterial b.
bronchovascular b.
central bronchovascular b.
common b.
fascicular b.
fiberoptic b.
Flechsig b.
b. function
Gierke respiratory b.
Gowers b.
His b.
b. of His
intercostal neuromuscular b.
James b.
Keith sinoatrial b.
b. of Kent accessory bypass fiber
Kent-His b.
maculoneural b.
Mahaim b.
main b.
middle perforating collagen b.
neurovascular b.
Pick b.
pigmented villonodular b. (PVB)
Probst callosal b.
Schultze b.
sinoatrial b.
b. of Stanley Kent
Thorel b.
vascular b.
b. of Vicq d'Azyr
bundle-branch
b.-b. heart block
b.-b. reentry (BBR)
Bunge amputation
bunion formation
bunk-bed fracture
Bunsen-type valve
Burdach
column of B.
B. tract
burden
body b.
maximum permissible body b.
tumor b.
Bureau of Radiological Health (BRH)
Burger scalene triangle
Burgess below-knee amputation
Burke syndrome
Burke-type metaphyseal dysplasia
Burkhalter-Reyes method of phalangeal fracture
Burkitt-like lymphoma (BLL)
Burkitt lymphoma
burn boutonnière deformity
burned-out
b.-o. colon
b.-o. mucosa
b.-o. tabes
b.-o. tumor
b.-o. tumor of testis
Burnett
B. applicator
B. cylinder
B. mouth positioning device
burning
selective hole b.
Burns
B. ligament
B. space
burnuous
sign of the b.
bursa, pl. **bursae**
Achilles b.
adventitious b.
anserine b.
bicipitoradial b.
Brodie b.
calcaneal b.
deltoid b.
b. exostotica
b. of Fabricius
Fleischmann b.
flexor b.
gastrocnemius b.
gastrocnemius-semimembranosus b.
iliopsoas b.
infrapatellar b.
intermediate b.
intermetatarsophalangeal b.
intraligamentous b.
intratendinous b.
ischiogluteal b.
Luschka b.
Monro b.

NOTES

bursa *(continued)*
olecranon b.
omental b.
plantar b.
popliteus b.
prepatellar b.
radial b.
retrocalcaneal b.
semimembranosus b.
subacromial b.
subacromial-subdeltoid b.
subdeltoid b.
subscapular b.
suprapatellar b.
synovial b.
trochanteric b.
ulnar b.
bursal
b. calcification
b. flap
b. fluid
b. inflammation
b. osteochondromatosis
b. sac
bursitis
anserine b.
bicipital b.
calcaneal b.
calcific b.
chronic retrocalcaneal b.
cubital b.
iliopsoas b.
infracalcaneal b.
intermetatarsophalangeal b.
intertubercular b.
ischial b.
ischiogluteal b.
olecranon b.
patellar b.
pes anserinus b.
posterior calcaneal b.
prepatellar b.
pseudotrochanteric b.
radiohumeral b.
retrocalcaneal b.
septic b.
subacromial b.
subacromial-subdeltoid b.
subdeltoid b.
Tornwaldt b.
trochanteric b.
bursography
bursolith
burst
b. fracture
b. fracture of atlas
b. injury
respiratory b.
burst-forming unit
bursting dislocation
Burton sign
Burwell-Charnley
B.-C. classification of fracture reduction
B.-C. fracture reduction classification
Buschke-Löwenstein tumor
Buschke-Ollendorff syndrome
busulfan lung damage
butanol
^{11}C b.
butanol-extractable iodine (BEI)
Butcher staging classification
butterfly
b. breast shadow
b. coil
b. configuration
b. fracture
b. fracture fragment
b. glioblastoma
b. glioma
b. lymphoma
b. pattern
b. pattern of infiltrate
b. vertebra
buttock sign
button
aortic b.
Carrel b.
duodenal b.
full-thickness Carrel b.
Kistner tracheal b.
patellar b.
b. sequestrum eosinophilic granuloma
b. sequestrum skull
subdural b.
b. toe amputation
tracheal "B" b.
buttoned device
buttonhole
b. deformity
b. fracture
b. mitral stenosis
b. opening
radiopaque wire of counteroccluder b.
b. rupture
b. tear
buttressing
medial femoral b.
buttress plate
butyl iminodiacetic acid (BIDA)
BV2 needle
BVAD
biventricular assist device

BVR
basal vein of Rosenthal
BVS
biventricular support system
bypass (BP)
biliοenteric b.
biliointestinal b. (BIB)
biliopancreatic b. (BPB)
brachial b.
cardiopulmonary b.
b. circuit
b. graft
jejunoileal b. (JIB)
temporary aortic shunt b.
byproduct material
byssinosis
byte mode
Byzantine arch palate
B-zone small lymphocytic lymphoma

NOTES

C
carbon
coulomb
C angle
C to E amplitude of mitral valve
C sign
^{11}C
carbon-11
^{11}C acetate
^{11}C acetate imaging agent
^{11}C butanol
^{11}C butanol imaging agent
^{11}C carbon monoxide
^{11}C carbon monoxide imaging agent
^{11}C carfentanil
^{11}C carfentanil imaging agent
^{11}C deoxyglucose
^{11}C deoxyglucose imaging agent
^{11}C flumazenil
^{11}C flumazenil imaging agent
^{11}C imaging agent
^{11}C L-159
^{11}C L-884
^{11}C L-159 imaging agent
^{11}C L-884 imaging agent
^{11}C L-methylmethionine
^{11}C L-methylmethionine imaging agent
^{11}C lumazenil
^{11}C methionine
^{11}C methoxystaurosporine
^{11}C methoxystaurosporine imaging agent
^{11}C N-methylspiperone
^{11}C N-methylspiperone imaging agent
^{11}C N-methylspiroperidol
^{11}C N-methylspiroperidol imaging agent
^{11}C nomifensine
^{11}C nomifensine imaging agent
^{11}C palmitate
^{11}C palmitate imaging agent
^{11}C palmitic acid radioactive
^{11}C palmitic acid radioactive imaging agent
^{11}C raclopride
^{11}C raclopride imaging agent
^{11}C thymidine
^{11}C thymidine imaging agent
^{12}C
carbon-12
^{13}C
carbon-13
^{14}C
carbon-14
C1-C5 segments of internal carotid artery
C-60 teletherapy
^{45}Ca
calcium-45
^{45}Ca imaging agent
CA15-3 antigen radioimmunoassay imaging agent
CABBS
computer-assisted blood background subtraction
cable
FlexStrand c.
CABS
Cacchione syndrome
cachexia
cancer c.
lymphatic c.
CAD
computer-aided diagnostics
cadaveric renal transplant
cadmium (Cd)
c. iodide detector
Caffey
C. disease
C. hyperostosis
Caffey-Kempe syndrome
Caffey-Silverman disease
cage
bony thoracic c.
Faraday c.
osseocartilaginous thoracic c.
threaded fusion c. (TFC)
CAH
congenital adrenal hyperplasia
Cahoon method
caisson disease
cake
c. kidney
omental c.
calamus scriptorius
calcaneal
c. apophysitis
c. articular surface
c. avulsion fracture
c. bone
c. bursa
c. bursa inflammation
c. bursitis
c. displaced fracture
c. inclination angle
c. pitch
c. pitch angle

calcaneal *(continued)*
c. process
c. spur
c. stress fracture
c. tendon
c. tubercle
c. tuberosity
calcanei (*gen. and pl. of* calcaneus)
calcaneocavus
c. foot
pes c.
talipes calcaneus c.
talipes cavus c.
calcaneoclavicular ligament
calcaneocuboid
c. articulation
c. joint
c. ligament
calcaneofibular ligament
calcaneonavicular
c. coalition
c. ligament
calcaneoplantar angle
calcaneotibial
c. fusion
c. ligament
calcaneovalgocavus
calcaneovalgus
c. flatfoot
pes c.
calcaneovarus deformity
calcaneus, gen. and pl. **calcanei**
c. altus
c. deformity
pes c.
sulcus calcanei, sulcus of c.
talipes c.
tendo c.
thalamic fracture of c.
calcar
c. avis
c. femorale
c. pedis
pivot of c.
calcareous
c. degeneration
c. deposit
c. infiltrate
c. metastasis
calcarine
c. artery
c. cortex
c. fissure
c. sulcus
calciferous canal
calcific
c. arteriosclerosis
c. artery
c. bicuspid valvular stenosis
c. bursitis
c. cochleitis
c. density
c. matrix
c. round body
c. senile aortic valvular stenosis
c. spur
c. tendonitis
calcificans
liponecrosis macrocystica c.
liponecrosis microcystica c.
calcification
abdominal diffuse c.
abdominal vascular c.
abdominal wall c.
adrenal c.
alimentary tract c.
aneurysmal wall c.
annular c.
anterior spinal ligament c.
aortic arch c.
aortic valve c.
arachnoid granulation c.
arterial c.
arteriovascular c.
basal ganglia c.
c. of basal ganglion
basketlike c.
benign breast c.
bladder wall c.
branching c.
breast popcorn c.
bursal c.
cardiac c.
carotid artery c.
cartilage c.
casting breast c.
cerebral c.
chicken-wire c.
c. of choroid plexus
choroid plexus c.
coarse c.
conglomerate c.
coronary artery c.
costal cartilage c.
curvilinear c.
dentate nuclei c.
dermal breast c.
diffuse abdominal c.
disk c.
dural c.
dystrophic soft tissue c.
eggshell c.
eggshell breast c.
eggshell nodal c.
falx c.
female genital tract c.

fetal intraabdominal c.
fine c.
fingertip c.
flaky c.
flocculent focus of c.
focal alimentary tract c.
focus of c.
free body c.
genital tract c.
glial tumor c.
gyriform c.
habenular commissure c.
heart valve c.
hepatic c.
idiopathic pleural c.
inadequate calvarial c.
inadequate cranial c.
intervertebral cartilage c.
intervertebral disk c.
intraabdominal c.
intraabdominal fetal c.
intracardiac c.
intracranial physiologic c.
intraductal c.
intraocular c.
involutional breast c.
irregular c.
isolated clustered c.'s
kidney c.
laminated c.
layering c.
ligamentous c.
c. line
linear c.
liver c.
lobular breast c.
lung popcorn c.
lymph node eggshell c.
male genital tract c.
malignant breast c.
medial collateral ligament c.
medullary c.
mesenteric c.
metastatic soft tissue c.
mitral ring c.
mitral valve c.
Mönckeberg c., Moenckeberg c.
mottled c.
mulberry-type c.
multiple pulmonary c.'s
myocardial c.
c. of myocardium
needle-shaped breast c.
neoplastic c.
node c.
normal c.
oyster-pearl breast c.
pancreatic c.
paraarticular c.
paraspinal c.
parietal pericardial c.
pathologic intracranial c.
pearl-like breast c.
Pellegrini-Stieda c.
periarticular c.
pericardial c.
periductal c.
peritendinous c.
periventricular c.
phlebolith-like c.
pineal gland c.
plaquing c.
pleomorphic c.
pleural c.
popcorn c.
poppy seedlike c.
premature c.
psammomatous c.
punctate c.
railroad track heart c.
renal c.
retroperitoneal c.
rice-like muscle c.
ring-and-arc c.
rod-shaped c.
scrotal c.
sebaceous gland c.
secondary c.
sella turcica c.
semilunar c.
c. sign
skin c.
splenic c.
stippled c.
subannular c.
suprasellar mass c.
sutural c.
target c.
teacup breast c.
thrombus c.
thyroid adenoma c.
tramline cortical c.
tram-track cortical c.
tram-track ductus arteriosus c.

NOTES

calcification *(continued)*
tram-track gyral c.
tram-track renal cortical necrosis c.
tumoral c.
urinary bladder wall c.
valvular leaflet c.
vascular abdominal c.
venous c.
visceral pericardial c.
wall c.
calcified
c. annulus
c. aorta
c. aortic valve
c. astrocytoma
c. brain mass
c. cartilage
c. cyst
c. density structure
c. ductus arteriosus
c. fetus
c. fibroadenoma
c. fibroid
c. free fragment
c. granuloma
c. intracranial mass
c. kidney mass
c. lesion
c. lung nodule
c. medullary defect
c. metastasis
c. nodularity
c. pericardium
c. pineal body
c. pineal gland
c. plaque
c. renal mass
c. sclerosis
c. sequestra of low signal intensity
c. thrombus
c. wall of aneurysm
calciform lobe
calcifying
c. epithelioma of Malherbe
c. Malherbe epithelioma
c. metastasis
calcinosis
c. circumscripta
cutis c.
generalized c.
interstitial c.
tumoral c.
c. universalis
calcis
os c.
trigonum c.
Calcitite bone
calcium
c. bile soap
c. bilirubinate stone
c. crystal
c. debris
c. deposit
fenoprofen c.
c. hydroxyapatite
c. infiltrate
intracardiac c.
c. ipodate
c. layering
milk of c.
c. pyrophosphate deposition disease (CPPD)
c. pyrophosphate dihydrate deposition disease
sedimented c.
c. sign
c. tungstate
calcium-45 (^{45}Ca)
c. imaging agent
calcium-47 imaging agent
calcium/oxyanion-containing particle
calcospherite
calculated
c. clearance time
c. image
c. resistance
calculation
bayesian c.
body surface area c.
Cerenkov c.
contrast-to-noise c.
gap c.
Monte Carlo c.
multiplane dosage c.
radiation dosimetry c.
signal-to-noise c.
spectrophotometric c.
volume implant c.
calculi (*pl. of* calculus)
calculogram
calculography
calculous
c. cholecystitis
c. cirrhosis
calculus, pl. **calculi**
alvine c.
articular c.
biliary c.
branched c.
bronchial c.
cat's eye c.
decubitus c.
echogenic c.
encysted c.
fibrin c.

gallbladder c.
gastric hemic c.
hemic c.
hepatic c.
impacted c.
intestinal c.
intrahepatic biliary c.
joint c.
kidney c.
lacteal c.
lucent c.
lung c.
mammary c.
metabolic c.
mulberry c.
nephritic c.
nonopaque c.
obstructive c.
opaque c.
pancreatic c.
pocketed c.
primary vesical c.
prostatic c.
radiopaque vesical c.
renal c.
salivary c.
spermatic c.
staghorn c.
Steinstrasse c.
stomach c.
stonelike c.
ureteral c.
uric acid c.
urinary bladder c.
urinary tract c.

Caldani ligament

Caldwell
C. method
C. occipitofrontal view
C. position
C. projection
C. view

Caldwell-Moloy
C.-M. classification
C.-M. method

calf
c. band
c. vein thrombosis

CALGB
CALGB (Cancer and Leukemia Group B) trial

caliber
bronchial c.
internal c.
luminal c.
medium c.
modest c.
narrow c.
normal bladder c.
spinal cord c.
tracheal c.
vessel c.
c. of vessel
wide c.

calibrated leak

calibration
absolute-peak efficiency c.
E-dial c.
c. failure artifact
film density c.
c. method

calibrator
accuracy c.

caliceal
c. abnormality
c. blunting
c. clubbing
c. dilatation
c. diverticulum
c. nephrostolithotomy
c. system

calices (*pl. of* calix)

caliectasis
focal c.
localized c.

californium

californium-252 (**^{252}Cf**)

calix, calyx, pl. **calices**
cupping of the c.
funny-looking c.
major c.
minor c.
renal c.
spiderlike c.
c. tube

Callander amputation

callosal
c. area
c. dysgenesis
c. formation
c. gyrus
c. lesion
c. sulcus

NOTES

callosomarginal
c. artery
c. fissure
callosum
corpus c.
rostrum of corpus c.
splenium of corpus c.
callous
callus
bony c.
bridging c.
central c.
definitive c.
c. deposit
endosteal c.
ensheathing c.
external c.
exuberant c.
florid c.
c. formation
fracture c.
intermediate c.
permanent c.
provisional c.
tumoral c.
c. weld
Calot triangle
calvaneovalgus
pes c.
calvaria, pl. **calvariae**
calvarial bone
calve
septal cusp of c.
Calvé disease
Calvé-Legg-Perthes disease
Calvé-Perthes disease
Calve vertebra plane
calyx (*var. of* calix)
camelback sign
camera
ADAC gamma c.
Anger c.
Anger scintillation c.
APEX 409, 415 c.
Biad c.
CeraSPECT c.
CID c.
Cidtech c.
cine c.
Circon video c.
Digirad gamma c.
DSI c.
dual-head gamma c.
Elscint dual-detector cardiac c.
four-head c.
gamma c.
GE gamma c.
GE single-detector SPECT-capable c.
GE Starcam single-crystal tomographic scintillation c.
Haifa c.
Helix c.
integral uniformity scintillation c.
Isocon c.
Israel c.
Medx c.
multicrystal gamma c.
multiformat c.
Orthicon c.
Picker c.
pinhole c.
Pixsys FlashPoint c.
positron scintillation c.
radioisotope c.
R&F c.
rotating gamma c.
Scinticore multicrystal scintillation c.
scintillation c.
Siemens gamma c.
slip-ring c.
SP6 c.
Starcam c.
Technicare c.
Trionix c.
triple-head c.
Vertex c.
video display c.
Vision c.
cameral fistula
Cameron method
Campbell ligament
Camp-Coventry position
Camper
C. chiasma
C. fascia
C. ligament
C. line
Camp-Gianturco method
Camp grid cassette
camptocormia
camptodactyly
camptomelic dysplasia
Camurati-Engelmann disease
CAMV
congenital anomaly of mitral valve
canal
abdominal c.
accessory c.
acoustic c.
adductor c.
Alcock c.
alimentary c.
alveolar c.

alveolodental c.
ampulla of semicircular c.
anal c.
anterior condylar c.
anterior semicircular c.
antropyloric c.
arachnoid c.
Arantius c.
archenteric c.
Arnold c.
arterial c.
atrial c.
atrioventricular c.
auditory c.
basipharyngeal c.
Bernard c.
Bichat c.
biliary c.
birth c.
bony semicircular c.
Böttcher c., Boettcher c.
Braun c.
Breschet c.
calciferous c.
caroticotympanic c.
carotid c.
carpal c.
caudal c.
central spinal c.
cerebrospinal c.
cervical c.
cervicoaxillary c.
ciliary c.
Civinini c.
Cloquet c.
cochlear c.
common atrioventricular c.
complex atrioventricular c.
condylar c.
condyloid c.
connecting c.
Corti c.
Cotunnius c.
craniopharyngeal c.
crural c.
c. of Cuvier
Cuvier c.
c. decompression
deferent c.
diploic c.
Dorello c.
Dupuytren c.
endocervical c.
endometrial fluid in c.
ethmoid c.
eustachian c.
external auditory c.
facial nerve c.
fallopian c.
femoral medullary c.
Ferrein c.
flexor c.
Fontana c.
galactophorous c.
ganglionic c.
Gartner c.
gastric c.
genital c.
gray horns in spinal c.
greater palatine c.
gubernacular c.
Guyon c.
gynecophoric c.
Hannover c.
haversian c.
hemal c.
Henle c.
Hensen c.
Hering c.
hernial c.
Hirschfeld c.
His c.
Huguier c.
Hunter c.
Huschke c.
hyaloid c.
hydrops c.
hypoglossal c.
iliac c.
incisive c.
inferior dental c.
infraorbital c.
inguinal c.
interfacial c.
internal auditory c.
intersacral c.
intestinal c.
intramedullary c.
Jacobson c.
Kovalevsky c.
c. of Kovalevsky
lacrimal c.
lateral semicircular c.
Löwenberg c., Loewenberg canal

NOTES

canal *(continued)*
lumbar c.
lumbosacral c.
lymphatic c.
mandibular c.
marrow c.
mastoid c.
maxillary c.
medullary c.
mental c.
Müller c.
musculotubal c.
narrowing of spinal c.
nasal c.
nasolacrimal c.
nasopalatine c.
neural c.
neurenteric c.
notochordal c.
c. of Nuck
Nuck c.
olfactory c.
optic c.
orbital c.
palatine c.
palatomaxillary c.
palatovaginal c.
paraurethral c.
parturient c.
pelvic c.
pericardioperitoneal c.
perivascular c.
persistent common atrioventricular c.
persistent complete atrioventricular c. (PCAVC)
petrous carotid c.
pharyngeal c.
pleural c.
pleuropericardial c.
pleuroperitoneal c.
portal c.
posterior semicircular c.
principal artery of pterygoid c.
pterygoid c.
pterygopalatine c.
pudendal c.
pulmoaortic c.
pulp c.
pyloric c.
recurrent c.
Reichert c.
Richet tibioastragalocalcaneal c.
Rivinus c.
root c.
Rosenthal c.
sacculocochlear c.
sacculoutricular c.
sacral c.
Santorini c.
c. of Scarpa
Schlemm c.
c. of Schlemm
scleral c.
semicircular c.
c. septum
sheathing c.
small internal auditory c.
Sondermann c.
sphenopalatine c.
sphenopharyngeal c.
spinal cord c.
c. stenosis
Stensen c.
Stilling c.
c. of stomach
subsartorial c.
Sucquet-Hoyer c.
supraorbital c.
target c.
tarsal c.
temporal c.
Theile c.
tibial medullary c.
tight spinal c.
Tourtual c.
tubal c.
tubotympanic c.
umbilical c.
uniting c.
urogenital c.
uterine c.
uterocervical c.
uterovaginal c.
utriculosaccular c.
vaginal c.
Van Hoorne c.
ventricular c.
Verneuil c.
vertebral c.
vesicourethral c.
vestibular c.
vidian c.
Volkmann c.
vomerine c.
vomerorostral c.
vomerovaginal c.
vulvouterine c.
zygomaticofacial c.
zygomaticotemporal c.

Canale-Kelly
C.-K. classification of talar neck fracture
C.-K. talar neck fracture classification

canalicular
c. duct
c. sphincter
canaliculus, pl. **canaliculi**
apical c.
auricular c.
bone c.
cochlear c.
haversian c.
innominate c.
canalization
Canavan disease
Canavan-van Bogaert-Bertrand disease
cancellated bone
cancellation
fat-water signal c.
cancellization
cancellous
c. bone chip
c. hematopoietic marrow
c. osteoid osteoma
c. screw
c. tissue
cancer
adrenal gland c.
aerodigestive c.
androgen-independent prostate c.
aniline c.
appendiceal c.
asbestos-related lung c.
biliary tract c.
bladder c.
bone c.
Boorman classification of gastric c.
bowel c.
brain c.
breast c.
buccal mucosal c.
c. cachexia
cecal c.
clay pipe c.
colloid c.
colon c.
colorectal c.
conjugal c.
contact c.
cystic c.
dendritic c.
dye worker's latent c.
c. embolus
encephaloid c.
endobronchial c.
endometrial c.
epidermoid c.
epithelial ovarian c.
esophageal c.
extrapulmonary small cell c.
gastric c.
gastric remnant c.
gastrointestinal c.
genitourinary c.
gingival c.
glandular c.
hard palate c.
head and neck c.
hepatic flexure c.
hepatobiliary c.
hepatocellular c.
hereditary nonpolyposis colorectal c. (HNPCC)
hormone-receptor negative c.
hormone-resistant prostate c. (HRPC)
hypopharyngeal c.
inflammatory breast c. (IBC)
intracystic breast c.
intrahepatic biliary c.
invasive breast c.
locoregional breast c.
malignant breast c.
melanotic c.
metastatic urothelial c.
Muir-Torre of hereditary nonpolyposis colon c.
multifocal breast c.
nasopharyngeal c.
node-negative c.
node-positive breast c.
noncomedo breast c.
noninvasive breast c.
non-small-cell lung c. (NSCLC)
opposite breast c.
palpatory T-stage prostate c.
pancreatic c.
paranasal sinus c.
perforating colorectal c.
pharyngeal wall c.
pipe smoker's c.
piriform sinus c.
pitch worker's c.
platinum-resistant ovarian c.
postcricoid pharyngeal c.
primary c.
prostate c.

NOTES

cancer *(continued)*
radiation-induced c.
rectal c.
rectosigmoid c.
recurrent c.
renal c.
resectable colorectal c.
retromolar trigone c.
salivary gland c.
scar c.
skin c.
small bowel c.
small-cell cribriform c.
small intestine c.
soft palate c.
splenic flexure c.
stump c.
subareolar c.
suture line c.
telangiectatic c.
testicular c.
testis c.
thyroid c.
tongue c.
tonsil c.
transitional cell c.
transitional kidney cell c.
transitional urinary bladder cell c.
transition ureteral cell c.
tubular c.
c. of unknown primary (CUP)
unresectable colorectal c.
urothelial c.
varicoid esophageal c.
vocal cord c.
cancerization
field c.
candelabra
c. artery
sylvian c.
candela lithotripsy
candida esophagitis
candle-flame osteolysis
candle-wax appearance of bone
candle wax drippings
candy-cane appearance of GI tract
caniocervical junction
cannon
c. bone
C. point
C. ring
C. segmentation
Cannon-Boehm point
cannula, pl. **cannulas, cannulae**
metallic tip c.
ultrasonic lithotripter c.
cannulated
c. artery
c. central vein
percutaneously c.
cannulation
aortic c.
arterial c.
atrial c.
bicaval c.
direct caval c.
endoscopic retrograde pancreatic duct c.
left atrial c.
ostial c.
retrograde c.
selective c.
single-cannula atrial c.
subselective c.
two-stage venous c.
venoarterial c.
venous c.
venovenous c.
Canon scanner
Cantelli sign
canthus
outer c.
Cantrell
pentalogy of C.
cap
apical c.
azygos hematoma c.
cartilaginous c.
duodenal c.
fibrous c.
hilar c.
left pleural apical hematoma c.
phrygian c.
pleural apical hematoma c.
pyloric c.
thin fibrous c.
capacious vein
capacitance
electric energy c.
capacitator
MOS c.
capacitive interaction
capacity
bladder c.
closing c.
cranial c.
decreased vital c.
diffusing c.
functional bladder c.
functional residual c.
gastric c.
lung c.
residual volume/total lung c. (RV/TLC)

respiratory c.
secretory c.
small urinary bladder c.
total lung c.
vasodilatory c.
vital c. (VC)
cap-and-anchor plate
Capener
triangle of C.
capholunate arthritic collapse wrist
capillary, pl. **capillaries**
c. angioma
arterial c.
bile c.
c. blood flow
c. blood volume
c. bronchiectasis
c. bud
c. congestion
continuous c.
c. density
c. embolus
c. endothelium
c. filling
c. filling time
c. hemangioblastoma
c. hemangioma
c. hemorrhage
c. hydrostatic pressure
c. lake
c. leak
c. leak syndrome
c. loop
lymph c.
c. lymphangioma
c. lymphatic space invasion
c. malformation
Meigs c.
c. perfusion
c. permeability
c. permeability edema
c. pneumonia
c. pulsation
c. refill
c. resistance test
ruptured c.
sinusoidal c.
c. telangiectasia
telangiectasia brain c.
c. tube
c. valve
c. vein
venous c.
c. vessel
c. wall
c. wedge pressure
capillary-lymphatic malformation (CLM)
capital
c. epiphysis (CE)
c. epiphysis angle
c. epiphysis angle of Wiberg
c. extension
c. femoral epiphysis
c. flexor
c. fragment
capitate
c. bone
c. facet
c. fracture
c. hamate joint
c. soft spot
capitellar fracture
capitellum (*var. of* capitulum), pl. **capitula, capitella**
capitis
fovea c.
capitolunate
c. angle
c. joint
capitular epiphysis
capitulum, capitellum, pl. **capitula**
c. costae
c. fibulae
c. humeri
c. mandibulae
c. radiale humeri fracture
c. radii
c. ulnae
Caplan syndrome
capping
apical c.
capsular
c. attachment
c. contracture
c. imbrication
c. infarct
c. insertion
c. ligament
c. ligament rupture
c. plane
c. reefing
c. space
c. thickening
c. thrombosis

NOTES

capsule
adrenal c.
articular c.
auditory c.
Bowman c.
cartilage c.
cricoarytenoid articular c.
cricothyroid articular c.
dorsal c.
external c.
facet c.
fatty renal c.
fibrous renal c.
Gerota c.
glenoid labrum c.
Glisson c.
hepatic c.
Heyman-Simon c.
internal c.
joint c.
limb of anterior c.
c. of liver
liver c.
medial carpal c.
metatarsophalangeal c.
organ c.
otic c.
plantar c.
posterolateral c.
prostate c.
redundant c.
renal c.
rim of c.
splenic c.
suprasellar c.
talonavicular c.
thyroid c.
tissue c.
tumor c.
volar c.
wrist c.
capsulitis
adhesive c.
capsulocaudate infarct
capsulolabral complex
capsuloma
capsuloperiosteal envelope
capsuloputaminal infarct
capsuloputaminocaudate infarct
Captopril renal scan
Captopril-stimulated renal imaging
capture
boron neutron c.
cross-section c.
electron c.
gamma-ray c.
K c.
caput medusae
Carabello sign
carbogen
c. radiosensitizer
c. radiosensitizer imaging agent
carbon (C)
c. dioxide (CO_2)
c. dioxide laser
double-bonded c.
c. fiber-reinforced plastic
c. imaging agent
c. metabolism
carbon-11 (^{11}C)
carbon-12 (^{12}C)
carbon-13 (^{13}C)
c. spectroscopy
carbon-14 (^{14}C)
carbonated saline solution imaging agent
carbone dioxide generator
carbon-loaded thermoluminescent dosimeter
carbon-load thermoluminescent dosimetry
carbuncle
renal c.
Carcassonne ligament
carcinogenesis
radiation c.
carcinoid
atypical c.
colorectal c.
c. GI tract
c. rule of 1/3
c. syndrome
thymic c.
c. tumor
carcinoma, pl. **carcinomata, carcinomas**
acinar pancreatic cell c.
acinic cell c.
acinous cell c.
adenocystic c.
adenoid cystic lung c.
adenoid squamous cell c.
adnexal c.
adrenal c.
adrenocortical c.
aldosterone-producing c.
aldosterone-secreting c.
alveolar basal cell c.
alveolar mucosal c.
ameloblastic c.
ampullary c.
anaplastic thyroid c.
apocrine c.
apple-core c.
aryepiglottic fold c.
Bartholin gland c.
basal cell c.

bile duct c.
bilharzial c.
bladder c.
breast c.
bronchial c.
bronchiolar c.
bronchoalveolar c.
bronchogenic c.
cavitary squamous cell c.
cavitating c.
cecal c.
cerebriform c.
cholangiocellular c.
chorionic c.
choroid plexus c.
colloid c.
colonic c.
colorectal c.
comedo-basal cell c.
corpus c.
cortisol-producing c.
cribriform c.
cylindrical c.
cylindromatous c.
cystic basal cell c.
cystic renal cell c.
differentiated c. (DC)
distal bile duct c. (DBDC)
ductal papillary c.
ductal in situ breast c.
Edmondson grading system for hepatocellular c.
embryonal cell c.
embryonal testicular cell c.
c. en cuirasse
endobronchial c.
endometrial adenosquamous c.
endometrioid ovarian c.
epidermal c.
epidermoid bone c.
epidermoid lung c.
epiglottic c.
epithelial-myoepithelial c.
esophageal c.
ethmoid sinus c.
exophytic c.
c. ex pleomorphic adenoma
extensive intraductal c. (EIC)
extrahepatic bile duct c.
fallopian tube c.
false cord c.
fibrolamellar hepatocellular c.
FIGO stage c.
International Federation of Gynecology and Obstetrics stage carcinoma
flat colorectal c.
focal lobular c.
follicular thyroid c.
gallbladder c.
gastric c.
gastric stump c.
gastroesophageal junction c.
gelatinous c.
genital c.
giant cell lung c.
glandular c.
glans c.
glottic c.
granulosa cell c.
hepatic c.
hepatocellular c. (HCC)
hyopharyngeal c.
hypernephroid c.
infantile embryonal c.
infiltrating ductal c.
intraductal c.
jugular node metastatic c.
juvenile embryonal c.
Kulchitsky cell c. (KCC)
large-cell undifferentiated c.
laryngeal c.
lenticular c.
leptomeningeal c.
linitis plastica c.
lobular c.
lung c.
maxillary sinus c.
medullary breast c.
medullary thyroid c.
meibomian gland c.
Merkel cell c.
mesometanephric c.
metachronous transitional cell c.
metaplastic c.
metastatic c.
micropapillary c.
Ming classification of gastric c.
moderately well-differentiated c.
mucin-hypersecreting c.
mucinous breast c.
mucin-producing c.
mucoepidermoid c.
mucoepidermoid lung c.

NOTES

carcinoma *(continued)*
mucous c.
multicentric basal cell c.
napkin-ring c.
nasopharyngeal c. (NPC)
nasopharyngeal squamous cell c.
necrotic renal cell c.
neuroendocrine small-cell c.
nevoid basal-cell c.
nodulo-ulcerative basal-cell c.
nonislet cell c.
non-small-cell c.
oat-cell c.
occult papillary c.
osteoid c.
ovarian c.
Paget c.
pancreatic c.
papillary breast c.
papillary renal cell c.
papillary serous c.
papillary thyroid c.
paranasal sinus c.
parathyroid c.
perforated c.
periampullary c.
peripheral c.
pharyngeal wall c.
pigmented basal cell c.
piriform sinus c.
polypoid c.
postcricoid c.
posterior pharyngeal wall c.
preinvasive c.
prickle cell c.
primary hepatocellular c.
primary intraosseous c.
primary neuroendocrine small cell c.
c. of prostate
prostatic c.
pulmonary c.
rectal c.
rectosigmoid c.
recurrent c.
renal cortical c.
renal pelvic urothelial c.
residual c.
retinoblastoma hereditary human c.
salivary gland c.
scar c.
schistosomal bladder c.
schneiderian c.
scirrhous breast c.
sclerosing basal cell c.
sclerosing hepatic c. (SHC)
sebaceous c.
secretory c.
serous c.
sessile nodular c.
sigmoid c.
signet ring cell c.
sinonasal c.
c. in situ
small-cell lung c. (SCLC)
small-cell undifferentiated c.
small round cell c.
solid circumscribed breast c.
solid and papillary pancreatic c.
spiculated c.
sporadic colorectal c.
squamous cell c.
string cell c.
subglottic c.
superficial basal cell c.
superficial depressed c.
superficial spreading esophageal c.
superficial spreading stomach c.
supraglottic c.
sweat gland c.
synchronous transitional cell c.
terminal c.
thymic c.
thyroid c.
tonsillar c.
trabecular c.
transitional cell c. (TCC)
transverse colon c.
tripartite duodenal c.
tubular breast c.
undifferentiated c. (UC)
undifferentiated nasopharyngeal c.
urachal c.
ureteral c.
uterine cervix c.
uterine corpus c.
uterine papillary serous c. (UPSC)
vaginal c.
varicoid c.
verrucous c.
villous c.
vulvar c.
vulvovaginal c.
Walker c.
well-circumscribed c.
well-differentiated c.
wolffian duct c.

carcinomatosa

carcinomatosis
lymphangitic c.
lymphatic c.
peritoneal c.
c. peritonei

carcinomatosum

carcinomatous
c. implant

c. myelopathy
c. myopathy
c. neuromyopathy
c. subacute cerebellar degeneration

carcinosarcoma
embryonal c.
esophageal c.
renal c.
Walker c.

carcinosis
abdominal c.

carcinostatic

Card
Novus Medical Image C.

Cardarelli sign

Carden amputation

cardia
crescent of c.
gastric c.
patulous c.

cardiac
c. anomaly
c. antrum
c. apex
c. atrial shunt
c. blood pool imaging
c. border
c. branch
c. calcification
c. catheterization
c. catheterization imaging
c. chamber
c. cirrhosis
c. compression
c. congestion
c. contractility
c. creep
c. decompensation
c. decompression
c. decortication
c. denervation
c. diameter
c. dilatation
c. edema
c. effusion
c. ejection fraction
c. failure
c. fibroma
c. fibrosarcoma
c. filling pressure
c. fossa
c. frontal area
c. ganglion
c. gated MR angiography
c. gated PGSE (pulsed-gradient spin-echo) sequence
c. gated respiration
c. gated study
c. gating
c. gating compensation
c. hamartoma
c. hemangioma
c. hypertrophy
c. hypokinesis
c. impression
c. impression on liver
c. index (CI)
c. infarct
c. insufficiency
c. inversion
c. irradiation
c. irritability
c. ischemia
c. laminography
c. lipoma
c. long axis view
c. lung
c. lymphangioma
c. mapping
c. margin
c. monitor
c. MRI
c. muscle
c. muscle fiber
c. muscle inflammation
c. myxoma
c. node
c. notch
c. obstruction
c. orifice
c. osteosarcoma
c. output (CO, Q)
c. output echocardiography
c. output measurement
c. overload
c. perforation
c. PET
c. plexus
c. polyp
c. position
c. positron emission tomography imaging
c. pumping ability
c. radiation syndrome

C

NOTES

cardiac *(continued)*
c. radiography
c. radiography imaging
c. recovery
c. reserve
c. rhabdomyoma
c. rhabdomyosarcoma
c. rupture
c. sarcoma
c. scan
c. scintigraphy
c. scintigraphy ejection fraction
c. segment
c. segmental bronchus
c. series
c. shadow
c. shape
c. shock
c. short axis view
c. silhouette
c. silhouette enlargement
c. silhouette snowman configuration
c. situs invertus
c. situs solitus
c. skeleton
c. sling
c. standstill
c. steady state
c. stomach
c. stress test
c. tamponade
c. teratoma
c. thrombosis
c. tumor
c. valve
c. valve mucoid degeneration
c. valvular lesion
c. vasculature
c. vein
c. ventricle aneurysm
c. waist
c. wall motion
c. wall motion imaging
cardinal
c. event
c. finding
c. ligament
c. point
c. sign
c. vein
Cardio3DScope imaging system
cardioangiography
blood pool radionuclide c.
CardioCamera imaging system
cardiochalasia
Cardio-Conray
cardiocutaneous syndrome
Cardio Data MK3 Holter scanner
cardiodiaphragmatic angle
cardiodilator
cardiodynia
cardioesophageal (CE)
c. junction
cardiofacial
c. defect
c. syndrome
cardiogenesis
cardiogenic
c. embolic stroke
c. embolus
c. plate
c. pulmonary edema
c. shock heart
Cardiografin
C. sodium imaging agent
cardiogram
derived value on apex c. (dD/dt)
ultrasonic c. (UCG)
Cardio-Green
C.-G. imaging agent
cardiohepatic
c. angle
c. triangle
cardiohepatomegaly
cardioinhibitory response
cardiointegram (CIG)
cardiokymography (CKG)
Cardiolite
C. heart imaging scan
C. imaging agent
C. scan imaging
technetium-tagged C.
C. Tl-201
cardiomegaly
alcoholic c.
borderline c.
boxlike c.
familial c.
funnel-like c.
globular c.
hypertensive c.
iatrogenic c.
idiopathic c.
cardiomotility
cardiomyopathic degeneration
cardiomyopathy
alcoholic dilated c.
amyloidotic c.
arrhythmogenic right ventricular c.
beer drinker's beriberi c.
concentric hypertrophic c.
congenital dilated c.
congestive c.
constrictive c.
degenerative c.
diabetic c.

diffuse symmetric hypertrophied c.
dilated c. (DCM)
end-stage c.
familial hypertrophic c. (FHC)
Friedreich ataxic c.
hypertrophic c. (HCM)
hypertrophic obstructive c. (HOC, HOCM)
idiopathic dilated c. (IDC)
idiopathic restrictive c.
infantile c.
infarctoid c.
infectious c.
infiltrative c.
ischemic congestive c.
left ventricular c.
metabolic c.
mucopolysaccharidosis c.
myotonia atrophica c.
noncoronary c.
nonischemic congestive c.
nonobstructive c.
obliterative c.
obscure c.
obstructive hypertrophic c.
peripartum dilated c.
postmyocarditis dilated c.
postpartum c.
primary c.
restrictive c.
right-sided c.
right ventricular c.
secondary c.
tachycardia-induced c.
thyrotoxicotic c.
toxic c.

cardionecrosis
cardionephric
cardioneural
cardiophrenic
c. angle
c. junction
c. right-angle mass

cardiopneumatic
cardioptosis
Wenckebach c.

cardiopulmonary
c. abnormality
c. bilharziasis
c. bypass
c. disease
c. edema
c. insufficiency
c. obesity
c. support system

cardiopyloric
cardiorenal disease
cardiorespiratory sign
cardiorrhexis
Cardioscint
cardiosclerosis
cardioselective agent
cardiospasm
cardiosplenic syndrome
Cardiotec imaging agent
CardioTek imaging
cardiothoracic
c. index
c. ratio (CT, CTR)
c. trauma

cardiothymic shadow
cardiothyrotoxicosis
cardiotocogram
cardiotocography imaging
cardiovalvular
cardiovascular
c. accident (CVA)
c. adverse effect
c. anomaly
c. computed tomographic scanner (CVCT)
c. disease (CD, CVD)
c. imaging technique
c. malformation
c. radioisotope scan and function imaging
c. radiology
c. renal disease
c. shadow
c. shunt
c. silhouette
c. system

cardioverter-defibrillator
automatic implantable c.-d. (AICD)

carditis
acute lethal c.
Lyme c.

carfentanil
^{11}C c.

caries
dental c.
radiation c.

carina, pl. **carinae**
mainstem c.

NOTES

carina *(continued)*
sharp c.
c. of trachea
carinal angle
cariniform cartilage
carious teeth
Carleton spot
C-arm
C.-a. fluoroscopy
MINI 6000 C.-a.
C.-a. portable x-ray unit
Carman
C. meniscal sign
C. sign
Carman-Kirklin meniscus sign
Carnesale-Stewart-Barnes hip dislocation classification
Carnett sign
Carnoy solution
Caroli disease
caroticocavernous fistula
caroticoclinoid ligament
caroticojugular spine
caroticotympanic
c. artery
c. canal
carotid
c. angiography
c. artery
c. artery aneurysm
c. artery arteritis
c. artery bifurcation
c. artery calcification
c. artery-cavernous sinus fistula
c. artery disease
c. artery dissection trauma
c. artery ischemia
c. artery kinking
c. artery occlusion
c. artery plaque
c. artery stenosis
c. atherosclerosis
c. atherosclerotic disease
c. bifurcation atheroma
c. blowout syndrome
c. body
c. body tumor
c. bulb
c. bulb baroreceptor
c. canal
c. cavernous fistula (CCF)
c. cavernous syndrome
c. cerebral arteriography
c. circulation
c. cistern
c. disobliteration
c. dissection string sign
c. distribution TIA
c. duct
c. duplex imaging
c. duplex study
c. duplex ultrasonography
c. duplex ultrasound
c. ejection time
c. endarterectomy
external c.
c. foramen
c. ganglion
c. gland
c. groove
internal c.
c. occlusive disease
c. phonoangiography
c. plaque hematoma
c. plexus
c. pulse peak
c. pulse tracing
c. pulse upstroke
c. sheath
c. sheath adenoma
c. shudder
c. sinus
c. sinus hypersensitivity
c. sinus imaging
c. sinus syncope
c. sinus syndrome (CSS)
c. siphon
c. sonography
c. space
c. space mass
c. triangle
c. tubercle
c. vein
c. velocity
c. wall
carotid-carotid venous bypass graft
carotid-cavernous
c.-c. fistula occlusion
c.-c. sinus fistula
carotid-dural fistula
carotid-ophthalmic aneurysm
carotid-subclavian transposition
carpal
c. arch
c. articular surface
c. bone anatomy
c. bone stress fracture
c. boss
c. box
c. canal
c. coalition
c. deviation
c. groove
c. navicular
c. navicular bone
c. navicular fracture

c. row
c. scaphoid bone fracture
c. sign
c. tunnel
c. tunnel projection
c. tunnel syndrome
c. tunnel view
c. wrist angle

Carpentier ring

carpet
c. lesion
c. lesion of colon
c. polyp

carpi (*pl. of* carpus)

carpometacarpal
c. articulation
c. fusion
c. joint (CMC)
c. joint fracture
c. ligament

carpophalangeal joint

carporadial articulation

carpus, pl. **carpi**
cuneiform bone of c.
ulnar translocation of the c.

Carrel
C. button
triangulation of C.

carrier
^{67}Ga GABA uptake c.
radionuclide c.

carrier-free
c.-f. radioisotope
c.-f. separation
c.-f. separation process

carrier-mediated transport system

Carrington
C. disease

carrot-shaped trachea

Carr-Purcell (CP)
C.-P. sequence

Carr-Purcell-Meiboom-Gill (CPMG)
C.-P.-M.-G. echo train
C.-P.-M.-G. sequence

carrying angle

Carswell grape

Carter equation

Carter-Rowe view

cartesian
c. reference coordinate system
c. reference coordinate voxel array

cartilage
absent bronchial c.
accessory nasal c.
alar c.
annular c.
aortic c.
arthrodial c.
articular c.
c. articulation
arytenoid c.
attenuated intercarpal articular c.
auditory c.
auricular c.
basilar c.
c. bone
branchial c.
bronchial annular c.
c. calcification
calcified c.
c. capsule
cariniform c.
ciliary c.
circumferential c.
conchal c.
connecting c.
corniculate c.
costal c.
costal intraarticular c.
cricoid c.
cricothyroid c.
cuneiform c.
elastic c.
ensiform c.
epiglottic c.
epiphyseal c.
facet c.
falciform c.
fibroelastic c.
fibrous c.
flaking of c.
floating c.
free flap of c.
hyaline articular c.
interarticular c.
c. joint space
c. lacuna
laryngeal c.
liplike projections of c.
loss of elasticity of c.
c. matrix
osteoarthritic c.
patellofemoral articular c.

NOTES

cartilage *(continued)*
physeal c.
pitted c.
pulmonary c.
quadrangle c.
roughened c.
scored c.
semilunar c.
shelling off of c.
softening of c.
sternal c.
c. stroma
swelling of c.
tag of c.
thinned c.
thyroid c.
tracheal c.
triradial c.
triradiate c.
unossified c.
xiphoid c.
Y c.
yellow c.
cartilage-containing giant cell tumor
cartilage-forming bone tumor
cartilaginous
c. acetabulum
c. anlage
c. bar
c. cap
c. cap of phalangeal head
c. degeneration
c. disk
c. endplate
c. epiphysis
c. growth plate
c. growth plate disorder
c. hamartoma
c. joint surface
c. lesion
c. metaplasia
c. node
c. nodule
c. ring
c. septum
c. soft-tissue tumor
c. synchondrosis
c. tissue
cartographic projection
cartwheel fracture
Carvallo sign
CAS
coronary artery scan
coronary artery spasm
CAS imaging
cascade
abdominal c.
diagnostic c.
gamma c.
c. stomach
caseous
c. necrosis
c. pneumonia
Casper plate
Casser
C. ligament
C. muscle
casserian
c. ligament
c. muscle
cassette
Adrian-Crooks type c.
book c.
Camp grid c.
cast
egg c.'s
halo c.
plaster c.
Castaneda thrombolytic brush
Castellani disease
Castellino sign
casting breast calcification
Castleman disease
CAT
chloramphenicol acetyl transferase
computerized axial tomography
catamenial pneumothorax
cataract
radiation c.
catarrhal pneumonia
catastrophe
vascular c.
CAT-CAM
contoured adduction trochanteric-controlled alignment method
CAT-CAM conversion
catechol-O-methyltransferase
cathartic colon
catheter
Achiever balloon dilatation c.
Ackrad balloon-bearing c.
ACS balloon c.
angulated c.
balloon-tipped angiographic c.
Berman angiographic c.
BPS spinal angiographic c.
braided diagnostic c.
central venous c. (CVC)
Chemo-Port c.
c. cholangiogram
cholangiographic c.
c. coiling sign
coil-tipped c.
conductance c.
Derek Harwood-Nash series of c. (DHN1, 2, 3)

eight-lumen esophageal
  manometry c.
ERCP c.
exit site of c.
expandable access c.
FAST balloon c.
c. fixation
fluid-filled c.
helium-filled balloon c.
Hickman indwelling c.
Hickman tunneled c.
HSG c.
hysterosalpingography c.
c. impact artifact
indwelling Foley c.
Infuse-a-Port c.
c. insertion
intraarterial chemotherapy c.
intraluminal ultrasound c.
intravascular ultrasound c.
ITC radiopaque balloon c.
jugular c.
c. kinking
c. mapping
micromanometer-tip c.
c. migration
multiaccess c. (MAC)
multielectrode impedance c.
c. obstruction
peripherally inserted central c.
  (PICC)
peritoneal dialysis c.
c. placement
c. position
Raaf Cath vascular c.
radiofrequency-generated thermal
  balloon c.
c. sheath
solid-state manometry c.
temporary pacing c.
c. tip
c. tip hockey-stick appearance
c. tip motion
c. tip motion artifact
c. tip position
c. tip position artifact
ventriculography c.
water-infusion esophageal
  manometry c.
c. whip artifact
c. with preformed curves
Z-Med balloon c.
Zucker c.

catheter-associated bacteremia
catheter-borne sector transducer
catheter-directed
c.-d. fenestration
c.-d. interventional procedure
catheter-induced
c.-i. coronary artery spasm
c.-i. embolus
c.-i. pulmonary artery hemorrhage
c.-i. subclavian vein thrombosis
c.-i. thromboembolization
catheterization
antegrade c.
cardiac c.
catheter-securing technique
catheter-skin interface
catheter-tipped manometer
catheter-tissue contact
cathode ray
cathode-ray tube (CRT)
CathTrack catheter locator system
cation
paramagnetic c.
cat phantom
cat's
c. eye calculus
c. tail configuration
cauda, pl. **caudae**
c. equina
c. equina compression
c. equina syndrome (CES)
caudad
c. projection
caudal
c. branch
c. canal
c. direction
c. flexure
c. ligament
c. pharyngeal complex
c. pons
c. projection
c. regression
c. sheath
c. tilt
c. vertebra
c. view
caudal-cranial angulation
caudate
c. body

NOTES

C

caudate *(continued)*
c. lobe
c. lobe of liver
c. nucleus
c. process
c. vein
c. volume
caudocranial
c. projection
c. view
caudothalamic groove
cauliflower appearance
cauliflower-shaped filling defect
cause-specific survival (CSS)
caustic esophagitis
Causton method
cava (*pl. of* cavum)
azygos continuation of inferior vena c.
bilateral superior vena c.
collapsed inferior vena c.
duplicated inferior vena c.
inferior vena c. (IVC)
infrahepatic vena c.
juxtarenal c.
membranous obstruction of inferior vena c.
paired inferior vena c.
persistent left inferior vena c.
persistent left superior vena c.
redirection of inferior vena c.
retrohepatic vena c.
sinus of vena c.
superior bilateral vena c.
superior vena c. (SVC)
suprahepatic vena c.
transposition of inferior vena c.
vena c.
cavagram
caval
c. filter
c. fold
c. lymph node
c. opening
c. tourniquet
c. valve
cavalry bone
CAVB
complete atrioventricular block
cavernoma
brain c.
portal vein c.
cavernosa
cavernosography
corpora c.
cavernosometry
cavernous
c. angioma
c. angiosarcoma
c. brain angiography
c. brain hemangioma
c. groove
c. internal carotid artery
c. lymphangioma
c. malformation
c. plexus
c. portal vein transformation
c. sinus
c. sinus aneurysm
c. sinus fistula
c. sinus lesion
c. sinus meningioma
c. sinus syndrome
c. tissue
c. transfer of portal vein
c. transformation of portal vein
c. tumor
c. urethra
caviar lesion
cavitary
c. dilatation
c. fluid
c. infiltrate
c. lung lesion
c. mass
c. mesenteric lymph node syndrome
c. prostatitis
c. small bowel lesion
c. squamous cell carcinoma
c. tuberculosis
cavitate
cavitating
c. carcinoma
c. lung metastasis
c. lung nodule
c. neoplasm
c. pattern
c. pneumonia
cavitation
collapse c.
lobar c.
pulmonary c.
stable c.
transient c.
cavity
abdominal c.
abdominopelvic c.
absorption c.
acetabular c.
air c.
amnionic c.
ancyroid c.
c. of aneurysm

axillary c.
banana-shaped uterine c.
body c.
Bragg-Gray c.
buccal c.
chest c.
cleavage c.
coexistent c.
cotyloid c.
cranial c.
crown c.
dome-shaped roof of pleural c.
endometrial c.
epamniotic c.
epidural c.
funnel-shaped c.
glenoid c.
grape-skin lung c.
greater sac of peritoneal c.
intraperitoneal c.
joint c.
lesser sac of peritoneal c.
lung c.
marrow c.
Meckel c.
medullary c.
midcarpal joint c.
miniature uterine c.
multiple thin-walled lung c.'s
nasal c.
orbital c.
pericardial c.
peritoneal c.
pleural c.
popliteal c.
pulmonary c.
resection c.
retroperitoneal c.
saclike c.
septum pellucidum c.
sigmoid c.
sinonasal c.
sinus c.
subarachnoid c.
subchondral cystic c.
subdural c.
surgically created resection c.
synovial c.
syringohydromyelic c.
syrinx c.
thin-walled lung c.
thoracic c.
trigeminal c.
tubular c.
tympanic c.
uterine c.
ventricular c.
c. volume
c. wall

cavoatrial junction

cavogram

cavography

cavovalgus
pes c.
talipes c.

cavovarus
c. deformity
pes c.

cavum, pl. **cava**
c. vergae

cavus
c. deformity
global c.
local c.
pes c.
posttraumatic c.
talipes c.

Cayler syndrome

CBCL
cutaneous B cell lymphoma

CBD
common bile duct

CBDE
common bile duct exploration

CBF
cerebral blood flow

CBFV
coronary blood flow velocity

CBI
convergent beam irradiation
CBI stereotactic ring

CBT
corticobulbar tract

CBV
cerebral blood volume

CBV/CBF
cerebral blood volume/cerebral blood flow
CBV/CBF ratio

C-C
convexoconcave
C-C heart valve

cc
cubic centimeter

NOTES

CCA
common carotid artery
CCAM
congenital cystic adenomatoid malformation
CCD
central collodiaphyseal
CCD angle
CCD photodetector
CCF
carotid cavernous fistula
CCI
Cronqvist cranial index
CCRT
computer-controlled conformal radiation therapy
CCT
cranial computed tomography
CCTA
coronal computed tomographic arthrography
CD
cardiovascular disease
cluster of differentiation
Crohn disease
Cd
cadmium
CDAI
Crohn disease activity index
CDC
Crohn disease of colon
CDCA
chenodeoxycholic acid
CDH
congenital dislocation of hip
congenital dysplasia of hip
CDI
color Doppler imaging
CDRPan digital x-ray system
CE
capital epiphysis
cardioesophageal
CE angle of Wiberg
CE junction
CEAker imaging agent
cebocephaly
ceca (*pl. of* cecum)
cecal
c. appendage
c. appendix
c. bar
c. bar sign
c. bascule
c. cancer
c. carcinoma
c. deformity
c. filling defect
c. fold
c. foramen
c. hernia
c. ileus
c. recess
c. serosa
c. sphincter
c. volvulus
cecocutaneous fistula
cecostomy
percutaneous c.
CECT
contrast-enhanced computed tomography
cecum, pl. **ceca**
antimesocolic side of c.
coned c.
kidney-shaped distended c.
c. mobile
subhepatic c.
Cedell
C. fracture
C. fracture of talus
Cedell-Magnusson
C.-M. arthritis classification
C.-M. classification of arthritis
Ceelen-Gellerstedt syndrome
CE-FAST
contrast-enhanced fast-acquisition in a steady state
CE-FAST scan
Cegka sign
celery stalk sign
celiac
c. angiography
c. arteriography
c. artery
c. artery aneurysm
c. artery compression syndrome
c. axis
c. axis syndrome
c. block
c. disease
c. ganglion
c. ganglion block
c. lymph node
c. lymph node metastasis
c. and mesenteric arteriography imaging
c. plexus
c. sprue
c. trunk
celiectasia
celioma
celioscopy
celiotomy
cell
epithelial c.
ethmoid air c.
^{111}In-labeled white blood c.

c. preparation bone marrow uptake
red blood c. (RBC)
technetium-tagged red blood c.
c. tumor
white blood c. (WBC)

cell-dose threshold
CellSeek technology
cellular
c. binding site
c. embolus
c. fibroadenoma
c. tumor

cellule formation
cellulitis
orbital c.

celomic
c. metaphysis
c. pouch

CEM
central extensor mechanism

Cemax/Icon scanner
Cemax PACS platform
cement
bone c.
c. line
c. mantle
orthopedic c.
radiopaque bone c.
residual c.

cemental fracture
cementation
cementifying fibroma
cementinoma
cementoblastoma
cementoma
gigantiform c.

cementoossifying fibroma
cementosis
cementum
Cencit surface scanner
center
accessory ossification c.
anechoic c.
bone c.
cortical c.
diaphyseal c.
elbow bone c.
emetic c.
enlargement with low-density lymph node c.
epiphyseal fetal bone c.
epiphyseal ossification c.
femoral ossification c.
fetal epiphyseal bone c.
c. line artifact
lucent c.
ossification c.
swallowing c.
tibial tubercle ossification c.
window c.

center-edge angle of Wiberg
centering ring
Center of Metabolic and Experimental Imaging
centigray (cGy)
centimeter (cm)
cubic c. (cc)

CentoRx imaging agent
central
c. amaurosis
c. aorta
c. aortic pressure
c. artery
c. axis depth dose
c. blood volume
c. bone
c. bronchovascular bundle
c. callus
c. canal stenosis
c. cavity of cerebrum
c. cementifying fibroma
c. cerebellar fissure
c. channel
c. chondrosarcoma
c. collodiaphyseal (CCD)
c. collodiaphyseal angle
c. dislocation
c. extensor mechanism (CEM)
c. fat signal intensity
c. fatty hilum
c. fibrosarcoma
c. fracture
c. groove
c. gyrus
c. hemorrhagic component
c. herniation
c. high-signal intensity stripe
c. hilar structure
c. horn
c. intraluminal saturation stripe
c. intrasubstance signal intensity
c. lesion
c. lung distance (CLD)
c. lymph node

NOTES

central *(continued)*
c. medullary bone lesion
c. motor pathways disease
c. necrosis
c. nervous system (CNS)
c. nervous system hemorrhage
c. nervous system tumor
c. neurofibromatosis
c. neurogenic hyperventilation
c. nidus of high-intensity marrow
c. ossifying fibroma
c. osteosarcoma
c. pancreatic lesion scar
c. perforation
c. perineal tendon
c. pit
c. placenta previa
c. pneumonia
c. point artifact
c. pontine
c. pontine myelinolysis
c. ray (CR)
c. return
c. rhomboid attachment
c. sacral line (CSL)
c. sinus lipomatosis
c. solitary papilloma breast
c. spinal canal
c. spinal stenosis
c. splanchnic venous thrombosis (CSVT)
c. sulcus
c. tegmental tract (CTT)
c. tendon diaphragm
c. vein
c. venous catheter (CVC)
c. venous drainage
c. venous line position
c. venous pressure (CVP)
c. venous pressure line
centralis
fovea c.
centrally ordered phase encoding
centrally uninhibited bladder
centriacinar emphysema
centriciput
centrifugation
discontinuous density gradient c.
centrilobular
c. congestion
c. distribution
c. emphysema
c. lesion
c. micronodule
c. necrosis
c. region of liver
c. shadow
centroblast
centroblastic lymphoma
centrocyte-like
c.-l. type
centrocytic lymphoma
centrocytoid
centromere
centrum
c. commune
c. ovale
c. semiovale
c. semiovale pattern
cephalad
c. direction
cephalhematoma (*var. of* cephalohematoma)
cephalic
c. angle
c. angulation
c. flexure
c. index
c. pole
c. presentation
c. presentation of fetus
c. tilt view
c. triangle
c. vein
c. ventricle
cephalization of blood flow
cephalocaudad length
cephalocele
occipital c.
oral c.
sincipital c.
cephalofacial proportionality
cephalogram
c. imaging
cephalohematocele
cephalohematoma, cephalhematoma
parietal c.
cephalomedullary nail fracture
cephalometer
Bertillon c.
cephalometric
c. analysis
c. angle
c. radiograph
cephalometrics
cephalometry
ultrasonic c.
cephalopelvic disproportion (CPD)
cephalopelvimetry
cephalostat
cephalosyndactyly
Vogt c.
CeraSPECT camera
ceratocricoid ligament
cercaria

cerclage
Shirodkar c.
cerebella (*pl. of* cerebellum)
cerebellar
c. anaplasia
c. aplasia
c. apoplexy
c. artery
c. astrocytoma
c. atrophy
c. attachment
c. cortex
c. cystic mass
c. degeneration
c. disease
c. ectopia
c. epidermoid
c. fiber
c. gliosarcoma
c. hemisphere
c. hemorrhage
c. hypoperfusion
c. hypoplasia
c. infarct
c. notch
c. pathway
c. peduncle
c. peg
c. sarcoma
c. syndrome
c. tonsil
c. tonsillar herniation
c. tract
c. uvula
c. vermis
c. view
c. volume
cerebelli
falx c.
gyrus c.
mediastinum c.
tentorium c.
vallecula c.
cerebellolabyrinthine artery
cerebellomedullary cistern
cerebelloolivary degeneration
cerebellopontine
c. angle (CPA)
c. angle meningioma
c. angle tumor
c. cistern
c. cisternography
c. recess
cerebelloretinal
c. hemangioblastoma
c. hemangioblastomatosis
cerebellorubral tract
cerebellorubrospinal tract
cerebellospinal tract
cerebellotegmental tract
cerebellothalamic tract
cerebellum, pl. **cerebella**
amygdala of c.
basal ganglia of c.
dentate nucleus of c.
flocculonodular lobe of c.
Gowers bundle in c.
midline c.
petrosal c.
towering c.
cerebra (*pl. of* cerebrum)
cerebral
c. abscess
c. amaurosis
c. amyloid angiopathy
c. aneurysm
c. angiography
c. anoxia
c. apotentiality
c. aqueduct
c. arteriography
c. arteriosclerosis
c. arteriovenous fistula
c. arteriovenous malformation
c. artery
c. artery infarct
c. artery stenosis
c. astrocytoma
c. blood flow (CBF)
c. blood vessel
c. blood volume (CBV)
c. blood volume/cerebral blood flow (CBV/CBF)
c. blood volume/cerebral blood flow ratio (CBV/CBF ratio)
c. blood volume map
c. brain death
c. calcification
c. circulation
c. circulation time
c. commissure
c. congestion
c. contusion

NOTES

cerebral *(continued)*
c. convexity
c. convolution
c. cortex
c. cortical vein sign
c. CT venography
c. cyst
c. dominance
c. dysfunction
c. edema
c. fat embolus
c. fissure
c. flexure
c. gigantism
c. glioma
c. gyri interdigitation
c. hemiatrophy
c. hemidecortication
c. hemisphere
c. hemorrhage
c. herniation
c. hypoperfusion
c. hypotension
c. infundibulum
c. ischemia
c. ischemic event
c. lesion
c. lymphoma
c. malformation classification
c. mantle
c. metabolic oxygen consumption
c. metabolic rate of oxygen ($CMRO_2$)
c. metabolism
c. metastasis
c. neuroblastoma
c. nocardiosis
c. nodule
c. operculum
c. palsy pathological fracture
c. parenchyma
c. peduncle
c. perfusion SPECT imaging
c. perfusion SPECT scan
c. perfusion study
c. pneumography
c. pneumonia
c. porosis
c. radionecrosis
c. revascularization
c. ridge
c. salt wasting
c. shunt
c. sinovenous occlusion
c. SPECT
c. steal syndrome
c. sulcus
c. surface
c. surface atrophy
c. thrombophlebitis
c. vasculature
c. vasoreactivity
c. vein
c. venous sinus
c. ventricle
c. ventricular shunt connector
c. ventriculogram
c. vesicle
c. Whipple disease
c. white matter hypoplasia

cerebri
choana c.
commotio c.
contusio c.
falx c.
fornix c.
gliomatosis c.
gyri c.
hypophysis c.
mediastinum c.
pseudotumor c. (PTC)

cerebriform
c. carcinoma

cerebritis
sinusitis c.

cerebrohepatorenal syndrome (CHRS)

cerebromacular degeneration (CMD)

cerebromeningeal intracerebral hemorrhage

cerebropontocerebellar pathway

cerebrospinal
c. canal
c. fluid (CSF)
c. fluid circulation
c. fluid-containing lesion
c. fluid fistula
c. fluid flow measurement
c. fluid leak
c. fluid leakage
c. fluid leak study
c. fluid obstruction
c. fluid pathway
c. fluid shunt function
c. fluid volume

cerebrotendinous xanthomatosis

cerebrovascular
c. accident (CVA)
c. aneurysmal clip
c. insufficiency
c. insult
c. malformation
c. occlusive disease
c. stroke

cerebrum, pl. **cerebra**
central cavity of c.
cistern of lateral fossa of c.

cortex of c.
degenerative disease in c.
c. demyelination
c. dysmyelination
first ventricle of c.
great vein of c.
lateral ventricle of c.
second ventricle of c.
third ventricle of c.

Cerenkov
C. calculation
C. count
C. counter
C. measurement
C. radiation
C. radiation production
C. scintillation analysis

Ceretec
C. brain imaging
C. radioisotope imaging agent
^{99m}Tc C.
technetium-99m Ceretec
technetium-99m C. (^{99m}Tc Ceretec)

cerium
c. silicate imaging agent

ceroid
c. gallbladder granuloma

Cerrobend block

cervical
c. adenocarcinoma
c. adenopathy
c. aorta
c. aorta syndrome
c. aortic arch
c. artery
c. canal
c. cord
c. cord lesion
c. CT
c. disk
c. disk disease
c. disk herniation
c. disk syndrome
c. dorsal outlet syndrome
c. dysplasia
c. enlargement
c. esophagostomy
c. esophagus
c. eversion
c. facet dislocation
c. fascia
c. flexure
c. fusion of spine
c. ganglion
c. heart
c. interbody fusion
c. intervertebral foraminal magnetic resonance phlebography
c. intraepithelial neoplasm
c. kink syndrome
c. length
c. loop
c. lordosis
c. lordotic curvature
c. lymph node
c. magnetic resonance phlebography (CMRP)
c. meningocele
c. mover ligament
c. muscle
c. musculature
c. myelography
c. myelopathy
c. nerve root
c. neural foramen
c. osteophyte
c. outlet
c. pain syndrome
c. paratracheal lymph node
c. pleura
c. plexus
c. polyp
c. pregnancy
c. rib
c. rib syndrome
c. sarcoma
c. sinus
c. spine
c. spine curve
c. spine dens view
c. spine fracture
c. spine fusion
c. spine injury
c. spine spondylosis
c. stenosis
c. stroma
c. structure
c. synostosis
c. syringomyelia
c. thymic cyst
c. triangle
c. tumor
c. vein

NOTES

cervical *(continued)*
c. vertebra
c. vesicle
cervicitis
cervicoaxillary canal
cervicocerebral
cervicocranium
cervicography
cervicomedullary
c. junction
c. kink
cervicooccipital fusion
cervicothoracic
c. ganglion
c. junction
c. sagittal scout image
cervicothoracolumbar
cervicotrochanteric fracture
cervigram
cervix
Cockscomb appearance of c.
incompetent c.
c. uteri
uterine c.
c. of uterus
CES
cauda equina syndrome
cesarean section
cesium
c. chloride imaging agent
c. implant
c. iodide input phosphor
c. needle
c. therapy
cesium-137 (^{137}Cs)
Céstan-Chenais syndrome
cestodic tuberculosis
Cetacaine
CF
circumflex
CF artery
^{252}Cf
californium-252
CFD
color-flow Doppler
CFI
color flow imaging
CFR
coronary flow reserve
CFT
crystal field theory
CGI
common gateway interface
CGR biplane angiographic system
cGy
centigray
Chachoua staging system
Chaddock sign
chain
branched c.
c. cystogram
internal mammary lymphatic c.
J c.
jugulodigastric c.
kappa light c.
c. of lakes deformity
c. of lakes filling defect
c. of lakes sign
lambda light c.
Markov c.
obturator nodal c.
sympathetic c.
chair
Pigg-O-Stat x-ray c.
SPECTurn c.
chalasia
chalky
c. bone
challenge
solid bolus c.
chamber
abnormal dimensions of cardiac c.
cardiac c.
cloud c.
c. compression
defective communication between cardiac c.'s
c. dilatation
c. enlargement
false aneurysmal c.
c. of heart
infundibular c.
ionization c.
irradiation c.
left atrial c.
left ventricular c.
personal ionization c.
pocket c.
reduced compliance of c.
reentrant well c.
right atrial c.
right ventricular c.
rudimentary outlet c.
rudimentary ventricular c.
Storm Von Leeuwen c.
c. volume
well-type ionization c.
Wilson cloud c.
Chamberlain procedure
Chamberlain-Towne view
champagne
c. glass iliac wing
c. glass pelvis
c. glass ureter
champagne-bottle legs

chance
c. equivalent
Chance spinal fracture
Chandra-Khetarpal syndrome
change
arthritic talonavicular c.'s
atherosclerotic c.
bony c.
consolidative c.
cystic c.
degenerative osseous c.
dystrophic c.
E:A c.
epithelial degenerative c.
Fairbanks c.'s
fibrocystic c.
fibrotic c.
fMRI signal c.
focal degenerative c.
hydropic c.'s
interstitial c.
interval c.
ischemic c.'s
lytic c.
nonspecific c.'s
onion bulb c.'s
osteoarthritic c.
papillary apocrine c.
paroxysmal c.
pathophysiologic c.'s
pelvicaliceal c.'s
postbiopsy c.
posttherapy c.
postthoracotomy c.
precancerous c.
prediverticular c.
pre-slip c.
pseudo-Pelger-Huet c.
pulmonary parenchymal c.'s
radiation-induced c.
radiation-related ischemic c.
reciprocal c.'s
residual interstitial c.'s
residual limb-shaped c.
roentgenographic c.
senescent c.
senile c.
serial c.'s
signal c.
spinal endplate c.
spondylitic c.
spongiform c.
vasomotor c.
changer
Elema roll-film c.
film c.
Franklin c.
Puck cutfilm c.
Puck film c.
rapid film c.
Sanchez-Perez automatic film c.
Sanchez-Perez cassette c.
Schonander film c.
serial film c.
Chang staging
channel
aberrant vascular c.
blood c.
central c.
collateral venous c.
deep venous c.
enlarged vascular c.
false c.
gastric c.
haversian c.
c. of Lambert
Lambert c.
lymphatic c.
pancreaticobiliary common c.
pyloric c.
c. pyloric ulcer
surface epithelium vascular c.
thread-and-streaks vascular c.'s
true c.
vascular c.
chaotic heart
Chaoul voltage x-ray tube
Chaput
C. fracture
C. tubercle
CHAR
continuous hyperfractionated accelerated radiotherapy
characteristic
contrast transfer c.
c. curve
echo c.
c. emission
excitatory pulse c.
c. finding
generator c.
receiver operating c.'s
suspension c.'s

NOTES

characteristic *(continued)*
tip dispersion c.
c. x-ray
characterization
tissue c.
charcoal
dextran-coated c.
Charcot
C. arthropathy
C. chondroma
C. cirrhosis
C. deformity
C. foot
C. joint
C. spine
C. triad
Charcot-Bouchard intracerebral microaneurysm
Charcot-Leyden crystal
Charcot-Marie-Tooth (CMT)
C.-M.-T. disease
charge
c. coupled device
technical c.
charge-coupled device scanner
charged
c. particle
c. particle equilibrium
charged-particle
c.-p. irradiation
c.-p. radiosurgery
Charnley centering ring
CHART
continuous hyperfractionated accelerated radiation therapy
chart
Segre c.
x-ray tube rating c.
chase
bolus c.
peripheral bolus c.
Chassaignac
C. muscle
C. space
Chassard-Lapine
C.-L. method
C.-L. position
C.-L. projection
C.-L. view
Chauffard point
chauffeur's fracture
Chausse
C. method
C. view
Chaussier
C. line
C. projection
C. view
CHB
complete heart block
CHD
common hepatic duct
congenital heart defect
congenital heart disease
coronary heart disease
arachnodactyly CHD
Check-Flo
C.-F. sheath
checkrein deformity
check rein ligament
check-valve
c.-v. mechanism
c.-v. sheath
Chédiak-Steinbrinck-Higashi syndrome
cheek bone
cheese
c. handler's disease
c. handler's lung
myometrium swiss c.
c. washer's disease
c. washer's lung
cheesy pneumonia
cheirolumbar
cheiromegaly
cheirospasm
chelate
B-19036 c.
Cr-HIDA c.
gadolinium c.
Gd-HIDA c.
chelonian pneumonia
chemical
c. dosimeter
c. pneumonia
c. pneumonitis
c. potential energy
c. pulmonary edema
c. ray
c. shift
c. shift artifact
c. shift imaging technique
c. shift phenomena artifact
c. shift selective (CHESS method, CHESS)
c. shift selective suppression technique
chemically induced dynamic nuclear polarization
chemical-selective
c.-s. fat saturation imaging
c.-s. fat-saturation MR
chemical-shift
c.-s. imaging (CSI)
c.-s. ratio
chemiluminescence
chemisorb

chemisorption
chemistry
anomalous serum c.
nuclear c.
radiopharmaceutical c.
chemodectoma
adrenal c.
chest c.
chemoembolization
hepatic c.
therapeutic c.
transcatheter arterial c.
transcatheter oily c.
chemoirradiation
concomitant c.
chemomodification
Chemo-Port
C.-P. catheter
C.-P. perivena catheter system
chemoradiation
adjuvant c.
c. therapy
chemoradiotherapy
high-dose c.
chemoreceptor tumor
chemoresistant tumor
chemotherapy
adjuvant c.
combination c.
continuous intravenous infusion c.
CT-guided intraarterial c.
chemotherapy-related myeloid suppression
chemsat fat suppression
chenodeoxycholic acid (CDCA)
Chen-Smith image coder
cherubism
CHESS
chemical shift selective
CHESS method
chest
alar c.
barrel c.
blast c.
c. cavity
c. chemodectoma
cobbler's c.
cylindrical c.
dirty c.
c. empyema
expiratory c.
c. film
flail c.
c. fluke lung
c. fluoroscopy
foveated c.
funnel c.
globular c.
hollow c.
jail-bar c.
keeled c.
narrow c.
paralytic c.
phthinoid c.
pigeon c.
pneumonectomy c.
pterygoid c.
c. radiology
c. sail sign
symmetric c.
tetrahedron c.
c. tube
c. view
c. wall
c. wall hamartoma
c. wall lateral xeromammogram
c. wall lesion
c. wall mesenchymoma
c. wall neuroblastoma
c. wall paradoxical motion
c. wall retraction
c. wall rhabdomyosarcoma
c. wave sign
c. x-ray (CXR)
Chester disease
chevron
c. bone
c. fracture
c. fusion
CHF
congenital hepatic fibrosis
congestive heart failure
CHI
closed head injury
Chiari
C. formation
C. I–II malformation
Chiari-Budd syndrome
Chiari-Foix-Nicolesco syndrome
chiasm
c. of digits of hand
optic c.

NOTES

chiasma
Camper c.
cistern of c.
chiasmal
c. compression
c. lesion
chiasmatic
c. cistern
c. defect
c. groove
chiasmatic-hypothalamic pilocytic astrocytoma
Chiba percutaneous cholangiogram
Chicago disease
chickenpox pneumonia
chicken-wire calcification
Chilaiditi
C. sign
C. syndrome
Child classification of esophageal varices
childhood
c. fracture
c. osteomyelitis
c. rhabdomyosarcoma
chimera
radiation c.
chimney-shaped
c.-s. aortic arch
c.-s. high aortic arch
Chinese fluke liver
chin muscle
chin-occiput piece
chip
bone c.
cancellous bone c.
corticocancellous bone c.
c. fracture
chiropractic
c. film
c. treatment fracture
chisel fracture
Chloramine T
chloramphenicol acetyl transferase (CAT)
chlordiazepoxide
chlorhexidine
chloride
benzalkonium c.
magnesium c.
manganese c.
polyvinyl c.
stannous c.
strontium-89 c.
thallium-201 c.
triphenyltetrazolium c. (TTC)
chloriodized oil
chloroma
bone c.
gastric c.
kidney c.
choana cerebri
choanal
c. atresia
c. polyp
chocolate
c. joint effusion
c. sauce abscess
cholangiectasis
extrahepatic c.
cholangiocarcinoma
extrahepatic c.
intrahepatic c.
peripheral c. (PCC)
Cholangiocath
cholangiocatheter
cholangiocellular carcinoma
cholangiodrainage
cholangiodysplastic pseudocirrhosis
cholangiofibromatosis
cholangiogram
balloon c.
catheter c.
Chiba percutaneous c.
common duct c.
contrast selective c.
cystic duct c.
drip-infusion c. (DIC)
endoscopic retrograde c. (ERC)
fine-needle transhepatic c. (FNTC)
HASTE MR c.
half-Fourier acquisition single-shot turbo spin echo magnetic resonance cholangiogram
intraoperative c.
intravenous c.
magnetic resonance c. (MRC)
operative c.
Oriental c.
percutaneous transhepatic c. (PTC, PTHC)
recurrent pyogenic c. (RPC)
serial c.
single-shot MR c.
transhepatic c. (THC)
transjugular c.
T-tube c. (TTC)
cholangiographic catheter
cholangiography
cystic duct c.
c. imaging
intravenous c.
percutaneous c.
percutaneous transhepatic c. (PTHC)

cholangiohepatitis
Oriental c.
cholangiolithiasis
cholangiopancreatography
endoscopic retrograde c. (ERCP)
magnetic resonance c. (MRCP)
cholangiopathy
AIDS-related c.
cholangiovenous communication
cholangitic biliary cirrhosis
cholangitis
acute nonsuppurative ascending c.
acute obstructive c.
acute suppurative ascending c.
AIDS c.
ascending c.
chronic nonsuppurative destructive c.
fibrous obliterative c.
intrahepatic sclerosing c.
nonsuppurative ascending c.
nonsuppurative destructive c.
primary sclerosing c.
progressive suppurative c.
pyogenic c.
recurrent pyogenic c.
sclerosing c.
secondary sclerosing c.
septic c.
suppurative ascending c.
Cholebrine
C. imaging agent
cholecystectasia
cholecystectomy
cholecystenteric fistula
cholecystitis
acalculous c.
acute c.
calculous c.
chronic c.
emphysematous c.
gangrenous c.
gaseous c.
lipid c.
perforated c.
c. with cholelithiasis
xanthogranulomatous c.
cholecystocholangiography
cholecystocholangitis
cholecystocholedochal fistula
cholecystocolic fistula
cholecystoduodenal
c. fistula
c. ligament
cholecystoduodenocolic
c. fistula
c. fold
cholecystogram
Graham-Cole c.
oral c. (OCG)
cholecystography
cholecystojejunostomy
cholecystokinetic food
cholecystolithiasis
cholecystomegaly
cholecystopaque
cholecystopathy
cholecystoptosis
cholecystosis
hyperplastic c.
cholecystosonography
cholecystostomy
percutaneous transhepatic c.
ultrasound-guided percutaneous c.
choledochal
c. cyst
c. sphincter
choledochal-colonic fistula
choledochocele
choledochocholedochostomy
choledochoduodenal
c. fistula
c. junctional stenosis
choledochojejunostomy stricture
choledocholithiasis
choledochopancreatic ductal junction
choledochoscope
choledochous duct
cholelith, chololith
cholelithiasis
cholecystitis with c.
cholelithoptysis
cholescintigraphy
cholestasis, cholestasia
intrahepatic c.
cholestatic liver disease
cholesteatoma
attic c.
congenital c.
ear c.
GU tract c.
inflammatory c.
pars flaccida c.

NOTES

cholesteatoma *(continued)*
pars tensa c.
primary acquired c.
primary CNS c.
primary temporal bone c.
secondary acquired c.
cholesterinosis, cholesterolosis
cholesterol
c. debris
c. ear cyst
c. ear granuloma
c. embolus
c. gallbladder polyp
c. gallstone
I-labeled c.
c. pneumonia
c. pneumonitis
c. stone
cholesterol-containing brain lesion
cholesterolosis (*var. of* cholesterinosis)
cholioangiopancreatography
Cholografin
C. meglumine imaging agent
chololith (*var. of* cholelith)
Cholovue
chondral
c. defect
c. fracture
c. fragment
chondrification
chondritis
chondroblastic osteosarcoma
chondroblastoma
benign c.
chondrocalcinosis
familial c.
chondrocyte
c. degeneration
epiphyseal c.
regenerative c.
chondrodiastasis
chondrodysplasia
metaphyseal c.
c. punctata
Schmid-like metaphyseal c.
chondrodystrophia
c. calcificans congenita
c. fetalis
chondrodystrophy
chondroectodermal dysplasia
chondrofibroma
chondrogenic tumor
chondroid
c. matrix
c. syringoma
c. tissue
chondroitin
c. sulfate iron colloid-enhanced MRI
c. sulfate iron colloid-enhanced MR imaging
chondrolipoma
chondrolysis
posttraumatic c.
chondroma
Charcot c.
extraskeletal c.
joint c.
juxtacortical c.
soft tissue c.
chondromalacia
c. patellae
patellar c.
ulnar c.
chondromatosis
Henderson-Jones c.
secondary c.
synovial c.
chondromatous hamartoma
chondromyofibroma
chondromyxoid fibroma (CMF)
chondromyxoma
chondromyxosarcoma
chondronecrosis
chondroosteodystrophy
chondrophyte
chondroporosis
chondrosarcoma
central c.
endosteal c.
exostotic c.
extraskeletal mesenchymal c.
mesenchymal c.
myxoid extraskeletal c.
parosteal c.
peripheral c.
chondrosarcomatosis
chondrosteoma
chondrosternal junction
chondroxiphoid ligament
chop amputation
Chopart
C. ankle dislocation
C. fracture
C. fracture-dislocation
C. hindfoot amputation
C. joint
Chopper-Dixon fat suppression imaging
choppy sea sign
Choquet fuzzy integral
choracobrachialis
chord
multiple c.'s
chorda, pl. **chordae**

basal c.
cleft c.
commissural c.
first-order c.
c. magna
second-order c.
strut c.
chordae tendineae cordis
chordae tendineae rupture
third-order c.
chordae Willisii
chordal rupture
chordocarcinoma
chordoepithelioma
chordoma
sacral c.
sacrococcygeal c.
c. of sacrum
sphenooccipital c.
spinal c.
vertebral c.
chordosarcoma
chorea
Huntington c. (HC)
rheumatic c.
Chorex
chorioallantoic placenta
chorioamnionic
c. elevation
c. separation
chorioangioma
choriocarcinoma
esophageal c.
gestational c.
nongestational c.
ovarian c.
primary ovarian c.
testicular c.
choriodecidua
choriodecidual reaction
chorionic
c. carcinoma
c. disk
c. gonadotropin
c. sac
c. tissue
chorionicity
choristoma
middle ear c.
renal c.
choroid
c. glomera
c. plexus
c. plexus blush
c. plexus calcification
c. plexus carcinoma
c. plexus cyst
c. plexus neoplasm
c. plexus papilloma
c. point
c. vein
choroidal
c. fissure
c. hemangioma
lateral posterior c. (LPCh)
medial posterior c. (MPCh)
c. melanoma
c. osteoma
c. pericallosal artery
c. ring
choroidal-hippocampal fissure complex
choroidea
tela c.
choroideum
glomus c.
Choron
Christian brachydactyly
Christmas
C. tree appearance
C. tree sign
chromaffin
c. paraganglioma
c. tumor
chromaffinomatosis
chromagranin
chromate
sodium c.
chromated ^{51}Cr serum albumin imaging agent
chromatogram
chromatographic separation
chromatography
anti-idiotypic affinity c.
DEAE-Sephadex A-25 c.
gas-liquid phase c. (GLPC)
high-performance liquid c.
high-performance size-exclusion c.
high-pressure liquid c.
ion-exchange c.
paper c.
chromically inflamed gallbladder
chromic phosphate ^{32}P colloidal suspension
chromium (Cr)

NOTES

chromium *(continued)*
c. imaging agent
c. phosphate
chromophobe
kidney carcinoma c.
pituitary adenoma c.
chronic
c. abdominal inflammation
c. airway obstruction
c. alveolar infiltrate
c. atelectasis
c. atrophic duodenitis
c. atrophic pyelonephritis
c. breast abscess
c. calcifying pancreatitis
c. cerebral ischemia
c. cholecystitis
c. communicating hydrocephalus
c. constrictive state
c. cystic mastitis
c. diffuse confluent lung opacity
c. diffuse reticulation
c. diffuse sclerosing alveolitis
c. diverticulitis
c. duodenal ileus
c. edema
c. eosinophilic pneumonia
c. esophagitis
c. extrinsic allergic alveolitis
c. fibrosing alveolitis
c. fibrosing mesenteritis
c. fissure
c. functional instability
c. gastric atony
c. gastritis
c. glomerulonephritis
c. heart failure
c. hemodynamic overload
c. hepatitis
c. hereditary nephritis
c. humoral rejection
c. hydronephrosis
c. hypertrophic emphysema
c. idiopathic intestinal pseudoobstruction (CIIP)
c. ileus duodenum
c. infantile hyperostosis
c. insufficiency of vein
c. interstitial lung disease sign
c. interstitial pneumonia
c. interstitial salpingitis
c. interstitial simulating air-space lung disease
c. irritation
c. ischemic brain infarct
c. lung thromboembolism
c. lung transplant rejection
c. lymphocytic leukemia
c. lymphocytic thyroiditis
c. mediastinitis
c. mesenteric ischemia
c. multifocal ill-defined lung opacity
c. necrotizing aspergillosis
c. nonsuppurative destructive cholangitis
c. obstructive emphysema
c. obstructive lung disease (COLD)
c. obstructive pancreatitis
c. obstructive pulmonary disease (COPD)
c. obstructive uropathy
c. overuse syndrome
c. parenchymal hemorrhage
c. partial epilepsy
c. passive congestion
c. peptic ulcer
c. periaortitis
c. peripheral arterial disease (CPAD)
c. phase
c. pleurisy
c. pneumonitis
c. posttraumatic aortic pseudoaneurysm
c. recurrent dislocation
c. recurrent multifocal oseomyelitis
c. recurrent sialadenitis
c. renal failure
c. renal failure amyloidosis
c. renal infarct
c. renal transplant rejection
c. renal vein thrombosis
c. reserve flow
c. respiratory decompensation
c. retrocalcaneal bursitis
c. simple silicosis
c. sinusitis
c. sprain
c. subdural hematoma (CSDH)
c. subperitoneal sclerosis
c. tamponade
c. testicular torsion
c. tuberculous emphysema
c. ulcerative colitis (CUC)
c. venous insufficiency
c. venous stasis
c. venous statis syndrome
chronologic age
chronotherapy
adjuvant c.
chronotropic
c. assessment exercise protocol
c. incompetence
chronotropy

CHRS
cerebrohepatorenal syndrome
Churg-Strauss syndrome
Chvostek-Weiss sign
chyle
c. cistern
effused c.
c. leak
c. vessel
chyli
cisterna c.
chylocele
nonfilarial c.
chyloma
chylothorax
postoperative c.
chylous
c. ascites
c. effusion
c. fistula
Chymodiactin
chymopapain
CI
cardiac index
continuous imaging
Ci
curie
cicatricial
c. kidney
c. stricture
cicatrization
cicatrizing phase
CID camera
Cidtech camera
CIG
cardiointegram
cigarroa formula
CIIP
chronic idiopathic intestinal pseudoobstruction
ciliary
c. canal
c. cartilage
c. ganglionic plexus
c. ligament
c. ring
c. vein
ciliated border
ciliospinal center of Budge
cine
c. camera
c. CT
c. CT imaging
c. CT scanner
c. film
c. fistulogram
c. gradient-echo MR imaging
c. gradient-echo sequence
c. left ventriculogram
c. loop
c. magnetic resonance function image
c. magnetic resonance imaging
c. magnetic resonance tagging
C. Memory with color flow Doppler imaging
c. mode
c. MRI
parallel c.
c. phase contrast (PC) imaging
c. projector
c. view
c. view imaging
cineangiocardiography
cineangiogram
ventricular c.
cineangiography
aortic root c.
axial c.
biplane c.
coronary c.
radionuclide c.
selective coronary c.
Sones technique for c.
cinearteriography
Judkins selective left coronary c.
cine-based viewing
cinecardioangiography
cine-cyclic method
cinedefecogram
cine-encoded image
cineesophagogram
cinefluorography
biplane c.
cinefluoroscopy
valve c.
cine-loop
cine-MR
breath-hold c.-M.
cinepharyngoesophagogram
cinephlebography
cineportography
cineradiographic view

NOTES

C

cineradiography
c. imaging
cinereum
tuber c.
cineroentgenofluorography
cineroentgenography
cineurography
cineventriculogram
cineventriculography
cingula (*pl. of* cingulum)
cingulate
c. gyrus
c. herniation
c. sulcus
cinguli
gyrus c.
cingulum, pl. **cingula**
cipher
transposition c.
Cippaux-Smirak arch index
circadian
c. continuous infusion
c. event recorder
c. pattern
c. periodicity
c. variation
circle
anastomotic arterial c.
arterial c.
articular vascular c.
c. loop biliary drainage
c. of Vieussens
c. of Weber
c. of Willis
c. of Willis aneurysm
c. wire nephrostomy
Circon video camera
circuit
anticoincidence c.
application-specific integrated c. (ASIC)
arrhythmia c.
ASIC c.
bridge c.
bypass c.
coincidence c.
doubly broadband triple-resonance NMR probe c.
macroreentrant c.
magnetoresistive sensor c.
microreentrant c.
phototube output c.
quad resonance NMR probe c.
reentry c.
shunting c.
triple-resonance NMR probe c.
circular
c. dichroism spectroscopy
c. fold
c. lesion
c. muscle
c. plane
c. polarization wave
c. sinus
c. supracondylar amputation
c. syncytium
circulares
plicae c.
circularly polarized coil
circulating blood volume
circulation
allantoic c.
arrested c.
balanced c.
bronchial collateral c.
carotid c.
cerebral c.
cerebrospinal fluid c.
codominant c.
c. collapse
collateral mesenteric c.
compensatory c.
cutaneous collateral c.
derivative c.
devoid of c.
c. disturbance
extracardiac collateral c.
extracorporeal c.
extracranial carotid c.
extracranial cerebral c.
c. failure
fetal c.
greater c.
high-impedance c.
c. hyperkinetic syndrome
intervillous c.
intracranial c.
Korotkoff test for collateral c.
microvascular c.
peripheral c.
persistent fetal c.
placental c.
portosystemic collateral c.
posterior fossa c.
pulmonary arterial c.
reduced c.
c. shock
spiderweb c.
c. stasis
systemic arterial c.
thebesian c.
c. time (CT)
uteroplacental c.
venous c.
vertebrobasilar c.
c. volume

circulator
sequential c.
circulatory
c. arrest
c. compromise
c. embarrassment
c. impairment
circumaortic
c. left renal vein
circumcaval ureter
circumference
femur length to abdominal c. (FL/AC, FL/AC ratio)
fetal abdominal c.
fetal head c.
c. of fetal head
fetal thoracic c.
head c. (HC)
thoracic c.
circumferential
c. cartilage
c. echodense layer
c. extremity coil
c. fibrocartilage
c. fracture
c. lamella
c. shortening
c. thickening
c. venous stenosis
circumflex (CF, CX)
c. artery (CF artery, CX artery)
c. branch
c. coronary artery
c. coronary system
c. groove artery
humeral c.
left c. (LCF, LCX)
c. retroesophageal arch
c. vein
c. vessel
circummarginate placenta
circummesencephalic cistern
circumscribed
c. edema
c. infiltrate
c. lesion
c. mass
c. pleurisy
circumscripta
calcinosis c.
osteoporosis c.
circumscript aneurysm
circumventricular organ
cirrhosis
acholangic biliary c.
acute juvenile c.
alcoholic c.
atrophic c.
biliary c.
Budd c.
calculous c.
cardiac c.
Charcot c.
cholangitic biliary c.
congestive c.
Cruveilhier-Baumgarten c.
cryptogenic c.
decompensated alcoholic c.
diffuse c.
end-stage c.
fatty c.
focal biliary c.
frank c.
glabrous c.
Hanot c.
hepatic c.
hypertrophic c.
Indian childhood c.
juvenile c.
liver c.
c. of liver
lung c.
macrolobular c.
medionodular c.
metabolic c.
microlobular c.
micronodular c.
multilobular c.
nutritional c.
obstructive biliary c.
periportal c.
pipestem c.
porta c.
posthepatic c.
postnecrotic c.
primary biliary c.
progressive familial c.
pulmonary c.
secondary biliary c.
septal c.
stasis c.
Todd c.
toxic c.

NOTES

cirrhosis *(continued)*
unilobular c.
vascular c.
cirrhotic
c. gastritis
c. inflammation
c. liver
c. nodule
cirsoid
c. aneurysm
c. placenta
cistern
ambient wing of the quadrigeminal c.
anterior interhemispheric c.
basal arachnoid c.
basilar c.
carotid c.
cerebellomedullary c.
cerebellopontine c.
c. of chiasma
chiasmatic c.
chyle c.
circummesencephalic c.
crural c.
c. effacement
great c.
increased basilar c.
c. indium
interpeduncular c. (IPC)
c. isotope
c. of lamina terminalis
c. of lateral fossa of cerebrum
mesencephalic c.
opticochiasmatic c.
c. oxygen
parasellar c.
c. of Pecquet
perimesencephalic c.
pontine c.
posterior c.
prepontine c.
quadrigeminal plate c. (QPC)
c. radioisotope
subarachnoid c.
suprasellar subarachnoid c.
sylvian c.
c. of Sylvius
trigeminal c.
cisterna
c. chyli
c. magna
c. magna effacement
cisternal
c. herniation
c. puncture
cisternogram
CT c.
metrizamide CT c.
cisternography
air c.
cerebellopontine c.
gas CT c.
c. imaging
isotopic c.
Katzman infusion of radionuclide c.
metrizamide computed tomography c. (MCTC)
oxygen c.
Pantopaque c.
radioisotope c.
radionuclide c.
Citelli angle
citrate
ferrous c.
gallium-67 c.
manganese c.
CIVI
continuous intravenous infusion
Civinini
C. canal
C. ligament
CKG
cardiokymography
CKG imaging
^{11}C-labeled
^{11}C-l. cocaine
^{11}C-l. cocaine imaging agent
^{11}C-l. fatty acid
^{11}C-l. fatty acids imaging agent
^{14}C lactose breath test
Clado
C. band
C. ligament
C. point
Clarke
C. arch angle
C. column
Clarke-Hadefield syndrome
Clark malignant melanoma classification
Clarkson scatter-summation algorithm
classic
c. carpal tunnel view
c. interstitial pneumonia
classical osteosarcoma
classification
AAOS acetabular abnormalities c.
acromioclavicular injury c.
Aitken acromioclavicular injury c.
Altman c.
American Spinal Cord Injury Association c.
Amstutz c.

anatomic brain c.
Anderson-D'Alonzo odontoid fracture c.
Ann Arbor c.
AO ankle fracture c.
AO-Danis-Weber ankle fracture c.
Arco c.
Bayne radial agenesis c.
Berndt-Harty talar lesion staging c.
Bigliani c.
Bleck metatarsus adductus c.
Bosniak c.
Boyd-Griffin trochanteric fracture c.
brain anatomy c.
brain tumor c.
Broders tumor index c.
Brooker periarticular heterotopic ossification c.
Burwell-Charnley fracture reduction c.
Butcher staging c.
Caldwell-Moloy c.
Canale-Kelly talar neck fracture c.
Carnesale-Stewart-Barnes hip dislocation c.
Cedell-Magnusson arthritis c.
cerebral malformation c.
Clark malignant melanoma c.
CNS anomaly c.
CNS tumor c.
Colonna hip fracture c.
congenital heart disease c.
Copeland-Kavat metatarsophalangeal dislocation c.
Couinaud c.
Danis-Weber ankle fracture c.
D'Antonio acetabular c.
DeBakey aortic c.
Delbet hip fracture c.
Denis c.
Denis c. of spinal injury (A–E)
Dickhaut-DeLee discoid meniscus c.
distance-based block c.
Essex-Lopresti calcaneal fracture c.
Evans intertrochanteric fracture c.
Fartland supracondylar fracture c.
Fielding-Magliato subtrochanteric fracture c.
fracture c.
Fränkel spinal cord injury c.
Freeman calcaneal fracture c.
Fries score for rheumatoid arthritis c.
Frykman distal radius fracture c.
Garden femoral neck fracture c.
Gawkins talar neck fracture c.
Gertzbein seatbelt injury c.
Glasscock-Jackson c.
Goldsmith & Woodburne c.
Grantham femur fracture c.
Gumley seatbelt injury c.
Gustilo-Anderson tibial plafond fracture c.
Hahn-Steinthal capitellum fracture c.
Hansen fracture c.
Hardy-Clapham sesamoid c.
Herbert-Fisher fracture c.
Hinchey c.
Hohl tibial condylar fracture c.
Holdsworth spinal fracture c.
Hughston Clinic injury c.
Hunt-Hess aneurysm c.
Hunt-Kosnik c.
Hyams grading of esthesioneuroblastoma c.
Ingram-Bachynski hip fracture c.
Jahss dislocation c.
Jeffery radial fracture c.
Jones c.
Judet epiphyseal fracture c.
Kalamchi-Dawe congenital tibial deficiency c.
Kernohan brain tumor c.
Key-Conwell pelvic fracture c.
Kiel non-Hodgkin lymphoma c.
Kilfoyle condylar fracture c.
Kimura c.
Kistler subarachnoid hemorrhage c.
Klatskin tumor c.
Kocher-Lorenz capitellum fracture c.
Kostuik-Errico spinal stability c.
Kyle fracture c.
Lauge-Hansen ankle fracture c.
Mason radial fracture c.
Mazur ankle evaluation c.
McCabe-Fletcher c.
McLain-Weinstein spinal tumor c.
Melone distal radius fracture c.
Merland perimedullary arteriovenous fistula c.
Meyer-McKeever tibial fracture c.

NOTES

classification *(continued)*
Michels c.
Milch elbow fracture c.
Mitchell c.
Modic disk abnormality c.
mulberry type c.
Müller humerus fracture c.
multiaxial c.
Neer-Horowitz humerus fracture c.
Nevaiser frozen shoulder c.
Newman radial fracture c.
Nurick spondylosis c.
NYHA congestive heart failure c.
O'Brien radial fracture c.
Ogden epiphyseal fracture c.
Olerud and Molander fracture c.
osteoarthritis grading c.
Ovadia-Beals tibial plafond fracture c.
Papile c.
Pauwel femoral neck fracture c.
pineal gland tumor c.
Pipkin femoral fracture c.
pneumoconiosis c.
Poland epiphyseal fracture c.
Potter c.
primary CNS tumor c.
Ratliff avascular necrosis c.
REAL c.
Revised European-American Lymphoma c.
rickets c.
Riemann c.
Riordan club hand c.
Riseborough-Radin intercondylar fracture c.
Robson staging c.
Rockwood acromioclavicular injury c.
Rowe calcaneal fracture c.
Rowe-Lowell fracture-dislocation c.
Ruedi-Allgower tibial plafond fracture c.
Runyon c.
Russell-Rubinstein cerebrovascular malformation c.
Sage-Salvatore acromioclavicular joint injury c.
Sakellarides calcaneal fracture c.
Salter-Harris fracture c.
Salter-Harris-Rang epiphyseal fracture c.
Schatzker fracture c.
Seinsheimer femoral fracture c.
Shelton femur fracture c.
Shimada histopathologic c.
Smith sesamoid position c.
Snyder c.
soft tissue lesion c.
SOMA c.
Sorbie calcaneal fracture c.
Stanford aortic dissection c.
Steinberg c.
Steinbrocker rheumatoid arthritis c.
Steinert epiphyseal fracture c.
Steward-Milford fracture c.
talocalcaneal index c.
Thompson-Epstein femoral fracture c.
Todani c.
Tronzo intertrochanteric fracture c.
Trunkey fracture c.
Vostal radial fracture c.
Watanabe discoid meniscus c.
Watson-Jones c.
Werner c.
WHO c.
Wiberg patellar types c.
Wilkins radial fracture c.
Winquist-Hansen femoral fracture c.
Wiseman c.
Wolfe breast carcinoma c.
Working Formulation c.
World Health Organization c.
Zickel fracture c.
Zlotsky-Ballard acromioclavicular injury c.

clasticus
conus c.

Claude syndrome

claudication of jaw

claustrum, pl. **claustra**

clavicle
absence of outer end of c.
destruction of medial end of c.
penciling of the distal c.

clavicular
c. birth fracture
c. facet
c. head of sternocleidomastoid
c. notch
c. osteitis condensans

clavipectoral
c. fascia
c. triangle

clavus
interdigital c.

clawfoot deformity

clawhand
c. deformity

clawtoe deformity

clay
c. pipe cancer
c. shoveler's fracture

Claybrook sign

CLC
Clerc-Levy-Cristeco syndrome
CLD
central lung distance
clean shadow
clear
c. cell neoplasm of ovary
enemas until c.
c. kidney cell sarcoma
c. zone
clearance
c. curve
c. half-time
isotope c.
multicompartment c.
c. phase ventilation scan
radioactive xenon c.
radioaerosol c.
renal c.
clear cell sarcoma
cleavage
c. cavity
c. fracture
plane of c.
c. tear
cleaved cell lymphoma
Cleaves
C. method
C. position
cleaving
plaque c.
Cleeman sign
cleft
anal c.
branchial c.
c. chorda
coronal c.
c. face syndrome
facial c.
first visceral c.
gill c.
Hahn c.
intergluteal c.
interinnominoabdominal c.
intranuclear c.
intravertebral body vacuum c.
lateral facial c.
median facial c.
median lip c.
meniscal c.
c. mitral valve
neural arch c.
pudendal c.
radiolucent c.
retrosomatic c.
spinal cord c.
splenic c.
synaptic c.
vacuum c.
ventricular c.
clefting
ectrodactyly-ectodermal dysplasia-c. (EEC)
cleidocranial
c. dysostosis
c. dysplasia
Cleland
C. ligament
C. ligament in the hand
Clements-Nakayama position
clenched fist view
Cleopatra view
Clerc-Levy-Cristeco syndrome (CLC)
clinical
c. complete response
c. correlation
c. diagnosis
c. feature
c. parameter
c. partial response
c. target volume (CTV)
clinicopathological analysis
CliniGlove
clinodactyly
clinoid
c. aneurysm
c. ligament
c. plate
c. process
clinoparietal line
clip
aneurysmal c.
cerebrovascular aneurysmal c.
hemostatic c.
c. ligation of aneurysm
metallic c.
sternal c.
surgical c.
clipping of aneurysm
clitoris
bifid c.
clival meningioma
clivus, pl. **clivi**
Blumenbach c.

NOTES

clivus *(continued)*
c. meningioma tumor
c. metastasis
clivus-canal angle
CLL
CLM
capillary-lymphatic malformation
cloaca, pl. **cloacae**
bone formation c.
cloacal
c. anomaly
c. exstrophy
c. formation
c. malformation
c. plate
cloacogenic carcinoma of the anorectum
cloaking
perivascular c.
clockwise whirlpool sign
cloning
subtraction c.
clonogen
c. number
clonogenicity
C loop
duodenal C. l.
C. l. of duodenum
Cloquet
C. canal
C. fascia
hyaloid canal of C.
C. inguinal lymph node
C. ligament
C. space
close apposition
closed
c. conducting loop
c. core transformer
c. dislocation
c. exstrophy
c. flap amputation
c. fontanelle
c. fracture
c. head injury (CHI)
c. pneumothorax
c. reduction
c. spinal dysraphism
closed-break fracture
closed-fist configuration
closed-loop intestinal obstruction
closed-mouth view
close-up view
closing
c. capacity
c. slope
c. velocity
c. volume
c. volume lung
closure
abrupt vessel c.
aortic c. (AC)
growth center c.
incomplete c.
native aortic valve c.
physeal c.
premature valve c.
sandwich patch c.
threatened vessel c.
tricuspid valve c.
valve c.
velopharyngeal c.
clot
agonal c.
autologous blood c.
blood c.
internal c.
intramural c.
isoechoic c.
marantic c.
mural c.
passive c.
plastic c.
preformed c.
c. retraction
subarachnoid c.
subdural c.
clot-filled lumen
clothesline injury
clothing artifact
cloud
c. chamber
electron c.
clouding
alveolar c.
cloudy swelling of heart
cloverleaf
c. deformity
c. plate
c. skull
cloverleaf-shaped lumen
clubbed
c. finger
c. penis
clubbing
caliceal c.
clubfoot deformity
clubhand deformity
club-shaped conus
clumsy-hand syndrome
cluneal nerve
cluster
c. of differentiation (CD)
c. of grapes kidney
c. of grapes lung
K-means c.
clustered microcalcification

clustering algorithm
Clutton painful joint
clysis
Clysodrast
cm
centimeter
CMC
carpometacarpal joint
CMD
cerebromacular degeneration
corticomedullary differentiation
CMF
chondromyxoid fibroma
CMOS
complementary metal oxide semiconductor
CMR
congenital mitral regurgitation
$CMRO_2$
cerebral metabolic rate of oxygen
CMRP
cervical magnetic resonance phlebography
CMT
Charcot-Marie-Tooth
C/N
contrast-to-noise ratio
C/N ratio
CNS
central nervous system
CNS amyloidosis
CNS anomaly classification
CNS ataxia-telangiectasia
CNS cortical hamartoma
CNS cysticercosis
CNS empyema
CNS fibromuscular dysplasia
CNS ghost tumor
CNS juvenile pilocytic astrocytoma
CNS multifocal tumor
CNS teratoma
CNS tumor classification
CO
cardiac output
CO_2
carbon dioxide
CO_2 angiography
CO_2 cylinder
CO_2 generator
CO_2 insufflation
CO_2 laser
CO_2 negative contrast medium
CO_2 retention
Co
cobalt
^{57}Co
cobalt-57
^{58}Co
cobalt-58
^{60}Co
cobalt-60
coagulation
disseminated intravascular c.
c. necrosis
coagulopathy
intravascular consumption c.
coal
c. macule
c. miner's lung
c. worker's lung
c. worker's pneumoconiosis
coalescence
coalescent granuloma
coalition
bony c.
calcaneonavicular c.
carpal c.
fibrous c.
intercarpal c.
lunate-triquetral c.
Minaar classification of c.
osseous c.
talocalcaneal c.
target c.
tarsal c.
c. view
coanalgesic
coaptation
c. plate
c. point
coapted leaflet
coarctation
abdominal aortic c.
c. of aorta
aortic c.
asymptomatic c.
atypical subisthmic c.
congenital isthmic c.
isthmic c.
juxtaductal aortic c.
localized c.
postductal aortic c.
preductal aortic c.

NOTES

coarctation *(continued)*
reversed c.
c. syndrome
coarcted
c. segment
coarse
c. bronchovascular markings
c. calcification
c. lung reticulation
c. nodularity
coast
c. of California café-au-lait spot
c. of Maine café-au-lait spot
coating of aneurysm
Coats disease
coaxial
c. steering
coaxial-needle method
cobalt (Co)
c. megavoltage machine
c. pneumopathy
radioactive c.
c. radioactive source
cobalt-57 (^{57}Co)
cobalt-58 (^{58}Co)
cobalt-60 (^{60}Co)
c. beam
c. gamma knife radiosurgical treatment
cobalt-chromium-molybdenum (Co-Cr-Mo)
cobalt-chromium-molybdenum alloy metal implant
cobalt-chromium-tungsten-nickel alloy metal implant (Co-Cr-W-Ni alloy implant metal)
Cobb
C. measurement
C. measurement of scoliosis
C. method of measuring kyphosis
C. scoliosis angle
C. syndrome
cobbler's
c. chest
c. chest syndrome
cobblestone
c. appearance
c. appearance of bile duct
c. appearance of the colon
c. appearance duodenum
c. appearance eosinophilic gastroenteritis
c. appearance esophagus
c. appearance lymphoma
c. appearance stomach
c. degeneration
c. ileum
c. lissencephaly
c. mucosa
c. pattern
cobblestoning
c. sign
cobra-head
c.-h. anastomosis
c.-h. appearance
c.-h. effect
c.-h. ureter
cobweb
c. appearance
c. pattern
cocaine
^{11}C-labeled c.
coccidioidoma
coccidioidomycosis
bone c.
disseminated c.
latent c.
lung c.
Posadas-Wernicke c.
primary c.
progressive c.
secondary c.
coccygeal
c. appendage
c. body
c. bone
c. ganglion
c. gland
c. ligament
c. plexus
c. sinus
c. spine
c. vertebra
c. whorl
coccygeopubic diameter
coccygeus
coccyx
c. bone
c. fracture
cochlea, pl. **cochleae**
c. aplasia
single-cavity c.
cochlear
c. anatomy
c. aqueduct
c. canal
c. canaliculus
c. duct
c. hearing loss
c. implant
c. labyrinth
c. lesion
c. nerve
c. otosclerosis
c. recess
c. root

cochleariform process
cochleate uterus
cochleitis
calcific c.
ossifying c.
Cockayne syndrome
Cockett vein
cocking injury
cock-robin position
cockscomb
c. appearance
C. appearance of cervix
c. papilloma
cock-up
c.-u. deformity
c.-u. deformity of toe
Co-Cr-Mo
cobalt-chromium-molybdenum
Co-Cr-Mo alloy metal implant
Co-Cr-W-Ni alloy implant metal
cocurrent flow-related enhancement
COD
computerized optical densitometry
coded-aperture imaging
coder
Chen-Smith image c.
ICS c.
improved Chen-Smith coder
codfish
c. deformity
c. vertebra
Codivilla extension
Codman
C. angle
C. sign
C. triangle
C. tumor
codominant
c. circulation
c. system
c. vessel
coefficient
absorption c.
apparent diffusion c.
attenuation c.
beta-spectra shapefactor c.
c. conversion
curve fit c.
diffusion c.
effective mass attenuation c.
Fourier c.
linear absorption c.
linear attenuation c.
mass attenuation c.
Ostwald solubility c. (Λ)
partition c.
reflection c.
stiffness c.
uniform attenuation c.
c. of variation (c.v.)
viscosity c.
coeur
c. en sabot
coexistent cavity
coffee-bean appearance
coffee-ground material
coffee worker's lung
coffin bone
Cogan
C. lid twitch sign
C. syndrome
cogwheel sign
coherence
phase c.
coherent scattering
coil
aneurysmal c.
birdcage head c.
c. blockade
body c.
breast c.
butterfly c.
circularly polarized c.
circumferential extremity c.
c. closure of coronary artery fistula
collagen-filled interlocking detachable c.
crossed c.
custom-curved c.
detachable c.
detector c.
double breast c.
embedding of stent c.
endoanal c.
endorectal c.
endoscopic quadrature radiofrequency c.
endovascular c.
fat-suppressed body c.
field-profiling c.
flexible surface c.
Gianturco occlusion c.
Gianturco-Wallace-Anderson c.

NOTES

C

coil *(continued)*
Gianturco-Wallace-Anderson c.
Gianturco-Wallace-Chuang c.
Gianturco wool-tufted wire c.
Golay c.
gradient sheet c.
Guglielmi detachable c. (GDC)
head c.
Helmholtz c.
immediately detachable c.
interlocking detachable c.
c.'s of intestine
intrarectal c.
intravascular c.
in vitro evaluation of c.
linearly polarized c.
liver c.
c. loading
local c.
local gradient c.
Medrad Mrinnervu endorectal colon probe c.
modified birdcage c.
neck c.
opposed loop-pair quadrature NMR c.
orthogonal radiofrequency c.
parallel data acquisition c.
pelvic phased-array c.
phased-array surface c.
phased-array torso c.
planar circular c.
platinum c.
posterior neck surface c.
proximal c.
quadrature cervical spine c.
quadrature radiofrequency receiver c.
quadrature T/L (terminal latency) surface c.
radiofrequency c. (RFC)
radiofrequency transmitter-receiver c.
receive-only circular surface c.
receiver c.
right ventricular c.
saddle c.
c. selection
sensing c.
shim c.
shoulder surface c.
solenoid surface c.
stainless steel c.
steel c.
surface c.
three-axis gradient c.
thrombogenic c.
torso phased-array c. (TPAC)
transmit-receive c.
transmitter c.
c. vascular stent
volume c.
whole-volume c.
wool c.

coiled-spring
c.-s. appearance
c.-s. pattern

coiling
c. of anastomosis
c. of aneurysm

coil-tipped catheter

coil-to-vessel diameter

coin
c. artifact
fracture en c.
c. lesion
c. lesion of lung

coincidence circuit

coincidence-summing correction

coin-on-edge vertebra

Coiter muscle

Colapinto
C. sheath

Colbert method

Colcher-Sussman method

COLD
chronic obstructive lung disease

cold
c. breast abscess
c. defect
c. defect renal scintigraphy
c. lesion
c. nodule thyroid
c. spine abscess
c. spot
c. spot myocardial imaging
c. thyroid nodule

colectasia

Cole sign

coli
haustra c.
melanosis c.
pneumatosis c.

colic
c. artery
biliary c.
cytomegalovirus (CMV) c.
episodic c.
c. impression
c. omentum
c. plexus
renal c.
c. sphincter
c. surface
c. vein

Colinet-Caplan syndrome

colitis
chronic ulcerative c. (CUC)
Crohn c.
c. cystica profunda
familial ulcerative c.
focal c.
fulminant c.
fulminating ulcerative c.
granulomatous transmural c.
hemorrhagic c.
ischemic c.
myxomembranous c.
neutropenic c.
c. polyposa
pseudomembranous c.
radiation-induced c.
regional c.
single-stripe c. (SSC)
spastic c.
transmural c.
ulcerative c. (UC)
c. ulcerosa gravis
collagen
c. disease arthritis
c. fiber separation
c. fibril
c. fragmentation
c. tissue proliferation
c. vascular disease (CVD)
collagen-filled interlocking detachable coil
collagenosis
mediastinal c.
collagenous
c. structure
c. tissue
collapse
acute vertebra c.
c. cavitation
circulation c.
jugular venous pressure c.
scapholunate advanced c. (SLAC)
scapholunate arthritic c. (SLAC)
subchondral c.
vertebral c.
vertebral body c.
collapsed
c. cava sign
c. distal ileum
c. inferior vena cava
c. lobe
c. lung
c. lung field
c. subpectoral implant
collapse-related vacuum phenomenon
collapsing cord sign
collar
c. bone
implant c.
periosteal bone c.
periportal c.
c. sign
collarbone
collar-button
c.-b. abscess
c.-b. appearance
c.-b. chest lesion
c.-b. ulcer
collateral
c. arcade
c. blood flow
c. blood supply
c. branch
c. circulation in compression of artery
c. edema
c. eminence
c. fissure
c. hyperemia
c. ligament
c. ligament of knee
c. mesenteric circulation
c. sulcus
c. system
c. trigone
c. venous channel
c. vessel
collateralization
collecting
c. system
c. system atony
c. system filling defect
c. system opacification
c. tube
c. tubule
c. vessel
collection
abdominal air c.
abdominal gas c.
air c.
anechoic fluid c.
c. of contrast material
crescentic c.
EAA c.

NOTES

C

collection *(continued)*
extraalveolar air c.
extraaxial fluid c.
extracerebral fluid c.
fluid c.
gas c.
hypoechoic fluid c.
intratendinous fluid c.
list mode data c.
pancreatic fluid c.
periarticular fluid c.
pericholecystic fluid c.
perifascial fluid-like c.
perinephric fluid c.
peripancreatic fluid c.
pleural fluid c.
posttraumatic subcapsular hepatic fluid c.
saccular c.

collective paramagnetism

Colles
C. fascia
C. fracture
C. ligament
C. space

Collet-Sicard syndrome

Collett analysis

colli
fibromatosis c.
pterygium c.

collicular fracture

colliculus, gen. and pl. **colliculi**
anterior c.
brachium of c.
facial c.
inferior c.
plicae colliculi
posterior c.
seminal c.
superior c.

Collier sign

collimating system

collimation
c. CT
detector c.
dynamic multileaf c.
electronic c.
c. imaging
lead c.
c. scanning
secondary c.
skin c.
tertiary c.
c. width

collimator
APC-3 c.
APC-4 c.
converging c.
diverging c.
dual-shaped c.
Eureka c.
c. exchange effect
fan-beam c.
heart-shaped c.
c. helmet
high-resolution multileaf c.
Leur-par c.
long-bore c.
low-energy c.
Machlett c.
medium-energy c.
Micro-Cast c.
multileaf c. (MLC)
multirod c.
parallel-hole medium sensitivity c.
pinhole c.
c. plugging pattern
c. scattering
slant hole c.
Summit LoDose c.
triple-leaf c.

colliquative necrosis

collision
c. detecting
c. tumor

collodiaphyseal
central c. (CCD)

colloid
c. adenocarcinoma
c. adenoma
^{198}Au c.
gold-198 colloid
c. cancer
c. carcinoma
c. cystic tumor
c. cyst of third ventricle
c. degeneration
c. goiter
gold-198 c. (^{198}Au colloid)
mini-microaggregated albumin c. (MMAA)
c. oncotic pressure (COP)
radioactive c.
radiogold c.
c. shift
c. shift on scan
sulfur c.
^{99m}Tc sulfur c.
technetium-99m albumin c.
technetium-99m mini-microaggregated albumin c.
technetium-99m sulfur c.

colloidal
c. brain cyst
c. chromic phosphorus

c. radioactive gold
c. suspension

colocolic
c. anastomosis
c. fistula
c. intussusception

colocutaneous fistula

colography
CT c.

Colombo count

colon
accessory sign c.
angiodysplasia of c.
anterior band of c.
ascending c.
barium-filled c.
burned-out c.
c. cancer
carpet lesion of c.
cathartic c.
cobblestone appearance of the c.
coned-down appearance of c.
Crohn disease of c. (CDC)
c. cutoff sign
c. cyst duplication
descending c.
distal c.
double-tracking c.
c. duplication
epithelial c.
fecal-filled c.
free band of c.
giant c.
hepatodiaphragmatic interposition of c. (HDIC)
hypoganglionosis of c.
iliac c.
inflammation of c.
intramural air in c.
irritable c.
jejunization of c.
c. kinking
knuckle of c.
lateral reflection of c.
left c.
c. margin
mesosigmoid c.
midsigmoid c.
pelvic c.
perisigmoid c.
proximal c.
c. pseudostricture
right c.
c. saw tooth sign
sigmoid c.
spastic c.
thumbprinting appearance of the c.
transverse c.
unused c.
c. whirl sign

colonic
c. activity
c. adenoma
c. adenomatous polyp
c. air
c. apple-core lesion
c. carcinoma
c. carpet lesion
c. dilatation
c. distention
c. diverticular hemorrhage
c. diverticulitis
c. diverticulosis
c. diverticulum
c. duplication cyst
c. evacuation
c. filling defect
c. fistula
c. flexure
c. gas composition
c. hamartomatous polyp
c. haustra
c. ileus
c. involvement of endometriosis
c. lead-pipe appearance
c. loop
c. motility
c. mucosal excretion
c. myenteric plexus
c. narrowing
c. necrosis
c. neoplasm
c. obstruction
c. perforation
c. pit
c. pseudoobstruction
c. saddle lesion
c. spasm
c. stricture
c. ulcer
c. urticaria pattern
c. varix
c. volvulus

NOTES

C

Colonlite
C. bowel preparation
Colonna hip fracture classification
colonography
computed tomographic c. (CTC)
CT c.
colonopathy
fibrosing c.
colonoscopic polypectomy
colonoscopy
virtual c.
coloproctitis
coloptosis
color
c. amplitude imaging
c. Doppler imaging (CDI)
c. Doppler recording
c. Doppler signal
c. Doppler ultrasound
c. duplex interrogation
c. duplex ultrasound
c. flow imaging (CFI)
c. gain
c. power transcranial Doppler sonography
c. power transcranial Doppler ultrasound
c. space conversion
c. space interpolation
c. space interpolator
color-coded
c.-c. duplex sonography
c.-c. duplex ultrasound
c.-c. pulmonary blood flow imaging
c.-c. real-time sonography
c.-c. real-time ultrasound
colorectal (CR)
c. adenoma
c. anastomosis
c. cancer
c. cancer endoscopy
c. carcinoid
c. carcinoma
c. duplication
c. hemorrhage
c. lymphoma
c. mucosa
c. polyp
color-flow
c.-f. Doppler (CFD)
c.-f. Doppler imaging
c.-f. Doppler real-time 2-D blood flow imaging
c.-f. Doppler sonography
c.-f. duplex imaging
c.-f. duplex scan
c.-f. imaging Doppler echocardiography
c.-f. mapping
colorimetric
c. color reproduction
c. test
ColorMark
coloscopy
endocervical canal c.
colosigmoid resection
colostomy
barium enema through c.
barium injection through c.
diverting c.
fecal diversion c.
colovaginal fistula
colovesical fistula
colpocele
colpocephaly
colpoptosis
colposcopy
colpostat applicator
column
anal c.
anterior gray c.
branchial efferent c.
c. of Burdach
Clarke c.
contrast medium c.
corrugated air c.
dye c.
extraction c.
c. extraction method
Gowers c.
head of barium c.
intermediolateral gray c.
Lissauer c.
c. mode sinogram image
c. of Morgagni
renal c.
thoracolumbar spine c.
variceal c.
vertebral c.
weighted spin-echo c.
columnar-lined esophagus
columnar metaphysis
columning of dye
columnization of contrast material
column-mode sinogram imaging
CoLyte bowel preparation
combination
c. chemotherapy
c. flow and pressure loads
combined
c. flexion-distraction injury and burst fracture
c. flexion phenomenon
c. leukocyte-marrow imaging

c. modality radiation therapy
c. multisection diffuse-weighted and hemodynamically weighted echoplanar MR
c. Myoscint/thallium imaging
c. pregnancy
c. radial-ulnar-humeral fracture
c. ^{99m}Tc-DMSA and ^{99m}Tc-DTPA scanning
c. thallium-Tc-HMPAO imaging

comb sign

comedo-basal cell carcinoma

comedocarcinoma

breast c.

comedomastitis

comet

c. tail

comet-tail

c.-t. artifact
c.-t. artifact gallbladder
c.-t. lung lesion sign
c.-t. sign

comitans

vena c., pl. venae comitantes

comma-shaped

c.-s. crus
c.-s. duodenum

comma tract of Schultze

commemorative sign

commencement of vessel

comminuted

c. bursting fracture
c. intraarticular fracture
c. teardrop fracture

Commission

Automic Energy C. (AEC)
Nuclear Regulatory C. (NRC)

commissural

c. attachment
c. chorda
c. function
c. leaflet
c. point

commissure

anterior c.
anterior commissure-posterior c. (AC-PC)
anteroseptal c.
cerebral c.
fused c.
gray c.
mitral valve c.
posterior c. (PC)
scalloped c.
tectum c.
valve c.
vestigial c.
white c.

Committee

Administration of Radioactive Substances Advisory C. (ARSAC)
C. of Radiation from Radioactive Medicinal Products (CRRMP)

common

c. atrioventricular canal
c. atrium
c. basal vein
c. bile duct (CBD)
c. bile duct bifurcation
c. bile duct diverticulum
c. bile duct exploration (CBDE)
c. bile duct obstruction
c. bile duct rat tail
c. bile duct spontaneous perforation
c. bile duct stone
c. bile duct stricture
c. bile duct target sign
c. bundle
c. cardinal vein
c. carotid artery (CCA)
c. carotid artery bifurcation
c. carotid plexus
c. cavity phenomenon
c. duct cholangiogram
c. duct dilatation
c. duct exploration
c. dural sac
c. extensor tendinosis
c. facial vein
c. femoral artery
c. gall duct
c. gateway interface (CGI)
c. hepatic artery
c. hepatic duct (CHD)
c. iliac artery
c. iliac lymph node
c. peroneal artery
c. pulmonary vein stenosis
c. synovial flexor sheath
c. tendinous ring
c. tendon

commotio cerebri

commune

centrum c.

NOTES

commune *(continued)*
mesenterium c.
persistent ostium atrioventriculare c.
communicating
c. artery
c. artery aneurysm
c. cavernous ectasia
c. fistula
c. hydrocephalus
c. syringomyelia
c. vein
c. vein incompetence
communication
asyndetic c.
cholangiovenous c.
interatrial c.
macrofistulous arteriovenous c.
medical ultrasound 3D portable, with advanced c. (MUSTPAC)
communis
extensor digitorum c. (EDC)
community-acquired pneumonia
Comolli sign
comorbid disease
compact
c. bone
c. island
companion
c. lymph node
c. shadow
c. vein
comparative value
comparison
beam quality c.
c. film
histopathologic c.
c. view
yield c.
compartment
anterior mediastinal c.
anterior tibial c.
deep posterior c.
DRUJ c.
distal radioulnar joint compartment
extensor c.
extracellular c.
extradural c.
extravascular c.
fifth c.
fourth c.
iliopsoas c.
infracolic c.
infratentorial c.
lateral c.
medial c.
midcarpal c.
patellofemoral c.
peribronchovascular interstitial c.
perirenal c.
plantar c.
posterior c.
posterolateral c.
posteromedial c.
radiocarpal c.
sixth c.
superficial posterior c.
supracolic c.
supramesocolic c.
c. syndrome
vascular c.
wrist extensor c.
compartmentalization
compartmental radioimmunoglobulin therapy
Compass
C. stereotactic frame
C. stereotactic frame system
compensated
c. composite spin-lock pulse
c. congestive heart failure
c. hydrocephalus
compensating filter
compensation
attenuation c.
cardiac gating c.
depth c.
flow c. (FC)
gradient c.
respiratory c.
scatter c.
second-order c.
section-select flow c.
supratentorial flow c.
time-gain c. (TGC)
compensator
multivane intensity modulation c. (MIMIC)
scattering foil c.
tissue deficit c.
compensatory
c. atrophy
c. capillary filling
c. circulation
c. deformity
c. emphysema
c. enlargement
c. enlargement of ventricle
c. hyperplasia
c. lobe hyperexpansion
c. nodular kidney hypertrophy
c. pause
competence of ureterovesical junction
competent ileocecal valve
competitive
c. adsorption
c. iron administration

complementary
c. hypertrophy
c. metal oxide semiconductor (CMOS)
complete
c. abortion
c. Achilles tendon rupture
c. atrioventricular block (CAVB)
c. atrioventricular dissociation
c. bladder emptying
c. bowel obstruction
c. congenital heart block
c. dislocation
c. duplication
c. fetal heart block
c. fracture
c. heart block (CHB)
c. lymphadenectomy
c. myelography
c. nerve lesion
c. occlusion
c. placenta previa
c. small bowel malrotation
c. stent expansion
c. transposition of great arteries
completed stroke
complex, pl. **complexes**
agyria pachygria c.
amygdaloid nuclear c.
ankle joint c.
c. anorectal fistula
anterior communicating artery c.
aperiodic c.
apical c.
arcuate c.
atrial c.
c. atrioventricular canal
auricular c.
biceps-labral c.
c. breast cyst
Buford c.
capsulolabral c.
caudal pharyngeal c.
choroidal-hippocampal fissure c.
complex blocking c.
compound dislocation c.
Dandy-Walker c.
diisocyanide-triisocyanide ^{99m}Tc c.
discoligamentous c.
Eisenmenger c.
epispadia exstrophy c.
c. extraperitoneal rupture
fabellofibular c.
fibrocartilage c.
foot-ankle c.
c. fracture
frontonasal dysplasia malformation c.
gadolinium c.
gallium-transferrin c.
gastrocnemius-soleus c.
gastroduodenal artery c.
Ghon c.
Ghon-Sachs c.
growth plate c.
hallux valgus-metatarsus primus varus c.
hindfoot joint c.
hippocampal-amygdaloid c.
hypoperfusion c.
hypovolemic c.
inferior glenohumeral ligament labral c. (IGLLC)
inverted-Y c.
Kirklin meniscal c.
labral capsular c.
labrum-ligament c.
c. lesion
ligamentous c.
limb-body wall c.
Lutembacher c.
mantle c.
c. mass
mastoid c.
medical collateral ligament c. (MCLC)
metal chelate c.
Michaelis c.
multiform ventricular c.
c. myxoma
nipple-areolar c.
ostiomeatal c.
outer annular/posterior longitudinal ligament c.
oxidized c.
pelvic mass c.
c. periosteal reaction
preintegration c.
primary c.
pulmonary sling c.
renal sinus c.
c. sclerosing lesion
sesamoid c.
shoulder labral capsular c.

NOTES

complex *(continued)*
c. simple fracture
sling ring c.
subluxation c.
superior olivary c.
syndesmotic ligament c.
tibiocalcaneal joint c.
transluminal coronary artery angioplasty c.
transposition c.
triangular fibrocartilaginous c. (TFCC)
VATER c.
ventricular premature c. (VPC)
vertebrobasilar c.
c. of vessels
VIII nerve c.
von Meyenburg c.

compliance
lung c.
c. randomized trial
reduced pulmonary c.

complicated
c. dislocation
c. fracture
c. pneumoconiosis
c. renal cyst
c. silicosis

component
anatomically graduated c. (AGC)
bottoming out of prosthetic c.
central hemorrhagic c.
dispersive c.
extensive intraductal c. (EIC)
extracellular matrix c.
frequency c.
keel of glenoid c.
markedly accentuated pulmonic c.
mitral c.
obstructive c.
secretory c.

composite
c. aortic valve
c. fracture
c. pulse
c. signal

composition
colonic gas c.
hydropic c.
renal stone mineral c.

compound
c. aneurysm
c. dislocation
c. dislocation complex
c. pregnancy
c. presentation
radiolabeled c.
c. skull fracture
thorium c.
titanium c.

compounding sterility test

compressed body

compression
aqueduct c.
c. atrophy
brachial artery c.
brachial plexus c.
brainstem c.
c. of breast
cardiac c.
cauda equina c.
chamber c.
chiasmal c.
coned-down spot c.
contrecoup c.
cord c.
c. device
external pneumatic calf c.
extrinsic bladder c.
fingerprint image c.
c. flexion injury
c. fracture
c. fracture of atlas
image c.
interfragmental c.
intrinsic c.
irreversible c.
magnification and spot c.
manual c.
multiplanar c.
nerve root c.
c. neuropathy
neurovascular c.
optic nerve c.
orbital mass c.
c. paddle
plaque c.
c. plate
c. plate and screw
radicular c.
c. ratio
root c.
c. sonography
spinal cord c.
spot c.
subchondral trabecular c.
symptomatic metastatic spinal cord c.
c. syndrome
thermal c.
c. ultrasonography
vascular esophageal c.
vascular tracheal c.
wavelet c.

compressive
c. atelectasis

c. edema
c. hyperextension injury
compromise
circulatory c.
respiratory c.
vascular c.
compromised
c. flow
c. respiratory status
c. ventricular function
Compton
C. coherent scattering densitometry
C. effect
C. electrons
C. scattering
C. scattering cross-section
C. scattering photons
C. suppression spectrometer
C. suppression spectrometry
C. wavelength
Compton-suppression system
Compuscan
C. Hittman computerized electrocardioscanner
C. Hittman computerized imaging
computed
c. ejection fraction
c. radiography (CR)
c. radiology (CR)
c. tomographic angiography (CTA)
c. tomographic bubble sign
c. tomographic colonography (CTC)
c. tomographic laser mammography
c. tomography (CT)
c. tomography angiographic portography (CTAP)
c. tomography arterial portography (CTAP)
c. tomography dose index (CTDI)
c. tomography scan (CT scan)
c. transmission tomography
c. transmission tomography imaging
computer
Aspect c.
Digitron DVI/DSA c.
c. method
c. subtraction technique
computer-aided
c.-a. diagnosis scheme
c.-a. diagnostics (CAD)
computer-assisted
c.-a. blood background subtraction (CABBS)
c.-a. intracranial navigation
c.-a. stereotactic resection
c.-a. volumetric stereotaxis
computer-controlled conformal radiation therapy (CCRT)
computer-generated
c.-g. artifact
c.-g. image
computerized
c. axial tomography (CAT)
c. cranial tomography
c. optical densitometry (COD)
C. Thermal Imaging system
c. tomographic hepatic angiography (CTHA)
c. tomographic holography (CTH)
c. tomography guidance
c. tomography-guided needle biopsy
c. transverse axial tomography (CTAT, CTAT imaging)
conal
c. cyst
c. papillary muscle
c. septum
c. ventricular septal defect
concatenation of shadows
Concato disease
concavity
concavoconvex
concealed
c. bypass tract
c. hemorrhage
c. penis
concentrated bile
concentration
hypertensive contrast c.
maximum permissible c.
methylene diphosphonate (MDP) c.
organ-specific c.
Poisson distributed activity c.
c. of radionuclide
synaptic dopamine c.
c. times time (C x T)
concentration-time curve
concentric
c. atherosclerotic plaque
c. contraction
c. fibroma
c. heart hypertrophy

NOTES

concentric *(continued)*
c. hernia
c. herniation
c. hourglass stenosis
c. hypertrophic cardiomyopathy
c. lamella
c. lesion
c. narrowing
c. reduction
concept
gooseneck c.
line integral c.
no-threshold c.
conception
retained products of c.
concha, pl. **conchae**
c. bullosa
nasal c.
conchal
c. cartilage
c. crest
concomitant
c. boost radiation therapy
c. chemoirradiation
c. defect
c. finding
c. infarct
c. pneumonia
c. tracheal injury
concordance
situs c.
concordant result
concretion
bile c.
fecal c.
concussion
brain c.
spinal c.
condensans
clavicular osteitis c.
conditioned reflex (CR)
conductance catheter
conducting bronchiole
conduction
c. block
interval intraatrial c.
nodal c.
c. ratio
reciprocating c.
retrograde ventriculoatrial c.
ventriculoatrial c.
zone of slow c. (ZSC)
conductive
c. development
c. hearing loss
c. loop
conductivity
tissue c.
vascular hydraulic c.
conductor
fiberoptic c.
c. resistivity
conduit
detour c.
ileal c.
intestinal c.
nonvalved c.
right ventricle-pulmonary artery c.
urinary c.
c. valve
valve c.
ventriculoarterial c.
condylar
c. angle
c. articulation
c. canal
c. emissary vein
c. flare
c. fossa
c. plate
c. skull hypoplasia
c. split fracture
c. translation
condyle
c. cord
external c.
femoral c.
lateral c.
mandibular c.
medial c.
occipital c.
tibial c.
condyloid
c. canal
c. joint
c. process
condyloma, pl. **condylomata**
c. urethra acuminata
condylus tertius
cone
arterial c.
c. beam
beveled electron beam c.
c. disk
c. epiphysis
medullary c.
parenchymal c.
transvaginal c.
c. of vignetting
cone-and-socket bone
cone-beam
c.-b. image
c.-b. reconstruction algorithm

coned
c. cecum
c. down
coned-down
c.-d. appearance of colon
c.-d. spot compression
c.-d. view
CO_2-negative imaging agent
confidence limit
configuration
back-to-back c.
batwing c.
beaklike c.
bilobed c.
biventricular c.
butterfly c.
cardiac silhouette snowman c.
cat's tail c.
closed-fist c.
cylindrical c.
dome-and-dart c.
double-halo c.
expansile c.
fishmouth mitral valve c.
geriatric c.
globular c.
Helmholtz c.
horizontal dipole c.
horseshoe c.
hourglass c.
inverted-Y c.
isosceles triangular c.
left ventricular c.
lock-washer c.
masslike c.
molar tooth c.
multilobular c.
reverse 3 c.
ringlike c.
rosary bead c.
sandwich c.
sawtooth c.
scalloped luminal c.
shepherd's crook c.
sigmoid-shaped c.
snowman heart c.
stellate c.
streak-like c.
surface c.
swallow-tail c.
tentorium keyhole c.
thoracic cage c.
tombstone pelvis c.
triple-peak cerebellum c.
unidurectional lead c.
water bottle heart c.
winged c.
wooden shoe c.
confinement
regional tumor c.
confluence
pulmonary c.
stellate c.
c. of vascular markings
confluens sinuum
confluent
c. areas of atelectasis
c. consolidation
c. fibrosis
c. infiltrate
confocal image
conformal
c. neutron and photon radiation therapy
c. radiation therapy (CRT)
congenita
amyotonia c.
arthrogryposis multiplex c.
chondrodystrophia calcificans c.
congenital
c. abnormality
c. absence of kidney
c. absence of pain
c. absence of pulmonary artery
c. absence of pulmonary valve
c. absence of thymus
c. adrenal hyperplasia (CAH)
c. adrenogenital syndrome
c. amputation
c. aneurysm of pulmonary artery
c. anomaly of mitral valve (CAMV)
c. aortic regurgitation
c. aortic sinus aneurysm
c. aortic valve stenosis
c. arteriosclerotic aneurysm
c. atelectasis
c. bar
c. biliary atresia
c. bipartite scaphoid
c. bronchiectasis
c. bronchogenic cyst
c. cardiac anomaly
c. cardiac tumor

NOTES

congenital *(continued)*
c. cerebral aneurysm
c. cholesteatoma
c. complete heart block
c. conotruncal anomaly
c. convex pes valgus
c. cystic adenomatoid malformation (CCAM)
c. cystic dilatation
c. cystic lesion of neck
c. cystic neck lesion
c. deformity
c. diaphragmatic hernia
c. diffuse fibromatosis
c. dilated cardiomyopathy
c. dislocation of hip (CDH)
c. disorder
c. duodenal obstruction
c. dysplasia of hip (CDH)
c. esophageal stenosis
c. Finnish nephrosis
c. fracture
c. gallbladder anomaly
c. generalized fibromatosis
c. glaucoma
c. goiter
c. heart block
c. heart defect (CHD)
c. heart disease (CHD)
c. heart disease classification
c. heart disease syndrome
c. heart malformation
c. hemiplegia
c. hepatic cyst
c. hepatic fibrosis (CHF)
c. hip dislocation
c. hip dysplasia
c. hippocampal sclerosis
c. hydrocele
c. hydrocephalus
c. hydronephrosis
c. insensitivity to pain
c. interruption of aortic arch
c. intestinal atresia
c. intracranial aneurysm
c. isthmic coarctation
c. kidney fibrosarcoma
c. laryngeal atresia
c. laxity of ligament
c. left-sided outflow obstruction
c. left ventricular aneurysm
c. liver fibrosis
c. lobar emphysema
c. lymphangiectasia
c. lymphangiectasia of intestine
c. lymphangiectasia lung
c. megacalix
c. megacolon
c. mesoblastic nephroma
c. mitral regurgitation (CMR)
c. mitral stenosis
c. muscular dystrophy
c. nasal mass
c. pancreatic anomaly
c. pericardial absence
c. pneumothorax
c. polyvalvular dysplasia
c. primary megaureter
c. pulmonary arteriovenous fistula
c. pulmonary artery aneurysm
c. pulmonary valve insufficiency
c. pulmonary venolobar syndrome
c. radioulnar synostosis
c. renal aneurysm
c. renal hypoplasia
c. renal osteodystrophy
c. ring
c. rubella pneumonitis
c. splenomegaly
c. stenosis of pulmonary vein
c. stippled epiphysis
c. subglottic stenosis
c. subpulmonic obstruction
c. subvalvular stenosis
c. symptomatic AV block
c. thyroid dyshormonogenesis
c. tracheobiliary fistula
c. tracheomalacia
c. urethral diverticulum
c. urethral stricture
c. valvular stenosis
c. vascular-bone syndrome (CVBS)
c. vascular malformation (CVM)
c. vertical talus
c. vesicoureteral reflux

congenitally
c. absent pericardium
c. corrected transposition
c. short esophagus

congested
c. kidney
c. pleura

congestion
active c.
asymmetric pulmonary c.
capillary c.
cardiac c.
centrilobular c.
cerebral c.
chronic passive c.
hepatic c.
hypostatic c.
c. index
intravascular c.
passive hepatic c.
passive vascular c.

pulmonary vascular c.
pulmonary venous c. (PVC)
splenic c.
symmetric pulmonary c.
vascular c.
venous heart c.

congestive
c. asymmetry
c. atelectasis
c. brain swelling
c. cardiomyopathy
c. cirrhosis
c. heart failure (CHF)
c. splenomegaly

conglomerate
c. calcification

conglutinating complement absorption test

congo
c. red
c. red test

congruence, congruency, congruity
c. angle
patellofemoral c.

congruent
c. articulation
c. point
c. reduction

conical
c. heart
c. mass

conjoined
c. cusp
c. nerve root anomaly
c. tendon
c. twins

conjugal cancer

conjugate
c. diameter
c. foramen
c. gradient
c. ligament
c. overshooting

conjunctival vein

conjunctivum
brachium c.

connecting
c. canal
c. cartilage
c. plate
c. tubule

connection
anomalous pulmonary venous c.
atrioventricular c.
corticocerebellar c.
partial anomalous pulmonary venous c.
partial pulmonary venous c.
rostral c.
slip-in c.
total anomalous pulmonary venous c.
total pulmonary venous c.
ventriculoarterial c.
wispy c.

connective
c. tissue
c. tissue disease
c. tissue fibrous tumor
c. tissue neoplasm
c. tissue proliferation
c. tissue septum

connector
cerebral ventricular shunt c.

conniventes
valvulae c.

Conn syndrome

conoid
c. ligament
c. process
c. tubercle

conotruncal congenital anomaly

conoventricular defect

Conrad-Bugg trapping of soft tissue in ankle fracture

Conrad-Crosby bone marrow biopsy needle

Conradi-Hünermann syndrome

Conradi line

Conray
C. 30, 43, 60, 280, 325, 400 imaging agent

consecutive dislocation

conservation surgery

console
Bruker c.
direct display c. (DDC)
Siemens Satellite CT evaluation c.

consolidated
c. infiltrate
c. lung

consolidation
air-space c.

NOTES

consolidation *(continued)*
alveolar c.
batwing lung c.
bilateral c.
confluent c.
dense c.
exudative c.
fracture line of c.
hemorrhage c.
ill-defined c.
lobar c.
lung parenchyma c.
nonhomogeneous c.
parenchymal c.
patchy air-space c.
peripheral c.
pulmonary c.
segmental bronchus c.
unilateral c.
consolidative
c. change
c. pneumonia
c. process
conspicuity
constant
air-kerma rate c.
decay c.
disintegration c.
equilibrium dissociation c.
equilibrium dose c.
maximum amplitude c.
radioactive c. (Λ)
c. tilt wave
time c.
transformation c.
T2 time c.
constellation
c. of findings
c. of symptoms
constituent
plaque c.
constitution
eunuchoid c.
constitutional
c. osteosclerosis
c. symptoms
constricting esophageal lesion
constriction
airway c.
c. band
c. band syndrome
ductal c.
hourglass c.
occult pericardial c.
postglomerular arteriolar c.
c. ring
supraannular c.
tangential c.
waistlike c.
constrictive
c. bronchiolitis
c. cardiomyopathy
c. pericarditis
construction artifact
consumption
cerebral metabolic oxygen c.
myocardial oxygen c.
oxygen c. (QO_2)
contact
bone-on-bone c.
c. B-scan ultrasound
c. cancer
catheter-tissue c.
c. effect
c. lateral view
poor screen/film c.
screen-film c.
stent-vessel wall c.
contained
c. aneurysmal rupture
c. aortic rupture
c. disk
c. leak
c. leak of aortic aneurysm
content
abdominal c.'s
bone mineral c. (BMC)
bowel c.'s
brain water c.'s
digestive tract c.'s
disk water c.
femoral triangular c.
gastric c.'s
herniated abdominal c.'s
intestinal c.'s
intravascular c.'s
macromolecular c.
overlying bowel c.
small bowel c.'s
tissue water c.
venous oxygen c.
contiguous
c. articular surfaces
c. image
c. loop
c. organ involvement
c. segment
c. slices
c. supramarginal gyrus
c. ventricular septal defect
continuation
azygos c.
interruption of inferior vena cava with azygos/hemiazygos c.

continuity
aortoseptal c.
c. of bone
bowel c.
pancreatic-enteric c.
continuous
c. capillary
c. diaphragm sign
c. hyperfractionated accelerated radiation therapy (CHART)
c. hyperfractionated accelerated radiotherapy (CHAR)
c. hyperthermic peritoneal perfusion
c. imaging (CI)
c. intravenous infusion (CIVI)
c. intravenous infusion chemotherapy
c. microinfusion device
c. mode
c. positive airway pressure (CPAP)
c. volumetric acquisition
c. wave (CW)
continuous-loop exercise echocardiography
continuous-wave
c.-w. (CW) Doppler ultrasonography
c.-w. Doppler
c.-w. Doppler echocardiography
c.-w. Doppler imaging
c.-w. Doppler recording
c.-w. laser system
c.-w. NMR
continuous-wave, high-frequency Doppler ultrasound system
contortus
pes c.
contour
convex outward c.
cupid's bow c.
diaphragmatic c.
double-diaphragm c.
c. extraction
irregular hazy luminal c.
isodose c.
lobulated c.
local bulge of kidney c.
local bulge renal c.
C. mammography system
c. mapping
patellar c.
reniform c.
S c.
sawtooth irregularity of bowel c.
scalloping c.
c. tilting compression mammography system
undulating c.
contoured
c. adduction trochanteric-controlled alignment method (CAT-CAM conversion, CAT-CAM)
c. tilting compression mammography
contour-following algorithm
contracted
c. bladder
c. bronchus
c. gallbladder
c. kidney
c. pelvis
contractile
c. function
c. pattern
c. reserve
c. ring dysphagia
c. stricture
c. work index
contractility
cardiac c.
c. index
myocardial c.
contraction
c. band necrosis
concentric c.
esophageal c.
kissing c.'s
nodal premature c.
peristaltic c.
phasic c.
premature nodal c. (PNC)
premature ventricular c. (PVC)
ringlike c.
c. stress test (CST)
uterine c.
ventricular premature c. (VPC)
ventricular segmental c.
contracture
bladder neck c.
capsular c.
c. deformity
Dupuytren c.
elbow c.
fixed flexion c.

NOTES

contracture *(continued)*
flexion c.
flexion-adduction c.
gastrocnemius/soleus c.
hip flexion c.
ischemic c.
joint c.
knee flexion c.
muscle c.
myocardial c.
myostatic c.
scar c.
secondary c.
soft tissue c.
Volkmann ischemic c.
web c.
contralateral
c. kidney
c. sign
c. vessel
contrast (*See* agent, material, medium)
c. administration
c. agent
c. angiography
c. aortography
c. arteriography
baby formula with ferrous sulfate c.
barium enema with air c.
blood oxygenation level-dependent c.
c. bolus
c. computed arthrotomography
CT scan with c.
dynamic susceptibility c. (DSC)
echo c.
c. enema
c. enhancement
c. esophagogram
extravasated c.
c. extravasation
ferric chloride c.
ferrioxamine methanesulfonate c.
Gd-DTPA with mannitol c.
image c.
c. inhomogeneity
c. injection
intraarticular c.
isoosmolar c.
c. laryngography
c. left atriography
c. loading
lymphangiographic c.
c. lymphangiography
magnetite albumin c.
magnetization transfer c. (MTC)
c. material
c. material instillation
c. media excretion
c. media leakage
c. media nephrotoxicity
c. medium
c. medium column
mineral oil c.
near-resonance spin-lock c.
c. nephropathy
nephropathy c.
nonionic iodinated c.
Nycomed c.
c. opacification
paramagnetic c.
phase c.
precipitated c.
c. precipitation
puddling of c.
purified water c.
radiographic c.
recent lymphangiographic c.
c. resolution
c. selective cholangiogram
c. sensitivity
short scale c.
spontaneous echo c.
subject c.
sucrose polyester c.
time to peak c. (TPC)
tissue c.
c. transfer characteristic
c. uptake
c. venography
c. ventriculogram
contrast-enhanced
c.-e. color Doppler
c.-e. computed tomography (CECT)
c.-e. CT
c.-e. dynamic snapshot
c.-e. echocardiography
c.-e. FAST
c.-e. fast-acquisition in a steady state (CE-FAST)
c.-e. imaging
c.-e. MR
c.-e. MR image
c.-e. power Doppler
c.-e. radiographic examination
c.-e. ultrasound
contrast-filled stomach
contrast-improvement factor
contrast-induced renal failure
contrast-to-noise
c.-t.-n. calculation
c.-t.-n. ratio (C/N)
contrecoup
c. compression
c. fracture

c. injury
c. mechanism
control
automatic exposure c. (AEC)
dynamic range c. (DRC)
fluoroscopic c.
image c.
locoregional c.
radiofrequency radiographic c.
radiographic c.
radiopharmaceutical quality c.
roentgenographic c.
scintigraphy quality c.
SPECT quality c.
Spli-Prest negative c.
Spli-Prest positive c.
time-varied gain c.
controlled ventricular response
controller
IMED Gemini PC-2 volumetric c.
contusio cerebri
contusion
bony c.
brain c.
cerebral c.
frontal lobe c.
lung c.
myocardial c.
osseous bone c.
c. pneumonia
pontine c.
pulmonary c.
rib c.
soft tissue c.
urinary bladder c.
conus
c. arteriosus medullaris
c. artery
c. branch ostia
c. clasticus
club-shaped c.
c. elasticus
c. eye
c. ligament
c. medullaris
c. medullaris lesion
c. medullaris position
c. septum
conventional
c. osteosarcoma
c. planar imaging (CPI)
c. pulse sequence
c. study
c. tomography
c. venography
conventionally fractionated stereotactic radiation therapy
convergence zone
convergent
c. beam irradiation (CBI)
c. color Doppler imaging
converging collimator
conversion
CAT-CAM c.
contoured adduction trochanteric-controlled alignment method
coefficient c.
color space c.
c. defect
c. efficiency
c. electron
fatty marrow endplate c.
c. ratio
spontaneous c.
thoracofemoral c.
converter
analog scan c.
analog-to-digital c.
digital scan c.
digital-to-analog c. (DAC)
motion-compensating format c.
multiplying digital-to-analog c. (MDAC)
real-time format c.
scan c.
convex
c. border of stomach
c. linear array
c. margin
c. outward contour
convexity
cerebral c.
frontocentral c.
c. meningioma
parietal c.
convexobasia
convexoconcave (C-C)
c. heart valve
convoluted
c. bone
c. T-cell lymphoma
c. tubule
convolution
Arnold c.

NOTES

convolution *(continued)*
ascending frontal c.
ascending parietal c.
Broca c.
cerebral c.
Gratiolet c.
Heschl c.
c. mask
occipitotemporal c.
Zuckerkandl c.
convolutional
c. impression
c. markings
c. pattern
Cookey-Tukey algorithm
Coolidge transformer
Coombs test
Cooper
C. droop
C. suspensory ligament
Coopernail sign
coordinate axis
coordinates for target lesion
coordination
meniscocondylar c.
COP
colloid oncotic pressure
COPD
chronic obstructive pulmonary disease
emphysematous COPD
Cope
C. biopsy needle
C. loop
C. method bronchogram
C. point
Copeland-Kavat metatarsophalangeal dislocation classification
coplanar
c. beam
c. contour point
copper (Cu)
c. (Cu) imaging agent
c. filtration
c. 7 intrauterine device
c. T intrauterine device
c. wire effect
copper-64 (^{64}Cu)
copper-67 (^{67}Cu)
copper-zinc (Cu/Zn)
c.-z. superoxide dismutase (Cu/Zn-SOD)
c.-z. superoxide dismutase imaging agent (Cu/Zn-SOD imaging agent)
coprecipitation
coprolith
coprostasis
cor
c. adiposum
c. arteriosum
c. biloculare
c. bovinum
c. dextrum
c. en cuirasse
c. mobile
c. pendulum
c. pulmonale
c. triatriatum
coracoacromial
c. arch
c. ligament
c. process
coracobrachialis
coracoclavicular
c. bar
c. joint
c. ligament
c. space
coracohumeral ligament
coracoid
c. fracture
c. notch
c. process
c. tip avulsion
c. tuberosity
coral
c. reef atheroma
c. thrombus
Corbin technique
cord
c. angioblastoma
anterior gray column of c.
anterior horns of spinal c.
anterolateral white matter of c.
c. astrocytoma
astrocytoma c.
c. atrophy
cervical c.
c. compression
condyle c.
dura mater of spinal c.
c. embarrassment
ependymoma c.
c. epidural extramedullary lesion
false vocal c.
fibrous c.
hemisection of spinal c.
hepatic c.
c. intradural extramedullary mass
c. intramedullary lesion
Lissauer tracts of spinal c.
medullary c.
meninges of spinal c.
mucoid degeneration of umbilical c.
multiple focal lesions of spinal c.
noncoiled umbilical c.

nuchal c.
posterior gray column of c.
c. presentation
pretendinous c.
c. prolapse
prolapse of umbilical c.
reactive cyst c.
ropelike c.
rostral spinal c.
c. sign
size of spinal c.
spermatic c.
spinal c.
split spinal c.
straight c.
c. structure
tethered spinal c.
thoracic spinal c.
three-vessel umbilical c.
transsection of spinal c.
true vocal c.
two-vessel umbilical c.
umbilical c.
velamentous insertion of c.
vocal c.
Weitbrecht c.
white commissure of spinal c.

cordate pelvis

cordiform pelvis

cordis
apex c.
atrium dextrum c.
atrium sinistrum c.
chordae tendineae c.
crux c.
ectopia c.
C. endovascular system
fetal ectopia c.
fossa ovalis c.
C. injector
C. multipurpose access port
C. sheath
ventriculus c.

cordlike
c. mass
c. trunk

cordocentesis
therapeutic c.

Cordonnier ureteroileal loop

cordotomy

corduroy
c. artery
c. artifact
c. cloth pattern

core
c. biopsy needle
bone c.
fibrovascular c.
c. needle biopsy

coregistration
morphological and physiological image c.

Corgonject

cork handler's lung disease

corkscrew
c. appearance
c. appearance of the esophagus
c. appearance of hepatic artery
c. appearance of small bowel
c. pattern
c. ureter
c. vessel

corn
apical c.
c. oil and ferric ammonium citrate imaging agent

corneal
c. facet
c. tube

Cornell protocol

corner
c. film
c. fracture
c. of knee
c. sign of Parke

cornflake esophageal motility study

corniculate
c. cartilage
c. tubercle

corniculopharyngeal ligament

cornu, pl. **cornua**
c. of sacrum
c. of uterus

cornual ectopic pregnancy

corona, pl. **coronae, coronas**
c. radiata

coronal
c. angulation
c. bending view
c. cleft
c. cleft vertebra

NOTES

coronal *(continued)*
c. computed tomographic arthrography (CCTA)
c. GRE MR image
c. maximum-intensity projection (MIPcor)
c. oblique technique
c. orientation
c. planar image
c. plane
c. reconstruction
c. reconstruction view
c. scan
c. section
c. slab
c. slice
c. suture
c. synostosis
c. view
coronary
c. angiography
c. arteriography
c. arteriosclerosis
c. arteriosystemic fistula
c. arteriovenous fistula
c. artery
c. artery aneurysm
c. artery bypass graft
c. artery bypass graft patency
c. artery calcification
c. artery cameral fistula
c. artery disease
c. artery dominance
c. artery ectasia
c. artery embolus
c. artery of heart
c. artery lesion
c. artery malformation
c. artery ostium
c. artery-pulmonary artery fistula
c. artery to right ventricular fistula
c. artery scan (CAS)
c. artery scan imaging
c. artery spasm (CAS)
c. artery steal
c. artery steal syndrome
c. artery stenosis
c. artery of stomach
c. artery tree
c. atherosclerosis
c. band
c. blood flow
c. blood flow velocity (CBFV)
c. bone
c. cineangiography
c. cusp
c. flow reserve (CFR)
c. groove
c. heart disease (CHD)
c. insufficiency
c. ischemia
c. ligament
c. luminal stenosis
c. maximum-intensity projection (MIPcor)
c. node
c. occlusion
c. orifice
c. ostial revascularization
c. ostial stenosis
c. perfusion gradient
c. perfusion pressure
c. plexus
proximal c. (PCS)
c. reserve flow (CRF)
c. sclerosis
c. sinus (CS)
c. sinus os
c. sinus ostium
c. sinus retroperfusion
c. sinus root
c. sinus of Valsalva
c. sinus valve
c. steal phenomenon
c. stenosis index (CSI)
c. sulcus
c. tendon
c. thrombosis (CT)
c. vascular resistance
c. vascular resistance index (CVRI)
c. vein
c. vessel anatomy
c. vessel aneurysm
c. vessel geometry
c. wedge pressure
coronary-subclavian steal syndrome
coronas (*pl. of* corona)
coronoid
c. fossa
c. process
c. process fracture
coronory artery anatomy
Coroskop C cardiac imaging system
corporis
uncus c.
corpus, pl. **corpora**
c. albicans cyst
anterior c.
c. callosum
c. callosum agenesis
c. callosum dysgenesis
c. callosum lipoma
c. callosum ring-enhancing lesion
c. carcinoma
corpora cavernosa penis
corpora cavernosography

c. cavernosonography imaging
corpora fornicis
c. hemorrhagicum
c. luteum cyst
c. luteum hematoma
c. Luysii
corpora restiformia
c. spongiosum
c. spongiosum penis
c. sterni
c. striatum
c. uteri
c. uterus

corpuscular radiation

corrected
c. sinus node recovery time
c. transposition of great arteries

correction
accidental c.
adaptive c.
attenuation c.
automatic motion c.
coincidence-summing c.
degree of c.
fuzzy logic contrast c.
inhomogeneity c.
multiilluminant color c.
Picker SPECT attenuation c.
scatter c.
summing c.
surface variable-attenuation c.
trend c.

correlation (CR)
c. algorithm (CR)
clinical c.
false-negative c.
functional c.
histologic c.
histopathologic CT c.
imaging-anatomic c.
imaging-pathologic c.
mammographic-histopathologic c.
morphological c.
pathologic c.
radiologic-anatomic c.
radiologic-pathologic c.
in vivo c.

correlative
c. diagnostic imaging
c. Doppler study

Correra line

Corrigan
C. pneumonia
C. sign

corrosive
c. esophagitis
c. gastritis

corrugated
c. air column
c. fat-pad surface

Cortenema retention enema

cortex, pl. **cortices**
adrenal c.
articular c.
auditory c.
bilateral orbital frontal c.
bone c.
calcarine c.
cerebellar c.
cerebral c.
c. of cerebrum
entorhinal c.
femoral c.
frontal c.
increased renal echogenicity c.
inner adrenal c.
lymphatic c.
mesial-frontal c.
motor c.
nonolfactory c.
opercular c.
orbitofrontal c.
ovarian c.
parastriate c.
parietal c.
patchy atrophy of renal c.
perirolandic parietal c.
peristriate c.
perisylvian c.
piriform c.
postrolandic parietal c.
premotor c.
primary auditory c.
primary visual c.
pyramidal layer of cerebral c.
rarefaction of c.
renal c.
renin-angiotensin-dependent outer c.
rolandic c.
sensorimotor c.
somatosensory c.
striate c.
visual c.

NOTES

Corti
- C. canal
- C. organ

cortical
- c. abrasion
- c. activity
- c. adenoma
- c. artery
- c. atrophy
- c. blush
- c. bone
- c. bone infarct
- c. bone lesion
- c. bone resorption
- c. branch
- c. center
- c. cerebellar degeneration
- c. defect
- c. deficit
- c. desmoid
- c. destruction
- c. dysfunction
- c. flattening
- c. fracture
- c. fragment
- c. gray matter
- c. hinge axis
- c. hyperintensity
- c. hyperostosis
- c. hypointensity
- c. intracerebral hemorrhage
- c. ischemia
- c. kidney arch
- c. kidney arteriography
- c. kidney necrosis
- c. margin
- c. motor area
- c. nephrocalcinosis
- c. nodular hyperplasia
- c. nodule
- c. notching
- c. osteoid osteoma
- c. plate
- c. renal cyst
- c. renal cyst syndrome
- c. rim nephrogram
- c. rim sign
- c. scarring of kidney
- c. scintigraphy
- c. signet ring shadow
- c. sulcus
- c. thinning
- c. thumb
- c. tissue
- c. transgression
- c. tuber
- c. vein
- c. vein sign
- c. vein thrombosis
- c. white matter
- c. window

corticale
- cryptostroma c.

corticated border

cortices (*pl. of* cortex)

corticobasal ganglionic degeneration

corticobulbar tract (CBT)

corticocallosal dysgenesis

corticocancellous
- c. bone
- c. bone chip
- c. strut

corticocerebellar connection

corticogram

corticography

corticomedullary
- c. differentiation (CMD)
- c. junction
- c. phase

corticopontine tract

corticorubral tract

corticospinal
- c. motor pathway
- c. pathway lesion
- c. tract (CST)
- c. tract sign

corticosteroid-induced osteoporosis

corticostriatospinal degeneration

corticotectal tract

cortisol-producing carcinoma

corundum smelter's lung

Corvisart syndrome

cosine transform

costa, pl. **costae**
- capitulum costae
- c. fluctuans decima
- c. retraction
- costae spuriae
- costae verae

costal
- c. angle
- c. bone
- c. cartilage
- c. cartilage calcification
- c. facet
- c. groove
- c. intraarticular cartilage
- c. margin
- c. margin syndrome
- c. notch
- c. osteoma
- c. pit
- c. pleura
- c. pleurisy
- c. process
- c. sulcus

c. surface
c. tubercle
c. tuberosity
costoaxillary vein
costocervical
c. artery
c. trunk
costochondral
c. joint
c. junction
c. junction separation
costochondritis
costoclavicular
c. ligament
c. line
c. maneuver
c. syndrome
c. test
costocolic
c. fold
c. ligament
costodiaphragmatic
c. margin
c. recess
c. recess of pleura
costolateral
costolumbar angle
costomediastinal
c. recess
c. sinus
costophrenic
c. angle
c. angle blunting
c. recess
c. septal line
c. sulcus
costosternal angle
costotransverse
c. foramen
c. joint
c. ligament
costovertebral
c. angle (CVA)
c. articulation
c. joint
costoxiphoid ligament
COSY H-1 MR spectroscopy
Cotrel-Dubousset system
cottage
c. loaf appearance
c. loaf deformity
Cotton
C. ankle fracture
cotton-ball appearance
Cotton-Berg syndrome
cotton fiber embolus
cotton-wool
c.-w. appearance
c.-w. spot
Cotunnius
C. canal
C. space
cotyloid
c. cavity
c. ligament
c. notch
couch view
cough
c. fracture of rib
c. resonance
coughing
c. sign
c. spasm
Couinaud classification
coulomb (C)
c. force
C. law
count
Cerenkov c.
Colombo c.
c. density
direct liquid scintillation c.
filament-nonfilament c.
lamellar body density (LBD) c.
counter
boron c.
Cerenkov c.
event c.
gamma-ray c.
gamma well c.
Geiger c.
Geiger-Müller c.
ionization c.
proportional c.
scintillation c.
well c.
whole-body c.
countercurrent
c. aortography
c. flow-related enhancement
counteroccluder
counterpulsation
balloon c.

NOTES

counterpulsation *(continued)*
diastolic c.
intraaortic balloon c.
mechanical c.
percutaneous intraaortic balloon c. (PIBC)
counterstimulation
counting
double-label c.
counts per second
couplet
ventricular premature contraction c.
coupling
dipole c.
dipole-dipole c.
dynamic c.
electric quadrupole c.
c. exchange
hyperfine c.
magnetic dipole-dipole c.
scalar c.
spin c.
spin-spin c.
static c.
Cournand arteriography needle
Cournand-Grino angiography needle
course
c. of artery
midlateral c.
relapsing c.
remitting c.
signal time c.
undulating c.
coursing of gas
Courvoisier
C. gallbladder
C. law
C. phenomenon
C. sign
Couvelaire uterus
covitary tuberculosis
cow
radioactive c.
cowhorn deformity
Cowley syndrome
cowl-shaped obstruction
Cowper
C. gland lesion
C. ligament
coxa, pl. **coxae**
c. adducta
c. brevis
c. flexa
c. magna
os coxae
c. plana
c. saltans
c. senilis
c. valga
c. valga deformity
c. vara
c. vara deformity
c. vara luxans
coxal bone
coxarthropathy
Postel destructive c.
coxitis fugax
Coyle trauma position
CP
Carr-Purcell
CPA
cerebellopontine angle
CPAD
chronic peripheral arterial disease
CPAP
continuous positive airway pressure
CPD
cephalopelvic disproportion
CPI
conventional planar imaging
cpm
cycles per minute
CPMG
Carr-Purcell-Meiboom-Gill
CPMG sequence
CPP
CPPD
calcium pyrophosphate deposition disease
CPPD arthritis of the hand
cps
cycles per second
CP sequence
CPT-11
CR
central ray
colorectal
computed radiography
computed radiology
conditioned reflex
correlation
correlation algorithm
crown-rump length
CR103
OncoScint C.
CR835
Cr
chromium
CR-39 nuclear tract detector
crabmeat-like appearance
crack
c. fracture
hairline c.
cracked-pot resonance
cracker
LeVeen plaque c.
plaque c.

cradle
alpha c.
CT scan c.
Spectrum DG-P pediatric c.
Cragg thrombolytic brush
Cramer-Rao minimum variance bound (CR-MVB)
Crampton
C. line
C. muscle
crania (*pl. of* cranium)
cranial
c. aneurysm
c. angled view
c. angulation
c. anomaly
c. base
c. bone
c. bone fixation plate
c. capacity
c. cavity
c. computed tomography (CCT)
c. flexure
c. fontanelle
c. foramen
c. fossa
c. granulomatous arteritis
c. irradiation
c. meningocele
c. nerve
c. nerve involvement
c. nerve neoplasm
c. nerve sign
c. nucleus
c. osteopetrosis
c. ridge
c. root
c. sinus
c. suture
c. ultrasound
c. vault
c. vertebra
c. vessel
craniectomy
keyhole-shaped c.
craniocaudal
c. projection
c. projection
c. view
craniocervical junction
craniofacial
c. angle
c. anomaly
c. dysjunction
c. dysjunction fracture
c. dysostosis
c. notch
c. pain syndrome
c. plexiform neurofibroma
c. remodeling
c. synostosis
craniolacunia
craniomandibular syndrome
craniometric point
cranioorbital deformity
craniopagus
craniopharyngeal
c. canal
c. duct
craniopharyngioma
adamantinomatous c.
ectopic c.
nasopharyngeal c.
cranioschisis
craniosclerosis
cranioskeletal dysplasia
craniospinal
c. axis
c. axis radiation therapy
c. hemangioblastoma
c. irradiation
craniostenosis, pl. **craniostenoses**
craniosynostosis, pl. **craniosynostoses**
craniotabes
craniotelencephalic dysplasia
craniotomy
c. defect
craniotrypesis
craniovertebral
c. angle
c. anomaly
c. junction
c. junction anatomy
cranium, pl. **crania**
c. bifidum
c. bifidum occultum
split c.
crankcase oil fluid
crater
ulcer c.
craterlike ulcer
Crawford suture ring
crazy paving pattern
Cr-chromate-labeled red cell technique

NOTES

CRE
cumulative radiation effect
crease
back c.
infragluteal c.
inframammary c.
inguinal c.
stellate c.
creep
cardiac c.
diaphragmatic c.
periosteal c.
creeping epithelialization
cremaster
cremasteric
c. artery
c. fascia
crescendo
c. TIA
crescent
air c.
c. artifact
c. of cardia
c. hip line
c. hip sign
c. lung sign
c. sign
crescentic
c. border
c. collection
c. lumen
c. submucosal fold
crescent-in-doughnut sign
crescent-shaped fibrocartilaginous disk
cress-correlation technique
CREST
calcinosis cutis, Raynaud phenomenon, esophageal motility disorder, sclerodactyly, and telangiectasia
CREST syndrome
crest
acoustic c.
acousticofacial c.
alveolar c.
ampullary c.
anterior iliac c.
arched c.
arcuate c.
articular c.
basilar c.
bilateral iliac c.
buccinator c.
conchal c.
deltoid c.
dental c.
ethmoidal c.
falciform c.
frontal c.
ganglionic c.
gingival c.
gyral c.
iliac c.
c. of the ilium
infundibuloventricular c.
intertrochanteric c.
posterior iliac c.
pubic c.
sacral c.
supraventricular c. (SVC)
terminal c.
tibial c.
urethral c.
cresyl blue
cretinism
goitrous c.
Creutzfeldt-Jakob disease
crevice
nonpolar c.
CRF
coronary reserve flow
Cr-heated RBC
Cr-HIDA
C.-H. chelate
C.-H. chelate imaging agent
cribriform
c. bone
c. carcinoma
c. fascia
c. pattern
c. plate
c. process
cricket bat shape
cricoarytenoid
c. articular capsule
cricoesophageal tendon
cricoid cartilage
cricopharyngeus, cricopharyngeal
c. achalasia
c. bar
c. diverticulum
c. ligament
c. muscle
c. sphincter
cricosantorinian ligament
cricothyreotomy
cricothyroid
c. articular capsule
c. cartilage
c. ligament
c. membrane
cricotracheal ligament
cri-du-chat syndrome
crinkle artifact

crinkling
mucosal c.
patch c.
crisscross heart
crista
c. supraventricularis
c. supraventricularis septal defect
criterion, pl. **criteria**
Biello criteria
error-sum c.
interpretive criteria
Jones criteria
morphologic criteria
Nyquist c.
PIOPED criteria
radiographic criteria
Schumacher criteria
Schwartz criteria
critical
c. coronary stenosis
c. dose table
c. lesion
c. organ
c. valvular stenosis
CRL
crown-rump length
Cr-labeled red cell technique
CR-MVB
Cramer-Rao minimum variance bound
Crohn
C. colitis
C. disease (CD)
C. disease activity index (CDAI)
C. disease of colon (CDC)
C. disease string sign
C. disease target sign
C. duodenitis
C. granulomatous enteritis
C. ileitis
C. ileocolitis
C. jejunitis
C. regional enteritis
Crohn-like lymphoid reaction
Cronkhite-Canada syndrome
Cronqvist cranial index (CCI)
cross-aortic
cross-chest impingement sign
cross-collateralization
cross-correlation technique
crossed
c. cerebellar diaschisis
c. coil
c. embolus
c. pyramidal tract
c. sciatica sign
crossed-coil design
crossed-fused renal ectopia
cross-filling
cross-fogging
crosshatch grid
cross ligament
crossover
c. of activity
femorofemoral c.
cross-pelvic collateral vessel
cross-section
bronchovascular anatomy c.-s.
c.-s. capture
Compton scattering c.-s.
elastic c.-s.
normalized c.-s.
pharynx c.-s.
thigh muscle c.-s.
vertebral c.-s.
cross-sectional
c.-s. area (CSA)
c.-s. area stenosis
c.-s. echocardiography
c.-s. imaging
c.-s. lung segment anatomy
c.-s. two-dimensional echocardiography
c.-s. ultrasonographic image
c.-s. zone
crosstable
c. lateral film
c. lateral projection
c. lateral view (CTLV)
crosstalk effect artifact
cross-union
Crouzon disease
CR/OV
OncoScint C.
crowded dentition
crowding of bronchovascular markings
Crowe pilot point
crown
c. artifact
c. cavity
halo c.
c. tubercle
crown-heel length
crown-rump length (CR, CRL)

NOTES

crow's
c. foot gallstone sign
CRRMP
Committee of Radiation from Radioactive Medicinal Products
CRT
cathode-ray tube
conformal radiation therapy
3D CRT
crucial angle of Gissane
cruciate
c. eminence
c. ligament
c. ligament injury
c. orientation
cruciatum cruris ligament
cruciform
c. eminence
c. ligament
crural
c. canal
c. cistern
c. cistern widening
c. fascia
c. fossa
c. ring
c. septum
c. sheath
c. triangle
crus, pl. **crura**
comma-shaped c.
c. cupula
c. of the diaphragm
diaphragmatic c.
displaced c.
c. dome
c. hiatus
lateral c.
left c.
medial c.
muscular c.
c. of penis
c. pericardium
c. phenomenon
c. pleura
right c.
crush
c. artifact
c. fracture
c. injury
c. kidney
c. preparation
c. syndrome
thoracic c.
"crushed eggshell" fracture
crushed tissue
Cruveilhier
C. fascia
C. joint
C. ligament
C. nodule
C. sign
C. ulcer
Cruveilhier-Baumgarten
C.-B. anomaly
C.-B. cirrhosis
crux
c. cordis
crypt
anal c.
enamel c.
epithelium c.
ileal c.
Lieberkühn c.
c. of Lieberkühn
Luschka c.
Morgagni c.
c. of Morgagni
cryptic vascular malformation (CVM)
cryptorchidism
cryptococcal spondylitis
cryptococcoma
cryptococcosis
AIDS c.
intracranial c.
cryptogenic
c. cirrhosis
c. fibrosing alveolitis
c. organizing pneumonia
cryptoscope
Satvioni c.
cryptostroma corticale
crystal
calcium c.
Charcot-Leyden c.
c. field theory (CFT)
hydroxyapatite c.
monosodium urate c.'s (MSU)
piezoelectric c.'s
pyrophosphate c.'s
scintillation c.
sodium iodide c.
CrystalEYES video system
crystal-induced arthrosis
crystallogram
crystallography
x-ray c.
CS
coronary sinus
^{137}Cs
cesium-137
CSA
cross-sectional area
CSDH
chronic subdural hematoma
Cserenkov effect

CSF
cerebrospinal fluid
CSF cytology
CSF-suppressed T2-weighted 3D MP-RAGE MR imaging
CSI
chemical-shift imaging
coronary stenosis index
CSI spectroscopy
CSI-enhanced MRI
CSIS-enhanced
C.-e. MRI
CSL
central sacral line
C-spine pseudosubluxation
CSS
carotid sinus syndrome
cause-specific survival
CST
contraction stress test
corticospinal tract
CSVT
central splanchnic venous thrombosis
CT
cardiothoracic ratio
circulation time
computed tomography
coronary thrombosis
CT angiogram lung sign
CT arteriography
CT arthrography
CT attenuation value
biphasic CT
bit CT
bone quantitative CT (BQCT)
CT bone window
CT bone window photography
CT bubble sign
cervical CT
cine CT
CT cisternogram
collimation CT
CT colography
CT colonography
contrast-enhanced CT
CT densitometer
CT densitometry
dual-energy CT
dual-isotope single-photon emission CT
dynamic CT
electron-beam CT
enhanced CT
expiratory CT
fast dynamic volumetric x-ray CT
CT halo lung sign
helical biphasic contrast-enhanced CT (HBCT)
helical thin-section CT
high spatial resolution cine CT
CT imaging error
indirect CT
CT Max 640 scanner
multiphasic CT
CT myelography
nonenhanced CT
CT number
CT peritoneography
quantitative spirometrically controlled CT
CT ratio
CT reconstruction image
CT scan
CT scan cradle
CT scan gantry
CT scan with contrast
CT sialography
single-photon emission CT
slip-ring CT
spiral volumetric CT
spirometrically controlled CT
stable xenon CT
CT stereotactic guide
surgical simulation CT
thallium-201 single-photon emission CT
thin-section CT
thin-slice CT
three-dimensional processed ultrafast CT
triphasic spiral CT
twin-beam CT
two-phase helical CT
ultrafast CT
CT unit
water-contrast CT
xenon-enhanced CT
Z-dependent CT
CT9000 scanner
CT9800 scanner
CTA
computed tomographic angiography
CT-aided volumetry

NOTES

CTAP
computed tomography angiographic portography
computed tomography arterial portography
CTAT
computerized transverse axial tomography
CTAT imaging
CTC
computed tomographic colonography
CTDI
computed tomography dose index
CT-directed
C.-d. biopsy
C.-d. hook-wire localization
CT-guided
C.-g. intraarterial chemotherapy
C.-g. needle aspiration
C.-g. needle biopsy
C.-g. percutaneous biopsy
C.-g. percutaneous endoscopic gastrostomy
C.-g. percutaneous excision
C.-g. stereotactic surgery
C.-g. transsternal core biopsy
C.-g. ultrasound
CTH
computerized tomographic holography
CTHA
computerized tomographic hepatic angiography
CTI
C. 933/04 ECAT scanner
C. PET scanner
CTLV
crosstable lateral view
CTMM
metrizamide-assisted computed tomography
CT/MRI-compatible stereotactic head frame
CT/MRI-defined
C.-d. tumor slice image
C.-d. tumor volume image
CTR
cardiothoracic ratio
C-TRAK hand-held gamma detector
CTT
central tegmental tract
CTV
clinical target volume
Cu
copper
^{62}Cu
^{62}Cu PTSM imaging agent
^{62}Cu pyruvaldehyde-bis-(4N-thiosemicarbazone) imaging agent
^{64}Cu
copper-64
^{67}Cu
copper-67
^{67}Cu imaging agent
cube vertex
cubic
c. centimeter (cc)
c. convolution interpolation
c. voxel
cubital
c. bone
c. bursitis
c. fossa
c. lymph node
c. tunnel
c. tunnel retinaculum
c. tunnel syndrome
cubitocarpal
cubitoradial
cubitus
c. valgus
c. valgus deformity
c. varus
c. varus deformity
cuboid
c. bone
c. fracture
c. squeeze technique
c. whip technique
cuboidal articular surface
cuboideonavicular ligament
cubonavicular joint
CUC
chronic ulcerative colitis
cue-based image analysis
cuff
c. abscess
aortic c.
atrial c.
inflow c.
musculotendinous c.
pressure c.
rectal muscle c.
right atrial c.
rotator c.
c. sign
suprahepatic caval c.
vaginal c.
cuffed endotracheal tube
cuffing
peribronchial c.
cuirasse
carcinoma en c.
cor en c.
cul-de-sac
Douglas c.-d.-s.
c.-d.-s. of Douglas

dural c.-d.-s.
free fluid c.-d.-s.

Culiner theory

Cullen sign

culpocephaly

culprit
c. lesion
c. stenosis
c. vessel

cumulative
c. dose
c. radiation effect (CRE)

cuneatus
funiculus c.

cuneiform
c. bone
c. bone of carpus
c. cartilage
c. fracture
c. fracture-dislocation
c. joint
c. lobe
c. mortise
c. tubercle

cuneocerebellar tract

cuneocuboid ligament

cuneonavicular ligament

CUP
cancer of unknown primary

cup
acetabular c.
hip replacement c.
migration of acetabular c.
prosthetic c.
retroversion of acetabular c.

cup-and-spill stomach

cupid's bow contour

cupola sign

cupping of the calix

cupula
crus c.
diaphragmatic c.
gas c.
pleural c.

curative irradiation

Curie
C. effect
C. law

curie (Ci)

curium

Curix Capacity Plus film processing system

curlicue ureter

curling
c. esophagus
C. ulcer

curly toe deformity

Curracino-Silverman syndrome

Currarino triad

currens
larva c.

current
beam c.
direct c. (DC)
eddy c.
gradient drive c.
ionization c.
c. leak
pulsing c.
tube c.
unmodulated radiofrequency c.
variable tube c.

curtain
subaortic c.

curvature
angular c.
c. anisotropy
anterior c.
backward c.
cervical lordotic c.
dorsal kyphotic c.
flattening of normal lordotic c.
gingival c.
kyphotic c.
lumbar c.
radius of c.
stomach c.

curve
area under the (concentration-time) c. (AUC)
biphasic c.
Bragg c.
brightness-time c.
catheter with preformed c.'s
cervical spine c.
characteristic c.
clearance c.
concentration-time c.
depth-dose c.
c. of duodenum
dye dilution c.
elimination c.
c. fit coefficient
flattening of normal lumbar c.

NOTES

curve *(continued)*
flow-time c.
fractionated dose-survival c.
Frank-Starling c.
free induction delay c.
full-width-at-half-maximum of lorentzian c.
gaussian c.
glow c.
H and D c.
Hurter and Driffield curve
Hurter-Driffield c.
Hurter and Driffield c. (H and D curve)
Hurter and Driffield photographic c.
indicator dilution c.
indocyanine dilution c.
isoclosed c.
isodose c.
lordotic c.
lorentzian c.
loss of sigmoid c.
lumbar lordotic c.
lung count c.
normal lordotic c.
pulmonary time activity c.
renal flow c.
renogram c.
ROC c.
receiver operating characteristic curve
sensitometric c.
sigmoid c.
signal intensity time c.
spline c.
Starling c.
stress-strain c.
superincumbent spinal c.
thoracic spine c.
time-activity c.
time-attenuation c.
time-density c.
time-intensity c.
ventricular function c.
videodensity c.
washout c.

curved
c. radiolucent line
c. vessel

curvilinear
c. calcification
c. defect
c. subpleural line
c. threshold shoulder

Cushing
C. disease
C. phenomenon
C. syndrome
C. triad
C. ulcer

cushingoid appearance

Cushing-Rokitansky ulcer

cushion
c. defect
endocardial c.

cusp
accessory c.
anterior c.
aortic c.
asymmetric closure of c.
conjoined c.
coronary c.
c. degeneration
dysplastic c.
c. fenestration
fibrocalcific c.
fishmouth c.
fusion of c.
intact valve c.
left coronary c.
left pulmonary c.
mitral valve c.
c. motion
noncoronary c.
perforated aortic c.
posterior c.
prolapse of right aortic valve c.
pulmonary valve c.
right coronary c.
ruptured aortic c.
semilunar valve c.
septal c.
c. shot
tricuspid valve c.
valve c.

custom-curved coil

custom shielding block

cut
c. and cine film
high-resolution coronal c.'s
off-center c.'s
tangential c.'s
tomographic c.'s

cutaneous
c. adenoma
c. angioma
c. B-cell lymphoma (CBCL)
c. collateral circulation
c. fissure
c. lateral branch
c. leukocytoclastic angitis
c. lymphoscintigraphy
c. nodule
c. pit
c. pneumocystosis

c. ridge
c. T-cell lymphoma
c. twig
c. vascular anomaly
c. vein
cut-film
c.-f. angiography
c.-f. technique
cuticular overgrowth
cutis calcinosis
cutoff
arterial c.
c. colon sign
Cuvier
canal of C.
C. canal
duct of C.
C. duct
Cu/Zn
copper-zinc
Cu/Zn-SOD
copper-zinc superoxide dismutase
Cu/Zn-SOD imaging agent
c.v.
coefficient of variation
CVA
cardiovascular accident
cerebrovascular accident
costovertebral angle
CVBS
congenital vascular-bone syndrome
CVC
central venous catheter
CVCT
cardiovascular computed tomographic scanner
CVD
cardiovascular disease
collagen vascular disease
CVIS imaging device
CVM
congenital vascular malformation
cryptic vascular malformation
CVP
central venous pressure
CVRI
coronary vascular resistance index
CW
continuous wave
C-wave pressure
CX
circumflex
CX artery
CXR
chest x-ray
C x T
concentration times time
cyanoacrylate
cyanocobalamin
c. Co (cobalt)
c. imaging agent
radioactive c.
cyanocobalamin Co 57
cyanocobalamin Co 58
cyanocobalamin Co 60
cyanotic kidney
cyberradiology
Cyberware system
Cybex ergometer
cycles
c. per minute (cpm)
c. per second (cps)
cycle time
cyclic
c. adenosine monophosphate
c. guanosine monophosphate
c. guanosine triphosphate
c. idiopathic edema
cycling
phase c.
cyclopia
cyclops lesion
cyclosporin nephrotoxicity
cyclotron
medical c.
multiparticle c.
negative-ion c.
positive-ion c.
C-Y color space
cylinder
Burnett c.
CO_2 c.
dome c.
Fletcher-Delclos dome c.
vaginal c.
cylindrical
c. bronchiectasis
c. carcinoma
c. chest
c. configuration
c. format
c. map projection

NOTES

cylindrical *(continued)*
c. projection map
c. thorax
cylindroid aneurysm
cylindroma
lung c.
c. parotis
cylindromatous carcinoma
cylindrosarcoma
cyllosis
Cyma line
Cyriax syndrome
cyst
acoustic c.
acquired hepatic c.
adnexal c.
adrenal c.
air c.
allantoic c.
amnionic inclusion c.
ampulla of Vater c.
aneurysmal bone c. (ABC)
apocrine c.
arachnoid brain c.
arachnoid spine c.
aryepiglottic c.
atypical renal c.
Baker c.
Bartholin gland c.
benign conal c.
bilateral arachnoid c.
bilateral choroid plexus c.
Blessig c.
bone implantation c.
brain c.
breast c.
bronchial cleft c.
bronchogenic c.
brown cell c.
calcified c.
cerebral c.
cervical thymic c.
choledochal c.
cholesterol ear c.
choroid plexus c.
colloidal brain c.
colonic duplication c.
complex breast c.
complicated renal c.
conal c.
congenital bronchogenic c.
congenital hepatic c.
corpus albicans c.
corpus luteum c.
cortical renal c.
cysticercus c.
Dandy-Walker c.
decidual c.
dental c.
dentigerous c.
dermoid ovarian c.
dorsal c.
dorsal enterogenous c.
duplication c.
echinococcal c.
endodermal c.
endometrial c.
endometriotic c.
enteric c.
enterogenous c.
entrapped ovarian c.
ependymal c.
epididymal c.
epidural arachnoid c.
epithelial c.
esophageal duplication c.
expansile aneurysmal bone c.
extraparenchymal c.
false splenic c.
first branchial cleft c.
fluid-filled c.
follicular ovarian c.
foregut c.
functional ovarian c.
ganglionic c.
Gartner duct c.
gastric duplication c.
gastrointestinal c.
hemorrhagic corpus luteum c.
hepatic c.
honeycomb c.
hydatid heart c.
hydatid lung c.
hydatid mediastinum c.
implantation c.
interhemispheric c.
interosseous c.
intracranial dermoid c.
intraduodenal choledochal c.
intramedullary epidermoid c.
intrameniscal c.
intraneural ganglion c.
intraosseous keratin c.
intraparenchymal c.
intrapulmonary bronchogenic c.
intrasellar Rathke cleft c.
intraspinal enteric c.
intratesticular c.
intrathoracic c.
intraventricular cryptococcal c.
joint c.
keratin testicular c.
kidney c.
Kimura-type choledochal c.
lipid c.
liver c.

lumbar synovial c.
lung c.
luteal c.
mammary c.
mediastinal bronchogenic c.
mediastinal dorsal enteric c.
meibomian c.
mesenteric c.
mesothelial c.
midline of brain c.
milk of calcium urinary tract c.
morgagnian c.
mucinous c.
mucous retention c.
müllerian duct c.
multilocular renal c.
multiple pulmonary c.'s
multiple thyroid c.'s
myxoid c.
nabothian c.
nasolabial c.
nasopharyngeal mucus retention c.
neoplastic c.
neuroenteric c.
noncommunicating c.
nonneoplastic c.
nuchal c.
odontogenic c.
oil c.
omental c.
omphalomesenteric duct c.
orbital blood c.
orbital chocolate c.
orbital dermoid c.
ovarian dermoid c.
ovarian follicular c.
ovarian image signature c.
ovarian retention c.
pancreatic c.
paraglenoid c.
paralabral c.
parameniscal c.
paramesonephric duct c.
paraovarian c.
parapelvic c.
parapharyngeal space c.
parathyroid c.
paratubal serous c.
paraurethral c.
parovarian c.
pelvic chocolate c.
pericaliceal c.
pericardial c.
perineural sacral c.
peripelvic c.
peritoneal inclusion c.
physiologic ovarian c.
pilonidal c.
pineal c.
pituitary c.
placental septal c.
pleural c.
pleuropericardial c.
pontine hydatid c.
popliteal c.
porencephalic c.
posterior fossa c.
postmenopausal adnexal c.
posttraumatic oil c.
posttraumatic spinal cord c.
primordial tooth c.
prostatic c.
pulmonary c.
pyelogenic c.
racemose c.
radicular c.
Rathke cleft c.
reactive spinal c.
c. rebound sign
rectal duplication c.
renal sinus c.
retention c.
retrocerebellar arachnoid c.
retroperitoneal c.
sacral c.
sebaceous c.
secondary archnoid c.
second branchial cleft c.
seminal vesicle c.
septal placenta c.
serous c.
simple bone c.
simple breast c.
simple cortical renal c.
small bowel duplication c.
solitary bone c.
spinal hydatid c.
splenic epidermoid c.
subarachnoid c.
subarticular c.
subchondral c.
subependymal c.
syndrome with multiple cortical renal c.

NOTES

cyst *(continued)*
synovial c.
synovium-filled degenerative c.
tailgut c.
talar dome c.
Tarlov c.
tarsal c.
tension c.
testicular c.
theca-lutein ovarian c.
thin-walled c.
thoracic duct c.
thymic c.
thyroglossal duct c.
thyroid c.
Todani type c.
Tornwaldt c.
traumatic bone c.
traumatic lipid c.
traumatic lung c.
tunica albuginea c.
umbilical cord c.
unicameral bone c.
unilocular c.
urachal c.
vaginal c.
wolffian c.

cystadenocarcinoma
mucinous c.
mucinous ovarian c.
ovarian serous c.
pseudomucinous c.
serous c.

cystadenofibroma
ovarian c.

cystadenoma
bile duct c.
biliary c.
glycogen-rich pancreatic c.
c. lymphomatosum
macrocystic c.
mucinous c.
ovarian c.
pancreas c.
papillary epididymal c.
serous c.
thyroid c.

cystectomy
radical c.

cystic
c. adenocarcinoma
c. adenomatoid malformation
c. airspace HRCT
c. appearance
c. arachnoiditis
c. area thyroid
c. artery
c. basal cell carcinoma
c. bone angiomatosis
c. breast disease
c. bronchiectasis
c. cancer
c. change
c. degeneration
c. dilatation
c. disease of breast
c. duct angiography
c. duct cholangiogram
c. duct cholangiography
c. duct lumen
c. duct remnant
c. duct remnant stone
c. duct stump
c. dysplasia
c. epididymis lesion
c. fibrosis
c. fistula
c. fluid
c. gall duct
c. ganglioglioma
c. glandular hyperplasia
c. glioma
c. goiter
c. hemangioblastoma
c. hygroma
c. hyperplasia photomicrograph
c. intracranial fetal lesion
c. intraparenchymal meningioma
c. kidney
c. kidney adenoma
c. kidney disease
c. liver lesion
c. lymph node
c. lysis
c. mass
c. mastitis
c. mastoplasia
c. medial necrosis
c. medionecrosis
c. mesothelioma
c. metastasis
c. myelomalacia
c. myelopathy
c. neck hygroma
c. neck lymphangioma
c. nephroma
c. orbital hygroma
c. osteofibromatosis
c. ovarian disease
c. ovary
c. partially differentiated nephroblastoma
c. pilocytic astrocytoma
c. pituitary adenoma
c. plexus
c. polyp

c. process
c. pulmonary emphysema
c. renal cell carcinoma
c. renal disease
c. rheumatoid arthritis
c. sac
c. splenic lesion
c. splenic neoplasm
c. structure
c. teratoma
c. tuberculosis
c. tumor
c. vein
c. wall

cystica
mastitis fibrosa c.
osteitis fibrosa c.
pyelitis c.
pyeloureteritis c.
ureteritis c.

cystic-choledochal junction

cysticercosis
CNS c.
parenchymal c.
subarachnoid c.

cysticercus cyst

cysticohepatic triangle

cystinosis
nephropathic c.

cystitis
AIDS c.
Cytoxan c.
emphysematous c.
interstitial c.
radiation c.
tuberculous c.

cystoatrial shunt

cystocarcinoma

cystocele
protrusion of c.

Cysto-Conray
C.-C. II contrast medium
C.-C. II imaging agent

cystoduodenal ligament

cystofibroma

Cystografin
C. contrast medium
C. imaging agent

cystogram
air c.
bead chain c.
chain c.
delayed c.
double voiding c.
excretory c.
postdrainage c.
postvoiding c.
radioisotope voiding c.
radionuclide c.
radiopharmaceutical voiding c.
retrograde c.
stress c.
triple-voiding c.
voiding c.

cystography
antegrade c.
c. imaging

Cystokon
C. imaging agent

cystopathy
diabetic c.

cystoplasty
ileocecal c.

cystoradiogram

cystosarcoma
c. phyllodes

cystoscopic urography

cystoscopy

cystosis
pancreatic c.

cystostomy

cystoureterogram

cystoureterography

cystourethrogram
voiding c. (VCU, VCUG)

cystourethrography

cystourethroscopy imaging

cyst-within-a-cyst

cytoarchitectonic abnormality

cytology
aspiration c.
CSF c.
fine-needle aspiration c.
imprint c.
nipple aspiration c.
scrape c.

cytomegalic inclusion disease

cytomegalovirus
c. (CMV) colic
c. encephalitis
c. esophagitis
c. interstitial pneumonitis
c. pneumonia
c. with microcephaly

C

NOTES

Cytomel
C. suppression
C. suppression test
cytometer
FACScan flow c.
cytometry
DNA flow c.
flow c.
image c.
multicolor flow c.
cytophotometry
DNA c.
cytotoxic edema of the gray matter
Cytoxan cystitis

D
dalton
D point
D signal
D1
diagonal branch #1
2D
2D B-mode ultrasound machine
2D color-coded imaging of blood flow
2D format
2D GRE dynamic protocol
2D J-resolved 1H MR spectroscopy
multislice FLASH 2D
2D portal image registration
2D pulsatility index mapping
2D resistance index mapping
2D sector scan
2D spatially selective radiofrequency pulse
2D time-of-flight technique
2D TOF
3D
3D conformal radiation therapy
3D connect operation
3D CRT
3D dose profile
3D elastic subtraction algorithm
3D freehand ultrasound
3D gadolinium-enhanced magnetic resonance angiography
3D image reconstruction
3D inflow MR angiography
3D magnetic resonance microscopy
3D magnetic source imaging
3D modeling
3D MRI data set
3D phase-contrast magnetic resonance angiography
3D plate
3D processed ultrafast computerized imaging
3D pulse design
3D radiation treatment planning
3D rendering
3D RODEO
3D RTP
3D spoiled gradient-recalled echo (GRE) sequence
3D stereotactic surface projection
3D surface anthropometry
3D surface digitizer
3D surface digitizer scanner
3D technique
3D time-of-flight magnetic resonance angiographic sequence
3D transesophageal echocardiographic sequence
3D turbo FLAIR
3D turbo fluid-attentuated inversion recovery
3D turbo SE imaging
3D ultrasound reconstruction imaging
D_{max}
maximum density
d,1-HMPAO imaging agent
DAC
digital-to-analog converter
Dacron-covered stent graft
dacryoadenitis
dacryocystocele
dacryocystogram
dacryocystography
d. imaging
radiopharmaceutical d.
dagger sign
Dagradi classification of esophageal varices
Dalen-Fuchs nodule
DALM
dysplasia with associated lesion or mass
dalton (D)
damage
busulfan lung d.
drug-induced pulmonary d.
endothelial d.
fatigue d.
focal d.
hemisphere d.
heroin lung d.
hypoxic brain d.
ischemic brain d.
methadone lung d.
methotrexate lung d.
myleran lung d.
nitrofurantoin lung d.
nitrosourea lung d.
physeal d.
procarbazine lung d.
projection fiber d.
propoxyphene lung d.
renal vascular d.
salicylate lung d.
seminiferous tubular d.
U-fiber d.
valvular d.
vascular cord d.
D'Amato sign

dammed-up cerebrospinal fluid
dampened
d. obstructive pulse
d. pulsatile flow
d. waveform
dampening
Doppler waveform d.
damping of catheter tip pressure
Damus-Kaye-Stancel (DKS)
D.-K.-S. anastomosis (DKS anastomosis)
dancer's
d. bone
d. foot malformation
d. fracture
Dance sign
Dandy-Walker
D.-W. complex
D.-W. cyst
D.-W. deformity
D.-W. malformation
D.-W. syndrome
D.-W. variant
dangling choroid plexus
Danis-Weber
D.-W. ankle fracture classification
D.-W. fracture
DANTE-selective
D.-s. pulse
DANTE sequence
D'Antonio
D. acetabular classification
D. classification of acetabular abnormality
DAP
real-time dose area product
Dardik Biograft
dark
d. lung
d. pixel value
d. region
d. signal intensity
d. signal intensity rim
darkfield
d. imaging
d. microscopy
darkroom error
Darrach-Hughston-Milch fracture
dartoic tissue
dartos muscle
darwinian tubercle
DAS
data-acquisition system
DASA
distal articular set angle
Daseler-Anson classification of plantaris muscle anatomy
dashboard fracture
data
d. acquisition
d. acquisition time
emission and transmission d.
radiology outcomes d.
d. set
d. spike detection error artifact
stereotactic d.
transmission d.
volumetric image d.
data-acquisition system (DAS)
data-clipping detection error artifact
dating
second-trimester gestational d.
third-trimester gestational d.
DATTA
Diagnostic and Therapeutic Technology Assessment
daughter
d. abscess
DES d.
d. isotope
Davidson shunt
Davies
D. endocardial fibrosis
D. endomyocardial fibrosis
Davies-Colley syndrome
Davis method
Dawbarn sign
Dawson finger
d'Azyr
bundle of Vicq d.
DBDC
distal bile duct carcinoma
DBM
demineralized bone matrix
DC
differentiated carcinoma
direct current
DC offset artifact
d.c.
DCA
directional color angiography
directional coronary atherectomy
DCBE
double-contrast barium enema
DCE-MRI
dynamic-contrast enhanced magnetic resonance imaging
DCIS
ductal carcinoma in situ
Van Nuys Prognostic Index for DCIS
DCM
dilated cardiomyopathy
DCS
distal coronary sinus

1D-CSI
one-dimensional chemical-shift imaging
DDC
direct display console
DDD
double-dose delay
dual-mode, dual-pacing, dual-sensing
dD/dt
derived value on apex cardiogram
DDFP
dodecafluoropentane
DDFP imaging agent
DDH
developmental dysplasia of hip
DE
dose equivalent
de
d. Broglie wavelength
d. la Camp sign
d. Lange syndrome
D. Martini-Balestra syndrome
d. Morsier syndrome
d. Musset sign
d. Mussey point
d. Mussey sign
d. novo
d. novo aneurysm
d. novo lesion
d. Quervain fracture
d. Quervain thyroiditis
dead
d. bone
d. bowel
d. space
d. tissue
DEAE-Sephadex A-25 chromatography
deafness
d., onychodystrophy, osteodystrophy, mental retardation (DOOR)
d., onychodystrophy, osteodystrophy, mental retardation syndrome
death
brain d.
cerebral brain d.
early fetal d.
fetal d.
imminent d.
intermediate fetal d.
late fetal d.
quadrant of d.
sudden cardiac d.
DeBakey
D. aortic classification
D. aortic dissection
deblurring technique
debris
atheromatous d.
atherosclerotic d.
bone d.
calcium d.
cholesterol d.
extraarticular d.
foreign d.
gelatinous d.
grumous d.
intimal d.
intraarticular d.
intraluminal d.
joint d.
necrotic d.
particulate d.
thallium d.
Debye-Scherrer photographic technique
decalcification
decalcified
d. bone marrow sample
d. dorsum sella
decannulation
decay
beta d.
branched d.
d. constant
energy d.
d. equation
exponential d.
free-induction d. (FID)
radioactive d.
repeated free-induction d.
d. scheme
d. series
d. time
decay-activating factor
deceleration-dependent block
deceleration time
decelerative injury
dechondrification
decidua
decidual
d. cyst
d. fissure
d. sac
deciduate placenta
deciduous

NOTES

decima
costa fluctuans d.
decimalized variance map
decision matrix
decoding
document image d. (DID)
Viterbi d.
decompensated
d. alcoholic cirrhosis
d. congestive heart failure
decompensation
cardiac d.
chronic respiratory d.
end-stage adult cardiac d.
end-stage fetal cardiac d.
hemodynamic d.
ischemic d.
respiratory d.
ventricular d.
decomposition
linear prediction with singular value d.
three-level Haar wavelet d.
decompression
arthroscopic d.
biliary d.
bony d.
canal d.
cardiac d.
endoscopic d.
d. of fracture
gastric d.
hydrostatic d.
intestinal d.
microvascular d. (MVD)
percutaneous transhepatic d.
peripheral nerve d.
portal d.
d. sickness
spinal cord d.
surgical d.
transduodenal endoscopic d.
transpedicular d.
tube d.
d. tube
variceal d.
venous d.
deconditioned exercise response
deconditioning
deconvolutional analysis
deconvolution technique
decortication
cardiac d.
heart d.
lung d.
decrease
split renal function d.
decreased
d. activity
d. attenuation
d. cerebral blood flow
d. closing velocity
d. E-to-F slope
d. intensity
d. peripheral vascular resistance
d. peristalsis
d. placenta size
d. pulmonary vascularity
d. stroke volume
d. systemic resistance
d. thyroid radiotracer uptake
d. tidal volume
d. uptake of radiotracer
d. vital capacity
decrement
scan d.
decryption algorithm
DecThreads software
decubitus
d. calculus
d. film
d. position
d. radiograph
d. ulcer
d. view
decussate
decussation
dedicated breast biopsy system
dedifferentiation
deep
d. arch
d. artery
d. cardiac plexus
d. collateral ligament
d. Doppler velocity interrogation
d. fascia
d. fascia of penis
d. interloop abscess
d. invasion
d. lymph vessel
d. muscle
d. myometrial invasion
d. to the nipple
d. pelvic abscess
d. perineal pouch
d. posterior compartment
d. sulcus sign
d. tumor
d. vein
d. vein system of leg
d. venous aplasia
d. venous channel
d. venous incompetence
d. venous insufficiency (DVI)
d. venous occlusion

d. venous thromboembolization
d. venous thrombosis (DVT)
d. white ischemia matter
d. white matter track

deep-seated
d.-s. lesion
d.-s. tumor

deep-shelled acetabulum

defecogram

defecography

defect
abdominal wall d.
anteroapical d.
aortic septal d.
aortopulmonary septal d.
atrial ostium primum d.
atrial septal d. (ASD)
atrioventricular canal d.
atrioventricular nodal septal d.
atrioventricular septal d.
bar d.
beneficial atrial septal d.
benign cortical d.
bile duct filling d.
bony d.
bridging d.
calcified medullary d.
cardiofacial d.
cauliflower-shaped filling d.
cecal filling d.
chain of lakes filling d.
chiasmatic d.
chondral d.
cold d.
collecting system filling d.
colonic filling d.
conal ventricular septal d.
concomitant d.
congenital heart d. (CHD)
conoventricular d.
contiguous ventricular septal d.
conversion d.
cortical d.
craniotomy d.
crista supraventricularis septal d.
curvilinear d.
cushion d.
developmental d.
discoid filling d.
duodenal filling d.
Eisenmenger d.
endocardial cushion ventricular septal d.
esophageal filling d.
extradural d.
extrinsic filling d.
extrinsic ureteral d.
fetal abdominal wall d.
fibrous cortical d.
fibrous medullary d.
fibrous metaphyseal-diaphyseal d.
field d.
filling d.
fixed intracavitary filling d.
fixed perfusion d.
flap valve ventricular septal d.
focal liver scintigraphic d.
focal plaquelike d.
frondlike filling d.
frontal d.
fusiform d.
fusion d.
gallbladder filling d.
gastric remnant filling d.
global cortical d.
gouge d.
hatchet d.
hernia d.
high d.
Hill-Sachs d.
hot d.
incisura d.
inferoapical d.
infracristal ventricular septal d.
infundibular ventricular septal d.
interatrial septal d.
intercalary d.
interventricular septal d. (IVSD)
intraarterial filling d.
intraatrial filling d.
intracavitary filling d.
intraductal breast filling d.
intraluminal filling d.
intramural filling d.
intravascular filling d.
intrinsic filling d.
inverted umbrella d.
ischemic d.
junctional cortical d.
junctional parenchymal kidney d.
juxtaarterial ventricular septal d.
juxtatricuspid ventricular septal d.
linear d.

NOTES

defect *(continued)*
lingular mandibular bony d. (LMBD)
lobulated filling d.
lucent d.
luminal d.
lung perfusion d.
luteal phase d.
malaligned atrioventricular septal d.
mapping of d.
mass d.
membranous ventricular septal d.
multiple colon filling d.'s
multiple small bowel filling d.'s
mural d.
muscular ventricular septal d.
napkin ring d.
neural tube d. (NTD)
nonexpansile well-demarcated multilocular bone d.
nonexpansile well-demarcated unilocular bone d.
nonsubperiosteal cortical d.
nonuniform rotational d. (NURD)
obstructive ventilatory d.
open neural tube d.
organification d.
osseous d.
osteocartilaginous d.
osteochondral d.
ostium primum atrial septal d.
ostium secundum atrial septal d.
pars interarticularis d.
partial atrioventricular canal d.
pear-shaped d.
pericardial d.
periinfarction conduction d. (PICD)
perimembranous ventricular septal d.
photopenic d.
plaquelike linear d.
plication d.
polypoid filling d.
porta hepatis d.
postcricoid d.
posteroapical d.
postinfarction ventriculoseptal d.
postoperative skull d.
punched-out bony d.
radial ray d.
radiolucent linear filling d.
Rastelli type A, B, C atrioventricular canal d.
resolving ischemic neurologic d.
restrictive ventilatory d.
reverse Hill-Sachs d.
reversible ischemic d.
right ventricular conduction d.
Roger ventricular septal d.
scan d.
scintigraphic perfusion d.
secundum atrial septal d.
segmental bone d.
segmental bronchus d.
septal d.
septation septal d.
septum transversum d.
sessile filling d.
single colonic filling d.
sinus venosus atrial septal d.
small bowel filling d.
soft tissue d.
solitary small bowel filling d.
spontaneous closure of d.
stellate d.
stomach filling d.
subcortical d.
subperiosteal cortical d.
subsegmental perfusion d.
superior caval d.
superior marginal d.
supracristal ventricular septal d.
Swiss cheese ventricular septal d.
thyroid organification d.
thyroid trapping d.
transient perfusion d.
trapping thyroid d.
triangular d.
trochlear d.
tumor d.
type I (supracristal) ventricular septal d.
type II (infracristal) ventricular septal d.
type IV (muscular) ventricular septal d.
ureteral filling d.
valvular cardiac d.
venous d.
ventilation d.
ventilation-perfusion d.
ventral hernia d.
ventricular septal d. (VSD)
wedge-shaped d.
wire-related d.

defective
d. communication between cardiac chambers
d. volume regulation delay

deferens
ductus d.
vas d., pl. vasa deferentia

deferent
d. canal
d. duct

deferential
d. artery
d. plexus
deficiency
Aitken femoral d.
d. disease
photon d.
proximal focal femoral d. (PFFD)
deficit
base d.
cortical d.
focal d.
lateralization d.
posterior column d.
reversible ischemic neurologic d. (RIND)
significant residual d.
space d.
definition
ground-glass d.
loss of d.
pseudopolyp d.
definitive
d. abnormality
d. callus
deflection
fracture simple and depressed full-scale d. (FSD)
intrinsic d.
deflector
tip d.
deformans
arthritis syphilitica d. (ASD)
arthrosis d.
osteitis d.
osteochondrodystrophia d.
Paget osteitis d.
spondylitis d.
spondylosis d.
deformity
Åkerlund d.
Alpine hunter's cap d.
angular d.
aortic valve d.
Arnold-Chiari d.
back-knee d.
bayonet d.
bell-and-clapper d.
biconcave d.
bifid thumb d.
bony d.
boutonnière d.
bowing d.
bull's eye d.
burn boutonnière d.
buttonhole d.
calcaneovarus d.
calcaneus d.
cavovarus d.
cavus d.
cecal d.
chain of lakes d.
Charcot d.
checkrein d.
clawfoot d.
clawhand d.
clawtoe d.
cloverleaf d.
clubfoot d.
clubhand d.
cock-up d.
codfish d.
compensatory d.
congenital d.
contracture d.
cottage loaf d.
cowhorn d.
coxa valga d.
coxa vara d.
cranioorbital d.
cubitus valgus d.
cubitus varus d.
curly toe d.
Dandy-Walker d.
digital d.
digitus flexus d.
dinner-fork d.
duodenal bulb d.
equinovalgus d.
equinovarus d.
equinovarus hindfoot d.
equinus d.
Erlenmeyer flask d.
eversion-external rotation d.
femoral head d.
flatfoot d.
flexible spastic equinovarus d.
flexion d.
foot d.
forefoot abduction d.
fracture d.
funnel chest d.
garden spade d.
genu valgum d.

D

NOTES

deformity *(continued)*
genu varum d.
gibbous d.
gooseneck outflow tract d.
gunstock d.
Haglund d.
hallus abductovalgus d.
hallux flexus d.
hallux malleus d.
hallux rigidus d.
hallux valgus d.
hallux varus d.
hammertoe d.
hatchet-head d.
Hill-Sachs d.
hindbrain d.
hindfoot d.
hockey-stick tricuspid valve d.
hourglass d.
humpback d.
Ilfeld-Holder d.
internal rotation d.
intrinsic minus d.
intrinsic plus d.
J-hook d.
joint d.
J-sella d.
keyhole d.
Kirner d.
kleeblatschädel d.
Klippel-Feil d.
knock-knee d.
lanceolate d.
lobster-claw d.
Madelung d.
mallet-finger d.
mermaid d.
metatarsus adductocavus d.
metatarsus adductovarus d.
metatarsus adductus d.
metatarsus atavicus d.
metatarsus latus d.
metatarsus primus varus d.
metatarsus varus d.
Michel d.
mitral valve d.
nasal tip d.
neuropathic midfoot d.
pannus d.
parachute mitral valve d.
pectus carinatum d.
pectus excavatum d.
pencil-in-cup d.
penciling d.
pencil-like d.
pencil-point metatarsal d.
perigastric d.
pes arcuatus clawfoot d.
pes cavus clawfoot d.
pes planovalgus d.
pes planus d.
phrygian cap d.
pigeon-breast d.
ping-pong ball d.
pistol-grip femur d.
planovalgus foot d.
plantar flexion-inversion d.
postoperative thoracic d.
procurvature d.
pseudo-Hurler d.
pulmonary valve d.
recurvatum d.
reduction d.
rockerbottom foot d.
rolled edge d.
rotational d.
rotoscoliotic d.
round back d.
round shoulder d.
saber-shin d.
sandal-gap d.
scimitar d.
seal-fin d.
shepherd's crook d.
snowman d.
spastic equinovarus d.
spastic hindfoot valgus d.
splayfoot d.
split foot d.
spondylitic d.
Sprengel d.
static foot d.
step-down shoulder d.
subtrochanteric varus d.
supination d.
supratip nasal tip d.
swan-neck finger d.
talus foot d.
thoracic d.
thumb-in-palm d.
torsional d.
trefoil d.
tricuspid valve d.
trigger finger d.
triphalangeal thumb d.
turned-up pulp d.
ulnar drift d.
valgus heel d.
varus d.
Velpeau d.
vertical talus foot d.
VISI d.
volarflexed intercalated segment instability deformity
Volkmann d.
wasp-tail d.

wedging d.
whistling d.
Whitehead d.
windblown d.
windswept d.

defuzzification algorithm

degassed tap water imaging agent

degenerated

d. fibroadenoma
d. tissue

degeneration

acquired hepatocerebral d.
angiolithic d.
articular cartilage d.
atheromatous d.
atrophic d.
ballooning d.
bony d.
brain d.
breast d.
calcareous d.
carcinomatous subacute cerebellar d.
cardiac valve mucoid d.
cardiomyopathic d.
cartilaginous d.
cerebellar d.
cerebelloolivary d.
cerebromacular d. (CMD)
chondrocyte d.
cobblestone d.
colloid d.
cortical cerebellar d.
corticobasal ganglionic d.
corticostriatospinal d.
cusp d.
cystic d.
disk d.
Doyne honeycomb d.
dystrophic d.
esophageal d.
fatty d.
fibrinous d.
fibroid d.
gliosis-induced microcystic d.
granulovacuolar d.
gray matter d.
heart d.
d. of heart
hepatic d.
hepatocerebral d.
hepatolenticular d.
Holmes cortical cerebellar d.
honeycomb d.
hyaline d.
hydropic d.
hypertensive vascular d.
hypertrophic olivary d.
intimal d.
intrameniscal mucoid d.
liquefaction d.
malignant d.
Menzel olivopontocerebellar d.
microcystic d.
mitral valve myxomatous d.
Mönckeberg d.
mucinous d.
mucoid umbilical cord d.
mucous d.
mural d.
muscular d.
myocardial cellular d.
myocardial fibrous d.
myxomatous d.
olivary d.
olivopontocerebellar d. (OPCD)
d. of pancreas
pancreatic d.
paraneoplastic cerebellar d.
parenchymatous cerebellar d.
paving-stone d.
primary progressive cerebellar d.
progressive d.
Regnauld-type great toe d.
renal tubular d.
retinal d.
retrograde d.
rim d.
sclerotic d.
secondary d.
senile d.
spinal d.
spinocerebellar d.
spongiform d.
spongy white matter d.
subacute combined spinal cord d.
testicular d.
thyroid d.
trabecular d.
traumatic d.
wear-and-tear d.
Zenker d.

degenerative

d. aortic aneurysm
d. arthritis

NOTES

degenerative *(continued)*
d. arthrosis
d. atrioventricular node disease
d. atrophy
d. brain disease
d. cardiomyopathy
d. cerebrum disease
d. dementia
d. disease in cerebrum
d. disk
d. disk disease
d. horizontal cleavage tear
d. joint disease (DJD)
d. liver
d. microcystic formation
d. narrowing
d. nuclear pattern
d. osseous change
d. osteoarthritis
d. spondylolisthesis
d. spondylosis
d. spur
d. spurring
degloving injury
deglutition
d. mechanism
muscle of d.
d. pneumonia
d. syncope
deglutitional paralysis
Degos disease
degradable starch microsphere
degradation
fibrinogen d.
d. of image
image quality d.
degraded
d. liver
d. photons
degranulation
degree
d. of correction
d. of inspiration
noncircularity d.
dehalogenation
Dehio test
dehiscence
bronchial d.
Killian d.
perivalvular d.
prosthesis d.
valve d.
dehiscent jugular bulb
Deiters tract
deivisum
pancreatic d.
Déjérine sign
Déjérine-Sottas hypertrophic polyneuropathy
Delarnette scanner
delay
defective volume regulation d.
double-dose d. (DDD)
echo d.
intraventricular conduction d.
phase d.
readout d.
regrowth d.
regular wedge d.
regurgitant flow d.
regurgitant lesion d.
temporal phase d.
d. time selection
delayed
d. bone age
d. bone imaging
d. closure of suture
d. cystogram
d. development
d. excretion of contrast medium
d. film
d. fracture union
d. gastric emptying
d. hydrocephalus
d. image
d. phase
d. phase of arteriography
d. pineal apoplexy
d. resolution of pneumonia
d. rupture spleen
d. small bowel transit
d. splenic rupture
d. transit time
d. transport of tracer
d. traumatic intracerebral hematoma (DTICH)
d. traumatic intracerebral hemorrhage (DTICH)
d. unilateral nephrogram
d. visualization
d. washout
Delbet
D. hip fracture classification
D. sign
deleterious effect
delivered total dose (DTD)
delivery
intracavitary d.
timed bolus d.
Delmege
D. sign
D. sign of tuberculosis
Delphian lymph node
DELTAmanager MedImage system

deltoid
- d. branch of posterior tibial artery
- d. bursa
- d. crest
- d. eminence
- d. fascia
- d. ligament
- d. tuberosity

deltoideopectoral
- d. triangle
- d. trigone

deltopectoral
- d. groove
- d. lymph node

demagnetization
- adiabatic d.
- d. field effect

demarcate

demarcation
- d. line
- nidus d.

dementia
- degenerative d.
- multiinfarct d. (MID)
- subcortical ischemic vascular d.

Demianoff sign

demifacet

demineralization
- bone d.
- d. from disease

demineralized
- d. bone matrix (DBM)
- d. bony structure

demise
- embryo d.
- d. of embryo
- d. of fetus
- imminent d.
- intrauterine d.

Demons-Meigs syndrome

demyelinating disease

demyelination
- brainstem d.
- cerebrum d.
- intramedullary d.
- large-fiber d.
- posterior column d.
- postinfectious d.
- segmental d.
- white matter d.

demyelinative disorder

DeMyer system of cerebral malformation

denatured
- d. Tc-RBC
- d. technetium Tc RBC imaging agent

dendritic
- d. cancer
- d. lesion
- d. spine

dendrocytoma
- disseminated dermal d.

denervated area

denervation
- d. atrophy
- autonomic d.
- cardiac d.
- sympathetic d.

Denis
- D. (A–E) classification of spinal fracture
- D. Browne classification of sacral fractures
- D. classification
- D. classification of spinal injury (A–E)

Denonvilliers
- D. fascia
- D. ligament

dens
- d. fracture
- d. view
- d. view of cervical spine

dense
- d. brain mass
- d. cerebral mass
- d. connective tissue
- d. consolidation
- d. echo
- d. enhancing brain lesion
- d. lung lesion
- d. metaphyseal band
- d. rib
- d. scar
- d. sigmoid sinus sign
- d. structure of bone
- d. vein sign

densitometer
- accuDEXA bone d.
- Achilles d.
- bone d.
- CT d.

D

NOTES

densitometer *(continued)*
- DEXA (dual-energy x-ray absorptiometry) d.
- DPX-IQ d.
- dual-photon d.
- Expert-XL d.
- Hologic 2000 d.
- Lunar DPX d.
- Lunar Expert d.
- Norland XR26 bone d.
- OsteoView digital bone d.
- pDEXA x-ray peripheral bone d.
- QDR-1500 bone d.
- QDR-2000 bone d.
- Sahara portable bone d.
- single-photon d.

densitometric measurement
densitometry
- Compton coherent scattering d.
- computerized optical d. (COD)
- CT d.
- dual-photon d.
- Norland bone d.
- photon d.

density
- air d.
- area of abnormal d.
- arterial linear d.
- asymmetric breast d.
- axial spin d.
- band of d.
- base d.
- bone mineral d. (BMD)
- calcific d.
- capillary d.
- count d.
- diffuse increase in breast d.
- diffuse reticular d.
- discrete perihilar d.
- d. discrimination
- double d.
- echo d.
- echo-spin d.
- energy flux d.
- d. equalization filter
- falx increased d.
- fat d.
- fibroglandular d.
- fluid d.
- focal asymmetric d.
- ground-glass d.
- hazy d.
- homogeneous soft tissue d.
- hydrogen spin d.
- ill-defined multifocal lung d.
- increased d.
- increased bone d.
- increased splenic d.
- integrated optical d. (IOD)
- ionization d.
- lamellar body d. (LBD)
- linear d.
- lung d.
- magnetic flux d.
- d. matrix theory
- maximum d. (D_{max})
- metallic d.
- mixed fat-water breast lesion d.
- mottled d.
- multiple pleural d.'s
- nodular d.
- optical d. (OD)
- patchy area of d.
- peak count d.
- perihilar d.
- periventricular d.
- photon d.
- pleural d.
- proton d.
- pulmonary d.
- radiographic d.
- radiolucent d.
- radiopaque d.
- reticulogranular pulmonary d.
- retroareolar d.
- retrocardiac d.
- ropy d.
- segmental lung d.
- soft tissue d.
- spicular d.
- spin d.
- strands of increased d.
- strandy d.
- streaks of increased d.
- streaky d.
- tissue d.
- tubular lung d.
- urographic d.
- variation in d.
- water d.
- wedge-shaped d.

densography
dental
- d. bulb
- d. caries
- d. crest
- d. cyst
- d. granuloma
- d. groove
- d. material
- d. neck
- d. polyp
- d. radiography
- d. ridge
- d. root
- d. sac

d. scan
d. shelf
d. tubercle
d. tubule
DentaScan
D. imaging
D. multiplanar reformation
dentate
d. fascia
d. fissure
d. fracture
d. gyrus
d. ligament
d. line
d. nuclei calcification
d. nucleus of cerebellum
d. suture
d. suture of skull
dentatoolivary pathway
dentatorubral-pallidoluysian atrophy
dentatothalamic tract
denticulate ligament
dentigerous cyst
dentin, dentinum
dentinal
d. sheath
d. tubule
dentinogenesis imperfecta
dentinum (*var. of* dentin)
dentition
crowded d.
dentoskeletal relationship
denture-supporting structure
Denuce ligament
denudation
area of d.
Denver ascites shunt
Denys-Drash tumor
deossification
band of d.
deoxygenated blood
deoxyglucose
^{11}C d.
deoxyribonucleic acid
dependence
quadratic d.
relaxation rate frequency d.
solvent water TI frequency d.
dependent
d. atelectasis
d. edema fluid resorption
d. extracellular fluid accumulation
d. lung
dephase-rephase magnitude subtraction technique
dephasing
d. gradient
intraluminal d.
intravoxel d.
odd-echo d.
rapid d.
signal d.
spin d.
depiction
magnetic resonance d.
d. of vasculature
d. in vivo
depletion
intravascular volume d.
depolarization
ventricular premature d. (VPD)
deposit
amyloid d.
arteriosclerotic d.
bony d.
calcareous d.
calcium d.
callus d.
endochondral bone d.
intramuscular hemosiderin d.
pericardium calcareous d.
deposition of tracer
depressed
d. diaphragm
d. ejection fraction
d. right ventricular contractile function
d. skull fracture
depression
bone marrow d.
fragment d.
hemidiaphragm d.
d. of left mainstem bronchus
marginal kidney d.
myocardial d.
d. of nasal bone
pacchionian d.
reciprocal d.
d. of renal margin
sinus node d.
spinal cord d.
translucent d.
ventricular d.

NOTES

depression-type intraarticular fracture
deprivation dwarfism
depth
d. compensation
d. dose
midplane d.
photon interaction d.
d. pulse
scatterer d.
signal d.
skin d.
target d.
depth-dose
d.-d. curve
d.-d. distribution
depth-pulse technique
depth-resolved surface coil spectroscopy (DRESS)
DER
dual-energy radiograph
derangement
disk d.
internal d.
longitudinal transarticular d.
derby-hat fracture
Derek Harwood-Nash series of catheter (DHN1, 2, 3)
derivative circulation
derived value on apex cardiogram (dD/dt)
dermal
d. bone
d. breast calcification
d. duct tumor
d. sinus tract
dermal–subcutaneous fat interface
dermoid
mediastinum d.
monodermal d.
ovarian d.
d. ovarian cyst
d. plug
spinal d.
d. tumor
derotate
derotation
DES
diethylstilbestrol
diffuse esophageal spasm
DES daughter
DES exposure
Desault
D. dislocation
D. fracture
D. sign
descended testis
descending
d. aorta dissection
d. colon
d. duodenum
left anterior d. (LAD)
d. septal artery
d. thoracic aorta
d. thoracic aortofemorofemoral (DTAF)
d. tract
descent
basal d.
epididymal d.
perineal d.
desert rheumatism
design
crossed-coil d.
3D pulse d.
factorial d.
pulse d.
Desilets introducer system
desmectasis
desmocytoma
desmofibromatosis
desmoid
cortical d.
d. lesion
periosteal d.
subperiosteal d.
d. tumor
desmoma
desmoplastic
d. infantile astrocytoma
d. small round-cell tumor (DSRCT)
desmosis
desmosome
d'Espine sign
desquamated epithelial breast hyperplasia
desquamative
d. fibrosing alveolitis
d. interstitial pneumonia (DIP)
destruction
bony d.
cortical d.
geographic bone d.
d. of medial end of clavicle
moth-eaten bone d.
mucosal d.
pattern of d.
permeative bone d.
sellar d.
d. of temporomandibular joint
temporomandibular joint d.
d. of tissue
trabecular d.
destructive
d. bone lesion
d. brucellar arthritis
d. interference technique

d. process
d. spondyloarthropathy
d. tumor

detachable coil

detail
exquisite d.
intraluminal d.
rib d.
suboptimal d.

detecting
collision d.
d. module

detection
annihilation coincidence d. (ACD)
early d.
d. echocardiography
magnetic resonance d.
occult d.
prospective investigation of pulmonary embolus d. (PIOPED)
quadrature d.
radioactivity d.
radwaste radioactivity d.
d. zone

detective quantum efficiency (DQE)

detector
annular d.
d. array
cadmium iodide d.
d. coil
d. collimation
CR-39 nuclear tract d.
C-TRAK hand-held gamma d.
digital x-ray d.
diode d.
Doppler ultrasonic blood flow d.
Doppler ultrasonic velocity d.
flame ionization d.
GE d.
Geiger-Müller d.
glass tract d.
HPGe d.
high-purity germanium detector
kinestatic charge d. (KCD)
Neoprobe radioactivity d.
passive track d.
phase-sensitive d.
quadrature phase d. (QPD)
scintillation d.
selenium-based digital d.
Si (Li) d.
sodium d.
solid-state d.
solid-state nuclear track d.
Wang-Binford edge d.
x-ray d.

Determann syndrome

determinant
sequential d.

determination
Budin-Chandler anteversion d.
d. of lung volume
particle size d.
void d.

detorsion
spontaneous d.

detour
d. conduit
d. sign

detritus

detrusor
d. areflexia
d. hyperreflexia
d. instability
d. muscle

Detsky modified cardiac risk index

deuterium
d. imaging agent
d. oxide

deuterium-tritium generator

deuteron

deuton

Deutschländer disease

devascularization
paraesophagogastric d.

developer artifact

development
branchial cleft d.
conductive d.
delayed d.
endocardial cushion d.
insulative d.
interval d.
lymphatic d.
pubertal d.

developmental
d. defect
d. dysplasia
d. dysplasia of hip (DDH)
d. groove
d. renal anomaly

Deventer
D. diameter
D. pelvis

NOTES

D

deviated mediastinum
deviation
angular d.
aortic d.
carpal d.
fracture d.
left axis d. (LAD)
mediastinal d.
radial d.
right axis d. (RAD)
rotary d.
septal d.
significant axis d.
standard d.
tracheal d.
ulnar d.
ureter d.
valgus d.
varus d.
device
abdominal left ventricular assist d. (ALVAD)
accuDEXA bone mineral density assessment d.
ACMI ulcer measuring d.
Apogee ultrasound d.
Arnoff external fixation d.
artificial left ventricular assist d.
beam-modifying d.
biventricular assist d. (BVAD)
BladderManager ultrasound d.
bone fixation d.
Bucky digital x-ray d.
Burnett mouth positioning d.
buttoned d.
charge coupled d.
compression d.
continuous microinfusion d.
copper 7 intrauterine d.
copper T intrauterine d.
CVIS imaging d.
diffracting Doppler transducer d.
Digital Add-On Bucky x-ray d.
directional atherectomy d.
DirectRay direct-to-digital x-ray capture d.
electrooptical d.
Elscint Planar d.
external fixation d.
halo d.
Hysterocath hysterosalpingography d.
Ilizarov d.
implantable vascular access d.
infrared-linked navigational d.
internal fixation d.
Intra-Dop intraoperative d.
intramedullary fixation d.
intrauterine contraceptive d. (IUD)
Kendall sequence compression d.
kinematic wrist d.
LaTeX d.
left ventricular assist d. (LVAD)
Leksell stereotactic d.
magnetic induction d.
Mammotome biopsy d.
nail-plate d.
Navarre interventional radiology d.
NMR LipoProfile d.
nonferromagnetic positioning d.
orthopedic fixation d.
OsteoAnalyzer d.
percutaneous atherectomy d.
PET balloon Simpson atherectomy d.
PGK (Panos G. Koutrouvelis, M.D.) stereotactic d.
Pigg-O-Stat immobilization d.
Ponomar transjugular clot-trapper d.
prosthetic d.
radiative hyperthermia d.
Rashkind double umbrella d.
right ventricular assist d. (RVAD)
Sideris buttoned double-disk d.
Simpson atherectomy d.
spinal fixation d.
stereotactic add-on d.
suction d.
superconducting quantum interference d. (SQUID)
synchronization d.
Telos radiographic stress d.
unbuttoning of d.
vascular access d.
venous access d.
ventricular assist d.
device-independent (DVI)
devitalized
d. portion of bone
d. tissue
devoid of circulation
DEXA
dual-energy x-ray absorptiometry
DEXA bone density scan imaging
DEXA (dual-energy x-ray absorptiometry) densitometer
DEXA scan
dexamethasone suppression test imaging
Dexter-Grossman classification of mitral regurgitation
dextran
Gd-DTPA-labeled d.
iron d.
dextran-coated charcoal
dextrocardia
dextroconcave

dextrogastria
dextroposition
dextropositioned aorta
dextrorotary
d. scoliosis
dextrorotoscoliosis
dextroscoliosis
dextrose 5% in water imaging agent
dextrotransposition of great arteries
dextrotropic
dextroversion
d. of heart
dextrum
cor d.
Deyerle sign
DFA
dorsiflexion angle
hallux dorsiflexion angle
DFI
disease-free interval
dye fluorescence index
DFP
diastolic filling pressure
DFS
disease-free survival
distraction-flexion staging
DFT
discrete Fourier transform
2DFT
two-dimensional Fourier transform
2DFT method
2DFT time-of-flight MR angiography
3DFT
three-dimensional Fourier transform
3DFT gradient-echo MR imaging
3DFT volume imaging
DGR
duodenogastric reflux
DI
diagnostic imaging
diabetic
d. cardiomyopathy
d. cystopathy
d. gastroparesis
d. nephropathy
diacondylar fracture
diagniol
diagnosis, pl. **diagnoses**
clinical d.
differential d.
empirical d.
noninvasive d.
pathologic d.
postoperative d.
preoperative d.
presumptive d.
radiologic d.
remote d.
roentgenographic d.
sonographic d.
tentative d.
ultrasound d.
working d.
Diagnost 120
diagnostic
d. angiography
d. cascade
computer-aided d.'s (CAD)
d. efficacy analysis
d. imaging (DI)
d. pneumothorax
d. procedure
d. radiation
d. radiology
d. radiopharmaceutical
d. range ultrasound
D. and Therapeutic Technology Assessment (DATTA)
d. ultrasound
diagonal
d. branch
d. branch #1 (D1)
d. branch of artery
d. conjugate diameter
diagram
Ladder d.
marker-channel d.
dialysis
d. fistula
d. shunt
d. tubing
diamagnetic
d. shift
d. substance
d. susceptibility
diamagnetism
Landau d.
diametaphyseal
diametaphysis
diameter
acetabular depth to femoral head d. (AD/FHD)
anterior sagittal d. (ASD)

NOTES

diameter *(continued)*
anterior-to-posterior sagittal canal d.
anteroposterior d.
aortic d. (AD)
aortic root d.
artery d.
Baudelocque d.
biischial d.
biparietal d. (BPD)
bispinous d.
bituberous d.
bronchial d.
cardiac d.
coccygeopubic d.
coil-to-vessel d.
conjugate d.
Deventer d.
diagonal conjugate d.
film d.
gestational sac d. (GS diameter)
GS d.
gestational sac diameter
increased anteroposterior d.
increment in luminal d.
intercristal d.
internal d. (ID)
internal conjugate d.
intertubercular d.
left anterior internal d. (LAID)
left ventricular internal d. (LVID)
Löhlein d., Loehlein d.
lumen d.
maximum anteroposterior d.
midsagittal d. (MSD)
minimal luminal d. (MLD)
minimal port d. (MPD)
narrow anteroposterior d.
oblique d.
orthonormal d.
pelvic d.
right ventricular internal d. (RVID)
sacropubic d.
spinal cord d.
stenosis d.
transverse pelvic d.
valve d.
vessel d.
yolk sac (YS) d.
diametric pelvic fracture
diamniotic pregnancy
diamond sign
diapedesis
diaphanography
diaphragm
above d. (AD)
accessory d.
antral mucosal d.
aperture d.
aponeurotic portion of d.
arcuate ligament of d.
below d. (BD)
Bucky d.
central tendon d.
d. collar sign
crus of the d.
depressed d.
dome of d.
duodenal d.
d. duplication
elevated d.
d. embryology
eventration of the d.
excursion of the d.
free air under d.
gastric d.
inferior vena cava d.
leaf of d.
median arcuate ligament of d.
muscular crus of d.
paralysis of d.
pelvic d.
polyarcuate d.
Potter-Bucky d.
respiratory d.
sella turcica d.
tenting of d.
thoracoabdominal d.
traumatic rupture of the d. (TRD)
urogenital d.
diaphragma sella
diaphragmatic
d. attenuation
d. border
d. contour
d. creep
d. crus
d. cupula
d. dome
d. echo
d. elevation
d. esophageal hiatus
d. eventration
d. fascia
d. hernia
d. ligament
d. lymph node
d. myocardial infarct (DMI)
d. paralysis
d. pericardium
d. pleura
d. pleurisy
d. rupture
d. segment
d. slip
d. surface

d. surface of heart
d. surface of liver
diaphyseal, diaphysial
d. aclasis
d. center
d. cortical mortise
d. dysplasia
d. fracture
d. lesion
d. ossification
d. sclerosis
diaphyseal-epiphyseal fusion
diaphysis, pl. **diaphyses**
diaphysitis
luetic d.
diaplasis
diarthrodial joint
diarthrosis
diaschisis
crossed cerebellar d.
ipsilateral cortical d.
Diasonics
D. ultrasound
D. ultrasound scanner
diastasis
d. of cranial bone
fracture d.
d. heart period
sutural d.
d. of suture
syndesmotic d.
tibiofibular d.
diastatic
d. fracture
d. lambdoid suture
diastematomyelia
spinal d.
diastolic
d. atrial volume
d. blood pressure
d. counterpulsation
d. depolarization phase
d. depolarization pulse
d. doming
d. filling period
d. filling pressure (DFP)
d. gating
d. gradient
d. heart failure
d. left ventricular index
d. notch impedance
d. overload
d. perfusion pressure
d. perfusion time
d. pressure-time index (DPTI)
d. pseudogating
d. regurgitant velocity
d. reserve
d. velocity ratio
Diastonics system
diastrophic
d. dwarfism
d. dysplasia
diathermic
d. loop
d. vascular occlusion
diathermy ultrasound
diathesis, pl. **diatheses**
hypertensive d.
diatrizoate
d. meglumine
d. meglumine imaging agent
d. meglumine radiopaque medium
methylglucamine d.
d. sodium imaging agent
diatrizoate-60 imaging agent
diatrizoic acid
diazepam imaging agent
DIC
drip-infusion cholangiogram
DIC microscopy
dicephalus
dichorionic, dichorial
d. diamniotic twin pregnancy
dichorionic-diamniotic twin
dichromate
d. dosimeter
d. dosimetry
Dickhaut-DeLee discoid meniscus classification
DICOM
Digital Imaging and Communications in Medicine interface
dicondylar fracture
Dicopac test
dicrotic notch
Dictaphone Digital Express clinical reporting system
DID
document image decoding
DIDA
diethyl iminodiacetic acid
dimethyl iminodiacetic acid
didactylism

NOTES

didelphia
uterine d.
didelphic uterus
didelphys
uterine d.
Didiee projection
diencephalic herniation
diencephalon, pl. **diencephala**
die-punch fracture
DIET
D. fast SE imaging
D. method of fat suppression
dietary rickets
diethylenetriamine pentaacetic acid
diethylenetriaminepentaacetic acid imaging agent (DTPA imaging agent)
diethyl iminodiacetic acid (DIDA)
diethylstilbestrol (DES)
Dieulafoy
D. lesion
D. triad
D. vascular malformation
difference
field-echo d.
differencing
d. fiber
d. filter
differential
d. diagnosis
d. diagnosis bone lesion
d. diagnostic lung mass feature
d. heart density sign
d. interference contrast microscopy (DIC microscopy)
renal function d.
d. renal function
scintillation camera linearity d.
scintillation camera uniformity d.
d. signal
d. uniformity
differentiated carcinoma (DC)
differentiation
cluster of d. (CD)
corticomedullary d. (CMD)
gray-white d.
liposarcomatous d.
nuclear annular d.
diffracting Doppler transducer device
diffraction
beam d.
high-resolution d.
high-temperature d.
low-temperature d.
d. pattern
d. peak
x-ray d.
diffuse
d. abdominal calcification
d. adenomyosis
d. aggressive lymphoma
d. aggressive polymorphous infiltrate
d. air-space disease
d. alveolar hemorrhage
d. alveolar interstitial infiltrate
d. aortic dilatation
d. aortomegaly
d. arterial ectasia
d. arteriolar spasm
d. bacterial nephritis
d. bilateral alveolar infiltrate
d. cerebral histiocytosis
d. cirrhosis
d. CNS sclerosis
d. dilation of the esophagus
d. distribution
d. edema
d. emphysema
d. enlargement of the thymus
d. esophageal spasm (DES)
d. fatty liver infiltrate
d. fibrocystic disease
d. fibrosis type
d. fine nodular lung disease
d. gallbladder wall thickening
d. ganglion
d. hepatic enlargement
d. hyperemia
d. idiopathic sclerosing hyperostosis (DISH)
d. idiopathic skeletal hyperostosis (DISH)
d. increase in breast density
d. infection
d. inflammation
d. intermediate lymphocytic lymphoma
d. interstitial pulmonary fibrosis (DIPF)
d. intimal thickening
d. irregularity
d. large-cell lymphoma
d. liver enlargement
d. lung uptake
d. lymphangioma
d. lymphocytic lymphoma
d. malignant peritoneal mesothelioma
d. mixed small- and large-cell lymphoma
d. mottling
d. mucosal polyposis
d. myelinoclastic sclerosis
d. narrowing
d. necrosis
d. necrotizing leukoencephalopathy

d. opacity
d. osteosclerosis
d. panbronchiolitis
d. pancreatitis
d. pattern
d. pericarditis
d. perivascular infiltrate
d. pleural thickening
d. pleurisy
d. pneumonia
d. pulmonary alveolar hemorrhage
d. reflector
d. reticular density
d. reticulonodular infiltrate
d. sarcomatosis
d. scleroderma
d. sclerosing alveolitis
d. signal hyperintensity
d. skeletal metastasis
d. small-cell lymphocytic lymphoma
d. spasm of the esophagus
d. spondylosis
d. stenosis
d. subarachnoid hemorrhage
d. symmetric hypertrophied cardiomyopathy
d. synovial lipoma
d. thymic enlargement
d. toxic goiter
d. ulcerative lesion
d. uterine enlargement
d. ventricular hypokinesis
d. white matter injury

diffuse, fine lung reticulation
diffusely swollen hemisphere
diffusing capacity
diffusion
anisotropically rotational d. (ARD)
d. coefficient
directional d.
d. factor
d. magnetic resonance imaging
molecular d.
d. pulse sequence
restricted d.
spectral d.
d. spectroscopy
spin d.
thermal d.
d. time
translational d.

diffusion-sensitive sequence
diffusion-weighted
d.-w. image
d.-w. MR imaging
d.-w. pulse sequence
d.-w. scanning

diffusum
papilloma d.

digastric
d. fossa
d. groove
d. impression
d. muscle
d. notch
d. triangle

DiGeorge syndrome
digestive
d. system
d. tract
d. tract contents
d. tube

DiGimard syndrome
Digirad gamma camera
digiscope
Direx d.

digit
accessory d.
arthrodesed d.
binary d.
fibroosseous pseudotumor of d.
flail d.
photoplethysmographic d.
replanted d.
sausage d.
supernumerary d.
syndactylization of d.

digital
D. Add-On Bucky image acquisition system
D. Add-On Bucky x-ray device
d. amputation
d. aponeurosis
d. archive
d. artery of foot
d. artery of hand
d. beam attenuation
d. branch
d. celiac trunk angiography
d. deformity
d. ejection fraction
D. Equipment system
d. fluoroscopy
d. fossa

NOTES

digital *(continued)*
d. free hepatic venography
d. frequency analysis
d. gray scale
d. holography system
d. imaging and communications in medicine
D. Imaging and Communications in Medicine interface (DICOM)
d. imaging processing (DIP)
d. imaging processing algorithm (DIP algorithm)
d. livedo reticularis infarct
d. mammographic system
d. mammography
d. markings
d. neuroma
d. parabola
d. plethysmography
d. process of fat
d. radiography (DR)
d. radiography imaging
d. ray
d. rectal evacuation
d. road mapping
d. rotational angiography (DRA)
d. runoff
d. sampling rate
d. scan converter
d. storage
d. subtraction
d. subtraction angiography (DSA)
d. subtraction aortography
d. subtraction arteriography (DSA)
d. subtraction film
d. subtraction pulmonary angiogram
d. subtraction rotational angiography
d. subtraction ventriculogram
d. tomosynthesis
D. Traumex system
d. unraveling
d. vascular imaging (DVI, DVI mode)
d. vein
d. videoangiography
d. video gastrointestinal radiography
d. x-ray detector

digitally
d. fused CT and radiolabeled imaging
d. fused CT and radiolabeled monoclonal antibody SPECT image
d. reconstructed radiograph (DRR)

digital-to-analog converter (DAC)

digiti (*pl. of* digitus)

digitization

digitized
d. CT slice
d. slices
d. spinography

digitizer
3D surface d.
multiple jointed d.
multisensor structured light range d.
Polhemus 3 d.
Scanmaster DX x-ray film d.

digitorum
extensor d.

Digitron
D. digital subtraction imaging system
D. DVI/DSA computer

digitus, pl. **digiti**
d. annularis
d. flexus deformity
digiti manus
d. medius
d. minimus
d. pedis
d. primus
d. secundus
d. valgus
d. varus

dihydropyrimidine dehydrogenase activity

dihydroxyphenalalanine imaging agent (DOPA imaging agent)

diiodotyrosine (DIT)

diisocyanide-triisocyanide ^{99m}Tc complex

diisopropyl iminodiacetic acid (DISIDA)

dilatation, dilation
alveolar d.
d. of aneurysm
annular d.
aortic root d.
arterial d.
ascending aorta d.
balloon d.
beaded ductal d.
bile duct d.
biliary d.
bowel loop d.
bronchial d.
bronchiolar d.
caliceal d.
cardiac d.
cavitary d.
chamber d.
colonic d.
common duct d.
congenital cystic d.
cystic d.
diffuse aortic d.

distal ureteral d.
ductal d.
Eder-Puestow d.
esophageal d.
extrahepatic biliary cystic d.
fusiform d.
gaseous d.
gastric d.
hepatic web d.
d. and hypertrophy
idiopathic pulmonary artery d.
idiopathic right atrial d.
intestinal d.
intrahepatic biliary cystic d.
intrahepatic biliary ductal d.
intrahepatic biliary tract d.
intraluminal d.
junctional d.
left ventricular d.
megacolon d.
multiple mural d.
mural d.
myocardial d.
pancreatic duct d.
paradoxical colon d.
percutaneous transluminal balloon d.
periportal sinusoidal d.
poststenotic d.
prestenotic d.
probe d.
prognathic d.
pulmonary artery d.
pulmonary trunk idiopathic d.
pulmonary valve stenosis d.
rectal d.
respiratory bronchiolar d.
right ventricular d.
saccular d.
stress-induced left ventricular d.
sulcus d.
d. of sulcus
thickened irregular small bowel fold d.
thickened smooth small bowel fold d.
tortuous vein d.
transient left ventricular d.
transluminal d.
d. of ureter
ureteral d.
vein d.
d. of ventricle
ventricular wall d.
Virchow-Robin space d.
Wirsung d.

dilated
d. aortic root
d. bile duct
d. bowel loop
d. bronchus
d. cardiomyopathy (DCM)
d. collateral vein
d. dry small bowel
d. duodenum
d. fetal bowel
d. gallbladder
d. intercavernous sinus
d. loops of bowel
d. myocardium
d. pulmonary artery
d. pulmonary trunk
d. rete testis
d. ureter
d. ventricle
d. wet small bowel

dilator
angiographic Teflon d.
balloon d.

dilution
isotopic d.

DIMAQ
D. integrated ultrasound system
D. integrated ultrasound workstation

dimeglumine
gadopentetate d. (Gd-DTPA)

dimension
abnormal heart chamber d.
absolute artery d.
aortic root d.
arterial d.
axial d.
intraluminal d.
intrathoracic d.
left ventricular diastolic d. (LVdd, LVDD)
left ventricular end-diastolic d. (LVEDD)
left ventricular end-systolic d. (LVESD)
left ventricular internal diastolic d. (LVIDd, LVIDD)
luminal d.

NOTES

dimension *(continued)*
right ventricular d. (RVD)
spleen d.
dimethyl iminodiacetic acid (DIDA)
dimethylsuccinic acid (DMSA)
diminished
d. lung volume
d. marrow signal intensity
d. systemic perfusion
diminutive vessel
dimple
blind d.
d. of bone
pretibial d.
dinner-fork deformity
diode
d. detector
infrared light-emitting d.
d. laser
d. measurement
Zener d.
diodine
diodone
Diodrast
D. imaging agent
Dionosil
D. imaging agent
dioxide
carbon d. (CO_2)
thorium d.
DIP
desquamative interstitial pneumonia
digital imaging processing
distal interphalangeal
DIP algorithm
DIP articulation
DIP joint
dip
d. phenomenon
septal d.
dip-and-plateau phenomenon
DIPF
diffuse interstitial pulmonary fibrosis
2,5-diphenyloxazole (PPO)
diphosphonate
methylene d. (MDP)
diplegia spinalis brachialis traumatica
diploic
d. canal
d. vein
diplomyelia
diplopia
dipolar
d. broadening
d. interaction
dipole
d. coupling
electric d.
d. field
magnetic d.
dipole-dipole
d.-d. coupling
d.-d. interaction
d.-d. relaxation rate
diprosopus
diprotrizoate imaging agent
dipygus
dipyridamole
d. echocardiography
d. echocardiography imaging
d. echocardiography test
d. handgrip imaging
d. handgrip test
d. infusion imaging
d. infusion test
d. technetium-99m-2-methoxy isobutyl
d. technetium-99m-2-methoxy isobutyl isonitrile
d. thallium-201
d. thallium-201 imaging
d. thallium-201 scintigraphy
d. thallium stress imaging
d. thallium ventriculogram
d. tomographic thallium stress test
direct
d. caval cannulation
d. current (DC)
d. current generator
d. current offset artifact
d. display console (DDC)
d. embolus
d. Fourier transformation imaging
d. fracture
d. immunofluorescence analysis
d. inguinal hernia
d. liquid scintillation count
d. needle puncture
d. puncture MR phlebogram
d. puncture phlebography
d. pyramidal tract
d. radioiodination
d. ray
d. visualization
direction
aboral d.
anterior-posterior flow d.
caudal d.
cephalad d.
mediolateral flow d.
phase-encoding d.
superior-inferior flow d.
directional
d. atherectomy device
d. color angiography (DCA)

d. coronary atherectomy (DCA)
d. diffusion

directly
d. coupled sample changer system
d. observed therapy

director
grooved d.

DirectRay direct-to-digital x-ray capture device

Direx
D. digiscope
D. Thermex
D. Tripter

dirty
d. acoustic shadowing
d. chest
d. fat
d. fat sign
d. mass
d. necrosis

disappearance
d. frequency
d. slope

disappearing fetus

disarticulation
hip d.

disc (*var. of* disk)

discectomy (*var. of* diskectomy)

discernible venous motion

discharge
nipple d.
sympathetic d.
vaginal d.

discharging tubule

disci (*pl. of* discus)

discitis

discogram (*var. of* diskogram)

discography (*var. of* diskography)

discoid
d. atelectasis
d. chest mass
d. filling defect
d. kidney
d. lateral meniscus
d. meniscus
d. shadow

discoligamentous complex

discontinuous
d. density gradient
d. density gradient centrifugation

discordant
d. nodule thyroid
d. thyroid nodule
d. twin

discrepancy
biomechanics of limb length d.
leg-length d. (LLD)
limb-length d. (LLD)

discreta
porokeratosis plantaris d.

discrete
d. bleeding source
d. Fourier transform (DFT)
d. hyperintense focus
d. hyperintense signal intensity
d. lesion
d. mass
d. perihilar density
d. subaortic stenosis
d. subvalvular aortic stenosis (DSAS)
d. tumor

discriminant analysis

discriminate

discrimination
density d.

discus, pl. **disci**

disease, pl. **diseases**
acquired cystic kidney d.
acquired renal cystic d.
active parenchymal d.
Addison d.
adrenal medullary d.
adrenocortical d.
adult polycystic kidney d.
advanced cortical d.
air-space d.
alcoholic liver d. (ALD)
Alexander d.
allergic d.
allogeneic d.
alloimmune d.
Alpers d.
alveolar d.
Alzheimer d. (AD)
amyloid oral cavity d.
angiomatous d.
anterior horn cell d.
aortic valvular d. (AVD)
aortoiliac obstructive d. (AIOD)
apical distribution lung d.
arterial degenerative d.
arteriosclerotic cardiovascular d. (ASCVD)

D

NOTES

disease *(continued)*
arteriosclerotic heart d. (ASHD)
arteriosclerotic occlusive d.
arteriosclerotic peripheral vascular d.
arteriosclerotic renal d.
asbestos-related pleural d.
atheroembolic renal d.
atheroocclusive d.
atherosclerotic cardiovascular d. (ASCVD)
atherosclerotic carotid artery d. (ACAD)
atherosclerotic pulmonary vascular d. (ASPVD)
Ayerza d.
Bamberger-Marie d.
Bannister angioedema d.
Banti d.
Barlow d.
Barrett d.
basilar distribution lung d.
basilar-vertebral artery d.
Batten d.
Bazin d.
Beau d.
Beauvais d.
Beemer d.
benign asbestos-related pleural d.
benign breast d. (BBD)
Bielschowsky-Jansky d.
biliary tract d.
Binswanger d.
black lung d.
Blount d.
Bornholm d.
Bouchard d.
Bouillaud d.
Bourneville d.
Bourneville-Pringle d.
Bouveret d.
brain d.
brainstem d.
breast d.
Brinton d.
Brodie d.
bronchial type B d.
bronchiolar d.
Bruck d.
Budlinger-Ludlof-Laewen d.
Buerger thromboangiitis obliterans d.
bullous lung d.
Caffey d.
Caffey-Silverman d.
caisson d.
calcium pyrophosphate deposition d. (CPPD)
calcium pyrophosphate dihydrate deposition d.
Calvé d.
Calvé-Legg-Perthes d.
Calvé-Perthes d.
Camurati-Engelmann d.
Canavan d.
Canavan-van Bogaert-Bertrand d.
cardiopulmonary d.
cardiorenal d.
cardiovascular d. (CD, CVD)
cardiovascular renal d.
Caroli d.
carotid artery d.
carotid atherosclerotic d.
carotid occlusive d.
Carrington d.
Castellani d.
Castleman d.
celiac d.
central motor pathways d.
cerebellar d.
cerebral Whipple d.
cerebrovascular occlusive d.
cervical disk d.
Charcot-Marie-Tooth d.
cheese handler's d.
cheese washer's d.
Chester d.
Chicago d.
cholestatic liver d.
chronic interstitial simulating air-space lung d.
chronic obstructive lung d. (COLD)
chronic obstructive pulmonary d. (COPD)
chronic peripheral arterial d. (CPAD)
Coats d.
collagen vascular d. (CVD)
comorbid d.
Concato d.
congenital heart d. (CHD)
connective tissue d.
cork handler's lung d.
coronary artery d.
coronary heart d. (CHD)
Creutzfeldt-Jakob d.
Crohn d. (CD)
Crouzon d.
Cushing d.
cystic breast d.
cystic kidney d.
cystic ovarian d.
cystic renal d.
cytomegalic inclusion d.
deficiency d.
degenerative atrioventricular node d.

degenerative brain d.
degenerative cerebrum d.
degenerative disk d.
degenerative joint d. (DJD)
Degos d.
demineralization from d.
demyelinating d.
Deutschländer d.
diffuse air-space d.
diffuse fibrocystic d.
diffuse fine nodular lung d.
disk d.
diskogenic d.
disseminated d.
diverticular colon d.
Dubin-Sprinz d.
duodenal peptic ulcer d.
Duroziez mitral stenosis d.
eccentric plaque d.
embolic d.
emphysematous type A d.
end-stage lung d.
end-stage renal d.
Engelmann d.
Engel-Recklinghausen d.
eosinophilic lung d.
Erb d.
EtOH-associated liver d.
exanthematous d.
extracranial carotid artery occlusive d.
extramammary Paget d.
Fabry d.
Fahr-Volhard d.
Fairbank d.
Fallot d.
Farber d.
Favre d.
Fenwick d.
fibrocystic breast d.
fibrocystic lung d.
Flatau-Schilder d.
flax dresser's d.
Fleischer d.
focal fibrous breast d.
focal intestinal inflammatory d.
focal lung d.
Fong d.
Forestier d.
Freiberg d.
Freiberg-Kohler d.
Friedrich d.
fulminant course of d.
Gairdner d.
Gandy-Nanta d.
Garré d.
gastroesophageal reflux d. (GERD)
Gaucher d.
Gee-Herter d.
Gee-Thaysen d.
generalized interstitial d.
Gerstmann-Straussler-Sheinker d.
gestational nonmetastatic trophoblastic d.
gestational trophoblastic d. (GTD)
Gilchrist d.
Glénard d.
glial d.
global cardiac d.
glycogen storage d.
Gorham d.
Graves orbital d.
Graves thyroid d.
Gull d.
Hagner d.
Hajdu-Cheney d.
hard metal d.
heart d.
Heberden d.
Heckathorn d.
Henderson-Jones d.
hepatic vein d.
hepatobiliary d.
hepatocellular d.
hepatocerebral d.
heterogeneous system d.
Hirschsprung d.
Hodgkin d.
Hodgson d.
Hoffa d.
Horton d.
Huchard d.
Hunter d.
Huppert d.
hydatid d.
hydroxyapatite deposition d. (HADD)
hypertensive cardiovascular d.
hypertensive renal d.
hypertensive vascular d.
idiopathic eosinophilic lung d.
idiopathic inflammatory bowel d.
idiopathic mural endomyocardial d.
ileocolic d.

NOTES

D

disease *(continued)*
iliac atherosclerotic occlusive d.
immunoproliferative small intestine d. (IPSID)
inactive granulomatous d.
infantile polycystic kidney d.
inflammatory bowel d.
interfollicular Hodgkin d.
interstitial bronchiolitic respiratory d.
interstitial lung d.
intimal atherosclerotic d.
intradural inflammatory d.
intrahepatic pigment stone d.
intramedullary bony d.
intrapulmonary d.
intrarenal arterial d.
intrasynovial d.
intrauterine cytomegalic inclusion d.
intrinsic pulmonary d.
ischemic bowel d.
Jaffe-Lichtenstein d.
Jagziekte d.
Jansen d.
Jeune d.
juvenile autosomal recessive polycystic d.
juvenile Paget d.
Kahler d.
Kawasaki d.
Keshan d.
Kikuchi d.
Kikuchi-Fujimoto d.
Kimura d.
Kinnier-Wilson d.
Köhler d.
Köhler-Pellegrini-Stieda d.
Krabbe d.
Kugelberg-Welander d.
Kümmel d.
Kussmaul-Maier d.
kyphoscoliotic heart d.
labyrinthine d.
Lamy-Bienenfeld d.
Lane d.
Langer d.
Langer-Saldino d.
Larsen-Johannson d.
Legg-Calvé-Perthes d. (LCP)
Legg-Calvé-Waldenström d.
Leigh d.
leptomeningeal d.
Lhermitte-Duclos d.
Lichtenstein-Jaffe d.
Ligman-Sacks endocarditis d.
liver hydatid d.
Lobstein d.
localized air space d.
localized cystic kidney d.
lower lung d.
Lyme d.
lymphocyte-predominance Hodgkin d. (LPHD)
MacLean-Maxwell d.
macronodular lung d.
Maffucci d.
Majewski d.
Majocchi d.
maple bark d.
marble bone d.
Marchiafava-Bignami d.
Marie-Bamberger d.
Marie-Strumpell d.
Marie-Tooth d.
Martin d.
McArdle d.
McKusick d.
medullary cystic d.
Meigs d.
Ménétrier d.
mesenteric Weber-Christian d.
metabolic bone d.
metastatic d.
micrometastatic d.
micronodular lung d.
microvascular d.
Mikulicz d.
miliary lung d.
Miller d.
Milroy d.
Milton angioedema d.
mixed connective tissue d. (MCTD)
mixed restrictive-obstructive lung d.
Mondor d.
Mounier-Kuhn d.
multicentric Castleman d.
multiple gland d.
Münchmeyer d.
mushroom picker's d.
myocardial deposition d.
myocardial granulomatous d.
Naumoff d.
neonatal wet lung d.
Niemann-Pick d.
Nievergelt d.
nodal d.
nodular lung d.
nodular sclerosis Hodgkin d.
nodular thyroid d.
no evidence of d. (NED)
nonatherosclerotic d.
Norrie d.
obstructive airway d.
obstructive lung d.
obstructive pulmonary d. (OPD)

occlusive cerebrovascular d.
occlusive vascular brain d.
Ollier d.
olycystic ovarian d.
optic chiasm d.
organic brain d. (OBD)
Ormond d.
Osgood-Schlatter d.
Osler d.
Osler-Weber-Rendu d.
Paas d.
Paget jaw d.
Paget temporal bone d.
pancreatic d.
Panner d.
parenchymal lung d.
Parenti-Fraccaro d.
Payr d.
Pel-Ebstein d.
Pelizaeus-Merzbacher d.
Pellegrini-Stieda d.
pelvic inflammatory d. (PID)
peptic ulcer d. (PUD)
pericardial d.
perihilar lung d.
periodontal d.
peripheral air-space d.
peripheral arterial d.
peripheral lung d.
peripheral vascular d. (PVD)
Perthes d.
Petit d.
Peyronie d.
Pfaundler-Hurler d.
Pfeiffer d.
Pick d.
platinum-resistant d.
pleural d.
polycystic kidney d.
polycystic liver d.
polycystic ovarian d. (PCOD)
polycystic renal d.
Pompe d.
popliteal artery occlusive d.
posttransplant coronary artery d.
Pott d.
precancerous d.
prediverticular d.
Preiser d.
progressive d.
pseudo-Whipple d.
pulmonary collagen vascular d. (PCVD)
pulmonary embolic septic d.
pulmonary interstitial d.
pulmonary thromboembolic d.
Pyle d.
Quincke angioedema d.
radiation-induced liver d. (RILD)
radiation pericardial d.
ragpicker's d.
Raynaud d.
reactive airways d. (RAD)
Reiter d.
renal cystic d.
renal parenchymal d.
renal sinus d.
Rendu-Osler-Weber d.
renovascular d.
residual d.
respiratory bronchiolitis-associated interstitial lung d. (RB-ILD)
restrictive lung d.
restrictive myocardial d.
reticulonodular lung d.
reversible airways d.
rheumatic arthritis-associated interstitial lung d.
rheumatic heart d.
rheumatic valvular d.
ribbing d.
Riley-Day d.
Ruysch d.
sacroiliac d.
Sanfilippo d.
Scheie d.
Scheuermann d.
Schilder d.
Schmid d.
Schmitt d.
Schmorl d.
secretory breast d.
Sever d.
severe acute liver d.
Shaver d.
silo filler's d.
Simmond d.
Sinding-Larsen-Johansson d. (SLJD)
single-vessel d.
Sipple d.
slim d.
Sly d.
snufftaker's pituitary d.

NOTES

D

disease *(continued)*
stable d.
Stickler d.
Still d.
Strümpell-Lorrain d.
Strümpell-Marie d.
Sturge-Weber d.
subarachnoid metastatic d.
Swediaur d.
synchronous d.
Taussig-Bing d.
Thiemann d.
three-vessel coronary d.
thromboembolic d. (TED)
thromboembolic lung d.
thyrocardiac d.
thyroid d.
tibial artery d.
tibioperoneal occlusive d.
Touraine-Solente-Gole d.
transhepatic biliary d.
Trevor d.
ulcer d.
upper lung d.
upper respiratory tract d.
valvular d. (VD)
valvular heart d.
van Bogaert-Canavan d.
van Neck d.
Vaquez d.
vascular occlusive d.
venous thromboembolic d. (VTED)
vertebrobasilar d.
von Gierke d.
von Hippel-Lindau d. (VHL)
Voorhoeve d.
Waldenström d.
Warburg d.
Weber-Christian breast d.
Weil d.
Werdnig-Hoffmann d.
Werner d.
Westphal-Strümpell d.
wet lung d.
white matter d.
Wilson bone d.
Winiwarter-Buerger d.
Winwarter-Manteuffel-Buerger d.
woolsorter's inhalation d.

disease-free
d.-f. interval (DFI)
d.-f. survival (DFS)
d.-f. vessel

DISH
diffuse idiopathic sclerosing hyperostosis
diffuse idiopathic skeletal hyperostosis

dishpan fracture

DISI
dorsal intercalated segmental instability

DISIDA
diisopropyl iminodiacetic acid
Tc-99 DISIDA
technetium-99m DISIDA
technetium-99m DISIDA (Tc-99 DISIDA)

disintegration
d. constant
myofibrillar d.
nuclear d.
radioactive d.
spontaneous d.

disjointing

disk, disc
acromioclavicular joint d.
anal d.
d. of ankle
articular d.
atrial d.
d. ballooning
Bardeen primitive d.
biconcave d.
Bowman d.
d. bulge
bulging d.
d. calcification
cartilaginous d.
cervical d.
chorionic d.
cone d.
contained d.
crescent-shaped fibrocartilaginous d.
d. degeneration
degenerative d.
d. derangement
d. disease
d. displacement
distal radioulnar d.
embryonic d.
d. of endocardium
epiphyseal d.
extruded d.
d. extrusion
fibrocartilaginous d.
fibrous ring of d.
fixation d.
d. fragment
frayed d.
golfer's elbow on d.
growth d.
H d.
hard d.
Hensen d.
herniated intervertebral d. (HID)
d. herniation
hydrodynamic potential of d.

I d.
interarticular d.
d. interspace
intervertebral d.
invertebral d.
isotropic d.
kidney d.
d. lesion
locking d.
lumbar d.
lumbosacral d.
mandibular d.
d. margin
massive herniated d.
d. maturation
Merkel tactile d.
midline herniation of d.
Molnar d.
noncontained d.
occult residual herniated d.
d. ossification
placental d.
d. plication
d. poppet
protruded d.
d. protrusion
ruptured d.
Schiefferdecker d.
sequestered d.
d. sequestration
slipped intervertebral d.
soft d.
d. space
d. space height
d. space infection
sternoclavicular joint d.
tactile d.
temporomandibular joint d.
thoracic d.
thoracolumbar vertebral d.
triangular d.
vacuum d.
vertebral d.
d. water content
d. water signal
Winchester d.
Z d.

diskectomy, discectomy
percutaneous automated d.
same-day microsurgical arthroscopic lateral-approach laser-assisted (SMALL) fluoroscopic d.

diskitis
septic d.

disklike atelectasis

diskogenic disease

diskogram, discogram
intervertebral d.
intranuclear d.

diskography, discography

diskoligamentous injury

diskovertebral infection

disk-space narrowing

disk-thecal sac interface

disk-to-magnetic
d.-t.-m. field
d.-t.-m. field orientation

disk-type valve

dislocated
d. hip
d. knee

dislocation
anterior d.
anteroinferior d.
atlantooccipital d.
axial carpal d.
Bankart d.
bayonet d.
Bell-Dally cervical d.
Bennett d.
bilateral intrafacetal d.
boutonnière d.
bursting d.
central d.
cervical facet d.
Chopart ankle d.
chronic recurrent d.
closed d.
complete d.
complicated d.
compound d.
congenital hip d.
consecutive d.
Desault d.
divergent d.
dysplasia d.
facet d.
d. fracture
fracture d.
frank d.
gamekeeper's habitual d.
glenohumeral d.
Hill-Sachs d.
hip d.

D

NOTES

dislocation *(continued)*
hyperextension d.
incomplete d.
interfacetal d.
interphalangeal d.
irreducible dorsal d.
isolated d.
Jahss classification of metatarsophalangeal joint d.
joint d.
Kienböck d., Keinboeck
Lisfranc d.
lunate d.
midcarpal d.
milkmaid's elbow d.
Monteggia d.
Nélaton d.
open d.
Otto pelvis d.
partial d.
d. of patella
patellar d.
pathologic d.
perilunar d.
perilunate carpal d.
posterior fracture d.
primitive d.
radiocarpal d.
recent d.
recurrent d.
rotational d.
scapholunate d.
shoulder d.
simple d.
Smith d.
subastragalar d.
subspinous d.
swivel d.
tibiotarsal d.
transradial styloid perilunate d.
transscaphoid perilunate d.
traumatic d.
triquetrolunate d.
unilateral interfacetal d.
unilateral intrafacetal d.
upward and backward d.
upward lens d.
volar d.
wrist d.

dislodgement
partial d.

dismutase
superoxide d.

disobliteration
carotid d.

disofenin
technetium-99m d.

disorder
angiitis-granulomatosis d.
angiocentric immunoproliferative d.
articular hand d.
articular wrist d.
bullous d.
cartilaginous growth plate d.
congenital d.
demyelinative d.
drug-induced bullous d.
esophageal motility d.
evacuation d.
functional d.
gastric motor d.
intractable bleeding d.
metabolic bone d.
motility d.
myeloproliferative d.
myotonic d.
neurocutaneous d.
neurogenic d.
nonspecific esophageal motility d. (NEMD)
patellofemoral d.
pulmonary lymphoid d.
right-left d.
sexual differentiation d.
systemic d.
vascular d.

disorientation
right-left d.

dispenser
film d.

dispersing agent

dispersion
gradient-induced phase d.
intravoxel phase d.
d. mode

dispersive component

disphenoid extraction

displaced
d. crus
d. crus sign
d. fat pad sign
d. fracture
d. fracture fragment
d. fragment of bone
d. gallbladder
d. left ventricular apex
d. vertebra

displacement
arterial brain d.
atlantoaxial rotary d.
d. of bowel gas
brainstem d.
d. of brain vessel
disk d.
Ellis Jones peroneal d.

d. field-fitting MR imaging
inferior d.
d. of interhemispheric fissure
left apexcardiogram, calibrated d. (LACD)
mediastinum d.
palmar d.
radial epiphyseal d.
retroperitoneal fat stripe d.
rotational d.
superolateral d.
tracheal d.

display
A-mode d.
B-mode d.
dynamic volume-rendered d.
image d.
M-mode d.
multiparametric color composite d.
multiplanar d. (MPD)
pseudocolor B-mode d.
real-time d.
segmentation method for real-time d.
shaded-surface d. (SSD)
static image d.
d. system

disproportion
cephalopelvic d. (CPD)
fetal-pelvic d.
fetal ventricular heart d.
fiber-type d.
ventricular d.

disproportionate upper septal thickening

disrupted plaque

disruption
anastomotic d.
annular d.
anterior labral d.
bony d.
d. of duct
epiglottic d.
facet capsule d.
ligamentous d.
myofascial d.
perivalvular d.
retinacular d.
skeletal d.
supraspinous ligament d.
trabecular d.
traumatic aortic d.

dissecans
osteochondritis d.
osteochondrosis d.

dissecting
d. abdominal aneurysm
d. aortic aneurysm
d. aortic hematoma
d. basilar artery aneurysm
d. intracranial aneurysm
d. intramural hematoma

dissection
aneurysmal d.
aortic d.
arterial wall d.
d. of artery
axial joint d.
DeBakey aortic d.
descending aorta d.
esophageal d.
extensive d.
extracapsular d.
extrapericardial d.
familial aortic d.
groin d.
intimal-medial d.
medial d.
sentinel node d.
sharp d.
spiral d.
spontaneous carotid d.
spontaneous coronary artery d. (SCAD)
Stanford type B aortic d.
subintimal d.
d. tubercle
vertebral arterial d.

disseminata
osteopathia condensans d.

disseminated
d. CNS histoplasmosis
d. coccidioidomycosis
d. dermal dendrocytoma
d. disease
d. inflammation
d. intravascular coagulation
d. intravascular coagulation of blood
d. lipogranulomatosis
d. necrotizing leukoencephalopathy
d. sclerosis
d. tuberculosis

D

NOTES

dissemination
lymphogenous d.
d. pattern
Disse space
dissociation
complete atrioventricular d.
electromechanical d. (EMD)
interference d.
scapholunate d.
dissociative instability
dissolution of gallstone
distal
d. acinar emphysema
d. aortic arch
d. aortic arch aneurysm
d. articular set angle (DASA)
d. bile duct
d. bile duct carcinoma (DBDC)
d. blind stomach
d. branch
d. bulbar septum
d. carpal row
d. circumflex marginal artery
d. colon
d. common bile duct obstruction
d. convoluted tubule
d. coronary perfusion pressure
d. coronary sinus (DCS)
d. duodenum
d. esophageal ring
d. femoral epiphyseal fracture
d. femur
d. humoral fracture
d. ileitis
d. interphalangeal (DIP)
d. interphalangeal joint
d. interphalangeal joint articulation
d. intestinal obstruction syndrome
d. leg cross section
d. lobular emphysema
d. occlusal distention
d. predominantly sensory polyneuropathy
d. radial fracture
d. radioulnar disk
d. radioulnar joint (DRUJ)
d. radioulnar joint compartment (DRUJ compartment)
d. radioulnar subluxation
d. rectal adenocarcinoma (DRA)
d. reference axis (DRA)
d. runoff
d. runoff vessel
d. segment
d. shift
d. small bowel
d. splenorenal shunt
d. surface
d. tibial physis
d. ureteral dilatation
distalward
distance
acromiohumeral d.
central lung d. (CLD)
Doppler-derived stroke d.
film tube d.
focal film d. (FFD)
focal spot-to-object d.
focus object d. (FOD)
focus-skin d. (FSD)
interarch d.
intercaudate d.
interlaminar d.
internuclear d.
interopercular d.
interorbital d.
interpedicular d.
interridge d.
interslice d.
interspinous d.
interuncal d.
object-film d. (OFD)
source-film d. (SFD)
source-skin d. (SSD)
source-surface d. (SSD)
source-to-image receptor d. (SID)
source-tray d. (STD)
surface d.
target-film d. (TFD)
target-skin d. (TSD)
widened teardrop d.
distance-based block classification
distant
d. metastasis
d. spread
distend
distended
d. abdomen
d. gallbladder
d. kidney
d. stomach
d. vein
distensibility
aortic d.
distensible
distention, distension
abdominal d.
azygos vein d.
bladder d.
bowel d.
colonic d.
distal occlusal d.
gaseous d.
gastric d.
hydraulic d.
intestinal d.

jugular venous d.
passive venous d.
pelvicaliceal d.
rectal d.
ureteral d.
venous d.
vesical d.
distinction
loss of d.
distorted anatomy
distortion
bronchial d.
focal d.
geometric d.
image d.
d. of limitations of image reconstruction algorithm artifact
pincushion d.
pituitary stalk d. (PSD)
radiographic pincushion d.
S d.
spiculated d.
Y-shaped d.
distraction
bifocal manipulation with d.
d. of fracture
d. gap
d. hyperflexion injury
d. of joint
joint d.
d. osteogenesis
physeal d.
segment d.
small-step d.
soft tissue d.
distraction-flexion staging (DFS)
distribution
anatomic d.
anomalous d.
centrilobular d.
depth-dose d.
diffuse d.
dose d.
gaussian d.
geometric d.
homogeneous thallium d.
inhomogeneous tracer d.
interstitial lung disease d.
loop d.
lung infiltrate d.
mottled d.
peribronchial d.
perivascular d.
Poisson d.
radioactivity d.
rapid d.
reverse d.
rimlike calcium d.
spectral noise d.
stocking-glove d.
symmetric d.
thallium-201 uptake and d.
trace element d.
d. transformer
uniform d.
unusual marrow d.
distributive shock
disturbance
architectural d.
d. of articulation
circulation d.
disturbed orientation
disuse
d. atrophy
lesser atrophy of d.
d. osteoporosis
d. syndrome
DIT
diiodotyrosine
diuretic
d. renal imaging
d. renal scan
divergent
d. dislocation
d. ray projection
d. spiculated pattern
diverging
d. collimator
d. meniscus
diversion
biliopancreatic d.
urinary d.
diversity segment
divertculum, diverticula (*pl. of* diverticulum)
acquired urethral d.
diverticular
d. abscess
d. colon disease
d. prostatitis
diverticulitis
acute d.
bladder d.
chronic d.

NOTES

D

diverticulitis *(continued)*
colonic d.
Meckel d.
sigmoid d.
diverticulosis
colonic d.
intramural esophageal d.
jejunal d.
tracheal d.
diverticulum, pl. **diverticula**
arachnoid d.
bladder d.
caliceal d.
colonic d.
common bile duct d.
congenital urethral d.
cricopharyngeal d.
divisional block d.
dorsal d.
ductus d.
duodenal intraluminal d.
esophageal d.
fallopian tube d.
false d.
fourth ventricle d.
functional d.
gallbladder d.
Ganser d.
gastric d.
giant sigmoid d.
Graser d.
hepatic d.
Hutch d.
hypopharyngeal d.
interaorticobronchial d.
interbronchial d.
intestinal d.
intraluminal duodenal d. (IDD)
intramural d.
inverted Meckel d.
jejunal d.
jejunoileal d.
juxtapapillary d.
Kirchner d.
Kommerell d.
Kumeral d.
Meckel d.
metanephric d.
midesophageal d.
d. of Nuck
Nuck d.
paraureteral d.
penile urethra d.
perforated d.
periampullary d.
pharyngoesophageal d.
pulsion d.
pyelocaliceal d.
Rokitansky d.
roofless fourth ventricle d.
sigmoid d.
small bowel d.
stomach d.
thoracic pulsion d.
thoracic root sleeve d.
traction d.
urachal d.
urethral d.
urinary bladder d.
Vater d.
vesical d.
Zenker d.
diverting
d. colostomy
d. stoma
divided dose
diving goiter
division
mandibular d.
maxillary d.
ureteral d.
divisional
d. block
d. block diverticulum
divisionary line
divisum
pancreas d.
divopontocerebellar atrophy
divot
Dixon method of phase unwrapping
dizygotic twin
DJD
degenerative joint disease
DJJ
duodenojejunal junction
DKS
Damus-Kaye-Stancel
DKS anastomosis
D-loop
ventricular D.-l.
D.-l. ventricular situs
DLT
dose-limiting toxicity
D-malposition of aorta
DMI
diaphragmatic myocardial infarct
DMPE
^{99m}Tc-bis-dimethylphosphonoethane
DMSA
dimethylsuccinic acid
technetium-99m DMSA
DNA
D. cytophotometry
D. flow cytometry
D. microinjection technique

DNET
dysembryoplastic neuroepithelial tumor
DNP
dynamic nuclear polarization
DNR
dose nonuniformity ratio
Dobbhoff feeding tube
dobutamine
d. stress echocardiography
d. thallium angiography
DOBV
double-outlet both ventricles
documentary arteriography
document image decoding (DID)
document-recognition algorithm
Dodd
D. perforating group of veins
D. perforating vein group
dodecafluoropentane (DDFP)
d. imaging agent (DDFP imaging agent)
Dodge
D. area-length method for ventricular volume
D. method for ejection fraction
D. principle
Doerner-Hoskins distribution law
Doge cap sign
doigt en lornette
dolastatin 15
dolens
phlegmasia cerula d.
dolichocephaly
dolichocolon
dolichoectasia
dolichoesophagus
dolichopellic pelvis
dolichosigmoid
dolichostenomelia
DOLV
double-outlet left ventricle
domain
dose rate d.
extracellular d.
Fourier d.
frequency d.
magnetic d.
spatial frequency d.
time d.
dome
d. of aneurysm
anterior talar d.
atrial d.
bladder d.
crus d.
d. cylinder
d. of diaphragm
diaphragmatic d.
d. fracture
d. of liver
liver d.
shoulder d.
talar d.
d. of urinary bladder
weightbearing acetabular d.
dome-and-dart configuration
dome-shaped
d.-s. heart
d.-s. roof of pleural cavity
dominance
cerebral d.
coronary artery d.
dominant
anatomically d.
d. follicle
d. hemisphere
d. hemisphere infarct
d. hemisphere lesion
d. left coronary artery
d. left coronary artery system
d. right coronary artery
d. right coronary artery system
d. vessel
doming
diastolic d.
d. of leaflet
d. of valve
donor
d. graft
d. heart
d. heart-lung block
d. site
d. twin
donut (*var. of* doughnut)
Dooley, Caldwell and Glass method
DOOR
deafness, onychodystrophy, osteodystrophy, mental retardation
DOOR syndrome
doorbell sign
DOPA imaging agent
doped water
Doplette monitor

NOTES

D

Doppler
D. angle
D. ankle systolic pressure
D. assessment
D. blood flow monitor
D. blood flow velocity signal
D. blood pressure
color-flow D. (CFD)
D. color-flow imaging
D. color-flow mapping
continuous-wave D.
D. continuous-wave echocardiography
contrast-enhanced color D.
contrast-enhanced power D.
duplex B-mode D.
D. echocardiography
D. effect
D. equation
D. flow echocardiographic probe
D. flow index
D. flowmetry
D. flow probe study
D. flow signal enhancement
D. frequency shift
gray-scale D.
high-frequency D. (HFD)
D. image
D. insonation
D. interrogation
intraoperative D.
D. kidney
D. ovary signal
periorbital bidirectional D.
D. phenomenon
D. physics
pocket D.
power D.
D. pulse
pulsed-wave D.
D. pulsed-wave echocardiography
range-gated pulsed D.
real-time D.
renal D.
D. Resistive Index (DRI)
D. shift frequency
D. shift principle
D. sonography
spectral D.
D. spectral analysis
D. spectral waveform
D. study of blood flow
D. tissue imaging (DTI)
transcranial D. (TCD)
D. tricuspid regurgitation
D. ultrasonic blood flow detector
D. ultrasonic fetal heart monitor
D. ultrasonic velocity detector
D. ultrasonic velocity detector segmental plethysmography
D. ultrasonography
D. ultrasonography imaging
D. ultrasound
D. ultrasound segmental blood pressure testing
D. venous examination
D. venous imaging
D. VWF
D. waveform
D. waveform analysis
D. waveform dampening

Doppler-derived stroke distance

Dorello canal

Dorendorf
D. sign
D. sign of aortic arch aneurysm

dormancy
tumor d.

Dornier
D. HM3 lithotripter
D. HM4 lithotripter
D. scanner

Dor reconstruction

dorsal
d. artery
d. artery of penis
d. aspect
d. branch
d. capsule
d. column sign
d. cyst
d. decubitus position
d. dermal sinus
d. diverticulum
d. enteric fistula
d. enteric sinus
d. enterogenous cyst
d. induction
d. induction error
d. intercalated segmental instability (DISI)
d. interossei
d. kyphotic curvature
d. meningocele
d. metacarpal ligament
d. muscle
d. nerve of penis
d. pancreas
d. pancreatic bud
d. penile vein
d. plate
d. point
d. primary ramus
d. ramus of spinal nerve
d. recumbent position
d. ridge

d. rim
d. rim distal radial fracture
d. root entry zone (DREZ)
d. root entry zone lesion
d. root ganglion (DRG)
d. scapular
d. spinal cord horn
d. spine
d. spinocerebellar tract
d. subaponeurotic space
d. subcutaneous space
d. talar beak
d. talonavicular bone
d. tubercle
d. vertebra
d. wing fracture
d. wrist ligament

dorsale
os supratrochleare d.

dorsalis
funiculus d.
d. pedis
tabes d.

dorsalward

dorsi
latissimus d.

dorsiflexion
d. angle (DFA)
d. view

dorsiflexor

dorsispinal vein

dorsoanterior

dorsocephalad

dorsolateral
d. aspect
d. tract

dorsoplantar
d. aspect
d. talometatarsal angle
d. talonavicular angle
d. view

dorsoposterior

dorsoradial

dorsorostral

dorsosacral position

dorsum
d. pedis
d. of penis
d. sellae
d. sellae atrophy

DORV
double-outlet right ventricle

dose
absorbed d. (AD)
adult d.
air d.
average radiation d.
bioeffect d. (BED)
biologically equivalent d. (BED)
bolus d.
bone marrow d.
boost d.
central axis depth d.
cumulative d.
delivered total d. (DTD)
depth d.
d. distribution
divided d.
effective d.
epilation d.
equivalent d.
d. equivalent (DE)
erythema d.
exit d.
exposure d.
fractionated d.
^{67}Ga higher d.
gonadal d.
gray radiation absorbed d. (Gy rad)
incremental d.
integral d.
iodine d.
isoeffect d.
joule radiation-absorbed d.
lethal d.
matched peripheral d. (MPD)
maximum permissible d. (MPD)
mean central d. (MCD)
median lethal d.
medical internal radiation d. (MIRD)
minimum tolerance d.
multiple scan average d. (MSAD)
nominal standard d. (NSD)
d. nonuniformity ratio (DNR)
normalized average glandular d.
optimum d.
percentage depth d. (PDD)
radiation-absorbed d. (RAD)
rad surface d. (RSD)
d. rate domain
reference d.
scatter d.
skin d.

NOTES

D

dose *(continued)*
table of radiation d.
tapering d.
tissue tolerance d. (TTD)
tracer d.
tumor lethal d. (TLD)
dose-limiting toxicity (DLT)
dose-surface histogram
dose-time relationship
dose-volume
d.-v. histogram (DVH)
d.-v. relationship
dosimeter
carbon-loaded thermoluminescent d.
chemical d.
dichromate d.
Gardray d.
high-dose film d.
LiF thermoluminescence d.
pencil d.
pocket d.
silicon diode d.
sucrose d.
thermoluminescent d. (TLD)
ultraviolet fluorescent d.
Victoreen d.
dosimetric penumbra
dosimetry
adjacent field x-ray d.
beam's-eye view d.
carbon-load thermoluminescent d.
dichromate d.
electron d.
four-field x-ray d.
free-radical d.
Fricke d.
high-dose film d.
large-field x-ray d.
LiF thermoluminescence d.
marrow d.
medical internal radiation d. (MIRD)
phantom d.
polymer d.
radiation d.
single x-ray d.
thermoluminescence d.
transmission d.
x-ray d.
Dos Santos aortography needle
dot
subpleural d.
dot-and-dash pattern
Dotter effect
dottering effect
double
d. aortic arch
d. aortic arch of Edwards
d. appendix
d. arch aorta
d. autograft
d. breast coil
d. camelback sign of knee
d. coronary orifice
d. decidual sac
d. density
d. density heart
d. emission
d. fracture
d. gallbladder
d. helical CT scan
d. injection
d. inversion recovery sequence
d. kidney
d. label
d. lumen
d. outflow
d. outlet right ventricle syndrome
d. outline
d. penis
d. pleurisy
d. pneumonia
d. reverse alpha sigmoid loop
d. systolic apical impulse
d. tracking of barium
d. track sign
d. uterus
d. vagina
d. voiding cystogram
d. wall sign
double-arc
d.-a. gallbladder shadow
d.-a. lung shadow sign
double-ball sign
double-barrel
d.-b. aorta
d.-b. esophagus
d.-b. lumen
d.-b. shotgun sign
double-bleb sign
double-bonded carbon
double-bubble
d.-b. appearance
d.-b. duodenal sign
d.-b. shadow
d.-b. sign
double-bulb appearance
double-camelback sign
double-channel
d.-c. endoscope
d.-c. sign
double-contrast
d.-c. arthrography
d.-c. arthrotomography of shoulder
d.-c. barium enema (DCBE)
d.-c. barium meal

d.-c. barium study
d.-c. enema
d.-c. examination
d.-c. laryngography
d.-c. radiograph
d.-c. technique
double-cortex sign
double-delta sign
double-density sign
double-diaphragm contour
double-dose
d.-d. delay (DDD)
d.-d. gadolinium imaging
double-duct sign
double-echo
d.-e. three-point Dixon method fat suppression
d.-e. three-point Dixon suppression method
double-exposed rib
double-exposure drift artifact
double-flanged valve sewing ring
double-fragment sign
double-freeze technique
double-fungus-ball wall sign
double-halo
d.-h. appearance
d.-h. configuration
d.-h. sign
double-helical CT imaging
double-helix
d.-h. acquisition
d.-h. prostatic stent
double-inlet
d.-i. left ventricle
d.-i. single ventricle
d.-i. ventricle anomaly
double-J
d.-J. ureteral stent
double-label counting
double-lesion sign
double-line hip sign
double-lumen
d.-l. breast implant
d.-l. endoprosthesis
double-mouthed uterus
double-outlet
d.-o. both ventricles (DOBV)
d.-o. left ventricle (DOLV)
d.-o. right ventricle (DORV)
double-phase technetium-99m sestamibi imaging
double-pigtail endoprosthesis
double-populated detector ring
double-spin echo proton spectroscopy
double-spiral CT arterial portography
double-stem silicone lesser MP implant
double-strand scission
double-target liver sign
double-throw
single-pole d.-t. (SPDT)
double-tracking colon
double-track pylorus sign
double-umbrella technique
double-vessel sign
double-walled fibroserous sac
double-wire atherectomy technique
doubly broadband triple-resonance NMR probe circuit
doughnut, donut
d. kidney
d. lesion
d. magnet
d. ring
d. sign
sonolucent d.
d. transformer
doughy mass
Douglas
D. back method for determining cardiac output
D. cul-de-sac
cul-de-sac of D.
D. fold
D. ligament
pouch of D.
D. rectouterine pouch
Dow
D. hollow fiber analyzer
D. method for measuring cardiac output
dowager's hump
dowel
iliac d.
down
coned d.
downhill varix
downscatter
downstaging
axillary tumor d.
downstream sampling method
Down syndrome
downward
d. displacement of apical impulse

NOTES

downward *(continued)*
d. slope
d. vergence
Doyne honeycomb degeneration
DPA
dual-photon absorptiometry
dP/dt
peak dP/dt
DPR
dynamic planar reconstructor
DPTI
diastolic pressure-time index
DPX-IQ densitometer
DQE
detective quantum efficiency
DR
digital radiography
DRA
digital rotational angiography
distal rectal adenocarcinoma
distal reference axis
drain
external ventricular d. (EVD)
radiopaque d.
retroperitoneal d.
rubber d.
sump d.
drainage
aberrant venous d.
anomalous d.
biliary d.
central venous d.
circle loop biliary d.
extrapleural d.
gaseous d.
guided d.
internal biliary d.
nephrostomy d.
pancreatic pseudocyst d.
percutaneous abscess d. (PAD)
percutaneous antegrade biliary d.
pulmonary venous d.
spontaneous d.
suction d.
total anomalous pulmonary venous d. (TAPVD)
transhepatic d.
transvaginal ultrasound-guided d.
tube d.
venous d.
ventricular d.
draining
d. sinus
d. with venous pressure
draped aorta
Drash syndrome
DRC
dynamic range control
DRC algorithm
Drennan metaphyseal-epiphyseal angle
DRESS
depth-resolved surface coil spectroscopy
Dressler postmyocardial infarction syndrome
DREZ
dorsal root entry zone
DREZ lesion
DRG
dorsal root ganglion
DRI
Doppler Resistive Index
Driffield
Hurter and D. (H and D)
drift
field d.
radial d.
drifting wedge pressure
drink
effervescent d.
drip
drip-infusion cholangiogram (DIC)
drippings
brain candle d.
candle wax d.
driven
d. equilibrium Fourier transform
d. equilibrium Fourier transform technique
dromedary hump
droop
Cooper d.
drooping
d. lily appearance
d. lily kidney sign
d. lily sign
d. shoulder
drop
d. finger
d. foot
d. heart
d. metastasis
d. metastasis in thecal sac
d. shoulder
d. test for pneumoperitoneum
drop-lock ring
dropsy
drowned
d. lung
d. newborn syndrome

DRR
digitally reconstructed radiograph
drug
adjuvant analgesic d.
d. administration
antimony antimotility d.
d. fraction
macromolecular d.
slow-channel blocking d.
d. tolerance
drug-induced
d.-i. bone marrow suppression
d.-i. bullous disorder
d.-i. drug resistance
d.-i. erythematous lupus
d.-i. esophagitis
d.-i. nephrotoxicity
d.-i. pneumonitis
d.-i. pulmonary damage
drug-resistant tumor
DRUJ
distal radioulnar joint
DRUJ compartment
drum
d. spur
Drummond
marginal artery of D.
D. marginal artery
D. sign
D. sign of aortic aneurysm
drumstick phalanx
dry
d. bowel preparation
d. bronchiectasis
E-Z CAT D.
d. laser imaging
d. pleurisy
d. swallow
dryer system
Drystar dry imager
DryView laser imaging system
DSA
digital subtraction angiography
digital subtraction arteriography
DSAS
discrete subvalvular aortic stenosis
DSC
dynamic susceptibility contrast
DSC MR imaging
D-shaped vessel lumen
DSI camera
DSR
dynamic spatial reconstructor
DSR scanner
DSRCT
desmoplastic small round-cell tumor
DTAF
descending thoracic aortofemorofemoral
DTD
delivered total dose
DTI
Doppler tissue imaging
DTICH
delayed traumatic intracerebral hematoma
delayed traumatic intracerebral hemorrhage
D-to-E
D.-t.-E. slope
D.-t.-E. slope on echocardiography
DTPA
D. imaging agent
indium-111 D.
D. renography
^{99m}Tc D.
technetium-99m DTPA
ytterbium-169 D.
dual
d. atrioventricular node pathway
d. blood supply
d.-echo DIET fast spin-echo imaging
d. gradient-recalled echo (GRE) pulse sequence
d. intracoronary scintigraphy
d. isotope imaging
d. isotope scanning
d. lookup table
d. photons
d. plate
d. screen/dual emulsion system
d. transverse linear-array sonogram
d. ventricle
dual-balloon method
dual-coil imaging
dual-contrast study
dual-demand pacing mode
dual-echo sequence
dual-energy
d.-e. CT
d.-e. linear accelerator
d.-e. radiograph (DER)
d.-e. subtraction

NOTES

dual-energy *(continued)*
d.-e. x-ray absorptiometry (DEXA, DXA)
d.-e. x-ray absorptiometry densitometer
dual-head
d.-h. gamma camera
d.-h. gamma camera system
d.-h. SPECT
dual-isotope
d.-i. single-photon emission CT
d.-i. SPECT
dual-lookup table algorithm
dual-mode, dual-pacing, dual-sensing (DDD)
dual-phase
d.-p. scan
d.-p. ^{99m}Tc-sestamibi imaging
dual-photon
d.-p. absorptiometry (DPA)
d.-p. densitometer
d.-p. densitometry
dual-shaped collimator
Dubin-Johnson
D.-J. phenomenon
D.-J. syndrome
Dubin-Sprinz disease
Duchenne
D. muscular dystrophy
D. sign
duct
aberrant intrahepatic bile d.
accessory hepatic d.
accessory pancreatic d.
alveolar d.
amnionic d.
arborization of d.'s
arterial d.
asymmetric bile d.
Bartholin d.
beaded bile d.
beaded hepatic d.
beaded pancreatic d.
d. of Bellini
bile d.
biliary d.
Botallo d.
branchial d.
bucconeural d.
canalicular d.
carotid d.
d. cell adenocarcinoma
choledochous d.
cobblestone appearance of bile d.
cochlear d.
common bile d. (CBD)
common gall d.
common hepatic d. (CHD)
craniopharyngeal d.
Cuvier d.
d. of Cuvier
cystic gall d.
deferent d.
dilated bile d.
disruption of d.
distal bile d.
duodenal end of dorsal d.
duodenal end of main d.
efferent d.
ejaculatory d.
endolymphatic d.
excretory d.
extrahepatic bile d.
extralobular terminal d.
focally dilated d.
frontonasal d.
fusiform widening of d.
galactophorous d.
gall d.
Gartner d.
genital d.
hepatic d.
Hering d.
His d.
hypophysial Rathke d.
infundibulum of bile d.
interlobular bile d.
intrahepatic bile d.
intralobular terminal d.
involution of d.
lacrimal d.
lactiferous d.
lollipop-tree bile d.
d. lumen
lymph d.
lymphatic d.
main pancreatic d. (MPD)
main papillary d. (MPD)
mammary d.
middle extrahepatic bile d.
müllerian d.
nasofrontal d.
nasolacrimal d.
nipplelike common bile d.
normal caliber d.
d. obstruction
obstruction of d.
omphalomesenteric d.
pancreatic d.
paramesonephric d.
paraurethral d.
parotid d.
percutaneous dilatation of biliary d.
perforation of common bile d.
perilobular d.
preampullary portion of bile d.

prepapillary bile d.
prostatic d.
proximal part of dorsal d.
pruned-tree-appearance bile d.
pseudocalculus bile d.
Rathke d.
rat-tail common bile d.
right hepatic d.
Rivinus d.
ruptured thoracic d.
Santorini d.
d. of Santorini
solitary dilated d.
sphincter of bile d.
spontaneous perforation of common bile d.
Stensen d.
submandibular d.
subvesical d.
terminal bile d.
thoracic d.
thyroglossal d.
Vater d.
vitelline d.
Wharton d.
Wirsung d.
d. of Wirsung
wolffian d.

ductal
d. adenoma
d. aneurysm
d. arch
d. architecture
d. breast microcalcification
d. carcinoma in situ (DCIS)
d. constriction
d. dilatation
d. ectasia
d. epithelial hyperplasia
d. epithelium
d. pancreatic adenocarcinoma
d. papillary carcinoma
d. papilloma
d. pattern
d. remnant
d. in situ breast carcinoma

ductectatic
d. mucinous cystic neoplasm
d. mucinous tumor

ductogram
mammary d.

ductography

ductular

ductule

ductus, pl. **ductus**
d. aneriosus
d. arteriosus
d. arteriosus aneurysm
d. arteriosus occlusion
d. arteriosus patency
d. deferens
d. deferens artery
d. diverticulum
d. infundibulum
recanalized d.
d. venosus
d. venosus patency
window d.

Dulcolax
D. bowel preparation

dullness
left border of cardiac d. (LBCD)
triangular area of d.

dumbbell
d. brain mass
d. lesion
d. needle
d. neurofibroma
d. shape
d. tumor

dumbbell-shaped shadow

dumbbell-type neuroblastoma

dummy source

dumping
d. stomach
d. syndrome

Duncan
D. placenta
D. ventricle

Duncan-Hoen method

Dunlap, Swanson and Penner method

Dunlop-Shands view

duodenal
d. adenocarcinoma
d. artery
d. atresia
d. bulb
d. bulb apex
d. bulb deformity
d. button
d. cap
d. C loop
d. diaphragm
d. duplication

NOTES

duodenal *(continued)*
d. end of dorsal duct
d. end of main duct
d. erosion
d. filling defect
d. fossa
d. gastrinoma
d. hernia
d. hourglass stenosis
d. impression
d. intraluminal diverticulum
d. leiomyosarcoma
d. ligament
d. loop
d. lumen
d. narrowing
d. papilla
d. peptic ulcer disease
d. polyp
d. segment
d. sphincter
d. stricture
d. stump
d. sweep
d. teardrop appearance
d. terminus
d. ulcer
d. varix
d. vein
d. villus
d. wall hamartoma
d. web
duodenal-gastric outlet obstruction
duodenitis
chronic atrophic d.
Crohn d.
erosive d.
hemorrhagic d.
duodenobiliary
d. pressure gradient
d. reflux
duodenocolic fistula
duodenogastric reflux (DGR)
duodenogastroesophageal reflux
duodenogastroscopy
retrograde d. (RDG)
duodenography
hypotonic d.
d. imaging
duodenojejunal
d. angle
d. flexure
d. fold
d. fossa
d. junction (DJJ)
d. recess
d. sphincter
duodenojejunitis
duodenomesocolic fold
duodenopancreatic
d. fistula
d. reflux
duodenorenal ligament
duodenum
chronic ileus d.
C loop of d.
cobblestone appearance d.
comma-shaped d.
curve of d.
descending d.
dilated d.
distal d.
d. extrinsic pressure effect
first portion of d.
d. inversum
d. malignant tumor
d. megabulbus
mobile d.
onion-shaped dilatation of d.
scarified d.
scarred d.
second portion of d.
supravaterian d.
suspensory muscle of d.
third portion of d.
water-trap d.
d. water-trap
widened sweep d.
windsock appearance of d.
Duografin
D. imaging agent
duplex
d. B-mode Doppler
d. B-mode ultrasound
d. carotid imaging
d. carotid ultrasound
d. Doppler imaging
d. echocardiography
d. pulsed Doppler sonography
d. pulsed Doppler ultrasound
d. scanner
d. screening test
d. ultrasonography
d. ultrasound analysis
d. ultrasound carotid artery
d. ultrasound error
d. uterus
duplicated
d. inferior vena cava
d. renal collecting system
duplication
d. anomaly
colon d.
colon cyst d.
colorectal d.
complete d.

d. cyst
diaphragm d.
duodenal d.
esophageal d.
foregut d.
gallbladder d.
hindgut d.
incomplete ureteral d.
inferior vena cava d.
d. of left kidney
partial ureter d.
renal d.
d. of right kidney
thoracoabdominal d.
ureteral d.

DuPont
D. Cronex x-ray film
D. Rare Earth imaging system
D. scanner

Dupré muscle

Dupuytren
D. canal
D. contracture
D. fracture
D. sign

dura
attenuated d.
bulging d.
effacement of d.
lamina d.
d. mater
d. mater of brain
d. mater of spinal cord
d. mater venous sinus

dural
d. arachnoid lymphoma
d. arteriovenous fistula
d. arteriovenous malformation
d. artery
d. attachment
d. calcification
d. cul-de-sac
d. ectasia
d. fold
d. hematoma
d. impingement
d. root pouch
d. sac
d. sac effacement
d. sheath
d. sinus occlusion
d. sinus thrombosis
d. sinus thrombosis infarct
d. tail
d. tear
d. trail sign
d. venous sinus
d. venous sinus thrombosis

Dürck node

Duret
D. hemorrhage
D. lesion

Durham flatfoot

durocutaneous fistula

Duroliopaque

Duroziez
D. mitral stenosis disease
D. sign

durum
heloma d.
papilloma d.

DUS
dynamic ultrasound of shoulder

Dusard syndrome

Duverney
D. foramen
D. fracture
D. gland
D. muscle

DVH
dose-volume histogram

DVI
deep venous insufficiency
device independent
digital vascular imaging
DVI mode
DVI Simpson AtheroCath

DVT
deep venous thrombosis

dwarfism
achondroplastic d.
acromelic d.
Amsterdam d.
bird-headed d.
deprivation d.
diastrophic d.
late-onset d.
lethal d.
Lorain-Lévi d.
mesomelic d.
metatrophic d.
micromelic d.
nonlethal d.
pituitary d.

NOTES

D

dwarfism *(continued)*
renal d.
rhizomelic d.
Russell-Silver d.
thanatophoric d.
Walt Disney d.
dwarf pelvis
dwell position
Dwyer correction of scoliosis
DXA
dual-energy x-ray absorptiometry
Dy
dysprosium
Dycal base
dyclonine
Dy-DTPA-BMA imaging agent
dye
d. column
columning of d.
d. dilution curve
d. extravasation
fill and spill of d.
d. fluorescence index (DFI)
indentation of myelography d.
indocyanine green d.
d. injection technique
d. laser system
lipophilic d.
d. punch fracture
d. reduction spot test
d. uptake
d. worker's latent cancer
^{166}Dy generator
Dyke-Davidoff-Masson syndrome
Dynabead
Dynal M450 magnetic beads
dynamic
d. aorta
d. axial fixator
d. beat filtration
d. bolus
d. bolus tracking technique
d. computed tomography
d. conformal therapy
d. contrast-enhanced MRI
d. contrast-enhanced subtraction MR imaging
d. contrast-enhanced subtraction study
d. coupling
d. CT
d. enhancement
d. entrapment of vertebral artery
d. filtering
d. hammer toe
d. ileus
d. image
d. lineshape effect
d. lung
d. multileaf collimation
d. nuclear polarization (DNP)
d. pedobarography
d. planar reconstructor (DPR)
d. pulmonary hyperinflation
d. radiation therapy
d. radiotherapy
d. range
d. range control (DRC)
d. range control algorithm (DRC algorithm)
d. scintigraphy imaging
d. series
d. snapshot
d. spatial reconstructor (DSR)
d. stabilizer
d. stereotactic radiosurgery
d. subaortic stenosis
d. susceptibility contrast (DSC)
d. susceptibility contrast magnetic resonance imaging (DSC MR imaging)
d. tagging magnetic resonance angiography
d. ultrasound of shoulder (DUS)
d. volume imaging
d. volume-rendered display
d. volumetric SPECT
d. wedge
dynamic-contrast enhanced magnetic resonance imaging (DCE-MRI)
dynamite heart
Dynapix
Dynarad portable imaging system
dynode
dynography
dysarthria syndrome
dysautonomia
familial d.
dyschezia
dyschondroplasia
dyschondrosteosis
dyschromia
dyscollagenosis
dyscrasic fracture
dysembryoplastic neuroepithelial tumor (DNET)
dysfunction
bladder d.
bowel and bladder d.
brain d.
cerebral d.
cortical d.
frontal lobe d.
hepatocellular d.
left ventricular d. (LVD)
neurogenic bladder d.

neuromuscular d.
oropharyngeal d.
papillary muscle d. (PMD)
positional d.
renal d.
salivary gland d.
sinoatrial node d.
sinus node d.
small airway d.
swallowing d.
testis d.
valvular d.
ventilatory d.
ventricular d.
voiding d.

dysfunctional
d. kidney
d. ventricle

dysgenesis
alar d.
anorectal d.
callosal d.
corpus callosum d.
corticocallosal d.
epiphyseal d.
gonadal d.
hindbrain d.
mixed gonadal d.
ovarian d.
renal tubular d.
thyroid d.
tubular d.

dysgenetic
d. kidney
d. syndrome

dysgerminoma
brain d.
mediastinum d.
ovarian d.
pineal d.

dyshormonogenesis
congenital thyroid d.

dysjunction
craniofacial d.

dyskeratosis, pl. **dyskeratoses**
kidney d.

dyskinesia, dyskinesis
bile duct d.
biliary d.
regional d.

dyskinetic
d. segmental wall motion
d. segmental wall motion abnormality
d. septum

dysmaturity
pulmonary d.

dysmorphism
lobar d.

dysmotile esophagus

dysmotility
esophageal d.

dysmyelination
cerebrum d.

dysmyelopoietic syndrome

dysosteogenesis

dysostosis, pl. **dysostoses**
cleidocranial d.
craniofacial d.
epiphyseal d.
mandibulofacial d.
metaphyseal d.
d. multiplex
mutational d.

dysphagia
contractile ring d.
esophageal d.
d. inflammatoria
liquid food d.
d. lusoria
d. nervosa
oropharyngeal d.
d. paralytica
postvagotomy d.
preesophageal d.
progressive d.
sideropenic d.
soft food d.
solid food d.
d. spastica
vallecular d.
d. valsalviana

dysplasia
acetabular residual d.
acromelic d.
acropectorovertebral d.
arteriohepatic d.
asphyxiating thoracic d.
bone d.
bronchopulmonary d. (BPD)
Burke-type metaphyseal d.
camptomelic d.
cervical d.
chondroectodermal d.

NOTES

dysplasia *(continued)*
cleidocranial d.
CNS fibromuscular d.
congenital hip d.
congenital polyvalvular d.
cranioskeletal d.
craniotelencephalic d.
cystic d.
developmental d.
diaphyseal d.
diastrophic d.
d. dislocation
ectrodactyly-ectodermal d.
endocardial d.
epiarticular osteochondromatous d.
epiphyseal d.
d. epiphysealis hemimelica
d. epiphysealis multiplex
epiphysealis punctua d.
external auditory canal d.
familial arterial fibromuscular d.
fetal musculoskeletal d.
fibromuscular d.
fibrous d.
fibrous temporal bone d.
foot d.
frontonasal d.
hip d.
Jansen metaphyseal d.
lethal bone d.
lethal musculoskeletal d.
mammary d.
McKusick-type metaphyseal d.
mesodermal d.
mesomelic d.
metaphyseal d.
metatrophic d.
Meyer d.
micromelic d.
microscopic cortical d.
Mondini d.
monostotic fibrous d.
multicystic d.
multiple epiphyseal d.
Namaqualand hip d.
neuroectodermal d.
nonlethal d.
OAV d.
oculoauriculovertebral dysplasia
obstructive renal d.
oculoauriculovertebral d. (OAV dysplasia)
odontoid d.
osseous d.
osteofibrous d.
Pena-Vaandrager metaphyseal d.
periapical cemental d.
perimedial d.
periosteal d.
polyostotic fibrous d.
polypoid d.
Potter d.
progressive diaphyseal d.
pulmonary valve d. (PVD)
renal artery fibromuscular d.
retinal d.
retroareolar d.
rhizomelic d.
right ventricular d.
Scheibe d.
Schmid-type metaphyseal d.
sheetlike d.
short limb d.
skeletal d.
Sponastrine d.
spondyloepiphyseal d.
Streeter d.
testis d.
thanatophoric d.
thoracic d.
thymic d.
tricuspid valve d.
ventricular d.
ventriculoradial d.
d. with associated lesion or mass (DALM)

dysplastic
d. cerebellar gangliocytoma
d. cusp
d. kidney
d. liver nodule
d. meniscus
d. pulmonary valve

dyspnea on exertion

dysprosium (Dy)
d. analog
d. HP-DO3A imaging agent

dysprosium-DTPA

dysprosium-holmium (^{166}Dy-166Ho) in vivo generator

dysraphism
closed spinal d.
occult spinal d.

dysrhythmia of fetal heart

dyssynergia, dyssynergy
biliary d.
Ramsay Hunt cerebellar myoclonic d.
regional d.
segmental d.

dystocia
fetal d.
shoulder d.

dystonia

dystonic reaction

dystopia

dystrophic
- d. change
- d. degeneration
- d. soft tissue calcification

dystrophy
- adiposogenital d.
- bone d.
- congenital muscular d.
- Duchenne muscular d.
- infantile thoracic d.
- limb-girdle muscular d.
- muscular d.
- neuraxonal d.
- oculopharyngeal d.
- reflex sympathetic d.
- Sudeck d.
- sympathetic d.

NOTES

E
E plane
E point of cardiac apex pulse
E point on echocardiography
E point to septal separation (EPSS)
E sign
E sign on x-ray
E trisomy
E:A
E. change
E. wave ratio
EAA
extraalveolar air
EAA collection
Eagle-Barrett syndrome
ear
e. cholesteatoma
frontal horn Mickey Mouse e.
e. implant
inner e.
middle e.
early
e. bone scintigraphy
e. detection
e. echo
e. fetal death
e. opening of valve
e. osteoarthritis
e. osteomyelitis
e. pneumonitis
e. repolarization pattern
e. stromal invasion
e. systolic peak
e. venous filling
early-phase termination
Eastman Kodak scanner
EasyGuide Neuro
Eaton
E. agent
E. agent pneumonia
EBA
extrahepatic biliary atresia
EBCT
electron-beam computed tomography
EBDA
effective balloon-dilated area
EBER
Epstein-Barr-encoded RNA
EBIORT
electron-beam intraoperative radiotherapy
EBRT
external beam radiation therapy
Ebstein
E. angle
E. anomaly
E. lesion
E. malformation
E. malformation of tricuspid valve
E. sign
EBT
electron beam tomography
eburnated bone
eburnation
bony e.
trapezium-metacarpal e. (TME)
ECA
external carotid artery
ECAF
extension corner avulsion fracture
E.CAM dual-head emission imaging system
ECAT
emission computer-assisted tomography
eccentric
e. atherosclerotic plaque
e. atrophy
e. axis of rotation of the ankle
e. coronary artery
e. epicenter
e. ledge
e. left ventricular hypertrophy
e. medullary bone lesion
e. narrowing
e. plaque disease
e. restenosis lesion
e. stenosis
e. vessel
eccentrically placed lumen
eccentricity index
ecchondroma
eccrine angiomatous hamartoma
ECE
extracapsular extension
ECG, EKG
ECG trigger
ECG-gated
E.-g. multislice
E.-g. multislice MR imaging
E.-g. spin echo
E.-g. spin-echo MR imaging
ECG-synchronized digital subtraction angiography
ECG-triggered, flow-compensated gradient echo image
echinococcal cyst
echinococcosis
alveolar e.
bone e.

echinococcosis *(continued)*
liver e.
lung e.
echo
amphoric e.
asymmetric e.
atrial e.
bright e.
e. characteristic
e. contrast
e. delay
e. delay time (TE, T-E)
dense e.
e. density
diaphragmatic e.
early e.
ECG-gated spin e.
endometrial e.
even distribution of e.'s
fast-field e.'s
fast-field e. (FFE)
fast spin e. (FSE)
fast spin e. (FSE)
fat-suppressed spin e.
field e.
e. FLASH MR
fuzzy e.
generation e.
gradient-recalled e. (GRE)
gradient-refocused e. (GRE)
Hahn spin e.
half-Fourier acquisition single-shot turbo-spin e. (HASTE)
hepatic pattern e.
high-amplitude e.
highly mobile e.
highly reflective e.
homogeneous e.
e. imaging
inhomogeneous e.
internal e.
linear e.
low-amplitude internal e.
low-level e.
magnitude preparation-rapid acquisition gradient e. (MP-RAGE)
median level e.
metallic e.
multiplanar gradient-recalled e.
navigator e.
offset radiofrequency spin e.
out-of-phase gradient e.
partial saturation spin e. (PSSE)
particulate e.
e. pattern
pencil-beam navigator e.'s
pulsed-gradient spin e. (PGSE)
radiofrequency spin e.
e. reflectivity
renal sinus e.
e. rephasing
reverberation e.
e. reverberation
ring-down e.
salvo of e.'s
shower of e.'s
e. signature
simulated e.
sludge-like intraluminal e.
smokelike e.
solid e.
sonographic e.
e. space
specular e.
spin e.
spin-echo using repeated gradient e.'s
standard single e.
stimulated e.
supraventricular venous e.
swirling smokelike e.'s
symmetric e.
e. texture
thick e.
e. time (TE, T-E)
e. train
turbo-spin e. (TSE)
T1-weighted spin e.
ultrasonographic e.
ventricular e.
echoaortography
echocardiogram
e. adenosine
echocardiographic
e. automated border
e. gating
echocardiography
ambulatory Holter e.
A-mode e.
aortic root e.
aortic valve e.
apical five-chamber view e.
apical two-chamber view e.
automated border detection by e.
biplane transesophageal e.
blood pool radionuclide e.
B-mode e.
cardiac output e.
color-flow imaging Doppler e.
continuous-loop exercise e.
continuous-wave Doppler e.
contrast-enhanced e.
cross-sectional e.
cross-sectional two-dimensional e.
detection e.

dipyridamole e.
dobutamine stress e.
Doppler e.
Doppler continuous-wave e.
Doppler pulsed-wave e.
D-to-E slope on e.
duplex e.
epicardial Doppler e.
E point on e.
exercise e.
Feigenbaum e.
fetal e.
four-chamber e.
H-mode e.
hypokinesis on e.
e. imaging
intracardiac e. (ICE)
intracoronary contrast e.
intraoperative cardioplegic
  contrast e.
Meridian e.
mitral valve e.
M-mode e.
multiplanar transesophageal e.
myocardial contrast e. (MCE)
myocardial perfusion e.
parasternal long-axis view e.
parasternal short-axis view e.
pharmacologic stress e.
postcontrast e.
postexercise e.
postinjection e.
postmyocardial infarction e.
precontrast e.
preinjection e.
premyocardial infarction e.
pulsed Doppler transesophageal e.
pulsed-wave (PW) Doppler e.
real-time e.
resting e.
sector e.
sector scan e.
septal wall motion on e.
short-axis view e.
stress e.
subcostal short-axis view e.
subxiphoid view e.
supine bicycle stress e.
three-dimensional transesophageal e.
transesophageal e. (TEE)
transthoracic e. (TTE)
transthoracic three-dimensional e.
transthoracic-three-dimensional e.
two-chamber e.
two-dimensional e.
ultrasound e.
ventricular wall motion e.

echodense
e. layer
e. pattern
e. valve

echoencephalography

echoendoscope
Olympus GF-UM2, GF-UM3 e.
Olympus VU-M2 e.
Olympus XIF-UM3 e.

echo-free
e.-f. area
e.-f. central zone
e.-f. layer
e.-f. space

EchoGen
E.-enhanced ultrasound
E. ultrasound imaging agent

echogenic
e. calculus
e. fetal bowel
e. liver
e. liver metastasis
e. mass
e. nodule
e. noise
e. periphery
e. plaque
e. plug
e. ring sign
e. solid lesion
e. tumor

echogenicity
brightly increased renal
  parenchymal e.
focally increased renal e.
generalized increased liver e.
increased e.
internal e.
normal e.
parenchymal e.
periventricular e. (PVE)

echogram
mitral valve e.

echographer

echography
B-mode e.

NOTES

E

echography *(continued)*
ophthalmic biometry by ultrasound e.
transrectal e.
transvaginal e.
echoic
echoicity
echolucent
e. pattern
e. plaque
EchoMark
echonography
echopenic liver metastasis
echophonocardiography
M-mode e.
echoplanar
e. FLAIR imaging
e. imaging (EPI)
e. imaging method
e. MRA imaging
e. pulse sequence
echo-spin density
echo-tagging technique
echotexture
internal e.
mottled e.
echo-train
e.-t. length (ETL)
e.-t. value
Echovar Doppler system
Echovist imaging agent
ECIDP
intracranial epidural pressure
Eck fistula
eclampsia
eclamptic
eclipse effect lung
ECRB
extensor carpi radialis brevis
ECRB muscle
ECRL
extensor carpi radialis longus
ECRL muscle
ECS
electrocerebral silence
ECT
emission computed tomography
ectasia
alveolar e.
annuloaortic e.
e. of aorta
basilar artery e.
benign duct e.
bilateral ductal e.
communicating cavernous e.
coronary artery e.
diffuse arterial e.
ductal e.
dural e.
mammary duct e.
renal tubular e.
tubular e.
vascular colon e.
ectatic
e. aneurysm
e. aortic valve
e. bronchus
e. carotid artery
e. emphysema
ectocardia
ectomesenchyme
ectopia
benign cerebellar e.
cerebellar e.
e. cordis
crossed-fused renal e.
gallbladder e.
longitudinal renal e.
posterior pituitary gland e.
testicular e.
tonsillar e.
ectopic
e. ACTH syndrome
e. anus
e. beat
e. bone growth
e. craniopharyngioma
e. focus
e. gallbladder
e. impulse
e. intraluminal gallstone
e. kidney
e. meningioma
e. nevus
e. ossification
e. pancreas
e. parathyroid
e. parathyroid adenoma
e. parathyroid syndrome
e. pinealoma
e. pregnancy (EP)
e. spleen
e. testis
e. thymus
e. thyroid tissue
e. ureter
e. ureterocele
e. wall motion abnormality
ectrodactyly-ectodermal
e.-e. dysplasia
e.-e. dysplasia-clefting (EEC)
e.-e. dysplasia-clefting syndrome
ECU
extensor carpi ulnaris
ECU muscle

EDAMS
encephaloduroarteriomyosynangiosis
EDAS
encephaloduroarteriosynangiosis
EDB
extensor digitorum brevis
EDB muscle
EDC
extensor digitorum communis
EDC muscle
eddy
e. current
e. current artifact
e. current mapping
e. formation
e. ringing artifact
edema
acute interstitial lung e.
acute pulmonary e.
air-space e.
alveolar pulmonary e.
angioneurotic e.
antral e.
bone marrow e.
brain e.
brainstem e.
breast e.
bronchial mucosal e.
bronchiolar e.
brown e.
bullous e.
capillary permeability e.
cardiac e.
cardiogenic pulmonary e.
cardiopulmonary e.
cerebral e.
chemical pulmonary e.
chronic e.
circumscribed e.
collateral e.
compressive e.
cyclic idiopathic e.
diffuse e.
e. of epididymis
fetal scalp e.
fingerprint e.
e. fluid
focal e.
frank pulmonary e.
fulminant pulmonary e.
generalized pulmonary e.
gravitational e.
gut e.
high-altitude pulmonary e. (HAPE)
hypervolemic pulmonary e.
idiopathic e.
ileocecal e.
inflammatory e.
intercellular e.
interstitial pulmonary e.
intracompartmental e.
laryngeal e.
leg e.
liver e.
local e.
localized e.
lung e.
lymphatic e.
malignant brain e.
massive ovarian e.
massive pulmonary hemorrhagic e.
mild e.
negative image pulmonary e.
e. neonatorum
nephrotic e.
nerve root e.
neurogenic pulmonary e.
noncardiogenic pulmonary e.
orbital e.
osmotic e.
ovarian e.
paroxysmal pulmonary e.
passive e.
patchy e.
e. pattern
pericholecystic e.
pericystic e.
perihilar e.
perineoplastic e.
periorbital e.
peripheral e.
peritumoral e.
perivascular e.
permeability pulmonary e.
placental e.
preosteonecrosis marrow e.
pulmonary e.
reactive marrow e.
reexpansion pulmonary e.
renal e.
reperfusion lung e.
solid e.
stasis e.
stomal e.

NOTES

edema *(continued)*
subchondral marrow e.
subcutaneous e.
subglottic e.
supraglottic e.
terminal e.
testicular posttraumatic e.
thalamic e.
trace e.
umbilical cord e.
unilateral pulmonary e.
vasogenic e.
venous e.
vernal e.
visceral e.
white matter e.
edematous
e. brain
e. bronchus
e. gallbladder
e. kidney
e. pancreatitis
e. pleura
e. tissue
edentulous
Eder-Puestow dilatation
edge
boundary e.
e. effect
e. enhancement
leading e.
ligament reflecting e.
ligament shelving e.
liver e.
e. misalignment artifact
patellar e.
e. response function (ERF)
e. ringing
e. ringing artifact
sawtooth e.
shelving e. of Poupart ligament
sternal e.
tentorial e.
trailing e.
ulcer with heaped-up e.'s
edge-boundary artifact
edge-detection angiography
edge-enhanced error diffusion algorithm
edge-region pixel
EDH
epidural hematoma
E-dial calibration
Edison
E. effect
E. fluoroscope
EDL
extensor digitorum longus
EDL muscle
Edmondson grading system for hepatocellular carcinoma
EDQ
extensor digiti quinti
EDQ muscle
EDR
effective direct radiation electrodermal response
EDTA
ethylenediaminetetraacetic acid
EDTMP
ethylenediamine tetramethylene phosphoric acid
EDTMP imaging agent
Edwards
double aortic arch of E.
Edward syndrome
EDXRF spectrometer
EEC
ectrodactyly-ectodermal dysplasia-clefting
EEC syndrome
EEG
electroencephalography
EF
ejection fraction
effaced collecting system
effacement
architectural e.
cistern e.
cisterna magna e.
e. of dura
dural sac e.
mesencephalic cistern e.
nerve root sheath e.
pelvocaliceal e.
e. of sulcus
sulcus e.
ventricle e.
e. of ventricle
effect
abscopal e.
adverse e.
Anrep e.
artifact e.
attenuation e.
Auger e.
Bayliss e.
beam-hardening e.
bilateral vagotomy e.
blood oxygenation level-dependent e.
Bohr e.
BOLD e.
Bowditch e.
bronchodilator e.
bronchomotor e.
bronchospastic e.

cardiovascular adverse e.
cobra-head e.
collimator exchange e.
Compton e.
contact e.
copper wire e.
Cserenkov e.
cumulative radiation e. (CRE)
Curie e.
deleterious e.
demagnetization field e.
Doppler e.
Dotter e.
dottering e.
duodenum extrinsic pressure e.
dynamic lineshape e.
edge e.
Edison e.
first-pass e.
flow-related enhancement e.
flow-void e.
gastrointestinal adverse e.
genitourinary adverse e.
halo e.
heel e.
hemispheral mass e.
hemodynamic e.
lag e.
Laplace e.
localized mass e.
Mach e.
Mach band e.
macromolecular hydration e.
magic angle e.
magnetization transfer e.
magnetohydrodynamic e.
masquerading e.
mass e.
mechanical dottering e.
missile e.
multilog e.
neurotoxic e.
nozzle e.
nuclear Overhauser e.
osmotic e.
outflow e.
Overhauser e.
oxygen e.
pad e.
paramagnetic e.
partial volume e.
phase e.
photoechoic e.
photoelectric e.
photographic e. (PE)
piezoelectric e.
priming e.
purse-stringing e.
radiation e.
reservoir e.
Russell e.
sausage segment e.
scalar e.
silver wire e.
sink e.
skin e.
skin-sparing e.
snowplow e.
sonic e.
star e.
susceptibility e.
systematic relaxation e.
teratogenic e.
thermal e.
time-of-flight e.
vagatomy e.
vasodilatory e.
Volta e.
Warburg e.
washboard e.
Wolff-Chaikoff e.

effective
e. balloon-dilated area (EBDA)
e. direct radiation electrodermal response (EDR)
e. dose
e. half-life
e. mass attenuation coefficient
e. pathlength (EPL)
e. pulmonary blood flow (EPBF)
e. pulmonic index
e. refractory period (ERP)
e. transverse relation time

effectiveness
relative biologic e. (RBE)

effector/target cell interaction

efferent
e. arteriolar resistance
e. digital nerve
e. duct
e. ductules of testis
e. loop
e. lymph vessel
e. view

NOTES

effervescent
e. agent
e. drink
efficacious
efficacy study
efficiency
absolute-peak e.
conversion e.
detective quantum e. (DQE)
full-energy peak e.
kidney extraction e.
quantum detection e. (QDE)
valvular e.
window e.
efficient relaxation time
effort
inspiratory e.
respiratory e.
shallow inspiratory e.
suboptimal e.
e. thrombosis
ventilatory e.
voluntary e. (VE)
effort-dependent
EFF probe
effused chyle
effusion
e. artifact
Baccelli sign of pleural e.
benign subdural e.
cardiac e.
chocolate joint e.
chylous e.
epidural e.
exudative pleural e.
fetal pleura e.
free pleural e.
hemorrhagic e.
inflammatory joint e.
ipsilateral pleural e.
joint e.
Karplus sign of pleural e.
Kellock sign of pleural e.
knee joint e.
layering e.
left-sided pleural e.
liquid pleural e.
loculated pleural e.
malignant pleural e.
massive pleural e.
milky e.
noninflammatory joint e.
parapneumonic e.
pericardial e. (PE)
peritoneal e.
pleural e.
pleuropericardial e.
pseudochylous e.
serofibrinous pericardial e.
serous e.
e. shadow
subdeltoid bursal e.
subdural e.
subpleural e.
subpulmonic e.
taut pericardial e.
transient pleural e.
transudative pleural e.
tuberculous e.
turbid e.
unilateral pleural e.
EFW
estimated fetal weight
EG
esophagogastric
Egan
E. mammography
E. technique
Egawa sign
egg casts
egg-on-its-side heart
egg-shaped orbit
eggshell
e. border of aneurysm
e. breast calcification
e. calcification
e. calcification of lymph node
e. nodal calcification
egress of blood
Egyptian splenomegaly
EHL
electrohydraulic lithotripsy
extensor hallucis longus
EHL muscle
EHM
extrahepatic metastasis
EHT
electrohydrothermo electrode
EIC
extensive intraductal carcinoma
extensive intraductal component
eigenvector
e. analysis
principal e.
eight-ball hemorrhage
eighth nerve tumor
eight-lumen esophageal manometry catheter
Eindhoven magnet
einsteinium (Es)
einsteinium-255 (^{255}Es)
Einthoven triangle
EIP
extensor indicis proprius
EIP muscle

Eisenmenger
E. complex
E. defect
E. reaction
E. syndrome
EIT
electrical impedance tomography
ejaculatory duct
ejection
e. fraction (EF)
e. fraction by first-pass technique
e. phase index
e. time (ET)
EJV
external jugular vein
EKG (*var. of* ECG)
electrocardiogram
Eklund
E. technique
E. view
EKY
electrokymogram
El-Ahwany classification of humeral supracondylar fractures
elastance
maximum ventricular e.
elastic
e. cartilage
e. cross section
e. recoil of artery
e. stable intramedullary nailing (ESIN)
e. subtraction algorithm
e. subtraction spiral CT angiography
elasticity
elasticum
pseudoxanthoma e.
elasticus
conus e.
elastofibroma
elastography
magnetic resonance e. (MRE)
elastomyofibrosis
elastosis
elbow
baseball pitcher's e.
e. bone center
boxer's e.
e. contracture
e. coronal scan
floating e.
e. fracture
golfer's e.
javelin thrower's e.
e. joint
milkmaid's e.
nursemaid's e.
pulled e.
reverse tennis e.
tennis e.
thrower's e.
wrestler's e.
elbow-patella syndrome
elective
e. arteriography
e. lymphadenectomy
electric
e. dipole
e. energy capacitance
e. generator
e. induction
e. interaction
e. joint fluoroscopy
e. joint fluoroscopy imaging
e. quadrupole coupling
e. stimulation
e. syringe
electrical
e. activity
e. circulatory arrest
e. impedance tomography (EIT)
e. potential energy
electrically activated implant
electrocardiogram (EKG)
resting e.
signal-averaged e. (SaECG)
e. tracing
e. trigger
electrocardiogram-gated
e.-g. MRI
e.-g. MRI imaging
e.-g. SPECT
electrocardiogram-synchronized digital subtraction angiography
electrocardiographic
e. gating
e. variant
electrocardiography
electrocardiography-gated echoplanar imaging
electrocardiophonogram

NOTES

electrocardioscanner
Compuscan Hittman computerized e.
electrocautery
endoluminal radiofrequency e.
monopolar radiofrequency e.
electrocerebral silence (ECS)
electrode
e. array
electrohydrothermo e. (EHT)
monitoring e.
e. monitoring
patch e.
polarographic needle e.
subcutaneous array e.
electrodesiccation
electrodiagnostic imaging
electroencephalography (EEG)
high-resolution e.
intracranial e.
quantitative e. (QEEG)
electrogastrogram
electrogram
RVA e.
electrohydraulic
e. fragmentation
e. lithotripsy (EHL)
e. shockwave lithotripsy (ESWL)
electrohydrothermo electrode (EHT)
electrokymogram (EKY)
electrokymograph
electrolytic reduction
electromagnet
structured coil e.
electromagnetic (EM)
e. absorption
e. blood flow imaging
e. blood flow study
e. (EM) field
e. energy
e. field
e. flow probe
e. focusing field probe (EFF probe)
e. interference (EMI)
e. interference scan
e. modeling
e. radiation
e. radiation exposure
e. spectrum
e. unit (emu)
e. wave
electromechanical dissociation (EMD)
electrometer
electromotive force (emf)
electromyogram
electron
e. arc technique
e. arc therapy
Auger e.'s
backscatter e.'s
e. beam
e. beam boost
e. beam therapy
e. beam tomography (EBT)
e. bolus
bound e.'s
e. capture
e. cloud
Compton e.'s
conversion e.
e. dosimetry
emission e.
e. equilibrium loss
excited e.'s
e. flow
e. flux
free e.'s
e. gun
internal conversion e.
K e.'s
L e.'s
e. linear accelerator
e. microscopy
e. multiplier tube
e. orbit
orbital e.'s
oscillating e.'s
e. paramagnetic resonance (EPR)
e. paramagnetic resonance (EPR) spatial imaging
positive e.
e. radiography
e. radiography imaging
recoil e.'s
secondary e.'s
e. spin
e. spin resonance (ESR)
e. theory
transition e.'s
valence e.
e. valence
e. volt (eV, ev)
electron-beam
e.-b. boost field
e.-b. computed tomography (EBCT)
e.-b. CT
e.-b. CT scanner
e.-b. intraoperative radiotherapy (EBIORT)
electroneuromyography
electronic
e. collimation
e. independent beam steering
e. magnification
e. portal imaging
electron-photon field matching

electron-positron pair
electron-volt (eV, ev)
electrooculographic analysis
electrooptical device
electropherogram
electrophilic radioiodination
electrophysiologic mapping
electroradiology
electroradiometer
electroscope
electrospray ionization mass spectroscopy
electrostatic
e. generator
e. imaging
e. imaging system
e. potential
electrostimulation
electrovectorcardiogram
electrovectorcardiography
Elema roll-film changer
element
blowout lesion of posterior vertebral e.
estrogen-response e.
fibroglandular e.
neoplastic destruction of spinal e.
picture e.
e. subluxation
volume e.
voxel e.
elementary fracture
elephant ears pelvis
elephantiasis neuromatosa
elevated
e. diaphragm
e. gradient
e. pressure
elevation
bilateral diaphragmatic e.
chorioamnionic e.
diaphragmatic e.
periosteal e.
unilateral diaphragmatic e.
elevatus
hallux e.
ELF
extremely low frequency
elimination
e. curve
e. half-life
e. kinetics
Ellestad protocol
ellipsoid
e. joint
e. lesion
elliptical
e. lumen
ellipticity index
Ellis
E. Jones peroneal displacement
E. line
E. sign
E. technique for Barton fracture
Ellis-Garland line
Ellis-van Creveld syndrome
elongated
e. aorta
e. heart
e. mass
e. structure
elongation
aortic e.
e. and tortuosity
e. of ventricle
eloquent areas of brain
ELPS
excessive lateral pressure syndrome
Elscint
E. dual-detector cardiac camera
E. Excel 905 scanner
E. MR scanner
E. Planar device
E. system
E. Twin CT scanner
Elsner syndrome
Elston-Scharff-Bloom-Richardson
E.-S.-B.-R. histologic grade system
EM
electromagnetic
emanation
actinium e.
radium e.
thorium e.
emanatorium
emanon
emanotherapy
embarrassment
circulatory e.
cord e.
nerve root e.
respiratory e.
embedding of stent coil
emboli (*pl. of* embolus)

NOTES

embolic
e. aneurysm
e. cerebral infarct
e. disease
e. event
e. necrosis
e. obstruction
e. occlusion
e. phenomenon
e. pneumonia
e. shower
e. stroke
embolism
embolization transcatheter therapy
embolus, pl. **emboli**
air e.
amnionic fluid e.
arterial e.
atheromatous e.
bacillary e.
bile pulmonary e.
bland e.
bone marrow e.
cancer e.
capillary e.
cardiogenic e.
catheter-induced e.
cellular e.
cerebral fat e.
cholesterol e.
coronary artery e.
cotton fiber e.
crossed e.
direct e.
fat e.
fibrin platelet e.
foam e.
foreign body e.
hematogenous e.
infective e.
intracranial e.
intraluminal e.
lymphogenous e.
massive e.
e. migration
miliary e.
multiple emboli
obturating e.
occluding spring e.
oil e.
pantaloon e.
paradoxical cerebral e.
peripheral e.
plasmodium e.
polyurethane foam e.
prosthetic valve e.
pulmonary e. (PE)
pulmonary venous-systemic air e.
pulmonary venous-systemic air e.
pyemic e.
recurrent e.
renal cholesterol e.
retinal e.
retrograde e.
riding e.
saddle e.
septic e.
septic pulmonary e.
silent cerebral e.
straddling e.
submassive pulmonary e.
therapeutic e.
thrombus e.
trichinous e.
tumor e.
venous thrombosis e.
visceral e.
embryo
adnexal e.
demise of e.
e. demise
e. size
embryogenesis
embryology
airway e.
e. of airway
breast e.
diaphragm e.
genital tract e.
reproductive tract e.
urogenital e.
embryonal
e. adenoma
e. carcinosarcoma
e. cell carcinoma
e. liver sarcoma
e. ovary teratoma
e. rhabdomyosarcoma
e. testicular cell carcinoma
e. tumor
e. vein
embryonic
e. anastomosis
e. aortic arch
e. branchial arch
e. disk
e. ovary
e. period
e. sac
e. truncus arteriosus
e. tumor
e. umbilical vein
embryopathy
EMD
electromechanical dissociation
EMED scanner

emetic center
EMF
endomyocardial fibrosis
emf
electromotive force
EMI
electromagnetic interference
EMI CT 500 scanner
EMI scan
EMI 7070 scanner
EMI unit
eminence
arcuate e.
articular e.
collateral e.
cruciate e.
cruciform e.
deltoid e.
facial e.
frontal e.
genital e.
hypothenar e.
iliopectineal e.
iliopubic e.
intercondylar e.
malar e.
medial e.
occipital e.
parietal e.
pyramidal e.
thenar e.
thyroid e.
tibial intercondylar e.
emissary
e. sphenoidal foramen
e. vein
emission
characteristic e.
e. computed tomography (ECT)
e. computer-assisted tomography (ECAT)
double e.
e. electron
filament e.
gamma e.
induced acoustic e.
photoelectric e.
e. probability
radioactive e.
e. range
spectral e.
thermonic e.
e. and transmission data
emitter
alpha-particle e.
Auger-electron e.
gamma e.
emphysema
alveolar duct e.
atrophic e.
bronchiolar e.
bullous e.
centriacinar e.
centrilobular e.
chronic hypertrophic e.
chronic obstructive e.
chronic tuberculous e.
compensatory e.
congenital lobar e.
cystic pulmonary e.
diffuse e.
distal acinar e.
distal lobular e.
ectatic e.
false e.
focal-dust e.
gangrenous e.
gastric e.
generalized e.
giant bullous e.
glass blower's e.
hypoplastic e.
idiopathic unilobar e.
increased markings of e.
infantile lobar e.
interlobular e.
interstitial lung e.
intestinal e.
intramural gastric e.
irregular e.
linear e.
liquefactive e.
lobar e.
localized obstructive e.
lung e.
mediastinal e.
neck e.
necrotizing e.
neonatal cystic pulmonary e.
nonbacterial gastric e.
obstructive e.
orbital e.
oxygen-dependent e.

NOTES

emphysema *(continued)*
panacinar e.
panlobular e.
paracicatricial e.
paraseptal e.
pericicatricial e.
perifocal e.
postoperative e.
postsurgical e.
proximal acinar e.
pulmonary interstitial e. (PIE)
pulmonary subcutaneous encephalitis e.
restrictive pulmonary e.
scar e.
senile e.
skeletal e.
small-lunged e.
subcutaneous e.
substantial e.
surgical e.
traumatic e.
unilateral lobar e.
vesicular e.
emphysematosa
vaginitis e.
emphysematous
e. bleb
e. bulla
e. cholecystitis
e. COPD
e. cystitis
e. expansion
e. gastritis
e. lung
e. pyelitis
e. pyelonephritis (EPN)
e. type A disease
empirical
e. diagnosis
e. method
empty
e. collapsed lung
e. gestational sac
e. heart
e. sella
e. sella syndrome
emptying
complete bladder e.
delayed gastric e.
gastric e. (GE)
incomplete bladder e.
oropharyngeal e.
e. time
tortuous e.
empyema
brain e.
chest e.
CNS e.
epidural e.
gallbladder e.
Hawkins accordion-type e.
interlobar e.
latent e.
left-sided e.
loculated e.
metapneumonic e.
e. necessitatis
pericardial e.
e. pleura
pleural e.
pulsating e.
right-sided e.
spinal e.
subdural e.
synpneumonic e.
thoracic e.
tuberculous e.
E-MRI
extremity MRI
emu
electromagnetic unit
emulsion film
Emulsoil bowel preparation
en
e. bloc
e. bloc excision
e. bloc resection
e. face view
e. passage feeder artery
enalaprilat-enhanced renography
enamel
e. crypt
e. lamella
enarthrosis
encapsulated
e. brain abscess
e. fat-containing lesion
e. fluid
e. gas bubble
e. mass
e. neoplasm
e. radioactive seed
e. subdural hematoma
encased heart
encasement
vascular e.
ventricular e.
encephalic
e. angioma
e. vesicle
encephalitis, pl. **encephalitides**
brainstem e.
bronzed sclerosing e.
cytomegalovirus e.
HIV e.

listeria e.
postinfectious e.
subacute e.
encephaloarteriography
encephalocele
frontoethmoidal e.
frontosphenoidal e.
occipital e.
parietal e.
sphenoethmoidal e.
sphenoidal e.
sphenomaxillary e.
sphenoorbital e.
sphenopharyngeal e.
transethmoidal e.
encephaloclastic
e. lesion
e. porencephaly
encephalocystocele
encephaloduroarteriomyosynangiosis (EDAMS)
encephaloduroarteriosynangiosis (EDAS)
encephalodysplasia
encephalogram
encephalography
air e.
A-mode e.
gamma e.
encephaloid
e. cancer
encephalolith
encephaloma
encephalomalacia
macrocystic e.
microcystic e.
neonate e.
encephalomyelitis
acute disseminated e. (ADEM)
postinfectious e. (PIE)
encephalomyelopathy
encephalomyopathy
mitochondrial e.
encephalopathia subcorticalis progressiva
encephalopathy
anoxic e.
Binswanger e.
hypertensive e.
hypoxic ischemic e.
ischemic e.
subcortical arteriosclerotic e.
subcortical atherosclerotic e.
encephalotrigeminal
e. angiomatosis
e. syndrome
encerclage
enchondral
e. bone formation
e. ossification
enchondroma
enchondromatosis
multiple e.
enchondrosarcoma
encoded-Fourier
encoding
centrally ordered phase e.
frequency e.
gradient e.
e. gradient
one-dimensional phase e.
ordered phase e.
phase e.
position e.
reordering of phase e.
respiratory ordered phase e. (ROPE)
respiratory sorted phase e.
spatial e.
wavelet e.
encroachment
bony e.
foraminal e.
luminal e.
soft tissue canal e.
encrustation
bile e.
encryption
e. algorithm
e. scheme
encysted
e. calculus
e. pleurisy
end
e. of atrial systole
bone e.
e. bud
e. bulb
e. exhalation
e. expiration
fimbriated e.
e. inhalation
e. organ resistance
e. plate
e. point

NOTES

E

end *(continued)*
e. of saturated bombardment (EOSB)
seen on e.
e. systole (ES)
endarterectomized segment
endarterectomy
carotid e.
e. and coronary artery bypass graft
extraluminal e.
surgical e.
transluminal e.
endarteritis obliterans
end-diastolic
e.-d. aortic-left ventricular pressure gradient
e.-d. imaging
e.-d. polar map
e.-d. pressure
e.-d. pressure-volume relation
e.-d. velocity measurement
e.-d. volume
e.-d. volume index
end-expiratory
e.-e. lung volume
e.-e. pressure
end-inspiratory pressure
endoanal
e. coil
e. MR imaging
e. sonography
e. ultrasound
Endobile
endobrachyesophagus
endobronchial
e. cancer
e. carcinoma
e. Kaposi sarcoma
e. lesion
e. metastasis
e. obstruction
e. tube
e. tuberculosis
e. tumor
endocardial, endocardiac
e. activation mapping
e. catheter mapping
e. cushion
e. cushion development
e. cushion malformation
e. cushion ventricular septal defect
e. dysplasia
e. fibroelastosis
e. fibrosis
e. plaque
e. pressure
e. sclerosis
e. trabeculation
e. volume
endocarditis
aortic valve e.
atypical verrucous e.
bacterial e.
Löffler e.
Löffler fibroplastic e.
marantic e.
subacute bacterial e. (SBE)
thrombotic e.
endocardium
disk of e.
wafer of e.
endocatheter ruler
endocavitary
e. applicator system
e. irradiation
endocervical
e. canal
e. canal coloscopy
e. mucosa
endochondral
e. bone
e. bone deposit
endochondroma
endocranium
endocrine
e. gland
e. imaging
e. tumor
endocyst
endodermal
e. cyst
e. pouch
e. sinus
e. sinus ovarian tumor
e. sinus testis tumor
endodiascope
endodiascopy
endoergic reaction
endofluoroscopic technique
endofluoroscopy
flexible e.
percutaneous e.
rigid e.
endogenous
e. callus formation
e. lipid pneumonia
Endografin
endoluminal
e. radiofrequency electrocautery
e. sonography
endolymphatic
e. duct
e. hydrops
e. sac
e. stromal myosis

endometria (*pl. of* endometrium)
endometrial
e. adenocanthoma
e. adenosquamous carcinoma
e. anatomy
e. canal fluid
e. cancer
e. cavity
e. chemical-shift imaging
e. cyst
e. echo
e. fluid in canal
e. hyperplasia
e. island
e. jet washings
e. polyp
e. secretory adenocarcinoma
e. stromal sarcoma
e. thickness
endometrioid
e. ovarian carcinoma
e. tumor
endometrioma
endometriosis
bladder e.
colonic involvement of e.
GI tract e.
gynecologic e.
e. interna
sciatic e.
studding of e.
ureteral e.
endometriotic cyst
endometritis
inflammatory e.
endometrium, pl. **endometria**
FIGO staging of adenocarcinoma of e.
inactive e.
e. menstrual phase
postmenopausal e.
proliferative phase e.
secretory phase e.
thickened irregular e.
endomyelography
endomyocardial
e. fibroplasia
e. fibrosis (EMF)
endoneural
endoneurium
end-on vessel
endopelvic fascia
endophlebitis
endoprosthesis
biliary e.
double-lumen e.
double-pigtail e.
large-bore bile duct e.
self-expanding metallic e.
Wallstent biliary e.
endopyelotomy
endorectal
e. coil
e. ileal pouch
e. surface-coil MR imaging
e. ultrasonography
end-organ response
endosalpingosis
endoscope
double-channel e.
endoscopic
e. decompression
e. laser
e. procedure
e. quadrature radiofrequency coil
e. retrograde cholangiogram (ERC)
e. retrograde cholangiopancreatography (ERCP)
e. retrograde pancreatic duct cannulation
e. retrograde pancreatography
e. retrograde parenchymography (ERP)
e. sonography
e. ultrasonography
e. ultrasound (EUS)
e. washing pipe
endoscopy
colorectal cancer e.
gastrointestinal e.
percutaneous e.
upper gastrointestinal e.
virtual e.
endoskeleton
endosonography
rectal e.
transduodenal e.
transgastric e.
vaginal e.
endosonoscopy
endosteal
e. callus
e. chondrosarcoma

NOTES

endosteal *(continued)*
e. revascularization
e. surface
endosteoma
endosteum
endothelia (*pl. of* endothelium)
endothelial
e. damage
e. hypoplasia
e. injury
e. myeloma
e. surface
endothelialization
endothelialized vascular graft
endotheliomatous meningioma
endothelium, pl. **endothelia**
arterial e.
capillary e.
pulmonary capillary e.
squamous e.
endothoracic fascia
endothorax
tension e.
endotracheal (ET)
e. intubation
e. tube
endovaginal
e. sonography
e. ultrasonography
endovascular
e. aortic graft
e. coil
e. flow wire study
e. stent-graft
e. technique
e. ultrasonography
e. ultrasound
endplate
cartilaginous e.
hyaline cartilage e.
e. sclerosis
vertebral body e.
endpoint
measurable e.
stress e.
end-pressure artifact
end-stage
e.-s. adult cardiac decompensation
e.-s. cardiomyopathy
e.-s. cirrhosis
e.-s. fetal cardiac decompensation
e.-s. lung disease
e.-s. rejection
e.-s. renal disease
e.-s. renal failure (ESRF)
end-systolic
e.-s. polar map
e.-s. pressure (ESP)
e.-s. pressure/end-systolic volume (ESP/ESV)
e.-s. pressure-volume relation
e.-s. residual volume
e.-s. reversal
e.-s. volume (ESV)
e.-s. volume index (ESVI)
e.-s. wall index (ESWI)
e.-s. wall index/end-systolic volume index (ESWI-ESVI)
e.-s. wall index/end-systolic volume ratio (ESWI-ESVI ratio)
end-viewing transducer
enema
air-contrast e.
air-contrast barium e. (ACBE)
analeptic e.
barium e. (BE)
blind e.
contrast e.
Cortenema retention e.
double-contrast e.
double-contrast barium e. (DCBE)
full-column barium e.
Gastrografin e.
Harris flush e.
hydrocortisone e.
hydrogen peroxide e.
Hypaque e.
mesalamine e.
methylene blue e.
nuclear e.
phosphate e.
phosphosoda e.
retention e.
Rowasa e.
single-contrast barium e.
small bowel e.
therapeutic barium e.
water-soluble contrast e.
enemas until clear
energy
average positron e.
beam e.
binding e.
chemical potential e.
e. decay
electrical potential e.
electromagnetic e.
e. fluence
e. flux density
gravitational potential e.
kinetic e.
laser e.
e. level
low-photon e.
mechanical potential e.
nuclear e.

photon e.
quantum e.
radiant e.
radiation e.
radiofrequency e.
e. resolution
e. spectrum
e. subtraction
thermal e.
e. transfer
e. transfer process
treatment e.
variable e.
e. wave
e. wavelength
e. window

Engel alakalinity

Engelmann disease

Engel-Recklinghausen disease

engorged
e. collecting system
e. tissue
e. vein

enhanced
e. CT
e. CT scan
e. glycolysis
e. imaging

Enhance deblurring method

enhancement
acoustic e.
bolus contrast e.
bright contrast e.
cocurrent flow-related e.
contrast e.
countercurrent flow-related e.
Doppler flow signal e.
dynamic e.
edge e.
evanescent e.
exercise-induced contrast e.
e. factor
flow-related e.
gadolinium e.
gyral brain e.
heterogeneous isodense e.
inhomogeneous e.
isodense e.
e. morphology
multislice flow-related e.
nodular e.
nonhomogeneous e.
PALA e.
N-phosphonoacetyl-*l*-aspartic acid
paradoxical e.
paramagnetic contrast e.
e. pattern
peak e.
peripheral e.
peritoneal e.
proton relaxation e.
pulmonary nodule e.
punctate e.
radiation e.
rapid acquisition with relaxation e. (RARE)
real-time e.
rim e.
ring of e.
e. ring
ring e.
scan with contrast e.
signal e.
sulcal e.
time-of-flight e.
vascular MR contrast e.

enhancing
e. brain lesion
e. mass
e. nodule
e. ventricular margin

enlarged
e. cardiac silhouette
e. frontal horn
e. gallbladder
e. heart
e. kidney
e. liver
e. presacral space
e. thyroid gland
e. vascular channel
e. vertebral foramen
e. vestibular aqueduct syndrome

enlargement
air-space e.
aortic e.
azygos vein e.
biventricular e.
bony e.
bulbous e.
cardiac silhouette e.
cervical e.
chamber e.
compensatory e.

E

NOTES

enlargement *(continued)*
diffuse hepatic e.
diffuse liver e.
diffuse thymic e.
diffuse uterine e.
e. of epididymis
epiglottic e.
extraocular muscle e.
global renal e.
hilar gland e.
hilar lymph node e.
iliopsoas compartment e.
e. of lacrimal gland
left atrial e. (LAE)
lymph node e.
mediastinal lymph node e.
optic nerve e.
panchamber e.
papilla of Vater e.
e. of parotid gland
pituitary gland e.
placenta e.
right atrial e. (RAE)
right ventricular e. (RVE)
e. of sella
sella e.
sulcal e.
thymic e.
e. of uterus
e. of ventricle
ventricular e.
e. of vertebral body
e. of vertebral foramen
e. with low-density lymph node center
enostosis
ensheathing callus
ensiform
e. appendix
e. cartilage
e. process
enteral alimentation
enteric
e. cyst
e. fistula
e. plexus
e. stricture
enteritis
Crohn granulomatous e.
Crohn regional e.
e. follicularis
radiation e.
regional e.
enterobiliary
enterocele
e. sac
enteroclysis
enterococcus, pl. **enterococci**
enterocolic fistula
enterocolitis
granulomatous e.
Hirschsprung-associated e. (HAEC)
necrotizing e.
neutropenic e.
enterocutaneous fistula
enterocystoma
enteroenteral fistula
enterogenous
e. cyst
e. cyst of ampulla of Vater
enteroinsular axis
enterolith
enteropathica
acrodermatitis e.
enteropathy-associated T-cell lymphoma
enteroperitoneal abscess
enteroptosis
enteroscopy
small bowel e. (SBE)
enterospinal fistula
enterourethral fistula
enterovaginal fistula
enterovesical fistula
enthesis
enthesopathic transformation
enthesophyte
plantar calcaneal e.
subacromial e.
entorhinal cortex
entrance block
entrapment
artery e.
gas e.
guide wire e.
lateral e.
median nerve e.
nerve e.
e. neuropathy
patellar e.
posterior interosseous nerve (PIN) e.
soft tissue e.
suprascapular nerve e.
e. syndrome
ulnar nerve e.
entrapped
e. ovarian cyst
e. plantar sesamoid bone
entry
e. flap
e. point
e. slice phenomenon artifact
e. tear
e. zone
entry-slice phenomenon

envelope
capsuloperiosteal e.
fascial e.
soft tissue e.
synovial e.
environmental
e. factor
e. plutonium
enzyme
angiotensin-converting e. (ACE)
enzyme-multiplied immunoassay technique
EOSB
end of saturated bombardment
eosinophilic
e. brain adenoma
e. granuloma
e. infiltrate
e. lung
e. lung disease
e. pneumonia
EP
ectopic pregnancy
excretory phase
epactal bone
epamniotic cavity
EPB
extensor pollicis brevis
EPB muscle
EPBF
effective pulmonary blood flow
ependymal cyst
ependymitis
bacterial e.
e. granularis
ependymoblastoma
ependymoma
anaplastic e.
brain e.
brainstem e.
e. cord
malignant e.
myxopapillary e.
spinal cord e.
subcutaneous sacrococcygeal myxopapillary e.
ephemeral pneumonia
EPI
echoplanar imaging
epiarterial bronchus
epiarticular osteochondromatous dysplasia
epicardial
e. attachment
e. coronary artery
e. Doppler echocardiography
e. Doppler flow sector transducer
e. fat pad
e. imaging
e. implantation
e. Kaposi sarcoma
e. mapping
e. space
e. surface
e. tension
e. volume
epicardium
epicenter
eccentric e.
epicolic lymph node
epicondylar
e. fracture
e. fracture of humerus
e. ridge
epicondyle
humeral e.
medial e.
epicondylitis
lateral e.
medial e.
epicondyloolecranon ligament
epicortical lesion
epicranial aponeurosis
epidermal
e. carcinoma
e. ridge
epidermoid
acquired e.
black e.
e. bone carcinoma
e. cancer
e. carcinoma of vulva
cerebellar e.
e. lung carcinoma
e. mediastinum
e. spine
e. tumor
white e.
epidermoidoma
incisural e.
intradural e.
prepontine white e.
epididymal
e. cyst

NOTES

epididymal *(continued)*
e. descent
e. fibrosarcoma
epididymis, pl. **epididymides**
appendix of e.
body of e.
edema of e.
enlargement of e.
inflammation of e.
interstitial congestion of e.
e. lesion
ligament of e.
lobule of e.
postvasectomy change in e.
sinus of e.
tail of e.
epididymitis
epididymography
e. imaging
epididymoorchitis
epidural
e. abscess
e. angiolipoma
e. arachnoid cyst
e. blood
e. blood patch
e. cavernous hemangioma
e. cavity
e. effusion
e. empyema
e. extramedullary lesion
e. fibrosis
e. hematoma (EDH)
e. hemorrhage
e. implant
e. infusion
e. lipoma
e. lipomatosis
e. lymphoma
e. mass
e. pneumatosis
e. space
e. steroid injection
e. venography
e. venous plexus
epidurogram
epidurography
magnetic resonance e.
epigastric
e. angle
e. fold
e. fossa
e. hernia
e. lymph node
e. vein
epigastrium
epiglottic
e. carcinoma
e. cartilage
e. disruption
e. enlargement
e. fold
e. tubercle
epiglottitis
bacterial e.
epignathus
epihyal
e. bone
e. ligament
epihyoid bone
epilarynx
epilation dose
epilepsy
chronic partial e.
structural e.
temporal lobe e.
epileptic focus
epileptogenic
e. focus
e. lesion
e. zone
epipericardial ridge
epiphrenic bulge
epiphyseal
e. arrest
e. cartilage
e. cartilage plate
e. chondroblastic growth
e. chondrocyte
e. coxa vara
e. disk
e. dysgenesis
e. dysostosis
e. dysplasia
e. exostosis
e. fetal bone center
e. growth plate
e. hematopoietic marrow
e. hyperplasia
e. hypertrophy
e. ischemic necrosis
e. lesion
e. line
e. ossification center
e. osteochondroma
e. overgrowth
e. plate fracture
e. plate injury
e. slip fracture
e. slippage
e. tibial fracture
epiphysealis punctua dysplasia
epiphyseolysis
femoral head e.

idiopathic e.
juvenile e.
epiphysis, pl. **epiphyses**
annular e.
atavistic e.
e. avulsion
ball-and-socket e.
balloon e.
e. bone
bone lesion e.
capital e. (CE)
capital femoral e.
capitular e.
cartilaginous e.
cone e.
congenital stippled e.
familial avascular necrosis of phalangeal e.
femoral capital e.
hypertrophy of e.
ossifying e.
osteochondrotic separation of epiphysis
Perthes e.
pressure e.
ring e.
slipped capital femoral e. (SCFE)
slipped upper femoral e. (SUFE)
tibial e.
traction e.
epiphysitis
juvenile e.
vertebral e.
epiploia
epiploic
e. appendage
e. appendicitis
e. appendix
e. foramen
epipteric bone
epirenal septum
episcleral
e. space
e. vein
episode
ischemic e.
mitochondrial myopathy, encephalopathy, lactic acidosis, and stroke-like e.'s (MELAS)
silent ischemic e.
episodic colic
epispadia exstrophy complex
Epistar
E. perfusion technique
E. subtraction
E. subtraction angiography
episternal bone
epitendineum
epithalamus
epithelia (*pl. of* epithelium)
epithelial
e. cell
e. colon
e. colonic polyp
e. cyst
e. degenerative change
e. hyperplasia
e. malignancy
e. neoplasm
e. ovarian cancer
e. spleen
e. tumor
epithelialization
creeping e.
epithelial-myoepithelial carcinoma
epithelioid
e. angiomatosis
e. granuloma
e. hemangioendothelioma
e. hemangioma
e. leiomyoma
e. malignant mesothelioma
e. osteosarcoma
e. sarcoma
epithelioma
calcifying Malherbe e.
epitheliosis
infiltrating breast e.
epitheliotropism
epithelium, pl. **epithelia**
atypical e.
Barrett e.
e. crypt
ductal e.
normal ovarian surface e. (NOSE)
papilla of columnar e.
squamous metaplasia white e.
surface e.
tumor of surface e.
white e.
epitrochlear
e. lymph node
epituberculous infiltrate

E

NOTES

epitympanic
e. recess (EPR)
e. space
epitympanum
EPL
effective pathlength
extensor pollicis longus
EPL muscle
EPN
emphysematous pyelonephritis
eponychium
epoöphoron
Eppendorf
E. pO_2 histograph
EPR
electron paramagnetic resonance
epitympanic recess
EPSS
E point to septal separation
Epstein-Barr-encoded RNA (EBER)
EQP
extensor quinti proprius
equal in intensity
equalization
histogram e.
pressure e.
e. of pressure
scan e.
equalized diastolic pressure
equation
Bohr e.
Bragg e.
Carter e.
decay e.
Doppler e.
Fick e.
Hamiltonian e.
Kety e.
Larmor e.
linear-quadratic e.
Nernst e.
Schroedinger e.
Solomon-Bloembergen e.
Stewart-Hamilton e.
Teichholz e.
transformer e.
equilibrium
charged particle e.
e. dissociation constant
e. dose constant
e. factor
e. magnetization
e. MUGA imaging
e. MUGA scan
e. phase
e. point
radioactive e.
e. radionuclide angiocardiography
e. radionuclide angiocardiography technique
e. radionuclide angiography
secular e.
state e.
thermal e.
transient e.
e. view
equina
cauda e.
equinovalgus
e. deformity
pes e.
equinovarus
e. deformity
e. hindfoot deformity
pes e.
talipes e.
equinus
e. deformity
pes e.
equipment artifact
equivalent
chance e.
e. dose
dose e. (DE)
meconium ileus e.
equivocal finding
Erb
E. area
E. disease
E. injury
E. point
E. sign
Erb-Duchenne-Klumpke
E.-D.-K. injury
E.-D.-K. injury to brachial plexus
Erb-Duchenne paresis
erbium-171
erbium-YAG
ERC
endoscopic retrograde cholangiogram
ERCP
endoscopic retrograde cholangiopancreatography
ERCP catheter
ERCP imaging
ERCP manometry
Erdheim
E. cystic medial necrosis
E. cystic medionecrosis
E. I syndrome
E. tumor
ERE
external rotation in extension
erect
e. position

e. radiograph
e. view
erecta
luxatio e.
erector spinae
ERF
edge response function
external rotation in flexion
ergometer
bicycle e.
Cybex e.
ergonovine test
Erichsen sign
Erlenmeyer flask deformity
erosion
articular e.
e. of articular surface
bony e.
bronchial e.
duodenal e.
e. of epiphyseal bone
focal cartilage e.
gastric antral e.
graft-enteric e.
infraspinatus insertion e.
linear e.
marginal e.
mouse ear e.
odontoid e.
osteoclastic e.
pedicle e.
plaque e.
rat-bite e.
salt-and-pepper duodenal e.
stomach varioliform e.
tumor e.
varioliform e.
erosive
e. duodenitis
e. gastritis
e. gastritis target sign
e. gingivitis
e. osteoarthritis
eroticism, erotism
brachioproctic e.
ERP
effective refractory period
endoscopic retrograde parenchymography
erratum
anatomic moment e.
error
CT imaging e.
darkroom e.
e. diffusion method
dorsal induction e.
duplex ultrasound e.
flow-related phase e.
Hausdorff e.
interobserver e.
intraobserver e.
isocenter placement e.
magnification e.
mean-square e.
photoreceptor fractional velocity e.
positioning e.
preparation e.
quantization e.
raster spacing e.
relative e.
sampling e.
sensing e.
size estimation e.
spatial frequency e.
error-sum criterion
eruption
rhythmic paradoxical e.
ERV
expiratory reserve volume
erythema
e. dose
e. of joint
e. threshold
erythrocyte
technetium-99m heat-denatured e.
ES
end systole
Es
einsteinium
^{255}Es
einsteinium-255
escalation
escape
e. of air into lung connective tissue
e. beat
e. interval
escape-capture rhythm
escape-peak ratio
ESIN
elastic stable intramedullary nailing
esophageal
e. achalasia pattern
e. apple-core lesion
e. A ring

NOTES

E

esophageal *(continued)*
e. atresia
e. balloon technique
e. body
e. B ring
e. cancer
e. carcinoma
e. carcinosarcoma
e. choriocarcinoma
e. contractile ring
e. contraction
e. degeneration
e. dilatation
e. dissection
e. diverticulum
e. duplication
e. duplication cyst
e. dysmotility
e. dysphagia
e. fibroadenoma
e. filling defect
e. fold
e. function imaging
e. groove
e. hernia
e. hiatus
e. impression
e. inflammation
e. inlet
e. leiomyoma
e. leiomyomatosis
e. leiomyosarcoma
e. lumen
e. lung
e. manometry
e. motility
e. motility disorder
e. mucosal nodule
e. mucosal ring
e. muscular ring
e. narrowing
e. neoplasm
e. obstruction
e. obturator airway
e. opening
e. perforation
e. peristalsis
e. peristaltic pressure
e. plaque
e. plexus
e. pseudosarcoma
e. reflux
e. rupture
e. shunt
e. spasm
e. stenosis
e. stent
e. stricture
e. tear
e. transition zone
e. transit time
e. tumor
e. ulcer
e. variceal sclerosis
e. varix
e. vein
e. vestibule
e. web
e. window

esophagectomy
transhiatal e. (THE)
transthoracic e.

esophagi (*pl. of* esophagus)

esophagitis
acute e.
AIDS-related e.
candida e.
caustic e.
chronic e.
corrosive e.
cytomegalovirus e.
drug-induced e.
herpes e.
HIV e.
peptic e.
pill e.
reflux e. (RE)
Sonnenberg classification of erosive e.
viral e.

esophagogastric (EG)
e. fat pad
e. intubation
e. junction
e. orifice
e. tamponade

esophagogastrostomy

esophagogram
air e.
barium e.
barium-water e.
contrast e.
radionuclide e.

esophagography
e. imaging

esophagojejunostomy

esophagorespiratory fistula

esophagoscopy

esophagospasm

esophagostomy
cervical e.
palliative e.

esophagotracheal fistula

esophagus, pl. **esophagi**
abnormal fold e.
abnormal peristalsis e.

achalasia of e.
aperistaltic e.
A ring of e.
atonic e.
Barrett e.
bird beak e.
B ring of e.
cervical e.
cobblestone appearance e.
columnar-lined e.
congenitally short e.
corkscrew appearance of the e.
curling e.
diffuse dilation of the e.
diffuse spasm of the e.
double-barrel e.
dysmotile e.
extrinsic impression of the e.
foreign body in e.
intramural rupture of the e.
long smooth narrowing e.
middle third of thoracic e.
muscular ring e.
nutcracker e.
rat-tail e.
rosary beading e.
scleroderma of e.
shaggy e.
shish kebab e.
spastic e.
thoracic e.
tortuous e.
upper thoracic e.
Z-line of e.

ESP
end-systolic pressure

ESP/ESV
end-systolic pressure/end-systolic volume
ESP/ESV ratio

ESR
electron spin resonance

ESRF
end-stage renal failure

essential osteolysis

Essex-Lopresti
E.-L. calcaneal fracture classification
E.-L. joint depression fracture

ester
iodipamide ethyl e.

esthesioneuroblastoma

esthesioneurocytoma

esthesioneuroepithelioma

estimated fetal weight (EFW)

estimation
bayesian image e. (BIE)
fractional moving blood volume e.
frequency e.
magnetic resonance volume e.
stereologic method of volume e.
volume e.

estradiol
^{18}F e.

estrogen-producing tumor

estrogen-response element

ESV
end-systolic volume

ESVI
end-systolic volume index

ESWI
end-systolic wall index

ESWI-ESVI
end-systolic wall index/end-systolic volume index
ESWI-ESVI ratio

ESWL
electrohydraulic shockwave lithotripsy
extracorporeal shockwave lithotripsy

ET
ejection time
endotracheal

etanidazole imaging agent

etching
track e.

ETF
extension teardrop fracture

ethanol (EtOH)
absolute e.

ethidium bromide

Ethiodane
E. contrast medium

ethiodized
e. oil

Ethiodol
E. contrast medium
E. imaging agent

ethmocephaly

ethmoid
e. air cell
e. bone
bulla e.
e. canal
e. sinus
e. sinus carcinoma

NOTES

ethmoidal
e. artery
e. bulla
e. crest
e. foramen
e. groove
e. labyrinth
e. meningoencephalocele
e. notch
e. process
e. vein
ethmoidolacrimal suture
ethmoidomaxillary suture
ethmovomerine plate
Ethodian imaging agent
ethyl
^{18}F-labeled polyfluorinated e.
ethylenediaminetetraacetic acid (EDTA)
ethylenediamine tetramethylene phosphoric acid (EDTMP)
etidronate
rhenium-186 e.
technetium-99m e.
ETL
echo-train length
E-to-F
E.-t.-F. slope
E.-t.-F. slope of valve
E-TOF (electron time-of-flight) detecting module
EtOH
ethanol
EtOH-associated liver disease
ETT
exercise tolerance test
EU
excretory urography
euchromatin
eukinesis
eunuchoid constitution
Eureka collimator
europium-activated barium fluorohalide
EUS
endoscopic ultrasound
eustachian
e. canal
e. tube
e. valve
euthyroid sick syndrome
eV, ev
electron-volt
electron volt
Evac-Q-Kit
Evac-Q-Kwik bowel preparation
evacuation
colonic e.
digital rectal e.
e. disorder
e. pouchography
precipitate e.
e. proctography
evaluation
e. of glucose metabolism
e. of mass mammography
evanescent enhancement
Evans
E. blue imaging agent
E. fracture classification system
E. intertrochanteric fracture classification
Evans-D'Angio staging system
EVD
external ventricular drain
even distribution of echoes
even-echo rephasing
event
adverse e.
cardinal e.
cerebral ischemic e.
e. counter
embolic e.
inciting e.
ischemic e.
main timing e. (MTE)
morbid e.
precipitating e.
e. recorder
true e.
eventration
e. of the diaphragm
diaphragmatic e.
eversion
e. of ankle
cervical e.
e. sprain
eversion-external rotation deformity
evidence
scintigraphic e.
evolution
stroke in e.
Evolution XP scanner
evolving
e. hematoma
e. myocardial infarct
e. stroke
evulsion
Ewald
E. node
E. test meal
Ewart sign
Ewing
E. sarcoma
E. tumor
exacerbation
exact framing

exaggerated
e. craniocaudal lateral (XCCL)
e. craniocaudal view
exametazime imaging agent
examination
barium e.
contrast-enhanced radiographic e.
Doppler venous e.
double-contrast e.
^{67}Ga e.
gated exercise e.
gray-scale e.
image-acquisition gated e.
limited e.
neuroradiologic e.
postglucose loading e.
reinjection thallium stress e.
rest-redistribution e.
self-breast e. (SBE)
stress gated blood pool cardiac e.
stress-redistribution e.
stress-rest-reinjection e.
suboptimal e.
T1-weighted spin-echo e.
T2-weighted spin-echo e.
unsuppressed e.
venous Doppler e.
in vivo e.
exanthematous disease
excavation
saucer-shaped e.
excavatum
pectus e.
excessive
e. callus formation
e. joint play
e. lateral pressure syndrome (ELPS)
exchange
air e.
coupling e.
intestinal gas e.
narrowing e.
proton-proton magnetization e.
pulmonary gas e.
spin e.
excimer
e. (excited dimer) laser
e. laser system
XeCl (xenon chloride) e.
excision
CT-guided percutaneous e.
en bloc e.
large loop e.
excitation
fast acquisition multiple e.
e. function
e. function measurement
magnetization-prepared rapid gradient echo-water e. (MP-RAGE-WE)
nonuniform e.
number of e.'s (NEX)
e. profile
quadrature e.
rebound e.
selective e.
slice-selective e.
supernormal e.
tailored e.
tilted optimized nonsaturating e. (TONE)
uniform TR (repetition time) e.
variable-angle uniform signal e. (VUSE)
variable flip-angle e.
volume-selective e.
wave of e.
excitation-spoiled
e.-s. fat-suppressed T1-weighted SE image
excitatory
e. lesion
e. pulse characteristic
excited
e. atoms
e. electrons
exclusion
subtotal gastric e.
exclusion-HPLC technique
excrescence
bony e.
papillary e.
excrescentic thickening of the optic nerve
excretion
ammonium e.
colonic mucosal e.
contrast media e.
^{67}Ga e.
uptake and e.
urinary e.
vicarious contrast e.

NOTES

excretory
e. cystogram
e. duct
e. intravenous pyelography
e. phase (EP)
e. urography (EU)
e. urography imaging
excursion of the diaphragm
exencephaly
exenteration
anterior e.
pelvic e.
exercise
e. echocardiography
e. first-pass LVEF
flexion and extension e.'s
e. image
e. index
e. intolerance
e. load
e. LV function
modified stage e.
e. oximetry
e. radionuclide angiocardiography
e. radionuclide ventriculogram
e. strain gauge venous plethysmography
e. stress-redistribution scintigraphy
e. thallium scintigraphy
e. thallium-201 stress imaging
e. thallium-201 stress test
e. thallium-201 tomography
e. tolerance test (ETT)
exercise-induced
e.-i. bronchoconstriction
e.-i. contrast enhancement
e.-i. transient myocardial ischemia
exertion
Borg scale of treadmill e.
dyspnea on e.
exertional rhabdomyolysis
exhalation
end e.
exit
e. block
e. dose
e. site of catheter
e. wound
Exner plexus
exocardia
exoccipital bone
exoergic reaction
exogenous
e. invasion
e. lipoid pneumonia
e. obesity
exophthalmic goiter
exophytic
e. adenocarcinoma
e. carcinoma
e. fibroid
exostosis, pl. **exostoses**
blocker's e.
bony e.
epiphyseal e.
hypertrophic e.
impingement e.
marginal e.
multiple hereditary exostoses
osteocartilaginous e.
pelvic e.
retrocalcaneal e.
tackler's e.
traction e.
turret e.
exostotica
bursa e.
exostotic chondrosarcoma
expandable access catheter
expanded
e. lung
e. polytetrafluoroethylene (e-PTFE) graft
expanding
e. cavernous sinus brain lesion
e. intracranial mass
expansile
e. aneurysmal bone cyst
e. aortic segment
e. configuration
e. lytic lesion
e. mass
e. multilocular bone lesion
e. multilocular osteolysis
e. osteoblastoma
e. rib lesion
e. unilocular well-demarcated bone lesion
expansion
complete stent e.
emphysematous e.
fluid e.
infarct e.
lung e.
peripheral e.
rapid fluid e.
stent e.
expenditure
resting energy e.
Expert-XL densitometer
expiration
end e.
flow-limited e.
quantitative CT during e.
e. view

expiratory
- e. attenuation
- e. chest
- e. computed tomography
- e. CT
- e. film
- e. flow
- inspiratory to e. (I:E)
- e. phase
- e. reserve volume (ERV)
- e. resistance
- e. view

exploration
- common bile duct e. (CBDE)
- common duct e.

explosion fracture

explosive follicular hyperplasia

exponential
- e. decay
- e. kinetics
- e. shape

expoSURE

exposure
- e. angle
- asbestos e.
- bone-tendon e.
- DES e.
- e. dose
- electromagnetic radiation e.
- intraperitoneal e.
- magnetic radiation e.
- e. meter
- operator e.
- overcouch e.
- radiation e.
- e. variation

expression vector

exquisite detail

exsanguinating hemorrhage

exstrophy
- e. of bladder
- bladder e.
- cloacal e.
- closed e.
- urinary bladder e.

extended
- e. field of view
- e. pattern
- e. radical mastectomy

extended-field irradiation therapy

extension
- angle of greatest e. (AGE)
- basal e.
- Buck e.
- capital e.
- Codivilla e.
- e. corner avulsion fracture (ECAF)
- external rotation in e. (ERE)
- extraaxial e.
- extracapsular e. (ECE)
- extranodal tumor e.
- extrascleral e.
- hilar e.
- e. injury
- e. injury of spine
- internal rotation in e. (IRE)
- intracavitary e.
- medial e.
- metaphyseal e.
- parenchymal e.
- parietal e.
- radiolucent operating room table e.
- subligamentous e.
- suprasellar e.
- e. teardrop fracture (ETF)
- thrombus e.
- e. of tumor
- tumor e.
- e. view

extensive
- e. anterior myocardial infarct
- e. bilateral pneumonia
- e. dissection
- e. head injury
- e. intraductal carcinoma (EIC)
- e. intraductal component (EIC)

extensor
- e. apparatus
- e. carpi radialis brevis (ECRB)
- e. carpi radialis brevis muscle
- e. carpi radialis longus (ECRL)
- e. carpi radialis longus muscle
- e. carpi ulnaris (ECU)
- e. carpi ulnaris muscle
- e. carpi ulnaris sheath
- e. compartment
- e. digiti quinti (EDQ)
- e. digiti quinti muscle
- e. digitorum
- e. digitorum brevis (EDB)
- e. digitorum brevis muscle
- e. digitorum communis (EDC)
- e. digitorum communis muscle
- e. digitorum longus (EDL)

NOTES

E

extensor *(continued)*
e. digitorum longus muscle
e. hallucis longus (EHL)
e. hallucis longus muscle (EHL muscle)
e. indicis
e. indicis proprius (EIP)
e. indicis proprius muscle
e. mechanism
e. pollicis brevis (EPB)
e. pollicis brevis muscle
e. pollicis longus (EPL)
e. pollicis longus muscle
e. quinti proprius (EQP)
e. retinaculum
e. tendon
ulnar e.
extensor-supinator group
extensus
hallux e.
exteriorization
externa
otitis e.
theca e.
external
e. acoustic foramen
e. anal sphincter
e. artifact
e. auditory canal
e. auditory canal atresia
e. auditory canal dysplasia
e. auditory meatus
e. band
e. beam irradiation
e. beam radiation
e. beam radiation therapy (EBRT)
e. beam with tandem
e. biliary fistula
e. callus
e. capsule
e. carotid
e. carotid artery (ECA)
e. carotid steal syndrome
e. condyle
e. ear mass
e. ear neoplasm
e. elastic lamina
e. fixation
e. fixation device
e. gamma dose reconstruction
e. heat generating source
e. hemorrhage
e. hernia
e. iliac artery
e. iliac lymph node
e. iliac stenosis
e. inguinal ring
e. jugular system
e. jugular vein (EJV)
e. looping technique
e. malignant otitis
e. oblique aponeurosis
e. oblique muscle
e. orthovoltage irradiation
e. os
e. pneumatic calf compression
e. pudendal vein
e. ring apex
e. rotation in extension (ERE)
e. rotation in flexion (ERF)
e. rotation view
e. scanning
e. snapping hip
e. urethral orifice
e. urethral sphincter
e. ventricular drain (EVD)
e. wire fixation
e. x-ray therapy
externum
os tibiale e.
externus
obturator e.
extinction phenomenon
extirpation
e. of saphenous vein
tumor e.
extraadrenal
e. chromaffin tissue
e. paraganglioma
e. site
extraalveolar
e. air (EAA)
e. air collection
extraarachnoid
e. injection
e. myelography
extraarticular
e. debris
e. fracture
e. hip fusion
e. posterior ossification
e. resection
extraaxial
e. cavernous hemangioma
e. CNS lesion
e. extension
e. fluid collection
e. low-attenuation lesion
e. space
e. tumor
extracapsular
e. ankylosis
e. dissection
e. extension (ECE)
e. fracture

e. ligament
e. metastasis
extracardiac
e. anomaly
e. collateral circulation
e. mass
extracavitary
e. infected graft
e. prosthetic arterial graft
extracellular
e. compartment
e. domain
e. fluid
e. fluid volume
e. matrix
e. matrix component
e. space
extracerebral
e. aneurysm
e. cavernous angioma
e. fluid collection
e. hematoma
e. intracranial glioneural hamartoma
extrachorialis
placenta e.
extrachorial placenta
extracompartmental tumor
extracorporeal
e. circulation
e. irradiation
e. membrane oxygenation
e. membrane oxygenator
e. photochemotherapy
e. shock wave
e. shockwave lithotripsy (ESWL)
extracorticospinal tract
extracranial
e. aneurysm
e. carotid artery atherosclerosis
e. carotid artery occlusive disease
e. carotid circulation
e. carotid system
e. cerebral circulation
e. cerebral vasculature
e. mass lesion
e. vertebral artery
e. vessel
extraction
automatic e.
e. catheter atherectomy
e. column
contour e.
disphenoid e.
first-pass e.
first-pass thallium e.
fringe skeleton e.
e. generator
e. method
solid phase e.
stone e.
vacuum e.
vascular segmentation and e.
extradural
e. abscess
e. anastomosis
e. artery
e. brain hematoma
e. compartment
e. defect
e. hemorrhage
e. space
e. tumor
e. vertebral plexus
e. vertebral plexus of vein
extraembryonic mesoderm
extrafascial hysterectomy
extrafollicular blast
extragonadal seminoma
extrahepatic
e. bile duct
e. bile duct carcinoma
e. biliary atresia (EBA)
e. biliary cystic dilatation
e. binary obstruction
e. cholangiectasis
e. cholangiocarcinoma
e. lesion
e. metastasis (EHM)
e. portal hypertension
e. portal vein tributary
e. primary malignant tumor
e. stone
extraintestinal
extralobar sequestration
extralobular
e. connective tissue
e. stroma
e. terminal duct
extraluminal
e. air
e. contrast medium
e. endarterectomy
e. gas
e. hemorrhage

E

NOTES

extramammary Paget disease
extramedullary
e. hemangioma
e. involvement
e. leukemic plasmacytoma
e. tumor
extraneous material
extranodal
e. follicular lymphoma
e. proliferation
e. site
e. tumor extension
extraoctave fracture
extraocular
e. muscle
e. muscle enlargement
extraosseous
e. Ewing sarcoma
e. osteosarcoma
extraovarian mass
extraparenchymal cyst
extrapelvic malignancy
extrapericardial dissection
extraperitoneal
e. bladder rupture
e. fascia
e. fat
e. organ
extrapleural
e. drainage
e. hemorrhage
e. pneumothorax
e. space
extrapolation
half-scan with e. (HE)
extrapontine myelinolysis
extrapulmonary
e. bronchus
e. sequestration
e. small cell cancer
e. tuberculosis
extrapyramidal
e. reaction
e. system
e. tract
e. tract sign
extrarenal renal pelvis
extrascleral extension
extraskeletal
e. chondroma
e. mesenchymal chondrosarcoma
e. osteosarcoma
extrasphincteric anal fistula
extra-stiff guide wire
extrasynovial
extratesticular
e. lesion
e. tumor
extrathecal nerve root
extrathoracic
e. metastasis
e. obstruction
extrauterine
e. gestation
e. pelvic mass
e. pregnancy
extravaginal testicular torsion
extravasated
e. blood
e. contrast
extravasation
bile e.
blood e.
contrast e.
dye e.
fluid e.
intravascular content e.
joint fluid e.
e. of radiopaque fluid
radiopaque fluid e.
renal transplant urine e.
secondary e.
spontaneous urinary e.
urinary e.
extravascular
e. compartment
e. fluid
e. granuloma
e. mass
e. pressure
extraventricular
e. obstructive hydrocephalus
extravesical
e. infrasphincteric ectopic ureter
e. opacification
extravital ultraviolet
extremely
e. low frequency (ELF)
e. low-frequency field
extreme micromelia
extremity
e. gigantism
e. hemangioma
left lower e. (LLE)
lower e. (LE)
e. malformation
e. MRI (E-MRI)
e. osteosarcoma
e. rhabdomyosarcoma
upper e. (UE)
extrinsic
e. allergic alveolitis
e. bladder compression
e. cellular parameter
e. esophageal impression
e. field uniformity

e. filling defect
e. foot muscle
e. impression of the esophagus
e. lesion
e. ligament
e. malignant obstruction
e. sick sinus syndrome
e. sphincter
e. stomach impression
e. ureteral defect

extrude

extruded
e. disk
e. disk fragment

extrusion
disk e.

extubate

extubation

exuberant
e. atheroma formation
e. callus
e. granulation tissue
e. synovium

exudative
e. bronchiolitis
e. consolidation
e. pleural effusion
e. pleurisy
e. stage
e. tuberculosis

ex vivo magnetic resonance imaging

eye
conus e.
e. exposure limit
fetal e.
intraconal portion of the e.
e. myositis
raccoon e.
e. trauma

eye-ear plane

eyelet
rod e.

eye-view
e.-v. 3D conformal radiation therapy
c.-v. 3D-CRT radiation thcrapy

E-Z CAT Dry

E-Z-EM cut biopsy needle

E-Z-Paque barium suspension

NOTES

E

F
female
fluorine
F point of cardiac apex
F18
fludeoxyglucose F.
^{18}F
^{18}F 2-deoxyglucose uptake
^{18}F estradiol
^{18}F estradiol imaging agent
^{18}F fludeoxyglucose imaging agent
^{18}F fluorodeoxyglucose
^{18}F fluorodeoxyglucose imaging agent
^{18}F fluoro-DOPA
^{18}F fluoro-DOPA imaging agent
^{18}F fluoroisonidazole imaging agent
^{18}F fluorotamoxifen
^{18}F fluorotamoxifen imaging agent
^{18}F L-DOPA imaging agent
^{18}F N-methylspiperone
^{18}F N-methylspiperone imaging agent
^{18}F spiperone
^{18}F spiperone imaging agent
^{18}F uptake
f
farad
frequency
F-1200 fluorescence spectrophotometer
F-2000 fluorescence spectrophotometer
F-4500 fluorescence spectrophotometer
Fab
^{131}I-labeled monoclonal F.
fabella
os f.
fabellofibular
f. complex
f. ligament
Fabricius
bursa of F.
Fabry disease
face presentation
facet, facette
f. arthropathy
articular f.
atlas f.
bilateral locked f.'s
capitate f.
f. capsule
f. capsule disruption
f. cartilage
clavicular f.
corneal f.
costal f.
f. dislocation
flat f.
f. fusion
hamate f.
inferior medial f.
f. joint
f. joint arthritis
f. joint injection
f. joint vacuum
jumped f.
Lenoir f.
locked f.
lunate f.
occlusal f.
scaphoid f.
squatting f.
superior articular f.
superior costal f.
f. surface of vertebra
f. syndrome
transverse costal f.
f. tropism
facetal imbrication
facetectomy
faceted gallstone
facette (*var. of* facet)
facial
f. abnormality
f. artery
f. asymmetry
f. bipartition
f. bone
f. cleft
f. colliculus
f. eminence
f. fracture
f. hemangioma
f. nerve
f. nerve anatomy
f. nerve canal
f. nerve paralysis
f. plexus
f. root
f. schwannoma
f. thickening
f. triangle
f. vein
faciale
facialis
facies ossea
facile synthesis
Facility
National Biomedical Tracer F. (NBTF)
facioauriculovertebral syndrome

faciostenosis
FACNM
Fellow of the American College of Nuclear Medicine
FACNP
Fellow of the American College of Nuclear Physicians
FACR
Fellow of the American College of Radiologists
FACScan
fluorescence-activated cell sorter
FACScan flow cytometer
FACSVantage cell sorter
FACT
focused appendix computed tomography
factitious regurgitation
factor
accelerator f.
activation f.
anisotropy f.
automotility f.
blocking f.
breast cancer risk f.
contrast-improvement f.
decay-activating f.
diffusion f.
enhancement f.
environmental f.
equilibrium f.
filling f.
Fletcher f.
gamma f.
geometry f.
growth f.
Hageman f. (HF)
inciting f.
incremental risk f.
kerma-to-dose conversion f.
magnification f. (MF)
Mayneord F f.
net magnetization f.
off-axis f. (OAF)
overrelaxation f.
peak scatter f.
protection f.
quality f. (QF)
radiation weighting f.
relative conversion f.
releasing f.
scatter degradation f.
screen-intensifying f. (IF)
therapeutic gain f. (TGF)
tissue inhomogeneity f.
tissue weighting f.
wedge f.
factorial design
Fahr-Volhard disease
failed
f. back surgery syndrome (FBSS)
f. back syndrome (FBS)
f. pregnancy
f. valve
failing
f. ovary syndrome
f. pregnancy
failure
acute heart f.
acute renal f. (ARF)
acute respiratory f. (ARF)
adrenal f.
backward heart f.
brittle bone f.
cardiac f.
chronic heart f.
chronic renal f.
circulation f.
compensated congestive heart f.
congestive heart f. (CHF)
contrast-induced renal f.
decompensated congestive heart f.
diastolic heart f.
end-stage renal f. (ESRF)
fetal heart f.
forward heart f.
frank congestive f.
fulminant hepatic f. (FHF)
functional classification of congestive heart f.
graft f.
heart f. (HF)
heart power f.
hepatic f.
high-output circulatory f.
high-output heart f.
intractable heart f.
intrauterine cardiac f.
intrauterine heart f.
irreversible organ f.
kidney f.
left-sided heart f.
left ventricular f.
liver f.
low-output heart f.
Mamm-Aire heart f.
multiple organ f.
neonatal cardiac f.
neonatal heart f.
ovulatory f.
passive congestive f.
pituitary f.
posttransplant acute renal f.
prerenal f.
pulmonary f.
refractory congestive heart f.
renal f.

respiratory f.
right-sided heart f.
right ventricular f.
systolic heart f.
time to distant f. (TTDF)
time to local f. (TTLF)
time-to-treatment f.
TIPS f.
ventilatory f.
ventricular f.

failure-free survival (FFS)
Fairbank disease
Fairbanks changes
Fajersztajn crossed sciatic sign
falces (*pl. of* falx)
falciform
f. cartilage
f. crest
f. fold
f. ligament
f. ligament sign
f. process
falcine meningioma
falcotentorial meningioma
falcula
falcular
fallen lung sign
fallopian
f. canal
f. ligament
f. pregnancy
f. tube
f. tube carcinoma
f. tube diverticulum
f. tube mass
f. tube occlusion
falloposcopy
Fallot
F. disease
pentalogy of F.
F. syndrome
F. tetrad
tetralogy of F. (TOF)
trilogy of F.
fallout
signal f.
false
f. aneurysm
f. aneurysmal chamber
f. ankylosis
f. bundle-branch block
f. channel
f. colonic obstruction
f. color scale
f. cord carcinoma
f. diverticulum
f. emphysema
f. frequency
f. hypoechogenicity
f. knot
f. localizing sign
f. lumen
f. negative ratio
f. pelvis
f. positive ratio
f. pregnancy
f. rib
f. sac
f. splenic cyst
f. steal
f. vertebra
f. vocal cord
false-negative
f.-n. correlation
f.-n. result
false-positive result
falx, pl. **falces**
f. artery
f. calcification
f. cerebelli
f. cerebri
fenestration of f.
f. fenestration
increased density of f.
f. increased density
familial
f. adenomatous polyposis (FAP)
f. adenomatous polyposis syndrome
f. amyotrophic lateral sclerosis
f. aortic dissection
f. arterial fibromuscular dysplasia
f. atresia
f. avascular necrosis of phalangeal epiphysis
f. cardiomegaly
f. cavernous malformation
f. cerebral ferrocalcinosis
f. chondrocalcinosis
f. colorectal polyposis
f. dysautonomia
f. dysplastic nevus syndrome
f. fibromuscular dysplasia of artery
f. gastrointestinal polyposis
f. goiter

NOTES

familial *(continued)*
f. heart block
f. hypertrophic cardiomyopathy (FHC)
f. hypertrophy (FHC)
f. hypophosphatemic rickets
f. idiopathic acroosteolysis
f. intestinal polyposis
f. intestinal pseudoobstruction
f. juvenile polyposis
f. multiple polyposis
f. myxoma
f. onychoosteodysplasia
f. polyposis syndrome
f. ulcerative colitis
f. varicose vein
fan
f. angle
f. beam
f. sign
fan-beam
f.-b. collimator
f.-b. formula
f.-b. projection
f.-b. reconstruction
Fanconi-Hegglin syndrome
fan-shaped
f.-s. mesentery
f.-s. view
FAP
familial adenomatous polyposis
farad (f)
Faraday
F. cage
F. law
F. shield
F. shielded resonator
Farber
F. disease
F. syndrome
far field
farmer's lung
Fartland supracondylar fracture classification
fascia, pl. **fasciae, fascias**
anal f.
antebrachial f.
anterior rectus f.
axillary f.
bicipital f.
brachial f.
f. of breast
broad f.
buccopharyngeal f.
Buck f.
Camper f.
cervical f.
clavipectoral f.
Cloquet f.
Colles f.
cremasteric f.
cribriform f.
crural f.
Cruveilhier f.
deep f.
deltoid f.
Denonvilliers f.
dentate f.
diaphragmatic f.
endopelvic f.
endothoracic f.
extraperitoneal f.
Gerota f.
iliac f.
infraspinous f.
investing f.
f. lata
lateral conal f.
lateral oblique f.
lateroconal f.
lumbar f.
medial geniculate f.
obturator internus f.
palmar f.
parietal pelvic f.
pelvic f.
perineal f.
pharyngobasilar f.
prepectoral f.
prevertebral f.
psoas f.
quadratus femoris f.
rectal f.
renal f.
retromammary f.
rim of f.
f. of Scarpa
Scarpa f.
Sibson f.
spigelian f.
subcutaneous f.
superficial temporalis f.
superficial temporoparietal f.
supraanal f.
thoracolumbar f.
transversalis f.
umbilicovesical f.
vesical f.
visceral pelvic f.
Waldeyer f.
Zuckerkandl f.
fascial
f. band
f. envelope
f. incisor
f. margin necrosis

f. plane
f. rent
f. sheath
f. stranding
f. tract

fascicle
synovium-lined f.
tibioligamentous f.
triquetroscaphoid f.
triquetrotrapezoid f.

fascicular
f. block
f. bundle
f. sarcoma

fasciculata
zona f.

fasciculation
tongue f.

fasciculus, pl. **fasciculi**
arcuate f. (AF)
Gowers f.
lenticular f.
longitudinal f.
longitudinalis medialis f.
mamillothalamic f.
medial longitudinal f. (MLF)
occipitofrontal f.
superior longitudinal f.
superior occipitofrontal f.

fasciitis
fulminant f.
necrotizing f.
f. ossificans
palmar f.
f. panniculitis
f. panniculitis syndrome
plantar f.
pseudosarcomatous f.
scrotal f.

fasciogram

fasciolar gyrus

fasiculoventricular bypass tract

FAST
FAST balloon catheter
contrast-enhanced FAST
FAST pulse sequence
reduced-acquisition matrix FAST
RF-spoiled FAST
T1-weighted FAST

fast
f. acquisition multiple excitation
f. adiabatic trajectory in steady state (FATS)
f. cardiac phase contrast cine imaging
f. dynamic volumetric x-ray CT
f. exchange-cellular suspension
f. exchange-soft tissue
f. Fourier imaging
f. Fourier spectral analysis
f. Fourier transform (FFT)
f. Fourier transformation
f. Fourier transform (FFT) image
f. fractionation
f. gradient-echo (GE) sequence
f. imaging with steady-state free precession (FISP)
f. low-angle shot (FLASH)
f. multiplanar inversion recovry (FMPIR) imaging
f. multiplanar spoiled gradient-recalled imaging (FMPSPGR imaging)
f. neutron
f. neutron radiation therapy
f. PC cine MR sequence with echoplanar gradient
f. routine production
f. scan magnetic resonance imaging
f. short tau inversion recovery
f. spin echo (FSE)
f. spin echo (FSE)
f. spin echo MR imaging
f. spin echo (SE) and fast inversion recovery (IR) imaging
f. spin-echo (SE) train
f. spin echo T2-weighted image
f. spoiled gradient-recalled MR imaging
f. STIR

fast-array processor

fast-breeder reactor

Fastcard

fast-field
f.-f. echo (FFE)
f.-f. echoes

fast-FLAIR technique

fast-flow
f.-f. lesion
f.-f. malformation
f.-f. vascular anomaly

fastigiobulbar tract

fast-neutron radiation therapy

NOTES

F

fast-scan magnetic resonance
fat
abdominal f.
anterior epidural f.
bony glenoid marrow f.
f. breast necrosis
f. density
digital process of f.
dirty f.
f. embolism syndrome (FES)
f. embolus
extraperitoneal f.
f. heart-pad sign
herniated preperitoneal f.
f. herniation
intraabdominal f.
ischiorectal pad of f.
f. island
lipid content of storage f.
f. lobule
f. lung herniation
mediastinal f.
mesocolonic f.
f. metabolism
microvesicular f.
f. pad
f. pad impingement syndrome
peribursal f.
pericolonic f.
perigastric f.
perihilar f.
perinephric f.
perineural f.
perirectal f.
perirenal f.
phagocytized f.
f. plane
posterior epidural f.
preperitoneal f.
prerenal f.
properitoneal f.
protruding f.
radiolucent f.
renal sinus f.
retromammary f.
f. signal intensity
subcutaneous f.
f. suppression
f. suppression pulse
tumoral f.
ventral epidural f.
fatal dose of radiation
fat-containing
f.-c. breast lesion
f.-c. mass
fat-density
f.-d. area
f.-d. line
fat-fluid
f.-f. density interface
f.-f. level
fatigue
f. damage
f. fracture
fat-pad sign
FATS
fast adiabatic trajectory in steady state
fat-selective presaturation
fat-spared
f.-s. area in fatty liver
f.-s. area in pancreas
fat-suppressed
f.-s. body coil
f.-s. gadolinium-enhanced imaging
f.-s. spin echo
f.-s. three-dimensional spoiled gradient-echo FLASH MR imaging
f.-s. T2-weighted fast spin-echo sequence
f.-s. T2-weighted FSE technique
fatty
f. acid metabolism
f. cirrhosis
f. degeneration
f. filum
f. filum terminale
f. halo
f. heart
f. infiltrate
f. intima streak
f. kidney
f. liver
f. marrow
f. marrow endplate conversion
f. meal
f. meal sonogram (FMS)
f. meal sonography (FMS sonography)
f. mesentery
f. necrosis
f. plaque
f. prostatic tissue
f. renal capsule
f. soft tissue tumor
f. streak atherosclerosis
fat-water
f.-w. interface
f.-w. out of phase
f.-w. signal cancellation
fat/water
f. chemical shift imaging
f. signal separation
fauces
anterior pillar of f.
arch of f.

faucial pillar
fault
sagittal plane f.
faulty
f. preparation
f. radiofrequency shielding
f. radiofrequency shielding artifact
f. union
faveolate
Favre disease
fawn-tail sign
FB
foreign body
FBM
fetal breathing movement
FBP
filtered back-projection
FBP method
FBS
failed back syndrome
FBSS
failed back surgery syndrome
FC
flow compensation
FCR
flexor carpi radialis
FCR 9501HQ high-resolution storage phosphor imaging agent
FCR muscle
FCS
FCS series
FCS view
FDA
Food and Drug Administration
FDG
fluorine-18-fluorodeoxyglucose
fluorodeoxyglucose
18-fluorodeoxyglucose
FDG myocardial imaging
FDG positron emission tomography
FDG SPECT
FDG uptake
FDG-blood flow mismatch
FDG-labeled positron imaging
^{18}FDG PET scan
FDI
first digital interosseous
frequency domain imaging
FDI muscle
FDI ultrasound
FDL
flexor digitorum longus
FDL muscle
FDP
flexor digitorum profundus
FDP muscle
^{18}FDP PET
FDQB
flexor digiti quinti brevis
FDQB muscle
FDS
flexor digitorum superficialis
FDS muscle
^{52}Fe
iron-52
^{55}Fe
iron-55
^{59}Fe
iron-59
feathery appearance
feature
clinical f.
differential diagnostic lung mass f.
geriatric f.'s
mammographic f.
mongoloid f.'s
proctographic f.'s
febrile granulocytopenia
fecal
f. concretion
f. diversion colostomy
f. fistula
f. impaction
f. incontinence
f. material
f. obstruction
f. residue
f. stone
f. tumor
fecal-filled colon
fecalith
fecaloid
fecaloma
fecaluria
feces
impacted f.
inspissated f.
semiliquid f.
feculence
feculent
Federici sign

F

NOTES

feedback
breathing f.
real-time respiratory f.
feeder
f. artery
f. vein
feeding
f. artery of aneurysm
f. branch
f. branch of artery
f. mean arterial pressure (FMAP)
f. vessel
feeding-vessel sign
FEER
field-echo sequence with even-echo rephasing
feet (*pl. of* foot)
Fe-Ex orogastric tube magnet
Feigenbaum echocardiography
feign tumor
Feiss line
Feist-Mankin position
Feldaker syndrome
Feldkamp algorithm
Fellow
F. of the American College of Nuclear Medicine (FACNM)
F. of the American College of Nuclear Physicians (FACNP)
F. of the American College of Radiologists (FACR)
F. of the Faculty of Radiologists (FFR)
Felson
silhouette sign of F.
Felty syndrome
female (F)
f. genital tract calcification
f. genital tract rhabdomyosarcoma
intersex f.
f. pelvis
f. pseudohermaphroditism
f. urethra
feminine aorta
feminization
testicular f.
feminizing
f. adrenal tumor
f. testes syndrome
femora (*pl. of* femur)
femoral
f. antetorsion
f. anteversion
f. artery
f. artery approach
f. articulation
f. bone
f. capital epiphysis
f. condylar shaving
f. condyle
f. cortex
f. fossa
f. head
f. head amputation
f. head deformity
f. head epiphyseolysis
f. head vascularity
f. hernia
f. intertrochanteric fracture
f. ligament
f. medullary canal
f. neck
f. neck fracture
f. nerve
f. ossification center
f. physeal scar
f. plate
f. plexus
f. retrotorsion
f. retroversion
f. ring
f. runoff angiography
f. runoff arteriography
self-articulating f. (SAF)
f. septum
f. shaft
f. shaft axis
f. shaft fracture
f. sheath
slipped capital f.
f. supracondylar fracture
f. torsion V angle
f. triangle
f. triangular content
f. tuberosity
f. vein
f. vein percutaneous insertion
f. venous approach
f. view
femorale
calcar f.
femoris
biceps f.
quadratus f.
quadriceps f.
rectus f.
tensor fasciae f.
femorocerebral catheter angiography
femorocrural graft
femorodistal popliteal bypass graft
femorofemoral
f. bypass graft
f. crossover
femorofemoropopliteal
femoropatellar joint

femoroperoneal in situ vein bypass graft
femoropopliteal
f. artery
f. atheromatous stenosis
f. bypass graft
f. Gore-Tex graft
f. outflow system
f. thrombosis
f. vessel
femorotibial
f. angle (FTA)
f. bypass graft
femtoliter (fL)
femur, pl. **femora**
apex of f.
body of f.
distal f.
greater trochanter of f.
head of f.
isthmus of f.
f. length (FL)
f. length to abdominal circumference (FL/AC, FL/AC ratio)
lesser trochanter of f.
neck of f.
nutrient artery of f.
proximal f.
fencer's bone
fender fracture
fenestra, pl. **fenestrae**
fenestral otosclerosis
fenestrated
f. compression plate
f. sheath
f. tube
fenestration
aortopulmonary f.
apical f.
balloon catheter f.
catheter-directed f.
cusp f.
f. of dissecting aneurysm
falx f.
f. of falx
interchordal space f.
fenoldopam mesylate
fenoprofen calcium
fentanyl
Fenwick disease
Fe_3O_4
magnetite
Ferguson
F. angle
F. view
Fergusson method for measuring scoliosis
Feridex
F. MRI contrast agent
fermium (Fm)
fermium-255 (^{255}Fm)
ferpentetate
technetium-99m f.
Ferrein
F. canal
F. foramen
F. ligament
ferric
f. ammonium citrate-cellulose paste
f. chloride contrast
ferrioxamine methanesulfonate contrast
ferrite
ferritin-labeled yttrium
ferrocalcinosis
familial cerebral f.
ferromagnetic
f. artifact
f. material
f. microembolization
f. microembolization treatment
f. microsphere
f. relaxation
ferrous citrate
ferruginous body
Fertinex
ferumoxides-enhanced MR imaging
ferumoxsil imaging agent
FES
fat embolism syndrome
flame emission spectroscopy
fetal
f. abdominal circumference
f. abdominal cystic mass
f. abdominal wall
f. abdominal wall defect
f. abnormality
f. adenoma
f. age
f. amputation
f. aortic flow volume
f. ascites
f. asphyxia

NOTES

fetal *(continued)*
f. biophysical profile score
f. bowel obstruction
f. BPS
f. bradycardia
f. breathing movement (FBM)
f. cardiac anomaly
f. cardiosplenic syndrome
f. chest anomaly
f. circulation
f. CNS anomaly
f. cystic adenomatoid malformation
f. cystic fibrosis
f. death
f. death in utero
f. dystocia
f. echocardiographic view
f. echocardiography
f. echocardiography in utero
f. ectopia cordis
f. epiphyseal bone center
f. eye
f. femoral length
f. foot length measurement
f. fracture
f. gallbladder
f. gastrointestinal anomaly
f. goiter
f. growth acceleration
f. growth retardation
f. hand malformation
f. head circumference
f. heart
f. heart anomaly
f. heart failure
f. hydrops
f. hypomineralization
f. intraabdominal calcification
f. kidney lobation
f. liver biopsy
f. lobe
f. lobulation
f. long bone measurement
f. lung hypoplasia
f. lymphoid tissue
f. mensuration
f. mesenchymal tumor
f. mesenchymal tumor of kidney
f. midface
f. movement (FM)
f. musculoskeletal dysplasia
f. musculoskeletal system
f. neck anomaly
f. neck pseudomembrane
f. period
f. placenta
f. pleura effusion
f. pole
f. pyelectasis
f. renal function
f. renal hamartoma
f. renal obstruction
f. scalp edema
f. skin biopsy
f. small parts
f. sonography
f. spine
f. stress test
f. swallowing
f. thoracic circumference
f. tone
f. ultrasonography
f. ultrasound
f. urinary tract anomaly
f. urogenital tract
f. uterus
f. ventricular heart disproportion
f. ventriculomegaly
f. weight

fetalis
chondrodystrophia f.
hydrops f., fetal hydrops
nonimmune hydrops f.

fetal-pelvic
f.-p. disproportion
f.-p. index

feticide

fetography

fetoliter

fetometry

fetus
amorphous f.
calcified f.
cephalic presentation of f.
demise of f.
disappearing f.
growth-retarded f.
hypomineralization in f.
impacted f.
intrauterine f.
malpositioned f.
maturity of f.
multiple f.'s
nonviable f.
paper-doll f.
papyraceus f.
f. papyraceus
parasitic f.
placenta of f.
postterm f.
previable f.
retained dead f.
skeletal dysplasia in f.
small-for-gestational-age f.
small parts of f.
stunted f.

syndactyly in f.
tissue of f.
trisomic f.
viable f.

fever
fracture f.
Mediterranean f.
polymer fume f.
rheumatic f.
San Joaquin Valley f., San Joaquin fever

FF
filtration fraction

FFA
free fatty acid

FFD
focal film distance

FFE
fast-field echo

FFR
Fellow of the Faculty of Radiologists

FFS
failure-free survival

FFT
fast Fourier transform

FHB
flexor hallucis brevis
FHB muscle

FHC
familial hypertrophic cardiomyopathy
familial hypertrophy

FHF
fulminant hepatic failure

FI
full scan with interpolation
FI method
FI projection

fiber
annular f.
asbestos f.'s
association f.
atrio-His f.
bundle of Kent accessory bypass f.
cardiac muscle f.
cerebellar f.
differencing f.
long f.'s
Mahaim and James f.'s
Müller f.'s
muscle f.
myocardial f.
myoclonus epilepsy associated with ragged red f.'s (MERRF)
nodoventricular bypass f.
onionskin configuration of collagenous f.
parasympathetic f.'s
pontocerebellar f.
postganglionic gray f.'s
postganglionic sympathetic f.'s
precharred f.
Purkinje f.'s
Sharpey f.'s
skeletal muscle f.
sling muscle f.
U f.
unmyelinated nerve f.

fiber-bundle striation

fiberglass pneumoconiosis

fiberoptic
f. bronchogram
f. bundle
f. conductor
f. light source
f. taper
f. video glasses

fiber-shortening velocity

fiber-type disproportion

Fibonacci search scheme

fibril
collagen f.

fibrillary

fibrillation
atrial f.

fibrin
f. calculus
f. mass
f. platelet embolus
f. sleeve stripping

fibrinogen
f. degradation
iodinated I-125 f.
labeled f.
radiolabeled f.
technetium labeled f.

fibrinoid necrosis

fibrinolytic treatment

fibrinopurulent pleurisy

fibrinous
f. degeneration
f. inflammation
f. pleurisy

NOTES

F

fibrinous *(continued)*
f. pneumonia
f. polyp
fibrin-split product
fibroadenolipoma
breast f.
fibroadenoma
f. of breast
breast f.
calcified f.
cellular f.
degenerated f.
esophageal f.
giant breast f.
hyalinized breast f.
involuting f.
juvenile f.
fibroadenomatosis
breast f.
fibroadipose tissue
fibroareolar tissue
fibroblastic
f. meningioma
f. osteosarcoma
fibroblastoma
perineural f.
fibroblast radiosensitivity
fibrocalcific
f. cusp
f. residual
fibrocalcification
fibrocartilage
avascular f.
circumferential f.
f. complex
intraarticular plate of f.
labral f.
triangular f. (TFC)
fibrocartilaginous
f. disk
f. labrum
f. meniscus
f. nodule
f. overgrowth
f. pad
f. ridge
f. ring
f. scar
f. tissue
f. volar plate
fibrocaseous
fibrochondrogenesis
fibrocollagenous connective tissue
fibrocongestive splenomegaly
fibrocystic
f. breast
f. breast disease
f. breast syndrome
f. change
f. lung disease
f. residual
fibrodysplasia ossificans progressiva
fibroelastic
f. band
f. cartilage
fibroelastoma
f. of heart valve
papillary f.
fibroelastosis
endocardial f.
fibroepithelial
f. papilloma
f. polyp collecting system
f. urethral polyp
fibroepithelioma
urinary tract f.
fibrofatty
f. breast tissue
f. layer
f. plaque
fibrogenesis imperfecta ossium
fibroglandular
f. density
f. element
f. tissue
fibrohistiocytic lesion
fibrohistiocytoma
fibrohistiocytosis
fibroid
f. adenoma
calcified f.
f. degeneration
exophytic f.
f. heart
intramural f.
f. lung
f. myocarditis
pedunculated uterine f.
f. polyp
submucosal f.
subserosal f.
f. tumor
uterine f.
f. uterus
fibrointimal hyperplasia
fibrolamellar
f. hepatocarcinoma
f. hepatocellular carcinoma
fibroleiomyoma, pl. **fibroleiomyomata**
fibrolipoma
filum terminale f.
neural f.
fibrolipomatosis
pelvic f.
renal pelvic f.

fibrolipomatous
f. hamartoma nerve
f. nerve hamartoma
fibroma
ameloblastic f.
aponeurotic f.
benign pleural f.
cardiac f.
cementifying f.
cementoossifying f.
central cementifying f.
central ossifying f.
chondromyxoid f. (CMF)
concentric f.
giant cell f.
f. of heart
heart f.
irritation f.
juvenile aponeurotic f.
juvenile ossifying f.
meningeal f.
f. molle
f. molle gravidarum
f. molluscum
f. myxomatodes
nonossifying f.
nonosteogenic f.
ossifying bone f.
ossifying skull f
osteogenic bone f.
ovarian f.
periosteal f.
peripheral ossifying f.
periungual f.
polypoid f.
psammomatoid ossifying f.
recurrent digital f.
scrotal f.
senile f.
Shope f.
sinonasal psammomatoid ossifying f.
soft tissue f.
subcutaneous f.
telangiectatic f.
ungual f.
fibroma-thecoma tumor of ovary
fibromatoid
fibromatosis
abdominal f.
aggressive infantile f.
f. colli
congenital diffuse f.
congenital generalized f.
infantile digital f.
juvenile f.
multicentric f.
multiple congenital f.
musculoaponeurotic f.
palmar f.
penile f.
plantar f.
fibromatous
fibromuscular
f. band
f. dysplasia
f. lesion
f. pelvic floor
f. ridge
f. subaortic stenosis
f. tissue
fibromyoma, pl. **fibromyomata**
fibromyositis
fibromyxoma
kidney f.
odontogenic f.
f. pleura
pleural f.
fibronodular
f. infiltrate
fibroosseous
f. attachment
f. lesion
f. pseudotumor of digit
f. tunnel
fibroosteoma of the tooth
fibroplasia
adventitial f.
endomyocardial f.
intimal f.
medial f.
perimedial f.
retrolental f.
fibroplastic
f. process
f. proliferation
fibroproductive tuberculosis
fibroretractive
fibrosa
hepatica f.
osteitis f.
fibrosarcoma
ameloblastic f.
bone f.

NOTES

F

fibrosarcoma *(continued)*
cardiac f.
central f.
congenital kidney f.
epididymal f.
infantile f.
inflammatory f.
periosteal f.
f. variant
fibrosclerotic
fibrosed muscle
fibroserous pericardial sac
fibrosing
f. alveolitis
f. arachnoiditis
f. colonopathy
f. cryptogenic alveolitis
f. inflammation
f. inflammatory pseudotumor
f. mediastinitis
f. mesenteritis
f. mesothelioma
f. piecemeal necrosis
f. tissue
fibrosis
acute diffuse interstitial f.
alcoholic f.
annular f.
arachnoid f.
asbestos-induced pleural f.
basilar f.
benign meningeal f.
bone marrow f.
breast f.
confluent f.
congenital hepatic f. (CHF)
congenital liver f.
cystic f.
Davies endocardial f.
Davies endomyocardial f.
diffuse interstitial pulmonary f. (DIPF)
endocardial f.
endomyocardial f. (EMF)
epidural f.
fetal cystic f.
focal f.
hepatic f.
horseshoe f.
hyalinized fibroadenoma with f.
idiopathic interstitial f.
idiopathic pulmonary f. (IPF)
interstitial diffuse pulmonary f.
interstitial prematurity f.
interstitial pulmonary f. (IPF)
intraalveolar f.
intralobular f.
leptomeningeal f.
f. of lung
mediastinal f.
meningeal f.
mural endomyocardial f.
nodal f.
nodular subepidermal f.
noncirrhotic portal f. (NCPF)
nonnodular f.
pancreatic cystic f.
perialveolar f.
periaortic f.
peribronchial f.
pericentral f.
periductal f.
peridural f.
perihilar f.
perimuscular f.
perineural f.
periportal f.
periureteral f.
perivascular f.
pipestem f.
portal f.
portal-to-portal f.
postinflammatory pulmonary f.
postradiation f.
posttraumatic f.
primary retroperitoneal f.
progressive interstitial pulmonary f.
progressive massive f.
progressive nodular pulmonary f.
progressive perivenular alcoholic f. (PPAF)
pulmonary idiopathic f.
pulmonary interstitial idiopathic f.
pulmonary vein f.
radiation-induced f. (RIF)
replacement f.
retroperitoneal f. (RPF)
secondary retroperitoneal f.
subadventitial f.
subintimal f.
subserosal f.
Symmers f.
transmural f.
fibrosum
adenoma f.
molluscum f.
pericardium f.
fibrosus
annulus f.
lacertus f.
fibrothorax
fibrotic
f. cavitating pattern
f. change
f. honeycombing
f. island

f. kidney
f. plaque
f. residual
f. scarring
f. tissue

fibrous
f. ankylosis
f. attachment
f. band
f. bar
f. bone lesion
f. cap
f. cartilage
f. coalition
f. connective tissue
f. connective tissue tumor
f. cord
f. cortical defect
f. dysplasia
f. dysplasia ossificans progressiva
f. GI tract polypoid lesion
f. goiter
f. hamartoma
f. histiocytoma
f. intima plaque
f. mastitis
f. medullary defect
f. meningioma
f. metaphyseal-diaphyseal defect
f. nodular pattern
f. nodule
f. nonunion
f. obliterative cholangitis
f. osteoma
f. pericardium
f. plaque atherosclerosis
f. pleural adhesion
f. pneumonia
f. polypoid lesion
f. renal capsule
f. ring
f. ring of disk
f. scar tissue
f. septum
f. sheath
f. skeleton
f. temporal bone dysplasia
f. tissue hyperplasia
f. trigone
f. tubercle
f. tumor pleura
f. union
f. urinary tract polyp
f. web

fibrovascular
f. core
f. polyp
f. stalk
f. tissue

fibroxanthoma
malignant f.
multiple f.'s
pediatric f.

fibroxanthosarcoma

fibula, gen. and pl. **fibulae**
apex of f.
capitulum fibulae
malleolus fibulae
nutrient artery of f.
proximal f.

fibular
f. articular surface
f. collateral ligament
f. fracture
f. lymph node
f. notch
f. physis
f. sesamoid bone
f. vein

fibulocalcaneal space

fibulotalar ligament

fibulotalocalcaneal (FTC)
f. ligament

Ficat
F. avascular necrosis staging
F. stage of avascular necrosis

Ficat-Marcus grading system

Fick
F. cardiac index
F. equation
F. law
F. method
F. method for cardiac output
F. position
F. principle

Ficoll gradient

FID
free-induction decay

fiducial
f. alignment system
f. movement

field
f. alignment
blocked vertex f.

NOTES

field *(continued)*
Brodmann cytoarchitectonic f.
f. cancerization
collapsed lung f.
f. defect
dipole f.
disk-to-magnetic f.
f. drift
f. echo
electromagnetic f.
electromagnetic (EM) f.
electron-beam boost f.
f. emission tube
extremely low-frequency f.
far f.
fringe f., fringing f.
Gibbs random f.
f. gradient
gradient magnetic f.
harmonic f.
helmet f.
high-powered f. (hpf)
insonifying wave f.
involved f.
large-hinge angle electron f.
f. lock
lower lung f.
lung f.
magnetic f.
mantle f.
Markov random f.
mid-lung f.
near f.
oscillating magnetic f.
perturbing magnetic f.
f. phenomenon
radiofrequency (RF) electromagnetic f.
rotational f.
skimming of magnetic f.
spade f.
static magnetic f.
stationary f.
stippling of lung f.
stray neutron f.
f. strength
tangential breast f.
tesla (T) f.
time-varying magnetic f.
f. uniformity
upper lung f.
f. variation
f. of view (FOV)
f. of view imaging

field-echo
f.-e. difference
f.-e. imaging
f.-e. sequence with even-echo rephasing (FEER)
f.-e. sum

field-fitting
f.-f. analysis
f.-f. technique

Fielding-Magliato
F.-M. classification of subtrochanteric fractures
F.-M. subtrochanteric fracture classification

field-of-view imaging

field-profiling coil

Fiessinger-Leroy-Reiter syndrome

Fiessinger-Leroy syndrome

fifth
f. compartment
f. cranial nerve
f. intercostal space
f. rib
f. ventricle

fighter's fracture

FIGO
F. stage carcinoma
F. staging of adenocarcinoma of endometrium

figure-3 sign

figure-of-eight
f.-o. abnormality
f.-o. cardiac configuration silhouette
f.-o. sign

filament
f. emission
f. transformer

filament-nonfilament count

file
Indian f.

filiform
f. appendix
f. polyp
f. polyposis

filigree pattern

filipuncture

filler block

filling
augmented f.
capillary f.
compensatory capillary f.
f. defect
f. defect collecting system
early venous f.
f. factor
late venous f.
passive f.
peak f.
f. pressure
rapid f. (RF)
reduced f.

retrograde f.
subintimal f.
ureteral f.
venous f.
ventricular f.
vessel f.
zero f.

fill and spill of dye

film (*See* film, projection, radiograph, scan, view, x-ray)
f. alternator
anteroposterior (AP) f.
biplane axial f.
bitewing f.
f. changer
chest f.
chiropractic f.
cine f.
comparison f.
corner f.
crosstable lateral f.
cut and cine f.
decubitus f.
delayed f.
f. density calibration
f. diameter
digital subtraction f.
f. dispenser
DuPont Cronex x-ray f.
emulsion f.
expiratory f.
flat plate f.
f. fog
gamma f.
GLP7 f.
f. graininess
grid f.
f. hangers
high-contrast f.
horizontal beam f.
kidneys, ureter, and bladder f.
Knuttsen bending f.
late f.
lateral cervical spine f.
lateral decubitus f.
latitude f.
limited f.
low-contrast f.
low-dose f.
manual subtraction f.
nitrocellulose f.
normal chest f.
oblique f.
occlusal f.
outside f.
overhead f.
overpenetrated f.
PA and lateral f.'s
panoramic x-ray f.
photo-plotter f.
plain f.
Polaroid f.
port f.
portable chest f.
posteroanterior chest f.
postevacuation f.
postvoiding f.
preliminary f.
prone f.
radiochromic f.
right or left lateral decubitus f.
scout f.
f. screen contact test
screen type f.
sequential f.'s
serial subtraction f.'s
silver halide f.
simulation f.
skull f.
f. slippage
f. speed
spot f.
stress f.
suboptimal f.
f. subtraction
subtraction f.
supine f.
survey f.
f. tube distance
UP7 f.
upright chest f.
weightbearing f.
wide-latitude f.
working f.

film-based viewing

filmless
f. catheterization laboratory
f. imaging
f. radiography

filter
bandpass f.
bird's nest f.
bowtie f.
caval f.

F

NOTES

filter *(continued)*
compensating f.
density equalization f.
differencing f.
flattening f.
Greenfield f.
helix f.
high-pass f.
inherent f.
Kalman f.
K-edge f.
low-pass f.
f. mold
nitinol f.
nitinol inferior vena cava f.
rhodium f.
sigma f.
spatial f.
temporal f.
translation-invariant f.
wall f.
wedge f.
Wiener MRI f.
Wratten 6B f.

filtered
f. back-projection (FBP)
f. back-projection method

filtering
dynamic f.
low-pass f.
phase f.

filtration
beam f.
copper f.
dynamic beat f.
f. fraction (FF)
glomerular f.
postbeat f.
supplemental beam f.

filum
fatty f.
f. terminale
f. terminale fibrolipoma

fimbriated
f. end

finding
angiographic f.
auscultatory f.
cardinal f.
characteristic f.
concomitant f.
constellation of f.'s
equivocal f.
focal lateralizing f.
lateralizing f.
no discernible f.
pathognomonic f.
roentgenographic f.
salient physical f.
scanty f.
secondary sonographic f.
specious f.
spurious f.

fine
f. calcification
f. reticular pattern

fine-needle
f.-n. aspiration
f.-n. aspiration cytology
f.-n. puncture
f.-n. transhepatic cholangiogram (FNTC)

fine-speckled appearance

finger
base of f.
baseball f.
bolster f.
bony tuft of f.
clubbed f.
Dawson f.
drop f.
football f.
f. fracture
hippocratic f.
index f.
jammed f.
jersey f.
little f.
long f.
f. lucent lesion
mallet f.
middle f.
f. opposition
overlapping f.
pedicle f.
pulley of f.
pulp of f.
replantation of f.
f. resorption of terminal tuft
ring f.
sausage f.
spade f.
speck f.
spider f.
stoved f.
tapered f.
trigger f.
f. of tumor
f. web
webbed f.

finger-in-glove
f.-i.-g. mucous plug
f.-i.-g. pattern
f.-i.-g. sign

fingerized hypoplastic thumb

fingerlike
f. mucus plug
f. mucus plugging
f. projection
f. villus
fingerprint
f. edema
f. image compression
f. pattern
fingertip
f. amputation
f. calcification
f. lesion
f. pad
f. sign
Finkelstein sign
firearm injury
firing
f. of ectopic atrial focus
f. temperature
firm
f. mass
f. neoplasm
Firooznia
threshold of F.
first
f. branchial arch
f. branchial cleft cyst
f. carpal row
f. cuneiform bone
f. diagonal branch artery
f. digital interosseous (FDI)
f. digital interosseous muscle (FDI muscle)
f. duodenal sphincter
f. major diagonal branch
f. metatarsal angle
f. metatarsal head (FMH)
f. obtuse marginal artery
f.-order chorda
f. parallel pelvic plane
f. portion of duodenum
f. ray instability
f. rib
f. septal perforator branch
f. temporal gyrus
f. trimester hemorrhage
f. ventricle of cerebrum
f. visceral cleft
first-degree
f.-d. AV block
f.-d. heart block
first-fifth intermetatarsal angle
first-order reaction
first-pass
f.-p. cardiac perfusion
f.-p. effect
f.-p. extraction
f.-p. MUGA
f.-p. myocardial perfusion imaging
f.-p. myocardial perfusion MR
f.-p. radionuclide angiography
f.-p. radionuclide exercise angiocardiography
f.-p. radionuclide ventriculogram
f.-p. study
f.-p. technique
f.-p. thallium extraction
f.-p. ventriculogram
f.-p. view
first-second intermetatarsal angle
first-set
f.-s. phenomenon
f.-s. rejection
first-trimester
f.-t. bleeding
f.-t. nuchal translucency
f.-t. placenta
Fischer
F. ring
F. sign
Fischgold
F. bimastoid line
F. biventer line
Fisher exact test
fish-flesh appearance
fishmeal worker's fresh lung
fishmouth
f. amputation
f. configuration of mitral valve
f. cusp
f. mitral stenosis
f. mitral valve configuration
f. vertebra
fishnet sign
fish-scale gallbladder
fishtail
f. tear
f. vertebra
fishtank granuloma
FISP
fast imaging with steady-state free precession
FISP pulse sequence

NOTES

Fissinger-Rendu syndrome
fission
f. product
f. track analysis
f. track analysis of urine
fissula
ante fenestram f.
fissural thickening
fissuration
fissure
abdominal f.
accessory f.
anal f.
f. of annulus
f. in ano
anterior interhemispheric f.
anterior median f.
antitragohelicine f.
auricular f.
azygos f.
brain f.
bulging lung f.
calcarine f.
callosomarginal f.
central cerebellar f.
cerebral f.
choroidal f.
chronic f.
collateral f.
cutaneous f.
decidual f.
dentate f.
displacement of interhemispheric f.
f. fracture
glaserian f.
hepatic f.
hippocampal f.
horizontal f.
incomplete pulmonary f.
inferior accessory f.
inferior orbital f.
interhemispheric f. (IHF)
interlobar f.
lateral f.
ligamentum venosum f.
liver f.
longitudinal f.
lung f.
main f.
major f.
minor f.
nasopalatal f.
oblique f.
occipital f.
oral f.
orbital f.
palpebral f.
portal f.
rolandic f.
f. of Rolando
f. sign
studded f.
superior orbital f.
supraorbital f.
sylvian f.
f. of Sylvius
transitional zone f.
umbilical f.
widened superior orbital f.
fissured atheromatous plaque
fisting
rectal f.
fistula, pl. **fistulae, fistulas**
abdominal f.
anal f.
f. in ano
anorectal f.
aorta-left ventricular f.
aorta-right ventricular f.
aortic sinus f.
aortic sinus to right ventricle f.
aortocaval f.
aortoduodenal f.
aortoenteric f.
aortoesophageal f.
aortopulmonary f.
aortosigmoid f.
arterial-arterial f.
arterial-portal f.
arteriobiliary f.
arterioportobiliary f.
arteriosinusoidal f.
arteriosinusoidal penile f.
arteriovenous f.
biliary f.
biliary-cutaneous f.
biliary-duodenal f.
biliary-enteric f.
bilioenteric f.
Blom-Singer tracheoesophageal f.
BP f.
branchial f.
Brescia-Cimino f.
bronchobiliary f.
bronchocavitary f.
bronchocutaneous f.
bronchoesophageal f.
bronchopleural f.
bronchopulmonary f.
cameral f.
caroticocavernous f.
carotid artery-cavernous sinus f.
carotid cavernous f. (CCF)
carotid-cavernous sinus f.
carotid-dural f.
cavernous sinus f.

cecocutaneous f.
cerebral arteriovenous f.
cerebrospinal fluid f.
cholecystenteric f.
cholecystocholedochal f.
cholecystocolic f.
cholecystoduodenal f.
cholecystoduodenocolic f.
choledochal-colonic f.
choledochoduodenal f.
chylous f.
coil closure of coronary artery f.
colocolic f.
colocutaneous f.
colonic f.
colovaginal f.
colovesical f.
communicating f.
complex anorectal f.
congenital pulmonary arteriovenous f.
congenital tracheobiliary f.
coronary arteriosystemic f.
coronary arteriovenous f.
coronary artery cameral f.
coronary artery-pulmonary artery f.
coronary artery to right ventricular f.
cystic f.
dialysis f.
dorsal enteric f.
duodenocolic f.
duodenopancreatic f.
dural arteriovenous f.
durocutaneous f.
Eck f.
enteric f.
enterocolic f.
enterocutaneous f.
enteroenteral f.
enterospinal f.
enterourethral f.
enterovaginal f.
enterovesical f.
esophagorespiratory f.
esophagotracheal f.
external biliary f.
extrasphincteric anal f.
fecal f.
f. formation
gastric f.
gastrocolic f.
gastrocutaneous f.
gastroduodenal f.
gastrointestinal f.
gastrojejunocolic f.
genitourinary f.
graft-enteric f.
hepatic arteriovenous f.
hepatic artery-portal vein f.
hepatopleural f.
hepatoportal biliary f.
horseshoe f.
H-type tracheoesophageal f.
hyperdynamic AV f.
ileosigmoid f.
intersphincteric anal f.
intracranial arteriovenous f.
intradural arteriovenous f.
intradural retromedullary arteriovenous f.
intrahepatic arterial-portal f.
intrahepatic AV f.
intrapulmonary arteriovenous f.
jejunocolic f.
labyrinthine f.
Mann-Bollman f.
mediastinal f.
mesenteric f.
metroperitoneal f.
microvenoarteriolar f.
mucous f.
orofacial f.
pancreatic cutaneous f.
pancreaticopleural f.
paraprosthetic-enteric f.
parietal f.
perineovaginal f.
persistent bronchopleural f.
pilonidal f.
pleural f.
pleurocutaneous f.
postbiopsy renal AV f.
premedullary arteriovenous f.
pulmonary arteriovenous f.
radial artery to cephalic vein f.
radiation f.
rectal f.
rectovaginal f.
rectovesical f.
respiratory-esophageal f.
retroperitoneal f.
spinal dural arteriovenous f.
splanchnic AV f.

NOTES

fistula *(continued)*
splenic AV f.
splenobronchial f.
suprasphincteric f.
TE f.
thoracic f.
tracheobiliary f.
tracheobronchial f.
tracheobronchoesophageal f.
tracheoesophageal f. (TEF)
f. tract study
transdural f.
transsphincteric anal f.
trigeminal cavernous f.
ureteral f.
ureterocutaneous f.
ureteroperitoneal f.
ureterovaginal f.
urethrovaginal f.
urinary f.
vaginal f.
venobiliary f.
vesical f.
vesicovaginal f.
vitelline f.
fistulogram
cine f.
venous f.
fistulography
fistulous tract
fit
smoothed curve f.
fitting
peak f.
Fitz-Hugh and Curtis syndrome
five-view
f.-v. chest x-ray
fixation
f. articulation
atlantoaxial rotary f.
catheter f.
f. disk
external f.
external wire f.
intramedullary f.
intrapedicular f.
metallic rod f.
open reduction and internal f. (ORIF)
f. of scoliosis
screw f.
spinal f.
suprasyndesmotic f.
transsyndesmotic screw f.
triangular external ankle f.
wire f.
fixator
dynamic axial f.
f. muscle
fixed
f. airway obstruction
f. coronary obstruction
f. flexion contracture
f. hammer toe
f. intracavitary filling defect
f. mass
f. perfusion defect
f. pulmonary valvular resistance
f. segment of bowel
f. shaped coplanar or nonplanar radiation beam bouquet
f. third-degree AV block
fixed-beam portal
fixed-grid stereologic method
fixed-orifice aortic stenosis
FL
femur length
fL
femtoliter
flabby heart
^{18}F-labeled
^{18}F-l. derivatives of m-tyrosine
^{18}F-l. HFA-134a
^{18}F-l. HFA-134a imaging agent
^{18}F-l. polyfluorinated ethyl
^{18}F-l. polyfluorinated ethyl imaging agent
FL/AC
femur length to abdominal circumference
FL/AC ratio
flaccid
Flack sinoatrial node
flag
Rudick red f.
flail
f. air
f. chest
f. digit
f. foot
f. joint
f. mitral valve
f. shoulder
FLAIR
fluid-attenuated inversion recovery
3D turbo FLAIR
FLAIR echoplanar imaging
FLAIR-FLASH
fluid-attenuated inversion recovery-fast low-angle shot
FLAIR-FLASH imaging
FLAK
flow artifact killer
FLAK technique

flake
f. fracture
f. fracture of hamate
flaking of cartilage
flaky calcification
flame
f. appearance
f. emission spectroscopy (FES)
f. ionization detector
flange
shaft f.
flank
f. bone
f. pain
f. stripe
f. stripe sign
flap
bone f.
bursal f.
entry f.
foramen ovale f.
intimal f.
Karapandzic f.
liver f.
lytic area bone f.
necrotic f.
osteoplastic f.
pedicle f.
pericardial f.
pleural f.
postangioplasty intimal f.
scapular f.
scimitar-shaped f.
subclavian f.
f. tear
f. valve ventricular septal defect
flaplike valve
flap-valve mechanism
flare
condylar f.
metaphyseal f.
f. phenomenon
tibial f.
trochanteric f.
flared ilium
FLASH
fast low-angle shot
FLASH 3D pulse sequence
FLASH image
FLASH magnetic resonance imaging
flashlamp-pulsed dye laser
flash photolysis
flask
vascular f.
flask-shaped
f.-s. heart
f.-s. ulcer
flat
f. bone
f. colorectal carcinoma
f. diastolic slope
f. facet
f. neck vein
f. pelvis
f. plate
f. plate of abdomen
f. plate film
f. time-intensity profile
Flatau-Schilder disease
flat-field imaging
flatfoot
calcaneovalgus f.
f. deformity
Durham f.
flat-hand test
flat-panel megavoltage imager
flattened
f. arch
f. duodenal fold
f. E-to-F slope
f. longitudinal arch of foot
flattening
cortical f.
f. filter
f. of gyrus
f. of normal lordotic curvature
f. of normal lumbar curve
flat-top
f.-t. bladder
f.-t. talus
flava (*pl. of* flavum)
flaval ligament
flavone acetic acid
flavum, pl. **flava**
ligamentum f.
pleating of ligamentum f.
flawed
f. image
f. imaging
flax dresser's disease
Flechsig
F. bundle
F. tract

F

NOTES

Fleckinger view
Fleck sign
fleecy mass
Fleet
F. bowel preparation
fleeting lung infiltrate
Fleischer disease
Fleischmann bursa
Fleischner
F. position
F. sign
F. syndrome
Fletcher
F. afterloader
F. factor
F. rule of irradiation tolerance
Fletcher-Delclos dome cylinder
Fletcher-Suit-Delclos tandem
Fletcher-Suit system for radium therapy
fleur-de-lis pattern
fleurette
flexa
coxa f.
flexible
f. biopsy needle
f. cardiac valve
f. endofluoroscopy
f. nephroscope
f. spastic equinovarus deformity
f. surface coil
f. surface-coil-type resonator (FSCR)
flexion
angle of greatest f. (AGF)
f. contracture
f. deformity
f. and extension exercises
f. and extension views
external rotation in f. (ERF)
internal rotation in f. (IRF)
f. maneuver
f. teardrop fracture
f. view
flexion-adduction contracture
flexion-burst fracture
flexion-compression fracture
flexion-distraction
f.-d. fracture
f.-d. injury
flexion-extension plane
flexion-rotation injury
flexor
f. bursa
f. canal
capital f.
f. carpi radialis (FCR)
f. carpi radialis muscle (FCR muscle)
f. carpi ulnaris
f. carpi ulnaris aponeurosis
f. digiti minimi
f. digiti minimi brevis
f. digiti quinti brevis (FDQB)
f. digiti quinti brevis muscle
f. digitorum brevis
f. digitorum longus (FDL)
f. digitorum longus muscle
f. digitorum profundus (FDP)
f. digitorum profundus muscle (FDP muscle)
f. digitorum superficialis (FDS)
f. digitorum superficialis muscle
f. hallucis brevis (FHB)
f. hallucis brevis muscle (FHB muscle)
f. hallucis longus
f. palmar plate
f. pollicis brevis
f. pollicis longus
f. retinaculum
f. tendon
f. tendon sheath
f. tenosynovitis
flexor-pronator muscle group
FlexStent
Gianturco-Roubin F.
FlexStrand cable
flexure
caudal f.
cephalic f.
cerebral f.
cervical f.
colonic f.
cranial f.
duodenojejunal f.
hepatic f.
left colonic f.
right colonic f.
sigmoid f.
splenic f.
flight
time of f. (TOF)
FlimFax teleradiology system
Flint Colon Injury Scale
flip
f. angle
spin f.
tristimulus value f.
value f.
flip-angle image
flip-flop sign
flipper hand
floating
f. arch fracture
f. cartilage
f. elbow

f. gallbladder
f. gallbladder stone
f. gallstone
f. kidney
f. knee
f. leaflet
f. ligament
f. liver
f. organ
f. osteophyte
f. patella
f. prostate
f. rib
f. spleen
f. teeth
f. thumb
f. villus

floccular fossa
flocculation of barium
flocculent focus of calcification
flocculonodular
f. lobe
f. lobe of cerebellum
f. tumor

Flocks-Kadesky system
Flood
F. ligament

flood section
floor
bladder f.
fibromuscular pelvic f.
inguinal f.
f. of mouth
f. of the orbit
pelvic f.
sellar f.
f. of ventricle

floppy
f. aortic valve
f. mitral valve
f. valve syndrome

floppy-thumb sign
Flo-Rester vessel occluder
florid
f. callus
f. cardiac tamponade
f. duct lesion
f. follicular hyperplasia
f. reactive periostitis

flottant
flow
absolute blood f.
aliased f.
altered blood f.
anatomic shunt f.
antegrade bile f.
antegrade blood f.
antegrade diastolic f.
aortic f. (AF)
f. arrest
f. artifact killer (FLAK)
autoregulation of cerebral blood f.
azygos blood f.
backward f.
bile f.
blood f.
capillary blood f.
cephalization of blood f.
cerebral blood f. (CBF)
cerebral blood volume/cerebral blood f. (CBV/CBF)
chronic reserve f.
collateral blood f.
f. compensation (FC)
compromised f.
f. of contrast material
coronary blood f.
coronary reserve f. (CRF)
f. cytometric DNA measurement
f. cytometry
f. cytometry sample preparation
f. cytometry technique
dampened pulsatile f.
2D color-coded imaging of blood f.
decreased cerebral blood f.
Doppler study of blood f.
f. effect artifact
effective pulmonary blood f. (EPBF)
electron f.
expiratory f.
fluid f.
forward f.
Ganz formula for coronary sinus f.
great cardiac vein f. (GCVF)
hepatofugal f.
hepatopetal f.
high-velocity f.
hyperemic f.
inspiratory f.
intercoronary collateral f.
intrarenal arterial f.
laminar f.

NOTES

flow *(continued)*
left-to-right f.
local bone blood f.
low-velocity f.
lung-volume loop f.
maintenance of f.
f. mapping technique
microcirculatory blood f.
midexpiratory tidal f.
mitral valve f.
mixed petal-fugal f.
f. mode ultrafast computed tomography
myocardial blood f. (MBF)
peak velocity of blood f.
peripheral blood f.
petal-fugal f.
f. phenomenon
physiologic shunt f.
plug f.
Poiseuille f.
portal f.
f. portion of bone scan
protodiastolic reversal of blood f.
pulmonary blood f. (PBF)
pulmonic output f.
pulmonic versus systemic f.
f. quantification
f. rate
f. redistribution
redistribution of pulmonary vascular f.
regional cerebral blood f. (rCBF)
regional myocardial blood f.
regurgitant pandiastolic f.
regurgitant systolic f.
relative shunt f.
resistance blood f.
resting regional myocardial blood f.
restoration of f.
retrograde systolic f.
reversed vertebral blood f. (RVBF)
sluggish f.
stasis of blood f.
f. study
supratentorial cerebral blood f.
systemic blood f. (SBF)
systemic output f.
time-averaged f.
tissue f.
total cerebral blood f. (TCBF)
f. tract
transmitral f.
tricuspid valve f.
turbulent blood f.
turbulent intraluminal f.
unequal pulmonary blood f.
uterine blood volume f.
f. velocity
f. velocity profile
f. velocity signal
f. velocity waveform
f. void
f. void pattern
f. volume
zero net f.

flow-compensated
f.-c. gradient-echo sequence
f.-c. image

flow-compromising lesion
flow-dependent obstruction
flow-encoding gradient
Flower bone
flow-induced artifact
flowing
f. anterior vertebra ossification
f. spin

FloWire Doppler ultrasound
flow-limited expiration
flow-limiting
f.-l. lesion
f.-l. stenosis

flowmeter
Parks bidirectional Doppler f.

flowmetry
blood f.
Doppler f.
laser Doppler f. (LDF)
Narcomatic f.
Parks 800 bidirectional Doppler f.
pulsed Doppler f.
Statham electromagnetic f.

flow-on gradient-echo image
flow-related
f.-r. enhancement
f.-r. enhancement artifact
f.-r. enhancement effect
f.-r. phase error

flow-sensitive MR imaging
flow-time curve
flow-void effect
flow-volume loop
Fluckiger syndrome
fluctuant mass
fluctuation
Poisson noise f.

fludeoxyglucose F18
fluence
energy f.
f. profile

fluffy
f. infiltrate
f. margins
f. periosteal reaction
f. rarefaction

fluid
abdominal collection of f.
f. accumulation
amnionic f.
anechoic f.
articular f.
ascitic f.
bloodless f.
broad band of pleural f.
bursal f.
cavitary f.
cerebrospinal f. (CSF)
f. collection
crankcase oil f.
cystic f.
dammed-up cerebrospinal f.
f. density
edema f.
f. embolic agent
encapsulated f.
endometrial canal f.
f. expansion
extracellular f.
f. extravasation
extravasation of radiopaque f.
extravascular f.
f. flow
free abdominal f.
free cul-de-sac f.
free peritoneal f.
high-signal intratendinous collection of f.
increased interstitial f.
f. intake
f. interface
interstitial f.
intestinal f.
intraperitoneal f.
joint f.
leakage of cerebrospinal f.
f. level
loculated pleural f.
f. overload
pelvic f.
pericardial f.
pericerebral f.
pericholecystic f.
perigraft f.
peritoneal cavity f.
pleural f.
prostatic f.
f. resorption
retained fetal lung f.
f. retention
f. sequestration
serosanguineous f.
silicone f.
f. space
spinal f.
subgaleal cerebrospinal f.
subphrenic f.
subpulmonic f.
synovial f.
transudative pericardial f.
f. vascular occluding agent
f. volume
f. wave

fluid-attenuated
f.-a. inversion recovery (FLAIR)
f.-a. inversion recovery-fast low-angle shot (FLAIR-FLASH)

fluid-filled
f.-f. area
f.-f. bronchogram
f.-f. catheter
f.-f. cyst
f.-f. kidney mass
f.-f. loop of bowel
f.-f. sac

fluid-flow artifact

fluid-fluid level

fluidification

fluke
liver f.
lung f.
f. lung
Oriental lung f.

flumazenil
^{11}C f.

fluorescein
f. angiography
f. sodium
f. uptake

fluorescence
f. spectroscopy

fluorescence-activated cell sorter (FACScan)

fluorescent
f. screen

Fluorescite injection

Fluorets ophthalmic strip

fluoride
f. ion-positron emission tomography (F-18-PET)

F

NOTES

fluoride *(continued)*
lithium f. (LiF)
yttrium lithium f. (YLF)
fluorine (F)
f. imaging agent
fluorine-18
fluorine-19
f. spectroscopy
fluorine-18-labeled glucose
fluorine-8-fluorodeoxyglucose
fluorine-18-fluorodeoxyglucose (FDG)
Fluor-I-Strip
Fluor-I-Strip-AT
fluoro-6-thia-heptadecanoic acid
fluorocaptopril
fluorocarbon-based ultrasound contrast agent
fluorochloride
barium f.
fluorochrome
^{18}fluoro-deoxy-D-glucose
^{18}f. PET
^{18}f. positron emission tomography (^{18}FDP PET)
fluorodeoxyglucose (FDG)
^{18}F f.
f. imaging agent
18-fluorodeoxyglucose (FDG)
fluorodeoxyglucose-6-phosphate
fluorodeoxyuridine
fluoro-DOPA
^{18}F f.-D.
fluorography
spot-film f.
fluorohalide
europium-activated barium f.
fluorometer
96-well scanning f.
fluorometry
image intensification f.
two-plane f.
fluoromibolerone
fluoromisonidazole
Fluoroplex
FluoroPlus
F. angiography
F. angiography imaging
F. angiography system
F. Roadmapper digital fluoroscopy
F. Roadmapper digital fluoroscopy imaging
F. Roadmapper digital fluoroscopy system
fluoropropylepidepride
fluoroptic thermometry system
fluoropyrimidine
fluororoentgenography
FluoroScan C-arm fluoroscopy
fluoroscope
Edison f.
fluoroscopic
f. assistance
f. control
f. guidance
f. imaging
f. localization
f. pushing technique
f. road-mapping technique
f. view
fluoroscopy
airway f.
biplane f.
C-arm f.
chest f.
digital f.
electric joint f.
FluoroPlus Roadmapper digital f.
FluoroScan C-arm f.
image-amplified f.
mobile f.
Orca C-arm f.
portable C-arm image intensifier f.
rapid scan f.
real-time CT f.
region-of-interest f.
simultaneous f.
video f.
fluoroscopy-guided
f.-g. condylar lift-off
f.-g. condylar lift-off imaging
f.-g. subarachnoid phenol block
f.-g. subarachnoid phenol block therapy
fluorosis
fluorotamoxifen
^{18}F f.
fluorotropapride
fluorotyrosine
FluoroVision
flush
f. aortogram imaging
f. aortography
flutter
atrial fetal f.
flux
electron f.
improved photon f.
magnetic f.
photon f.
fluxionary hyperemia
fly-through viewing
FM
fetal movement
Fm
fermium

^{255}**Fm**
fermium-255
FMAP
feeding mean arterial pressure
FMH
first metatarsal head
F-misonidazole
FMPSPGR imaging
fMRA
functional magnetic resonance angiography
fMRI
functional magnetic resonance imaging
fMRI signal change
FMS
fatty meal sonogram
FMS sonography
FNH
follicular nodular hyperplasia
FNTC
fine-needle transhepatic cholangiogram
foam
f. embolus
focal
f. alimentary tract calcification
f. area of hemorrhage
f. area of hypometabolism
f. asymmetric density
f. asymmetry
f. atrophy
f. attenuation
f. bacterial nephritis
f. biliary cirrhosis
f. bone sclerosis
f. caliectasis
f. cartilage erosion
f. cerebral ischemia
f. cerebral syndrome
f. cold liver lesion
f. colitis
f. cortical hyperplasia
f. damage
f. deficit
f. degenerative change
f. dilatation of air space
f. distortion
f. eccentric stenosis
f. edema
f. endocardial hemorrhage
f. esophageal narrowing
f. fat necrosis
f. fatty infiltration of liver
f. fibrocartilaginous dysplasia of tibia
f. fibrosis
f. fibrous breast disease
f. film distance (FFD)
f. gallbladder wall thickening
f. gigantism
f. hemispheric lesion
f. hepatic necrosis
f. hot liver lesion
f. hydronephrosis
f. hyperinflation
f. inflammation
f. interstitial infiltrate
f. intestinal inflammatory disease
f. intimal thickening
f. ischemic lesion
f. lateralizing finding
f. length
f. limb abnormality
f. liver lesion
f. liver scintigraphic defect
f. lobular carcinoma
f. lung disease
f. mass
f. moderate rejection
f. neurologic sign
f. nodular hyperplasia
f. organizing pneumonia
f. pancreatitis
f. parenchymal brain lesion
f. perivascular infiltrate
f. plaquelike defect
f. pleural plaque
f. pool
f. pooling of tracer
f. pyloric hypertrophy
f. renal hypertrophy
f. skin infarct
f. splenic lesion
f. spot (FS)
f. spot blur
f. spot-to-film angle
f. spot-to-object distance
f. tumor
f. ulcer
f. uptake
f. wall motion abnormality
f. white matter signal abnormality
f. zone (FZ)
focal-dust emphysema

NOTES

focally
f. decreased renal neoplasm
f. dilated duct
f. increased renal echogenicity
focus, pl. **foci**
Assmann f.
atrial f.
basal ganglia echogenic f.
f. of calcification
discrete hyperintense f.
ectopic f.
epileptic f.
epileptogenic f.
firing of ectopic atrial f.
hemorrhagic f.
hyperintense f.
hypermetabolic activity f.
inflammatory f.
junctional f.
mesial frontal f.
midline parasagittal f.
multiple f.
multizone transmit-receive f.
nodular hyperintense f.
f. object distance (FOD)
occipital f.
punctate hyperintense f.
radiolucent f.
satellite cartilaginous f.
Simon f.
f. of tumor
focused
f. appendix computed tomography (FACT)
f. grid
f. nuclear magnetic resonance (Fonar)
f. segmented ultrasound machine (FSUM)
focusing
zone f.
focus-skin distance (FSD)
FOD
focus object distance
fog
f. artifact
base f.
film f.
Fogarty
fogging phenomenon
foil
scattering f.
Foix-Alajouanine syndrome
Foix-Chavany-Marie syndrome
fold
abnormal esophageal f.
abnormal small bowel f.
accordion f.
adipose f.
alar f.
amnionic f.
aryepiglottic f.
caval f.
cecal f.
cholecystoduodenocolic f.
circular f.
costocolic f.
crescentic submucosal f.
Douglas f.
duodenojejunal f.
duodenomesocolic f.
dural f.
epigastric f.
epiglottic f.
esophageal f.
falciform f.
flattened duodenal f.
gastric f.
gastropancreatic f.
genital f.
giant gastric f.
glossoepiglottic f.
glossopalatine f.
gluteal f.
Guérin f.
haustral f.
Hensing f.
hepatopancreatic f.
hidebound small bowel f.
ileocecal f.
ileocolic f.
inferior transverse rectal f.
inframammary f.
inguinal f.
Kerckring f.
Kohlrausch f.
lateral umbilical f.
longitudinal esophageal f.
medical umbilical f.
mucosal f.
Nélaton f.
palatopharyngeal f.
paraduodenal f.
f. pattern
pericardial f.
peritoneal f.
pleuroperitoneal f.
prepyloric f.
rectal f.
rectouterine f.
f. of Rindfleisch
rugal f.
sacrogenital f.
semilunar f.
sentinel f.
sickle-shaped f.

sigmoid f.
skin f.
spiral f.
submucosal circular f.
superior duodenal f.
superior transverse rectal f.
tethered small bowel f.
thickened duodenal f.
thickened gastric f.
thickened nodular irregular small bowel f.
thickened stomach f.
thickened straight small bowel f.
transverse esophageal f.
uteric f.
ventricular f.
ventriculoinfundibular f.
vestigial f.

folded
f. fundus of gallbladder
f. lung
f. step ramp

folding potential analysis

foldover
image f.

Folex

folium vermis

Folius muscle

follicle
aggregated lymphatic f.
anovular ovarian f.
ascendant f.
atretic ovarian f.
dominant f.
gastric lymphatic f.
geographic f.
graafian f.
intestinal f.
inverse f.
luteinized unruptured f.
f. lysis
malpighian f.
nabothian f.
primordial f.
ruptured f.
thyroid f.
unruptured f.

follicular
f. bronchiectasis
f. bronchiolitis
f. bronchitis
f. center-cell lymphoma
f. gastritis
f. involution
f. mixed small cleaved lymphoma
f. mucinosis
f. nodular hyperplasia (FNH)
f. ovarian cyst
f. pattern
f. phase
f. predominantly large cell lymphoma
f. predominantly small cell lymphoma
f. salpingitis
f. thyroid adenoma
f. thyroid carcinoma

follicularis
enteritis f.

followthrough
small bowel f. (SBFT)
upper GI with small bowel f.
f. view

Follutein

Fonar
focused nuclear magnetic resonance
Fonar Stand-Up MRI imaging
Fonar Stand-Up MRI scanner
Fonar system

Fong disease

Fontan

Fontana canal

fontanelle, fontanel
anterior f.
anterolateral f.
bregmatic f.
bulging f.
closed f.
cranial f.
frontal f.
fused f.
Gerdy f.
mastoid f.
occipital f.
open f.
overriding sutures of f.
posterior f.
posterolateral f.
sagittal f.
sphenoid f.
tense f.
triangular f.

Food
F. and Drug Administration (FDA)

NOTES

food
f. bolus
f. bolus obstruction
cholecystokinetic f.
foot, pl. **feet**
abnormal position of f.
arch of f.
f. architecture
arcuate artery of f.
ball of f.
calcaneocavus f.
Charcot f.
f. deformity
digital artery of f.
drop f.
f. dysplasia
flail f.
flattened longitudinal arch of f.
f. fracture
Friedreich f.
hollow f.
large-vessel disease of diabetic f.
lateral spring ligament of f.
Madura f.
march f.
perforating artery of f.
phalanges of f.
planovalgus f.
f. plate
f. revascularization
rocker-bottom f.
valgus f.
varus f.
foot-ankle complex
football
f. finger
f. sign
footballer's ankle
footling presentation
footprint analysis
foot-progression angle (FPA)
foramen, pl. **foramina**
alveolar f.
anterior condyloid f.
anterior palatine f.
anterior sacral f.
aortic f.
apical f.
arachnoidal f.
base of skull f.
Bichat f.
blind f.
Bochdalek f.
f. of Bochdalek
Botallo f.
brain mass in jugular f.
carotid f.
cecal f.
cervical neural f.
conjugate f.
costotransverse f.
cranial f.
Duverney f.
emissary sphenoidal f.
enlarged vertebral f.
enlargement of vertebral f.
epiploic f.
ethmoidal f.
external acoustic f.
Ferrein f.
Froesch f.
frontal f.
greater palatine f.
greater sciatic f.
great sacrosciatic f.
Huschke f.
Hyrtl f.
intertransverse f.
interventricular f.
intervertebral f.
jugular f.
f. lacerum
lesser sciatic f.
f. of Luschka
Magendie f.
f. magnum
f. magnum herniation
mandibular f.
mastoid f.
f. of Morgagni
Morgagni f.
neural f.
nutrient f.
obturator f.
optic f.
f. ovale
f. ovale flap
ovale skull base of f.
f. ovale valve
palatine f.
parietal f.
petrosal f.
restrictive bulboventricular f.
Retzius f.
f. rotundum
sacral f.
sacrosciatic f.
f. spinosum
spinous f.
Stensen f.
stylomastoid f.
sublabral f.
superior maxillary f.
supraorbital f.
thebesian f.
f. transversarium

f. venosum
vertebral f.
f. of Vesalius
Weitbrecht f.
f. of Winslow
zygomaticofacial f.

foraminal
f. encroachment
f. node
f. space
f. stenosis

force
coulomb f.
electromotive f. (emf)
pascals of f.
reserve f.
rotational f.
shearing f.
stroke f.
tensile f.
torsional impaction f.
transverse plane f.

forced
f. expiratory volume
f. flexion injury

force-frequency relation

forceful parasternal motion

force-length relation

force-velocity relation

forearm
f. amputation
f. fracture

forebrain

forefoot
f. abduction deformity
f. angulation
narrowing of f.

foregut
bronchopulmonary f.
f. cyst
f. duplication

foreign
f. body (FB)
f. body embolus
f. body in esophagus
f. body granuloma
f. body ingestion
f. body upper airway obstruction
f. debris
f. material artifact

Forel
H field of F.

forensic radiology

foreshortening
annular f.

Forestier
F. bowstring sign
F. disease

forking
aqueductal f.
f. of sylvian aqueduct

form
ring-shaped f.

Formad kidney

format
cylindrical f.
2D f.
hemodynamic f.
slice f.
three-dimensional f.
two-dimensional f.

formation
batwing f.
beaklike osteophyte f.
bone f.
bony callus f.
brainstem reticular f.
bulla f.
bunion f.
callosal f.
callus f.
cellule f.
Chiari f.
cloacal f.
degenerative microcystic f.
eddy f.
enchondral bone f.
endogenous callus f.
excessive callus f.
exuberant atheroma f.
fistula f.
glomeruloid f.
Gothic arch f.
hematoma f.
heterotopic bone f.
hippocampal f.
honeycomb f.
hooklike osteophyte f.
image f.
intracavitary clot f.
lateral reticular f.
marginal osteophyte f.
mesencephalic reticular f.
microcystic f.

NOTES

formation *(continued)*
midbrain reticular f. (MRF)
mural thrombus f.
myelin ball f.
neointima f.
new bone f.
nipplelike osteophyte f.
osteophyte f.
palisade f.
pannus f.
paramedian pontine reticular f.
periosteal new bone f.
pontine parareticular f. (PPRF)
pseudointimal f.
pseudopod f.
reticular f. (RF)
reticular activating f.
ruffled border f.
saccular f.
scar f.
semilunar bone f.
sparsity of bone f.
spur f.
subperiosteal new bone f.
thrombus f.
tophus f.
vesical stone f.
forme tardive
forming
formula, pl. **formulas, formulae**
bayesian f.
Boyd f.
cigarroa f.
fan-beam f.
rapid dissolution f. (RDF)
Forney syndrome
fornicatus
gyrus isthmus f.
forniceal rupture
fornicis
corpora f.
fornix, pl. **fornices**
f. cerebri
f. of vagina
vaginal f.
Forrester syndrome
forward
f. flow
f. heart failure
f. positioning of head
f. stroke volume (FSV)
f. subluxation
f. transport
f. triangle method
f. velocity
forward-angle light scattering
fossa, pl. **fossae**
acetabular f.
adipose f.
amygdaloid f.
anconeal f.
antecubital f.
anterior recess of ischiorectal f.
articular f.
axillary f.
bony f.
cardiac f.
condylar f.
coronoid f.
cranial f.
crural f.
cubital f.
digastric f.
digital f.
duodenal f.
duodenojejunal f.
epigastric f.
femoral f.
floccular f.
gallbladder f.
glenoid f.
Gruber f.
hyaloid f.
hypoglossal f.
hypophyseal f.
iliac f.
infraspinous f.
infrasternal f.
infratemporal f.
intercondylar f.
intercondyloid f.
interpeduncular f.
intratemporal f.
ischiorectal f.
Jobert f.
Landzert f.
f. of Landzert
mandibular f.
meningioma of posterior f.
mesentericoparietal f.
middle cranial f.
f. navicularis
olecranon f.
f. ovalis
f. ovalis cordis
ovarian f.
paraduodenal f.
pararectal f.
paravesical f.
patellar f.
pituitary f.
popliteal f.
posterior pituitary f.
pterygoid f.
pterygopalatine f.
radial f.

rectouterine f.
retroappendiceal f.
rhomboid f.
f. of Rosenmüller
sphenoidal f.
subscapular f.
supraclavicular f.
f. of Sylvius
Sylvius f.
temporal f.
Treitz f.
uterovesical f.
valve of navicular f.
f. of Waldeyer
Waldeyer f.

four-artery sign
four-chamber
f.-c. apical view
f.-c. echocardiography
f.-c. hypertrophy
f.-c. plane
four-dimensional
f.-d. image
f.-d. imaging
four-fiber therapy
four-field
f.-f. technique
f.-f. x ray dosimetry
four-head camera
four-hour delayed thallium imaging
Fourier
F. analysis
F. coefficient
F. direct transformation imaging
F. discrete transformation
F. domain
F. imaging technique
F. multislice modified KWE direct imaging
F. optical theory
F. pulsatility index
F. transfer
F. transform
F. transformation reconstruction
F. transformation zeugmatography
F. transform infrared spectroscopy
F. transform NMR spectrometry
F. transform Raman spectroscopy
F. two-dimensional imaging
F. two-dimensional projection reconstruction
Fourier-acquired
F.-a. steady-state technique
F.-a. steady-state technique pulse sequence (FAST pulse sequence)
Fourier-encoded
Fourmentin thoracic index
four-part fracture
four-quadrant bar pattern
fourth
f. branchial arch
f. branchial cleft pouch
f. compartment
f. cranial nerve
f. intercostal space
f. parallel pelvic plane
f. turbinated bone
f. ventricle
f. ventricle diverticulum
f. ventricle tumor
four-vessel
f.-v. arteriography
f.-v. cerebral angiography
four-view
f.-v. chest x-ray
f.-v. wrist survey
FOV
field of view
FOV imaging
fovea
f. capitis
f. centralis
f. inferior
foveal fat pad
foveated chest
foveola
gastric f.
Fowler position
Fox sign
FP
frontopolar
FP artery
FPA
foot-progression angle
F-18-PET
fluoride ion-positron emission tomography
fractal analysis
fractal-based method
fraction
active emptying f.
area-length method for ejection f.
blood flow extraction f.

NOTES

fraction *(continued)*
blunted ejection f.
cardiac ejection f.
cardiac scintigraphy ejection f.
computed ejection f.
depressed ejection f.
digital ejection f.
Dodge method for ejection f.
drug f.
ejection f. (EF)
filtration f. (FF)
gallbladder ejection f.
global ejection f.
globally depressed ejection f.
interval ejection f.
Kennedy method for calculating ejection f.
left atrial active-emptying f.
left ventricular ejection f. (LVEF)
Maddahi method of calculating right ventricular ejection f.
myofibril volume f.
one-third ejection f.
oxygen extraction f. (OEF)
radionuclide ejection f.
regional ejection f.
regurgitant f.
resting left ventricular ejection f.
right ventricular ejection f. (RVEF)
shunt f.
S-phase f.
systolic ejection f.
Teichholz ejection f.
thermodilution ejection f.
unattached f.'s
ventricular ejection f.
well-preserved ejection f.

fractional
f. area
f. moving blood volume
f. moving blood volume estimation
f. myocardial shortening
f. shortening (FS)
f. shortening of left ventricle

fractionated
f. dose
f. dose-survival curve
f. external beam irradiation
f. external beam radiation therapy
f. stereotactic radiation therapy

fractionation
accelerated f.
fast f.
quasi-accelerated f.
S-phase f.

fracture (fx) (*See* fracture-dislocation)
abduction f.
abduction-external rotation f.
acetabular f.
acetabular posterior wall f.
acetabular rim f.
acute avulsion f.
adduction f.
agenetic f.
Aitken classification of epiphyseal f.'s
alveolar bone f.
anatomic f.
Anderson-Hutchins tibial f.
angulated f.
ankle mortise f.
annular f.
anterior column f.
anterolateral compression f.
AO classification of ankle f.
apophyseal f.
arch f.
articular mass separation f.
articular pillar f.
artificial f.
Ashhurst-Bromer classification of ankle f.'s
f. of astragalus
Atkin epiphyseal f.
atlas f.
atrophic f.
avulsion chip f.
avulsion stress f.
axial compression f.
axis f.
backfire f.
Bankart f.
Barton f.
Barton-Smith f.
basal neck f.
basal skull f.
baseball finger f.
basilar femoral neck f.
basilar skull f.
basocervical f.
bayonet position of f.
beak f.
bedroom f.
bending f.
Bennett comminuted f.
bicondylar T-shaped f.
bicondylar Y-shaped f.
bicycle spoke f.
bimalleolar ankle f.
bipartite f.
f. blister
blow-in f.
blowout f.
bone f.
boot-top f.
Bosworth f.

both-bone f.
both-column f.
bowing f.
boxer's punch f.
Boyd type II f.
f. bracing
bronchial f.
bucket-handle pelvic f.
buckle f.
bumper f.
bunk-bed f.
Burkhalter-Reyes method of phalangeal f.
burst f.
butterfly f.
buttonhole f.
calcaneal avulsion f.
calcaneal displaced f.
calcaneal stress f.
f. callus
f. callus loading
Canale-Kelly classification of talar neck f.
capitate f.
capitellar f.
capitulum radiale humeri f.
carpal bone stress f.
carpal navicular f.
carpal scaphoid bone f.
carpometacarpal joint f.
cartwheel f.
Cedell f.
cemental f.
central f.
cephalomedullary nail f.
cerebral palsy pathological f.
cervical spine f.
cervicotrochanteric f.
Chance spinal f.
Chaput f.
chauffeur's f.
chevron f.
childhood f.
chip f.
chiropractic treatment f.
chisel f.
chondral f.
Chopart f.
circumferential f.
f. classification
clavicular birth f.
clay shoveler's f.
cleavage f.
f. in close apposition
closed f.
closed-break f.
coccyx f.
Colles f.
collicular f.
combined flexion-distraction injury and burst f.
combined radial-ulnar-humeral f.
comminuted bursting f.
comminuted intraarticular f.
comminuted teardrop f.
complete f.
complex f.
complex simple f.
complicated f.
composite f.
compound skull f.
compression f.
condylar split f.
congenital f.
Conrad-Bugg trapping of soft tissue in ankle f.
contrecoup f.
coracoid f.
corner f.
coronoid process f.
cortical f.
Cotton ankle f.
crack f.
craniofacial dysjunction f.
crush f.
"crushed eggshell" f.
cuboid f.
cuneiform f.
dancer's f.
Danis-Weber f.
Darrach-Hughston-Milch f.
dashboard f.
decompression of f.
f. deformity
Denis (A–E) classification of spinal f.
Denis Browne classification of sacral f.'s
dens f.
dentate f.
depressed skull f.
depression-type intraarticular f.
de Quervain f.
derby-hat f.

NOTES

fracture *(continued)*
Desault f.
f. deviation
diacondylar f.
diametric pelvic f.
diaphyseal f.
f. diastasis
diastatic f.
dicondylar f.
die-punch f.
direct f.
dishpan f.
dislocation f.
f. dislocation
displaced f.
distal femoral epiphyseal f.
distal humoral f.
distal radial f.
distraction of f.
dome f.
dorsal rim distal radial f.
dorsal wing f.
double f.
Dupuytren f.
Duverney f.
dye punch f.
dyscrasic f.
El-Ahwany classification of humeral supracondylar f.'s
elbow f.
elementary f.
Ellis technique for Barton f.
f. en coin
f. en rave
epicondylar f.
epiphyseal plate f.
epiphyseal slip f.
epiphyseal tibial f.
Essex-Lopresti joint depression f.
explosion f.
extension corner avulsion f. (ECAF)
extension teardrop f. (ETF)
extraarticular f.
extracapsular f.
extraoctave f.
facial f.
fatigue f.
femoral intertrochanteric f.
femoral neck f.
femoral shaft f.
femoral supracondylar f.
fender f.
fetal f.
f. fever
fibular f.
Fielding-Magliato classification of subtrochanteric f.'s
fighter's f.
finger f.
fissure f.
flake f.
flexion-burst f.
flexion-compression f.
flexion-distraction f.
flexion teardrop f.
floating arch f.
foot f.
forearm f.
four-part f.
f. fragment
f. fragment separation
f. frame
Freiberg f.
frontal f.
Frykman radial f.
fulcrum f.
Gaenslen f.
Galeazzi f.
f. gap
Garden femoral neck f.
Gartland classification of humeral supracondylar f.
glenoid rim f.
Gosselin f.
Grantham classification of femoral f.
greater trochanteric femoral f.
greater tuberosity f.
greenstick f.
grenade thrower's f.
gross f.
growth plate f.
Guérin f.
gunshot f.
Gustilo-Anderson open clavicular f.
gutter f.
Hahn-Steinthal f.
hairline f.
hamate tail f.
hand f.
hangman's f.
Hansen classification of f.'s
Hawkins classification of talar f.'s
head-splitting humeral f.
healing f.
heat f.
hemicondylar f.
hemitransverse f.
Henderson f.
Herbert scaphoid bone f.
Hermodsson f.
hickory-stick f.
Hill-Sachs posterolateral compression f.
hockey-stick f.

Hoffa f.
Holstein-Lewis f.
hook of the hamate f.
hoop stress f.
horizontal maxillary f.
humeral condylar f.
humeral head-splitting f.
humeral physeal f.
humeral supracondylar f.
Hutchinson f.
hyperextension teardrop f.
hyperflexion teardrop f.
ice skater's f.
idiopathic f.
ileofemoral wing f.
impacted subcapital f.
impacted valgus f.
implant f.
impression f.
incomplete f.
indented f.
indirect f.
inflammatory f.
infraction f.
Ingram-Bachynski classification of hip f.'s
insufficiency f.
intercondylar femoral f.
intercondylar humeral f.
intercondylar tibial f.
internally fixed f.
interperiosteal f.
intertrochanteric four-part f.
intraarticular calcaneal f.
intraarticular proximal tibial f.
intracapsular femoral neck f.
intraoperative f.
intraperiosteal f.
intrauterine f.
inverted-Y f.
ipsilateral femoral neck f.
ipsilateral femoral shaft f.
irreducible f.
ischioacetabular f.
Jefferson burst f.
Jefferson cervical f.
Jeffery classification of radial f.'s
joint depression f.
Jones f.
Jones classification of diaphyseal f.'s
juvenile Tillaux f.
juxtaarticular f.
juxtacortical f.
Key-Conwell classification of pelvic f.'s
Kilfoyle classification of condylar f.'s
knee f.
Kocher f.
labral and anterior inferior glenoid rim f.
LaGrange classification of humeral supracondylar f.'s
laryngeal f.
lateral column calcaneal f.
lateral condylar humeral f.
laterally displaced f.
lateral malleolar f.
lateral tibial plateau f.
lateral wedge f.
Lauge-Hansen classification of ankle f.'s
Laugier f.
Le Fort fibular f.
Le Fort mandibular f.
Le Fort-Wagstaffe f.
lesser trochanteric f.
f. line
linear skull f.
f. line of consolidation
Lisfranc f.
local compression f.
local decompression f.
long bone f.
longitudinal f.
long oblique f.
loose f.
lorry driver's f.
low-energy f.
low-T humerus f.
lumbar spine f.
lunate f.
Maisonneuve fibular f.
malar f.
Malgaigne pelvic f.
malleolar f.
mallet f.
malunited f.
mandibular f.
marginal f.
Mathews classification of olecranon f.'s
maxillary f.

F

NOTES

fracture *(continued)*
maxillofacial f.
medial column calcaneal f.
medial epicondyle f.
medial malleolar f.
metacarpal f.
metaphyseal f.
metatarsal f.
Meyers-McKeever classification of tibial f.'s
midfacial f.
midfoot f.
midshaft f.
midwaist scaphoid f.
Milch classification of humeral f.'s
milkman's f.
minimally displaced f.
Moberg-Gedda f.
molar tooth f.
monomalleolar f.
Monteggia f.
Montercaux f.
Moore f.
Mouchet f.
multangular ridge f.
multipartite f.
multiple f.'s
multiray f.
nasal f.
nasoorbital f.
navicular body f.
navicular hand f.
naviculocapitate f.
f. of necessity
neck f.
Neer-Horowitz classification of humeral f.'s
neoplastic f.
neural arch f.
neurogenic f.
neuropathic f.
neurotrophic f.
Newman classification of radial neck and head f.'s
nightstick f.
nonarticular radial head f.
noncontiguous f.
nondisplaced f.
nonphyseal f.
nonrotational burst f.
f. nonunion
nonunited f.
nutcracker f.
oblique spiral f.
O'Brien classification of radial f.'s
obturator avulsion f.
occipital condyle f.
occult f.
odontoid condyle f.
Ogden classification of epiphyseal f.'s
olecranon tip f.
one-part f.
open f.
open-book f.
open-break f.
orbital blowout f.
orbital floor f.
osteochondral slice f.
osteoporotic f.
overlapping f.
Pais f.
panfacial f.
Papavasiliou classification of olecranon f.'s
paratrooper's f.
parry f.
pars interarticularis f.
patellar sleeve f.
pathologic f.
pedicle f.
pelvic insufficiency f.
pelvic rim f.
pelvic ring f.
pelvic straddle f.
penetrating f.
perforating f.
periarticular f.
peripheral f.
periprosthetic f.
peritrochanteric f.
phalangeal diaphyseal f.
physeal plate f.
Piedmont f.
pillar f.
pillion f.
pillow f.
pilon ankle f.
ping-pong f.
Pipkin classification of femoral f.'s
pisiform f.
plafond f.
plaque f.
plastic bowing f.
plateau tibia f.
Poland classification of epiphyseal f.'s
pond f.
Posada f.
posterior arch f.
posterior element f.
posterior ring f.
posterior wall f.
postirradiation f.
Pott ankle f.
pressure f.

pronation-abduction f.
pronation-eversion f.
proximal femoral f.
proximal humeral f.
proximal tibial metaphyseal f.
pseudo-Jefferson f.
puncture f.
pyramidal f.
Quinby classification of pelvic f.'s
radial head f.
radial neck f.
radial styloid f.
radiographically occult f.
f. reduction
resecting f.
retrodisplaced f.
reverse Barton f.
reverse Colles f.
reverse Monteggia f.
rib f.
ring f.
ring-disrupting f.
Riseborough-Radin classification of intercondylar f.
Rockwood classification of clavicular f.
Rolando f.
rotational burst f.
Ruedi-Allgower tibial plafond f.
f. running length of bone
sacral insufficiency f. (SIF)
sacroiliac f.
Sakellarides classification of calcaneal f.'s
Salter-Harris classification of epiphyseal f.'s
Salter I–IV f.
sandbagging f.
scaphoid hand f.
scottie dog f.
seatbelt f.
secondary f.
segmental bronchus f.
Segond f.
Seinsheimer classification of femoral f.'s
senile subcapital f.
sentinel f.
SER-IV f.
  supination, external rotation type IV fracture
shaft f.
shear f.
Shepherd f.
short oblique f.
sideswipe f.
silver fork f.
f. simple and depressed full-scale deflection (FSD)
simple skull f.
f. site
skier's f.
Skillern f.
skull f.
sleeve f.
slice f.
Smith f.
Sorbie classification of calcaneal f.
sphenoid bone f.
spinal f.
spinous process f.
spiral oblique f.
splintered f.
split compression f.
split-heel f.
splitting f.
spontaneous f.
sprain f.
Springer f.
sprinter's f.
stability of f.
stable f.
stairstep f.
stellate skull f.
stellate undepressed f.
stepoff of f.
Stieda f.
straddle f.
strain f.
stress f.
strut f.
subcapital f.
subchondral f.
subcutaneous f.
subperiosteal f.
subtrochanteric f.
supination-adduction f.
supination-eversion f.
supination, external rotation type IV f. (SER-IV fracture)
supracondylar femoral f.
supracondylar humeral f.
supracondylar Y-shaped f.
surgical neck f.

NOTES

fracture *(continued)*
T f.
talar avulsion f.
talar dome f.
talar neck f.
talar osteochondral f.
T condylar f.
teacup f.
teardrop burst f.
teardrop-shaped flexion-compression f.
temporal bone f.
tension f.
testis f.
thalamic f.
Thompson-Epstein classification of femoral f.'s
thoracic spine f.
thoracolumbar junction f.
three-part f.
f. threshold
through-and-through f.
thrower's f.
Thurston Holland f.
tibial bending f.
tibial condyle f.
tibial diaphyseal f.
tibial open f.
tibial pilon f.
tibial plafond f.
tibial plateau f.
tibial shaft f.
tibial triplane f.
tibial tuberosity f.
tibiofibular f.
Tillaux f.
Tillaux-Chaput f.
Tillaux-Kleiger f.
toddler's f.
tongue f.
tongue-type intraarticular f.
torsional f.
torus f.
total f.
total condylar depression f.
trabecular f.
tracheal f.
traction f.
trampoline f.
transcaphoid f.
transcapitate f.
transcervical femoral f.
transchondral talar f.
transcondylar f.
transepiphyseal f.
transhamate f.
transiliac f.
transsacral f.
transscaphoid dislocation f.
transtriquetral f.
transverse comminuted f.
transversely oriented endplate compression f.
transverse maxillary f.
transverse process f.
trapezium f.
traversing the f.
trimalleolar ankle f.
triplane f.
tripod f.
triquetral f.
Tronzo classification of intertrochanteric f.'s
trophic f.
T-shaped f.
tuft f.
two-part f.
ulnar f.
uncinate process f.
undepressed skull f.
undisplaced f.
unicondylar f.
unilateral f.
unimalleolar f.
unstable f.
ununited f.
upper thoracic spine f.
vertebral body f.
vertebral compression f.
vertebral plana f.
vertebral wedge compression f.
vertical shear f.
volar rim distal radial f.
Volkmann f.
Vostal classification of radial f.'s
V-shaped f.
Wagstaffe f.
Walther f.
Watson-Jones classification of tibial tubercle avulsion f.'s
Weber C f.
wedge compression f.
wedge flexion-compression f.
"western boot" in open f.
Wilkins classification of radial f.'s
willow f.
Wilson f.
Winquist-Hansen classification of femoral f.'s
Y f.
Y-T f.
Zickel f.
f. zone
zygomaticomalar complex f.
zygomaticomaxillary f.

fractured
f. bronchus
f. kidney
f. vertebra
fracture-dislocation
Chopart f.-d.
cuneiform f.-d.
Galeazzi f.-d.
intermediate cuneiform f.-d.
pedicolaminar f.-d.
perilunate f.-d. (PLFD)
Fraenkel typhus nodule
fragile bone
fragilitas ossium
fragment
alignment of fracture f.
anteroinferior triangular f.
articular f.
avulsed fracture f.
bone f.
f. of bone
butterfly fracture f.
calcified free f.
capital f.
chondral f.
cortical f.
f. depression
disk f.
displaced fracture f.
extruded disk f.
fracture f.
free disk f.
free-floating cartilaginous f.
iodine-125-labeled f.
jagged bone f.'s
Klenow f.
loose f.
major fracture f.
malunion of fracture f.'s
metallic f.
nonunion of fracture f.'s
osteochondral f.
overriding of fracture f.'s
retropulsed fracture f.
smear f.
Spengler f.
technetium-99m antimyosin Fab f.
torsion of fracture f.
union of fracture f.'s
fragmentation
f. of apophysis
f. of barium
collagen f.
electrohydraulic f.
meniscal f.
f. myocarditis
f. therapy
unilateral f.
fragmentocytosis
frame
adduction f.
Balkan fracture f.
Brown-Roberts-Wells f.
Compass stereotactic f.
CT/MRI-compatible stereotactic head f.
fracture f.
ISAH stereotactic immobilization f.
Komai stereotactic head f.
Laitinen stereotactic head f.
Leksell D-shaped stereotactic f.
Leksell-Elekta stereotactic f.
Malcolm-Lynn C-RXF cervical retractor f.
pelvic fracture f.
radiolucent spine f.
Radionics CRW stereotactic head f.
f. of reference
Reichert-Mundinger-Fischer stereotactic f.
robotics-controlled stereotactic f.
stereotactic head f.
stereotactic localization f.
Stryker f.
frameless
f. stereotactic digital subtraction angiography
f. stereotactic guidance
f. stereotaxy
framing
exact f.
Frank
F. sign
F. vectorcardiography
frank
f. breech presentation
f. cirrhosis
f. congestive failure
f. disk herniation
f. dislocation
f. hemorrhage
f. lesion
f. necrosis

NOTES

F

frank *(continued)*
f. pulmonary edema
f. rupture
Fränkel
F. classification system
F. sign
F. spinal cord injury classification
white line of F.
F. white line
Frankfort
F. horizontal plane
F. line
F. mandibular incisor angle
F. mandibular notch
Franklin changer
Frank-Starling
F.-S. curve
F.-S. mechanism
F.-S. relation
Franz sign
fraternal twin
Fraunfelder technique
Fraunhofer zone
frayed
f. disk
f. metaphysis
f. string appearance
Frederick-Miller tube
free
f. abdominal fluid
f. air
f. air passage
f. air under diaphragm
f. band of colon
f. band of colon band
f. body
f. body calcification
f. cul-de-sac fluid
f. disk fragment
f. electrons
f. fatty acid (FFA)
f. flap of cartilage
f. fluid cul-de-sac
f. gas bubble
f. hepatic venography
f. induction delay curve
f. intraperitoneal air
f. intraperitoneal gas
f. knee joint
f. path
f. pericardial space
f. peritoneal fluid
f. pertechnetate (TcO^{4-})
f. pleural effusion
f. precession
f. radical
f. reflux
f. subphrenic gas
f. wall tract
free-floating
f.-f. cartilaginous fragment
f.-f. meniscus
f.-f. retinaculum
free-fragment disk herniation
freehand
f. interventional sonography
f. interventional ultrasound
free-induction
f.-i. decay (FID)
f.-i. signal
freely movable mass
Freeman calcaneal fracture classification
free-radical
f.-r. dosimetry
freezing phenomenon
Freiberg
F. disease
F. fracture
F. infraction
Freiberg-Kohler disease
French
F. T-tube
frenulum of valve
frequency (f)
f. analysis
angular f.
f. component
disappearance f.
f. domain
f. domain image
f. domain imaging (FDI, FDI ultrasound)
Doppler shift f.
f. encoding
f. estimation
extremely low f. (ELF)
false f.
halftone f.
f. intensification
Larmor f.
Nyquist f.
offset f.
f. offset
peak repetition f. (PRF)
pelvic mass f.
precessional f.
pulse repetition f.
f. range
raster f.
resonance f.
resonant f.
respiratory f.
rotational f.
f. separation
spatial f.

f. spectrum
f. synthesizer
vibration f.
frequency-encoded gradient
frequency-related peak
frequency-selective
f.-s. fat saturation
f.-s. inversion
f.-s. pulse
Fresnel zone plate
Freund anomaly
Frey syndrome
friability
friable
f. annulus
f. artery
f. lesion
f. mass
f. mucosa
f. thickened degenerated intima
f. tumor
f. vegetation
f. wall
Fricke
F. dosimetry
F. gel
friction neuritis
Friedel Pick syndrome
Friedländer pneumonia
Friedman
F. method
F. position
Friedreich
F. ataxic cardiomyopathy
F. foot
F. phenomenon
F. sign
Friedrich disease
Fries score for rheumatoid arthritis classification
Frimodt-Moller syndrome
fringe
f. field
moiré f.
f. of osteophyte
f. skeleton extraction
synovial f.
f. thinning algorithm
fringing field
FRODO technique
Froesch foramen
frogleg
f. lateral projection
f. lateral view
f. position
f. view of the hips
froglike appearance
Frohse
arcade of F.
F. ligamentous arcade
Froment paper sign
frond
villous f.
frondlike
f. appearance
f. filling defect
frontal
f. abscess
f. arteriovenous malformation
f. artery
f. bone
f. bossing
f. bossing of Parrot
f. cephalometric radiograph
f. cortex
f. crest
f. defect
f. eminence
f. fontanelle
f. foramen
f. fracture
f. gyrus
f. horn
f. horn of lateral ventricle
f. horn Mickey Mouse ear
f. lobe
f. lobe contusion
f. lobe dysfunction
f. lobe infarct
f. lobe lesion
f. lobe sign
f. lobe tumor
f. nerve
f. notch
f. plane
f. plane growth abnormality
f. plane loop
f. plane vectorcardiography
f. plate
f. pole
f. process
f. sinus
f. sinus mucocele

NOTES

frontal *(continued)*
f. sulcus
f. suture
f. vein
f. view
frontier ulcer
frontocentral convexity
frontoethmoidal
f. encephalocele
f. giant cell reparative granuloma
f. mucocele
f. suture
frontolacrimal suture
frontomaxillary suture
frontonasal
f. duct
f. dysplasia
f. dysplasia malformation complex
f. process
f. suture
frontoorbital advancement
frontoparietal
f. arteriovenous malformation
ascending f. (ASFP)
f. suture
frontopolar (FP)
f. artery (FP artery)
f. point
frontopontine tract
frontosphenoidal
f. encephalocele
f. process
frontosphenoid suture
frontotemporal (FT)
f. atrophy
f. muscle
f. tract
frontozygomatic suture
Frostberg-3 sign
Frostberg inverted-3 sign
frostbite
frosted liver
frothy colonic mucosa
Frouin
quadrangulation of F.
frozen
f. hemithorax
f. joint
f. pelvis
f. shoulder
FRP
functional refractory period
Frykman
F. distal radius fracture classification
F. radial fracture
FS
focal spot
fractional shortening
FS (frequency-shifted) burst MR imaging
FS method
FS projection
FSCR
flexible surface-coil-type resonator
FSD
focus-skin distance
fracture simple and depressed full-scale deflection
FSE
fast spin echo
FSU
functional subunit
FSUM
focused segmented ultrasound machine
FSV
forward stroke volume
FT
frontotemporal
FTA
femorotibial angle
FTC
fibulotalocalcaneal
FTC ligament
Fuchs
F. adenoma
F. odontoid view
F. position
F. principle
fugax
coxitis f.
Fuji
F. AC2 storage phosphor computed radiology system
F. FCR9000 computed radiology system
fulcrum
f. fracture
joint f.
Ful-Glo ophthalmic strip
fulguration
nephroscopic f.
full
f. bladder ultrasound
f. cervical spine series (FCS series)
f. cervical spine view (FCS view)
f. lateral position
f. scan with interpolation (FI)
f. scan with interpolation method (FI method)
f. scan with interpolation projection (FI projection)
f. thickness
f. width at half maximum (FWHM)
full-bladder ultrasound technique

full-blown cardiac tamponade
full-body echoplanar system imager
full-column
f.-c. barium enema
f.-c. view
full-energy peak efficiency
Fuller earth pneumoconiosis
full-field digital mammography system
full-intensity needle
full-length view
full-line scanning
full-scan
f.-s. method (FS method)
f.-s. projection (FS projection)
full-thickness
f.-t. button of aortic wall
f.-t. Carrel button
f.-t. infarct
f.-t. tear
full-to-empty VAD mode
full-volume loop spirometry
full-wave
f.-w. rectification
f.-w. rectifier
full-width at half-maximum
full-width-at-half-maximum of lorentzian curve
fulminant
f. cerebral lymphoma
f. colitis
f. course of disease
f. fasciitis
f. hepatic failure (FHF)
f. hydrocephalus
f. pulmonary edema
f. tuberculosis
fulminating ulcerative colitis
function
abnormal tubular f.
atrial-phase volumetric f.
brain f.
bundle f.
cerebrospinal fluid shunt f.
commissural f.
compromised ventricular f.
contractile f.
depressed right ventricular contractile f.
differential renal f.
edge response f. (ERF)
excitation f.
exercise LV f.
fetal renal f.
gaussian f.
global ventricular f.
gonadal f.
harmonic f.
impaired renal f.
leaflet f.
left atrial f.
left ventricular systolic/diastolic f.
left ventricular systolic pump f.
line spread f. (LSF)
line-spread f. (LSF)
midbrain f.
modulation transfer f. (MTF)
myocardial contractile f.
pharyngoesophageal f.
point-spread f. (PSR)
rectosigmoid f.
regional left ventricular f.
reserve cardiac f.
rest left ventricular f.
rest right ventricular f.
right atrial f.
right and left atrial phasic volumetric f.
right ventricular systolic/diastolic f.
Shepp-Logan filter f.
sinusoid reference f.
stress perfusion and rest f.
swallowing f.
systolic f.
time activity f.
tubular f.
velocity distribution f. (F(v))
ventricular contractility f. (VCF)
volumetric f.
Zeeman hamiltonian f.
functional
f. abnormality
f. aerobic impairment
f. bladder capacity
f. bowel syndrome
f. brain imaging
f. classification of congestive heart failure
f. correlation
f. disorder
f. diverticulum
f. hyperlordosis
f. hypertrophy
f. magnetic resonance angiography (fMRA)

F

NOTES

functional *(continued)*
f. magnetic resonance imaging (fMRI)
f. marrow
f. MRI
f. neuroimaging
f. ovarian cyst
f. paraganglioma
f. reentry
f. refractory period (FRP)
f. residual capacity
f. scoliosis
f. sphincter
f. spin echo imaging
f. subunit (FSU)
f. units of spine
f. ureteral obstruction
functioning
f. neoplasm
f. nodule
f. pituitary adenoma
fundal
f. placenta
f. portion of gallbladder
fundi (*pl. of* fundus)
fundic-antral junction
fundic metaphysis
fundiform ligament
fundoplication
Nissen f.
fundus, pl. **fundi**
f. of aneurysm
aneurysmal f.
bald gastric f.
bladder f.
f. of gallbladder
gallbladder f.
gastric f.
saddle-shaped uterine f.
stomach f.
urinary bladder f.
f. uteri
uterine f.
vaginal f.
Funduscein injection
fungal
f. hypha
f. plaque
f. pneumonia
fungating
f. tumor
fungoides
Alibert-Bazin form of mycosis f.
tumor d'emblee mycosis f.
fungus ball
funic souffle
funicular
f. inguinal hernia
f. souffle
funiculus
f. cuneatus
f. dorsalis
f. gracilis
f. medullae spinalis
f. ventralis
funnel
f. chest
f. chest deformity
funnel-like cardiomegaly
funnel-shaped
f.-s. cavity
f.-s. pelvis
funny-looking calix
Fürbringer sign
furifosmin
technetium-99m f.
furosemide imaging agent
furrier's lung
fused
f. ankle
f. commissure
f. fontanelle
f. kidney
f. papillary muscle
f. physis
f. rib
f. vertebrae
fusiform
f. aneurysm
f. bronchiectasis
f. defect
f. dilatation
f. gyrus
f. malformation
f. mass
f. narrowing of arteries
f. shadow
f. swelling
f. thickening
f. widening of duct
fusion
ankle f.
anterior cervical f. (ACF)
atlantooccipital f.
bony f.
calcaneotibial f.
carpometacarpal f.
cervical interbody f.
cervical spine f.
cervicooccipital f.
chevron f.
f. of cusp
f. defect
diaphyseal-epiphyseal f.

extraarticular hip f.
facet f.
Hatcher-Smith cervical f.
image f.
interbody f.
interphalangeal f.
intersegmental laminar f.
interspinous process f.
intraarticular knee f.
joint f.
Kellogg-Speed lumbar spinal f.
metatarsocuneiform joint f.
metatarsophalangeal joint f.
multilevel f.
nuclear f.
occipitoatlantoaxial f.
occipitocervical f.
pantalar f.
f. plate
posterior lumbar interbody f. (PLIF)
posterior spine f. (PSF)
sacroiliac joint f.
spinal f.
talar body f.
talocrural f.
tibiocalcaneal f.
tibiotalocalcaneal f.
transfibular f.
two-stage f.
vertebral f.

fuzzy
f. echo
f. logic contrast correction
f. rules
f. set theory

F(v)
velocity distribution function

FWHM
full width at half maximum

fx
fracture

FZ
focal zone

NOTES

Ga
gallium
^{68}Ga
gallium-68
^{67}Ga, Ga-67
gallium-67
^{67}Ga bone scan
^{67}Ga examination
^{67}Ga excretion
^{67}Ga GABA uptake carrier
^{67}Ga higher dose
gadobenate dimeglumine imaging agent
gadobenic acid imaging agent
gadobutrol imaging agent
gadodiamide
g. imaging agent
gadolinium (Gd)
g. chelate
g. complex
g. cyclohexanediaminetetraacetic acid (Gd-CDTA)
g. enhancement
g. ethylenediaminetetraacetic acid (Gd-EDTA)
g. iron
g. oxide imaging agent
g. scan
g. sucralfate
g. tetraazacyclododecanetetraacetic acid (Gd-DOTA)
g. texaphyrin
gadolinium-153
gadolinium-diethylenetriamine pentaacetic acid
gadolinium-DTPA (Gd-DTPA)
gadolinium-enhanced
g.-e. MR imaging
g.-e. T1-weighted axial image
gadopentetate
g. dimeglumine (Gd-DTPA)
gadopentetic acid
gadopentolate-polylysine
gadoteridol (Gd-HP-DO3A)
g. imaging agent
gadoversetamide imaging agent
Gaeltec catheter-tip pressure transducer
Gaenslen
G. fracture
G. sign
Gaertner (*var. of* Gärtner)
Gaffney joint
gain
accelerated phase g.
brightness g.
color g.
phase g.
power g.
quadratic phase g.
swept g.
time-compensated g.
time compensation g.
time-varied g. (TVG)
Gairdner disease
Gaisbock syndrome
galactocele
galactogram
mammary g.
galactography
galactophoritis
galactophorous
g. canal
g. duct
Galant sign
galea aponeurotica
galeal extension of tumor
Galeazzi
G. fracture
G. fracture-dislocation
G. sign
Galen
great cerebral vein of G.
G. Scan scanner
G. teleradiology system
G. vein aneurysm
G. ventricle
galenic venous malformation
Gallannaugh bone plate
Gallavardin phenomenon
gallbladder
g. adenoma
g. agenesis
g. bed
bilobed g.
blunt trauma g.
body of g.
g. calculus
g. carcinoma
chromically inflamed g.
comet-tail artifact g.
contracted g.
Courvoisier g.
dilated g.
displaced g.
distended g.
g. diverticulum
double g.
g. duplication
g. ectopia
ectopic g.
edematous g.

gallbladder *(continued)*
g. ejection fraction
g. empyema
enlarged g.
fetal g.
g. filling defect
fish-scale g.
floating g.
folded fundus of g.
g. fossa
fundal portion of g.
fundus of g.
g. fundus
gangrene g.
g. gravel
g. halo sign
hourglass constriction of g.
g. hydrops
g. hypoplasia
g. ileus
g. imaging
g. infundibulum
g. lift
mobile g.
multiseptated g.
neck of g.
nonvisualization of g.
pearl necklace g.
g. perforation
g. polyp
porcelain g.
porcine g.
g. rim sign
g. septation
g. series (GBS)
shrunken g.
g. size
g. sludge
small g.
stasis g.
g. stone
strawberry g.
g. study
thick-walled g.
thin-walled g.
g. torsion
g. trauma
g. ultrasound
g. villus
g. wall
g. wall abscess
wandering g.
gallbladder-vena cava line
gall duct
Gallie H-graft
gallium (Ga)
g. bone scintigraphy
g. imaging agent
g. imaging in bone
g. lung imaging
g. lung scintigraphy
g. nitrate
g. scan
g. tumor scintigraphy
g. uptake
gallium-67 (^{67}Ga, Ga-67)
g. citrate
gallium-68 (^{68}Ga)
gallium-67-labeled leukocytes
gallium-avid thymic hyperplasia
gallium-transferrin complex
gallstone
asymptomatic g.
cholesterol g.
dissolution of g.
ectopic intraluminal g.
faceted g.
floating g.
gas-containing g.
g. ileus
innocent g.
intraluminal g.
laminated g.
layered g.
layering of g.'s
g. migration
mulberry g.
opacifying g.
radiolucent g.
retained g.
silent g.
solitary g.
symptomatic g.
GALT
gut-associated lymphoid tissue
gamekeeper's
g. habitual dislocation
g. thumb
gamma (γ)
g. camera
g. cascade
g. emission
g. emitter
g. encephalography
g. factor
g. film
g. heating
g. irradiation
g. knife
g. knife radiosurgery
g. probe
g. radiation
g. ray
g. ray attenuation
g. signal
g. spectrometric analysis
g. tocopherol (γ-T)

g. transverse colon loop
g. unit
g. well counter
gamma-aminobutyrate
gamma camera
rotating g. c.
single-head rotating g. c.
gamma-detection probe
gamma-emitting isotope
gammagram
gamma-ray
g.-r. capture
g.-r. counter
g.-r. spectrometer
g.-r. spectrum
Gammex
G. RMI DAP (dose-area product) meter
G. RMI scanner
Gamna-Gandy
G.-G. body
G.-G. nodule
G.-G. nodule
Gamna nodule
Gandy-Nanta disease
ganglia (*pl. of* ganglion)
gangliocytic paraganglioma
gangliocytoma
dysplastic cerebellar g.
ganglioglioma
cystic g.
infantile g.
intracerebral g.
gangliolysis
radiofrequency g.
ganglioma
intracerebral g.
ganglion, pl. **ganglia, ganglions**
aberrant g.
acousticofacial g.
Acrel g.
aorticorenal g.
auditory g.
auricular g.
basal g.
calcification of basal g.
cardiac g.
carotid g.
celiac g.
g. cell tumor
cervical g.
cervicothoracic g.
coccygeal g.
diffuse g.
dorsal root g. (DRG)
gasserian g.
geniculate g.
intraarticular g.
intraosseous g.
ipsilateral basal g.
otic g.
palmar g.
paravertebral g.
periosteal g.
petrosal g.
posterior root g.
prevertebral g.
pterygopalatine g.
radiocapitellar joint g.
g. ridge
Scarpa g.
g. of Scarpa
sensory g.
soft tissue g.
sphenopalatine g.
spinal g.
submandibular g.
superior cervical g.
superior mesenteric g.
sympathetic g.
trigeminal g.
uterine cervical g.
vestibular g.
Wrisberg cardiac g.
ganglioneuroblastoma
ganglioneurofibromatosis
mucosal g.
ganglioneuroma
adrenal g.
ganglionic
g. canal
g. crest
g. cyst
ganglions (*pl. of* ganglion)
gangrene
g. gallbladder
g. of lung
gangrenous
g. cholecystitis
g. emphysema
g. pneumonia
g. tissue
Ganser diverticulum

NOTES

gantry
g. angulation
CT scan g.
g. room
g. rotation
g. tilt
Gantzer muscle
Ganz formula for coronary sinus flow
gap
air g.
Bochdalek g.
g. calculation
g. conduction phenomenon
distraction g.
fracture g.
intersection g.
interslice g.
Garcin syndrome
Garden
G. angle
G. femoral neck fracture
G. femoral neck fracture classification
garden spade deformity
Gardner
G. bone syndrome
G. GI tract syndrome
Gardner-Diamond syndrome
Gardray dosimeter
gargoylism
Pfaundler-Hurler g.
Garland
G. brain sign
G. syndrome
G. triad
G. triangle
garland
g. sign
Garn method
Garré
G. disease
sclerosing osteomyelitis of G.
Garren-Edwards gastric bubble (GEG bubble)
Garth view
Gartland classification of humeral supracondylar fracture
Gartner
G. canal
G. duct
G. duct cyst
Gärtner, Gaertner
G. phenomenon
gas, pl. **gases**
abdominal g.
accumulation of g.
aneurysmal wall g.
bile duct g.
biliary tree g.
bowel g.
g. bubble
g. collection
coursing of g.
g. CT cisternography
g. cupula
g. density line
displacement of bowel g.
g. entrapment
extraluminal g.
free intraperitoneal g.
free subphrenic g.
genital tract g.
hyperpolarized ^{129}Xe g.
inhalation of radioactive xenon g.
g. insufflation
intestinal g.
intrahepatic portal vein g.
intramural g.
intrauterine g. (IUG)
natural neon g.
overlying bowel g.
g. pattern
paucity of bowel g.
portal venous g.
pulmonary g.
radiopaque xenon g.
scrotal g.
small bowel g.
soft tissue g.
subcutaneous tissue g.
superimposed bowel g.
g. target
urinary tract g.
g. ventilation imaging
g. ventilation study
g. volume
gas-bloat syndrome
gas-containing
g.-c. gallstone
g.-c. stone
gaseous
g. cholecystitis
g. dilatation
g. distention
g. drainage
g. mediastinography
g. oxygen artifact
gases (*pl. of* gas)
gas-fluid level
gasless abdomen
gas-liquid phase chromatography (GLPC)
gasserian
g. ganglion
g. ganglion tumor
gastral mesoderm

gastrectomy
gastric
g. adenopapillomatosis
g. air bubble
g. antral erosion
g. antrum
g. artery
g. atony
g. atrophy
g. bypass surgery (GBS)
g. canal
g. cancer
g. capacity
g. carcinoma
g. cardia
g. channel
g. chloroma
g. contents
g. decompression
g. diaphragm
g. dilatation
g. distention
g. diverticulum
g. duplication cyst
g. emphysema
g. emptying (GE)
g. emptying imaging
g. emptying scan
g. fistula
g. fold
g. foveola
g. fundus
g. groove
g. hamartomatous polyposis
g. hemic calculus
g. hemorrhage
g. hernia
g. heterotopia
g. hypersecretion
g. impression
g. insufficiency
g. intramural-extramucosal lesion
g. leiomyoma
g. leiomyosarcoma
g. lumen
g. lung
g. lymphatic follicle
g. lymph node
g. lymphoma
g. metastasis
g. motor disorder
g. mucosa imaging
g. mucosal pattern
g. narrowing
g. omentum
g. outlet obstruction
g. outline
g. partition
g. pit
g. plexus
g. pneumatosis
g. polyp
g. pool
g. pouch
g. pseudolymphoma
g. pull-through procedure
g. reflux of bile
g. remnant
g. remnant cancer
g. remnant filling defect
g. residual
g. rugae
g. sclerosis
g. secretion
g. stump
g. stump carcinoma
g. surface
g. transit time
g. transposition
g. ulcer (GU)
g. varix
g. vein
g. volvulus
g. window
g. xanthoma
gastrica
area g.
gastrinoma
duodenal g.
gastritis
acute erosive g. (AEG)
AIDS-related g.
alcoholic g.
antral g.
atrophic g.
bile reflux g.
chronic g.
cirrhotic g.
corrosive g.
emphysematous g.
erosive g.
follicular g.
giant hypertrophic g.
hypertrophic g.

NOTES

gastritis *(continued)*
necrotizing g.
phlegmonous g.
pseudomembranous radiation g.
g. radiation
reflux g.
zonal g.
gastrocardiac syndrome
gastrocnemial ridge
gastrocnemius
g. bursa
g. muscle
gastrocnemius-semimembranosus bursa
gastrocnemius-soleus
g.-s. complex
g.-s. junction
g.-s. muscle group
gastrocnemius/soleus contracture
gastrocolic
g. fistula
g. ligament
g. omentum
gastrocutaneous fistula
gastrodiaphragmatic ligament
gastroduodenal
g. artery
g. artery complex
g. fistula
g. junction
g. lumen
g. lymph node
g. mucosal prolapse
g. orifice
gastroduodenitis
gastroduodenoscopy
gastroduodenostomy
Billroth I, II g.
gastroenteritis
acute g. (AGE)
cobblestone appearance eosinophilic g.
gastroenterocolitis
gastroenterogenous rickets
gastroenteroptosis
gastroenterostomy
percutaneous g.
g. stoma
gastroepiploic
g. arcade
g. artery
g. lymph node
g. vein
g. vessel
gastroesophageal (GE)
g. angle
g. (GE) junction
g. incompetence
g. junction carcinoma
g. junction stricture
g. reflux (GER)
g. reflux disease (GERD)
g. variceal plexus
Gastrografin
G. enema
G. imaging agent
G. swallow
gastrohepatic
g. bare area
g. ligament
g. ligament node
g. omentum
gastrointestinal (GI)
g. adverse effect
g. bleed (GI bleed)
g. bleeding
g. cancer
g. cyst
g. endoscopic ultrasound
g. endoscopy
g. fetal anomaly
g. fistula
g. hemorrhage
g. lymphoma
g. malignancy
g. motility imaging
g. plaque
g. renal transplant hemorrhage
g. scintigraphy
g. series
g. stoma
g. stromal tumor (GIST)
g. syndrome
g. tract (GI tract)
g. tract adenocarcinoma
g. tract obstruction
g. ulcer
upper g. (UGI)
gastrointestinal-associated lymphoid tissue
gastrojejunal
g. mucosal prolapse
gastrojejunocolic fistula
gastrojejunostomy
Billroth I, II g.
gastrolienal ligament
GastroMARK
G. oral contrast medium
G. oral imaging agent
gastroomental lymph node
gastropancreatic
g. fold
g. ligament
gastroparesis
diabetic g.
gastropathy
hyperplastic g.

gastropexy
gastrophrenic ligament
gastroplasty (GP)
Gastroport
gastroptosis
gastroschisis
gastroscope
Pentax EUP-EC124 ultrasound g.
gastroscopy
gastrosphincteric pressure gradient
gastrosplenic
g. ligament
g. omentum
gastrostomy
CT-guided percutaneous endoscopic g.
percutaneous endoscopic g. (PEG)
radiologic percutaneous g.
g. tube
gastrotomy
Gastrovist
G. contrast medium
G. imaging agent
gastrulation
gate array
gated
g. blood pool angiography
g. blood pool scintigraphy
g. blood pool ventriculogram
g. cardiac blood pool imaging
g. 3D reconstruction
g. equilibrium blood pool scanning
g. equilibrium cardiac blood pool imaging
g. equilibrium radionuclide angiography
g. exercise examination
g. imaging study
g. inflow magnetic resonance
g. inflow technique
g. magnetic resonance imaging
g. nuclear angiography
g. nuclear ventriculogram
g. planar study
g. radionuclide angiocardiography
g. radionuclide ventriculogram
g. RNA
g. single-photon emission computed tomography (GSPECT)
g. SPECT myocardial perfusion imaging
g. view
gating
cardiac g.
diastolic g.
echocardiographic g.
electrocardiographic g.
heartbeat g.
peripheral g.
respiratory g.
retrospective g.
systolic g.
Gaucher
G. disease
G. splenomegaly
gauge
gauss
gaussian
g. curve
g. distribution
g. dose-volume histogram
g. function
g. line
g. line saturation
g. mode profile laser beam
g. smoothing
Gavard muscle
Gawkins talar neck fracture classification
Gaynor-Hart
G.-H. method
G.-H. position
GBM
glioblastoma multiforme
glomerular basement membrane
GBS
gallbladder series
gastric bypass surgery
GCT
germ-cell tumor
GCTTS
giant cell tumor of the tendon sheath
GCVF
great cardiac vein flow
Gd
gadolinium
Gd-153 imaging agent
Gd-BOPTA/Dimeg imaging agent
GDC
Guglielmi detachable coil
Gd-CDTA
gadolinium cyclohexanediaminetetraacetic acid

NOTES

Gd-DOTA
gadolinium tetraazacyclododecanetetraacetic acid
Gd-DOTA contrast medium
Gd-DOTA-enhanced subtraction dynamic study
Gd-DTPA
gadolinium-DTPA
gadopentetate dimeglumine
Gd-DTPA radioisotope
Gd-DTPA with mannitol contrast
Gd-DTPA-BMA
Gd-DTPA/Dimeg imaging agent
Gd-DTPA-enhanced turbo FLASH MRI
Gd-DTPA-labeled
G.-D.-l. albumin
G.-D.-l. dextran
Gd-EDTA
gadolinium ethylenediaminetetraacetic acid
Gd-enhanced imaging agent
Gd-EOB-DTPA imaging agent
Gd-FMPSPGR imaging
Gd-HIDA chelate
Gd-HP-DO3A
gadoteridol
Gd-HP-DO3A imaging agent
Gd oxide contrast medium
Gd-Tex
GE
gastric emptying
gastroesophageal
General Electric
GE Advance PET scanner
GE CT Advantage scanner
GE CT Hi-Speed Advantage system
GE CT Max scanner
GE CT Pace scanner
GE 8800 CT/T scanner
GE detector
GE gamma camera
GE Genesis CT scanner
GE GN 500-MHz scanner
GE GN300 7.05-T/89-mm bore multinuclear spectrometer
GE 9800 high-resolution CT scanner
GE HiSpeed Advantage helical CT scanner
GE MR Max scanner
GE MR Signa scanner
GE MR Vectra scanner
GE NMR spectrometer
GE Omega 500-MHz scanner
GE Pace CT scanner
GE QE 300-MHz scanner
GE Signa 5.4 Genesis MR imager
GE Signa 5.5 Horizon EchoSpeed MR imager
GE Signa 4.7 MRI scanner
GE Signa MR system
GE Signa 5.2 scanner
GE Signa 1.5-T magnet
GE Signa 1.5-T scanner
GE Signa 5.2 with SR-230 three-axis EPI gradient upgrade scanner
GE single-axis SR-230 echoplanar scanner
GE single-axis SR-230 echoplanar system
GE single-detector SPECT-capable camera
GE SPECT
GE Spiral CT scanner
GE Starcam single-crystal tomographic scintillation camera
GE 1.5-T system
GE Vectra MR scanner
Gee-Herter disease
Gee-Thaysen disease
GEG bubble
Gehan methodology
Geiger counter
Geiger-Müller (G-M)
G.-M. counter
G.-M. detector
G.-M. tube
gel
acoustic g.
Fricke g.
ultrasound g.
gelatinous
g. ascites
g. brain pseudocyst
g. carcinoma
g. debris
g. hematoma
g. tissue
gelatin phantom
gemellary pregnancy
gemellus, pl. **gemelli**
gemistocytic astrocytoma
gemistocytoma
General Electric (GE)
generalisata
platyspondyly g.
generalized
g. angiofollicular lymph node hyperplasia
g. arteriosclerosis
g. breast hyperplasia
g. calcinosis
g. capillary leak

g. cortical hyperostosis
g. cortical hyperstasis
g. emphysema
g. hamartomatosis
g. increased liver echogenicity
g. interstitial disease
g. lymphadenopathy syndrome
g. lymphangiectasia
g. osteoarthritis
g. pulmonary edema
g. seizure

general pattern matching
generation echo
generator
anterior current (AC) g.
carbone dioxide g.
g. characteristic
CO_2 g.
deuterium-tritium g.
direct current g.
^{166}Dy g.
dysprosium-holmium (^{166}Dy-166Ho) in vivo g.
electric g.
electrostatic g.
extraction g.
high-voltage g.
^{166}Ho in vivo g.
molybdenum-99 g.
molybdenum-technetium g.
nuclide g.
pizoelectric g.
polyphase g.
6-pulse, 3-phase g.
12-pulse, 3-phase g.
radionuclide g.
resonance g.
spark gap g.
supervoltage g.
Triphasix g.
Van de Graaf g.
video signal g.
x-ray g.

generator-produced ^{188}Re
genial
g. tubercle
g. tubercle of mandible

geniculate
g. body
g. branch
g. ganglion
g. ganglion schwannoma

geniculocalcarine tract
geniculocalvarium
geniculostriate tract
geniculum
genioglossus muscle
genital
g. canal
g. carcinoma
g. duct
g. eminence
g. fold
g. groove
g. ligament
g. ridge
g. tract
g. tract calcification
g. tract embryology
g. tract gas

genitalia
ambiguous g.

genitalis
genitoinguinal ligament
genitourinary (GU)
g. adverse effect
g. anomaly
g. cancer
g. fistula
g. injury
g. reflex
g. rhabdomyosarcoma
g. tract
g. tract trauma
g. tuberculosis

Gennari
band of G.
G. band
line of G.
stripe of G.
G. stripe

genomic instability
genu, pl. **genua**
g. recurvatum
g. valgum
g. valgum deformity
g. varum
g. varum deformity

geode
geographic
g. bone destruction
g. follicle
g. lesion

G

NOTES

geographic *(continued)*
g. pattern
g. skull
geography
brain g.
geometric
g. blur
g. distortion
g. distribution
g. optimization algorithm
g. unsharpness
geometry
coronary vessel g.
g. factor
Golay g.
scintillation camera g.
slice g.
geophagia
g. artifact
GER
gastroesophageal reflux
GERD
gastroesophageal reflux disease
Gerdy
G. fontanelle
G. interatrial loop
G. interauricular loop
G. ligament
G. tubercle
G. tubercle in knee
Gerhardt
G. sign
G. triangle
geriatric
g. configuration
g. features
germanate-68
bismuth g.
German horizontal plane
germ-cell tumor (GCT)
germinal
g. bleed matrix
g. pole
germinolysis
subependymal g.
germinoma
intracranial g.
mediastinum g.
multicentric g.
pineal g.
suprasellar hemorrhagic g.
Gerota
G. capsule
G. fascia
G. method
Gerstmann-Straussler-Sheinker disease
Gertzbein
G. classification of seatbelt injury
G. seatbelt injury classification
gestation
extrauterine g.
intrauterine g.
multiple g.
normal g.
triplet g.
gestational
g. age
g. choriocarcinoma
g. nonmetastatic trophoblastic disease
g. sac (GS)
g. sac abnormality
g. sac diameter (GS diameter)
g. sac measurement
g. trophoblastic disease (GTD)
g. trophoblastic neoplasm
g. trophoblastic tumor
geyser sign
GGO
ground-glass opacification
GHA
glucoheptanoic acid
GHCH
giant hepatic cavernous hemangioma
Ghon
G. complex
G. node
G. primary lesion
G. tubercle
Ghon-Sachs complex
ghost
g. image
red cell g.
separation of g.'s (SEP)
g. vertebra
ghosting artifact
GHz
gigahertz
GI
gastrointestinal
GI bleed
Imagent GI
GI tract
GI tract amyloidosis
GI tract endometriosis
GI tract lipoma
GI tract lymphoid hyperplasia
GI tract mastocytosis
GI tract scintigraphy
GI tract trauma
GI tract tuberculosis
giant
g. brain aneurysm
g. breast fibroadenoma

g. bullous emphysema
g. cell adenocarcinoma
g. cell astrocytoma
g. cell carcinoma of thyroid gland
g. cell fibroma
g. cell interstitial pneumonia (GIP)
g. cell lung carcinoma
g. cell monstrocellular sarcoma
g. cell reparative granuloma
g. cell sarcoma
g. cell tumor
g. cell tumor doughnut sign
g. cell tumor of the tendon sheath (GCTTS)
g. colon
g. duodenal ulcer
g. follicle lymphoma
g. follicular hyperplasia
g. gastric fold
g. hepatic cavernous hemangioma (GHCH)
g. hyperplasia lymph node
g. hypertrophic gastritis
g. left atrium
g. limb of Robertson
g. osteoid osteoma
g. peptic ulcer
g. sigmoid diverticulum
g. villous adenoma

giant-cell

Gianturco
G. occlusion coil
G. wool-tufted wire coil

Gianturco-Roubin
G.-R. FlexStent

Gianturco-Wallace-Anderson coil

Gianturco-Wallace-Chuang coil

gibbous deformity

Gibbs
G. phenomenon
G. phenomenon artifact
G. random field
G. sampling

Gibbs-Donnan law

gibbus
thoracic g.

GiCi-400 Invader

Gierke respiratory bundle

gigahertz (GHz)

gigantiform
g. cementoma

gigantism
cerebral g.
extremity g.
focal g.

Gilbert sign

Gilchrist disease

gill
g. arch skeleton
g. cleft
G. lesion

Gillette
G. joint
G. suspensory ligament

Gillies suture

Gimbernat ligament

gingival
g. cancer
g. crest
g. curvature
g. septum
g. space

gingivitis
erosive g.
necrotizing ulcerative g.

gingivobuccal groove

gingivodental ligament

gingivolabial groove

GIP
giant cell interstitial pneumonia

girdle
limb g.
pectoral g.
pelvic g.
shoulder g.

Girdlestone arthroplasty

girth
abdominal g.

Gissane
G. angle
crucial angle of G.

GIST
gastrointestinal stromal tumor

glabella

glabrous cirrhosis

gladiolus

gladiomanubrial

gland
absorbent g.
accessory thyroid g.
admaxillary g.
adrenal g.
Albarran g.

NOTES

gland *(continued)*
alveolar g.
anteprostatic g.
aortic g.
apical g.
apocrine sweat g.
aporic g.
arterial g.
arteriococcygeal g.
axillary sweat g.
Bartholin g.
Brunner g.
bulbocavernous g.
bulbourethral g.
calcified pineal g.
carotid g.
coccygeal g.
Duverney g.
endocrine g.
enlarged thyroid g.
enlargement of lacrimal g.
enlargement of parotid g.
giant cell carcinoma of thyroid g.
globate g.
glomiform g.
haversian g.
hilar g.
interscapular g.
lacrimal g.
Littré g.
lymph g.
mammary g.
Montgomery g.
mucosal g.
ovary g.
pancreas g.
paramediastinal g.
paraurethral g.
parotid g.
periurethral g.
pineal g.
pituitary g.
prostate g.
salivary g.
Stensen g.
subaortic g.
sublingual g.
submandibular g.
submaxillary g.
substernal thyroid g.
supernumerary parathyroid g.
suprarenal g.
testicular g.
thymus g.
thyroid g.
urethral g.
g. volume
Wharton g.

glandular
g. cancer
g. carcinoma
g. proliferation

glans
g. carcinoma
g. penis

glare
imaging chain veiling g.
scatter and veiling g. (SVG)
veiling g.

glaserian fissure

Glasgow sign

glass
g. blower's emphysema
g. eye artifact
hepatic test of G.
quartz g.
g. ray
g. tract detector
vita g.

Glasscock-Jackson classification

glasses
fiberoptic video g.

glaucoma
congenital g.
primary g.

Glazunov tumor

Gleason grade

Glénard disease

Glenn
G. anastomosis
G. shunt

glenohumeral
g. dislocation
g. instability
g. joint
g. ligament

glenoid
g. cavity
g. fossa
g. labral ovoid body
g. labrum
g. labrum capsule
g. labrum injury
g. ligament
g. ovoid mass
g. point
g. process
g. rim
g. rim fracture
g. surface

glial
g. brain tumor
g. disease
g. nodule
g. scarring

g. stranding
g. tumor calcification
Glidewire
long taper/stiff shaft G.
Radiofocus G.
gliding joint
glioblast
glioblastoma
butterfly g.
multicentric g.
g. multiforme (GBM)
glioma
anaplastic cerebral g.
brainstem g.
butterfly g.
cerebral g.
cystic g.
high-grade g.
hypothalamic g.
intracranial g.
low-grade g.
malignant g.
multicentric malignant g.
nonanaplastic g.
optic nerve g.
pathognomonic signthalamic infiltrating g.
pontine g.
pontocerebellar g.
recurrent high-grade malignant g.
rolandoparietal g.
spinal cord g.
supratentorial g.
temporooccipital g.
thalamic g.
gliomatosis
g. cerebri
g. peritonei
glioneural hamartoma
gliosarcoma
cerebellar g.
gliosis
astrocytic g.
ischemic g.
progressive subcortical g.
reactive g.
g. of sylvian aqueduct
gliosis-induced microcystic degeneration
Glisson capsule
global
g. cardiac disease
g. cavus
g. cerebral hypoperfusion
g. cerebral ischemia
g. cortical defect
g. ejection fraction
g. hypokinesis
g. hypometabolism
g. myocardial ischemia
g. renal enlargement
g. tissue loss
g. ventricular function
g. wall motion abnormality
globally depressed ejection fraction
globate gland
globe
optic g.
globe-orbit relationship
globi (*pl. of* globus)
globoid heart
globular
g. cardiomegaly
g. chest
g. configuration
g. meningioma
g. tumor
g. valve
globus, pl. **globi**
g. hystericus
g. major
g. minor
g. pallidus
glomangioma
glomera
choroid g.
glomerular
g. basement membrane (GBM)
g. filtration
g. filtration agent
g. filtration rate
g. lesion
g. nephritis
glomeruli (*pl. of* glomerulus)
glomerulocytoma
glomeruloid formation
glomerulonephritis
acute g.
chronic g.
membranous g.
necrotizing g.
proliferative g.
segmental necrotizing g.
glomerulopathy

NOTES

G

glomerulosa
zona g.
glomerulosclerosis
glomerulus, pl. **glomeruli**
glomiform gland
glomus
body g.
g. body tumor
g. choroideum
g. of choroid plexus
g. jugulare
g. jugulare tumor
g. neck tumor
g. tympanicum
g. vagale
glomus-type arteriovenous malformation
glossectomy
total g.
glossitis, pl. **glossitides**
glossoepiglottic
g. fold
g. ligament
glossopalatine fold
glossopharyngeal nerve
glottic
g. carcinoma
g. larynx
g. narrowing
glottis, pl. **glottides**
glove
optic g.
g. phenomenon
g. phenomenon artifact
radiation-attenuating surgical g.'s
gloved-finger sign
glow curve
GLP7 film
GLPC
gas-liquid phase chromatography
glucagon imaging agent
glucagonoma
glucamoma
Glucarate imaging agent
gluceptate
technetium-99m g.
glucoheptanate
glucoheptanoate
^{99m}Tc g.
technetium-99m glucoheptanoate
technetium-99m g. (^{99m}Tc glucoheptanoate)
glucoheptanoic acid (GHA)
Glucophage
glucose
fluorine-18-labeled g.
g. metabolism
Glukor
glutamate spectroscopy
gluteal
g. bonnet
g. fold
g. line
g. lymph node
g. ridge
gluteus
g. maximus
g. medius
g. minimus
glycerolphosphorylcholine (GPC)
glycogen-rich pancreatic cystadenoma
glycogen storage disease
glycol
polyethylene g.
glycolysis
enhanced g.
glycoprotein-secreting adenoma
G-M
Geiger-Müller
G-M counter
GMN
gradient moment nulling
GMR
gradient moment reduction
gradient moment rephasing
gradient motion rephasing
gnathic osteosarcoma
goblet-shaped pelvis
Godwin tumor
Goethe bone
goiter
adenomatous g.
Basedow g.
colloid g.
congenital g.
cystic g.
diffuse toxic g.
diving g.
exophthalmic g.
familial g.
fetal g.
fibrous g.
intrathoracic g.
iodide g.
iodine-deficiency g.
lingual g.
multinodular g.
nodular g.
parenchymous g.
retrotracheal g.
retrovascular g.
simple g.
substernal g.
suffocative g.
thyroid g.
toxic multinodular g.
toxic nodular g.

vascular g.
wandering g.
goitrous cretinism
Golay
G. coil
G. geometry
gold
colloidal radioactive g.
radioactive g.
g. radioactive source
g. seeds
g. standard
gold-198 (^{198}Au)
g. colloid (^{198}Au colloid)
Goldblatt
G. kidney
G. phenomenon
Golden
motility of G.
S sign of G.
Goldenhar syndrome
golden pneumonia
gold-195m radionuclide
Goldsmith & Woodburne classification
Goldthwait sign
golfer's
g. elbow
g. elbow on disk
golf-hole ureteral orifice
Goll tract
GoLYTELY bowel preparation
Gombault-Philippe tract
gonad
indifferent g.
gonadal
g. artery
g. dose
g. dysgenesis
g. function
g. neoplasm
g. stroma
g. stromal tumor
g. venography
gonadoblastoma
gonadotroph cell adenoma
gonadotropin
chorionic g.
gonadotropin-secreting adenoma
gonial angle
Gonic
goniometer
Sceratti g.
gonion
gonion-gnathion plane
gonorrheic perihepatitis
Goodpasture syndrome
goose foot tendon
gooseneck
g. concept
g. outflow tract deformity
g. shape
g. sign
Gordon
G. knee phenomenon
G. sign
Gordon-Brostrom single-contrast arthrography
Gore-Tex patch
Gorham
G. disease
G. syndrome
Gorham-Stout syndrome
Gorlin
G. formula for aortic valve area
G. formula for mitral valve area
G. method for cardiac output
Gosling pulsatility index
Gosselin fracture
Gosset
spiral band of G.
Gothic arch formation
Gottron sign
Gottschalk staging
gouge defect
Gould Statham pressure transducer
Gouley syndrome
gout
articular g.
tophaceous g.
gouty
g. arthritis
g. arthropathy
g. node
g. tophus
Gowers
G. bundle
G. bundle in cerebellum
G. column
G. fasciculus
G. phenomenon
G. sign
G. syndrome
G. tract

NOTES

G

GP
gastroplasty
GPC
glycerolphosphorylcholine
graafian
g. follicle
g. vesicle
Grace method of ratio of metatarsal length
gracile
g. bone
g. habitus
gracilis
funiculus g.
g. tendon
grade
Gleason g.
histologic g.
Hyams g.
osteoarthritis g.
placental g.
Scharff-Bloom-Richardson g.
g. 1–3 signal intensity
graded
g. compression sonography technique
g. compression ultrasound
g. infusion
gradient
g. acquisition
g. across valve
g. amplifier
g. amplitude
aortic outflow g.
aortic valve g. (AVG)
aortic valve peak instantaneous g.
aortic valve pressure g.
arteriovenous pressure g.
atrioventricular g.
biliary-duodenal pressure g.
bipolar g.
brain-core g.
g. compensation
conjugate g.
coronary perfusion g.
dephasing g.
diastolic g.
discontinuous density g.
g. drive current
duodenobiliary pressure g.
g. echo MR with magnetization transfer
elevated g.
g. encoding
encoding g.
end-diastolic aortic-left ventricular pressure g.
fast PC cine MR sequence with echoplanar g.
Ficoll g.
field g.
flow-encoding g.
frequency-encoded g.
gastrosphincteric pressure g.
hepatic venous pressure g.
holosystolic g.
imaging g.
instantaneous g.
left ventricular outflow pressure g.
linear g.
g. linearity
g. magnetic field
magnetic field g. (MFG)
maximal estimated g.
mean mitral valve g.
mean systolic g.
mitral valve g.
g. moment nulling (GMN)
g. moment reduction (GMR)
g. moment rephasing (GMR)
g. motion rephasing (GMR)
negligible pressure g.
nonisotropic g.
oscillating g.
outflow tract g.
peak diastolic g.
peak instantaneous g.
peak pressure g.
peak right ventricular-right atrial systolic g.
peak systolic g. (PSG)
peak-to-peak pressure g.
peak-to-pressure g.
perfusion g.
phase-encoding g.
portosystemic g.
pressure-flow g.
pullback pressure g.
pulmonary artery to right ventricle diastolic g.
pulmonary outflow g.
pulmonic valve g.
g. pulse
pulsed g.
readout g.
rephasing g.
residual g.
g. reversal
right ventricular to main pulmonary artery pressure g.
g. scheme
g. selection
sensitizing g.
g. sheet coil
slice selection g.

spoiler g.
stenotic g.
subvalvular g.
g. system
systolic g.
thoracoabdominal g.
g. timing
transaortic systolic g.
translesional g.
transmitral g.
transpulmonic g.
transstenotic g.
transtricuspid valve diastolic g.
transvalvular pressure g.
tricuspid valve g.
velocity g.
ventricular g.
washout g.
g. waveform
X g.
Z g.

gradient-echo (GE SPECT)
g.-e. axial image
g.-e. cine technique
g.-e. coronal image
g.-e. flow imaging
g.-e. imaging sequence
magnetization prepared 3D g.-e.
g.-e. method
g.-e. MR imaging
g.-e. phase imaging
g.-e. pulse sequence
g.-e. recall technique
g.-e. sequence imaging
g.-e. three-dimensional Fourier transform volume imaging

gradient-echo-phase image
gradient-encoded image
gradient-induced phase dispersion
gradient-recalled
g.-r. acquisition in a steady state (GRASS)
g.-r. echo (GRE)
g.-r. echo image

gradient-refocused echo (GRE)
gradient-reversal fat suppression method
gradient-to-noise imaging
graft
aortic g.
aorticorenal g.
aortic tube g.
aortofemoral bypass g.
aortoiliac bypass g.
aortoplasty with patch g.
arterial bypass g.
autogenous vein bypass g.
autologous patch g.
autologous vein g.
axillary-axillary bypass g.
axillary-brachial bypass g.
axillary-femoral bypass g.
axillary-femorofemoral bypass g.
axillobifemoral bypass g.
bifemoral g.
bifurcation g.
bilateral myocutaneous g.
bone g.
bone-tendon-bone g.
Brescia-Cimino g.
bypass g.
carotid-carotid venous bypass g.
coronary artery bypass g.
Dacron covered stent g.
donor g.
endarterectomy and coronary artery bypass g.
endothelialized vascular g.
endovascular aortic g.
expanded polytetrafluoroethylene (e-PTFE) g.
extracavitary infected g.
extracavitary prosthetic arterial g.
g. failure
femorocrural g.
femorodistal popliteal bypass g.
femorofemoral bypass g.
femoroperoneal in situ vein bypass g.
femoropopliteal bypass g.
femoropopliteal Gore-Tex g.
femorotibial bypass g.
H g.
hepatorenal saphenous vein bypass g.
iliac-renal bypass g.
ilioprofunda bypass g.
infected thrombosed g.
infrainguinal vein bypass g.
inlay g.
interbody bone g.
internal thoracic artery g.
interposition g.
g. interstice
intraabdominal arterial bypass g.

G

NOTES

graft *(continued)*
ITA g.
jump vein g.
g. kinking
limb of bifurcation g.
loop g.
occluded g.
g. occlusion
onlay g.
osseous g.
g. patency
patency of vein g.
pedicle bone g.
polytetrafluoroethylene (PTFE) g.
prosthetic femoral distal g.
g. rejection
g. revascularization
reversed vein g.
g. roof impingement
saphenous vein g.
saphenous vein bypass g.
Sauvage filamentous velour g.
sequence bypass g.
g. shrinkage
in situ g.
snake g.
splenorenal arterial bypass g.
g. stenosis
straight interposition g.
subcutaneous arterial bypass g.
suprailiac aortic mesenteric g.
synthetic vascular bypass g.
transluminally placed stented g.
Varivas loop g.
vascular bypass g.
vein g.
venous interposition g.

graft-enteric
g.-e. erosion
g.-e. fistula

Graham-Burford-Mayer syndrome

Graham-Cole
G.-C. cholecystogram
G.-C. test

grain handler's lung

graininess
film g.

Grancher
G. sign
G. triad

grand mal seizure

Grandy method

Granger
G. line
G. projection
G. view

Grantham
G. classification of femoral fracture
G. femur fracture classification

granular
g. breast-cell myoblastoma
g. kidney
g. lung-cell myoblastoma
g. sella-cell myoblastoma

granularis
ependymitis g.

granulation
arachnoid g.
pacchionian g.
g. stenosis
g. tissue

granulocyte
antibody-labeled circulating g.

granulocytopenia
febrile g.

granuloma, pl. **granulomata**
actinic g.
apical g.
beryllium g.
bilharzial g.
button sequestrum eosinophilic g.
calcified g.
ceroid gallbladder g.
cholesterol ear g.
coalescent g.
dental g.
eosinophilic g.
epithelioid g.
extravascular g.
fishtank g.
foreign body g.
frontoethmoidal giant cell reparative g.
giant cell reparative g.
Hodgkin g.
hyalinizing g.
inguinal g.
lethal midline g.
lung g.
g. lung
malarial g.
mediastinal g.
midline g.
Mignon g.
miliary g.
noncaseating g.
paracoccidioidal g.
periapical g.
pseudopyogenic g.
pulmonary hyalinizing g.
reparative giant cell g.
reticulohistiocytic g.
rheumatic g.
root end g.

sarcoid g.
sea urchin g.
silicotic g.
sperm g.
stellate g.
swimming pool g.
thorium dioxide g.
tuberculous g.
umbilical g.
xanthomatous g.
zirconium g.

granulomatosis
allergic g.
bronchocentric g.
limited Wegener g.
lymphomatoid g.
mainline g.
Miescher g.
necrotizing respiratory g.
organic g.
pulmonary mainline g.
Wegener g.

granulomatous
g. brain abscess
g. enterocolitis
g. ileitis
g. inflammation of bronchus
g. lesion of sinus
g. lymphoma
g. pneumonia
g. pneumonitis
subacute g.
g. transmural colitis
g. uveitis

granulomonocyte
granulomonocytic
granulosa
g. cell carcinoma
pyoderma g.

granulosa-theca cell tumor
granulovacuolar degeneration
grape
Carswell g.

grape-like vesicle
grape-skin lung cavity
graph
spin-phase g.

graphite fibrosis of lung
Graser diverticulum
Grashey
G. method
G. position
G. shoulder view

grasping technique
GRASS
gradient-recalled acquisition in a steady state
GRASS MR imaging
GRASS pulse sequence
spoiled GRASS (SPGR)

Gratiolet convolution
Graupner method
gravel
gallbladder g.

Graves
G. orbital disease
G. thyroid disease

gravida
gravidarum
fibroma molle g.

gravid uterus
gravis
colitis ulcerosa g.
myasthenia g.

gravitational
g. edema
g. potential energy

Grawitz tumor
gray (Gy)
g. commissure
g. hepatization stage of pneumonia
g. horns in spinal canal
g. lung
g. matter
g. matter abnormality
g. matter degeneration
g. matter heterotopia
g. radiation absorbed dose (Gy rad)
g. reticular
g. scale
g. unit
g. to white matter activity ratio
g. to white matter utilization ratio

gray-bone-cortex sign
gray-level
g.-l. histogram
g.-l. spacing
g.-l. thresholding

gray-scale
g.-s. Doppler
g.-s. examination
g.-s. image
g.-s. imaging

NOTES

gray-scale *(continued)*
g.-s. range
g.-s. sonography
g.-s. ultrasonography
g.-s. ultrasound
Grayson ligament
gray-white
g.-w. differentiation
g.-w. matter contrast ratio
g.-w. matter junction
gray/white matter interface
GRE
gradient-recalled echo
gradient-refocused echo
GRE breath-hold hepatic imaging
GRE gadolinium-chelate enhanced imaging
GRE magnetic resonance imaging
great
g. cardiac plexus
g. cardiac vein
g. cardiac vein flow (GCVF)
g. cerebral vein of Galen
g. cerebral vein of Galen aneurysm
g. cistern
g. sacrosciatic foramen
g. toe sesamoid bone
g. vein of cerebrum
g. vessels
g. vessel transposition
greater
g. arc injury
g. circulation
g. curvature of stomach
g. curvature ulcer
g. multangular bone
g. multangular ridge
g. omentum
g. palatine canal
g. palatine foramen
g. pelvis
g. peritoneal sac
g. petrosal
g. sac of peritoneal cavity
g. saphenous system
g. saphenous vein
g. sciatic foramen
g. sciatic notch
g. sigmoid notch
g. sphenoid wing
g. superficial petrosal nerve
g. trochanter
g. trochanter of femur
g. trochanteric femoral fracture
g. tubercle
g. tuberosity
g. tuberosity fracture
green
indocyanine g.
Greene
G. biopsy set
G. sign
Greenfield
G. filter
G. vena cava filter system
Green-Joynt sign
greenstick
g. fracture
GRE-in
G.-i. image
G.-i. imaging
grenade thrower's fracture
grenz ray
GRE-out
G.-o. image
G.-o. imaging
Greulich
G. and Pyle atlas
G. and Pyle bone age standard
G. and Pyle skeletal maturation staging
Grey Turner sign
grid
crosshatch g.
g. film
focused g.
localization g.
Lysholm g.
megavoltage g.
oscillating g.
g. ratio
g. technique
g. therapy
Griesinger sign
griffe
simian g.
Griffith point
Grisel syndrome
Grocco sign
Grocott methenamine silver
groin
g. dissection
g. hit
g. mass
groove
alveolingual g.
alveolobuccal g.
alveololabial g.
anal intersphincteric g.
anterior interventricular g.
anterolateral g.
anteromedian g.
arterial g.
atrioventricular g.
auriculoventricular g.

basilar g.
bicipital g.
bronchial g.
buccal g.
carotid g.
carpal g.
caudothalamic g.
cavernous g.
central g.
chiasmatic g.
coronary g.
costal g.
deltopectoral g.
dental g.
developmental g.
digastric g.
esophageal g.
ethmoidal g.
gastric g.
genital g.
gingivobuccal g.
gingivolabial g.
Harrison g.
infraorbital g.
interatrial g.
intercollicular g.
intercondylar g.
intertubercular g.
interventricular g.
labial g.
lacrimal g.
Liebermeister g.
meningeal artery g.
middle meningeal artery g.
neural g.
paravertebral g.
patellar g.
posterior interventricular g.
radial neck g.
Ranvier g.
sagittal g.
Sibson g.
spindle colonic g.
supraorbital g. (SOG)
trochlear g.
trochleocapitellar g.
ulnar g.
urethral g.
venous g.
Verga lacrimal g.
vertebral g.
Waterston g.

grooved director

grooving of articular surface

gross

g. fracture
g. lesion
g. tumor
g. tumor volume (GTV)

Grossman

G. principle
G. scale for regurgitation
G. sign

ground

g. plate
g. state

ground-glass

g.-g. attenuation
g.-g. definition
g.-g. density
g.-g. infiltrate
g.-g. opacification (GGO)
g.-g. opacity
g.-g. osteoporosis
g.-g. ovary pattern
g.-g. pattern

group

Dodd perforating vein g.
extensor-supinator g.
flexor pronator muscle g.
gastrocnemius-soleus muscle g.
interosseous muscle g.
iodinated tyrosine g.
g. viewing

growth

g. acceleration
g. arrest line
g. center of bone
g. center closure
g. disk
ectopic bone g.
epiphyseal chondroblastic g.
g. factor
g. hormone-producing adenoma
g. impairment
lepidic g.
morphologic g.
nutrient artery g.
papillomatous g.
g. parameter
g. plate
g. plate abscess
g. plate arrest
g. plate complex

NOTES

G

growth *(continued)*
g. plate fracture
g. plate injury
g. plate widening
g. retardation
spinal g.
targetoid g.
twin pregnancy discordant g.
Virchow law of skull g.
growth-retarded fetus
Gruber
G. fossa
G. suture
grumous
g. debris
g. tissue
Grüntzig, Gruentzig
G. PTCA technique
Grynfeltt triangle
GS
gestational sac
GS diameter
GSA imaging agent
Gsell-Erdheim syndrome
GSPECT
gated single-photon emission computed tomography
GSW
gunshot wound
GSWH
gunshot wound to head
GTD
gestational trophoblastic disease
GTF-A
Olympus Gastrocamera G.-A.
GTV
gross tumor volume
GU
gastric ulcer
genitourinary
GU tract cholesteatoma
GU tract tuberculosis
guarding sign
gubernacular canal
gubernaculi
pars infravaginalis g.
Gubler
G. line
G. tumor
Guenzberg (*var. of* Günzberg)
Guérin
G. fold
G. fracture
G. sinus
Guglielmi detachable coil (GDC)
guidance
active biplanar MR imaging g.
angioscopic g.
biplanar MR imaging g.
computerized tomography g.
fluoroscopic g.
frameless stereotactic g.
indirect ultrasound g.
mammographic g.
radiologic g.
sonographic g.
g. system selection
ultrasonic g.
guide
CT stereotactic g.
guided
g. biopsy
g. coaxial balloon catheter system
g. drainage
guideline
MIR g.'s
string g.
guide wire, guidewire
angiographic g. w.
basket g. w.
g. w. entrapment
g. w. exchange technique
extra-stiff g. w.
hydrophilic g. w.
open-ended g. w.
Terumo g. w.
through-and-through g. w.
tip-deflecting g. w.
torque control g. w.
torsional attenuating diameter g. w.
Wholey steerable g. w.
guiding
g. sheath
g. shot
Guillain-Barré syndrome
Guilland sign
guillotine rib
guilt screen
Gull disease
Gumley seatbelt injury classification
gumma, pl. **gummas, gummata**
g. of rib
gun
electron g.
Gunn crossing sign
gunshot
g. fracture
g. wound (GSW)
g. wound to head (GSWH)
Gunson method
gunstock deformity
Günzberg, Guenzberg
G. ligament
Gustilo-Anderson
G.-A. open clavicular fracture

G.-A. tibial plafond fracture classification

gut

aging g.
blind g.
g. edema
large g.
primitive g.
g. signature
small g.

gut-associated lymphoid tissue (GALT)

Guthrie muscle

gutter

g. fracture
lateral g.
left g.
paracolic g.
parapelvic g.
paravertebral g.
peritoneal g.
right g.
sacral g.
synovial g.

Guyon canal

Gy

gray
Gy rad

gymnast's wrist

gynecoid pelvis

gynecologic endometriosis

gynecomastia

gynecophoric canal

gyral

g. brain enhancement
g. crest
g. infarct

gyration

Gyratome

gyri (*pl. of* gyrus)

gyriform

g. calcification
g. pattern

gyromagnetic ratio

Gyroscan

G. S15 scanner

gyrus, pl. **gyri**

angular g. (AG)
annectant g.
ascending parietal g.
Broca g.
callosal g.
central g.
g. cerebelli
gyri cerebri
cingulate g.
g. cinguli
contiguous supramarginal g.
dentate g.
fasciolar g.
first temporal g.
flattening of g.
frontal g.
fusiform g.
Heschl transverse g.
hippocampal g.
g. hippocampi
inferior frontal g.
inferior temporal g.
infracalcarine g.
insular g.
g. isthmus fornicatus
lamination of g.
lateral occipitotemporal g.
lingual g.
marginal g.
medial occipitotemporal g.
middle frontal g.
middle temporal g.
occipital g.
occipitotemporal g.
olfactory g.
orbital g.
paracentral g.
parahippocampal g.
paraterminal g.
parietal g.
postcentral g.
posterior central g.
precentral g.
preinsular g.
quadrate g.
g. recti
short insular g.
subcallosal g.
subcollateral g.
superior frontal g.
superior parietal lobule g.
superior temporal g.
supracallosal g.
supramarginal g.
temporal g.
transverse temporal g.
Turner marginal g.
uncal g.

NOTES

gyrus *(continued)*
uncinate g.

H
Hauch
henry
Holzknecht unit
hydrogen
H band
H and D curve
H disk
H field of Forel
H graft
H rays
H1
halistatin-1
H1 imaging agent
H-1
H. MR spectroscopic imaging
H. MR spectroscopy
hν
photon
Haas
H. method
H. position
habenula
habenular commissure calcification
habenulopeduncular tract
habitus
body h.
gracile h.
large h.
twisted body h.
HADD
hydroxyapatite deposition disease
Hadlock table
hadron therapy
HAEC
Hirschsprung-associated enterocolitis
Haeckerman area
Hageman factor (HF)
Hagie pin
HAGL
humeral avulsion of the glenohumeral ligament
Haglund deformity
Hagner disease
Hahn
H. cleft
H. spin echo
Hahnemann University Hospital technique
Hahn-Steinthal
H.-S. capitellum fracture classification
H.-S. fracture
HAI
hepatic arterial infusion
Haifa camera
Haines-McDougall medial sesamoid ligament
hairbrush pattern
hairline
h. crack
h. fracture
hair-on-end periosteal reaction
hair-on-end of skull
hairpin
h. technique
h. vessel
hair-standing-on-end appearance
hairy heart
Hajdu-Cheney
H.-C. disease
H.-C. syndrome
Hale-Denver sign
Hale syndrome
half
h. axial view
h. Nex imaging
h. ring
half-axial projection
half-body radiation therapy
half-Fourier
h.-F. acquisition single-shot turbo spin echo magnetic resonance cholangiogram (HASTE MR cholangiogram)
h.-F. imaging (HFI)
h.-F. three-dimensional technique
h.-F. transformation technique
half-Fourier acquisition single-shot turbo-spin echo (HASTE)
half-intensity needle
half-life (HL)
antibody h.-l.
biologic h.-l.
effective h.-l.
elimination h.-l.
h.-l. layer
physical h.-l.
radioactive h.-l.
short h.-l.
half-maximum
full-width at h.-m.
half-moon
h. m. artifact
h.-m. patella
h.-m. shape
half-scan (HS)
h.-s. with extrapolation (HE)
h.-s. with extrapolation method
h.-s. with extrapolation projection

half-time
blood clearance h.-t.
clearance h.-t.
pressure h.-t.
halftone
h. banding
h. frequency
halftoning
iterative h.
half-value layer (HVL)
half-wedged field technique
halistatin-1 (H1)
h. imaging agent (H1 imaging agent)
Hallermann-Streiff-François syndrome
hallmark
radiofrequency radiographic h.
Hall sign
hallucal pronation
hallucis
adductor h.
hyperdynamic abductor h.
hallus abductovalgus deformity
hallux
h. abductovalgus
h. dorsiflexion angle (DFA)
h. elevatus
h. extensus
h. flexus deformity
h. interphalangeal joint
h. interphalangeus angle
intrinsic minus h.
h. limitus (HL)
h. malleus deformity
h. migration
h. rigidus
h. rigidus deformity
h. saltans
h. sesamoid bone
h. valgus (HV)
h. valgus angle (HVA)
h. valgus deformity
h. valgus interphalangeus angle
h. valgus-metatarsus primus varus complex
h. varus
h. varus deformity
halo
h. cast
h. crown
h. device
h. effect
fatty h.
hypoechoic h.
lucent h.
perinuclear h.
periventricular h.
h. ring
h. sign
h. sign of hydrops
sonolucent h.
subendometrial h.
h. vest
halogenated
h. pyrimidine
h. thymidine analog
h. thymidine analog radiosensitizer
hamartoma, pl. **hamartomata**
angiomatous lymphoid h.
astrocytic h.
benign fetal h.
bile duct multiple h.
breast h.
cardiac h.
cartilaginous h.
chest wall h.
chondromatous h.
CNS cortical h.
duodenal wall h.
eccrine angiomatous h.
extracerebral intracranial glioneural h.
fetal renal h.
fibrolipomatous nerve h.
fibrous h.
glioneural h.
hypothalamic h.
leiomyomatous kidney h.
lung h.
h. lung
lymphoid h.
mesenchymal liver h.
multiple bile duct hamartomas
myoid h.
pancreatic h.
pigmented iris h.
pulmonary h.
renal h.
retrorectal cystic h.
h. spleen
splenic h.
subcortical CNS h.
subependymal h.
tuber cinereum h.
vascular h.
ventromedial hypothalamic h.
hamartomatosis
generalized h.
hamartomatous
h. gastric polyp
h. lesion
hamate
h. arthritis
h. bone
h. facet

flake fracture of h.
h. tail fracture
hamburger vertebra
Hamiltonian equation
Hamilton-Stewart formula for measuring cardiac output
Hamman pneumopericardium sign
Hamman-Rich syndrome
hammered
h. brass appearance
h. silver appearance
h. silver skull
hammer-marked skull
hammertoe deformity
hammocking
h. of mitral valve leaflet
h. of valve
hammock ligament
hammock-like posterior bowing of mitral valve
Hampton
H. hump
H. line
H. maneuver
H. technique
H. view
hamstring
h. tendon
hamulus
pterygoideus h.
hand
apelike h.
h. arthritis scleroderma
bear's paw h.
bipenniform muscles of h.
Breuerton x-ray view of h.
chiasm of digits of h.
Cleland ligament in the h.
CPPD arthritis of the h.
digital artery of h.
flipper h.
h. fracture
hypothenar muscle groups of h.
h. injection
h. injection of contrast medium
opera-glass h.
h. osteoarthritis
phalanges of h.
spadelike h.
tangential layer of h.
trident h.
ulnar h.
vaginal ligament of h.
windswept h.
hand-agitated imaging agent
hand-foot syndrome
hand-held
h.-h. exploring electrode probe
h.-h. mapping probe
hand-instilled contrast material
handle
Amplatz radiolucent h.
hand-shaped bend
hand/wrist arthritis
hangers
film h.
hanging
h. fruit pattern
h. heart
h. hip
hanging-block technique
hangman's fracture
Hannover canal
Hanot cirrhosis
Hansen
H. classification of fractures
H. fracture classification
HAP
hepatic arterial phase
Hapad metatarsal arch
HAPE
high-altitude pulmonary edema
Harbitz-Mueller syndrome
HARC-C wavelet compression technique
hard
h. disk
h. disk herniation
h. metal disease
h. palate
h. palate cancer
h. papilloma
h. ray
hard-copy image
hardened
h. lung
h. pelvis
hardening
beam h.
bone h.
Hardy-Clapham
H.-C. classification of sesamoid bone
H.-C. sesamoid classification
Hardy-Vezine classification system

NOTES

H

Harkavy syndrome
harlequin eye sign
harmonic
h. field
h. function
h. imaging
harness
Pavlik h.
Harrington rod
Harris
H. band
H. flush enema
H. line
H. view
Harris-Beath axial hindfoot view
Harrison
H. groove
H. sulcus
Harrison-Stubbs method
HART
hyperfractionated accelerated radiation therapy
Hartmann
H. closure of rectum
H. point
H. pouch
Hart sign
harvested vein
harvester's lung
HASTE
half-Fourier acquisition single-shot turbo-spin echo
HASTE MR cholangiogram
Hatcher-Smith cervical fusion
hatchet
h. defect
h. sign
hatchet-head deformity
Hatle method to calculate mitral valve area
Hatt method
HAT-transformed imaging
Hauch (H)
Haudek niche
haunch bone
Hausdorff
H. error
H. metric measure
H. metric measurement
haustra (*pl. of* haustrum)
haustral
h. blunting
h. fold
h. indentation
h. markings
h. pattern
h. pouch
haustration
haustrum, pl. **haustra**
haustra coli
colonic haustra
haversian
h. canal
h. canaliculus
h. channel
h. fat pad
h. gland
Hawkins
H. accordion-type empyema
H. breast lesion localization needle
H. classification of talar fractures
H. inside-out nephrostomy set
H. inside-out nephrostomy technique
H. line
H. method
H. needle
H. one-stick needle
H. single-stick technique
Hawkins-Akins needle
Hayem-Widal syndrome
hay-fork sign
Haygarth node
hazard
sandbag h.
haze
hilar h.
hazy
h. density
h. infiltrate
HBCT
helical biphasic contrast-enhanced CT
HBCT imaging
H-benzapine imaging agent
HBI
hemibody irradiation
HC
head circumference
Huntington chorea
HC/AC ratio
HCC
hepatocellular carcinoma
HCM
hypertrophic cardiomyopathy
HCS
hematocystic spot
HCTA
helical computed tomographic angiography
H and D
Hurter and Driffield
HDI
high-definition imaging
HDI 5000 ultrasound imaging system

HDI 1000 ultrasound system
HDI 3000 ultrasound system

HDIC
hepatodiaphragmatic interposition of colon

HDR
high-dose rate

HE
half-scan with extrapolation

^{3}He
helium-3

^{4}He
helium-4

head
h. of barium column
cartilaginous cap of phalangeal h.
h. of the caudate nucleus
h. cheese sign
h. circumference (HC)
h. circumference to abdominal circumference ratio (HC/AC ratio)
circumference of fetal h.
h. coil
femoral h.
h. of femur
first metatarsal h. (FMH)
forward positioning of h.
gunshot wound to h. (GSWH)
h. of the humerus
h. injury (HI)
ischemic necrosis of femoral h. (INFH)
large fetal h.
long h.
metatarsal h.
MRI probe h.
h. and neck cancer
h. of the pancreas
pancreatic h.
radial h.
radial facing of metacarpal h.'s
h. of rib
h. shape
short h.
strawberry-shaped h.
terminal h.
transillumination of h.
h. trauma
ulnar h.
ulnar facing of metacarpal h.'s
ureter cobra h.

head-splitting humeral fracture

Heaf test

healing
bony h.
h. flare response
h. fracture
h. infarct
resorption phase of h.
h. ulcer

Health
Bureau of Radiological H. (BRH)

health physics

heart
abdominal h.
admixture lesion of h.
air-driven artificial h.
alcoholic h.
h. amyloidosis
angioreticuloendothelioma of h.
angiosarcoma of h.
h. anomaly
anterior border of h.
aortic opening of h.
apex of the h.
apical surface of h.
armored h.
artificial h.
h. asynchrony
athlete's h.
h. attack
axis of h.
balloon-shaped h.
base of h.
Baylor total artificial h.
beer h.
beriberi h.
h. block
boat-shaped h.
bony h.
booster h.
boot-shaped h.
h. border
bovine h.
bread-and-butter h.
bulb of h.
h. bulb
cardiogenic shock h.
cervical h.
chamber of h.
chaotic h.
cloudy swelling of h.
conical h.
coronary artery of h.

NOTES

H

heart *(continued)*
crisscross h.
h. decortication
degeneration of h.
h. degeneration
dextroversion of h.
diaphragmatic surface of h.
h. disease
dome-shaped h.
donor h.
double density h.
drop h.
dynamite h.
dysrhythmia of fetal h.
egg-on-its-side h.
elongated h.
empty h.
encased h.
enlarged h.
h. failure (HF)
fatty h.
fetal h.
fibroid h.
h. fibroma
fibroma of h.
flabby h.
flask-shaped h.
globoid h.
h. and great vessels
hairy h.
hanging h.
holiday h.
Holmes h.
horizontal h.
hyperdynamic h.
hyperkinetic h.
hyperthyroid h.
hypertrophied h.
hypokinesis of h.
hypoplastic right h.
hypothermic h.
inferior border of h.
inflammation of h.
intermediate h.
irritable h.
ischemic h.
left h.
left border of h.
left ventricle of h.
L-loop h.
h. and lung transplantation
luxus h.
h. lymphoma
lymphosarcoma of h.
malpositioned h.
massively enlarged h.
mesoversion of h.
mildly enlarged h.
movable h.
h. muscle necrosis
myxedema of h.
myxoma of h.
h. myxoma
one-ventricle h.
ovoid h.
ox h.
paracorporeal h.
parasternal view of h.
parchment h.
pear-shaped h.
pectoral h.
pendulous h.
h. position
posterior border of h.
h. power failure
h. pseudoaneurysm
pulmonary h.
Quain fatty degeneration of h.
h. rate reserve mechanism
h. remnant
resting h.
rhabdomyoma of h.
h. rhabdomyoma
right h.
right border of h.
right ventricle of h.
round h.
sabot h.
h. sac
h. scintigraphy
semihorizontal h.
semivertical h.
shoulder of h.
h. silhouette
single-outlet h.
snowman appearance of h.
soldier's h.
h. sounds
spastic h.
squared-off h.
sternocostal surface of h.
stone h.
h. stress test
h. stroke volume
superior border of h.
superoinferior h.
suspended h.
swinging h.
systemic h.
h. tamponade
Taussig-Bing congenital malformation of h.
teardrop h.
three-chambered h.
thrush breast h.
thymoma of h.

tiger h.
tiger lily h.
tobacco h.
total artificial h. (TAH)
h. transplant
transverse h.
Traube h.
triatrial h.
trilocular h.
h. tumor
univentricular h.
upstairs-downstairs h.
h. valve
h. valve calcification
h. valve leaflet
h. valve vegetation
venous h.
venting of h.
vertical h.
wandering h.
water-bottle h.

heartbeat gating
heart-lung transplant
heart-shaped
h.-s. collimator
h.-s. pelvis
h.-s. uterus
heart-to-background ratio
heart-to-lung ratio (HLR)
heat
h. fracture
h. unit (H.U.)
heat-damaged Tc-RBC
heater
resistance wire h.
heat-generating source
heating
gamma h.
hot-source h.
interstitial conductive h.
nonablative h.
ohmic h.
heave
h. and lift
sustained left ventricular h.
heavily penetrated view
heaving precordial motion
heavy
h. charged particle
h. hydrogen
h. ion medical accelerator in Chiba (HIMAC)
h. metal injection
h. water
heavy-charged particle Bragg peak radiosurgery
heavy-particle irradiation
Heberden
H. disease
H. node
H. sign
Hecht pneumonia
Heckathorn disease
Hector
tendon of H.
186-HEDP
rhenium 186-HEDP
Hedspa imaging agent
heel
black-dot h.
h. bone
h. effect
h. fat pad
h. pad thickening
Sorbol h.
h. spur
h. tendon
valgus h.
varus h.
Heerfordt syndrome
Hegglin syndrome
Heidenhain pouch
height
disk space h.
h. of vertebral body
Heim-Kreysig sign
Heineke-Mikulicz maneuver
Heinig view
Heister
valve of H.
Helbing sign
helical
h. biphasic computed tomography (HBCT imaging)
h. biphasic contrast-enhanced CT (HBCT)
h. computed tomographic angiography (HCTA)
h. computed tomography
h. CT holography
h. CT scanner
h. pattern
h. thin-section CT
h. thin-section CT scan

NOTES

helicine artery
Helios
H. diagnostic imaging
H. laser system
helium
hyperpolarized h.
h. ion beam
helium-3 (^{3}He)
helium-4 (^{4}He)
helium-cadmium laser
helium-filled balloon catheter
Helix
H. camera
H. multihead nuclear imaging system
helix
h. filter
helmet
collimator h.
h. field
Helmholtz
H. axis ligament
H. coil
H. configuration
helminthoma
heloma
h. durum
h. molle
Helweg tract
hemal
h. arch
h. canal
h. node
hemangioblastoma
capillary h.
cerebelloretinal h.
craniospinal h.
cystic h.
third ventricular h.
hemangioblastomatosis
cerebelloretinal h.
hemangioendothelial
h. bone
h. bone sarcoma
h. liver sarcoma
hemangioendothelioma
epithelioid h.
infantile h.
malignant h.
osseous h.
hemangioepithelioma
hemangiofibroma
hemangiolymphangioma
hemangioma, pl. **hemangiomata**
arteriovenous h.
bone capillary h.
brain calcification h.
capillary h.
cardiac h.
cavernous brain h.
choroidal h.
epidural cavernous h.
epithelioid h.
extraaxial cavernous h.
extramedullary h.
extremity h.
facial h.
giant hepatic cavernous h. (GHCH)
hepatic h.
infantile hepatic h.
intraarticular h.
intramuscular h.
liver capillary h.
lung h.
orbital h.
orbital capillary h.
osseous h.
pediatric h.
small bowel h.
soft tissue h.
splenic h.
subcutaneous h.
subglottic h.
synovial h.
trigeminal h.
umbilical cord h.
urinary bladder h.
vascular h.
venous h.
verrucous h.
hemangiomatosis
pulmonary capillary h.
hemangiopericytoma
meningeal h.
renal h.
hemangiosarcoma
liver h.
hemarthrosis
hematocele
scrotal h.
hematocystic spot (HCS)
hematogenous
h. embolus
h. osteomalacia
h. tuberculosis
hematologic parameter
hematoma
acute intramural h.
acute subdural h.
adrenal h.
h. of aneurysm
aneurysmal h.
axillary h.
balancing subdural h.
basal ganglia h.
bladder flap h.

bowel wall h.
brain h.
breast h.
carotid plaque h.
chronic subdural h. (CSDH)
corpus luteum h.
delayed traumatic intracerebral h. (DTICH)
dissecting aortic h.
dissecting intramural h.
dural h.
encapsulated subdural h.
epidural h. (EDH)
evolving h.
extracerebral h.
extradural brain h.
h. formation
gelatinous h.
hemispheral h.
infected pelvic h.
interhemispheric subdural h.
intermuscular h.
interstitial loculated h.
intracerebral h.
intracranial h.
intramural h.
intraparenchymal h.
intrarenal h.
intraventricular h.
isodense subdural h.
mediastinal h.
mural h.
nasal septum h.
nasopharyngeal h.
organized h.
parenchymal h.
perianal h.
periaortic mediastinal h.
pericardial h.
peridiaphragmatic h.
perigraft h.
perinephric h.
perirenal h.
posterior fossa h.
postoperative breast h.
primary intracerebral h.
rectal sheath h.
retromembranous h.
retroperitoneal h.
retropharyngeal h.
retroplacental h.
scalp h.
spontaneous h.
subacute subdural h.
subcapsular renal h.
subchorionic h.
subdural interhemispheric h.
subfascial h.
subgaleal h.
submembranous placental h.
subperiosteal h.
umbilical cord h.

hematomediastinum

hematopericardium

hematopoietically active bone marrow

hematopoietic reticulum

HemeSelect

hemiagenesis

hemianopsia
altitudinal h.

hemiarch

hemiatrophy
cerebral h.

hemiaxial view

hemiazygos vein

hemiblock
left anterosuperior h. (LASH)
left bundle branch h.

hemibody irradiation (HBI)

hemicardium

hemic calculus

hemicolon

hemicondylar fracture

hemicranium

hemidecortication
cerebral h.

hemidesmosome

hemidiaphragm
accessory h.
attenuation by h.
h. attenuation
h. depression
h. rupture
tenting of h.

hemidiaphragmatic

hemifacial
h. microsomia
h. spasm

hemiglossectomy

hemihypertrophy

hemilingual paresis

hemimandibulectomy

hemimeganencephaly

hemimelia

NOTES

H

hemimelica
dysplasia epiphysealis h.
hemimyelocele
hemiparesis
residual h.
hemiparkinsonism
hemipelvectomy
hemipelvis
hemiplegia
congenital h.
infantile h.
spinal h.
hemiscrotum
hemisection
spinal cord h.
h. of spinal cord
hemisensory syndrome
hemispheral
h. hematoma
h. mass effect
hemisphere
h. atrophy
cerebellar h.
cerebral h.
h. damage
diffusely swollen h.
dominant h.
left h.
h. lesion
mesial h.
right h.
h. stroke
swollen brain h.
hemispheric
h. infarct
h. vein
hemithorax, pl. **hemithoraces**
frozen h.
opacification of h.
h. opacification
hemithyroidectomy
hemitransverse fracture
hemitruncus
hemivertebra
balanced h.
unbalanced h.
hemivertebral
hemizygosity
HemoCue photometer
hemodynamic
h. alteration
h. assessment
h. decompensation
h. effect
h. format
h. impotence
h. index
h. pattern
h. penumbra
h. reserve impairment
h. response
hemodynamically
h. significant lesion
h. significant stenosis
h. weighted echoplanar MR imaging
hemolymph node
hemolytic splenomegaly
hemomediastinum
hemoperfusion
hemopericardium
hemoperitoneum
hemophilic pseudotumor
hemopleuropneumonia syndrome
hemopneumothorax
hemorrhage
abdominal h.
adrenal h.
alveolar h.
anastomotic h.
h. of aneurysm
aneurysmal h.
antepartum h.
arterial h.
basilar intracerebral h.
bladder h.
brainstem h.
brain stenosis h.
bulbar intracerebral h.
capillary h.
catheter-induced pulmonary artery h.
central nervous system h.
cerebellar h.
cerebral h.
cerebromeningeal intracerebral h.
chronic parenchymal h.
colonic diverticular h.
colorectal h.
concealed h.
h. consolidation
cortical intracerebral h.
delayed traumatic intracerebral h. (DTICH)
diffuse alveolar h.
diffuse pulmonary alveolar h.
diffuse subarachnoid h.
Duret h.
eight-ball h.
epidural h.
exsanguinating h.
external h.
extradural h.
extraluminal h.
extrapleural h.
first trimester h.

focal area of h.
focal endocardial h.
frank h.
gastric h.
gastrointestinal h.
gastrointestinal renal transplant h.
hypertensive brain h.
hypothalamic h.
infant gastrointestinal h.
internal capsule intracerebral h.
interstitial h.
intertrabecular h.
intraabdominal arterial h.
intracerebral h. (ICH)
intracranial h.
intraluminal h.
intramural arterial h.
intramural gastrointestinal tract h.
intraparenchymal h.
intraplaque h. (IPH)
intrapleural h.
intrapontine intracerebral h.
intrapulmonary h.
intratumoral h.
intraventricular h. (IVH)
intraventricular neonate h.
labyrinthine h.
life-threatening h.
lobar intracerebral h.
lower gastrointestinal h.
lung h.
massive exsanguinating h.
mediastinal h.
meningeal h.
neonatal choroid plexus h.
neonatal intracerebellar h.
neonatal intracranial h.
neonatal intraventricular h.
nonaneurysmal perimesencephalic subarachnoid h.
nondominant putaminal h.
nontraumatic epidural h.
old h.
parenchymal h.
periaqueductal h.
peribronchial h.
perigestational h.
perinephric space h.
perirenal h.
placental h.
h. plaque
plaque h.
pontine h.
postoperative mediastinal h.
posttraumatic h.
preplacental h.
pulmonary artery h.
putaminal h.
retrobulbar h.
retroperitoneal h.
retropharyngeal h.
salmon-patch h.
sentinel transoral h.
slit h.
small bowel h.
spinal epidural h. (SEH)
spinal subarachnoid h.
spinal subdural h. (SSH)
splinter h.
spontaneous renal h.
striate h.
subacute h.
subarachnoid h. (SAH)
subchorionic h.
subcortical intracerebral h.
subdural h. (SDH)
subependymal h.
subgaleal h.
submucosal h.
subperiosteal h.
subserosal h.
thalamic h.
traumatic meningeal h.
upper gastrointestinal h.
variceal h.
venous h.
ventricular intracerebral h.
vitreous h.

hemorrhagic
h. brain infarct
h. bronchopneumonia
h. colitis
h. consolidation of lung
h. corpus luteum cyst
h. duodenitis
h. effusion
h. focus
h. lesion
h. lung nodule
h. lung syndrome
h. metastasis
h. necrosis
h. pericarditis
h. pleurisy

NOTES

H

hemorrhagic *(continued)*
h. pneumonia
h. salpingitis
h. stroke
hemorrhagicum
corpus h.
hemorrhoidal plexus
hemostatic clip
hemothorax, pl. **hemothoraces**
Henderson fracture
Henderson-Jones
H.-J. chondromatosis
H.-J. disease
Henke
H. space
H. triangle
H. trigone
Henle
H. canal
jejunal interposition of H.
jejunal loop interposition of H.
ligament of H.
H. ligament
loop of H.
H. sheath
trapezoid bone of H.
Henning sign
Henry
master knot of H.
vertebral artery of H.
henry (H)
Henschke
H. afterloader
H. seed applicator
Hensen
H. canal
H. disk
H. node
H. plane
Hensing
H. fold
H. ligament
hen worker's lung
heparinization
systemic h.
hepar lobatum
hepatectomy
hepatic
h. abscess
h. adenoma
h. anaplastic sarcoma
h. angiography
h. angiomyolipoma
h. angiosarcoma
h. angle
h. angle sign
h. architecture
h. arterial infusion (HAI)
h. arterial phase (HAP)
h. arteriography
h. arteriovenous fistula
h. artery
h. artery anatomy
h. artery aneurysm
h. artery-portal vein fistula
h. artery pseudoaneurysm
h. artery stenosis
h. artery thrombosis
h. bed
h. calcification
h. calculus
h. capsule
h. carcinoma
h. chemoembolization
h. cirrhosis
h. congestion
h. cord
h. cyst
h. degeneration
h. 2,6-dimethyliminodiacetic acid (HIDA)
h. diverticulum
h. duct
h. ductal system
h. duct bifurcation
h. echo pattern
h. failure
h. fibrosis
h. fissure
h. flexure
h. flexure cancer
h. fungal infection
h. hemangioma
h. hilum
h. insufficiency
h. ligament
h. lipoma
h. lobe
h. lymph node
h. metabolism
h. metastasis
h. necrosis
h. neoplasm
h. nerve plexus
h. outflow tract
h. parenchyma
h. pattern echo
h. resistive artery index
h. sarcoidosis
h. sclerosis
h. sinusoid
h. steatosis
h. test of Glass
h. transplant
h. trauma
h. triad

h. tumor
h. vein
h. vein disease
h. vein portalization
h. vein thrombosis
h. venography
h. venous outflow
h. venous outflow obstruction
h. venous pressure gradient
h. venous system
h. web
h. web dilatation
h. wedge pressure (HWP)
hepatica fibrosa
hepatis
parenchymal peliosis h.
phlebectatic peliosis h.
porta h.
sagittal porta h.
hepatitis, pl. **hepatitides**
acute h.
chronic h.
neonatal h.
radiation h.
recurrent pyogenic h.
hepatization
lung h.
hepatobiliary
h. cancer
h. contrast agent
h. disease
h. ductal system imaging
h. pathway
h. scan
h. scintigraphy
h. tree
hepatoblastoma
hepatocarcinogenesis
hepatocarcinoma
fibrolamellar h.
hepatocellular
h. adenoma
h. cancer
h. carcinoma (HCC)
h. disease
h. dysfunction
hepatocerebral
h. degeneration
h. disease
hepatoclavicular view
hepatocolic ligament
hepatocystocolic ligament
hepatodiaphragmatic
h. interposition
h. interposition of colon (HDIC)
hepatoduodenal ligament
hepatoesophageal ligament
hepatofugal flow
hepatogastric ligament
hepatogastroduodenal ligament
hepatogram
hepatography
hepatoid adenocarcinoma
hepatoiminodiacetic
h. acid (HIDA)
h. acid scan
hepatojejunal anastomosis
hepatolenticular degeneration
hepatolienography
hepatolithiasis
hepatoma
hepatomalacia
hepatomegaly
hepatopancreatic fold
hepatopathy
hepatopctal flow
hepatophrenic ligament
hepatopleural fistula
hepatoportal
h. biliary fistula
h. sclerosis
hepatoptosis
hepatorenal
h. angle
h. ligament
h. pouch
h. recess
h. saphenous vein bypass graft
h. syndrome (HRS)
hepatosplenic
hepatosplenography
hepatosplenomegaly (HSM)
hepatoumbilical ligament
herald bleed
Herbert-Fisher
H.-F. fracture classification
Herbert scaphoid bone fracture
Hercules power injector
hereditary
h. amyloidosis
h. nonpolyposis colorectal cancer (HNPCC)
h. predisposition
Herendeen phenomenon

NOTES

H

Hering
H. canal
H. duct
H. phenomenon
hermaphroditism
true h.
Hermodsson
H. fracture
H. tangential projection
hernia, pl. **herniae**
abdominal wall h.
axial hiatal h.
Barth h.
Beclard h.
Bochdalek h.
broad ligament h.
cecal h.
concentric h.
congenital diaphragmatic h.
h. defect
diaphragmatic h.
direct inguinal h.
duodenal h.
epigastric h.
esophageal h.
external h.
femoral h.
funicular inguinal h.
gastric h.
hiatal h.
hiatus h.
Holthouse h.
incarcerated h.
incomplete h.
indirect inguinal h.
internal h.
interstitial h.
intrapericardial diaphragmatic h.
Lesgaft h.
lesser sac h.
Littré h.
lumbar h.
mediastinal h.
Morgagni h.
obturator h.
ovarian h.
pantaloon h.
paraduodenal h.
paraesophageal h.
parahiatal h.
paraileostomal h.
h. paralysis
parastomal h.
peritoneal h.
peritoneopericardial diaphragmatic h.
h. pouch
properitoneal h.
Richter h.
Rieux h.
rolling hiatal h.
h. rupture
scrotal h.
short esophagus-type hiatal h.
sliding hiatal h.
spigelian h.
strangulated inguinal h.
transient hiatal h.
traumatic diaphragmatic h.
Treitz h.
umbilical h.
ventral h.
hernial
h. aneurysm
h. canal
h. sac
herniated
h. abdominal contents
h. bowel
h. cerebellar tonsil
h. intervertebral disk (HID)
h. nucleus pulposus (HNP)
h. preperitoneal fat
herniation
h. of brain tissue
brain tissue h.
central h.
cerebellar tonsillar h.
cerebral h.
cervical disk h.
cingulate h.
cisternal h.
concentric h.
diencephalic h.
disk h.
fat h.
fat lung h.
foramen magnum h.
frank disk h.
free-fragment disk h.
hard disk h.
hippocampal h.
impending h.
intercervical disk h.
internal disk h.
intradural disk h.
intraspongy nuclear disk h.
lateral disk h.
lumbosacral intervertebral disk h.
nucleus pulposus h.
phalangeal h.
h. pit
posterolateral disk h.
soft disk h.
subfalcine h.
subligamentous disk h.
supraligamentous disk h.

temporal lobe h.
tentorial notch h.
thoracic disk h.
tonsillar h.
transtentorial h.
uncal h.

herniography
heroin lung damage
Herophili
torcular H.
herpes
h. esophagitis
h. zoster oticus
herpesvirus pneumonia
herringbone pattern
hertz (Hz)
Heryln-Werner-Wunderlich syndrome
Heschl
H. convolution
H. transverse gyrus
Hesselbach
H. ligament
H. triangle
heterocladic anastomosis
heterocyclic free radical
heterogeneous
h. appearance
h. carotid plaque
h. hyperattenuation
h. internal echo pattern
h. isodense enhancement
h. microdistribution
h. perfusion pattern
h. radiation
h. signal intensity
h. system disease
h. uptake
heterotaxia, heterotaxy
abdominal h.
h. syndrome
visceral h.
heterotopia
gastric h.
gray matter h.
heterotopic
h. bone
h. bone formation
h. gray matter
h. pancreas
h. pregnancy
h. scar ossification
h. white matter island

Hetzel forward triangle method for cardiac output
Heubner
H. artery
recurrent artery of H.
Hewlett-Packard
H.-P. color flow imager
H.-P. phased-array imaging
H.-P. phased-array imaging system
H.-P. scanner
H.-P. ultrasound
H.-P. ultrasound unit
Hexabrix
H. imaging agent
hexadactyly
hexametazime
hexamethylpropyleneamine oxime
Hey
H. amputation
H. ligament
Heyman-Simon
H.-S. capsule
H.-S. source
HF
Hageman factor
heart failure
HFA-134a
^{18}F-labeled H.
HFD
high-frequency Doppler
HFI
half-Fourier imaging
HGPT
hypoxantine-guanosine phosphoribosyl transferase
HGPT locus
H-graft
Gallie H.-g.
HI
head injury
hiatal hernia
hiatus
adductor h.
aortic h.
crus h.
diaphragmatic esophageal h.
esophageal h.
h. hernia
patulous h.
popliteal h.
h. semilunaris
Hibbs metatarsocalcaneal angle

NOTES

hibernating myocardium
hibernation
myocardial h.
hibernoma
Hickey
H. method
H. position
Hickman
H. indwelling catheter
H. line
H. tunneled catheter
hickory-stick fracture
HID
herniated intervertebral disk
HIDA
hepatic 2,6-dimethyliminodiacetic acid
hepatoiminodiacetic acid
HIDA imaging
HIDA scan
hidebound small bowel fold
hidradenitis
hierarchical
h. information
h. scanning pattern
HIFU
high-intensity focused ultrasound
high
h. arch
h. arched palate
h. cervical spinal cord lesion
h. defect
h. endothelial venule
h. filling pressure
h. interstitial pressure
h. jugular bulb (HJB)
h. lateral wall myocardial infarct
h. left main diagonal artery
h. linear energy transfer radiation
h. minute ventilation
h. normal
h. pontine lesion
h. reflectivity
h. right atrium (HRA)
h. small bowel obstruction
h. spatial resolution cine CT
h. spatial resolution mode
h. spin
h. takeoff
h. temporal resolution
h. temporal resolution mode
h. torque
h. velocity
h. wedge pressure
high-altitude pulmonary edema (HAPE)
high-amplitude
h.-a. echo
h.-a. impulse
high-attenuation
h.-a. stone
high-caliber, low-velocity handgun injury
high-contrast film
high-definition
h.-d. imaging (HDI)
h.-d. three-dimensional analysis
high-density
h.-d. barium
h.-d. barium imaging agent
h.-d. bile
h.-d. lesion
h.-d. linear array
h.-d. rim
h.-d. structure
high-dose
h.-d. chemoradiotherapy
h.-d. film dosimeter
h.-d. film dosimetry
h.-d. radiotherapy
h.-d. rate (HDR)
h.-d. therapy
high-dose-rate
h.-d.-r. (HDR) intracavitary radiation therapy
h.-d.-r. remote afterloading
high-energy
h.-e. bent-beam linear accelerator
h.-e. imaging
h.-e. proton
h.-e. trauma
highest turbinated bone
high-field
h.-f. open MRI scanner
h.-f. system
high-field-strength
h.-f.-s. MR imaging
h.-f.-s. scanner
high-frame-rate mode
high-frequency
h.-f. Doppler (HFD)
h.-f. Doppler (HFD) ultrasound
h.-f. Doppler ultrasound imaging
h.-f. miniature probe
h.-f. therapeutic ultrasound
h.-f. transducer
high-grade
h.-g. AV block
h.-g. glioma
h.-g. malignancy
h.-g. narrowing
h.-g. obstruction
h.-g. obstructive lesion
h.-g. partial tear
h.-g. proximal stenosis
h.-g. surface osteogenic sarcoma
h.-g. tumor

high-impedance circulation
high-intensity
h.-i. focused ultrasound (HIFU)
h.-i. lesion
h.-i. signal
h.-i. zone (HIZ)
high-kV technique
highly
h. mobile echo
h. reflective echo
h. vascular tumor
high-lying patella
Highmore
H. antrum
antrum cardiacum of H.
high-osmolar
h.-o. contrast agent (HOCA)
h.-o. medium (HOM)
high-osmolarity contrast medium (HOCM)
high-output
h.-o. circulatory failure
h.-o. heart failure
h.-o. state
high-pass filter
high-performance
h.-p. liquid chromatography
h.-p. size-exclusion chromatography
high-pitched signal
high-powered field (hpf)
high-pressure liquid chromatography
high-probability lesion
high-purity germanium detector (HPGe detector)
high-rate
h.-r. detect interval
h.-r. ventricular response
high-resolution
h.-r. B-mode imaging
h.-r. bone algorithm technique
h.-r. computed tomography (HRCT)
h.-r. coronal cuts
h.-r. CT imaging
h.-r. CT mammography
h.-r. 3DFT MR imaging
h.-r. diffraction
h.-r. 3D spoiled-grass image
h.-r. electroencephalography
h.-r. infrared imaging (HRI, HRI imaging)
h.-r. linear array transducer
h.-r. magnification
h.-r. multileaf collimator
h.-r. multisweep (HRMS)
h.-r. storage phosphor imaging
h.-r. transverse view image
h.-r. ultrasound
h.-r. ultrasound scanning
high-resolution, low-speed radiography
high-riding
h.-r. patella
h.-r. scapula
h.-r. third ventricle
high-sensitivity measurement
high-signal
h.-s. abnormality
h.-s. intratendinous collection of fluid
h.-s. lesion
h.-s. mass
high-signal-intensity yellow marrow
high-spatial-frequency reconstruction algorithm
high-spatial-resolution cine computed tomography (HSRCCT)
high-speed imaging
high-temperature diffraction
high-temporal-resolution cine computed tomography (HTRCCT)
high-velocity
h.-v. flow
h.-v. gunshot wound
h.-v. jet
h.-v. signal loss
high-voltage
h.-v. generator
h.-v. pulsed galvanic stimulation (HVPGS)
h.-v. transformer
hila (*pl. of* hilum)
Hilal
H. embolization apparatus
H. microcoil
hilar
h. adenopathy
h. area
h. artery
h. cap
h. cell tumor of ovary
h. comma sign
h. extension
h. gland
h. gland enlargement
h. haze

NOTES

hilar *(continued)*
h. kidney lip
h. lipoma
h. lymph node
h. lymph node enlargement
h. mass
h. plate
h. prominence
h. reaction
h. shadow
h. structure
h. tumor
h. vessel
h. waterfall sign
Hildreth sign
Hilgenreiner
H. angle
H. line
Hilight Advantage System CT scanner
Hillock arch
Hill-Sachs
H.-S. defect
H.-S. deformity
H.-S. dislocation
H.-S. posterolateral compression fracture
H.-S. shoulder lesion
Hill sign
Hilton
H. law
H. muscle
hilum, pl. **hila**
central fatty h.
hepatic h.
kidney h.
h. of kidney
lips of h.
h. of lung
lung h.
pulmonary h.
renal h.
splenic h.
waterfall h.
HIMAC
heavy ion medical accelerator in Chiba
HIMAC system
Hinchey classification
hindbrain
h. deformity
h. dysgenesis
hindfoot
h. deformity
h. instability
h. joint complex
h. valgus
hindgut
h. duplication
primitive h.
h. syndrome
Hine-Duley phantom
hinged implant
hinge joint
hip
h. bone
h. bump
h. capsule joint
congenital dislocation of h. (CDH)
congenital dysplasia of h. (CDH)
developmental dysplasia of h. (DDH)
h. disarticulation
dislocated h.
h. dislocation
h. doughnut sign
h. dysplasia
h. equator sign
external snapping h.
h. flexion contracture
frogleg view of the h.'s
hanging h.
h. hump
h. muscle cross section
h. pinning
h. pointer
h. protrusion
h. replacement
h. replacement cup
snapping h.
transient osteoporosis of h.
transient synovitis of h.
Hippel-Lindau syndrome
hippocampal
h. atrophy
h. fissure
h. formation
h. gyrus
h. herniation
h. infarct
h. magnetic resonance volumetry
h. sclerosis
h. sulcus
h. volume
hippocampal-amygdaloid complex
hippocampi
gyrus h.
hippocampus
hippocratic finger
hippuran
I h.
Hippuran imaging agent
Hipputope imaging agent
hip-to-ankle view
Hirschberg sign

Hirschfeld canal
Hirschsprung-associated enterocolitis (HAEC)
Hirschsprung disease
Hirtz method
His
H. angle
angle of H.
atrioventricular node of H.
atrioventricular opening of H.
H. band
bundle of H., His bundle
H. canal
H. duct
H. line
H. perivascular space
H. spindle
His-Haas muscle transfer
Hispeed CT scanner
Hi-Star midfield MRI system
histiocyte
sinusoidal h.
histiocytic
h. bone lymphoma
h. bone tumor origin
h. brain lymphoma
h. chest lymphoma
histiocytoma
angiomatoid malignant fibrous h.
atypical benign fibrous h.
benign fibrous h.
fibrous h.
malignant fibrous h. (MFH)
malignant fibrous osseous h.
myxoid malignant fibrous h.
primary pulmonary malignant fibrous h.
scrotal h.
histiocytosis
diffuse cerebral h.
Langerhans lung cell h.
sinus h.
histogram
dose-surface h.
dose-volume h. (DVH)
h. equalization
h. equalization algorithm
gaussian dose-volume h.
gray-level h.
hose-volume h.
integrated optical density h.
multisectional dose-volume h.
histograph
Eppendorf pO_2 h.
histologic
h. correlation
h. grade
histopathologic
h. comparison
h. CT correlation
histoplasmoma
histoplasmosis
disseminated CNS h.
lung h.
pulmonary h.
historadiography
history
remote h.
hit
groin h.
h. the pink
Hitachi
H. CT scanner
H. MR scanner
H. Open MRI system
H. Open MRI System scanner
H. 0.3-T unit scanner
H. ultrasound
hitchhiker's thumb
HIV
H. encephalitis
H. esophagitis
H. nephropathy
HIZ
high-intensity zone
HJB
high jugular bulb
HL
half-life
hallux limitus
HLA
horizontal long axial
HLA imaging
HLHS
hypoplastic left heart syndrome
HLR
heart-to-lung ratio
H-mode echocardiography
HNP
herniated nucleus pulposus
HNPCC
hereditary nonpolyposis colorectal cancer
Hobb view
hobnail liver

NOTES

Hoboken nodule
HOC
hypertrophic obstructive cardiomyopathy
HOCA
high-osmolar contrast agent
hockey-stick
h.-s. appearance of catheter tip
h.-s. appearance of the ureter
h.-s. deformity of tricuspid valve
h.-s. fracture
h.-s. tricuspid valve deformity
HOCM
high-osmolarity contrast medium
hypertrophic obstructive cardiomyopathy
Hodge plane
Hodgkin
H. disease
H. granuloma
H. tumor
Hodgson
H. aneurysmal dilatation of the aorta
H. disease
Hodson-type kidney
Hoffa
H. disease
H. fat pad
H. fracture
Hoffmann
H. atrophy
H. sign
Hofmeister anastomosis
Hohl tibial condylar fracture classification
hold
single breath-h.
Holdaway ratio
Holdsworth spinal fracture classification
holdup in flow of barium
hole pattern
hole-within-hole
h.-w.-h. appearance
h.-w.-h. bone lesion
holiday
h. heart
h. heart syndrome
Holl ligament
hollow
h. bone
h. chest
h. foot
h. organ
h. ribbon
h. structure
h. viscera
h. viscus
h. viscus injury
hollow-point bullet
Holman carotid slim sign
Holmes
H. cortical cerebellar degeneration
H. heart
H. syndrome
holmium
h. imaging agent
h. yttrium aluminum garnet laser (Ho:YAG laser)
holmium-166
holmium-YLF
holoacardia
holocord
h. hydromyelia
h. syringohydromyelia
Hologic
H. 2000 densitometer
H. QDR 1000-W dual-energy x-ray absorptiometry imaging
H. QDR 1000W dual-energy x-ray absorptiometry scanner
H. 2000 scanner
hologram
holography
computerized tomographic h. (CTH)
helical CT h.
h. imaging
medical h.
multiple-exposure volumetric h.
three-dimensional h.
volumetric multiplexed transmission h.
Voxgram multiple-exposure h.
holoprosencephaly
alobar h.
lobar h.
semilobar h.
holosystolic
h. gradient
h. mitral valve prolapse
holoventricle
Holstein-Lewis fracture
Holthouse hernia
Holt-Oram syndrome
Holzknecht
H. space
H. stomach
H. unit (H)
Holz phlegmon
HOM
high-osmolar medium
homeostasis
brain h.
Homerlok needle
Homer Mammalok needle
Homer-Wright rosette

homing
h. mechanism
h. molecule
homoartery
homogeneous
h. appearance
h. carotid plaque
h. echo
h. echo pattern
h. lesion
h. opacity
h. perfusion
h. radiation
h. signal intensity
h. soft tissue density
h. thallium distribution
homograft
aortic root h.
homology mapping
homonuclear spin system
homospoil
homovanillic acid
homuncular
homunculus
Honda
H. sign
H. sign appearance
honeycomb
h. cyst
h. degeneration
h. formation
h. lung
h. pattern
h. vertebra
honeycombed appearance
honeycombing
fibrotic h.
hood-shaped ureter
Hood syndrome
hooked
h. acromion
h. bone
hook of the hamate fracture
hooklike osteophyte formation
hookwire
hoop
h. stress
h. stress fracture
hoop-shaped loops of bowel
Hoover sign
Hope sign
Hopkins rod
Hopmann
H. papilloma
H. polyp
horizontal
h. beam film
h. boundary
h. dipole configuration
h. fissure
h. heart
h. lie
h. long axial (HLA imaging, HLA)
h. long axis slice
h. long axis SPECT image
h. maxillary fracture
h. overframing
h. plane
h. plane loop
h. position
h. striping
hormone-receptor negative cancer
hormone-resistant prostate cancer (HRPC)
horn
Ammon h.
anterior h.
central h.
dorsal spinal cord h.
enlarged frontal h.
frontal h.
iliac h.
lateral h.
meniscal h.
occipital h.
posterior gray h.
posterior spinal cord h.
projectile h.
spinal dorsal h.
splaying of frontal h.
temporal h.
uterine h.
h. of uterus
ventral h.
ventricular h.
Horner muscle
Horn sign
horseshoe
h. abscess
h. appearance
h. configuration
h. configuration of brain
h. fibrosis
h. fistula

NOTES

horseshoe *(continued)*
- h. kidney
- h. lung
- h. osteophyte
- h. placenta
- h. shape

Horsley anastomosis
Horton disease
hose-pipe appearance of terminal ileum
hose-volume histogram
hot
- h. area
- h. cathode x-ray tube
- h. caudate lobe
- h. contrast medium
- h. defect
- h. lesion
- h. light
- h. node
- h. spot
- h. spot artifact
- h. thyroid nodule

hot-cross-bun
- h.-c.-b. appearance
- h.-c.-b. skull

hot-nose sign
hot-source heating
hot-spot
- h.-s. heart imaging
- h.-s. myocardial imaging

hot-tip laser
hot-tipped laser probe
Hough transform (HT)
Hounsfield
- H. calcium density measurement unit
- H. number
- H. unit (HU)

hourglass
- h. bladder
- h. configuration
- h. constriction
- h. constriction of gallbladder
- h. deformity
- h. membrane
- h. pattern
- h. phalanx
- h. shape
- h. stenosis
- h. stomach
- h. tumor
- h. ventricle
- h. vertebra

hourglass-shaped lesion
House grading system
housemaid's knee
housing
- x-ray tube h.

Houston
- H. muscle
- valve of H.

^{166}Ho in vivo generator
Howell-Jolly body
Howship-Romberg sign
Howtek Scanmaster DX scanner
Ho:YAG laser
HP
- Profasi H.
- H. SONOS 5500 ultrasound imaging system

HPA
hypothalamic-pituitary-adrenal
- HPA axis

hpf
high-powered field

HPGe detector
HPV16-associated tumor
HPV18-associated tumor
HRA
high right atrium

HRCT
high-resolution computed tomography
- cystic airspace HRCT
- inhomogeneous lung attenuation HRCT
- interstitial nodule HRCT

HRI
high-resolution infrared imaging
- HRI imaging

HRMS
high-resolution multisweep

HRPC
hormone-resistant prostate cancer

HRS
hepatorenal syndrome

HS
half-scan

H/S
hysterosalpingogram
hysterosalpingography

HSG
hysterosalpingogram
hysterosalpingography
hysterosonography
- HSG catheter

H-shaped
- H.-s. vertebra
- H.-s. vertebral body

HSM
hepatosplenomegaly

HSR
hypersensitivity reaction

HSRCCT
high-spatial-resolution cine computed tomography

HSSG
hysterosalpingosonography
HT
Hough transform
HTRCCT
high-temporal-resolution cine computed tomography
H-type
H.-t. tracheoesophageal fistula
HU
Hounsfield unit
H.U.
heat unit
Huchard
H. disease
H. sign
Hudson attachment
Hueck ligament
Hueter fracture sign
Hughes-Stovin syndrome
Hughston
H. Clinic injury classification
H. view
Huguier canal
human
h. milk
h. serum-ABGd imaging agent
h. serum albumin
h. serum-albumin imaging agent
h. visual sensitivity weighting
Humegon
humeral
h. avulsion of the glenohumeral ligament (HAGL)
h. avulsion of the glenohumeral ligament (HAGL) lesion
h. bone
h. circumflex
h. condylar fracture
h. epicondyle
h. head-splitting fracture
h. length
h. line
h. mechanism
h. metaphysis
h. physeal fracture
h. ridge
h. supracondylar fracture
humeri (*pl. of* humerus)
humeroradial articulation
humeroulnar articulation
humerus, pl. **humeri**
capitulum humeri
epicondylar fracture of h.
head of the h.
surgical neck of h.
humidifier lung
hump
buffalo h.
h. and dip breast sign
dowager's h.
dromedary h.
Hampton h.
hip h.
Kump h.
humpback
h. deformity
Humphry
ligament of H.
H. ligament
hunchback
Kokopelli h.
hunger
air h.
Hunner ulcer
Hunter
H. canal
H. disease
H. ligament
hunterian ligation of aneurysm
Hunter-Schreger band
Hunter-Sessions
Hunt-Hess
H.-H. aneurysm classification
H.-H. aneurysm grading system
H.-H. subarachnoid hemorrhage scale
Huntington
H. chorea (HC)
H. rod insertion
H. sign
Hunt-Kosnik
H.-K. classification
H.-K. classification of aneurysm
Huppert disease
Hurst phenomenon
Hurter
H. and Driffield (H and D)
H. and Driffield curve (H and D curve)
H. and Driffield photographic curve
Hurter-Driffield curve
Hürthle cell adenoma

NOTES

Huschke
H. canal
H. foramen
H. ligament
Hutch diverticulum
Hutchinson
H. fracture
H. plaque
H. syndrome
H. teeth
Hutchinson-Gilford syndrome
Hutchinson-type neuroblastoma
Hutinel-Pick syndrome
Huygens principle
HV
hallux valgus
HVA
hallux valgus angle
HVL
half-value layer
HVPGS
high-voltage pulsed galvanic stimulation
HWP
hepatic wedge pressure
hyaline
h. arteriosclerosis
h. articular cartilage
h. cartilage endplate
h. degeneration
h. necrosis
hyalinized
h. breast fibroadenoma
h. fibroadenoma with fibrosis
hyalinizing granuloma
hyalocapsular ligament
hyaloid
h. artery
h. canal
h. canal of Cloquet
h. fossa
hyaloserositis
h. pleura
Hyams
H. grade
H. grading of esthesioneuroblastoma classification
hybrid
h. magnet
h. MRI imaging agent
h. probe
h. subtraction technique
hybridization probe
hybridization-subtraction technique
hybrid-RARE imaging
hydatid
alveolar h.
h. disease
h. heart cyst
h. lung cyst
h. mediastinum cyst
Morgagni h.
h. polyp
h. pregnancy
sessile h.
Virchow h.
Hydradjust IV table
hydramnios, hydramnion
hydraulic distention
hydrencephaly
hydrocalicosis
hydrocalyx
hydrocele
congenital h.
idiopathic h.
infantile h.
primary h.
secondary h.
hydrocephalic obstruction
hydrocephalocele
hydrocephalus
acquired h.
acute h.
asymptomatic h.
bilateral h.
chronic communicating h.
communicating h.
compensated h.
congenital h.
delayed h.
extraventricular obstructive h.
h. ex vacuo
fulminant h.
idiopathic h.
infantile h.
intraventricular obstructive h.
low-pressure h.
noncommunicating h.
nonobstructive h.
normal-pressure h.
normotensive h.
obstructive h.
occult h.
posthemorrhagic h.
postinfectious h.
posttraumatic h.
primary h.
progressive h.
secondary h.
symptomatic h.
unilateral h.
unshunted h.
hydrocolpocele
hydrocortisone enema
hydrodynamic potential of disk
hydroencephalocele

hydroencephalomeningocele
hydrogen (H)
 heavy h.
 h. peroxide enema
 h. peroxide imaging agent
 h. proton imaging
 h. spin density
hydrogen-1
hydrogen-2
hydrogen-3
hydrolysis in vivo
hydrolyzed technetium
hydroma (*var. of* hygroma)
hydrometra
hydrometrocolpos
hydromyelia
 holocord h.
hydromyoma
hydronephrosis
 acute h.
 chronic h.
 congenital h.
 focal h.
hydronephrotic kidney
hydropericardium
hydroperitoneum
hydrophilic
 h. guide wire
 h. nonflocculating barium
hydrophilicity
hydrophone
 needle h.
hydrophthalmos
hydropic
 h. changes
 h. composition
 h. degeneration
 h. villus
hydropneumothorax
 loculated h.
hydrops
 h. canal
 endolymphatic h.
 fetal h.
 h. fetalis
 gallbladder h.
 halo sign of h.
 labyrinthine h.
 nonimmune fetal h.
 semicircular canal h.
 transient gallbladder h.
 h. tubae profluens
hydropyonephrosis
hydrosalpinx
hydrostatic
 h. decompression
 h. pressure of blood
 h. reduction rule of 3
hydrosyringomyelia
hydrothorax
hydroureter
hydroureteronephrosis
hydroxyapatite
 air plasma spray h.
 calcium h.
 h. crystal
 h. deposition disease (HADD)
 h. implant
 h. rheumatism
hydroxyindole acetic acid
hygroma, hydroma, pl. **hygromata**
 cystic h.
 cystic neck h.
 cystic orbital h.
 pseudocystic h.
 subdural h.
hyoepiglottic ligament
hyoglossus muscle
hyoid
 h. arch
 h. bar
 h. bone
hyopharyngeal carcinoma
hyoscine butylbromide imaging agent
Hypaque
 H. contrast medium
 H. enema
 H. Meglumine contrast medium
 H. Meglumine imaging agent
 H. myelography
 H. Sodium contrast medium
 H. Sodium imaging agent
 H. swallow
Hypaque-76
 H. contrast medium
 H. imaging agent
Hypaque-Cysto
 H.-C. contrast medium
 H.-C. imaging agent
Hypaque-50 imaging agent
Hypaque-M
 H.-M. contrast medium
 H.-M. imaging agent
hyparterial bronchus

NOTES

Hyperab
hyperabduction
 h. maneuver
 h. syndrome
hyperactive peristalsis
hyperacute
 h. ischemic brain infarct
 h. lung transplant rejection
 h. myocardial infarct
 h. renal transplant rejection
 h. stroke
hyperaeration
hyperattenuation
 heterogeneous h.
hyperbaric oxygen
hypercalcemic supravalvular aortic stenosis
hypercellular marrow
hyperconcentration of contrast medium
hyperconvex nail
hyperdense
 h. brain lesion
 h. mass
 h. middle cerebral artery sign
 h. sinus secretion
 h. spleen
hyperdynamic
 h. abductor hallucis
 h. AV fistula
 h. heart
 h. right ventricular impulse
hyperechogenicity
hyperechoic
 h. area
 h. region
 h. renal medulla
 h. renal nodule
 h. splenic spot
hyperechoicity
hyperemia
 active h.
 arterial h.
 collateral h.
 diffuse h.
 fluxionary h.
 mucous membrane h.
 passive h.
 reactive h.
 subchondral marrow h.
 venous h.
hyperemic flow
hyperexpanded lobe
hyperexpansion
 compensatory lobe h.
hyperextensibility
 joint h.
 h. of joint
hyperextension
 h. dislocation
 h. injury
 h. of neck
 h. teardrop fracture
hyperfine coupling
hyperfixation
hyperflexion/hyperextension cervical injury
hyperflexion teardrop fracture
hyperfractionated
 h. accelerated radiation therapy (HART)
 h. radiation
 h. total body irradiation
hyperfractionation
hyperfunction
 adrenocortical h.
hypergastrinemia
hypergonadotropic hypogonadism
hyperinflation
 dynamic pulmonary h.
 focal h.
 pulmonary h.
hyperintense
 h. focus
 h. marrow space
 h. mass
 h. muscle
 h. periventricular brain lesion
 h. periventricular lesion
 h. ring sign
 h. signal
hyperintensity
 cortical h.
 diffuse signal h.
 incidental punctate white matter h.
 localized h.
 multifocal area of h.
 muscle h.
 punctate white matter h.
 sacral h.
 white matter signal h.
hyperkinetic
 h. heart
 h. segmental wall motion
 h. segmental wall motion abnormality
hyperlordosis
 functional h.
hyperlucent
 h. lung
 h. rib
hypermaturation
hypermetabolic
 h. activity focus
 h. nodule
 h. region

hypermobile
h. first ray
h. joint
h. kidney
hypermotility
hypermyelination
hypernephroid carcinoma
hypernephroma
hyperosmotic solution
hyperostosis
ankylosing h.
bony h.
Caffey h.
chronic infantile h.
cortical h.
diffuse idiopathic sclerosing h. (DISH)
diffuse idiopathic skeletal h. (DISH)
h. frontalis interna
generalized cortical h.
idiopathic cortical h. (ICH)
infantile cortical h.
h. of Morgagni
senile ankylosing h.
skeletal h.
skull h.
sternoclavicular h.
vertebral h.
HyperPACS system
hyperparathyroidism
persistent h.
primary h.
recurrent h.
secondary h.
tertiary h. (tHPT)
hyperperfusion
h. abnormality of liver
ictal h.
mesial h.
septal h.
hyperperistalsis
hyperplasia
adaptive h.
adenomatous h.
adrenal h.
adrenocortical h.
alveolar epithelial h.
angiofibroblastic h.
angiofollicular lymph node h.
angiolymphoid h.
antral G-cell h.
atypical ductal h. (ADH)
atypical lobular breast h.
atypical regenerative h.
benign prostatic h. (BPH)
bone marrow lymphoid h.
breast h.
Brunner gland h.
compensatory h.
congenital adrenal h. (CAH)
cortical nodular h.
cystic glandular h.
desquamated epithelial breast h.
ductal epithelial h.
endometrial h.
epiphyseal h.
epithelial h.
explosive follicular h.
fibrointimal h.
fibrous tissue h.
florid follicular h.
focal cortical h.
focal nodular h.
follicular nodular h. (FNH)
gallium-avid thymic h.
generalized angiofollicular lymph node h.
generalized breast h.
giant follicular h.
GI tract lymphoid h.
intimal h. (IH)
intravascular papillary endothelial h.
lipoid adrenal h.
localized angiofollicular lymph node h.
lung lymphoid h.
lymphoid h.
lymphonodular h.
medial h.
mucosal h.
myointimal h.
neointimal h.
neoplastic h.
nodular adrenal h.
nodular lymphoid h.
nodular regenerative h. (NRH)
paracortical h.
parathyroid h.
pituitary h.
plantar h.
polypoid lymphoid h.
prostatic h.

NOTES

hyperplasia *(continued)*
pseudoangiomatous stromal h. (PASH)
pseudointimal h. (PIH)
reactive follicular h.
reactive lymphoid h.
sclerosing duct h.
sinus h.
smooth h.
splenic h.
subadventitial h.
tenocyte h.
thymic h.
h. thymus
thyroid h.
torus h.
unicentric angiofollicular lymph node h.

hyperplastic
h. adenomatous polyp
h. bone
h. cholecystosis
h. colon polyp
h. gastric polyp
h. gastropathy
h. inflammation
h. lesion
h. stomach polyp
h. synovium
h. tissue

hyperpolarized
h. He-3 imaging agent
h. helium
h. ^{129}Xe gas
h. ^{129}Xe imaging agent

hyperreflexia
detrusor h.

hyperreninemic hypertension

hyperrugosity

hypersecretion
gastric h.
mucus h.

hypersegmentation
manubrium h.
h. of the manubrium

hypersensitivity
alveolar h.
carotid sinus h.
h. pneumonia
h. pneumonitis
h. reaction (HSR)
tracheobronchial h.

hypersignal

hypersplenism

hyperstasis
generalized cortical h.

hyperstimulation of ovary

hypertelorism

hypertension
acute thromboembolic pulmonary arterial h.
arterial h.
benign intracranial h.
extrahepatic portal h.
hyperreninemic h.
hypoxic pulmonary h.
idiopathic intracranial h.
idiopathic noncirrhotic portal h.
idiopathic portal h. (IPH)
h. injury
intracranial h.
persistent pulmonary h.
precapillary lung h.
primary pulmonary h. (PPH)
pulmonary h. (PHTN)
pulmonary arterial h.
pulmonary venous h.
refractory h.
renal transplant h.
renal vascular h. (RVH)
secondary h.
segmental portal h.
sinistral portal h.
suprahepatic h.
systemic arterial h.
systemic venous h.
systolic h.
venous h.

hypertensive
h. arteriosclerosis
h. brain hemorrhage
h. cardiomegaly
h. cardiovascular disease
h. contrast concentration
h. diathesis
h. encephalopathy
h. ischemic ulcer
h. left ventricular hypertrophy
h. lower esophageal sphincter
h. renal disease
h. stroke
h. vascular degeneration
h. vascular disease

hyperthermia
annular phased-array h.
interstitial h.
locoregional h.
microwave h.
h. probe
radiofrequency h.
radiotherapy with h.
radiotherapy without h.
volumetric interstitial h.

hyperthyroid heart

hypertonic airway

hypertransradiancy

hypertrophic
h. asymmetry
h. bladder
h. cardiomyopathy (HCM)
h. cirrhosis
h. duct network
h. exostosis
h. gastritis
h. inflammation
h. infundibular subpulmonic stenosis
h. marginal spur
h. marginal spurring
h. nonunion
h. obstructive cardiomyopathy (HOC, HOCM)
h. olivary degeneration
h. pulmonary osteoarthropathy
h. pyloric string sign stenosis
h. pyloric target sign stenosis
h. pylorus
h. subaortic stenosis
h. tissue
hypertrophicans
osteodermopathia h.
hypertrophied
h. heart
h. intima
h. myocardium
h. trigone
hypertrophy
adaptive h.
apical h. (AHC)
asymmetric septal h. (ASH)
asymptomatic h.
benign prostatic h. (BPH)
biatrial h.
biventricular h.
bladder h.
bone h.
Brunner gland h.
cardiac h.
compensatory nodular kidney h.
complementary h.
concentric heart h.
dilatation and h.
eccentric left ventricular h.
epiphyseal h.
h. of epiphysis
familial h. (FHC)
focal pyloric h.
focal renal h.
four-chamber h.
functional h.
hypertensive left ventricular h.
interatrial septal h.
left atrial h.
left ventricular h. (LVH)
ligamentous-muscular h.
lipomatous h.
muscular h.
myocardial cellular h.
olivary h.
panchamber h.
physiologic h.
pyloric h.
right atrial h.
right ventricular h. (RVH)
Romhilt-Estes score for left ventricular h.
scalenus anticus muscle h.
septal h.
septate h.
smooth-muscle h.
symmetric heart h.
trigeminal trigonal h.
trigonal h.
type A–C right ventricular h.
unilateral h.
ventricular h.
villous h.
Wigle scale for ventricular h.
hypervariable
h. region
h. sequence
hypervascular
h. arterialization
h. granulation tissue
h. liver metastasis
h. mediastinal mass
h. pancreatic tumor
hypervascularity
hyperventilation
autonomic h.
central neurogenic h.
hyperviscosity syndrome
hypervitaminosis A
hypervolemia
h. of pregnancy
hypervolemic pulmonary edema
hypha, pl. **hyphae**
fungal h.
hypoacousia
hypoaeration
hypoattenuation

NOTES

H

hypocellular marrow
hypochordal arch
hypocycloidal
h. ankle tomography
h. tomography
hypodense
h. area
h. basal ganglion brain lesion
h. mass
h. mesencephalic low-density brain lesion
hypodensity
periventricular h.
white matter h.
hypodiploid tumor
hypodiploidy
hypoechogenic
h. tumor
hypoechogenicity
false h.
hypoechoic
h. area
h. area of ultrasound
h. band
h. fluid collection
h. halo
h. layer
h. liver
h. mantle
h. renal sinus
h. rim
h. zone
hypofractionated
h. radiation
h. radiation therapy
hypofrontality
hypoganglionosis of colon
hypogastric
h. artery
h. plexus
hypogastrium
hypogenetic
h. lung
h. lung syndrome
hypoglossal
h. canal
h. fossa
h. nerve
h. nerve palsy
h. trigone
hypogonadism
hypergonadotropic h.
hypogonadotropic h.
hypogonadotropic hypogonadism
hypoinflation of the lung
hypointense
h. sella lesion
h. signal
h. signal inhomogeneity
hypointensity
cortical h.
hypokinesis, hypokinesia
apical h.
cardiac h.
diffuse ventricular h.
global h.
h. of heart
inferior wall h.
h. on echocardiography
regional h.
septal h.
wall h.
hypokinetic
h. left ventricle
h. segment
h. segmental wall motion
h. segmental wall motion abnormality
hypolucency of lung
hypometabolic area
hypometabolism
biparietotemporal h.
focal area of h.
global h.
hypomineralization
fetal h.
h. in fetus
hypoparathyroidism
idiopathic h.
secondary h.
hypoperfused state
hypoperfusion
acute alveolar h.
apical h.
cerebellar h.
cerebral h.
h. complex
global cerebral h.
peripheral h.
pulmonary h.
resting regional myocardial h.
septal h.
systemic h.
hypoperistalsis
h. syndrome
hypopharyngeal
h. cancer
h. diverticulum
h. tumor
hypopharynx
hypophosphatemic
h. osteomalacia
h. vitamin D refractory rickets
hypophyseal fossa
hypophysectomy

hypophysial
h. pouch
h. Rathke duct
hypophysis
h. cerebri
infundibulum of h.
hypophysitis
lymphoid h.
hypopituitarism
hypothalamic h.
hypoplasia
annular h.
aortic tract complex h.
ascending aorta h.
basiocciput h.
bone marrow h.
cerebellar h.
cerebral white matter h.
condylar skull h.
congenital renal h.
endothelial h.
fetal lung h.
gallbladder h.
left ventricular h.
lung h.
mandible h.
maxillary sinus h.
occipital condyle h.
optic nerve h.
pulmonary h.
radius h.
seminal vesicle h.
sinus h.
skeletal h.
transverse h.
tubular aortic h.
uterine h.
vermis h.
h. vermis
hypoplastic
h. aorta syndrome
h. aortic arch
h. emphysema
h. heart syndrome
h. heart ventricle
h. horizontal rib
h. left heart syndrome (HLHS)
h. left ventricle
h. left ventricle syndrome
h. lung
h. penis
h. right heart
h. right heart syndrome
h. right ventricle
h. subpulmonic outflow
h. thumb
h. tricuspid orifice
h. valve
hypopnea
obstructive h.
hyposensitive carotid sinus syndrome
hyposensitization
hypospadias
hyposplenism
hypostatic
h. bronchopneumonia
h. congestion
h. pneumonia
h. pulmonary insufficiency
hypotelorism
hypotension
arterial h.
cerebral h.
spontaneous intracranial h.
hypothalamic
h. glioma
h. hamartoma
h. hemorrhage
h. hypopituitarism
h. hypothyroidism
h. lesion
h. sulcus
hypothalamic-pituitary-adrenal (HPA)
h.-p.-a. axis
hypothalamic-pituitary axis
hypothalamic-pituitary-gonadal
h.-p.-g. axis
hypothalamohypophysial tract
hypothalamoneurohypophysial
h. axis
hypothalamus
anterior h.
rostral h.
h. tumor
hypothenar
h. eminence
h. muscle groups of hand
hypothermia
scalp h.
hypothermic
h. heart
h. perfusion
hypothesis
incessant ovulation h.

NOTES

H

hypothyroidism
bone h.
hypothalamic h.
primary h.
secondary h.
tertiary h.
hypotonic
h. bladder
h. duodenography
h. duodenography imaging
h. patient
hypovascular zone
hypovolemia trauma
hypovolemic
h. complex
h. shock
hypoxantine-guanosine phosphoribosyl transferase (HGPT)
hypoxemia
hypoxia
ischemic h.
relative h.
tumor h.
hypoxia-ischemia
hypoxic
h. brain damage
h. injury
h. ischemic encephalopathy
h. ischemic insult
h. pulmonary hypertension
h. pulmonary vasoconstriction
hypoxic/ischemic injury
Hyrtl
H. foramen
H. sphincter
hysterectomy
abdominal h.
extrafascial h.
radical abdominal h.
radical vaginal h.
supracervical h.
total abdominal h.
vaginal h.
Wertheim h.
hysteresis
hystericus
globus h.
Hysterocath hysterosalpingography device
hysterogram
hysterography
hysteromyoma
hysterosalpingo-contrast sonography
hysterosalpingogram (H/S, HSG)
hysterosalpingography (H/S, HSG)
h. catheter
h. imaging
hysterosalpingosonography (HSSG)
hysteroscopy
hysterosonography (HSG)
transvaginal h. (TVHS)
hysterotomy
hysterotubogram
hysterotubography
Hytrast
Hz
hertz

I
iodine
I disk
I hippuran
^{123}I
iodine-123
^{123}I heptadecanoic acid
I-123 OIH
^{125}I
iodine-125
^{125}I fibrinogen scan
^{125}I interstitial radiation implant
^{127}I
iodine-127
^{131}I
iodine-131
^{131}I serum albumin
^{132}I
iodine-132
IAB
IABP
intraaortic balloon pump
IADSA
intraarterial digital subtraction angiography
IAEA
International Atomic Energy Agency
IAS
interatrial septum
iatrogenic
i. avulsion
i. cardiomegaly
i. dural tear
i. perforation
i. ureteral injury
IAVB
incomplete atrioventricular block
I-B1 radiolabeled antibody injection radiation therapy
IBC
inflammatory breast cancer
IBM
I. field-cycling research relaxometer
I. NMR spectrometer
I. Speech Server clinical reporting system
IBTR
ipsilateral breast tumor recurrence
ICA
internal carotid artery
intracranial aneurysm
ICE
intracardiac echocardiography
ice
i. mapping
i. skater's fracture
iceberg
i. phenomenon
i. radiotherapy
ice-pick
i.-p. view
ICEUS
intracaval endovascular ultrasound
ice-water swallow
ICH
idiopathic cortical hyperostosis
intracerebral hemorrhage
ichorous pleurisy
ichthyosis
acquired i.
ICIS
imaging center information system
ICP
intracranial pressure
ICRP
International Commission on Radiation Protection
ICRT
intracoronary radiation therapy
ICRU
International Commission on Radiation Units and Measurements
ICRU 50 radiation therapy
ICRU reference point
ICS coder
ictal
i. hyperperfusion
i. phase study
i. technetium Tc-99m HMPAO (hexamethylpropyleneamine oxime) brain SPECT
ICUS
intracoronary ultrasound
ICV
internal cerebral vein
intracerebroventricular
ICV reservoir
ID
internal diameter
IDA
image display and analysis
iminodiacetic acid
IDA (iminodiacetic acid) scanning
IDC
idiopathic dilated cardiomyopathy
IDD
intraluminal duodenal diverticulum

identification
particle i.
peak i.
phase i.
topographic i.
idiopathic
i. amyloidosis
i. cardiomegaly
i. cortical hyperostosis (ICH)
i. dilated cardiomyopathy (IDC)
i. dilated pulmonary artery
i. edema
i. eosinophilic lung disease
i. epiphyseolysis
i. fibrous mediastinitis
i. fracture
i. gastric perforation
i. hydrocele
i. hydrocephalus
i. hypertrophic subaortic sclerosis (IHSS)
i. hypertrophic subaortic stenosis
i. hypoparathyroidism
i. inflammatory bowel disease
i. interstitial fibrosis
i. interstitial pneumonia
i. interstitial pneumonitis
i. intestinal pseudoobstruction
i. intracranial hypertension
i. medial aortopathy
i. megacolon
i. mural endomyocardial disease
i. noncirrhotic portal hypertension
i. obstruction
i. osteolysis
i. pleural calcification
i. portal hypertension (IPH)
i. pulmonary arteriosclerosis (IPA)
i. pulmonary artery dilatation
i. pulmonary fibrosis (IPF)
i. restrictive cardiomyopathy
i. right atrial dilatation
i. scoliosis
i. unilateral hyperlucent lung
i. unilobar emphysema
i. varicocele
idioventricular rhythm (IVR)
IDIS
intraoperative digital subtraction angiography
IDIS angiography system
IDK
internal derangement of the knee
IDM
infant of diabetic mother
idoxuridine (IUDR)
IDP
imidodiphosphonate
IDSA
intraoperative digital subtraction angiography
IDSI
IDSI scanner
iduronidase
IDXrad
I:E
inspiratory to expiratory
I:E ratio
IES
inferior esophageal sphincter
IF
screen-intensifying factor
IFT
inverse Fourier transform
IGLLC
inferior glenohumeral ligament labral complex
IH
intimal hyperplasia
IHA
intrahepatic atresia
IHF
interhemispheric fissure
^{192}I high-dose-rate remote afterloader
IHSS
idiopathic hypertrophic subaortic sclerosis
iiRAD DR1000C digital radiographic system
IJV
internal jugular vein
I-labeled
I.-l. cholesterol
I.-l. macroaggregated albumin
I.-l. rose bengal
^{131}I-labeled
^{131}I-l. human MoAb
^{131}I-l. monoclonal Fab
ILBBB
incomplete left bundle-branch block
ileal
i. atresia
i. conduit
i. crypt
i. inflow tract
i. loop
i. loopography
i. motility
i. neobladder
i. obstruction
i. pouch-anal anastomosis
i. spill
i. S pouch
i. stenosis
ileitis
backwash i.

Crohn i.
distal i.
granulomatous i.
obstructive dysfunctional i.
prestomal i.
regional i.
terminal i.

ileoanal pouch

ileocecal
i. cystoplasty
i. edema
i. fat pad
i. fold
i. insufficiency
i. junction
i. orifice
i. pouch
i. recess
i. syndrome
i. valve
i. valve abnormality

ileococcygeus muscle

ileocolic
i. artery
i. disease
i. fold
i. intussusception
i. lymph node
i. plexus
i. vein
i. vessel

ileocolitis
Crohn i.

ileocolostomy

ileoentectropy

ileofemoral
i. vein
i. wing fracture

ileogram

ileoileal intussusception

ileorectal anastomosis (IRA)

ileosacral (IS)

ileosigmoid fistula

ileostogram

ileostomy

ileotransverse colon anastomosis

ileum
antimesenteric border of distal i.
cobblestone i.
collapsed distal i.
hose-pipe appearance of terminal i.
jejunization of i.
terminal i.

ileus
adhesive i.
adynamic i.
adynamic/paralytic i.
cecal i.
chronic duodenal i.
colonic i.
dynamic i.
gallbladder i.
gallstone i.
localized i.
mechanical i.
meconium i.
nonobstructive i.
occlusive i.
paralytic i.
postoperative i.
reflex i.
spastic i.

Ilfeld-Holder deformity

ilia (*pl. of* ilium)

iliac
i. apophysitis
i. artery
i. artery aneurysm
i. artery stenosis
i. atherosclerotic occlusive disease
i. bifurcation
i. canal
i. cancellous bone
i. circumflex lymph node
i. colon
i. crest
i. dowel
i. fascia
i. fossa
i. fossa abscess
i. horn
internal i.
i. lesion
i. lymph node
i. plaque
i. spine
i. tubercle
i. tuberosity
i. vein
i. venography
i. vessel
i. wing

iliac-renal bypass graft

NOTES

iliacus
ilii
osteitis condensans i.
iliocaval
i. compression syndrome
i. junction
i. thrombus
i. tree
iliocostal muscle
iliofemoral
i. artery
i. ligament
i. thrombosis
i. triangle
i. vein
i. venous stenosis
ilioinguinal
i. lymph node
i. ring
i. syndrome
iliolumbar ligament
ilioneoureterocystotomy
iliopectineal
i. eminence
i. ligament
i. line
ilioprofunda bypass graft
iliopsoas
i. bursa
i. bursitis
i. compartment
i. compartment enlargement
i. muscle
i. muscle shadow
i. ring
i. sign
i. tendon
iliopubic
i. eminence
i. ligament
iliotibial (IT)
i. band
i. band friction syndrome
i. ligament
i. tract
iliotrochanteric ligament
ilium, pl. **ilia**
crest of the i.
flared i.
Ilizarov
I. device
I. ring
ill-defined
i.-d. consolidation
i.-d. mass
i.-d. multifocal lung density
illuminator
Mammo Mask i.
ILP
isolated limb perfusion
ILUS
intraluminal ultrasound
IM
intermetatarsal
intramedullary
IM joint
IM rod
IM rodding
IMA
inferior mesenteric artery
intermetatarsal angle
internal mammary artery
IMA pedicle
image (*See* imaging, film, projection, radiograph, radiography, scanning, scan, view, x-ray)
i. acquisition
i. acquisition gated scan imaging
aliasing i.
alignment and registration of 3D i.
i. amplifier
AMT-25-enhanced MR i.
i. analysis system
anterior planar i.
arterial flow-phase i.
artifact i.
attenuated i.
axial gradient echo i.
axial transabdominal i.
binary i.
blood pool phase i.
bone phase i.
bull's eye i.
calculated i.
cervicothoracic sagittal scout i.
cine-encoded i.
cine magnetic resonance function i.
column mode sinogram i.
i. compression
computer-generated i.
cone-beam i.
confocal i.
contiguous i.
i. contrast
contrast-enhanced MR i.
i. control
coronal GRE MR i.
coronal planar i.
cross-sectional ultrasonographic i.
CT/MRI-defined tumor slice i.
CT/MRI-defined tumor volume i.
CT reconstruction i.
i. cytometry
degradation of i.
delayed i.
diffusion-weighted i.

digitally fused CT and radiolabeled monoclonal antibody SPECT i.
i. display
i. display and analysis (IDA)
i. distortion
Doppler i.
dynamic i.
ECG-triggered, flow-compensated gradient echo i.
excitation-spoiled fat-suppressed T1-weighted SE i.
exercise i.
fast Fourier transform (FFT) i.
fast spin echo T2-weighted i.
FLASH i.
flawed i.
flip-angle i.
flow-compensated i.
flow-on gradient-echo i.
i. foldover
i. formation
four-dimensional i.
frequency domain i.
i. fusion
gadolinium-enhanced T1-weighted axial i.
ghost i.
gradient-echo axial i.
gradient-echo coronal i.
gradient-echo-phase i.
gradient-encoded i.
gradient-recalled echo i.
gray-scale i.
GRE-in i.
GRE-out i.
hard-copy i.
high-resolution 3D spoiled-grass i.
high-resolution transverse view i.
horizontal long axis SPECT i.
imaginary i.
immediate postflow i.
inhomogeneous i.
in-phase i.
i. intensification
i. intensification fluorometry
i. intensifier
intercondylar sagittal i.
intermediate i.
inversion recovery i.
large-field-of-view i.
lateral sagittal i.
localizing i.
longitudinal i.
magnetic susceptibility-weighted i.
magnetization transfer gradient-echo i.
magnitude i.
i. matrix
matrix i.
maximum intensity projection and source i.
midcoronal oblique i.
midplane sagittal i.
midsagittal MR i.
minimum intensity projection (MIP) i.
misleading i.
modulus i.
motion-triggered cine kinematic MR i.
multiecho axial i.
multiecho coronal i.
multiple planar gradient-recalled i.'s
native i.
negative i.
i. noise
nonmagnetization transfer gradient-refocused echo i.
nonsubtraction i.
opposed GRE i.
opposed-phase i.
i. Orthicon tube
overlapping i.'s
panoramic i.
parallel-tagged MR i.'s
parasagittal i.
phase i.
phase-contrast (PC) i.
phase-velocity i.
pinhole i.
plain-paper i.
planar left anterior oblique i.
postexercise i.
postintraarticular paramagnetic contrast injection T1-weighted i.
i. postprocessing error artifact
poststress i.
i. quality degradation
quasiradiographic i.
real-time echoplanar i.
i. reconstruction
i. recording system
recovery time i.
redistribution i.

NOTES

image *(continued)*
regional ejection fraction i.
registration and alignment of 3D i.'s
i. restoration algorithm
scout i.
scrambled i.
second-echo i.
sequential postcontrast MR i.
serial static i.
i. shading
short-axis i.
short tau inversion recovery (STIR) i.
short T1 inversion recovery (STIR) i.
silhouette i.
single-slice gradient-echo i.
spatial modulation of magnetization (SPAMM) i.
i. spatial resolution
spectral-spatial i.
spin-echo i.
spin-lock-induced T1-rho weighted i.
spot i.
static i.
stop-action i.
stress-and-rest i.
stress thallium i.
striations across i.
stroke count i.
stroke volume i.
subtraction i.
surface-projection rendering i.
survey-view i.
T2-gradient refocused i.
thick-slice i.
thin-collimation i.
thin-section axial i.
thin-slice i.
three-dimensional Fourier transform volume i.
transaxial i.
transcoronal STIR i.
T1-weighted coronal i.
T1-weighted fat-suppressed i. (T1FS)
T1-weighted i. (T1WI)
T2-weighted i. (T2WI)
T2-weighted sagittal oblique i.
T2-weighted spin-echo i.
two-dimensional gradient-encoded i.
two-dimensional portal i.
ultrasonic tomographic i.
unopposed i.
variance i.
velocity-encoded i.
ventilation i.
ventricular function equilibrium i.
vertical-long axial i.
i. volume
volume-rendered i.
volumetric i.
voxel-gradient rendering i.
zebra stripe i.

image-acquisition
i.-a. gated examination
i.-a. time

image-amplified fluoroscopy

image-degrading scattering

image-guided
i.-g. radiosurgery
i.-g. surgery
i.-g. therapy

ImageMASTER

Imagent
I. BP
I. GI
I. GI imaging agent
I. LN

imager
Acuson 128EP i.
Drystar dry i.
flat-panel megavoltage i.
full-body echoplanar system i.
GE Signa 5.4 Genesis MR i.
GE Signa 5.5 Horizon EchoSpeed MR i.
Hewlett-Packard color flow i.
Integris V3000 i.
Kodak Digital Science 3600 distributed medical i.
Kodak 1200 Digital Science medical i.
Magnetom SP MRI i.
NeuroScan 3D i.
Tesla magnetic resonance i.

image-reconstruction time

image-selected in vivo spectroscopy

imaginary
i. image
i. mode
i. number

imaging (*See* image, MRI)
3DFT gradient-echo MR i.
3DFT volume i.
3D magnetic source i.
3D processed ultrafast computerized i.
3D turbo SE i.
3D ultrasound reconstruction i.
acoustic i.
acute cerebral infarct i.
Adenoscan i.
adenosine echocardiography i.

adrenal i.
A-FAIR i.
air-contrast i.
air enema fluoroscopic i.
airway fluoroscopy i.
Aloka i.
amplitude i.
AMT-25-enhanced MR i.
angiography i.
anisotropically rotational diffusion i.
anisotropic 3D i.
annotated i.
antegrade pyelography i.
anterior planar i.
anthropometric i.
antifibrin antibody i.
aortography i.
aperiodic functional MR i.
arterial flow phase i.
arteriovenous shunt i.
arthrography i.
Artoscan MRI i.
A-scan i.
ascending contrast phlebography i.
Aspire continuous i.
ATL real-time Neurosector scan i.
attenuation i.
Aurora MR breast i.
axial grade echo i.
axial plane i.
axial transabdominal i.
balloon expulsion i.
balloon test occlusion i.
barium enema i.
barium swallow i.
beta-methyl-p-iodophenyl-pentadecanoic acid SPECT scan i.
Biad SPECT i.
bile duct scan i.
biliary tract CT scan i.
binary i.
black blood T2-weighted inversion-recovery MR i.
blood flow i.
blood oxygenation level-dependent i.
blood pool i.
blood pool phase i.
BMIPP SPECT scan i.
B-mode i.
body coil i.
body section radiography i.
bolus challenge i.
bone age i.
bone density i.
bone length i.
bone mineral content i.
bone phase i.
bone scintiscan i.
brain scan i.
breath-hold, contrast-enhanced 3D MR angiography scan i.
breath-hold T1-weighted MP-GRE MR i.
breath-hold ungated i.
breath-hold velocity-encoded cine MR i.
bright-field i.
bronchial provocation i.
bronchogram i.
B-scan i.
bull's eye i.
Captopril-stimulated renal i.
cardiac blood pool i.
cardiac catheterization i.
cardiac positron emission tomography i.
cardiac radiography i.
cardiac wall motion i.
Cardiolite scan i.
CardioTek i.
cardiotocography i.
cardiovascular radioisotope scan and function i.
carotid duplex i.
carotid sinus i.
CAS i.
celiac and mesenteric arteriography i.
i. center information system (ICIS)
Center of Metabolic and Experimental I.
cephalogram i.
cerebral perfusion SPECT i.
Ceretec brain i.
i. chain veiling glare
chemical-selective fat saturation i.
chemical-shift i. (CSI)
cholangiography i.
chondroitin sulfate iron colloid-enhanced MR i.
Chopper-Dixon fat suppression i.
cine CT i.
cine gradient-echo MR i.

NOTES

imaging *(continued)*
cine magnetic resonance i.
Cine Memory with color flow Doppler i.
cine phase contrast (PC) i.
cineradiography i.
cine view i.
cisternography i.
CKG i.
coded-aperture i.
cold spot myocardial i.
collimation i.
color amplitude i.
color-coded pulmonary blood flow i.
color Doppler i. (CDI)
color flow i. (CFI)
color-flow Doppler i.
color-flow Doppler real-time 2-D blood flow i.
color-flow duplex i.
column-mode sinogram i.
combined leukocyte-marrow i.
combined Myoscint/thallium i.
combined thallium-Tc-HMPAO i.
Compuscan Hittman computerized i.
computed transmission tomography i.
continuous i. (CI)
continuous-wave Doppler i.
contrast-enhanced i.
conventional planar i. (CPI)
convergent color Doppler i.
coronary artery scan i.
corpus cavernosonography i.
correlative diagnostic i.
cross-sectional i.
CSF-suppressed T2-weighted 3D MP-RAGE MR i.
CTAT i.
computerized transverse axial tomography
cystography i.
cystourethroscopy i.
dacryocystography i.
darkfield i.
delayed bone i.
DentaScan i.
DEXA bone density scan i.
dexamethasone suppression test i.
diagnostic i. (DI)
DIET fast SE i.
diffusion magnetic resonance i.
diffusion-weighted MR i.
digitally fused CT and radiolabeled i.
digital radiography i.
digital vascular i. (DVI, DVI mode)
dipyridamole echocardiography i.
dipyridamole handgrip i.
dipyridamole infusion i.
dipyridamole thallium-201 i.
dipyridamole thallium stress i.
direct Fourier transformation i.
displacement field-fitting MR i.
diuretic renal i.
Doppler color-flow i.
Doppler tissue i. (DTI)
Doppler ultrasonography i.
Doppler venous i.
double-dose gadolinium i.
double-helical CT i.
double-phase technetium-99m sestamibi i.
dry laser i.
DSC MR i.
dynamic susceptibility contrast magnetic resonance imaging
dual-coil i.
dual-echo DIET fast spin-echo i.
dual isotope i.
dual-phase ^{99m}Tc-sestamibi i.
duodenography i.
duplex carotid i.
duplex Doppler i.
dynamic-contrast enhanced magnetic resonance i. (DCE-MRI)
dynamic contrast-enhanced subtraction MR i.
dynamic scintigraphy i.
dynamic susceptibility contrast magnetic resonance i. (DSC MR imaging)
dynamic volume i.
ECG-gated multislice MR i.
ECG-gated spin-echo MR i.
echo i.
echocardiography i.
echoplanar i. (EPI)
echoplanar FLAIR i.
echoplanar MRA i.
electric joint fluoroscopy i.
electrocardiogram-gated MRI i.
electrocardiography-gated echoplanar i.
electrodiagnostic i.
electromagnetic blood flow i.
electronic portal i.
electron paramagnetic resonance (EPR) spatial i.
electron radiography i.
electrostatic i.
end-diastolic i.
endoanal MR i.

endocrine i.
endometrial chemical-shift i.
endorectal surface-coil MR i.
enhanced i.
epicardial i.
epididymography i.
equilibrium MUGA i.
ERCP i.
esophageal function i.
esophagography i.
excretory urography i.
exercise thallium-201 stress i.
ex vivo magnetic resonance i.
fast cardiac phase contrast cine i.
fast Fourier i.
fast multiplanar inversion recovry (FMPIR) i.
fast multiplanar spoiled gradient-recalled i. (FMPSPGR imaging)
fast scan magnetic resonance i.
fast spin echo MR i.
fast spin echo (SE) and fast inversion recovery (IR) i.
fast spoiled gradient-recalled MR i.
fat-suppressed gadolinium-enhanced i.
fat-suppressed three-dimensional spoiled gradient-echo FLASH MR i.
fat/water chemical shift i.
FDG-labeled positron i.
FDG myocardial i.
ferumoxides-enhanced MR i.
field-echo i.
field-of-view i.
field of view i.
filmless i.
first-pass myocardial perfusion i.
FLAIR echoplanar i.
FLAIR-FLASH i.
FLASH magnetic resonance i.
flat-field i.
flawed i.
flow-sensitive MR i.
FluoroPlus angiography i.
FluoroPlus Roadmapper digital fluoroscopy i.
fluoroscopic i.
fluoroscopy-guided condylar lift-off i.
flush aortogram i.
FMPSPGR i.
fast multiplanar spoiled gradient-recalled imaging
Fonar Stand-Up MRI i.
four-dimensional i.
four-hour delayed thallium i.
Fourier direct transformation i.
Fourier multislice modified KWE direct i.
Fourier two-dimensional i.
FOV i.
frequency domain i. (FDI, FDI ultrasound)
FS (frequency-shifted) burst MR i.
functional brain i.
functional magnetic resonance i. (fMRI)
functional spin echo i.
gadolinium-enhanced MR i.
gallbladder i.
gallium lung i.
gastric emptying i.
gastric mucosa i.
gastrointestinal motility i.
gas ventilation i.
gated cardiac blood pool i.
gated equilibrium cardiac blood pool i.
gated magnetic resonance i.
gated SPECT myocardial perfusion i.
Gd-FMPSPGR i.
i. gradient
gradient-echo flow i.
gradient-echo MR i.
gradient-echo phase i.
gradient-echo sequence i.
gradient-echo three-dimensional Fourier transform volume i.
gradient-to-noise i.
GRASS MR i.
gray-scale i.
GRE breath-hold hepatic i.
GRE gadolinium-chelate enhanced i.
GRE-in i.
GRE magnetic resonance i.
GRE-out i.
half-Fourier i. (HFI)
half Nex i.
harmonic i.
HAT-transformed i.
HBCT i.

NOTES

imaging *(continued)*
helical biphasic computed tomography
Helios diagnostic i.
hemodynamically weighted echoplanar MR i.
hepatobiliary ductal system i.
Hewlett-Packard phased-array i.
HIDA i.
high-definition i. (HDI)
high-energy i.
high-field-strength MR i.
high-frequency Doppler ultrasound i.
high-resolution B-mode i.
high-resolution CT i.
high-resolution 3DFT MR i.
high-resolution infrared i. (HRI, HRI imaging)
high-resolution storage phosphor i.
high-speed i.
HLA i.
horizontal long axial
H-1 MR spectroscopic i.
Hologic QDR 1000-W dual-energy x-ray absorptiometry i.
holography i.
hot-spot heart i.
hot-spot myocardial i.
HRI i.
high-resolution infrared imaging
hybrid-RARE i.
hydrogen proton i.
hypotonic duodenography i.
hysterosalpingography i.
image acquisition gated scan i.
infarct-avid i.
infrared i.
initial i.
in-phase GRE i.
intermediate i.
interventional i.
intracoronary i.
intracranial i.
intraoperative i.
intraperitoneal technetium sulfur colloid i.
intrathecal i.
intravascular ultrasound i.
intravenous fluorescein angiography i. (IVFA imaging)
^{111}In white blood cell i.
iodine fluorescence i.
iodomethyl-norcholesterol scintigraphy i.
irreversible compression of MR i.
Isocam scintillation i.
isotope hepatobiliary i.
isotope-labeled fibrinogen i.
isotope shunt i.
isotopic 3D i.
IVFA i.
intravenous fluorescein angiography imaging
KCD i.
511-keV high-energy i.
kidney function i.
kidney radionuclide i.
kidneys, ureter, and bladder i.
kinematic magnetic resonance i.
kinestatic charge detector i.
KUB i.
laser-polarized helium MR i.
limited i.
line i.
linear scan i.
lipid-polarized helium MR i.
lipid-sensitive MR i.
liver-spleen i.
localizing i.
loopogram i.
lower extremity i.
lower limb venography i.
low-field-strength MR i.
low-flip-angle gradient-echo i.
low-resolution i.
lung i.
lymphangiography i.
macromolecular contrast-enhanced MR i.
magic-angle spinning i.
Magnes 2500 whole-head i.
magnetic resonance i. (MRI)
magnetic resonance catheter i.
magnetic source i. (MSI)
magnetization and spin-lock transfer i.
magnetization transfer weighted i.
magnetoacoustic i.
malignant melanoma gallium i.
mammary ductogram i.
mammary galactogram i.
marker transit i.
mass i.
Matrix LR3300 laser i.
maxillofacial i.
maximum intensity projection i.
mediastinal cross-sectional i.
microscopic i.
microwave i.
middle-field-strength MR i.
midsagittal MR i.
miniature i.
minimum intensity projection i.
mirror i.
misleading i.

M-mode echocardiogram i.
MR i.
MRA i.
MR echoplanar i.
MRI-guided laser-induced interstitial i.
MUGA cardiac blood pool i.
multiecho i.
multiformatted i.
multimodality i.
multiorgan i.
multiplanar MR i.
multiplanar reformatted radiographic and digitally reconstructed radiographic i.
multiple-echo i.
multiple-gated blood pool i.
multiple-line scan i.
multiple-plane i.
multisection diffuse-weighted magnetic resonance i.
multishot echoplanar i.
multislice first-pass myocardial perfusion i.
multislice modified KEW direct Fournier i.
multitime point i.
multitracer i.
musculoskeletal i.
MUSTPAC ultrasound i.
myelography i.
myocardial infarct i.
myocardial perfusion i.
myocardial thallium i.
Myoscint i.
native tissue harmonic i. (NTHI)
navigated spin-echo diffusion-weighted MR i.
nephrostogram i.
nephrotomography i.
neurodiagnostic i.
neuroradiologic i.
newborn renal i.
nonavid infarct i.
noninvasive i.
nonsubtraction i.
nuclear bone i.
nuclear cardiovascular i.
nuclear gated blood pool i.
nuclear hepatobiliary i.
nuclear magnetic resonance i.
nuclear perfusion i.
oblique axial MR i.
oblique magnetic resonance i.
OCG i.
off-resonance saturation pulse i.
one-dimensional chemical-shift i. (1D-CSI)
one-shot echoplanar i.
on-line portal i.
opposed-phase GRE i.
opposed-phase MR i.
optical surface i. (OSI)
optimum-angle i.
oral cholecystogram i.
orthopantogram i.
orthoroentgenogram i.
out-of-phase GRE i.
oxygenation-sensitive functional MR i.
pancreas ultrasonography i.
pancreatography i.
panoramic i.
parallel hole i.
parallel-tag MR i.
paramagnetic enhancement accentuation by chemical shift i.
parathyroid ultrasonography i.
PASTA i.
PC i.
  phase-contrast imaging
percutaneous intracoronary angioscopy i.
perfusion MR i.
perfusion and ventilation lung i.
perfusion-weighted i.
perineogram i.
periorbital Doppler i.
peripheral vascular i.
peritoneogram i.
Persantine-thallium i.
PET i.
PET lung i.
PET metabolic i.
PET myocardial fatty acid i.
PET perfusion metabolism i.
PETT i.
phase-contrast i. (PC imaging)
phased-array body-coil MR i.
phased-array multicoil i.
phased-array surface coil MR i.
phase-dependent spectroscopic i.
phase-encode time-reduced acquisition sequence i.

NOTES

imaging *(continued)*
phase-offset multiplanar i.
phase-ordered multiplanar i.
phase-sensitive gradient-echo MR i.
phase velocity i.
photostimulable phosphor digital i.
pinhole i.
PIPIDA hepatobiliary i.
plain film i.
planar radionuclide i.
planar spin i.
planar thallium i.
i. plane
point i.
polarity-altered spectral-selective acquisition i.
POMP i.
positron i.
positron emission tomography i.
positron emission transaxial tomography i.
postcontrast MR i.
postdrainage i.
postexercise i.
postinjection i.
postmetrizamide CT i.
postoperative cholangiography i.
poststress i.
power Doppler i. (PDI)
precontrast i.
preoperative i.
pressure perfusion i.
pretherapy i.
projection-reconstruction i.
projection tract i.
protodensity MR i.
proton chemical shift i.
proton density-weighted i.
pseudodynamic MR i.
pullback i.
pulmonary perfusion i.
pulmonary ventilation i.
pulsed electron paramagnetic i.
pulsed magnetization transfer MR i.
pulse sequence echoplanar i.
pyelography i.
PYP i.
pyrophosphate i.
QCT i.
quantitative fluorescence i.
quantitative lung perfusion i.
quantitative spirometrically controlled CT i.
radioactive fibrinogen i.
radioactive iodine uptake i.
radiographically normal i.
radioisotope cisternography i.
radioisotope gallium i.
radioisotope indium-labeled white blood cell i.
radioisotope technetium i.
radionuclide gated blood pool i.
radionuclide milk i.
radionuclide renal i.
radionuclide renography i.
radionuclide thyroid i.
RAIU i.
rapid axial MR i.
rapid-sequence i.
^{82}Rb-based cardiac i.
real-time color Doppler i.
real-time 2D blood flow i.
real-time echocardiogram i.
reconstructed radiographic i.
reconstructive i.
rectilinear bone scan i.
redistribution myocardial i.
redistribution thallium-201 i.
regional ejection fraction i. (REFI)
renal angiography i.
renal CT i.
renal cyst i.
renal duplex i.
renal ultrasonography i.
renal venography i.
renogram i.
i. renogram
resting MUGA i.
rest myocardial perfusion i.
rest-redistribution i.
rest thallium-201 myocardial i.
reticuloendothelial i.
retrograde cystography i.
retrograde ureteropyelography i.
ring-type i.
rose bengal sodium I-131 biliary i.
rotating delivery of excitation off-resonance (RODEO) MR i.
rotating frame i.
row-mode sinogram i.
R-to-R i.
sagittal gradient-echo i.
sagittal oblique i.
sagittal T1 i.
sagittal transabdominal i.
saline-enhanced MR i.
scanogram i.
scintigraphic scan i.
scintillation i.
scout i.
scrambled i.
sector-scan echocardiography i.
segmental k-space turbo gradient-echo breath-hold sequence i.
segmenting dual-echo MR i.

selective excitation projection reconstruction i.
selenium-labeled bile acid i.
sensitive plane projection reconstruction i.
sequence echoplanar i.
sequence quantitative MR i.
sequential first-pass i.
sequential line i.
sequential plane i.
sequential point i.
sequential quantitative MR i.
serial contrast MR i.
serial duplex i.
serialography i.
serial static i.
sestamibi stress scan i.
shaded-surface display i. (SSD imaging)
short inversion recovery i.
short TI inversion recovery i.
shuntogram i.
sialography i.
SieScape ultrasound i.
silhouette i.
simultaneous volume i.
single-dose gadolinium i.
single-echo diffusion i.
single-slice modified KEW direct Fournier i.
single-voxel proton brain spectroscopy i.
sinus tract i.
sliding thin-slab maximum intensity projection CT i.
slip-ring i.
small field-of-view MR i.
SmartSpot high-resolution digital i.
sodium i.
Sones coronary arteriography i.
source i.
spastic electron paramagnetic resonance (EPR) i.
SPECT i.
spectamine brain i.
spectral Doppler i.
spin-echo cardiac i.
spin-echo magnetic resonance i.
spin-lock and magnetization transfer i.
spin-warp i.
SPIO i.
spirometrically controlled CT i.
splanchnic vascular i.
spleen ultrasonography i.
splenoportography i.
split-brain i.
spoiled gradient-echo i.
spot-film i.
SSD i.
  shaded-surface display imaging
stacked-scan i.
static 3D FLASH i.
steady-state free-precession i.
steady-state gradient-echo i.
STIR i.
stop-action i.
strain-rate MR i.
stress-redistribution i.
stress thallium-201 myocardial i.
stroke volume i.
i. study
subsecond FLASH i.
subtraction i.
superparamagnetic iron oxide i.
SureStart feature of Aspire continuous i.
survey-view i.
susceptibility-weighted MR i.
tagging cine MR i.
targeted i.
^{99m}Tc-HMPAO cerebral perfusion SPECT i.
TechneScan MAG3 i.
technetium stannous pyrophosphate i.
technetium-thallium subtraction i.
thallium-201 i.
thallium myocardial perfusion i.
thallium myocardial scan with SPECT i.
thallium rest-redistribution i.
thallium scintography i.
thallium stress i.
thick-slice i.
thin-collimation i.
thin-slice i.
three-dimensional fast low-angle shot i.
three-dimensional fast spin-echo magnetic resonance i.
three-dimensional Fourier i.
three-dimensional projection reconstruction i.

NOTES

imaging *(continued)*
three-phase i.
ThromboScan i.
through-transfer i.
thyroid ultrasonography i.
i. time
timed i.
time-of-flight i.
time-of-flight echoplanar i.
TIPS i.
tissue Doppler i.
TOF i.
tomographic i.
Toshiba Aspire continuous i.
total body scan i.
transabdominal i.
transaxial i.
transcervical catheterization of fallopian tube i.
transcranial real-time color Doppler i.
transesophageal Doppler color flow i.
transfer i.
transjugular intrahepatic portosystemic shunt i.
transluminal atherectomy i.
transluminal balloon angioplasty i.
transthoracic i.
transverse section i.
triple-dose gadolinium i.
triple-phase bone scan i.
true dynamic joint i.
TSPP i.
turbo FLAIR i.
turbo FLASH i.
T1-weighted coronal i.
T1-weighted sagittal i.
two-dimensional Fourier transformation i.
two-frame gated i.
two-phase computed tomographic i.
two-phase CT i.
UBM i.
ultrafast CT i.
ultrasonic tomographic i.
ultrasound backscatter microscopy i.
unenhanced MR i.
unsuppressed i.
urethrocystography i.
urography i.
vaginogram i.
variance i.
vascular flow i.
vectorcardiography i.
velocity-density i.
velocity-encoded cine MR i.
venography i.
venous i.
ventilation-perfusion i.
vertical-long axial i.
vesiculography i.
videofluoroscopic i.
video radiography i.
virtual reality i.
Vitrea 3D i.
in vivo He-3 MR i.
voiding cystourethrography i.
volume-rendered i.
volumetric i.
V/Q i.
wall-motion i.
water selective spin-echo i.
wavelet-encoded magnetic resonance i.
wet laser i.
white blood cell i.
whole-body scan i.
whole-body thallium i.
wide-beam scan i.
i. workstation
xenon-133 SPECT i.
xeroradiography i.
Xillix LIFE-GI fluorescence endoscopy i.
x-ray-sensitive vidicon i.

imaging-anatomic correlation
imaging-based stereotaxis
imaging-directed 3D volumetric information
imaging-pathologic correlation
Imagopaque
I. contrast medium
I. imaging agent

Imatron
I. C-150L EBCT scanner
I. C-1000 UFCT scanner
I. C-100 Ultrafast CT scanner
I. C-100XL CT scanner
I. Fastrac C-100 cine x-ray CT scanner
I. system

imbalance
biomechanical i.
i. of gain artifact
i. of phase artifact
ventilatory capacity-demand i.

imbrication
capsular i.
facetal i.

IMED Gemini PC-2 volumetric controller
IMI
inferior myocardial infarct

^{131}I-mIB6
monoiodobenzylguanidine

imidoacetic acid radioactive agent
imidodiphosphonate (IDP)
iminodiacetic acid (IDA)
immature
 i. bone
 i. ovarian teratoma
 skeletally i.
immediate
 i. postflow image
 i. postictal period
immediately detachable coil
immersion
 i. B-scan ultrasound
 i. technique
imminent
 i. death
 i. demise
immobilization
immobilizer
 shoulder i.
immovable joint
immune
 i. electron microscopy
 i. response
immunoblastic
 i. large-cell lymphoma
Immuno 1 Dpd assay automated bone-resorption test
immunologic injury
immunolymphoscintigraphy
immunomagnetic
 i. beads
 i. purging
Immunomedics system
immunoprecipitate
immunoproliferative small intestine disease (IPSID)
immunoradioassay
immunoreactivity
immunoscintigraphy
immunoscintimetry
immunostained surface
ImmuRAID antibody imaging agent
Immurait imaging agent
imodoacetic acid imaging agent
impacted
 i. calculus
 i. feces
 i. fetus
 i. subcapital fracture
 i. urethral stone
 i. valgus fracture
impaction
 anteromedial superior humeral head i.
 fecal i.
 lateral compartment i.
 i. lesion
 mucoid i.
 stone i.
impact velocity
impaired
 i. renal function
 i. renal perfusion
 i. tubular transit
 i. venous return
 i. ventilation-perfusion
impairment
 circulatory i.
 functional aerobic i.
 growth i.
 hemodynamic reserve i.
 inspiratory muscle function i.
 motor i.
 renal function i.
 sensory i.
Impax PACS system
impedance
 acoustic i.
 aortic i.
 diastolic notch i.
 i. matching
 i. MR phlebogram
 i. phlebography
 i. plethysmography (IPG)
 pulmonary arterial input i.
 pulmonary vascular bed i.
 respiratory modulation of vascular i.
 vascular i.
impending
 i. herniation
 i. myocardial infarct
imperfecta
 dentinogenesis i.
 osteogenesis i. (OI)
imperfect regeneration
imperforate
 i. aneurysm
 i. anus
impingement
 anterolateral i.
 dural i.
 i. exostosis

NOTES

impingement *(continued)*
graft roof i.
lateral i.
ligamentous i.
nerve root i.
outlet i.
posterior i.
posterosuperior glenoid i.
shoulder i.
sidewall i.
i. spur
syndesmotic i.
i. syndrome
talar i.
talofibular i.
triquetral i.
ulnolunate i.
impinging osteophyte
implant
biodegradable i.
bone i.
carcinomatous i.
cesium i.
cobalt-chromium-molybdenum alloy metal i.
cobalt-chromium-tungsten-nickel alloy metal i. (Co-Cr-W-Ni alloy implant metal)
cochlear i.
Co-Cr-Mo alloy metal i.
collapsed subpectoral i.
i. collar
double-lumen breast i.
double-stem silicone lesser MP i.
ear i.
electrically activated i.
epidural i.
i. fracture
hinged i.
hydroxyapatite i.
^{125}I interstitial radiation i.
interstitial i.
intracavitary i.
iridium-192 endobronchial i.
iridium-192 wire i.
malignant pleural i.
mammary i.
mechanically activated i.
metallic otologic i.
methyl methacrylate bead i.
ocular i.
open-cord tendon i.
otologic i.
palladium i.
^{103}Pd prostatic i.
penile i.
permanent interstitial i.
polymethyl methacrylate (PMMA) i.
prostate i.
prosthetic i.
retropectoral mammary i.
saline i.
silicone elastomer rubber ball i.
silicone wrist i.
single-lumen silicone breast i.
subpectoral i.
synthetic bone i.
temporary interstitial i.
total knee i.
transperineal i.
transvaginal i.
tumor i.
VDS i.
ventral derotating spinal implant
implantable
i. drug delivery system
i. infusion port
i. infusion pump
i. vascular access device
implantation
i. cyst
epicardial i.
percutaneous transperineal seed i.
peroral i.
radon seed i.
subxiphoid i.
transvenous i.
implanted
i. imaging opaque marker
i. pacemaker
impotence
arteriogenic i.
hemodynamic i.
vasogenic i.
impression
basilar i.
cardiac i.
colic i.
convolutional i.
digastric i.
duodenal i.
esophageal i.
extrinsic esophageal i.
extrinsic stomach i.
i. fracture
gastric i.
liver i.
renal i.
suprarenal i.
imprint
i. cytology
tissue i.
improved
i. Chen-Smith coder (ICS coder)
i. photon flux

improvement
interval i.
impulse
apical i.
bifid precordial i.
double systolic apical i.
downward displacement of apical i.
ectopic i.
high-amplitude i.
hyperdynamic right ventricular i.
jugular venous i.
nodal i.
prolonged left ventricular i.
sustained apical i.
systolic i.
undulant i.
IMRT
intensity-modulated radiation therapy
In
indium
^{111}In
indium-111
^{111}In imciromab pentetate
^{111}In murine monoclonal antibody Fab to myosin
^{111}In pentetreotide
^{111}In white blood cell imaging
in
i. situ
i. situ graft
i. situ pinning
i. toto
i. utero detection of cardiac anomaly
i. vitro evaluation of coil
i. vitro labeling
i. vivo
i. vivo balloon pressure
i. vivo correlation
i. vivo disposition study
i. vivo examination
i. vivo He-3 MR imaging
i. vivo labeling
i. vivo method
i. vivo microscopy
i. vivo proton MR spectroscopy
i. vivo stereologic assessment
i. vivo technique
In-111 oxine WBCs
inactivator
inactive
i. endometrium
i. granulomatous disease
i. mode
inadequate
i. bowel preparation
i. calvarial calcification
i. cardiac output
i. cranial calcification
i. runoff
i. visualization
inadvertent arterial injection
incarcerated
i. hernia
i. omentum
i. placenta
incarceration
incarial bone
incessant
i. ovulation
i. ovulation hypothesis
incidence
small angle double i.
incident
i. angle
i. ray
incidentaloma
adrenal i.
brain i.
incidental punctate white matter hyperintensity
incisive
i. bone
i. canal
incisor
fascial i.
i. teeth
incisura, incisure, pl. **incisurae**
i. angularis
aortic i.
i. defect
i. scapulae
stomach defect i.
incisural
i. epidermoidoma
i. sclerosis
inciting
i. event
i. factor
inclination of treadmill
inclinometer
incoherence
magnetic resonance spin i.
incoherent motion

NOTES

incompetence
aortic valvular i.
chronotropic i.
communicating vein i.
deep venous i.
gastroesophageal i.
mitral valve i.
myocardial i.
postphlebitic valvular i.
pulmonary i.
saphenous vein i.
sphincter i.
traumatic tricuspid i.
tricuspid i. (TI)
valvular i.
incompetent
i. cervix
i. ileocecal valve
i. perforator
incomplete
i. atrioventricular block (IAVB)
i. bladder emptying
i. closure
i. dislocation
i. fracture
i. fracture of bone
i. heart block
i. hernia
i. Kartagener syndrome
i. left bundle-branch block (ILBBB)
i. neurofibromatosis
i. obstruction
i. placenta previa
i. pulmonary fissure
i. resolution of pneumonia
i. right bundle-branch block (IRBBB)
i. stroke
i. tumor
i. ureteral duplication
incongruency
patellofemoral i.
incongruity
angle of i.
joint i.
incontinence
bladder i.
bowel i.
fecal i.
motor urge i.
stress i.
increased
i. activity
i. airway
i. anteroposterior diameter
i. attenuation
i. basilar cistern
i. bone density
i. carrying angle
i. central venous pressure
i. cerebrovascular resistance
i. density
i. density of falx
i. density spleen
i. echogenicity
i. echo signal
i. extracellular fluid volume
i. interstitial fluid
i. interstitial markings
i. intracranial pressure
i. intrapericardial pressure
i. isotope uptake
i. lateral joint space
i. left ventricular ejection time
i. markings of emphysema
i. myocardial oxygen requirement
i. outflow resistance
i. peripheral resistance
i. peristalsis
i. prominence of pulmonary vessels
i. pulmonary arterial pressure
i. pulmonary obstruction
i. pulmonary vascularity
i. pulmonary vascular markings
i. pulmonary vascular resistance
i. pulmonary vasculature
i. renal echogenicity cortex
i. skull thickness
i. splenic density
i. thyroid uptake
i. tracer uptake
i. uptake of radiotracer
i. ventricular afterload
increase in intensity
increasingly dense nephrogram
increment
i. in luminal diameter
i. of perfusion
incremental
i. dose
i. increases in treadmill speed
i. passive positioning method
i. risk factor
increta
placenta i.
incus, pl. **incudes**
i. bone
indentation
haustral i.
i. of myelography dye
semilunar i.
indented
i. fracture
i. fracture of skull
independent jaw

indeterminate age
indeterminatus
index, pl. **indices**
acetabular i.
amnionic fluid i.
angiographic muscle mass i.
ankle-arm i.
ankle-brachial i. (ABI)
apnea-hypopnea i. (AHI)
arch length i.
Ashman i.
Benink tarsal i.
bifrontal i.
biliary saturation i.
body mass i. (BMI)
Broca i.
bromodeoxyuridine labeling i.
cardiac i. (CI)
cardiothoracic i.
cephalic i.
Cippaux-Smirak arch i.
computed tomography dose i. (CTDI)
congestion i.
contractile work i.
contractility i.
coronary stenosis i. (CSI)
coronary vascular resistance i. (CVRI)
Crohn disease activity i. (CDAI)
Cronqvist cranial i. (CCI)
Detsky modified cardiac risk i.
diastolic left ventricular i.
diastolic pressure-time i. (DPTI)
Doppler flow i.
Doppler Resistive I. (DRI)
dye fluorescence i. (DFI)
eccentricity i.
effective pulmonic i.
ejection phase i.
ellipticity i.
end-diastolic volume i.
end-systolic volume i. (ESVI)
end-systolic wall i. (ESWI)
end-systolic wall index/end-systolic volume i. (ESWI-ESVI)
exercise i.
fetal-pelvic i.
Fick cardiac i.
i. finger
Fourier pulsatility i.
Fourmentin thoracic i.
Gosling pulsatility i.
hemodynamic i.
hepatic resistive artery i.
Insall-Salvati i.
ischemic i.
left ventricular end-diastolic volume i. (LVEDI)
left ventricular end-systolic volume i. (LVESVI)
left ventricular fractional shortening i.
left ventricular mass i. (LVMI)
left ventricular stroke work i. (LVSWI)
lithogenic i.
maturation i.
mean ankle-brachial systolic pressure i.
mean wall motion score i.
Mengert i.
metacarpal i.
mitral flow velocity i.
myocardial infarction recovery i. (MIRI)
myocardial jeopardy i.
myocardial O_2 demand i.
Nakata i.
O_2 consumption i.
patellofemoral i.
penile-brachial pressure i. (PBPI)
pipe-stemming of ankle-brachial i.
portal vein congestion i.
postexercise i. (PEI)
poststress ankle/arm Doppler i.
Pourcelot i.
predicted cardiac i.
profundal popliteal collateral i.
proliferative i.
pulmonary arterial resistance i.
pulmonary blood volume i. (PBVI)
pulmonary vascular resistance i. (PVRI)
pulmonic output i.
pulsatility i.
quantum mottle i.
renal resistive i.
resistive i. (RI)
resting ankle-arm pressure i. (RAAPI)
right and left ankle i.
right ventricular stroke work i. (RVSWI)

NOTES

index *(continued)*
Ritchie i.
i. of runoff resistance
runoff resistance i.
saturation i. (SI)
short-increment sensitivity i.
Singh osteoporosis i.
stroke i. (SI)
stroke volume i. (SVI)
stroke-work i. (SWI)
systemic arteriolar resistance i.
systemic output i.
systemic vascular resistance i. (SvO_2, SVRI)
systolic pressure-time i.
systolic toe/brachial i.
talocalcaneal i.
tension-time i. (TTI)
therapeutic i.
thoracic i.
thymidine labeling i. (TLI)
tritiated thymidine labeling i.
truncated arch i.
tubular fertility i.
valgus i.
venous distensibility i. (VDI)
wall-motion score i.
water perfusable tissue i.
widened anterior meningeal i.
Wood unit i.

Indian
I. childhood cirrhosis
I. file

Indiana pouch

indicator
i. dilution curve
i. dilution therapy
i. fractionation principle
xylol pulse i.

indicator-dilution method for cardiac output measurement

indices (*pl. of* index)

indicis
extensor i.

Indiclor
I. imaging agent

indifferent gonad

indirect
i. blood supply
i. computed tomography
i. CT
i. fracture
i. hernia sac
i. inguinal hernia
i. laryngoscopy
i. MR arthrography
i. ray
i. ultrasound guidance

indiscriminate lesion

indistinct liver sign

indium (In)
cistern i.
i. imaging agent

indium-111 (^{111}In)
i. antimyosin scintigraphy
i. DTPA
i. labeling
i. pentetreotide
i. satumomab pendetide
i. WBCs

indium-111-labeled
i.-l. leukocytes
i.-l. white blood cell scan

indium-111-oxime leukocytes

indocyanine
i. dilution curve
i. green
i. green angiography
i. green dye
i. green imaging agent

indoleamine

indolent
i. myeloma
i. radiation-induced rectal ulcer

Indomitable scanner

induced
i. acoustic emission
i. biopotential
i. pneumothorax
i. radioactivity
i. thrombosis of aortic aneurysm

inducibility basal state

inducible

inductance-capacitance (LC)

induction
dorsal i.
electric i.
magnetic i.
neuromuscular system electric i.
ovulation i.

inductive reactance (XL)

indurated
i. mass
i. tissue

indurative
i. mastopathy
i. necrosis
i. pleurisy
i. pneumonia

indwelling
i. Foley catheter
i. nonvascular shunt
i. stent

inelastic pericardium

inequality
- limb-length i.
- ventilation-perfusion i.

inexorable progression

^{111}In-Fab-DTPA

infant
- i. of diabetic mother (IDM)
- i. gastrointestinal hemorrhage
- profoundly obtunded i.

infantile
- i. arteriosclerosis
- i. cardiomyopathy
- i. coarctation of aorta
- i. cortical hyperostosis
- i. digital fibromatosis
- i. embryonal carcinoma
- i. fibrosarcoma
- i. ganglioglioma
- i. hemangioendothelial liver
- i. hemangioendothelioma
- i. hemangioendothelioma of liver
- i. hemiplegia
- i. hepatic hemangioma
- i. hydrocele
- i. hydrocephalus
- i. lobar emphysema
- i. myofibromatosis
- i. pneumonia
- i. polycystic kidney disease
- i. pylorospasm
- i. syndrome
- i. thoracic dystrophy
- i. uterus

infantile-onset spinocerebellar ataxia

infantilism
- intestinal i.

infarct, infarction
- acute ischemic brain i.
- acute myocardial i.
- acute renal i.
- age-indeterminate i.
- anemic i.
- anterior communicating artery distribution i.
- anterior myocardial i. (AMI)
- anterior septal myocardial i.
- anterior wall myocardial i.
- anteroinferior myocardial i.
- anterolateral myocardial i.
- anteroseptal myocardial i.
- apical-lateral wall myocardial i.
- apical myocardial i.
- arrhythmic myocardial i.
- atherothrombotic brain i.
- atrial i.
- basal ganglia i.
- bicerebral i.
- bilateral i.
- bland i.
- bone i.
- bowel i.
- brain i.
- brainstem i.
- capsular i.
- capsulocaudate i.
- capsuloputaminal i.
- capsuloputaminocaudate i.
- cardiac i.
- cerebellar i.
- cerebral artery i.
- chronic ischemic brain i.
- chronic renal i.
- concomitant i.
- cortical bone i.
- diaphragmatic myocardial i. (DMI)
- digital livedo reticularis i.
- dominant hemisphere i.
- dural sinus thrombosis i.
- embolic cerebral i.
- evolving myocardial i.
- i. expansion
- extensive anterior myocardial i.
- focal skin i.
- frontal lobe i.
- full-thickness i.
- gyral i.
- healing i.
- hemispheric i.
- hemorrhagic brain i.
- high lateral wall myocardial i.
- hippocampal i.
- hyperacute ischemic brain i.
- hyperacute myocardial i.
- impending myocardial i.
- inferior myocardial i. (IMI)
- inferolateral wall myocardial i.
- inferoposterior wall myocardial i.
- inferoposterolateral myocardial i.
- intestinal i.
- ischemic brainstem i.
- kidney i.
- lacunar brain i.
- lateral myocardial i.
- lobar renal i.

NOTES

infarct *(continued)*
marrow i.
medullary bone i.
mesencephalic i.
mesenteric i.
middle cerebral artery i.
multifocal i.
multiple cortical i.'s
muscle i.
myocardial i. (MI)
nonarrhythmic myocardial i.
nonembolic i.
nonfatal myocardial i.
non-Q-wave myocardial i.
nonseptic embolic brain i.
nontransmural myocardial i.
nonviable scar from myocardial i.
occipital lobe i.
occlusive mesenteric i.
old myocardial i.
omental i.
papillary muscle i.
paramedian i.
parenchymal i.
periventricular hemorrhagic i.
pituitary i.
placental i.
i. of pons
pontine i.
posterior cerebral territory i.
posterior wall myocardial i.
posterobasal wall myocardial i.
posteroinferior myocardial i.
posterolateral wall myocardial i.
postmyocardial i.
postmyocardiotomy i.
pulmonary i.
Q-wave myocardial i.
red i.
renal i.
right ventricular i.
rule out myocardial i. (ROMI)
segmental bowel i.
segmental omental i.
septal myocardial i.
septic pulmonary i.
severe i.
silent myocardial i.
sinoatrial node i.
i. size limitation
small bowel i.
small, deep, recent i. (SDRI)
spinal cord i.
splenic i.
subacute ischemic brain i.
subacute myocardial i.
subcortical i.
subendocardial i. (SEI)
subendocardial myocardial i.
temporal lobe i.
testicular i.
thalamic i.
thrombolysis in myocardial i. (TIMI)
thrombotic i.
transmural myocardial i.
traumatic i.
uncomplicated myocardial i.
uninfected i.
venous i.
ventral pontine i.
watershed brain i.
wedge-shaped i.
white matter i.

infarct-avid
i.-a. hot-spot scintigraphy
i.-a. imaging

infarcted
i. bowel
i. heart muscle
i. lung segment
i. scar
i. testis

infarction (*var. of* infarct)

infarct-localized asynergy

infarctoid cardiomyopathy

infected
i. aneurysm
i. bone
i. pelvic hematoma
i. thrombosed graft

infection
aortic graft i.
bone i.
buccal space i.
diffuse i.
diskovertebral i.
disk space i.
hepatic fungal i.
intraabdominal i.
masticator space i.
mycotic lung i.
nosocomial i.
opportunistic i.
opportunistic lung cavity i.
orbital i.
pelvic i.
pneumocystic i.
Pneumocystis carinii kidney i.
pulmonary parenchymal i.
renal fungal i.
respiratory tract i.
retroperitoneal i.
sacroiliac i.
salivary gland i.
spinal i.

subperiosteal i.
temporal space i.
tendon sheath space i.
vessel displacement brain i.

infectious
i. aortitis
i. bubbly bone lesion
i. cardiomyopathy
i. sacroiliitis
i. splenomegaly

infective
i. embolus
i. thrombosis

inferior
i. accessory fissure
i. apical aspect of the myocardium
i. aspect
i. border
i. border of heart
i. cardiac branch
i. cerebellar peduncle
i. colliculus
i. dental canal
i. displacement
i. dorsal radioulnar ligament
i. duodenal recess
i. epigastric artery
i. esophageal sphincter (IES)
i. extensor retinaculum
fovea i.
i. frontal gyrus
i. gemellus muscle
i. glenohumeral ligament labral complex (IGLLC)
i. jugular vein bulb
i. lobe
i. lobe bronchus
i. lobe of lung
i. margin of superior rib
i. medial facet
i. mediastinum
i. mesenteric artery (IMA)
i. mesenteric plexus
i. mesenteric vein
i. myocardial infarct (IMI)
i. ophthalmic vein
i. orbital fissure
i. parietal lobule
i. pole
i. pubic ramus
i. pulmonary ligament
i. pulmonary vein
i. quadriceps retinaculum
i. rectal vein
i. sagittal sinus (ISS)
i. spur
i. temporal gyrus
i. temporal lobule
i. thyroid vein
i. tip of scapula
i. transverse rectal fold
i. triangle sign
i. turbinated bone
i. vena cava (IVC)
i. vena cava diaphragm
i. vena cava duplication
i. vena cava obstruction
i. vena cava orifice
i. vena cava syndrome
i. vena cava transposition
i. venacavography
i. wall
i. wall akinesis
i. wall branch
i. wall hypokinesis
i. wall MI
i. wall motion

inferior-anterior count ratio

inferiormost

inferoapical
i. defect
i. segment
i. wall

inferobasal segment

inferolateral
i. displacement of apical beat
i. surface of prostate
i. wall myocardial infarct

inferolaterally

inferomedial

inferoposterior
i. segment
i. wall myocardial infarct

inferoposterolateral
i. myocardial infarct

INFH
ischemic necrosis of femoral head

infiltrate
active i.
acute alveolar i.
aggressive interstitial i.
aggressive perivascular i.
alveolar i.
apical i.

NOTES

infiltrate *(continued)*
basilar zone i.
benign i.
bilateral interstitial pulmonary i.
bilateral upper lobe cavitary i.
bone marrow i.
brachial plexus i.
bronchocentric inflammatory i.
butterfly pattern of i.
calcareous i.
calcium i.
cavitary i.
chronic alveolar i.
circumscribed i.
confluent i.
consolidated i.
diffuse aggressive polymorphous i.
diffuse alveolar interstitial i.
diffuse bilateral alveolar i.
diffuse fatty liver i.
diffuse perivascular i.
diffuse reticulonodular i.
eosinophilic i.
epituberculous i.
fatty i.
fibronodular i.
fleeting lung i.
fluffy i.
focal interstitial i.
focal perivascular i.
ground-glass i.
hazy i.
interstitial nonlobar i.
invasive angiomatous interstitial i.
linear i.
lung base i.
marrow i.
massive i.
meningeal i.
micronodular i.
migratory patchy i.
mottled i.
multifocal aggressive i.
mural i.
parasitic i.
patchy migratory i.
peribronchial i.
pericapsular fat i.
perihilar batwing i.
peripheral i.
perivascular i.
pneumonic i.
pulmonary parenchymal i.
pulmonic i.
punctate i.
recurrent fleeting i.
reticular i.
reticulonodular i.
retrocardiac i.
reverse peripheral bat-wing i.
soft i.
strandy i.
subcutaneous i.
sulfasalazine-induced pulmonary i.
transient i.
tuberculous i.

infiltrating
i. adenocarcinoma
i. breast epitheliosis
i. ductal carcinoma
i. lesion
i. lipoma
i. plaque

infiltration
myocardial i.
i. pattern
i. suture

infiltrative
i. astrocytoma
i. cardiomyopathy
i. lymphoma

infinitesimal Z spectrum

inflamed
i. bronchus
i. edematous bronchus
i. pleura

inflammation
abdominal i.
acute phase of i.
adhesive i.
alveolar septal i.
atrophic i.
i. of bone
i. of brain
bronchial i.
bursal i.
calcaneal bursa i.
cardiac muscle i.
chronic abdominal i.
cirrhotic i.
i. of colon
diffuse i.
disseminated i.
i. of epididymis
esophageal i.
fibrinous i.
fibrosing i.
focal i.
i. of heart
hyperplastic i.
hypertrophic i.
interstitial i.
lung i.
meningeal i.
mucosal i.
myocardial i.

necrotic i.
obliterative i.
parenchymatous i.
polyarticular symmetric tophaceous joint i.
proliferative i.
pseudomembranous i.
radionuclide i.
renal i.
retrodiskal temporomandibular joint pad i.
sclerosing i.
spinal i.
spleen i.
subacute i.
suppurative i.
thyroid gland i.
transmural i.
vein i.

inflammatoria
dysphagia i.

inflammatory
i. adhesion
i. aortic aneurysm
i. bowel disease
i. bowel disease arthritis
i. breast cancer (IBC)
i. cholesteatoma
i. colonic polyp
i. edema
i. endometritis
i. esophagogastric polyp
i. fibroid polyp
i. fibrosarcoma
i. focus
i. fracture
i. heart block
i. idiopathic orbital pseudotumor
i. intestinal pseudotumor
i. joint effusion
i. lesion
i. myofibroblastic tumor
i. polypoid mass
i. reaction
i. response syndrome
i. spleen
i. stomach polyp
i. synovial process

inflation
air i.
balloon i.
sequential balloon i.
simultaneous balloon i.

inflow
aortic i.
blood i.
i. cuff
i. disease progression
i. tract of left ventricle

influence
paramagnetic i.

information
hierarchical i.
imaging-directed 3D volumetric i.

infraapical

infracalcaneal bursitis

infracalcarine gyrus

infracardiac-type total anomalous venous return

infraclavicular
i. area
i. node
i. pocket

infracolic
i. compartment
i. midline

infracristal ventricular septal defect

infraction
i. fracture
Freiberg i.

infradiaphragmatic vein

infragastric infragenicular popliteal artery

infragenicular position

infrageniculate popliteal artery

infraglenoid
i. recess
i. tuberosity

infraglottic
i. larynx
i. space

infragluteal crease

infrahepatic
i. arteriography
i. vena cava

infrahilar area

infra-His block

infrahisian block

infrahyoid
i. lymph node

infrainguinal
i. bypass stenosis

NOTES

infrainguinal *(continued)*
i. revascularization
i. vein bypass graft
inframammary
i. crease
i. fold
i. syndrome
inframesocolic space
infranulcear lesion
infraorbital
i. canal
i. groove
i. margin (IOM)
infraorbitomeatal line (IOML)
infrapatellar
i. aspect
i. bursa
i. contracture syndrome (IPCS)
i. ligament
i. plica
i. tendon
i. view
infrapopliteal
i. artery occlusion
i. vessel
infrapulmonary
i. position
infrared
i. imaging
i. light
i. light-emitting diode
i. ray
i. spectrum
i. thermography
infrared-linked navigational device
infrarenal
i. abdominal aorta
i. abdominal aortic aneurysm
i. stenosis
infrascapular
infraspinatus
i. insertion erosion
i. muscle
i. tendon
infraspinous
i. fascia
i. fossa
infrasternal
i. angle
i. fossa
infratemporal fossa
infratentorial
i. compartment
i. Lindau tumor
i. syndrome
infraumbilical
i. mound
i. omphalocele
infravesical obstruction
infundibula (*pl. of* infundibulum)
infundibular
i. atresia
i. chamber
i. pulmonary stenosis
i. septum
i. stalk
i. subpulmonic stenosis
i. tumor
i. ventricular septal defect
infundibuloovarian ligament
infundibulopelvic ligament
infundibuloventricular crest
infundibulum, pl. **infundibula**
i. of bile duct
bile duct i.
cerebral i.
ductus i
gallbladder i.
i. of hypophysis
junctional i.
i. of kidney
os i.
pituitary i.
right ventricular i.
i. sign
tumor of i.
i. widening
Infuse-a-Port catheter
infuser
Ohio i.
infusion
balloon-occluded arterial i.
circadian continuous i.
continuous intravenous i. (CIVI)
epidural i.
graded i.
hepatic arterial i. (HAI)
intralymphatic i.
intraportal i.
isolated hepatic i.
isoproterenol i.
local streptokinase i.
pericardial i.
protracted venous i. (PVI)
retrograde coronary sinus i.
subcutaneous i.
i. transcatheter therapy
infusothorax
ingestion
foreign body i.
Ingram-Bachynski
I.-B. classification of hip fractures
I.-B. hip fracture classification
ingrowth
bone i.

peripheral perimeniscal capillary i.
porous i.

inguinal
i. bulge
i. canal
i. crease
i. floor
i. fold
i. granuloma
i. ligament
i. ligament syndrome
i. lymphadenectomy
i. lymph node
i. lymph node metastasis
i. ring
i. triangle
i. trigone

inguinale
papilloma i.

inhalation
i. bronchopneumonia
end i.
i. of krypton-77
i. pneumonia
i. of radioactive xenon gas
radioactive xenon gas i.
i. study
i. technique
i. tuberculosis

inhaled
i. oxygen
i. oxygen imaging agent
i. radionuclide

inherent filter

inhibited
atrial i. (AAI)

inhomogeneity
contrast i.
i. correction
hypointense signal i.
metaphyseal-diaphyseal low-signal-intensity red marrow i.
off-axis dose i.
signal intensity i.

inhomogeneous
i. echo
i. echo pattern
i. echo texture
i. enhancement
i. image
i. lung attenuation HRCT
i. tracer distribution

iniencephaly

^{111}In-InG

inion bump

initial
i. atelectasis
i. imaging

injection
air i.
AK-Fluor i.
barium i.
bolus intravenous i.
contrast i.
double i.
epidural steroid i.
extraarachnoid i.
facet joint i.
Fluorescite i.
Funduscein i.
hand i.
heavy metal i.
inadvertent arterial i.
intraamniotic i.
intraarterial i.
intracavernosal i.
intradermal i.
intramuscular fetal i.
intramuscular (IM) i.
intraperitoneal fetal i.
intravascular i.
intravenous fetal i.
intravenous (IV) bolus i.
ipsilateral i.
machine i.
manual i.
i. mass
Omnipaque i.
opacifying i.
percutaneous ethanol i.
i. port
power i.
i. of radionuclide
radionuclide i.
rest i.
retrograde i.
i. scan interval (ISI)
sclerosing i.
selective i.
selective arterial i.
serial i.
silicone i.
straight AP pelvic i.
subarachnoid i.

NOTES

injection *(continued)*
subdural contrast i.
test i.
ultrasonographically guided i.
venous i.
injector
auto i.
Cordis i.
Hercules power i.
Medrad contrast medium i.
Medrad power angiographic i.
power i.
pressure i.
PulseSpray i.
Renovist II i.
Taveras i.
injury
acute stretch i.
acute traumatic aortic i. (ATAI)
Ajmalin liver i.
Allman classification of acromioclavicular i.
anterior cruciate ligament i.
anterior urethral i.
aortic-brachiocephalic (ABC) i.
apophyseal i.
axial compression i.
ballistic i.
barked i.
bilateral incomplete ureteral i.
blunt i.
bony trabecular i.
brachial plexus birth i.
burst i.
cervical spine i.
closed head i. (CHI)
clothesline i.
cocking i.
compression flexion i.
compressive hyperextension i.
concomitant tracheal i.
contrecoup i.
cruciate ligament i.
crush i.
decelerative i.
degloving i.
diffuse white matter i.
diskoligamentous i.
distraction hyperflexion i.
endothelial i.
epiphyseal plate i.
Erb i.
Erb-Duchenne-Klumpke i.
extension i.
extensive head i.
firearm i.
flexion-distraction i.
flexion-rotation i.
forced flexion i.
genitourinary i.
Gertzbein classification of seatbelt i.
glenoid labrum i.
greater arc i.
growth plate i.
head i. (HI)
high-caliber, low-velocity handgun i.
hollow viscus i.
hyperextension i.
hyperflexion/hyperextension cervical i.
hypertension i.
hypoxic i.
hypoxic/ischemic i.
iatrogenic ureteral i.
immunologic i.
intercostal nerve i.
intraoperative gastrointestinal i.
intraperitoneal i.
inversion i.
irradiation i.
ischemic reperfusion i.
isolated airway i.
Klumpke brachial plexus i.
Kulkarni i.
labral i.
lateral bending i.
lateral compartment traumatic bony i.
lesser arc i.
lethal myocardial i.
Lisfranc i.
locked facet i.
low back i.
Maisonneuve i.
matrix i.
mechanism of i.
meniscal i.
metatarsal i.
midtarsal i.
mild head i.
motor vehicle i. (MVI)
myocardial reperfusion i.
needlestick i.
nerve i.
nonlethal myocardial ischemic i.
obstetric i.
overuse i.
penetrating lung i.
P-ER i.
pericarinal i.
perinatal i.
peripheral nerve i.
phrenic nerve i.
physeal i.

plexus i.
posterior cruciate ligament i.
posterior urethral i. (PUI)
posterolateral corner i.
postnatal i.
prenatal i.
pronation-abduction i.
pronation-external rotation i.
proximity i.
pulmonary parenchymal i.
radial vascular thermal i.
radiation-induced skin i.
rapid deceleration i.
rectal radiation i.
renal i.
repetitive strain i. (RSI)
repetitive stress i. (RSI)
Sage-Salvatore classification of acromioclavicular joint i.
seatbelt i.
sesamoid i.
severe head i.
I. Severity Scale (ISS)
I. Severity Score (ISS)
shearing white matter i.
skier's i.
softball sliding i.
soft tissue i.
solid viscus i
spinal cord i. (SCI)
straddle i.
strain-sprain i.
stress i.
subendocardial i.
superior labral anteroposterior (SLAP) i.
supination-adduction i.
supination-external rotation i.
supination-outward rotation i.
talofibular ligament i.
tensile i.
three-column i.
through-and-through i.
throwing arm i.
tracheobronchial i. (TBI)
transcutaneous crush i.
traumatic aortic i.
traumatic brain i. (TBI)
traumatic head i.
two-column i.
ultrasonic assessment of i.
unilateral locked facet i.
urethral straddle i.
valgus-external rotation i.
vesical i.
weightbearing rotational i.
whiplash i.
white matter shearing i.
windup i.
Zlotsky-Ballard classification of acromioclavicular i.

^{111}In-labeled
^{111}In-l. human nonspecific immunoglobulin G
^{111}In-l. leukocyte bone
^{111}In-l. white blood cell

inlay graft

inlet
esophageal i.
pelvic i.
thoracic i.
transaxial thoracic i.

inner
i. adrenal cortex
i. bright layer
i. ear
i. ear anatomy
i. ear atresia
i. ear mass
i. ear vestibule
i. stripe of Baillinger
i. table
i. table of the skull

innermost intercostal muscle

innervation
sympathetic i.

Innervision MR scanner

innocent gallstone

innocuous

innominate
i. absence of line
i. aneurysm
i. angiography
i. artery
i. artery buckling
i. artery compression syndrome
i. artery kinking
i. artery stenosis
i. bone
i. canaliculus
i. vein

Innovator Holter system

innumerable
i. small enhancing brain lesions
i. small enhancing cerebral nodule
inoperable brain tumor
inorganic phosphorus
In-pentetreotide scintigraphy
in-phase
i.-p. GRE imaging
i.-p. image
i.-p. sequence
in-plane vessel
Inrad HiLiter ultrasound-enhanced stylet
Insall ratio
Insall-Salvati
I.-S. index
I.-S. ratio
insertion
anomalous i.
Bosworth bone peg i.
capsular i.
catheter i.
femoral vein percutaneous i.
Huntington rod i.
ligamentous i.
percutaneous pin i.
tendinous i.
velamentous i.
insidious
i. onset
i. progression
insipidus
nephrogenic diabetes i.
insonation
angle of i.
Doppler i.
insonifying wave field
Inspec-100
inspiration
degree of i.
shallow i.
suspended i.
inspiratory
i. effort
i. to expiratory (I:E)
i. to expiratory ratio
i. flow
i. flow rate
i. increase in venous pressure
i. muscle function impairment
i. phase
i. reserve volume (IRV)
i. retraction
i. spasm
i. stridor
i. view
inspired air
inspissated
i. feces
i. material
i. meconium
instability
ankle i.
anterolateral rotary knee i.
articular i.
atlantoaxial i.
atraumatic, multidirectional, bilateral radial i. (AMBRI)
chronic functional i.
detrusor i.
dissociative i.
dorsal intercalated segmental i. (DISI)
first ray i.
genomic i.
glenohumeral i.
hindfoot i.
inversion i.
ischemic i.
joint i.
lateral rotatory ankle i.
ligamentous i.
microsatellite i.
midcarpal i.
nondissociative i.
osseous i.
perilunar i.
perilunate i.
phase i.
posterolateral rotatory i.
postlaminectomy i.
rotary ankle i.
rotational i.
rotatory i.
shoulder joint i.
spinal i.
i. of spine
subtalar i.
sympathetic vascular i.
truncal i.
varus-valgus i.
ventricular electrical i.
volarflexed intercalated segment i.
volar intercalated segment i.
instantaneous
i. enhancement rate
i. gradient
InstaScan scanner
instillation
contrast material i.
subarachnoid i.
instrument
Advanced Breast Biopsy I.
ionization i.

i. output
Sabouraud-Noiré i.

instrumentation
interspinous segmental spinal i. (ISSI)
I. Laboratory system

insufficiency
acute cerebrovascular i.
acute coronary i.
adrenal i.
aortic valvular i.
arterial i.
autonomic i.
basilar artery i.
brachial-basilar i.
cardiac i.
cardiopulmonary i.
cerebrovascular i.
chronic venous i.
congenital pulmonary valve i.
coronary i.
deep venous i. (DVI)
i. fracture
gastric i.
hepatic i.
hypostatic pulmonary i.
ileocecal i.
mesenteric vascular i.
mitral i. (MI)
muscular i.
myocardial i.
nonocclusive mesenteric arterial i.
nonrheumatic aortic i.
pad sign of aortic i.
parathyroid i.
postirradiation vascular i.
posttraumatic pulmonary i.
primary adrenal i.
pulmonary arterial flow i.
pulmonary valve i.
pulmonic i. (PI)
pyloric i.
renal i.
respiratory i.
rheumatic aortic i.
secondary venous i.
Sternberg myocardial i.
thyroid i.
transient ischemic carotid i.
tricuspid i. (TI)
uterine i.
uteroplacental i.
valvular aortic i.
vascular i.
velopharyngeal i.
venous i.
vertebrobasilar i. (VBI)

insufficient cochlear turn

insufflation
air i.
CO_2 i.
gas i.
mechanical i.
perirenal i.
tubal i.

insula, pl. **insulae**
roof of i.
i. root

insular
i. gyrus
i. lobe
i. region
i. region of brain
i. ribbon sign
i. triangle

insulative development

insulinoma

insult
aortic i.
bihemispheral i.
cerebrovascular i.
hypoxic ischemic i.
mechanical i.
myocardial i.
occlusive cerebrovascular i.
vascular i.

intact
i. valve cusp
i. ventricular septum

intake
fluid i.

integral
Choquet fuzzy i.
i. dose
systolic velocity-time i.
i. uniformity scintillation camera

integrated
i. optical density (IOD)
i. optical density histogram
i. reference air-kerma (IRAK)

Integris
I. 3000 scanner
I. V3000 imager

NOTES

integrity
spinal i.
intense uptake
intensification
frequency i.
image i.
intensified
i. radiographic imaging system (IRIS)
i. radiographic imaging system scanner
intensifier
image i.
portable C-arm i.
intensifying
i. screen
i. screen artifact
intensity
absolute dose i. (ADI)
amorphous high signal i.
beam i.
calcified sequestra of low signal i.
central fat signal i.
central intrasubstance signal i.
dark signal i.
decreased i.
diminished marrow signal i.
discrete hyperintense signal i.
equal in i.
fat signal i.
grade 1–3 signal i.
heterogeneous signal i.
homogeneous signal i.
increase in i.
intermediate signal i.
intrameniscal signal i.
juxtaarticular low signal i.
linear degenerative signal i.
low signal i.
marrow fat signal i.
maximal i.
pedicle signal i.
photostimulable luminescence i.
radiation i.
reduced signal i.
signal i. (SI)
site of maximal i.
spatial average-pulse average (SAPA) i.
spatial average-temporal average (SATA) i.
spatial peak-temporal average (SPTA) i.
temporal average i.
temporal peak i.
variable i.
vertebral body marrow signal i.
waterlike signal i.
i. windowing
intensity-modulated
i.-m. photon beam
i.-m. radiation therapy (IMRT)
intensive
i. care unit
i. therapy unit (ITU)
intentional reversible thrombosis
interaction
capacitive i.
dipolar i.
dipole-dipole i.
effector/target cell i.
electric i.
magnetic i.
mind-body i.
proton-electron dipole-dipole i.
interactive
i. electronic scalpel
i. gradient optimization
i. MR-guided biopsy
interaorticobronchial diverticulum
interarch distance
interarticular
i. cartilage
i. disk
i. ridge
interarticularis
pars i.
interatrial
i. baffle leak
i. communication
i. groove
i. septal defect
i. septal hypertrophy
i. septum (IAS)
i. transposition of venous return
interbody
i. bone graft
i. bone plug
i. fusion
interbronchial
i. diverticulum
i. mass
intercalary defect
intercalated segment
intercalating agent
intercalation
intercapital ligament
intercarpal
i. articular
i. articulation
i. coalition
i. joint
i. ligament
intercaudate distance
intercaval band

intercavernous
- i. anastomosis
- i. sinus

intercellular
- i. edema
- i. space

intercervical disk herniation
interchondral joint
interchordal space fenestration
interclavicular
- i. ligament
- i. notch

interclinoid ligament
intercollicular groove
intercom
- noise-reduction i.

intercomparison
- i. measurement
- i. measurement technique

intercondylar
- i. eminence
- i. femoral fracture
- i. fossa
- i. groove
- i. humeral fracture
- i. joint space
- i. notch
- i. roof
- i. sagittal image
- i. tibial fracture
- i. tubercle

intercondyloid fossa
intercornual ligament
intercoronary
- i. collateral flow
- i. steal syndrome

intercostal
- i. artery
- i. artery angiography
- i. lymph node
- i. muscle
- i. nerve
- i. nerve injury
- i. neuromuscular bundle
- i. retraction
- i. space
- i. vein
- i. vessel

intercostobrachial nerve
intercristal diameter
intercuneiform ligament
interdigital
- i. clavus
- i. ligament
- i. neoplasm
- i. neuroma

interdigitation
- cerebral gyri i.
- i. of vastus lateralis

interest
- region of i. (ROI)

interface
- acetabular-prosthetic i.
- acoustic i.
- air i.
- air–soft tissue i.
- bidirectional i.
- body i.
- bone-air i.
- bone-implant i.
- catheter-skin i.
- common gateway i. (CGI)
- dermal–subcutaneous fat i.
- Digital Imaging and Communications in Medicine i. (DICOM)
- disk-thecal sac i.
- fat-fluid density i.
- fat-water i.
- fluid i.
- gray/white matter i.
- joint i.
- lumen-intimal i.
- media-adventitia i.
- muscle-fat i.
- reactive i.
- shear i.
- socket/residuum i.
- socket-stump i.
- transducer-skin i.

interfacetal dislocation
interfacial canal
interference
- i. dissociation
- electromagnetic i. (EMI)
- i. screw
- slice i.

interferometry
- phase-shifting i.

interfibrosis
interfollicular Hodgkin disease
interfoveolar ligament
interfraction interval

NOTES

interfragmental compression
interfragmentary plate
intergluteal cleft
interhaustral septum
interhemispheric
i. asymmetry
i. cyst
i. fissure (IHF)
i. subdural hematoma
interictal
i. PET FDG study
i. phase
i. SPECT
i. SPECT study
i. spiking
interiliac lymph node
interinnominoabdominal cleft
interior surface of pancreas
interlacing
interlaminar
i. distance
interleaved
i. acquisition
i. axial slab
i. GRE sequence
i. imaging passes
i. inversion-readout segment
i. phase contrast technique
interleukin-3
iodine-125-labeled i.
interlobar
i. artery
i. empyema
i. fissure
i. pleurisy
i. septal line
i. septum
i. space
interlobular
i. bile duct
i. emphysema
i. lung septum
i. septal thickening
i. septum
i. tissue
i. vasculature
i. vessel
interlocking detachable coil
interloop abscess
intermaxillary
i. bone
i. spine
intermedia
massa i.
intermediate
i. bronchus
i. bursa
i. callus
i. coronary artery
i. coronary syndrome
i. CT slice
i. cuneiform bone
i. cuneiform fracture-dislocation
i. fetal death
i. heart
i. image
i. imaging
i. nerve of Wrisberg
i. ray
i. signal intensity
i. signal mass
intermediolateral
i. gray column
i. tract
intermedius
bronchus i.
nervus i.
vastus i.
intermesenteric
i. abscess
i. plexus
intermetacarpal articulation
intermetatarsal (IM)
i. angle (IMA)
i. joint
i. ligament
i. space
intermetatarsophalangeal
i. bursa
i. bursitis
intermittent
i. diffuse esophageal spasm
i. occlusion
i. sinus arrest
i. third-degree AV block
intermuscular
i. hematoma
i. septum
interna
endometriosis i.
hyperostosis frontalis i.
theca i.
internal
i. abdominal ring
i. aberrant carotid artery
i. auditory canal
i. auditory canal anatomy
i. auditory canal enhancing lesion
i. auditory meatus
i. band
i. biliary drainage
i. caliber
i. capsule
i. capsule intracerebral hemorrhage
i. carotid
i. carotid angiography

i. carotid artery (ICA)
i. carotid artery aneurysm
i. carotid balloon test
i. carotid system
i. cerebral vein (ICV)
i. cervical os
i. clot
i. collateral ligament
i. conjugate diameter
i. conversion electron
i. cyclotron target
i. derangement
i. derangement of the knee (IDK)
i. diameter (ID)
i. disk herniation
i. echo
i. echogenicity
i. echotexture
i. femoral rotation
i. fixation device
i. hernia
i. iliac
i. iliac artery
i. inguinal ring
i. intercostal muscle
i. intermuscular septum
i. jugular bulb
i. jugular triangle
i. jugular vein (IJV)
i. mammary artery (IMA)
i. mammary artery pedicle (IMA pedicle)
i. mammary lymphatic chain
i. mammary lymph node
i. mammary lymphoscintigraphy
i. oblique aponeurosis
i. oblique radiograph
i. pudendal artery
i. pudendal vessel
i. radiation therapy
i. retention mechanism
i. rotation deformity
i. rotation in extension (IRE)
i. rotation in flexion (IRF)
i. rotation view
i. snapping hip syndrome
i. thoracic artery (ITA)
i. thoracic artery graft
i. thoracic vein
i. tibial torsion (ITT)
i. tibiofibular torsion
i. urethral orifice
i. urethrotomy

internally fixed fracture

international
I. Atomic Energy Agency (IAEA)
I. Commission on Radiation Protection (ICRP)
I. Commission on Radiation Units and Measurements (ICRU)
I. Commission on Radiological Units
I. Federation of Gynecology and Obstetrics stage carcinoma (FIGO stage carcinoma)
i. reference preparation
i. standard (IS)

internervous plane

internuclear distance

internus
obturator i.

interobserver error

interopercular distance

interorbital distance

interossei
dorsal i.
palmar i.
plantar i.

interosseous
i. border
i. cyst
first digital i. (FDI)
i. membrane (IOM)
i. muscle
i. muscle group
i. nerve
i. ridge
i. space
i. talocalcaneal ligament

interparietal
i. bone
i. suture

interpectoral lymph node

interpedicular
i. distance
i. distance widening

interpediculate

interpeduncular
i. cistern (IPC)
i. fossa
i. notch
i. space

interperiosteal fracture

NOTES

interphalangeal
i. articulation
i. dislocation
distal i. (DIP)
i. fusion
i. joint
i. joint arthritis of great toe
interpleural space
interpolation
i. algorithm
color space i.
cubic convolution i.
full scan with i. (FI)
i. kernel
linear i.
nearest neighbor i.
prism i.
trilinear i.
interpolator
color space i.
Interpore bone replacement material
interposed
i. colon segment
i. colon segment obstruction
interposition
i. graft
hepatodiaphragmatic i.
soft tissue i.
interpretation
mirror-image i.
interpretive
i. criteria
i. variability
interpulse
i. interval
i. time
interridge distance
interrogation
color duplex i.
deep Doppler velocity i.
Doppler i.
pulse Doppler i.
radiation i.
transtelephonic ICD i.
interrupted
i. duct sign
i. periosteal reaction
interruption
aortic arch i.
i. of aortic arch
i. of inferior vena cava with azygos/hemiazygos continuation
i. of pulmonary artery
pulmonary artery i.
surgical venous i.
intersacral canal
interscapular gland
interscapulothoracic amputation
intersection gap
intersegmental
i. aberration
i. laminar fusion
i. tract
intersesamoid ligament
intersex
i. female
true i.
intersigmoid recess
interslice
i. distance
i. gap
interspace
ballooning of vertebral i.
disk i.
vertebral disk i.
wedging of vertebral i.
intersperse
interspersed lucency
intersphincteric
i. abscess
i. anal fistula
interspinal muscle
interspinous
i. distance
i. ligament
i. plane
i. process
i. process fusion
i. segmental spinal instrumentation (ISSI)
i. widening
interstice, pl. **interstices**
bone i.
graft i.
interstitial
i. afterloading nylon tube
i. atrophy
i. boost
i. bronchiolitic respiratory disease
i. calcinosis
i. change
i. conductive heating
i. congestion of epididymis
i. cystitis
i. diffuse pulmonary fibrosis
i. ectopic pregnancy
i. fluid
i. fluid hydrostatic pressure
i. fluid space
i. heat-generating source
i. hemorrhage
i. hernia
i. hyperthermia
i. hyperthermia treatment
i. implant
i. inflammation

i. laser photocoagulation
i. loculated hematoma
i. lung disease
i. lung disease distribution
i. lung disease with increased lung volume
i. lung emphysema
i. lung pattern
i. markings
i. meniscal tear
i. nephritis
i. nodule HRCT
i. nonlobar infiltrate
i. OB line sign
i. organizing pneumonia
i. pattern
i. plasma cell pneumonia
i. pneumonia air leak
i. pneumonitis
i. prematurity fibrosis
i. probe
i. prominence
i. pulmonary edema
i. pulmonary fibrosis (IPF)
i. radioactive colloid therapy
i. radioelement application
i. radiosurgery
i. radiotherapy
i. salpingitis
i. scarring
i. shadowing
i. tear pattern
i. template irradiation
i. therapy
i. thermoradiotherapy
i. tissue

interstitiospinal tract

interstitium
lung i.
pulmonary i.

intertarsal

interthalamic bridge

intertrabecular
i. hemorrhage
i. soft tissue

intertransverse
i. foramen
i. ligament
i. muscle

intertrochanteric
i. crest
i. four-part fracture
i. plate
i. ridge

intertubercular
i. bursitis
i. diameter
i. groove
i. plane

intertwin membrane

interuncal distance

interureteric ridge

interval
acromiohumeral i. (AHI)
i. articulation
atlantoaxial i.
atlantodens i. (ADI)
basion-axial i.
basion-dens i.
i. change
i. development
disease-free i. (DFI)
i. ejection fraction
escape i.
high-rate detect i.
i. improvement
injection scan i. (ISI)
interfraction i.
interpulse i.
i. intraatrial conduction
lucent i.
preejection i.
i. progression
prolonged i.
QRS i.
i. resolution
rotator i.
supracricoid i.
upper rate i.
ventriculoatrial i.

interventional
i. angiography
i. imaging
i. neuroradiology
i. procedure
i. radiography
i. radiology

intervention study

interventricular
i. block
i. foramen
i. groove
i. septal defect (IVSD)

NOTES

interventricular *(continued)*
i. septal rupture
i. septal thickness (IVST)
intervertebral
i. cartilage calcification
i. disk
i. disk calcification
i. disk narrowing
i. diskogram
i. disk space
i. disk space vacuum phenomenon
i. foramen
i. joint
i. ligament
i. notch
i. osteochondrosis
intervillous
i. circulation
i. lacuna
i. placental thrombosis
interzone
intestinal
i. atony
i. Behçet syndrome
i. bypass procedure
i. calculus
i. canal
i. carcinoid tumor
i. conduit
i. congenital atresia
i. contents
i. decompression
i. dilatation
i. distention
i. diverticulum
i. doughnut sign
i. emphysema
i. fluid
i. follicle
i. gas
i. gas exchange
i. gas pattern
i. hypoperistalsis syndrome
i. infantilism
i. infarct
i. intussusception
i. kinking
i. lipodystrophy
i. loop
i. lumen
i. lymphangiectasia
i. mesentery
i. metaphysis
i. metaplasia
i. necrosis
i. obstruction
i. perforation
i. polyposis
i. prolapse
i. pseudoobstruction syndrome
i. tract
i. tract malrotation
i. tube
i. ulcer
i. ureter
i. villous architecture
i. villus
i. wall
i. web
intestinalis
pneumatosis cystoides i.
intestine
blind i.
bullous emphysema of i.
coils of i.
congenital lymphangiectasia of i.
kink in i.
large i.
malrotation of i.
papillary adenoma of large i.
serous i.
small i.
intima
arterial i.
friable thickened degenerated i.
hypertrophied i.
pulmonary artery i.
tunica i.
intimal
i. arteriosclerosis
i. atherosclerosis
i. atherosclerotic disease
i. attachment of diseased vessel
i. debris
i. degeneration
i. fibroplasia
i. flap
i. hyperplasia (IH)
i. irregularity
i. proliferation
i. remodeling
i. tear
i. thickening
intimal-medial dissection
intimate attachment
intimomedial thickness
intolerance
exercise i.
intoxication
psychogenic water i.
systemic mercury i.
water i.
intraabdominal
i. abscess
i. arterial bypass graft
i. arterial hemorrhage

i. calcification
i. fat
i. fetal calcification
i. infection
i. mass
i. viscera
intraacetabular
intraacinar pulmonary artery
intraalveolar fibrosis
intraamniotic injection
intraaneurysmal thrombus
intraaortic
i. balloon assist
i. balloon counterpulsation
i. balloon pump (IABP)
intraarterial
i. chemotherapy catheter
i. digital subtraction angiography (IADSA)
i. filling defect
i. injection
i. stereotactic digital subtraction angiography
i. superselective nimodipine
i. thrombosis
i. thrombus
intraarticular
i. adhesion
i. calcaneal fracture
i. contrast
i. debris
i. ganglion
i. hemangioma
i. knee fusion
i. ligament
i. localized nodular synovitis
i. loose body
i. plate of fibrocartilage
i. proximal tibial fracture
i. radiopharmaceutical therapy
intraatrial
i. block
i. filling defect
i. reentry
i. thrombus
intraauricular muscle
intraaxial
i. brain lesion
i. brain tumor
i. varix
intracanalicular
i. irradiation
intracapsular
i. ankylosis
i. fat pad
i. femoral neck fracture
i. osteoid osteoma
intracardiac
i. calcification
i. calcium
i. echocardiography (ICE)
i. mass
i. pressure
i. thrombus
intracartilaginous
i. bone
i. ossification
intracaval
i. endovascular ultrasonography
i. endovascular ultrasound (ICEUS)
intracavernosal injection
intracavernous
i. carotid aneurysm
i. internal carotid artery
intracavitary
i. afterloading applicator
i. clot formation
i. delivery
i. extension
i. extension of tumor
i. filling defect
i. hyperthermia treatment
i. implant
i. irradiation
i. prostate ultrasonography
i. prostate ultrasound
i. radiation source
i. radiation therapy
i. radioactive colloid therapy
i. radioelement application
i. radiotherapy
i. radium
intracavity mass
intracellular
i. adhesion molecule
i. water
intracerebral
i. aneurysm
i. arteriovenous malformation
i. blood
i. ganglioglioma
i. ganglioma
i. hematoma
i. hemorrhage (ICH)

NOTES

intracerebral *(continued)*
i. hemorrhage trauma
i. lesion
i. lymphoma
i. tumor
i. vascular malformation
intracerebroventricular (ICV)
intrachondral bone
intracolonic Kaposi sarcoma
intracompartmental
i. edema
i. ischemia
i. tumor
intraconal
i. lesion
i. portion of the eye
intracondyloid
intracoronary
i. contrast echocardiography
i. imaging
i. radiation therapy (ICRT)
i. stenting
i. stent placement
i. thrombolytic therapy
i. ultrasound (ICUS)
intracortical
i. osteogenic sarcoma
i. osteosarcoma
intracranial
i. air
i. aneurysm (ICA)
i. arteriovenous fistula
i. arteriovenous malformation
i. berry aneurysm
i. carotid artery atherosclerosis
i. cavernous angioma
i. circulation
i. cryptococcosis
i. dermoid cyst
i. electroencephalography
i. embolus
i. epidural pressure (ECIDP)
i. fat prolapse
i. germinoma
i. glioma
i. hematoma
i. hemorrhage
i. hypertension
i. imaging
i. lipoma
i. mass
i. mass lesion
i. MR angiography
i. neoplasm
i. neuroblastoma
i. physiologic calcification
i. pneumocephalus
i. pressure (ICP)
i. seeding
i. shift
i. sinus thrombosis
i. tuberculoma
i. tumor
i. vascular abnormality
i. vascular lesion
i. vascular occlusion
i. vertebral artery
i. vessel
intractable
i. bleeding disorder
i. heart failure
i. ulcer
intracystic
i. breast cancer
i. breast papillary carcinoma in situ
intradermal
i. angioma
i. injection
intradiaphragmatic aortic segment
intradiskal
Intra-Dop intraoperative device
intraductal
i. breast filling defect
i. breast papillomatosis
i. bridge
i. calcification
i. carcinoma
i. mucin-producing tumor
i. papilloma
i. pressure
i. ultrasonography
intraduodenal choledochal cyst
intradural
i. abscess
i. arteriovenous fistula
i. disk herniation
i. epidermoidoma
i. extramedullary lesion
i. extramedullary mass
i. inflammatory disease
i. lipoma
i. nerve root
i. retromedullary arteriovenous fistula
i. spinal AVM
i. tumor
i. vessel
intraforaminal vein
intragastric bubble
intrahaustral contraction ring
intrahepatic
i. abscess
i. arterial-portal fistula
i. atresia (IHA)
i. AV fistula

i. bile duct
i. biliary calculus
i. biliary cancer
i. biliary cystic dilatation
i. biliary ductal dilatation
i. biliary neoplasm
i. biliary tract
i. biliary tract dilatation
i. biliary tree
i. biloma
i. cholangiocarcinoma
i. cholestasis
i. pigment stone disease
i. portal vein branch
i. portal vein gas
i. sclerosing cholangitis
i. stone

intra-His block

intrahisian block

intralabyrinthine

intralaminar thalamus

intraligamentary pregnancy

intraligamentous bursa

intralobar sequestration

intralobular
i. connective tissue
i. fibrosis
i. terminal duct

intraluminal
i. adenocarcinoma
i. air
i. debris
i. dephasing
i. detail
i. dilatation
i. dimension
i. duodenal diverticulum (IDD)
i. embolus
i. esophageal pressure
i. filling defect
i. flow phenomenon
i. foreign body
i. gallstone
i. hemorrhage
i. intubation
i. membrane
i. plaque
i. stomach mass
i. stone
i. thrombus
i. ultrasound (ILUS)
i. ultrasound catheter

intralymphatic
i. infusion
i. radioactivity administration

intramammary
i. lesion
i. lymph node

intramedullary (IM)
i. arteriovenous malformation
i. bony disease
i. canal
i. compartment neoplasm
i. cord lesion
i. demyelination
i. epidermoid cyst
i. fixation
i. fixation device
i. lipoma
i. marrow involvement
i. nail
i. rodding
i. spinal cord tumor
i. spinal lesion
i. tumor biopsy

intramembranous
i. bone
i. ossification

intrameniscal
i. cyst
i. mucoid degeneration
i. signal intensity

intramesenteric abscess

intramural
i. air in colon
i. arterial hemorrhage
i. clot
i. colonic air
i. coronary artery aneurysm
i. diverticulum
i. esophageal diverticulosis
i. esophageal pseudodiverticulosis
i. esophageal rupture
i. fibroid
i. filling defect
i. gas
i. gastric emphysema
i. gastrointestinal tract hemorrhage
i. hematoma
i. hematoma of aorta
i. leiomyosarcoma
i. mapping
i. mechanics
i. portion of distal ureter

NOTES

intramural *(continued)*
i. rupture of the esophagus
i. thrombus
i. tumor
i. tunnel
intramural-extramucosal stomach lesion
intramuscular
i. aortic segment
i. fetal injection
i. fluid pressure
i. hemangioma
i. hemosiderin deposit
i. (IM) injection
i. venous malformation
intramyocardially
intraneural ganglion cyst
intraneuronal neurofibrillary tangle
intranodal
i. architecture
i. block
i. myofibroblastoma
in-transit metastasis
intranuclear
i. cleft
i. diskogram
intraobserver error
intraocular
i. calcification
i. foreign body
i. lesion
i. melanoma
i. spread
Intra-Op autotransfusion system
intraoperative
i. arteriography
i. cardioplegic contrast echocardiography
i. cholangiogram
i. digital subtraction angiography (IDIS, IDSA)
i. Doppler
i. electrocortical stimulation (IOECS)
i. electrocortical stimulation mapping
i. fracture
i. gamma probe
i. gastrointestinal injury
i. high dose rate (IOHDR)
i. imaging
i. laser photocoagulation
i. pancreatography
i. radiation therapy (IORT)
i. radiography
i. radiotherapy
i. scanning technique
i. sonography (IOS)
i. ventriculogram
i. view
i. x-ray visualization
intraoral
i. cone irradiation
i. periapical radiography
i. swage technique
intraorbital air
intraosseous
i. abscess
i. arteriovenous malformation
i. bone lesion
i. desmoid tumor
i. ganglion
i. keratin cyst
i. lipoma
i. meningioma
i. osteosarcoma
i. vascular malformation
i. venography
i. wiring
intrapancreatic obstruction
intrapapillary terminus
intraparenchymal
i. blood
i. cyst
i. hematoma
i. hemorrhage
i. lymph node
i. meningioma
i. metastasis
intrapatellar fat pad
intrapedicular fixation
intrapericardial
i. bleeding
i. diaphragmatic hernia
i. patch lead placement
i. portion
i. pressure
intraperiosteal fracture
intraperitoneal
i. abscess
i. air
i. cavity
i. drug administration
i. exposure
i. fetal injection
i. fluid
i. hyperthermic perfusion (IPHP)
i. injury
i. pregnancy
i. rupture
i. rupture of bladder
i. technetium sulfur colloid imaging
i. viscera
intrapixel
i. sequential processing (IPSP)
i. sequential processing neuron evaluation method

intraplacental venous lake
intraplaque hemorrhage (IPH)
intrapleural
- i. hemorrhage
- i. pressure

intrapontine intracerebral hemorrhage
intraportal
- i. endovascular ultrasonography (IPEUS)
- i. infusion

intrapulmonary
- i. arteriovenous fistula
- i. barotrauma
- i. bronchogenic cyst
- i. bronchus
- i. disease
- i. hemorrhage
- i. pressure

intrarectal
- i. coil
- i. ultrasound

intrarenal
- i. arterial disease
- i. arterial flow
- i. collecting system
- i. hematoma
- i. pelvis
- i. reflux
- i. stenosis

intrascapular ligament
intrascrotal abscess
intrasellar
- i. brain mass
- i. lesion
- i. Rathke cleft cyst
- i. tumor

intrasinus air-fluid level
intraspinal
- i. adenoma
- i. enteric cyst
- i. lesion
- i. tumor

intraspongy nuclear disk herniation
intrastitial radiation source
intrasubstance cleavage tear
intrasynovial disease
intratemporal fossa
intratendinous
- i. bursa
- i. fluid collection
- i. rupture

intratendon sheath
intratentorial lipoma
intratesticular
- i. band
- i. cyst

intrathecal
- APT i.
- i. imaging
- i. root
- i. space

intrathoracic
- i. cyst
- i. dimension
- i. dislocation of shoulder
- i. fetal mass
- i. goiter
- i. Kaposi sarcoma
- i. low-attenuation mass
- i. pressure
- i. stomach
- i. thyroid
- i. trachea
- i. upper airway obstruction

intratracheal
intratumoral
- i. agent
- i. hemorrhage
- i. necrosis
- i. structure

intrauterine
- i. cardiac failure
- i. contraceptive device (IUD)
- i. cytomegalic inclusion disease
- i. demise
- i. fetus
- i. fracture
- i. gas (IUG)
- i. gestation
- i. growth restriction
- i. growth retardation (IUGR)
- i. heart failure
- i. membrane
- i. parabiotic syndrome
- i. pregnancy
- i. sac

intravaginal torsion
intravasation
- venous i.

intravascular
- i. clotting process
- i. coil
- i. congestion
- i. consumption coagulopathy

NOTES

intravascular *(continued)*
i. content extravasation
i. contents
i. filling defect
i. foreign body
i. injection
i. leiomyosarcoma
i. mass
i. MRI catheter-based technique
i. papillary endothelial hyperplasia
i. radiopharmaceutical therapy
i. sickling
i. space
i. stent
i. stenting
i. thrombosis
i. tumor thrombus
i. ultrasonography
i. ultrasound (IVUS)
i. ultrasound catheter
i. ultrasound imaging
i. volume depletion
i. volume status
intravenous
i. administration of contrast material
i. block
i. bolus
i. cholangiogram
i. cholangiography
i. digital subtraction angiography (IVDSA)
i. fetal injection
i. fluorescein angiography (IVFA)
i. fluorescein angiography imaging (IVFA imaging)
i. infusion line
i. injection of isotope
i. (IV) bolus injection
i. pyelography (IVP)
i. stereotactic digital subtraction angiography
i. urography (IVU)
intravenously
i. enhanced CT scan
i. enhanced MRI
intraventricular
i. aberration
i. block (IVB)
i. blood
i. brain tumor
i. conduction block
i. conduction delay
i. cryptococcal cyst
i. heart block
i. hematoma
i. hemorrhage (IVH)
i. mass
i. meningioma
i. neonate hemorrhage
i. neuroblastoma
i. neurocytoma
i. obstructive hydrocephalus
i. right ventricular obstruction
i. septum
i. systolic tension
intravertebral body vacuum cleft
intravesical
i. obstruction
i. stone
i. ureter
intravital ultraviolet
intravoxel
i. coherent motion
i. dephasing
i. incoherent motion
i. phase dispersion
intrinsic
i. cellular parameter
i. compression
i. deflection
i. energy resolution
i. field uniformity
i. field uniformity test
i. filling defect
i. foot muscle
i. ligament
i. minus deformity
i. minus hallux
i. plus deformity
i. pulmonary disease
i. sick sinus syndrome
i. spatial linearity
i. stenotic lesion
i. stomach wall lesion
i. vein graft stenosis
introducer
Tuohy-Borst i.
introitus
Intropaque
I. imaging agent
intubated small bowel series
intubation
endotracheal i.
esophagogastric i.
intraluminal i.
nasal i.
nasogastric i.
nasotracheal i.
oral i.
orotracheal i.
intussuscepted bowel
intussusception
appendiceal i.
bowel i.
colocolic i.

ileocolic i.
ileoileal i.
intestinal i.
jejunoduodenogastric i.
jejunogastric i.
rectal i.
retrograde jejunoduodenogastric i.
stomal i.
i. target sign
i. of vein
vein i.
venous i.

intussusceptum

intussuscipiens

Invader
GiCi-400 I.

invagination
basilar i.
i. skull base

invasion
arterial i.
blood vessel i.
capillary lymphatic space i.
deep i.
deep myometrial i.
early stromal i.
exogenous i.
mediastinal i.
neoplastic i.
occipital condyle i.
perineural i.
seminal vesicle i. (SVI)
transmural i.
tumoral i.
vascular i.

invasive
i. angiomatous interstitial infiltrate
i. assessment
i. breast cancer
i. lesion
i. malignant sheath tumor
i. pulmonary aspergillosis
i. radiological vascular procedure
i. surgical staging (ISS)
i. thermometry

inverse
i. comma appearance
i. follicle
i. follicle pattern
i. Fourier transform (IFT)
i. inspiratory-expiratory time ratio
i. radiotherapy technique

inverse-square law

inversion
i. ankle stress view
cardiac i.
frequency-selective i.
i. injury
i. injury of ankle
i. instability
isolated ventricular i.
magnetic i.
i. pulse
i. recovery
i. recovery image
i. recovery spin-echo (IRSE)
i. recovery spin-echo sequence
i. sprain
terminal i.
i. time (TI)
torcular-lambdoid i.
i. transfer
ventricular i.

inversion-eversion

inversion-recovery technique

inversum
duodenum i.

inversus
abdominal situs i.
situs viscerum i.

invertebral disk

inverted
i. Meckel diverticulum
i. nipple
i. pancreatic 3 sign
i. papilloma
i. pelvis
i. teardrop sign
i. umbrella defect

inverted-T
i.-T. appearance
i.-T. appearance mainstem bronchus

inverted-V sign

inverted-Y
i.-Y. block
i.-Y. complex
i.-Y. configuration
i.-Y. fracture

invertus
cardiac situs i.

investing fascia

invisible
i. light

NOTES

invisible *(continued)*
i. main pulmonary artery
i. spectrum
involucrum, pl. **involucra**
involuting fibroadenoma
involution
i. of duct
follicular i.
spontaneous i.
involutional breast calcification
involved-field
i.-f. radiation
i.-f. radiotherapy
involved field
involvement
arcuate fiber i.
axillary node i.
contiguous organ i.
cranial nerve i.
extramedullary i.
intramedullary marrow i.
lymph node i.
metastatic axillary i.
pagetoid epidermal i.
supraclavicular node i.
thalamotegmental i.
INVOS 2100 optical spectroscopy
Ioban prep
iobenzamic
i. acid
i. acid imaging agent
iobitridol
i. imaging agent
iobutoic acid
iocarmate meglumine
iocarmic
i. acid
i. acid imaging agent
iocetamate
iocetamic
i. acid
i. acid contrast medium
i. acid imaging agent
IOCM
isosmolar contrast medium
IOD
integrated optical density
iodamic acid
iodamide
iodamine meglumine imaging agent
iodatol
iodecol
iodide
i. goiter
potassium i.
propidium i.
radioactive i. (RAI)
sodium i. (NaI)
i. transport
iodinated
i. contrast material
i. contrast medium
i. I-131 aggregated albumin
i. I-125 fibrinogen
i. imaging agent
i. I-131 serum albumin
i. ^{125}I serum albumin
i. nanoparticle
i. tyrosine group
iodination
iodine (I)
i. allergy
butanol-extractable i. (BEI)
i. dose
i. fluorescence imaging
i. load
protein-bound i. (PBI)
radioactive i. (RAI)
i. radioactive source
i. scintigraphy
iodine-123 (^{123}I)
i. brain imaging spectamine
i. orthoiodohippurate (OIH)
i. thyroid
iodine-125 (^{125}I)
iodine-127 (^{127}I)
iodine-131 (^{131}I)
i. antiferritin
i. antiferritin treatment
i. metaiodobenzylguanidine
i. OIH
i. orthoiodohippurate
sodium iodide i.
i. thyroid
i. whole-body scan
iodine-132 (^{132}I)
iodine-deficiency goiter
iodine-125-labeled
i.-l. fragment
i.-l. interleukin-3
iodine-labeled product
iodine-to-particle ratio
iodipamide
i. ethyl ester
i. meglumine
i. meglumine imaging agent
methylglucamine i.
i. methylglucamine
iodixanol
iodized
i. oil
i. oil imaging agent
5-iodo-2-deoxyuridine imaging agent
5-iodoacetamidofluorescein imaging agent
iodoalphionic acid

iodobenzamide
iodochlorol
iodocholesterol
iododeoxyuridine (IUDR)
i. labeling
iododoxorubicin
Iodo-gen imaging agent
iodohippurate
i. sodium
i. sodium imaging agent
iodomethamate
i. sodium
i. sodium imaging agent
iodomethyl-norcholesterol-59 scintigraphy (^{59}NP scintigraphy)
iodomethyl-norcholesterol scintigraphy imaging
iodopanoic acid
iodophendylate
iodophthalein
i. sodium imaging agent
iodophylated chelates imaging agent
iodopyracet
Iodotope imaging agent
iodovinylestradiol
iodoxamate
i. meglumine
i. meglumine imaging agent
iodoxamic
i. acid
i. acid imaging agent
iodoxyl
IOECS
intraoperative electrocortical stimulation
IOECS mapping
ioglicate
ioglicic acid
ioglucol
ioglucomide
ioglunide
ioglycamic acid
ioglycamide
iogulamide
IOHDR
intraoperative high dose rate
iohexol
i. CT ventriculogram
i. imaging agent
IOM
infraorbital margin
interosseous membrane
iomide
IOML
infraorbitomeatal line
ion-bound water
ion-exchange chromatography
ionic
i. binding
i. monomer
i. paramagnetic contrast medium
i. paramagnetic imaging agent
i. polar valence
i. potassium
ionium
ionization
i. chamber
i. counter
i. current
i. density
i. instrument
i. potential
ionized atom
ionizing radiation
ionography
ion pump
iopamidol
i. imaging agent
Iopamiron 310, 370 imaging agent
iopanoate
iopanoic
i. acid
i. acid imaging agent
iopentol
i. nonionic imaging agent
iophendylate
i. imaging agent
iophenoxic acid
ioprocemic acid
iopromide
iopronic acid
iopydol
i. imaging agent
iopydone
i. imaging agent
IORT
intraoperative radiation therapy
IOS
intraoperative sonography
iosefamate
iosefamic
i. acid
i. acid imaging agent
ioseric acid
iosimide

NOTES

iosulamide
iosumetic acid
iotasul
ioteric acid
iotetric acid imaging agent
iothalamate
meglumine i.
i. meglumine imaging agent
i. sodium
i. sodium imaging agent
iothalamic acid
iothalmic acid imaging agent
iotrol
i. imaging agent
iotrolan
iotroxamide
iotroxic
i. acid
i. acid imaging agent
ioversol
i. imaging agent
ioxaglate
i. meglumine
i. meglumine imaging agent
i. sodium
i. sodium imaging agent
ioxaglic acid
ioxilan
i. with iohexol imaging agent
ioxithalamate
ioxithalamic acid
iozomic acid
IPA
idiopathic pulmonary arteriosclerosis
IPC
interpeduncular cistern
IPCS
infrapatellar contracture syndrome
IPEUS
intraportal endovascular ultrasonography
IPF
idiopathic pulmonary fibrosis
interstitial pulmonary fibrosis
IPG
impedance plethysmography
IPH
idiopathic portal hypertension
intraplaque hemorrhage
IPHP
intraperitoneal hyperthermic perfusion
ipodate
calcium i.
i. calcium imaging agent
i. sodium
i. sodium imaging agent
ipodic acid
ipomeanol
IPSID
immunoproliferative small intestine disease
ipsilateral
i. antegrade arteriography
i. antegrade site
i. basal ganglion
i. breast tumor recurrence (IBTR)
i. bundle-branch block
i. cerebellar sign
i. cortical diaschisis
i. corticospinal tract sign
i. downstream artery
i. femoral neck fracture
i. femoral shaft fracture
i. hemispheric carotid TIA
i. injection
i. lateral ventricle
i. pleural effusion
IPSP
intrapixel sequential processing
IPSP neuron evaluation method
IR
arrhythmia-insensitive flow-sensitive alternating I.
Ir
iridium
^{192}Ir
iridium-192
^{192}Ir ribbon
^{192}Ir seed therapy
^{192}Ir wire
^{194}Ir
iridium-194
IRA
ileorectal anastomosis
IRA-400 resin
IRAK
integrated reference air-kerma
IRBBB
incomplete right bundle-branch block
IRE
internal rotation in extension
Irex
I. Exemplar ultrasound
I. Exemplar ultrasound scanner
IRF
internal rotation in flexion
Iriditope
iridium (Ir)
i. imaging agent
i. needle
i. prosthesis
i. wire
iridium-192 (^{192}Ir)
i. endobronchial implant
i. wire implant
iridium-194 (^{194}Ir)

IRIS
intensified radiographic imaging system
IRIS scanner
iris-like stenosis
^{192}Ir-loaded stent
iron
i. accumulation in kidney
i. dextran
gadolinium i.
i. overload artifact
iron-52 (^{52}Fe)
iron-55 (^{55}Fe)
iron-59 (^{59}Fe)
iron-ascorbate-DTPA
technetium-99m i.-a.-D.
iron-transporting protein mechanism
irradiate
irradiated zinc
irradiation
abdominal i.
adjuvant i.
axillary i.
breast i.
cardiac i.
i. chamber
charged-particle i.
convergent beam i. (CBI)
cranial i.
craniospinal i.
curative i.
endocavitary i.
external beam i.
external orthovoltage i.
extracorporeal i.
fractionated external beam i.
gamma i.
heavy-particle i.
hemibody i. (HBI)
hyperfractionated total body i.
i. injury
interstitial template i.
intracanalicular i.
intracavitary i.
intraoral cone i.
low-intensity laser i. (LILI)
neutron i.
palliative i.
partial brain i.
phosphorus-32 intracavitary i.
i. pneumonia
proton i.
selective i.
stereotactic external-beam i. (SEBI)
stereotactic proton i.
template i.
i. tolerance
total body i. (TBI)
ultraviolet (UV) i.
vaginal code i.
whole-body i.
whole-brain i.
whole-breast i.
irreducible
i. dorsal dislocation
i. fracture
irregular
i. block
i. bone
i. border
i. calcification
i. emphysema
i. enchondral ossification
i. gallbladder wall thickening
i. hazy luminal contour
i. infrapatellar fat-pad sign
i. kidney
i. mass
irregularity
avulsive cortical i.
diffuse i.
intimal i.
luminal i.
sinus i. (SI)
irregularly shaped lesion
irreversible
i. airways obstruction
i. compression
i. compression of MR imaging
i. ischemia
i. narrowing of bronchioles
i. organ failure
irritability
atrial i.
cardiac i.
muscle i.
myocardial i.
nerve root i.
ventricular i.
irritable
i. bowel
i. bowel syndrome
i. colon
i. heart
i. stricture

NOTES

irritation
chronic i.
i. fibroma
sciatic nerve i.
irrotationally bound water
IRSE
inversion recovery spin-echo
IRSE sequence
IRV
inspiratory reserve volume
IS
ileosacral
international standard
ISAH
I. stereotactic immobilization frame
I. stereotactic immobilizing mask
ischemia
acute mesenteric i.
anoxic i.
balanced i.
brachiocephalic i.
brain i.
brainstem i.
cardiac i.
carotid artery i.
cerebral i.
chronic cerebral i.
chronic mesenteric i.
coronary i.
cortical i.
exercise-induced transient myocardial i.
focal cerebral i.
global cerebral i.
global myocardial i.
intracompartmental i.
irreversible i.
limb-threatening i.
mesenteric i.
myocardial i.
neonatal intracranial i.
nonlocalized i.
nonocclusive mesenteric i.
organ i.
periinfarction i.
provocable i.
radiation-induced i.
radiation-related i.
regional myocardial i.
regional transmural i.
remote i.
reversible myocardial i.
rostral brainstem i.
segmental bronchus i.
silent myocardial i.
stress-induced i.
subendocardial i.
talar dome i.
testicular i.
transient cerebral i.
transient myocardial i.
vertebrobasilar i.
zone of i.
ischemic
i. area
i. bowel
i. bowel disease
i. brain damage
i. brainstem
i. brainstem infarct
i. changes
i. colitis
i. congestive cardiomyopathy
i. contracture
i. decompensation
i. defect
i. encephalopathy
i. episode
i. event
i. gliosis
i. heart
i. hypoxia
i. index
i. instability
i. lesion
i. mesentery
i. necrosis
i. necrosis of femoral head (INFH)
i. reperfused myocardium
i. reperfusion injury
i. segment
i. time
i. ulcer
i. viable myocardium
i. zone
ischemically mediated mitral regurgitation
ischial
i. bone
i. bursitis
i. spine
i. tuberosity
i. weightbearing ring
ischioacetabular fracture
ischiocapsular ligament
ischiocavernosus muscle
ischiofemoral ligament
ischiogluteal
i. bursa
i. bursitis
ischiopagus
ischiopubic ramus
ischiorectal
i. abscess
i. fat pad
i. fossa

i. fossa lesion
i. fossa plane
i. pad of fat
ischiospongiosus muscle of penis
ischium
ascending ramus of i.
ramus of i.
transverse diameter between i.'s
ISG medical imaging workstation
Isherwood position
ISI
injection scan interval
ISIS spectroscopy
island
bone i.
bony i.
compact i.
endometrial i.
fat i.
fibrotic i.
heterotopic white matter i.
mucosal i.
Pander i.
Reil i.
i. of Reil
sclerotic calvarium bone i.
tissue i.
i. of tissue
islet pancreatic cell tumor
isoattenuation
isobar
isobutyl
dipyridamole technetium-99m-2-methoxy i.
Isocam
I. scintillation imaging
I. scintillation imaging system
I. SPECT imaging system
isocapnic hyperventilation-induced bronchoconstriction
isocenter
i. placement error
i. shift method
shoulder i.
single i.
isoclosed curve
Isocon camera
isodense
i. appearance
i. enhancement
i. mass
i. subdural hematoma
isodose
i. contour
i. curve
i. line
i. plan
i. shift method
i. width
isoechoic
i. clot
isoeffect dose
isoeffective bronchial mucosa
isoelectric
i. line
i. period
isoflurane
i. imaging agent
isoimmunization
rhodium i.
isointense
i. lesion
i. mass
i. soft tissue
isointensity
Isolar rod
isolated
i. airway injury
i. clustered calcifications
i. dislocation
i. dislocation of semilunar bone
i. hepatic infusion
i. limb perfusion (ILP)
i. tethered cord syndrome
i. ventricular inversion
isolation-perfusion technique
isoleucine
isomer
optical i.
isomeric transition
isomerism
atrial i.
isometric
i. contractile force ring
i. exercise stress test
i. transition
isonitrile
dipyridamole technetium-99m-2-methoxy isobutyl i.
isoosmolar contrast
Isopaque
I. contrast medium
I. imaging agent
isophil

NOTES

isoporosis
isopotential line
isoproterenol
i. infusion
isosceles triangular configuration
isosmolar contrast medium (IOCM)
isosulfan blue
isotonicity
isotope
i. bone scan
cistern i.
i. clearance
daughter i.
gamma-emitting i.
i. hepatobiliary imaging
intravenous injection of i.
labeling of the i.
i. meal
^{103}Pd i.
phosphorus i.
poorly concentrated i.
radioactive i.
rhenium i.
i. scintigraphy
short-range i.
i. shunt imaging
stable i.
strontium i.
i. uptake
i. venography
isotope-labeled fibrinogen imaging
isotopic
i. bone scanning
i. cisternography
i. dilution
i. 3D imaging
i. 3D study
i. lung scan
i. ratio
i. skeletal survey
i. volume study
isotretinoin
isotropic
i. disk
i. motion
i. resolution
i. tissue
i. voxel
isotropy
isotype
isovolumetric
i. contraction time
i. period
i. relaxation
isovolumic relaxation time (IVRT)
Isovue
I. nonionic imaging agent
Isovue-128 imaging agent
Isovue-250 imaging agent
Isovue-300 imaging agent
Isovue-370 imaging agent
Isovue M
Isovue-M 200, 300 imaging agent
Israel camera
ISS
inferior sagittal sinus
Injury Severity Scale
Injury Severity Score
invasive surgical staging
ISSI
interspinous segmental spinal instrumentation
isthmic
i. coarctation
i. spondylolisthesis
isthmus, pl. **isthmi, isthmuses**
i. aneurysm
aortic i.
i. of femur
pontine i.
renal i.
stenotic i.
temporal i.
thyroid i.
uterine i.
i. of uterus
i. of Vieussens
IT
iliotibial
IT band
ITA
internal thoracic artery
ITA graft
ITC radiopaque balloon catheter
iterative
i. algorithm
i. gradient optimization
i. halftoning
i. reconstruction
Ito cell sarcoma
ITT
internal tibial torsion
ITU
intensive therapy unit
IUD
intrauterine contraceptive device
lost IUD
IUDR
idoxuridine
iododeoxyuridine
IUG
intrauterine gas
IUGR
intrauterine growth retardation
asymmetric IUGR
late flattening IUGR

low-profile IUGR
mixed IUGR
symmetric IUGR

IV
IV Persantine
supination-external rotation IV (SER-IV)

Ivalon
I. particle
I. sponge

IVB
intraventricular block

IVC
inferior vena cava
solitary left IVC

IVDSA
intravenous digital subtraction angiography

Ivemark CHD syndrome

IV-enhanced MRI

IVFA
intravenous fluorescein angiography
IVFA imaging

IVH
intraventricular hemorrhage

ivory
i. bone
i. phalanx
i. vertebra

IVP
intravenous pyelography
rapid-sequence IVP
IVP rim sign

IVR
idioventricular rhythm

IVRT
isovolumic relaxation time

IVSD
interventricular septal defect

IVST
interventricular septal thickness

IVU
intravenous urography

IVUS
intravascular ultrasound

NOTES

J
joule
J chain
J junction
J loop
J sign
JA
jet area
Jaboulay amputation
Jaccoud sign
jacket
x-ray film j.
jackknife position
Jackson
J. sign
J. staging
J. staging system
Jacobson canal
Jaffe-Campanacci syndrome
Jaffe-Lichtenstein disease
jagged
j. bone fragments
j. osteophyte
Jagziekte disease
Jahss
J. classification of metatarsophalangeal joint dislocation
J. dislocation classification
jail-bar
j.-b. chest
j.-b. rib
jail-bars appearance
James bundle
jammed finger
Janeway lesion
Jansen
J. disease
J. metaphyseal dysplasia
Janus syndrome
Jarcho-Levin syndrome
Jarjavay ligament
Jatene transposition
jaundice
obstructive j.
javelin thrower's elbow
jaw
ameloblastoma of the j.
j. bone
claudication of j.
independent j.
j. osteosarcoma
J-coupled spin
Jefferson
J. burst fracture
J. cervical fracture
Jeffery
J. classification of radial fractures
J. radial fracture classification
jejunal
j. diverticulosis
j. diverticulum
j. interposition of Henle
j. leiomyosarcoma
j. loop
j. loop interposition of Henle
j. motility
j. obstruction
j. pouch
j. ulcer
jejunitis
Crohn j.
ulcerative j.
jejunization
j. of colon
j. of ileum
vascular j.
jejunocolic fistula
jejunoduodenogastric
j. intussusception
jejunogastric intussusception
jejunoileal
j. bypass (JIB)
j. diverticulum
j. shunt
jejunoileitis
ulcerative j.
jejunum
jelly-belly appearance
Jenet sign
jeopardized myocardium
jersey finger
jet
j. area (JA)
high-velocity j.
j. length (JL)
j. lesion
pressurized fluid j.
regurgitant j.
ureteral j.
Jeune
J. disease
J. syndrome
Jeune-Tommasi syndrome
Jewitt-Whitmore staging
JGA
juxtaglomerular apparatus

J-hook
J.-h. deformity
J.-h. deformity of distal ureter
JIB
jejunoileal bypass
JL
jet length
JNPA
juvenile nasopharyngeal angiofibroma
Jobert fossa
Jod-Basedow phenomenon
Johnson-Jahss classification of posterior tibial tendon tear
Johnson position
joint
acromioclavicular j.
ankle j.
j. ankylosis
apophyseal j.
j. arthrography
j. articular surface
j. articulation
atlantoaxial j.
bail-lock knee j.
ball-and-socket j.
basal j.
Budin j.
calcaneocuboid j.
j. calculus
capitate hamate j.
capitolunate j.
j. capsule
carpometacarpal j. (CMC)
carpophalangeal j.
j. cavity
Charcot j.
j. chondroma
Chopart j.
Clutton painful j.
condyloid j.
j. contracture
coracoclavicular j.
costochondral j.
costotransverse j.
costovertebral j.
Cruveilhier j.
cubonavicular j.
cuneiform j.
j. cyst
j. debris
j. deformity
j. depression fracture
destruction of temporomandibular j.
diarthrodial j.
DIP j.
j. dislocation
distal interphalangeal j.
distal radioulnar j. (DRUJ)
j. distraction
distraction of j.
j. effusion
elbow j.
ellipsoid j.
erythema of j.
facet j.
femoropatellar j.
flail j.
j. fluid
j. fluid extravasation
free knee j.
frozen j.
j. fulcrum
j. fusion
Gaffney j.
Gillette j.
glenohumeral j.
gliding j.
hallux interphalangeal j.
hinge j.
hip capsule j.
hyperextensibility of j.
j. hyperextensibility
hypermobile j.
IM j.
immovable j.
j. incongruity
j. instability
intercarpal j.
interchondral j.
j. interface
intermetatarsal j.
interphalangeal j.
intervertebral j.
j. kinematics
knee j.
j. laxity
lesser metatarsophalangeal j.
j. line
Lisfranc j.
lunotriquetral j.
Luschka j.
j.'s of Luschka
manubriosternal j.
metacarpophalangeal j. (MCPJ)
metatarsal j.
metatarsocuneiform j.
metatarsophalangeal j. (MTPJ)
j. mice
midcarpal j.
midtarsal j.
j. morphology
mortise j.
MTP j.
naviculocuneiform j.
near-anatomic position of j.
neuropathic tarsometatarsal j.

neurotrophic j.
occipitoaxial j.
osteolysis on both sides of j.
patellofemoral j.
PIP j.
pisotriquetral j.
pivot j.
j. play
primary cartilage j.
proximal interphalangeal j. (PIP, PIPJ)
proximal radioulnar j.
pulvinar hip j.
radiocapitellar j.
radiocarpal j.
radioscaphoid j.
radioulnar j.
Regnauld degeneration of MTP j.
sacrococcygeal j.
sacroiliac j.
saddle j.
scaphocapitate j.
scapholunate j.
scaphotrapeziotrapezoid j.
scapulothoracic j.
seagull j.
secondary cartilaginous j.
j. segment
sesamoidometatarsal j.
shoulder j.
SI j.
signal j.
Silastic finger j.
SL j.
slanting tibiotalar j.
j. space
j. space pseudowidening
sternal j.
sternoclavicular j.
sternocostal j.
sternomanubrial j.
STT j.
subtalar j.
surgeon's tarsal j.
j. survey
Swanson finger j.
j. swelling
symphysis cartilage j.
synovial diarthroidal j.
talocalcaneal j.
talocalcaneonavicular j.
talocrural j.
talofibular j.
talonavicular j.
tarsal j.
tarsometatarsal j.
temporomandibular j. (TMJ)
thoracic j.
tibiofibular j.
tibiotalar j.
j. tissue
transverse tarsal j.
trapeziometacarpal j.
trapezioscaphoid j.
trapeziotrapezoid j.
triquetrohamate j.
j.'s of trunk
UJ j.
uncovertebral joint
uncovertebral j. (UJ joint)
unstable j.
weightbearing j.
widened sacroiliac j.
j. widening
wrist j.
xiphisternal j.
zygapophyseal j.

joint-space narrowing

Joliot
J. method
J. sorption study

Jones
J. classification
J. classification of diaphyseal fractures
J. criteria
J. fracture
J. view

Jones-Mote reaction

Joubert syndrome

joule (J)
j. radiation-absorbed dose
j. shock

JPA
juvenile pilocytic astrocytoma

J-sella
J.-s. deformity

J-shaped
J.-s. anastomosis
J.-s. sella
J.-s. stomach
J.-s. tube
J.-s. ureter

NOTES

Jude
J. pelvic view
J. pelvic x-ray
Judet
J. epiphyseal fracture classification
J. view
Judkins
J. coronary arteriography
J. selective left coronary cinearteriography
J. technique
jugal
j. ligament
j. suture
jugular
j. bulb anomaly
j. catheter
j. compression maneuver
j. foramen
j. foramen schwannoma
j. foramen syndrome
j. foraminal mass
j. lymph node
j. megabulb
j. node metastatic carcinoma
j. process
j. sign
j. technique
j. tubercle
j. vein
j. vein thrombosis
j. venous distention
j. venous impulse
j. venous oxygen saturation
j. venous pressure
j. venous pressure collapse
jugulare
glomus j.
jugulodigastric
j. chain
j. node
juguloomohyoid lymph node
jump
j. sign
j. vein graft
jumped facet
jumper's knee
junction
anomalous craniovertebral j.
anorectal j.
aortic sinotubular j.
atlantooccipital j.
atriocaval j.
atrioventricular j.
beaked cervicomedullary j.
bird-beak taper at esophagogastric j.
bulbous costochondral j.
caniocervical j.
cardioesophageal j.
cardiophrenic j.
cavoatrial j.
CE j.
cervicomedullary j.
cervicothoracic j.
choledochopancreatic ductal j.
chondrosternal j.
competence of ureterovesical j.
corticomedullary j.
costochondral j.
craniocervical j.
craniovertebral j.
cystic-choledochal j.
duodenojejunal j. (DJJ)
esophagogastric j.
fundic-antral j.
gastrocnemius-soleus j.
gastroduodenal j.
gastroesophageal (GE) j.
gray-white matter j.
ileocecal j.
iliocaval j.
J j.
meniscocapsular j.
meniscosynovial j.
metaphyseal-diaphyseal j.
mucocutaneous j.
musculotendinous j.
myoneural j.
myotendinous j.
neuromuscular j.
occipitocervical j.
pancreaticobiliary ductal j.
pelviureteral j.
phrenovertebral j.
pontomedullary j.
pontomesencephalic j.
prostaticovesical j.
pyloroduodenal j.
rectosigmoid j.
saphenofemoral j.
sinotubular j.
splenoportal j.
squamocolumnar j.
sternochondral j.
supraspinatus musculotendinous j.
sylvian-rolandic j.
temporooccipital j.
temporoparietooccipital j.
tracheoesophageal j.
ureteropelvic j. (UPJ)
ureterovesical j. (UVJ)
uterovesical j.
venous j.
junctional
j. cortical defect

j. dilatation
j. epidermolysis bullosa
j. focus
j. infundibulum
j. parenchymal kidney defect
j. zone

Junghans pseudospondylolisthesis
Jung muscle
Jürgensen sign
juvenile

j. aponeurotic fibroma
j. autosomal recessive polycystic disease
j. breast papillomatosis
j. cirrhosis
j. embryonal carcinoma
j. epiphyseolysis
j. epiphysitis
j. fibroadenoma
j. fibromatosis
j. nasopharyngeal angiofibroma (JNPA)
j. nephronophthisis
j. orbital pilocytic astrocytoma
j. ossifying fibroma
j. osteoporosis
j. Paget disease
j. pelvis
j. pilocytic astrocytoma (JPA)
j. polyp
j. polyposis
j. rheumatoid arthritis
j. Tillaux fracture
j. T-wave pattern
j. xanthogranuloma

juvenilis

kyphosis dorsalis j.
osteochondrosis deformans j.

juxtaanastomotic stenosis
juxtaarterial ventricular septal defect
juxtaarticular

j. fracture
j. low signal intensity
j. osteoid osteoma

juxtaarticulation
juxtacortical

j. bone lesion
j. chondroma
j. fracture
j. osteogenic sarcoma

juxtacrural
juxtadiaphragmatic location
juxtaductal

j. aortic coarctation
j. coarctation of aorta

juxtaglomerular

j. apparatus (JGA)
j. tumor

juxtaintestinal node
juxtapapillary diverticulum
juxtaphrenic peak
juxtaposed rightward
juxtaposition

atrial appendage j.
j. of atrial appendage

juxtapyloric ulcer
juxtarenal

j. aortic aneurysm
j. aortic atherosclerosis
j. cava

juxtarestiform body
juxtatricuspid ventricular septal defect
juxtavesical

NOTES

K

potassium

K capture

K electrons

K shell

^{39}K

potassium-39

^{40}K

potassium-40

^{42}K

potassium-42

^{43}K

potassium-43

K4-81 imaging agent

Kadish

K. staging

K. staging system

Kager triangle

Kahler disease

Kalamchi-Dawe congenital tibial deficiency classification

Kalman filter

Kanavel sign

Kandel method

Kantor sign

kaolin pneumoconiosis

Kaplan-Meier method

Kaplan sign

Kaposi

K. epicardial sarcoma

K. sarcoma (KS)

kappa (κ)

k. meson

kappa light chain

Karapandzic flap

Karnofsky performance status (KPS)

Karplus

K. relationship

K. sign

K. sign of pleural effusion

Kartagener

K. syndrome

K. triad

Kasabach-Merritt

K.-M. phenomenon

K.-M. syndrome

Kast syndrome

Katayama syndrome

Katzman infusion of radionuclide cisternography

Katz-Wachtel

K.-W. phenomenon

K.-W. sign

Kawai bioptome

Kawasaki

K. disease

K. syndrome

Kayser-Fleischer ring

k-capture

KCC

Kulchitsky cell carcinoma

KCD

kinestatic charge detector

KCD imaging

Kearns-Sayre syndrome

K-edge filter

keel

k. of glenoid component

laryngeal k.

keeled chest

keel-like ridge

Keen sign

Kehr sign

Keith

K. node

K. sinoatrial bundle

Keith-Flack sinoatrial node

Kelley-Goerss Compass stereotactic system

Kellgren

K. arthritis

K. sign

Kellock

K. sign

K. sign of pleural effusion

Kellogg-Speed lumbar spinal fusion

Kemp-Elliot-Gorlin syndrome

Kendall sequence compression device

Kennedy

K. area-length method

K. ligament technique

K. method for calculating ejection fraction

Kensey-Nash lithotrite

Kent

bundle of Stanley K.

Kent-His bundle

keratin

k. pearl

k. testicular cyst

k. urinary tract ball

keratinizing squamous metaplasia

keratocyst

odontogenic k.

keratoma

Kerckring

K. fold

Kerckring *(continued)*
K. nodule
K. ossicle
Kerley
K. A lines
K. B lines
K. C lines
kerma
kinetic energy released in the medium
kerma-to-dose conversion factor
kernahorn notch
kernel
interpolation k.
k. of popcorn appearance
k. size
Kernig sign
Kernohan
K. brain tumor classification
K. notch phenomenon
Kerr sign
Keshan disease
ketamine
ketanserin
ketene
Kety equation
keV
k. gamma ray
511-k. high-energy imaging
Key-Conwell
K.-C. classification of pelvic fractures
K.-C. pelvic fracture classification
keyhole
k. deformity
keyhole-shaped craniectomy
keystone of calcar arch
kg
kilogram
Khan scatter analysis
kHz
kilohertz
kick
atrial k.
Kidner lesion
kidney
abdominal k.
k. abscess
absent k.
k. adenocarcinoma
k. adenoma
k. amyloidosis
k. anatomy
k. aneurysm
k. angiomyolipoma
k. anomaly
k. arteriosclerosis
arteriosclerotic k.
Ask-Upmark k.
atrophic k.
k. atrophy
bilateral large k.
bilateral small k.
blunt trauma k.
bunch of flowers in k.
cake k.
k. calcification
k. calculus
k. carcinoma chromophobe
k. chloroma
cicatricial k.
cluster of grapes k.
congenital absence of k.
congested k.
contracted k.
contralateral k.
cortical scarring of k.
crush k.
cyanotic k.
k. cyst
cystic k.
discoid k.
k. disk
distended k.
Doppler k.
double k.
doughnut k.
duplication of left k.
duplication of right k.
dysfunctional k.
dysgenetic k.
k. dyskeratosis
dysplastic k.
ectopic k.
edematous k.
enlarged k.
k. extraction efficiency
k. failure
fatty k.
fetal mesenchymal tumor of k.
k. fibromyxoma
fibrotic k.
floating k.
Formad k.
fractured k.
k. function imaging
k. function study
k. fungus ball
fused k.
Goldblatt k.
granular k.
k. hilum
hilum of k.
Hodson-type k.
horseshoe k.
hydronephrotic k.
hypermobile k.

k. infarct
infundibulum of k.
iron accumulation in k.
irregular k.
k. leiomyoma
lobe of k.
lobulated k.
long axis of k.
lower pole of k.
lumbar k.
lump k.
k. lymphoma
k. malrotation
k. mass growth pattern
medullary sponge k.
mesonephric k.
k. metastasis
movable k.
multicystic k. (MCK)
multicystic dysgenetic k.
multicystic dysplastic k. (MCDK)
mural k.
k. mycetoma
native k.
k. neurofibromatosis
nonfunctioning k.
k. oxalosis
Page k.
pancake k.
k. papillary blush
partially polycystic k.
pelvis of k.
k. pole
pole-to-pole length of k.
polycystic k.
porous k.
Potter type IV k.
k. pseudotumor
ptotic k.
putty k.
k. radionuclide imaging
Rose-Bradford k.
sacciform k.
k. scan
scarred k.
sclerotic k.
k. shadow
shattered k.
shriveled k.
sigmoid k.
k. sinus mass
k. size
sponge k.
k. stone
supernumerary k.
suspension of k.
thoracic k.
k. tomography
k. transplant
k. trauma
tree-barking k.
unicaliceal k.
unilateral large smooth k.
unilateral small k.
unipapillary k.
k.'s, ureter, and bladder film
k.'s, ureter, and bladder imaging
k.'s, ureters, bladder (KUB)
k. vessel
wandering k.

kidney-pancreas transplant

kidney-shaped

k.-s. distended cecum
k.-s. placenta

kidney-to-background ratio

Kiel non-Hodgkin lymphoma classification

Kienböck

K. dislocation
K. unit (X)

Kiernan space

Kikuchi disease

Kikuchi-Fujimoto disease

Kilfoyle

K. classification of condylar fractures
K. condylar fracture classification

Kilian

K. line
K. pelvis

killer

flow artifact k. (FLAK)

Killian dehiscence

kilogram (kg)

kilohertz (kHz)

kilovoltage

peak k. (pkV)
k. peak (kVp)

Kimmelstiel-Wilson syndrome

Kimura

K. classification
K. disease

Kimura-type choledochal cyst

NOTES

kinase C antiglioma monoclonal antibody imaging agent
kindling phenomenon
kinematic
- k. magnetic resonance imaging
- k. MRI study
- k. MR technique
- k. wrist device

kinematics
- joint k.

kinestatic
- k. charge detector (KCD)
- k. charge detector imaging

kinetic
- k. cervical spine
- k. energy
- k. energy released in the medium (kerma)
- k. parameter analysis
- k. perfusion parameter

kinetics
- elimination k.
- exponential k.
- sorption k.
- washout k.

kinetocardiogram
Kinevac
- K. imaging agent

King classification of thoracic scoliosis
King-Moe scoliosis
kinin
kininogen
kininogenase
kink
- k. artifact
- cervicomedullary k.
- k. in intestine
- Lane k.

kinked
- k. aorta
- k. bowel
- k. ureter

kinking
- aortic k.
- arterial k.
- blood vessel k.
- bowel k.
- bronchial k.
- k. of carotid artery
- carotid artery k.
- catheter k.
- colon k.
- graft k.
- innominate artery k.
- intestinal k.
- Lane k.
- patch k.

kinky-hair syndrome
Kinnier-Wilson disease
Kinsbourne syndrome
Kirchner diverticulum
Kirk distal thigh amputation
Kirklin
- K. meniscal complex
- K. sign

Kirner deformity
kissing
- k. artifact
- k. atherectomy technique
- k. contractions
- k. sequestra
- k. spine
- k. ulcer

kissing-balloon technique
kissing-cousin heart sign
Kistler subarachnoid hemorrhage classification
Kistner tracheal button
kite angle
kit prep
Klatskin
- K. tumor
- K. tumor classification

Klauder syndrome
***Klebsiella* pneumonia**
kleeblatschädel deformity
Kleffner-Landau syndrome
Klein
- K. muscle
- K. technique

Klein-Waardenburg syndrome
Klemm sign
Klenow fragment
Klinefelter syndrome (KS)
Klippel-Feil
- K.-F. deformity
- K.-F. sequence
- K.-F. syndrome

Klippel-Trenaunay syndrome
Klippel-Trenaunay-Weber-Rubashov syndrome
Klippel-Trenaunay-Weber syndrome
Klumpke
- K. brachial plexus injury
- K. paralysis
- K. paresis

K-means
- K.-m. cluster
- K.-m. clustering algorithm

knee
- anterior cruciate deficit of k.
- breaststroker's k.
- Brodie k.
- collateral ligament of k.
- corner of k.
- dislocated k.

double camelback sign of k.
k. flexion contracture
floating k.
k. fracture
Gerdy tubercle in k.
housemaid's k.
internal derangement of the k. (IDK)
k. joint
k. joint effusion
jumper's k.
k. knob
locked k.
motorcyclist's k.
posterolateral corner (PLC) of k.
reefing of medial retinaculum of k.
runner's k.
spontaneous osteonecrosis of k. (SONK)
k. view
wrenched k.

kneecap
knee-like bend
knife, pl. **knives**
gamma k.
roentgen k.
UltraCision ultrasonic k.

knob
absent aortic k.
aortic k.
blurring of aortic k.
knee k.
notched aortic k.

knobby process
knocked-down shoulder
knock-knee deformity
knot
false k.
surfer's k.
true umbilical cord k.

knuckle
aortic k.
k. bone
k. of colon
k. lung sign

knuckle-shaped
Knuttsen
K. bending film
K. bending roentgenogram

Koch
K. sinoatrial node
K. triangle
K. triangle apex

Kocher
K. anastomosis
K. dilatation ulcer
K. fracture
K. maneuver

Kocher-Cushing sign
Kocher-Lorenz capitellum fracture classification
Kodak
K. Digital Science 3600 distributed medical imager
K. 1200 Digital Science medical imager
K. software

Koeppe nodule
Koerber-Salus-Elschnig syndrome
Köhler
K. disease
K. line

Köhler-Pellegrini-Stieda disease
Kohlrausch fold
Kohn and Lambert pores
Kokopelli hunchback
Köllicker nucleus
Kolmogorov-Smirnov normality test
Komai stereotactic head frame
Kommerell diverticulum
Konica scanner
Konstram angle
Kontrast U imaging agent
Korányi-Grocco
K.-G. sign
K.-G. triangle

Kormed liver biopsy needle
Korotkoff
K. method
K. test for collateral circulation

Korsakoff syndrome
Kostuik-Errico spinal stability classification
Kouchoukos method
Kovalevsky
canal of K.
K. canal

KPS
Karnofsky performance status

Kr
krypton

NOTES

Krabbe
K. diffuse sclerosis
K. disease
K-radiation
Krause ligament
Kretschmann space
Kretztechnik
Krigel staging system
Krönlein orbitotomy
krypton (Kr)
k. laser
krypton-77
inhalation of k.
krypton-81
krypton-81m
k. radioactive imaging agent
KS
Kaposi sarcoma
Klinefelter syndrome
k-space
k.-s. matrix
k.-s. velocity mapping
KUB
kidneys, ureters, bladder
KUB imaging
KUB view
Kubelka-Munk theory
Kuchendorf method
Kugel
K. anastomosis
K. artery
Kugelberg-Welander
K.-W. disease
K.-W. juvenile spinal muscle atrophy
Kuhnt space
Kulchitsky cell carcinoma (KCC)
Kulkarni injury
Kumar, Welti and Ernst (KWE)
K. W. a. E. method
Kumeral diverticulum
Kümmel disease
Kump hump
Kupffer
K. cell sarcoma
Kürner septum
Kurtz-Sprague-White syndrome
Kurzbauer position
Kussmaul-Maier disease
Kussmaul sign
Kveim-Stilzbach test
kVp
kilovoltage peak
kVp meter
kwashiorkor
KWE
Kumar, Welti and Ernst
KWE method
Kyle fracture classification
kyllosis
kymography
kyphoscoliosis
kyphoscoliotic
k. heart disease
k. pelvis
kyphosis
Cobb method of measuring k.
k. dorsalis juvenilis
loss of thoracic k.
lumbar k.
lumbosacral k.
postlaminectomy k.
Scheuermann juvenile k.
thoracic k.
thoracolumbar k.
kyphotic
k. angulation
k. curvature
k. pelvis

Λ
Avogadro number
Ostwald solubility coefficient
radioactive constant
wavelength
L
liter
lumbar vertebra
L electrons
L shell
L-159
^{11}C L.
L-884
^{11}C L.
LA
left atrium
L/A
liver/aorta
LAA
left atrial appendage
left auricular appendage
LA/AR
left atrium/aortic root
LA/AR ratio
Labbé
L. triangle
L. vein
label
double l.
radioactive l.
radionuclide l.
single l.
triple l.
labeled
l. atom
l. fibrinogen
l. free fatty acid scintigraphy
l. leukocyte scan
l. positron
l. RBC
l. red blood cell sequestration
l. thyroxine
labeling
l. abnormality
antibody l.
indium-111 l.
iododeoxyuridine l.
l. of the isotope
microglobulin l.
pulse l.
radioactive l.
radioisotope l.
site-specific l.
technetium human serum albumin l.
technetium-99m antibody l.
technetium-tagged RBC l.
in vitro l.
in vivo l.
white blood cell l.
labial
l. groove
l. vein
labia majora
labile blood pressure
labor
premature l.
laboratory
filmless catheterization l.
l. simulation
labral
l. and anterior inferior glenoid rim fracture
l. capsular complex
l. fibrocartilage
l. injury
l. variant
labrum, pl. **labra**
acetabular l.
anterior glenoid l. (AGL)
articular l.
fibrocartilaginous l.
glenoid l.
labrum-ligament complex
labyrinth, labyrinthus
artery of l.
bony l.
cochlear l.
ethmoidal l.
Ludwig l.
membranous l.
osseous l.
renal l.
Santorini l.
vestibular l.
labyrinthine
l. artery
l. disease
l. fistula
l. hemorrhage
l. hydrops
l. structure
labyrinthitis ossificans
labyrinthus (*var. of* labyrinth)
LACD
left apexcardiogram, calibrated displacement
lacelike
l. appearance
l. trabecular pattern

laceration
bladder l.
brain l.
parenchymal l.
spinal cord l.
lacertus fibrosus
lacerum
foramen l.
Lachman sign
laciniate
l. ligament
l. ligament of ankle
lacrimal
l. artery
l. bone
l. canal
l. duct
l. gland
l. gland lesion
l. groove
l. mass
l. nerve
l. recess
l. sac
lactate proton
lactating breast
lacteal calculus
lactiferous
l. duct
l. sinus
lactoferrin production
lacuna, pl. **lacunae, lacunas**
bone l.
cartilage l.
intervillous l.
l. of Morgagni
Morgagni l.
osseous l.
penis l.
resorption l.
lacunaire
lacunar
l. abscess
l. brain infarct
l. ligament
l. node
l. skull
l. stroke
lacunas (*pl. of* lacuna)
lacune
LAD
left anterior descending
left axis deviation
Ladd band
Ladder diagram
ladderlike pattern
Lady Windermere syndrome
LAE
left atrial enlargement
Laënnec sign
laeve
LAFB
left anterior fascicular block
lag
l. effect
l. screw
Lagios classification system
LaGrange classification of humeral supracondylar fractures
LAID
left anterior internal diameter
Laimer
triangle of L.
Laitinen
L. CT guidance system
L. stereotactic head frame
lake
bile l.
capillary l.
intraplacental venous l.
lipid l.
maternal l.
musous l.
venous intraplacental l.
venous skull l.
Laks method
lambda (λ)
l. light chain
lambdoid
l. synostosis
lambdoidal cranial suture
Lambert
channel of L.
L. channel
L. projection
lamella, pl. **lamellae**
articular l.
basal l.
circumferential l.
concentric l.
enamel l.
lamellar
l. body density (LBD)
l. body density (LBD) count
l. bone
l. periosteal reaction
lamellated bone
lamina, pl. **laminae**
l. dura
external elastic l.
medullary l.
osseous spiral l.
l. papyracea
l. propria
vertebral l.

laminagram
laminagraphy (*var. of* laminography)
laminar
l. brain necrosis
l. flow
laminated
l. calcification
l. gallstone
l. intraluminal thrombus
lamination of gyrus
laminectomy
laminogram
laminography, laminagraphy
cardiac l.
laminotomy
lamp
Wood l.
Lamy-Bienenfeld disease
lanceolate deformity
Lancisi
L. muscle
L. sign
Landau diamagnetism
landmark
anatomic l.
bony skull l.
l. registration
Landolfi sign
Landsmeer ligament
Landzert
fossa of L.
L. fossa
Lane
L. band
L. disease
L. kink
L. kinking
Lanex medium screen
Langenbeck triangle
Langer
L. disease
L. line
Langerhans
L. body
L. lung cell histiocytosis
Langer-Saldino disease
Langoria sign
language area
Lanier clinical reporting system
Lannelongue ligament
lanthanic
lanthanide-induced shift
lanthanide metal
lanthanides
lanthanum
Lanz
L. line
L. point
LAO
left anterior oblique
LAO position
LAO projection
LAP
left atrial pressure
laparoscopic
l. contact ultrasonography (LCU)
l. contact ultrasound
l. Doppler probe
l. intracorporeal ultrasound (LICU)
l. ultrasound (LUS)
laparoscopy
laparotomy
L/A peak ratio
Laplace
L. effect
L. mechanism
Laquerriere-Perquin
L.-P. method
L.-P. projection
large
l. airway
l. airway narrowing
l. bowel
l. bowel obstruction
l. cleaved-cell lymphoma
l. colloidal particle
l. column of Bertin
l. duct papilloma
l. fetal head
l. field of view (LFV)
l.-for-dates uterus
l. for gestational age (LGA)
l. gut
l. habitus
l. intestine
l. loop excision
l. obtuse marginal branch
l. solid adrenal mass
l. spleen
l. thymus shadow
l. utricle
l. venous tributary
l. vestibule

NOTES

L

large-bore
l.-b. bile duct endoprosthesis
l.-b. magnet
l.-b. 0.6-T imaging system scanner
l.-b. 1.5-T imaging system scanner
large-caliber tube
large-cell
l.-c. lymphoma
l.-c. undifferentiated carcinoma
large-core technique
large-droplet fatty liver
large-fiber demyelination
large-field
l.-f. radiation therapy
l.-f. radiotherapy
l.-f. x-ray dosimetry
large-field-of-view image
large-hinge angle electron field
large-vessel
l.-v. disease of diabetic foot
l.-v. thrombosis
lariat sign
Larkin position
Larmor
L. equation
L. frequency
L. precession
Larsen-Johannson disease
larva currens
laryngeal
l. atresia
l. carcinoma
l. cartilage
l. edema
l. fracture
l. keel
l. nerve
l. nodule
l. papillomatosis
l. part of pharynx
l. polyp
l. skeleton
l. stridor
l. ventricle
l. vestibule
l. web
laryngectomy
supraglottic l.
vertical partial l.
larynges (*pl. of* larynx)
laryngis
aditus l.
laryngitis
laryngocele
laryngogram
laryngography
contrast l.
double-contrast l.
laryngomalacia
laryngopyocele
laryngoscopy
indirect l.
laryngotracheitis
laryngotracheobronchitis
acute l.
larynx, pl. **larynges**
appendix of ventricle of l.
glottic l.
infraglottic l.
supraglottic l.
ventricle of l.
vestibule of l.
Lasègue sign
laser
argon-pumped dye l.
l. beam
l. biliary lithotripsy
carbon dioxide l.
CO_2 l.
l. desiccation of thrombus
diode l.
l. Doppler flowmetry (LDF)
l. Doppler velocimetry
endoscopic l.
l. energy
l. energy absorption
excimer (excited dimer) l.
flashlamp-pulsed dye l.
helium-cadmium l.
holmium yttrium aluminum garnet l. (Ho:YAG laser)
hot-tip l.
Ho:YAG l.
holmium yttrium aluminum garnet laser
krypton l.
Lastec System angioplasty l.
microsecond pulsed flashlamp pumped dye l.
Nd:YAG l.
neodymium:yttrium-aluminum-garnet laser
pulsed infrared l.
pulsed metal vapor l.
l. sclerosis
Spectranetics excimer l.
l. system
TEC-2100 postioning l.
YAG l.
yttrium-aluminum-garnet l.
laser-assisted microvascular anastomosis
laser-Doppler flowmetry probe (LDF probe)
Laserflow Doppler probe

laser-induced
l.-i. thermography (LITT)
l.-i. thermotherapy (LITT)
laser-polarized
l.-p. helium MRI
l.-p. helium MR imaging
Laserprobe-PLR Plus
LASH
left anterosuperior hemiblock
Lasix renography
Laslett-Short syndrome
lasso sign
last
l. menstrual period (LMP)
l. normal vertebra (LNV)
Lastec System angioplasty laser
lata
fascia l.
snapping fascia l.
latae
tensor fasciae l.
Latarjet
nerve of L.
LATC
lateral talocalcaneal
late
l. effect analysis
l. effects of normal tissue (LENT)
l. effects of normal tissues score (LENT score)
l. effects toxicity score
l. false aneurysm
l. fetal death
l. film
l. flattening IUGR
l. graft occlusion
l. normal tissue sequela
l. phase
l. systolic bulge
l. systolic retraction
l. venous filling
latent
l. coccidioidomycosis
l. empyema
l. pleurisy
late-onset dwarfism
late-phase termination
lateral
l. aneurysm
l. anterior drawer stress view
l. arcuate ligament
l. aspect
l. band
l. basal segmental bronchus
l. bending injury
l. bending view
l. bending views of spine
l. border
l. cephalometric radiograph
l. cervical spine film
l. collateral ligament (LCL)
l. column calcaneal fracture
l. compartment
l. compartment impaction
l. compartment traumatic bony injury
l. conal fascia
l. condylar humeral fracture
l. condyle
l. corticospinal tract
l. costotransverse ligament
l. crus
l. decubitus film
l. decubitus position
l. decubitus radiograph
l. decubitus view
l. disk herniation
l. entrapment
l. epicondylitis
exaggerated craniocaudal l. (XCCL)
l. extension view
l. facial cleft
l. fissure
l. flexion view
l. geniculate body
l. gutter
l. horn
l. impingement
l. joint line
l. joint space
l. left anterior oblique position
l. lemniscus tract
l. lobe of prostate
l. lumbar meningocele
l. malleolar fracture
l. malleolus
l. mass
l. myocardial infarct
l. oblique fascia
l. oblique radiograph
l. oblique view
l. occipital sulcus
l. occipitotemporal gyrus
l. opposed beam

NOTES

lateral *(continued)*
l. patellofemoral angle
l. placenta previa
l. plantar metatarsal angle
l. posterior choroidal (LPCh)
l. precordium
l. projection
l. pterygoid muscle
l. pterygoid tendinous attachment
l. recess
l. recess stenosis
l. rectus muscle
l. reflection of colon
l. resolution
l. reticular formation
l. root
l. rotatory ankle instability
l. sagittal image
l. semicircular canal
l. sesamoid bone
l. shelf
l. sinus
l. skull radiograph
l. spinothalamic tract
l. spring ligament of foot
l. subluxation
l. talocalcaneal (LATC)
l. talocalcaneal angle
l. talocalcaneal ligament
l. talometatarsal angle
l. tarsometatarsal angle
l. temporal epileptogenic lesion
l. thoracic meningocele
l. tibial plateau fracture
l. tilt stress ankle view
l. tomography
l. ulnar collateral ligament (LUCL)
l. umbilical fold
l. ventricle
l. ventricle of cerebrum
l. ventricle trigone
l. wall refractive shadowing
l. web
l. wedge fracture

lateralis
interdigitation of vastus l.
meniscus l.
sinus l.
vastus l.

laterality

lateralization
l. deficit

lateralizing
l. finding
l. sign

laterally displaced fracture

lateroconal fascia

lateromedial
l. oblique view
l. projection

latex
Spli-Prest l.

LaTeX device

latissimus
l. dorsi
l. dorsi muscle

latitude film

lattice
l. relaxation time
l. vibration

latticework

Laubry-Pezzi syndrome

Laue
L. pattern
L. photographic technique

Lauenstein
L. and Hickey method
L. and Hickey projection

Lauge-Hansen
L.-H. ankle fracture classification
L.-H. classification of ankle fractures

Laugier
L. fracture
L. sign

Laurence-Moon-Biedl-Bardet syndrome

Laurence-Moon-Biedl syndrome

Laurin
L. angle
L. x-ray view

Lausanne stereotactic robot

Lauth ligament

lavage
oral colonic l. (OCL)

Law
L. position
L. view

law
Beer l.
Bragg l.
Coulomb l.
Courvoisier l.
Curie l.
Doerner-Hoskins distribution l.
Faraday l.
Fick l.
Gibbs-Donnan l.
Hilton l.
inverse-square l.
least-squares l.
Le Borgne l.
Lenz l.
Poiseuille l.
Rayleigh scattering l.

transformer l.
Wolff l.
Lawrence
L. method
L. position
lawrencium (Lr)
laxative
bulk l.
laxity
joint l.
ligamentous l.
varus stress l.
layer
basal l.
Bekhterev l.
boundary l.
bright l.
circumferential echodense l.
echodense l.
echo-free l.
fibrofatty l.
half-life l.
half-value l. (HVL)
hypoechoic l.
inner bright l.
parietal l.
seromuscular l.
sonolucent l.
subcuticular l.
subserosal l.
tenth-value l.
visceral l.
layered gallstone
layering
l. calcification
calcium l.
l. of contrast material
l. effusion
l. of gallstones
Lazarus sign
L/B
lesion-to-brain
L/B ratio
LBBB
left bundle-branch block
LBCD
left border of cardiac dullness
LBD
lamellar body density
LBP
low back pain
LC
inductance-capacitance
LCA
left coronary angiography
left coronary artery
LC-DCP
low-contact dynamic compression plate
LCF
left circumflex
LCIS
lobular carcinoma in situ
lck
LCL
lateral collateral ligament
LCP
Legg-Calvé-Perthes disease
LCT
liquid crystal thermography
LCU
laparoscopic contact ultrasonography
LCX
left circumflex
LDF
laser Doppler flowmetry
LDF probe
LE
lower extremity
Le
Lewis
Le Borgne law
Le Fort amputation
Le Fort fibular fracture
Le Fort mandibular fracture
Le Fort-Wagstaffe fracture
lead (Pb)
l. apron
l. apron shield
bipolar l.
l. collimation
l. eye shield
l. line
pacemaker l.
l. pellet marker
l. point
l. poisoning
precordial l.
leading edge
lead-pipe rigidity
lead-time bias
leaf of diaphragm
leafless tree appearance

NOTES

leaflet
anterior mitral valve l.
anterior motion of posterior mitral valve l.
anterior tricuspid l. (ATL)
anterior tricuspid valve l.
apposition of l.'s
arching of mitral valve l.
bowing of mitral valve l.
coapted l.
commissural l.
doming of l.
floating l.
l. function
hammocking of mitral valve l.
heart valve l.
mitral l.
l. motion
myxomatous valve l.
noncalcified mitral l.
posterior mitral l. (pML)
posterior mitral valve l. (PMVL)
posterior tricuspid l. (PTL, pTL)
pseudomitral l.
redundant aortic valve l.
redundant mitral valve l.
l. retraction
l. separation
septal l.
spoonlike protrusion of l.
systolic prolapse of mitral valve l.
valve l.

leaflike villus

leak
air l.
aortic paravalvular l.
baffle l.
blood l.
calibrated l.
capillary l.
cerebrospinal fluid l.
chyle l.
contained l.
current l.
generalized capillary l.
interatrial baffle l.
interstitial pneumonia air l.
light l.
mitral l.
paraprosthetic l.
paravalvular l.
periprosthetic l.
perivalvular l.
transient chyle l.

leakage
anastomotic l.
bile l.
blood-tumor-barrier l.
l. of cerebrospinal fluid
cerebrospinal fluid l.
contrast media l.
paraprosthetic l.
silicone implant l.

leaking
l. abdominal aortic aneurysm
l. vein

leaky valve

lean mass

least-squares
l.-s. algorithm
l.-s. law

least squares (LS)

leatherbottle stomach

leaves of mesentery

Leclercq test

ledge
eccentric l.

left
l. anterior chest wall wall
l. anterior descending (LAD)
l. anterior descending artery
l. anterior fascicular block (LAFB)
l. anterior hemiblock block
l. anterior internal diameter (LAID)
l. anterior oblique (LAO)
l. anterior oblique (LAO) view
l. anterior oblique position
l. anterior oblique projection
l. anterior oblique projection ventriculogram
l. anterosuperior hemiblock (LASH)
l. apexcardiogram, calibrated displacement (LACD)
l. atrial active-emptying fraction
l. atrial appendage (LAA)
l. atrial cannulation
l. atrial chamber
l. atrial end-diastolic pressure
l. atrial enlargement (LAE)
l. atrial function
l. atrial hypertrophy
l. atrial maximal volume
l. atrial myxoma
l. atrial pressure (LAP)
l. atrioventricular groove artery
l. atrium (LA)
l. atrium/aortic root (LA/AR)
l. atrium/aortic root ratio
l. auricle
l. auricular appendage (LAA)
l. axis deviation (LAD)
l. border of cardiac dullness (LBCD)
l. border of heart
l. bundle branch
l. bundle-branch block (LBBB)

l. bundle branch hemiblock
l. circumflex (LCF, LCX)
l. circumflex coronary artery
l. colon
l. colonic flexure
l. common carotid artery
l. common femoral artery
l. coronary angiography (LCA)
l. coronary artery (LCA)
l. coronary cusp
l. coronary plexus
l. coronary sinus
l. crus
l. gutter
l. heart
l. heart syndrome
l. hemisphere
l. hepatic vein (LHV)
l. iliac system
l. intercostal space (LICS)
l. internal mammary artery (LIMA)
l. internal mammary artery (LIMA) anastomosis
l. lateral projection
l. lobe of liver
l. lower extremity (LLE)
l. lower lobe (LLL)
l. lower lobe lesion
l. lower quadrant (LLQ)
l. main coronary artery (LMCA)
l. main stem bronchus
l. mid lung
l. parietal syndrome
l. pleural apical hematoma cap
l. posterior oblique (LPO)
l. posterior oblique position
l. posterior oblique projection
l. primary bronchus
l. pulmonary artery (LPA)
l. pulmonary cusp
l. pulmonary vein (LPV)
l. respiratory nerve
l. retroaortic renal vein
l. sternal border (LSB)
l. subclavian central venous
l. subclavian central venous pressure (LSCVP)
l. upper lobe (LUL)
l. upper lobe lesion
l. upper quadrant (LUQ)
l. upper quadrant abscess
l. ventricle
l. ventricle of heart
l. ventricular afterload
l. ventricular aneurysm
l. ventricular angiography
l. ventricular apex
l. ventricular assist device (LVAD)
l. ventricular asynergy
l. ventricular cardiomyopathy
l. ventricular cavity pressure
l. ventricular chamber
l. ventricular chamber volume
l. ventricular configuration
l. ventricular contraction pattern
l. ventricular diastolic dimension (LVdd, LVDD)
l. ventricular dilatation
l. ventricular dysfunction (LVD)
l. ventricular ejection fraction (LVEF)
l. ventricular ejection time (LVET)
l. ventricular end-diastolic dimension (LVEDD)
l. ventricular end-diastolic pressure (LVEDP)
l. ventricular end-diastolic volume
l. ventricular end-diastolic volume index (LVEDI)
l. ventricular end-systolic dimension (LVESD)
l. ventricular end-systolic volume index (LVESVI)
l. ventricular failure
l. ventricular fast filling time
l. ventricular filling pressure
l. ventricular fractional shortening index
l. ventricular free wall (LVFW)
l. ventricular functional shortening (LVFS)
l. ventricular function pressure
l. ventricular function wall motion
l. ventricular gated blood pool scan
l. ventricular hypertrophy (LVH)
l. ventricular hypertrophy with strain
l. ventricular hypoplasia
l. ventricular inflow tract obstruction
l. ventricular inflow volume (LVIV)

L

NOTES

left *(continued)*
l. ventricular internal diameter (LVID)
l. ventricular internal diastolic dimension (LVIDd, LVIDD)
l. ventricular internal dimension at end systole (LVIDs)
l. ventricular internal end-systole
l. ventricular loading
l. ventricular mass (LVM)
l. ventricular mass index (LVMI)
l. ventricular maximal volume
l. ventricular muscle
l. ventricular outflow pressure gradient
l. ventricular outflow tract (LVOT)
l. ventricular outflow tract obstruction (LVOTO)
l. ventricular outflow volume (LVOV)
l. ventricular peak systolic pressure
l. ventricular posterior superior process
l. ventricular posterior wall (LVPW)
l. ventricular preload
l. ventricular pressure (LVP)
l. ventricular regional wall motion
l. ventricular regional wall motion abnormality
l. ventricular slow filling time ($LVFT_2$)
l. ventricular strain pattern
l. ventricular stroke volume
l. ventricular stroke work (LVSW)
l. ventricular stroke work index (LVSWI)
l. ventricular support system
l. ventricular systolic/diastolic function
l. ventricular systolic functional reserve
l. ventricular systolic pressure (LVs pressure)
l. ventricular systolic pump function
l. ventricular systolic time interval ratio
l. ventricular wall (LVW)
l. ventriculogram (LVG)
left-dominant coronary anatomy
left-handedness
ventricular l.-h.
left-right asymmetry
left-sided
l.-s. empyema
l.-s. heart failure
l.-s. heart pressure
l.-s. pleural effusion
left-sidedness
bilateral l.-s.
left-side-down decubitus position
left-to-right
l.-t.-r. flow
l.-t.-r. shift
l.-t.-r. shunting of blood
leg
l. axis
baker's l.
bayonet l.
bowed l.'s
champagne-bottle l.'s
deep vein system of l.
l. edema
postphlebitic l.
scissoring of l.'s
l. shortening
tennis l.
Legg-Calvé-Perthes disease (LCP)
Legg-Calvé-Waldenström disease
leg-length discrepancy (LLD)
Leichtenstern sign
Leigh disease
leiomyoblastoma
leiomyoma, pl. **leiomyomata, leiomyomas**
epithelioid l.
esophageal l.
gastric l.
kidney l.
multiple vascular leiomyomas
pedunculated l.
renal l.
small bowel l.
stomach l.
urinary bladder l.
uterine l.
vascular l.
leiomyomatosis
esophageal l.
leiomyomatous kidney hamartoma
leiomyosarcoma
duodenal l.
esophageal l.
gastric l.
intramural l.
intravascular l.
jejunal l.
retroperitoneal l.
right atrial extension of uterine l.
small bowel l.
stomach l.
leiomyosarcomatosis
Leitner syndrome
Leksell
L. D-shaped stereotactic frame

L. gamma unit
L. stereotactic device
L. stereotactic system
L. technique

Leksell-Elekta stereotactic frame

lemniscus, pl. **lemnisci**
medial l.

lemon sign

Lenard ray tube

length
basic cycle l. (BCL)
basic drive cycle l. (BDCL)
Beatson combined ankle l.
cephalocaudad l.
cervical l.
crown-heel l.
crown-rump l. (CR, CRL)
echo-train l. (ETL)
femur l. (FL)
fetal femoral l.
focal l.
Grace method of ratio of metatarsal l.
humeral l.
jet l. (JL)
limb l.
pulse l.
sinus cycle l. (SCL)
track cone l.

length-biased sampling

length-time bias

Lennhoff sign

Lenoir facet

lens
acoustic l.
right-angled telescopic l.
Thorpe plastic l.

LENT
late effects of normal tissue
LENT paradigm
LENT score
LENT scoring system

lenticular
l. area
l. bone
l. carcinoma
l. fasciculus
l. loop
l. nucleus

lenticulostriate
l. artery
l. vessel

lentiform
l. bone
l. nucleus

lentigo maligna

Lenz law

Leonard-George
L.-G. method
L.-G. position

leontiasis ossea

lepidic growth

leptocyte

leptocytosis

leptomeningeal
l. artery
l. carcinoma
l. disease
l. fibrosis

leptomeninges

leptomeningitis

leptomeningoencephalitis

leptomyelolipoma

Leri
melorheostosis of L.
L. pleonosteosis
L. sign

Leriche syndrome

Leri-Layani-Weill syndrome

LES
lower esophageal sphincter

Lesch-Nyhan syndrome

Lesgaft
L. hernia
L. space
L. triangle

lesion
acute cerebellar hemispheric l.
admixture l.
adrenal l.
afferent nerve l.
ALPSA l.
anechoic l.
angiocentric immunoproliferative l.
angiocentric lymphoproliferative l.
angulated l.
annular constricting l.
anterior labroligamentous periosteal sleeve avulsion l.
anterior labrum periosteal sleeve avulsion l.
anterior parietal l.
anterochiasmatic l.
aortic arch l.

NOTES

L

lesion *(continued)*
aortic valve l.
apical l.
apophyseal l.
Armanni-Ebstein l.
atheromatous l.
atherosclerotic l.
atrophic brain l.
Baehr-Lohlein l.
Bankart l.
barrel-shaped l.
basal hypodense ganglia l.
benign bone l.
benign fibrous bone l.
benign lymphoepithelial l.
benign lymphoproliferative l.
benign vascular l.
Bennett l.
bifurcation l.
bilateral l.
bilobed polypoid l.
biparietal l.
bird's nest l.
black star breast l.
blastic l.
bleeding l.
blowout bone l.
Blumenthal l.
bone l.
bone marrow l.
Bracht-Wachter l.
brain l.
brainstem l.
breast l.
Brown-Séquard l.
bubbly bone l.
bulbourethral gland l.
bull's eye stomach l.
calcified l.
callosal l.
cardiac valvular l.
carpet l.
cartilaginous l.
cavernous sinus l.
caviar l.
cavitary lung l.
cavitary small bowel l.
central l.
central medullary bone l.
centrilobular l.
cerebral l.
cerebrospinal fluid-containing l.
cervical cord l.
chest wall l.
chiasmal l.
cholesterol-containing brain l.
circular l.
circumscribed l.
cochlear l.
coin l.
cold l.
collar-button chest l.
colonic apple-core l.
colonic carpet l.
colonic saddle l.
complete nerve l.
complex l.
complex sclerosing l.
concentric l.
congenital cystic neck l.
constricting esophageal l.
conus medullaris l.
coordinates for target l.
cord epidural extramedullary l.
cord intramedullary l.
coronary artery l.
corpus callosum ring-enhancing l.
cortical bone l.
corticospinal pathway l.
Cowper gland l.
critical l.
culprit l.
cyclops l.
cystic epididymis l.
cystic intracranial fetal l.
cystic liver l.
cystic splenic l.
deep-seated l.
dendritic l.
de novo l.
dense enhancing brain l.
dense lung l.
desmoid l.
destructive bone l.
diaphyseal l.
Dieulafoy l.
differential diagnosis bone l.
diffuse ulcerative l.
discrete l.
disk l.
dominant hemisphere l.
dorsal root entry zone l.
doughnut l.
DREZ l.
dumbbell l.
Duret l.
Ebstein l.
eccentric medullary bone l.
eccentric restenosis l.
echogenic solid l.
ellipsoid l.
encapsulated fat-containing l.
encephaloclastic l.
endobronchial l.
enhancing brain l.
epicortical l.

epididymis l.
epidural extramedullary l.
epileptogenic l.
epiphyseal l.
esophageal apple-core l.
excitatory l.
expanding cavernous sinus brain l.
expansile lytic l.
expansile multilocular bone l.
expansile rib l.
expansile unilocular well-demarcated bone l.
extraaxial CNS l.
extraaxial low-attenuation l.
extracranial mass l.
extrahepatic l.
extratesticular l.
extrinsic l.
fast-flow l.
fat-containing breast l.
fibrohistiocytic l.
fibromuscular l.
fibroosseous l.
fibrous bone l.
fibrous GI tract polypoid l.
fibrous polypoid l.
finger lucent l.
fingertip l.
florid duct l.
flow-compromising l.
flow-limiting l.
focal cold liver l.
focal hemispheric l.
focal hot liver l.
focal ischemic l.
focal liver l.
focal parenchymal brain l.
focal splenic l.
frank l.
friable l.
frontal lobe l.
gastric intramural-extramucosal l.
geographic l.
Ghon primary l.
Gill l.
glomerular l.
gross l.
hamartomatous l.
hemisphere l.
hemodynamically significant l.
hemorrhagic l.
high cervical spinal cord l.
high-density l.
high-grade obstructive l.
high-intensity l.
high pontine l.
high-probability l.
high-signal l.
Hill-Sachs shoulder l.
hole-within-hole bone l.
homogeneous l.
hot l.
hourglass-shaped l.
humeral avulsion of the glenohumeral ligament (HAGL) l.
hyperdense brain l.
hyperintense periventricular l.
hyperintense periventricular brain l.
hyperplastic l.
hypodense basal ganglion brain l.
hypodense mesencephalic low-density brain l.
hypointense sella l.
hypothalamic l.
iliac l.
impaction l.
indiscriminate l.
infectious bubbly bone l.
infiltrating l.
inflammatory l.
infranuclear l.
innumerable small enhancing brain l.'s
internal auditory canal enhancing l.
intraaxial brain l.
intracerebral l.
intraconal l.
intracranial mass l.
intracranial vascular l.
intradural extramedullary l.
intramammary l.
intramedullary cord l.
intramedullary spinal l.
intramural-extramucosal stomach l.
intraocular l.
intraosseous bone l.
intrasellar l.
intraspinal l.
intrinsic stenotic l.
intrinsic stomach wall l.
invasive l.
irregularly shaped l.
ischemic l.
ischiorectal fossa l.

NOTES

lesion *(continued)*
isointense l.
Janeway l.
jet l.
juxtacortical bone l.
Kidner l.
lacrimal gland l.
lateral temporal epileptogenic l.
left lower lobe l.
left upper lobe l.
lipomatous l.
liver bull's eye l.
l. localization
localized l.
Löhlein-Baehr l.
low-attenuation l.
low-density mesencephalic l.
lower motor neuron l.
lucent finger l.
lucent lung l.
lumbar spine l.
lunge l.
Lynch and Crues type 2 l.
lytic bone l.
macroscopic placental l.
malignant l.
Mallory-Weiss l.
mammographically suspicious l.
mass l.
medial longitudinal fasciculus l.
median nerve l.
mediastinal l.
mesencephalic low-density brain l.
mesenteric vascular l.
mesial temporal epileptogenic l.
metabolic l.
metachronous l.
metastatic l.
micropapillary l.
midbrain l.
midline l.
mixed bone l.
mixed fat-water density l.
mixed sclerotic and lytic bone l.
MLF l.
mongolian spotlike l.
Monteggia l.
mucosal l.
mulberry eye l.
multicentric lytic l.
multifocal enhancing brain l.
multilocular cystic l.
multiple lucent lung l.
multiple lytic bone l.'s
multiple osteosclerotic l.'s
multiple parotid gland l.'s
multiple stenotic l.'s
muscular l.
nail bed l.
napkin-ring annular l.
necrotic l.
needle localization of breast l.
neoplastic l.
neurogenic l.
neurologic bladder l.
neurovascular l.
nidus of l.
nodular l.
nondominant hemisphere l.
nonenhancing l.
nonexpansile multilocular bone l.
nonexpansile unilocular bone l.
noninvasive l.
nonmeningiomatous malignant l.
nucleus ambiguus l.
nucleus basalis l.
obstructive l.
occipital l.
occlusive l.
occult l.
ocular l.
onionskin l.
optic nerve l.
organic l.
osseous l.
osteoblastic l.
osteocartilaginous l.
osteochondral l.
osteolytic l.
osteosclerotic l.
ostial l.
outcropping of l.
oval-shaped breast l.
papillary l.
papular l.
papulonecrotic l.
paralabral l.
paraorbital l.
parasagittal l.
parasellar l.
parietal cortex l.
parietal lobe l.
parietooccipital l.
parosteal bone l.
patch l.
pedunculated l.
perforative l.
periapical l.
peripheral nerve l.
perisellar vascular l.
periventricular l.
permeative l.
Perthes l.
Perthes-Bankart l.
photon-deficient bone l.
plaquelike l.

polyostotic bone l.
polypoid l.
pontine l.
posterior column l.
posterior compartment l.
posterior fossa-foramen magnum l.
posterior language area l.
posterior vertebral elements blowout l.
prechiasmal optic nerve l.
presacral cystic l.
pretectal l.
primary l.
prostate hypoechoic l.
pulmonary l.
punched-out lytic bone l.
purulent l.
questionable l.
radial sclerosing l.
radiodense l.
radiofrequency l.
radiographic stability of l.
radiolucent l.
radiopaque l.
reactive lymphoid l.
rectal l.
rectosigmoid polypoid l.
recurrent l.
regurgitant l.
remote lower motor neuron l.
renal mass l.
resectable l.
retrochiasmal l.
reverse Hill-Sachs l.
rheumatic l.
rib l.
right lower lobe l.
right upper lobe l.
rim-enhancing l.
ring l.
ring-enhancing brain l.
root entry-zone l.
rotator cuff l.
round lucent l.
saddle l.
satellite l.
scirrhous l.
sclerosing l.
sclerotic l.
secondary l.
segmental bronchus l.
serial l.
sessile l.
sharply demarcated circumferential l.
sinonasal l.
sinusoidal l.
skeletal l.
skin l.
skip l.
SLAP l.
slow-flow l.
slowly developing l.
small bowel cavitary l.
solid splenic l.
solid thymic l.
solitary cold l.
solitary osteosclerotic l.
sonolucent cystic l.
space-occupying l.
spherical l.
spiculated scirrhous l.
spinal cord l.
spleen l.
splenic l.
spontaneous l.
squamous intraepithelial l.
stacked ovoid l.
stellate border breast l.
Stener l.
stenotic l.
stomach bull's eye l.
striatal l.
structural l.
subchondral l.
subcortical intracranial l.
submucosal l.
subtentorial l.
subtotal l.
superficial l.
superior labral anteroposterior (SLAP) l.
supranuclear l.
suprasellar low-density l.
supratentorial l.
suspicious l.
synchronous l.
systemic l.
tandem l.
target lung l.
tectal l.
telangiectatic l.
temporal lobe l.
testicular cystic l.

NOTES

lesion *(continued)*
thalamic l.
thoracic inlet l.
tight l.
total l.
trabeculated bone l.
transfer l.
transverse cord l.
trophic l.
tuberculous l.
tubular l.
tumorlike bone l.
tumor-mimicking breast l.
ulcerative l.
ulnar nerve l.
umbilical cord l.
uncommitted metaphyseal l.
unilateral l.
unilocular cystic l.
unilocular well-demarcated bone defect expansile l.
unresectable l.
unstable l.
upper motor neuron l.
valvular regurgitant l.
vascular l.
vasculitic l.
vegetative l.
vertebral expansile l.
visceral l.
Waldeyer ring l.
wedge-shaped l.
well-circumscribed l.
well-defined l.
white matter l.
white star breast l.
wide field l.
wire-loop l.
Wolin meniscoid l.
X, Y, and Z coordinates for target l.
lesion-to-background ratio
lesion-to-brain (L/B)
l.-t.-b. ratio (L/B ratio)
lesion-to-cerebrospinal fluid noise
lesion-to-muscle ratio
lesion-to-nonlesion count ratio
lesion-to-white matter noise
LESP
lower esophageal sphincter pressure
lesser
l. arc injury
l. atrophy
l. atrophy of disuse
l. curvature of stomach
l. curvature ulcer
l. metatarsophalangeal joint
l. multangular bone
l. muscle
l. omentum
l. pancreas
l. pelvis
l. peritoneal sac
l. petrosal
l. sac hernia
l. sac of peritoneal cavity
l. saphenous system
l. saphenous vein
l. sciatic foramen
l. sciatic notch
l. trochanter
l. trochanter of femur
l. trochanteric fracture
l. tubercle
l. tuberosity
Lesshaft space
LET
linear energy transfer
lethal
l. bone dysplasia
l. dose
l. dwarfism
l. midline granuloma
l. musculoskeletal dysplasia
l. myocardial injury
l. neoplasm
l. wasting syndrome
lettering artifact
leucine radical
LeukaScan imaging agent
leukemia
chronic lymphocytic l.
T-cell acute lymphoblastic l. (T-ALL)
leukemic bone line
leukocyte
autologous labeled l.'s
gallium-67-labeled l.'s
indium-111-labeled l.'s
indium-111-oxime l.'s
leukoencephalitis
acute hemorrhagic l.
leukoencephalopathy
diffuse necrotizing l.
disseminated necrotizing l.
multifocal l.
periventricular l.
postviral l.
progressive multifocal l. (PML)
radiation-induced l.
spongiform l.
leukomalacia
periventricular l. (PVL)
leukopenia
autoimmune l.

radiofreqency radiogenic l.
radiogenic l.
Leur-par collimator
levator
l. ani
l. muscle
l. palpebrae
l. palpebrae superioris
l. scapulae
l. span
l. veli palatini
LeVeen plaque cracker
level
air-fluid l.
attenuation l.
energy l.
fat-fluid l.
fluid l.
fluid-fluid l.
gas-fluid l.
intrasinus air-fluid l.
l. I obstetric ultrasound
pontine-medullary l.
significance l.
stairstep air-fluid l.
supraventricular l.
window l.
Zielke derotation l.
level-dependent
blood oxygenation l.-d.
Levenberg-Marquardt method
Levine sign
levoposition
levorotary scoliosis
levorotatory
levoscoliosis
levotransposition (L-transposition)
levoversion
Levovist
L. imaging agent
Lewis (Le)
L. angle
Leydig
L. cell adenoma
L. cell tumor
Leyla arm
LFV
large field of view
LGA
large for gestational age
low-grade astrocytoma
LGL
Lown-Ganong-Levine syndrome
LHB
long head of biceps
Lhermitte-Duclos disease
Lhermitte syndrome
LHV
left hepatic vein
Lian-Siguier-Welti venous thrombosis syndrome
Lichtenstein-Jaffe disease
LICS
left intercostal space
LICU
laparoscopic intracorporeal ultrasound
lidofenin
technetium-99m l.
lie
horizontal l.
longitudinal l.
posterior l.
transverse l.
Liebel-Flarsheim CT 9000 contrast delivery system
Lieberkühn
crypt of L.
L. crypt
Liebermeister groove
Liebow
usual interstitial pneumonia of L. (UIP)
lienis
sustentaculum l.
lienography
lienophrenic ligament
lienorenal ligament
Lieutaud trigone
LiF
lithium fluoride
LiF thermoluminescence dosimeter
LiF thermoluminescence dosimetry
life
half-l. (HL)
Life-Pack 5 cardiac monitor
life-threatening
l.-t. hemorrhage
l.-t. pneumothorax
lift
gallbladder l.
heave and l.
sternal l.

NOTES

lift-off
fluoroscopy-guided condylar l.-o.
ligament
abdominal triangular l.
accessory atlantoaxial l.
acromioclavicular l.
acromiocoracoid l.
adipose l.
alar l.
annular l.
anococcygeal l.
anterior cruciate l. (ACL)
anterior fibular l.
anterior inferior tibiofibular l.
anterior talofibular l. (ATF)
anterior tibiofibular l.
apical l.
Arantius l.
arcuate l.
arterial l.
atlantal l.
attenuated l.
auricular l.
avulsed l.
l. avulsion
axis l.
Bardinet l.
Barkow l.
beak l.
Bellini l.
Berry l.
Bertin l.
Bichat l.
bifurcated l.
l. of Bigelow
Bigelow l.
l. of Botallo
Botallo l.
Bourgery l.
broad l.
Brodie l.
Burns l.
calcaneoclavicular l.
calcaneocuboid l.
calcaneofibular l.
calcaneonavicular l.
calcaneotibial l.
Caldani l.
Campbell l.
Camper l.
capsular l.
Carcassonne l.
cardinal l.
caroticoclinoid l.
carpometacarpal l.
Casser l.
casserian l.
caudal l.
ceratocricoid l.
cervical mover l.
check rein l.
cholecystoduodenal l.
chondroxiphoid l.
ciliary l.
Civinini l.
Clado l.
Cleland l.
clinoid l.
Cloquet l.
coccygeal l.
collateral l.
Colles l.
congenital laxity of l.
conjugate l.
conoid l.
conus l.
Cooper suspensory l.
coracoacromial l.
coracoclavicular l.
coracohumeral l.
corniculopharyngeal l.
coronary l.
costoclavicular l.
costocolic l.
costotransverse l.
costoxiphoid l.
cotyloid l.
Cowper l.
cricopharyngeal l.
cricosantorinian l.
cricothyroid l.
cricotracheal l.
cross l.
cruciate l.
cruciatum cruris l.
cruciform l.
Cruveilhier l.
cuboideonavicular l.
cuneocuboid l.
cuneonavicular l.
cystoduodenal l.
deep collateral l.
deltoid l.
Denonvilliers l.
dentate l.
denticulate l.
Denuce l.
diaphragmatic l.
dorsal metacarpal l.
dorsal wrist l.
Douglas l.
duodenal l.
duodenorenal l.
epicondyloolecranon l.
l. of epididymis
epihyal l.

extracapsular l.
extrinsic l.
fabellofibular l.
falciform l.
fallopian l.
femoral l.
Ferrein l.
fibular collateral l.
fibulotalar l.
fibulotalocalcaneal l.
flaval l.
floating l.
Flood l.
FTC l.
fundiform l.
gastrocolic l.
gastrodiaphragmatic l.
gastrohepatic l.
gastrolienal l.
gastropancreatic l.
gastrophrenic l.
gastrosplenic l.
genital l.
genitoinguinal l.
Gerdy l.
Gillette suspensory l.
Gimbernat l.
gingivodental l.
glenohumeral l.
glenoid l.
glossoepiglottic l.
Grayson l.
Günzberg l.
Haines-McDougall medial sesamoid l.
hammock l.
Helmholtz axis l.
l. of Henle
Henle l.
l.'s of Henry and Wrisberg
Hensing l.
hepatic l.
hepatocolic l.
hepatocystocolic l.
hepatoduodenal l.
hepatoesophageal l.
hepatogastric l.
hepatogastroduodenal l.
hepatophrenic l.
hepatorenal l.
hepatoumbilical l.
Hesselbach l.
Hey l.
Holl l.
Hueck l.
humeral avulsion of the glenohumeral l. (HAGL)
Humphry l.
l. of Humphry
Hunter l.
Huschke l.
hyalocapsular l.
hyoepiglottic l.
iliofemoral l.
iliolumbar l.
iliopectineal l.
iliopubic l.
iliotibial l.
iliotrochanteric l.
inferior dorsal radioulnar l.
inferior pulmonary l.
infrapatellar l.
infundibuloovarian l.
infundibulopelvic l.
inguinal l.
intercapital l.
intercarpal l.
interclavicular l.
interclinoid l.
intercornual l.
intercuneiform l.
interdigital l.
interfoveolar l.
intermetatarsal l.
internal collateral l.
interosseous talocalcaneal l.
intersesamoid l.
interspinous l.
intertransverse l.
intervertebral l.
intraarticular l.
intrascapular l.
intrinsic l.
ischiocapsular l.
ischiofemoral l.
Jarjavay l.
jugal l.
Krause l.
laciniate l.
lacunar l.
Landsmeer l.
Lannelongue l.
lateral arcuate l.
lateral collateral l. (LCL)

NOTES

L

ligament *(continued)*
lateral costotransverse l.
lateral talocalcaneal l.
lateral ulnar collateral l. (LUCL)
Lauth l.
lienophrenic l.
lienorenal l.
limited proteoglycan matrix of l.
Lisfranc l.
Lockwood l.
longitudinal l.
lumbocostal l.
lunotriquetral interosseus l.
Luschka l.
Mackenrodt l.
macroscopic hemorrhage l.
Maissiat l.
Mauchart l.
Meckel l.
medial collateral l.
median arcuate l.
median cruciate l.
median umbilical l.
meniscofemoral l.
meniscotibial l.
metacarpoglenoidal l.
metacarpophalangeal l.
microscopic hemorrhage of l.
mucosal suspensory l.
natatory l.
naviculocuneiform l.
nuchal l.
occipitoatlantoaxial l.
occipitoaxial l.
odontoid l.
opacification of posterior longitudinal l.
orbicular l.
Osborne l.
ossification of the posterior longitudinal l.
ossified posterior longitudinal l.
ovarian suspensory l.
l. of ovary
palmar metacarpal l.
palmar radiocarpal l.
pectinate l.
pelvic l.
periodontal l.
peritoneal l.
Petit l.
Pétrequin l.
petroclinoid l.
phalangeal glenoidal l.
phrenicocolic l.
phrenicolienal l.
phrenicosplenic l.
phrenoesophageal l.
phrenogastric l.
phrenosplenic l.
pisohamate l.
pisometacarpal l.
pisounciform l.
pisouncinate l.
plantar l.
popliteal l.
posterior cruciate l. (PCL)
posterior inferior tibiofibular l.
posterior longitudinal l. (PLL)
posterior oblique l.
posterior talofibular l. (PTF ligament)
posterior tibiotalar l.
Poupart inguinal l.
pterygomandibular l.
pterygospinous l.
PTF l.
posterior talofibular ligament
pubocapsular l.
pubocervical l.
pubofemoral l.
puboprostatic l.
pubovesical l.
pulmonary l.
quadrate l.
radial collateral l.
radial metacarpal l.
radiate sternocostal l.
radiocarpal l.
radiolunotriquetral l.
radioscaphocapitate l.
radioscaphoid l.
radioscapholunate l.
reflected edge of Poupart l.
reflected inguinal l.
l. reflecting edge
retinacular l.
l. of Retzius
Retzius l.
rhomboid l.
right triangular l.
ring l.
Robert l.
round l.
Rouviere l.
l. of Rouviere
sacrodural l.
sacrospinous l.
sacrotuberous l.
Santorini l.
Sappey l.
scapholunate l. (LSS)
scaphotriquetral l.
l. of Scarpa
Schlemm l.
serous l.

sesamoid l.
sesamophalangeal l.
sheath l.
l. shelving edge
short radiolunate l.
Simonart l.
Soemmerring l.
sphenomandibular l.
spinoglenoid l.
spiral l.
splenocolic l.
splenorenal l.
spring l.
Stanley cervical l.
stellate l.
sternoclavicular l.
sternopericardial l.
stretched out l.
l. of Struthers
Struthers l.
stylohyoid l.
stylomandibular l.
stylomaxillary l.
superficial dorsal sacrococcygeal l.
superficial posterior sacrococcygeal l.
superficial transverse metacarpal l.
superficial transverse metatarsal l.
superior costotransverse l.
superior pubic l.
superior transverse scapular l.
suprascapular l.
supraspinous l.
suspensory l.
sutural l.
syndesmotic l.
synovial l.
talocalcaneal l.
talofibular l.
talonavicular l.
tarsal l.
tarsometatarsal l.
l. tear
tectoral l.
temporomandibular l.
Teutleben l.
Thompson l.
thyroepiglottic l.
thyrohyoid l.
tibial collateral l.
tibial sesamoid l.
tibiocalcaneal l.
tibiofibular l.
tibionavicular l.
torn meniscotibial l.
transverse atlantal l.
transverse carpal l.
transverse cervical l.
transverse crural l.
transverse genicular l.
transverse humeral l.
transverse intertarsal l.
transverse metacarpal l.
transverse metatarsal l.
transverse perineal l.
transverse tibiofibular l.
trapezoid l.
l. of Treitz
triangular l.
triquetrohamate l.
triquetroscaphoid l.
Tuffier inferior l.
ulnar collateral l. (UCL)
ulnocarpal l.
ulnolunate l.
ulnotriquetral l.
umbilical l.
urachal l.
uterine l.
uterosacral l.
uterovesical l.
vaginal l.
venous l.
ventral sacrococcygeal l.
ventral sacroiliac l.
ventricular l.
vertebropelvic l.
vesicosacral l.
vesicoumbilical l.
vesicouterine l.
vestibular l.
vocal l.
volar carpal l.
Walther oblique l.
Weitbrecht l.
Winslow l.
Wrisberg l.
xiphicostal l.
xiphoid l.
Y-shaped l.
Zaglas l.
Zinn l.

ligamenta (*pl. of* ligamentum)

NOTES

ligamentous
l. ankylosis
l. attachment
l. bouncing
l. box
l. calcification
l. complex
l. disruption
l. impingement
l. insertion
l. instability
l. laxity
l. luxation
l. strain
l. support
l. thickening
ligamentous-muscular hypertrophy
ligamentum, pl. **ligamenta**
l. arteriosum
l. flavum
l. flavum thickening
l. mucosum
l. nuchae
l. patellae
l. teres
l. teres notch
l. teres sign
l. venosum fissure
ligand
l. agent
light
l. bulb appearance
hot l.
infrared l.
invisible l.
l. leak
l. microscopy
l. pink lung
l. scanning
Wood l.
lighter-than-bile contrast agent
Lightwood syndrome
Ligman-Sacks endocarditis disease
LILI
low-intensity laser irradiation
Lilienfelds
L. method
L. position
Liliequist membrane
lily-pad sign
LIMA
left internal mammary artery
limb
l. absence
l. of anterior capsule
l. of bifurcation graft
l. bud
l. girdle
l. length
l. perfusion
l. reduction
l. reduction abnormality
l. reduction anomaly
Roux-en-Y l.
vertebral, anal, cardiac, tracheal, esophageal, renal l. (VACTERL)
limb-body wall complex
limb-girdle muscular dystrophy
limbic lobe
limb-length
l.-l. asymmetry
l.-l. discrepancy (LLD)
l.-l. inequality
limb-lengthening procedure
limb-threatening ischemia
limbus
l. fossae ovalis
l. vertebra
l. of Vieussens
limit
confidence l.
eye exposure l.
Nyquist l.
quantum l.
tracking l.
limitation
beam l.
infarct size l.
l. of joint motion
limited
l. examination
l. film
l. imaging
l. proteoglycan matrix of ligament
l. view
l. Wegener granulomatosis
limited-slice
l.-s. computed tomography
limitus
hallux l. (HL)
LINAC
linear accelerator
LINAC radiosurgery
Varian LINAC
Lincoln log vertebra
Linder sign
line
absence of innominate l.
absorption l.
acanthiomeatal l.
AC-PC l.
air-fluid l.
aneuploid cell l.
anorectal l.
anterior humeral l.
anterior junction l.

aortic vent suction l.
axillary l.
azygoesophageal l.
basilar l.
bimastoid l.
Blumensaat l.
branching l.
calcification l.
Camper l.
cement l.
central sacral l. (CSL)
central venous pressure l.
Chaussier l.
clinoparietal l.
Conradi l.
Correra l.
costoclavicular l.
costophrenic septal l.
Crampton l.
crescent hip l.
curved radiolucent l.
curvilinear subpleural l.
Cyma l.
demarcation l.
dentate l.
divisionary l.
Ellis l.
Ellis-Garland l.
epiphyseal l.
fat density l.
Feiss l.
Fischgold bimastoid l.
Fischgold biventer l.
l. focus principle
fracture l.
Fränkel white l.
Frankfort l.
gallbladder-vena cava l.
gas density l.
gaussian l.
l. of Gennari
gluteal l.
Granger l.
growth arrest l.
Gubler l.
Hampton l.
Harris l.
Hawkins l.
Hickman l.
Hilgenreiner l.
His l.
humeral l.
iliopectineal l.
l. imaging
infraorbitomeatal l. (IOML)
innominate absence of l.
l. integral concept
interlobar septal l.
intravenous infusion l.
isodose l.
isoelectric l.
isopotential l.
joint l.
Kerley A l.'s
Kerley B l.'s
Kerley C l.'s
Kilian l.
Köhler l.
Langer l.
Lanz l.
lateral joint l.
lead l.
leukemic bone l.
Linton l.
Looser l.'s
lorentzian l.
lower lung l.
low-intensity l.
lucent l.
Mach l.
McGregor l.
McKee l.
McRae l.
medial joint l.
median l.
Mees l.
Merkel cell carcinoma cell l.
Meyer l.
midaxillary l.
midclavicular l. (MCL)
midhumeral l.
midscapular l.
midspinal l.
midsternal l.
Moyer l.
Nélaton l.
oblique prescription l.
obturator l.
Ogston l.
Ohngren l.
orthogonal tag l.
l. pair
parallel M l.
parallel pitch l.

NOTES

line *(continued)*
paraspinal l.
pectinate l.
peripheral intravenous infusion l.
peripherally inserted central catheter (PICC) l.
Perkin l.
photon therapy beam l.
l. placement
pleural l.'s
pleuroesophageal l.
popliteal l.
posterior axillary l.
posterior junction l.
pronator quadratus l.
properitoneal fat l.
psoas l.
pubococcygeal l.
radiocapitellar l.
radiolucent crescent l.
raster l.
reference l.
resonance l.
l. of Retzius
Richter-Monroe l.
Rolando l.
Sappey l.
l. saturation
Schoemaker l.
semilunar l.
septal l.
l. shadow
l. shape
Shenton l.
Simpson white l.
skin l.
soleal l.
spectral l.
spinographic l.
l. spread function (LSF)
subchondral fracture l.
subclavian l.
subcutaneous fat l.
subpleural curvilinear l.
suture l.
transcondylar l.
transverse lucent metaphyseal l.
trough l.
twining l.
Ullmann l.
ventral venous pressure l.
vertebral body l.
Wagner l.
water density l.
Wegner l.
white l.
l. width
Z l.
zero l.

linea, pl. **lineae**
l. alba
l. semilunaris

linear
l. absorption coefficient
l. accelerator (LINAC)
l. accelerator isocenter motion
l. accelerator unit
l. amplifier
l. array-hydrophone assembly
l. array transducer
l. artifact
l. attenuation
l. attenuation coefficient
l. band of maximal radiolucency
l. calcification
l. defect
l. degenerative signal intensity
l. density
l. echo
l. electrode array
l. emphysema
l. energy transfer (LET)
l. erosion
l. gradient
l. infiltrate
l. interpolation
l. lucency
l. markings
l. measure
l. opacity
l. phased array
l. phosphates
l. photons
l. polarization
l. prediction with singular value decomposition
l. radiopacity
l. scan imaging
l. scanning
l. shadow
l. skull fracture
l. stenosis
l. tomography
l. ulcer

linearity
absolute l.
gradient l.
intrinsic spatial l.
lung l.
pulmonary l.
scintillation camera l.

linearization
perceptual l.

linearly polarized coil
linear-quadratic (LQ)
l.-q. equation
linebacker's arm
line-pair measurement
line-shape sensitivity
line-spread function (LSF)
lingual
l. artery
l. bone
l. goiter
l. gyrus
l. nerve
l. root
l. thyroid
l. tonsil
linguine breast sign
lingula, pl. **lingulae**
l. pulmonis
right middle lobe l.
lingular
l. artery
l. bronchus
l. division of the left lung
l. mandibular bony defect (LMBD)
l. nodule
l. orifice
l. pneumonia
lining
mucosal l.
linitis
l. plastica
l. plastica carcinoma
link
musculotendinous-osseous l.
Linsman water test
Linton line
Lintro-Scan
liothyronine sodium
LIP
lymphocytic interstitial pneumonia
lymphoid interstitial pneumonia
lip
hilar kidney l.
l.'s of hilum
l.'s of lateral sulcus
median cleft l.
osteophytic bone l.
posterior l.
lipid
l. cholecystitis
l. content of storage fat
l. cyst
l. fraction relaxation rate
l. lake
l. signal
l. zone
lipid-laden plaque
lipid-polarized helium MR imaging
lipid-rich material
lipid-sensitive
l.-s. MR
l.-s. MR imaging
lipiodol myelographic imaging agent
liplike projections of cartilage
lipoblastic
l. meningioma
l. sarcoma
lipoblastoma
lipocalcinogranulomatosis
lipodystrophy
intestinal l.
mesenteric l.
lipofibroadenoma
breast l.
lipogenic tumor
lipogranulomatosis
disseminated l.
lipohemarthrosis
lipoid
l. adrenal hyperplasia
l. endogenous pneumonia
l. pneumonitis
lipoleiomyoma
lipoma
l. arborescens
bone l.
brain l.
breast l.
cardiac l.
corpus callosum l.
diffuse synovial l.
epidural l.
GI tract l.
hepatic l.
hilar l.
infiltrating l.
intracranial l.
intradural l.
intramedullary l.
intraosseous l.
intratentorial l.
liver l.
l. macrodystrophia

L

NOTES

lipoma *(continued)*
mediastinum l.
pericallosal l.
soft tissue l.
spine l.
synovial diffuse l.
lipomatosa
macrodystrophia l.
lipomatosis
central sinus l.
epidural l.
mediastinal l.
l. mediastinum
multiple symmetrical l.
pancreatic l.
pelvic l.
peripelvic l.
renal sinus l.
sinus l.
soft tissue l.
lipomatous
l. hypertrophy
l. lesion
l. polyp
l. tissue
l. tumor
lipomyelomeningocele
lipomyeloschisis
liponecrosis
l. macrocystica calcificans
l. microcystica calcificans
lipophilic
l. dye
l. imaging agent
l. oxine-indium
l. sequestration system
liposarcoma
myxomatous l.
pleomorphic l.
retroperitoneal l.
liposarcomatous differentiation
liposclerotic mesenteritis
liposome
antibody-conjugated paramagnetic l. (ACPL)
lipotropin
Lipowitz metal
lipoxygenase
Lippes loop
lipping
osteophytic l.
liquefaction
l. degeneration
l. necrosis
liquefactive emphysema
liquid
l. crystal contact thermography
l. crystal thermogram
l. crystal thermography (LCT)
l. food dysphagia
l. pleural effusion
l. scintillation analysis
l. scintillation spectrometer
l. scintillation spectrometry
Liquipake
L. imaging agent
Lisch nodule
Lisfranc
L. amputation
L. dislocation
L. fracture
L. injury
L. joint
L. ligament
Lissauer
L. column
L. tract
L. tracts of spinal cord
lissencephaly, lissencephalia
cobblestone l.
lissencephaly-pachygyria spectrum
listeria encephalitis
Lister tubercle
list mode data collection
liter (L)
lithiasis
renal l.
lithium
l. fluoride (LiF)
lithium-7
lithogenic
l. bile
l. index
lithokelypedion
lithokelyphosis
litholysis
lithopedion
Lithostar nonimmersion lithotripter
lithotripsy
biliary l.
candela l.
electrohydraulic l. (EHL)
electrohydraulic shockwave l. (ESWL)
extracorporeal shockwave l. (ESWL)
laser biliary l.
microexplosion l.
rotational contact l.
ultrasonic l.
lithotripter, lithotriptor
Dornier HM3 l.
Dornier HM4 l.
Lithostar nonimmersion l.
Siemens Lithostar l.
Wolf Piezolith 2200 l.

lithotrite
Kensey-Nash l.
LITT
laser-induced thermography
laser-induced thermotherapy
Litten diaphragm phenomenon
little
l. finger
Little Leaguer shoulder
Littré
L. gland
L. hernia
Litzmann obliquity
liver
l. abscess
l. agenesis
alcoholic fatty l.
amiodarone l.
l. angiosarcoma
l. ascariasis
l. attenuation
bare area of l.
l. bed
biliary cirrhotic l.
brimstone l.
bronze l.
l. bull's eye lesion
l. calcification
l. capillary hemangioma
capsule of l.
l. capsule
cardiac impression on l.
caudate lobe of l.
l. cell adenoma
centrilobular region of l.
Chinese fluke l.
l. cirrhosis
cirrhosis of l.
cirrhotic l.
l. coil
l. cyst
degenerative l.
degraded l.
diaphragmatic surface of l.
l. dome
dome of l.
l. echinococcosis
echogenic l.
l. edema
l. edge
enlarged l.
l. enzyme test
l. failure
fat-spared area in fatty l.
fatty l.
l. fissure
l. flap
l. flap sign
floating l.
l. fluke
focal fatty infiltration of l.
frosted l.
l. function test
l. hemangiosarcoma
hobnail l.
l. hydatid disease
hyperperfusion abnormality of l.
hypoechoic l.
l. impression
infantile hemangioendothelial l.
infantile hemangioendothelioma of l.
large-droplet fatty l.
left lobe of l.
l. lipoma
l. lymphoma
l. mass
l. metastasis
nodular l.
nodule-in-nodule l.
noncirrhotic l.
l. parenchyma
polycystic l.
polylobar l.
potato l.
prominent l.
pyogenic l.
quadrate lobe of l.
right lobe of l.
l. ring sign
l. scan
l. scintigraphy
l. scintiphotography
l. segment
l. segment anatomy
shrunken l.
small-droplet fatty l.
l. span
l. spoke-wheel pattern
stasis l.
l. steatosis
sugar-icing l.
l. target sign
l. transplant

NOTES

liver *(continued)*
l. trauma
undersurface of l.
visceral surface of l.
wandering l.
waxy l.
liver/aorta (L/A)
l./a. peak ratio
liver-jugular sign
liver, kidneys, and spleen (LKS)
liverlike lung
liver/liver peak ratio (L/LP ratio)
liver-lung scan
Liverpool silicosis
liver-spleen
l.-s. imaging
l.-s. scan
Livierato abdominocardiac sign
Livingston triangle
LKS
liver, kidneys, and spleen
LL
lower lobe
LLD
leg-length discrepancy
limb-length discrepancy
LLE
left lower extremity
LLL
left lower lobe
L-loop
L.-l. heart
L.-l. ventricular situs
L-looping
L/LP ratio
LLQ
left lower quadrant
L-malposition of aorta
LMBD
lingular mandibular bony defect
LMCA
left main coronary artery
L-methylmethionine
^{11}C L.-m.
LMP
last menstrual period
LMR
localized magnetic resonance
LN
Imagent L.
LNV
last normal vertebra
load
combination flow and pressure l.'s
exercise l.
iodine l.
osmotic l.
predominant flow l.
rotatory l.
loading
axial weight l.
coil l.
contrast l.
fracture callus l.
left ventricular l.
longitudinal l.
peripheral l.
spike l.
l. technique
uniform l.
lobar
l. atelectasis
l. breast anatomy
l. bronchus
l. cavitation
l. consolidation
l. dysmorphism
l. emphysema
l. holoprosencephaly
l. intracerebral hemorrhage
l. lung atrophy
l. pneumonia
l. renal infarct
l. sclerosis
lobation
fetal kidney l.
persistent cortical kidney l.
lobatum
hepar l.
lobatus
ren l.
lobe
accessory l.
anterior l.
anterior tip of temporal l.
association cortex of parietal l.
azygos l.
l. of azygos vein
calciform l.
caudate l.
collapsed l.
cuneiform l.
fetal l.
flocculonodular l.
frontal l.
hepatic l.
hot caudate l.
hyperexpanded l.
inferior l.
insular l.
l. of kidney
left lower l. (LLL)
left upper l. (LUL)
limbic l.
lower l. (LL)

medial temporal l.
middle l. (ML)
occipital l.
orbital aspect of frontal l.
parietal l.
piriform l.
polyalveolar l.
prominent pyramidal thyroid l.
pulmonary l.
pyramidal l.
ratio of caudate to right hepatic l.
Riedel l.
right lower l. (RLL)
right middle l. (RML)
right upper l. (RUL)
Rokitansky l.
sequestered l.
spigelian l.
succenturiate placental l.
superior l.
temporal l.
thyroid l.
uncus of temporal l.
upper l. (UL)
wedge-shaped l.

lobectomy
sleeve l.

Lobstein disease

lobster-claw deformity

lobular
l. architecture
l. atelectasis
l. breast calcification
l. breast microcalcification
l. bronchiole
l. carcinoma
l. carcinoma in situ (LCIS)
l. lung atrophy
l. pattern
l. pneumonia

lobulated
l. border
l. contour
l. filling defect
l. kidney
l. mass
l. saccular appearance
l. tumor

lobulation
fetal l.

lobule
l. breast
l. of epididymis
fat l.
inferior parietal l.
inferior temporal l.
lung l.
l. lung
paracentral l.
primary pulmonary l.
Reid l.
secondary pulmonary l.
splenic l.

LOCA
low-osmolality contrast agent
low-osmolar contrast agent

local
l. bone blood flow
l. bulge of kidney contour
l. bulge renal contour
l. cavus
l. coil
l. compression fracture
l. decompression fracture
l. edema
l. gradient coil
l. metastasis
l. recurrence (LR)
l. streptokinase infusion

localization
autoradiographic l.
CT-directed hook-wire l.
fluoroscopic l.
l. grid
lesion l.
needle l.
needle-hookwire l.
off-axis point l.
placental l.
point l.
preoperative l.
radiopharmaceutical l.
radiotherapy l.
seizure l.
stereotactic l.
surface coil l.
l. technique
l. window
wire l.

localization-compression grid plate

localized
l. air space disease
l. angiofollicular lymph node hyperplasia

NOTES

L

localized *(continued)*
l. caliectasis
l. coarctation
l. cystic kidney disease
l. edema
l. fibrous mesothelioma
l. fibrous tumor of pleura
l. H1 spectroscopy
l. hyperintensity
l. ileus
l. lesion
l. lucent lung
l. lymphangioma
l. magnetic resonance (LMR)
l. mass effect
l. muscular atrophy
l. myeloma
l. necrosis
l. obstructive emphysema
l. osteopenia
l. osteoporosis
l. pleura tumor
l. shimming
l. uptake
localizer
axial l.
breast l.
T1-weighted axial l.
localizing
l. image
l. imaging
l. probe
l. sign
locally invasive tumor
location
juxtadiaphragmatic l.
lock
field l.
locked
l. facet
l. facet injury
l. knee
l. nuclear magnetization
locking
adiabatic off-resonance spin l.
l. disk
lock-washer configuration
Lockwood ligament
LOCM
low-osmolar contrast medium
locomotor pattern
locoregional
l. breast cancer
l. control
l. field radiotherapy
l. hyperthermia
loculated
l. empyema
l. hydropneumothorax
l. pleural effusion
l. pleural fluid
l. ventricle
locule
loculus, pl. **loculi**
locus
HGPT l.
scanning l.
Loeffler (*var. of* Löffler)
Loehlein diameter
Loehr-Kindberg syndrome
Loepp projection
Loewenberg canal
Löffler, Loeffler
L. endocarditis
L. fibroplastic endocarditis
L. pneumonia
L. syndrome
log
l. amplifier
logetronography
log-rank test
Löhlein-Baehr lesion
Löhlein diameter
lollipop
l. tree appearance
l. tree sign
lollipop-tree bile duct
long
l. axial oblique view
l. axis
l. axis acquisition
l. axis of bone
l. axis of kidney
l. axis ray
l. axis of spleen
l. axis view
L. Beach stereotactic robot
l. bone
l. bone fracture
l. bone pseudoarthrosis
l. fibers
l. finger
l. head
l. head of biceps (LHB)
l. oblique fracture
l. segmental diaphyseal uptake
l. segmental diaphyseal uptake bone scintigraphy
l. smooth esophageal narrowing
l. smooth narrowing esophagus
l. taper/stiff shaft Glidewire
l. tract
l. tract sign
l. TR/TE sequence
l. wavelength photolabel

long-axis
l.-a. parasternal view
l.-a. slice
long-bore collimator
long-cannula coaxial method
long-chain fatty acid
longitudinal
l. acoustic wave
l. arch
l. arteriography
l. axis
l. band
l. blood supply
l. B mode
l. esophageal fold
l. esophageal stricture
l. fasciculus
l. fissure
l. fracture
l. image
l. lie
l. ligament
l. loading
l. magnetization
l. muscle
l. narrowing
l. oval pelvis
l. raphe
l. recovery time
l. relaxation
l. relaxation time
l. relaxivity (R1)
l. renal ectopia
l. ridge
l. scan
l. split biceps tendon
l. taenia musculature
l. transarticular derangement
l. ultrasonic biometry
longitudinalis medialis fasciculus
longitudinally
long-scale imaging agent
long-standing
long-term patency
longum
vinculum l.
longus
adductor l.
l. colli muscle
extensor carpi radialis l. (ECRL)
extensor digitorum l. (EDL)
extensor hallucis l. (EHL)
extensor pollicis l. (EPL)
flexor digitorum l. (FDL)
flexor hallucis l.
flexor pollicis l.
palmaris l.
peroneus l.
loop
afferent l.
air-filled l.
alpha sigmoid l.
bowel l.
l. of bowel
capillary l.
cervical l.
cine l.
closed conducting l.
colonic l.
conductive l.
contiguous l.
Cope l.
Cordonnier ureteroileal l.
diathermic l.
dilated bowel l.
l. distribution
double reverse alpha sigmoid l.
duodenal l.
efferent l.
flow-volume l.
frontal plane l.
gamma transverse colon l.
Gerdy interatrial l.
Gerdy interauricular l.
l. graft
l. of Henle
horizontal plane l.
ileal l.
intestinal l.
J l.
jejunal l.
lenticular l.
Lippes l.
Meyer l.
Meyer-Archambault l.
N-shaped sigmoid l.
l. ostomy bridge
P l.
peduncular l.
pressure-volume l.
puborectalis l.
reentrant l.
rubber vessel l.
sagittal plane l.

NOTES

loop *(continued)*
sentinel l.
separation of bowel l.
sigmoid l.
small bowel l.
Stoerck l.
subclavian l.
T l.
transverse colon l.
vector l.
ventricular l.
vessel l.
l. of Vieussens
Vieussens l.
Waltman l.
loopogram imaging
loopography
ileal l.
loose
l. fracture
l. fragment
l. intraarticular body
l. shoulder
Looser
L. lines
L. transformation zone
L. zones
Looser-Milkman syndrome
LORAD StereoGuide
Lorain-Lévi dwarfism
lordosis
cervical l.
lumbar l.
reversal of cervical l.
spinal l.
thoracic l.
lordotic
l. aspect
l. curve
l. pelvis
l. position
l. view
lorentzian
l. curve
l. field mapping
l. line
l. line saturation
Lorenz sign
lornette
doigt en l.
lorry driver's fracture
loss
l. of bone mass
cochlear hearing l.
conductive hearing l.
l. of definition
l. of distinction
l. of elasticity of cartilage
electron equilibrium l.
global tissue l.
high-velocity signal l.
percentage signal intensity l. (PSIL)
retrocochlear hearing l.
segmental bone l.
sensorineural hearing l.
l. of sigmoid curve
signal l.
l. of thoracic kyphosis
time-of-flight signal l.
transformer l.
volume l.
lossy algorithm
lost IUD
lotus position
Louis
L. angle
sternal angle of L.
Louis-Bar syndrome
love test
low
l. back injury
l. back pain (LBP)
l. back syndrome
l. cardiac output
l. cardiac output syndrome
l. conus medullaris
l. metastatic potential
l. moderate rejection
l. normal
l. osmolality
l. right atrium (LRA)
l. septal right atrium
l. signal intensity
l. signal intensity artifact
l. signal intensity synchondrosis
l. small bowel obstruction
l. urethral pressure (LUP)
l. yield
low-amplitude internal echo
low-angle
l.-a. scattering
l.-a. shot technique
low-attenuation
l.-a. lesion
l.-a. mediastinal mass
l.-a. pulsation artifact
Low-Beers
L.-B. position
L.-B. projection
L.-B. syndrome
L.-B. view
low-contact dynamic compression plate (LC-DCP)

low-contrast
l.-c. film
l.-c. structure
low-density
l.-d. mesencephalic lesion
l.-d. rim
l.-d. ring
l.-d. structure
low-dose
l.-d. film
l.-d. film mammographic technique
l.-d. folic acid
l.-d. mammography
l.-d. screen-film technique
Löwenberg
L. canal
L. sign
low-energy
l.-e. collimator
l.-e. fracture
l.-e. photon attenuation measurement
l.-e. radiofrequency conduction hyperthermia treatment
Lowenthal tract
lower
l. basilar aneurysm
l. esophageal mucosal ring
l. esophageal narrowing
l. esophageal sphincter (LES)
l. esophageal sphincter pressure (LESP)
l. extremity (LE)
l. extremity arterial tree
l. extremity imaging
l. field visual sector
l. gastrointestinal hemorrhage
l. left sternal border
l. limb venography
l. limb venography imaging
l. lobe (LL)
l. lobe lung mass
l. lobe pneumonia
l. lobe reticulation
l. lung disease
l. lung field
l. lung line
l. moiety ureter
l. motor neuron
l. motor neuron lesion
l. pole
l. pole collecting system
l. pole of kidney
l. pole of patella
l. pole ureter
l. pulmonary lobe atelectasis
l. sternal border (LSB)
l. tract
Lower tubercle
low-field
l.-f. magnetic resonance
l.-f. MR angiography
low-field-strength MR imaging
low-flip-angle gradient-echo imaging
low-flow syndrome
low-grade
l.-g. astrocytoma (LGA)
l.-g. central osteogenic sarcoma
l.-g. glioma
l.-g. malignancy
l.-g. neoplasm
low-intensity
l.-i. laser irradiation (LILI)
l.-i. line
l.-i. pulsed ultrasound
low-level echo
low-lying placenta
Lown-Ganong-Levine syndrome (LGL)
low-osmolality contrast agent (LOCA)
low-osmolar
l.-o. contrast agent (LOCA)
l.-o. contrast material
l.-o. contrast medium (LOCM)
low-output heart failure
low-pass
l.-p. filter
l.-p. filtering
low-photon energy
low-pressure
l.-p. cardiac tamponade
l.-p. hydrocephalus
low-profile
l.-p. IUGR
l.-p. mitral valve
low-resistance spectral waveform
low-resolution imaging
low-signal-intensity
l.-s.-i. fibrous band
l.-s.-i. fibrous septum
l.-s.-i. peripheral band
l.-s.-i. replacement
low-signal mass
Lowsley lobar anatomy
low-temperature diffraction

NOTES

low-T humerus fracture
low-velocity flow
LPA
left pulmonary artery
LPAM
L-phenylalanine mustard
LPCh
lateral posterior choroidal
LPHD
lymphocyte-predominance Hodgkin disease
L-phenylalanine mustard (LPAM)
LPO
left posterior oblique
LPO position
LPV
left pulmonary vein
LQ
linear-quadratic
LQ ratio
LR
local recurrence
Lr
lawrencium
LRA
low right atrium
L-radiation
LS
least squares
lumbosacral spine
LSB
left sternal border
lower sternal border
LSCVP
left subclavian central venous pressure
LSF
line spread function
line-spread function
LSS
scapholunate ligament
L-transposition
levotransposition
L-tyrosine imaging agent
^{197}Lu
lutetium-177
lucency
interspersed l.
linear l.
sandlike l.
lucent
l. band
l. calculus
l. center
l. defect
l. finger lesion
l. halo
l. hilar notch
l. interval
l. line
l. lung lesion
Luciani-Wenckebach phenomenon
lucite
l. beam
l. beam spoiler
LUCL
lateral ulnar collateral ligament
Ludloff sign
Ludovici angle
Ludwig
L. angle
L. labyrinth
L. plane
lues
luetic
l. aortic aneurysm
l. aortitis
l. arteritis
l. diaphysitis
LUL
left upper lobe
lumazenil
^{11}C l.
lumbar
l. arteriography
l. artery
l. canal
l. curvature
l. disk
l. fascia
l. hernia
l. kidney
l. kyphosis
l. lordosis
l. lordotic curve
l. lymph node
l. myelography
l. nerve root
l. plexus
l. pneumencephalography
l. puncture
l. rib
l. root avulsion
l. scoliosis
l. spinal stenosis
l. spine
l. spine fracture
l. spine lesion
l. spine view
l. synovial cyst
l. thecoperitoneal shunt syndrome
l. transverse process
l. vertebra (L)
lumbarization
lumbarized spine
lumbocostal ligament
lumbocostoabdominal triangle

lumborum
quadratus l.
lumbosacral
l. agenesis
l. canal
l. dermal sinus
l. disk
l. intervertebral disk herniation
l. joint angle
l. kyphosis
l. myelography
l. plexus
l. series
l. spine (LS)
l. spine strain
l. trunk
lumbrical
lumen, pl. **lumina, lumens**
aortic l.
arterial l.
attenuated l.
bile duct l.
bowel l.
bronchial l.
clot-filled l.
cloverleaf-shaped l.
crescentic l.
cystic duct l.
l. diameter
double l.
double-barrel l.
D-shaped vessel l.
duct l.
duodenal l.
eccentrically placed l.
elliptical l.
esophageal l.
false l.
gastric l.
gastroduodenal l.
intestinal l.
mid-groove portion of lumina
occluded l.
patent l.
scalloped bowel l.
slitlike l.
slit-shaped vessel l.
star-shaped vessel l.
tracheal l.
true l.
vascular l.
lumen-intimal interface
lumenogram (*var. of* luminogram)
luminal
l. area
l. caliber
l. defect
l. dimension
l. encroachment
l. irregularity
l. narrowing
l. plaque
l. plaquing
l. plug
l. silhouette
l. stenosis
l. thrombosis
l. wall
luminance
luminogram, lumenogram
air l.
Lumiscan scanner
lumpectomy
lump kidney
lumpy appearance of lung
Lunar
L. DPX densitometer
L. Expert densitometer
L. scanner
lunate
avascular necrosis l.
l. bone
l. dislocation
l. facet
l. fracture
l. tilt
lunate-shaped trachea
lunate-triquetral coalition
lunatomalacia
Lunderquist
lung
l. abscess
acquired unilateral hyperlucent l.
l. adenocarcinoma
l. agenesis
air conditioner l.
air-filled l.
airless l.
l. air space
amiodarone l.
l. amyloidosis
l. ankylosis spondylitis
l. apex
l. aplasia

L

NOTES

lung *(continued)*
l. arch
l. architecture
arc welder's l.
artificial l.
atelectatic l.
azygos lobe of l.
l. base
base of l.
l. base infiltrate
bauxite fibrosis of l.
bilateral hyperlucent l.
bird breeder's l.
bird fancier's l.
bird handler's l.
black l.
bleomycin l.
blunt border of l.
brown induration of l.
bubbly l.
budgerigar fancier's l.
l. calculus
l. capacity
l. carcinoma
cardiac l.
l. cavity
cheese handler's l.
cheese washer's l.
chest fluke l.
l. cirrhosis
closing volume l.
cluster of grapes l.
coal miner's l.
coal worker's l.
l. coccidioidomycosis
coffee worker's l.
coin lesion of l.
collapsed l.
l. compliance
congenital lymphangiectasia l.
consolidated l.
l. contusion
corundum smelter's l.
l. count curve
l. cylindroma
l. cyst
dark l.
l. decortication
l. density
dependent l.
drowned l.
dynamic l.
l. echinococcosis
eclipse effect l.
l. edema
l. emphysema
emphysematous l.
empty collapsed l.
eosinophilic l.
esophageal l.
expanded l.
l. expansion
farmer's l.
fibroid l.
fibrosis of l.
l. field
fishmeal worker's fresh l.
l. fissure
fluke l.
l. fluke
folded l.
l. fungus ball
furrier's l.
gangrene of l.
gastric l.
grain handler's l.
granuloma l.
l. granuloma
graphite fibrosis of l.
gray l.
hamartoma l.
l. hamartoma
hardened l.
harvester's l.
l. hemangioma
l. hemorrhage
hemorrhagic consolidation of l.
hen worker's l.
l. hepatization
hilum of l.
l. hilum
l. histoplasmosis
honeycomb l.
horseshoe l.
humidifier l.
hyperlucent l.
hypogenetic l.
hypoinflation of the l.
hypolucency of l.
l. hypoplasia
hypoplastic l.
idiopathic unilateral hyperlucent l.
l. imaging
inferior lobe of l.
l. infiltrate distribution
l. inflammation
l. interstitium
left mid l.
light pink l.
l. linearity
lingular division of the left l.
liverlike l.
lobule l.
l. lobule
localized lucent l.
lumpy appearance of l.

l. lymphangiectasia
l. lymphangioma
l. lymphangiomyomatosis
l. lymphoid hyperplasia
l. lymphoma
malt worker's l.
maple bark stripper's l.
l. markings
mason's l.
l. mass
meat wrapper's l.
l. metastasis
miller's l.
miner's l.
mottled gray l.
l. mucormycosis
mushroom worker's l.
l. necrosis
l. nodularity
l. nodule
nondependent l.
l. opacity
l. overexpansion
l. overinflation
l. paragonimiasis
l. parenchyma
l. parenchyma consolidation
partial collapse of l.
l. perfusion
l. perfusion defect
l. perfusion radionuclide
l. periphery
pigeon fancier's l.
l. popcorn calcification
l. pseudocavitation
l. pseudolymphoma
pump l.
l. reexpansion
reexpansion of l.
reperfusion injury of postischemic l.
rheumatoid l.
right l.
root of l.
l. root
rounded border of l.
rudimentary l.
l. scan
l. scintigraphy
l. segmentation
septic l.
sequestered lobe of l.
sharp border of l.
l. shock
shock l.
shrunken l.
1-2-3 l. sign
silicotic fibrosis of l.
silo filler's l.
silver finisher's l.
silver polisher's l.
small cell carcinoma of l.
smoker's l.
solid edema of l.
l. starfish scar
static l.
l. stiffness
stiff noncompliant l.
l. stone
stretched l.
subsegment of l.
superior lobe of l.
surface tension of l.
Swyer-James unilateral hyperlucency of l.
l. talcosis
thatched-roof worker's l.
thresher's l.
l. torsion
l. transplant
l. transplant rejection
l. tuberculoma
l. tumor
l. underinflation
underinflation of l.
underventilated l.
unilateral hyperlucent l.
vanishing l.
l. varix
l. volume (V)
l. washout
welder's l.
well-inflated l.
wet l.
white l.
l. window
l. zone

lunge lesion
lung/heart ratio of thallium 201 activity
lung-volume loop flow
lunocapitate bone

NOTES

lunotriquetral
l. interosseus ligament
l. joint
lunula
LUP
low urethral pressure
lupus
drug-induced erythematous l.
pernio l.
l. pneumonitis
systemic erythematosus l.
LUQ
left upper quadrant
Luque rod
LUS
laparoscopic ultrasound
Luschka
L. bursa
L. crypt
foramen of L.
L. joint
joints of L.
L. ligament
L. muscle
sinuvertebral nerve of L.
lusoria
arteria l.
dysphagia l.
luteal
l. cyst
l. phase
l. phase defect
luteinized
l. unruptured follicle
Lutembacher
L. complex
L. syndrome
lutetium-177 (^{197}Lu)
lutetium tantalate
Lutkens sphincter
luxans
coxa vara l.
luxated bone
luxatio erecta
luxation
ligamentous l.
Luxtec fiberoptic system
luxury
l. perfusion
l. perfusion syndrome
luxus heart
Luys body
Luysii
corpus L.
LVAD
left ventricular assist device
LVD
left ventricular dysfunction
LVdd, LVDD
left ventricular diastolic dimension
LVEDD
left ventricular end-diastolic dimension
LVEDI
left ventricular end-diastolic volume index
LVEDP
left ventricular end-diastolic pressure
LVEF
left ventricular ejection fraction
exercise first-pass LVEF
LVESD
left ventricular end-systolic dimension
LVESVI
left ventricular end-systolic volume index
LVET
left ventricular ejection time
LVFS
left ventricular functional shortening
$LVFT_2$
left ventricular slow filling time
LVFW
left ventricular free wall
LVG
left ventriculogram
LVH
left ventricular hypertrophy
LVID
left ventricular internal diameter
LVIDd, LVIDD
left ventricular internal diastolic dimension
LVIDs
left ventricular internal dimension at end systole
LVIV
left ventricular inflow volume
LVM
left ventricular mass
LVMI
left ventricular mass index
LVOT
left ventricular outflow tract
LVOTO
left ventricular outflow tract obstruction
LVOV
left ventricular outflow volume
LVP
left ventricular pressure
LVPW
left ventricular posterior wall
LVs
LVs pressure
LVs system
LVSW
left ventricular stroke work

LVSWI
left ventricular stroke work index
LVW
left ventricular wall
Lyell syndrome
Lyme
L. carditis
L. disease
lympangiomyomatosis
lymph
l. capillary
l. duct
l. gland
l. node
l. node eggshell calcification
l. node enlargement
l. node involvement
l. node sinus
l. node syndrome
l. node tissue
l. plexus
l. vessel of prostate
lymphadenectomy
bilateral l.
complete l.
elective l.
inguinal l.
paraaortic l.
sentinel l.
lymphadenitis
regional granulomatous l.
lymphadenography
lymphadenopathy
angioblastic l.
angioimmunoblastic l.
axillary l.
benign l.
mesenteric l.
peripancreatic l.
persistent generalized l.
reactive l.
retrocrural l.
retroperitoneal l.
secondary axillary l.
superficial l.
l. syndrome
lymphangiectasia
congenital l.
generalized l.
intestinal l.
lung l.
primary pulmonary l.
pulmonary l.
secondary l.
lymphangiectasis
acquired intestinal l.
pulmonary cystic l.
lymphangiogram
lymphangiographic
l. contrast
l. imaging agent
lymphangiography
bipedal l.
contrast l.
l. imaging
pedal l.
lymphangiohemangioma
lymphangioleiomyomatosis
lymphangioma
capillary l.
cardiac l.
cavernous l.
cystic neck l.
diffuse l.
localized l.
lung l.
l. mesentery
neck l.
orbital l.
pancreatic cystic l.
retroperitoneal l.
simple capillary l.
lymphangiomatosis
pulmonary l.
lymphangiomyomatosis
lung l.
lymphangitic
l. carcinomatosis
l. metastasis
lymphangitis
lymphatic
l. cachexia
l. canal
l. carcinomatosis
l. channel
l. cortex
l. development
l. drainage pattern
l. duct
l. edema
l. malformation
l. mapping
l. medulla
l. metastasis

NOTES

lymphatic *(continued)*
l. network
l. obstruction
paracervical l.
prominent septal l.'s
l. sac
l. sarcoma
subpleural l.
l. tissue
l. trunk
l. vessel
lymphatica
pseudopolyposis l.
lymphaticum
angioma l.
Lymphazurin imaging agent
lymphedema
Meige l.
Nonne-Milroy l.
postmastectomy l.
lymphoblastic lymphoma
lymphoblastoma
lymphocele
renal transplant l.
lymphocyte-predominance Hodgkin disease (LPHD)
lymphocytic
l. interstitial pneumonia (LIP)
l. interstitial pneumonitis
l. plasmacytoid lymphoma
l. poorly differentiated lymphoma
l. well-differentiated lymphoma
lymphoepithelial
l. parotid tumor
lymphoepithelioma
salivary gland l.
lymphogenous
l. dissemination
l. embolus
l. metastasis
lymphogranuloma
Schaumann l.
venereal l.
lymphography
time-lapse quantitative computed tomography l.
lymphoid
l. hamartoma
l. hyperplasia
l. hypophysitis
l. interstitial pneumonia (LIP)
l. interstitial pneumonitis
l. polyp
l. ring
l. tissue
l. tumor
lymphokine
lymphoma
acute lymphoblastic l.
adult T-cell l.
African Burkitt l.
AIDS-related l.
anaplastic large-cell l. (ALCL)
angiocentric T-cell l.
angioimmunoblastic lymphadenopathy-like T-cell l.
angiotropic large cell l.
B-cell monocytoid l.
bone l.
brain l.
breast l.
Burkitt l.
Burkitt-like l. (BLL)
butterfly l.
B-zone small lymphocytic l.
centroblastic l.
centrocytic l.
cerebral l.
cleaved cell l.
cobblestone appearance l.
colorectal l.
convoluted T-cell l.
cutaneous B-cell l. (CBCL)
cutaneous T-cell l.
diffuse aggressive l.
diffuse intermediate lymphocytic l.
diffuse large-cell l.
diffuse lymphocytic l.
diffuse mixed small- and large-cell l.
diffuse small-cell lymphocytic l.
dural arachnoid l.
enteropathy-associated T-cell l.
epidural l.
extranodal follicular l.
follicular center-cell l.
follicular mixed small cleaved l.
follicular predominantly large cell l.
follicular predominantly small cell l.
fulminant cerebral l.
l. gallium scintigraphy
gastric l.
gastrointestinal l.
giant follicle l.
granulomatous l.
heart l.
histiocytic bone l.
histiocytic brain l.
histiocytic chest l.
immunoblastic large-cell l.
infiltrative l.
intracerebral l.
kidney l.

large-cell l.
large cleaved-cell l.
liver l.
lung l.
lymphoblastic l.
lymphocytic plasmacytoid l.
lymphocytic poorly differentiated l.
lymphocytic well-differentiated l.
macroglobulinemic l.
MALT l.
marginal zone l. (MZL)
marginal zone B-cell l.
mediastinal l.
mesencephalic cerebral l.
mesenteric l.
metastatic l.
metastatic testicular l.
mixed lymphocytic-histiocytic l.
mixed small and large cell l.
multifocal l.
noncleaved cell l.
non-Hodgkin l. (NHL)
non-Hodgkin chest l.
orbital l.
pancreatic l.
peripheral l.
perirenal l.
plasmablastic l.
pleomorphic T-cell l.
polypoid l.
primary bone l.
primary brain l.
primary CNS l.
primary cutaneous large B-cell l. (PCLBCL)
primary refractory Burkitt l.
pulmonary l.
pyothorax-associated pleural l.
recurrent l.
renal l.
retroperitoneal l.
Revised European-American L. (REAL)
secondary brain l.
secondary cutaneous large B-cell l. (SCLBCL)
sinonasal l.
skeletal l.
small B-cell l.
small cleaved-cell l.
small lymphocytic T-cell l.
spinal epidural l.
splenic B-cell l.
sporadic Burkitt l.
l. staging
systemic brain l.
T-cell lymphoblastic l.
thymic l.
thyroid l.
true histiocytic l.
T-zone l.
ulcerative l.
undefined l.
undifferentiated l.
undifferentiated non-Hodgkin l.
urinary bladder l.
vitreous l.
Waldeyer ring l.

lymphomasonography
primary l.

lymphomatoid granulomatosis

lymphomatosis

lymphomatosum
cystadenoma l.
papillary cystadenoma l.

lymphomatous
l. lymph node
l. mass

lymphonodular hyperplasia

lymphopneumatosis
peritoneal l.

lymphoreticular tissue

lymphosarcoma
l. of heart

LymphoScan
L. nuclear imaging system
L. nuclear imaging system scanner

lymphoscintigraphy
cutaneous l.
internal mammary l.
radiocolloid l.

Lynch and Crues type 2 lesion

lyoluminescence

lyophilized

lysate

Lyser
trapezoid bone of L.

Lysholm
L. grid
L. method

lysis
bony l.
cystic l.
follicle l.

NOTES

lysozyme
lytic
l. area
l. area bone flap
l. bone lesion
l. change
l. lesion of skull
l. osteolysis

μ
mu
μ meson
μA
microampere
μCi
microcurie
M
M. pattern
M. shell
m
meter
99m
Pertscan 99m
M1-M5 segments of middle cerebral artery
M1 segment aneurysm
mA
microampere
ma, mA
milliampere
MAA
macroaggregated albumin
technetium-99m MAA (^{99m}Tc MAA)
MAC
multiaccess catheter
Macalister muscle
maceration
Macewen sign
Mach
M. band
M. band effect
M. effect
M. line
machine
Brown-Bovari m.
cobalt megavoltage m.
2D B-mode ultrasound m.
focused segmented ultrasound m. (FSUM)
m. injection
Narco esophageal motility m.
neutron therapy m.
panoramic rotating m.
parallel virtual m. (PVM)
Philips ultrasound m.
remote control afterloading m.
Toshiba echocardiograph m.
Machlett collimator
Mackenrodt ligament
Mackenzie point
MacLean-Maxwell disease
Macleod syndrome
macrencephaly, macrenephalia
macroadenoma
pituitary m.
prolactin-secreting pituitary m.
macroaggregated
m. albumin (MAA)
m. albumin imaging agent
macrocalcification
macrocephalia, macrocephaly
macrocirculation
macrocolon
macroconidia
macrocyst
adrenocortical m.
macrocystic
m. adenoma
m. cystadenoma
m. encephalomalacia
m. neoplasm
m. pilocytic cerebellar astrocytoma
Macrodantin pneumonia
macrodystrophia
lipoma m.
m. lipomatosa
macrofistulous arteriovenous communication
macroglobulinemic lymphoma
macroglossia
macrolobular cirrhosis
macromolecular
m. content
m. contrast-enhanced MR imaging
m. drug
m. hydration effect
m. imaging agent
macronodular
m. lung disease
m. pattern
macrophage
alveolar m.
m. inflammatory protein (MIP)
phagocytic m.
macrophthalmia
macrophthalmos
macroreentrant circuit
macroscopic
m. hemorrhage ligament
m. magnetic moment
m. magnetization vector
m. placental lesion
macrosomia
Macrotec
M. imaging agent
MacSpect
M. real-time NMR station
M. real-time NMR workstation

macule
coal m.
maculoneural bundle
Maddahi method of calculating right ventricular ejection fraction
Madelung
M. deformity
M. neck
Madura foot
maduromycosis
Maestro
Maffucci
M. disease
M. syndrome
MAG
mercaptoacetyltriglycerine
Magendie
M. foramen
M. space
magenstrasse
Maggi biopsy needle
magic
m. angle effect
m. angle effect artifact
m. angle spinning NMR
magic-angle
m.-a. phenomenon
m.-a. spinning imaging
Magilligan technique for measuring neutral anteversion
magna
abnormal cisterna m.
arteria radicularis anterior m.
chorda m.
cisterna m.
coxa m.
mega cisterna m.
Magnascanner
Picker M.
Magna-SL scanner
Magnes
M. biomagnetometer
M. biomagnetometer system
M. 2500 whole-blood scanner
M. 2500 whole-head imaging
magnesium chloride
magnet
air-core m.
doughnut m.
Eindhoven m.
Fe-Ex orogastric tube m.
GE Signa 1.5-T m.
hybrid m.
"in the m."
large-bore m.
Magnex m.
m. mode
nonenclosed m.
open m.
Oxford m.
pancake MRI m.
passively shimmed superconducting m.
permanent m.
poor shimming of MRI m.
m. rate
resistive m.
m. response
shimmed m.
short-bore m.
superconducting m.
tubular m.
Walker m.
magnetic
m. anisotropy
m. bolus tracking
m. dipole
m. dipole-dipole coupling
m. dipole moment
m. domain
m. field
m. field gradient (MFG)
m. field perturbation
m. flux
m. flux density
m. induction
m. induction device
m. interaction
m. inversion
m. material
m. particulates
m. radiation exposure
m. resonance (MR)
m. resonance angiography (MRA)
m. resonance angiography-directed bypass procedure
m. resonance arthrography
m. resonance catheter imaging
m. resonance cholangiogram (MRC)
m. resonance cholangiopancreatography (MRCP)
m. resonance depiction
m. resonance detection
m. resonance elastography (MRE)
m. resonance enhancement pattern
m. resonance epidurography
m. resonance imaging (MRI)
m. resonance imaging-guided focused ultrasound sector transducer
m. resonance mammography (MRM)
m. resonance myelography
m. resonance needle tracking
m. resonance neurography (MRN)

m. resonance phase velocity mapping
m. resonance phlebography
m. resonance receptor agent
m. resonance sialography
m. resonance signal
m. resonance simulator
m. resonance spectroscopy (MRS)
m. resonance spin incoherence
m. resonance urography (MRU)
m. resonance venography
m. resonance volume estimation
m. shielding
m. source imaging (MSI)
m. susceptibility
m. susceptibility artifact
m. susceptibility-weighted image
m. tape storage

magnetism
nuclear m.

magnetite (Fe_3O_4)
m. albumin contrast
m. albumin imaging agent

magnetization
equilibrium m.
locked nuclear m.
longitudinal m.
net tissue m.
net transverse m.
m. precession angle
m. prepared 3D gradient-echo
rephased transverse m.
residual m.
rest m.
spatial modulation of m. (SPAMM)
m. and spin-lock transfer imaging
SSFP m.
m. transfer (MT)
m. transfer contrast (MTC)
m. transfer effect
m. transfer gradient-echo image
m. transfer ratio (MTR)
m. transfer technique
m. transfer weighted imaging
transverse m.

magnetization-prepared
m.-p. 3D gradient-echo sequence
m.-p. rapid acquisition gradient-echo sequence
m.-p. rapid gradient echo-water excitation (MP-RAGE-WE)

magnetoacoustic
m. imaging
m. MRI

magnetoencephalogram

magnetoencephalography (MEG)

magnetogyric ratio

magnetohydrodynamic effect

Magnetom
M. Open system
M. SP MRI imager
M. SP63 scanner
M. 1.5-T scanner
M. Vision MR system

magnetometer probe

magneton
Bohr m.

magnetopharmaceutical

magnetophosphene

magnetoresistive sensor circuit

Magnevist
M. imaging agent

Magnex
M. Alpha MR system
M. magnet
M. MR scanner

magnification (X)
m. angiography
electronic m.
m. error
m. factor (MF)
high-resolution m.
m. mammography
m. radiography
signal m.
spot m.
m. and spot compression
ultra-high m.
m. view

magnitude
m. image
m. of obliquity
m. preparation-rapid acquisition gradient echo (MP-RAGE)
m. reconstruction

magnum
foramen m.

magnus
adductor m.

Mahaim
M. bundle
M. and James fibers

Mahler sign

NOTES

main
m. bundle
m. energy substrate
m. fissure
m. glow peak
m. magnetic field inhomogeneity artifact
m. pancreatic duct (MPD)
m. papillary duct (MPD)
m. portal vein peak velocity (MPPv)
m. pulmonary artery (MPA)
m. sac
m. timing event (MTE)
m. tumor
mainline granulomatosis
mainstem
m. bronchus
m. carina
m. coronary artery
maintenance of flow
Maisonneuve
M. fibular fracture
M. injury
M. sign
Maissiat
M. band
M. ligament
M. tract
Majewski
M. disease
M. syndrome
Majocchi disease
major
m. aorticopulmonary collateral arteries
m. bronchus
m. calix
m. duodenal papilla
m. fissure
m. fracture fragment
globus m.
m. muscle
psoas m.
rhomboid m.
teres m.
majora
labia m.
majus
omentum m.
majuscula
Makar stricture
malabsorption
m. syndrome
Malacarne
M. antrum
M. space
malacoplakia (*var. of* malakoplakia)
maladie de Roger
malaise
malakoplakia, malacoplakia
renal parenchymal m.
malaligned atrioventricular septal defect
malalignment
patellar m.
rotational m.
malangulation
malar
m. bone
m. eminence
m. fracture
m. lymph node
malarial
m. granuloma
m. pneumonitis
Malcolm-Lynn C-RXF cervical retractor frame
mal de Meleda syndrome
maldescended testis
maldevelopment
pubic bone m.
maldistribution of ventilation and perfusion
male
m. genital tract calcification
m. pelvis
m. Turner syndrome
m. urethra
malformation
adenomatoid m.
angiographically occult intracranial vascular m. (AOIVM)
angiographically occult vascular m. (AOVM)
angiographically visualized vascular m. (AVVM)
anorectal m.
aortic arch m.
Arnold-Chiari m.
arterial m. (AM)
arterial lung m.
arteriovenous m. (AVM)
arteriovenous brain m.
arteriovenous colon m.
arteriovenous cord m.
arteriovenous intraosseous m.
arteriovenous kidney m.
bronchopulmonary foregut m.
capillary m.
capillary-lymphatic m. (CLM)
cardiovascular m.
cavernous m.
cerebral arteriovenous m.
cerebrovascular m.
Chiari I–II m.
cloacal m.

congenital cystic adenomatoid m. (CCAM)
congenital heart m.
congenital vascular m. (CVM)
coronary artery m.
cryptic vascular m. (CVM)
cystic adenomatoid m.
dancer's foot m.
Dandy-Walker m.
DeMyer system of cerebral m.
Dieulafoy vascular m.
dural arteriovenous m.
Ebstein m.
endocardial cushion m.
extremity m.
familial cavernous m.
fast-flow m.
fetal cystic adenomatoid m.
fetal hand m.
frontal arteriovenous m.
frontoparietal arteriovenous m.
fusiform m.
galenic venous m.
glomus-type arteriovenous m.
intracerebral arteriovenous m.
intracerebral vascular m.
intracranial arteriovenous m.
intramedullary arteriovenous m.
intramuscular venous m.
intraosseous arteriovenous m.
intraosseous vascular m.
lymphatic m.
mixed venous-lymphatic m.
Mondini m.
neural axis vascular m.
occult cerebral vascular m. (OCVM)
occult vascular brain m.
pulmonary arterial m.
pulmonary arteriovenous m.
retromedullary arteriovenous m.
Russell-Rubinstein classification of cerebrovascular m.
saccular m.
septal m.
sink-trap m.
slow-flow vascular m.
spinal vascular m.
telencephalic m.
valve m.
vascular m.
vein of Galen m.
venous vascular m.
Wyburn-Mason arteriovenous m.

malformed phlebectasia

Malgaigne

M. pelvic fracture

Malherbe

calcifying epithelioma of M.

maligna

lentigo m.

malignancy

aggressive m.
borderline m.
epithelial m.
extrapelvic m.
gastrointestinal m.
high-grade m.
low-grade m.
metastatic m.
mimicker of m.
pelvic m.
primary pulmonary m.
secondary m.
staging of m.
T-cell m.
m. threshold
uroepithelial m.
urogenital m.
vulvar m.

malignant

m. acetabular osteolysis
m. airway obstruction
m. angioblastoma
m. bone aneurysm
m. brain edema
m. breast calcification
m. breast cancer
m. degeneration
m. duodenal tumor
m. ependymoma
m. external otitis
m. fibrous histiocytoma (MFH)
m. fibrous histiocytoma of bone (MFH-B)
m. fibrous osseous histiocytoma
m. fibrous xanthoma
m. fibroxanthoma
m. gastric ulcer
m. glioma
m. hemangioendothelioma
m. lesion
m. mediastinum teratoid tumor
m. melanoma gallium imaging

NOTES

malignant *(continued)*
m. melanoma staging
m. melanoma target sign
m. meningioma
m. myeloid sarcoma
m. nephrosclerosis
m. osteoid
m. osteopetrosis
m. ovarian germ-cell tumor
m. ovarian teratoma tumor
m. pleomorphic adenoma
m. pleural effusion
m. pleural implant
m. pleural mesothelioma
m. polyp
m. small bowel tumor
m. teratoma
m. thymoma
m. urethral neoplasm
m. uveal melanoma
malignum
adenoma m.
mallei (*pl. of* malleus)
malleolar fracture
malleolus, pl. **malleoli**
m. bone
m. fibulae
lateral m.
medial m.
m. tibiae
mallet
m. finger
m. fracture
mallet-finger deformity
malleus, pl. **mallei**
Mallinckrodt
M. imaging agent
M. Institute of Radiology (MIR)
M. scanner
Mallory-Weiss
M.-W. esophageal tear
M.-W. lesion
M.-W. mucosal tear
M.-W. syndrome
malnutrition
malperfused
malperfusion
malpighian
m. body
m. follicle
m. vesicle
malpositioned
m. fetus
m. heart
m. testis
malrotation
complete small bowel m.
intestinal tract m.
m. of intestine
kidney m.
midgut volvulus with m.
partial small bowel m.
renal m.
small bowel m.
MALT
mucosa-associated lymphoid tissue
MALT lymphoma
malt worker's lung
malum
m. perforans pedis
malunion of fracture fragments
malunited fracture
Mamex DC mammography
mamillary
m. body
m. suture
m. system
mamillopeduncular tract
mamillotegmental tract
mamillothalamic
m. fasciculus
m. tract
Mamm-Aire heart failure
mammalation
mammaplasty (*var. of* mammoplasty)
mammary
m. artery
m. calculus
m. cyst
m. duct
m. duct ectasia
m. duct obstruction
m. ductogram
m. ductogram imaging
m. dysplasia
m. galactogram
m. galactogram imaging
m. gland
m. implant
m. parenchyma
m. tissue
m. tumorigenesis
Mammo
M. Mask illuminator
M. QC
M. QC mammography
mammogram
mammographic
m. evaluation of breast mass
m. feature
m. guidance
m. measurement
m. view box
mammographically suspicious lesion
mammographic-histopathologic correlation

mammography
baseline m.
computed tomographic laser m.
contoured tilting compression m.
digital m.
Egan m.
evaluation of mass m.
high-resolution CT m.
low-dose m.
magnetic resonance m. (MRM)
magnification m.
Mamex DC m.
Mammomat B m.
Mammo QC m.
microfocal spot m.
orthogonal projection m.
M. Quality Standards Act
radionuclide m.
screen-film m.
screening m.
Senographe 500-T m.
single-view oblique m.
spot compression magnification m.
stereotactic m.
m. technique
two-view film-screen m.
ultra-high magnification m. (UHMM)
ultrasound augmented m.
x-ray m.
Mammo-lock needle
Mammo-Lume
Mammomat
M. B mammography
mammoplasia
mammoplasty, mammaplasty
augmentation m.
postreduction m.
reduction m.
Mammorex
Mammospot
Mammotest
M. breast biopsy system
M. unit
mammotome
Biopsys m.
Mammotome biopsy device
Mammotrax
man
roentgen equivalent m. (REM)
Manchester
M. LDR implant system
M. ovoid
mandible
alveolar border of m.
angle of m.
genial tubercle of m.
m. hypoplasia
m. osteolysis
mandibulae
capitulum m.
mandibular
m. angle
m. canal
m. condyle
m. disk
m. division
m. foramen
m. fossa
m. fracture
m. lymph node
m. nerve
m. ramus
mandibularis
torus m.
mandibulofacial dysostosis
maneuver
Adson m.
costoclavicular m.
flexion m.
Hampton m.
Heineke-Mikulicz m.
hyperabduction m.
jugular compression m.
Kocher m.
Müller m.
Osler m.
pull m.
push m.
Rivero-Carvallo m.
scalene m.
squatting m.
temporal artery tap m.
transabdominal left lateral retroperitoneal m.
Valsalva m.
mangafodipir
m. trisodium
m. trisodium imaging agent
manganese (Mn)
m. acetate
m. chloride

NOTES

manganese *(continued)*
m. citrate
m. imaging agent
m. pneumonitis
m. sulfate
m. tetrasodium-meso-tetra (Mn-TPPS$_4$)
manganese-BOPTA
manifest
manifold
three-stopcock m.
Mankin method
Mann-Bollman fistula
mannitol and saline imaging agent
Mannkopf sign
manofluorography (MFG)
manometer
catheter-tipped m.
Riva-Rocci m.
manometric pattern
manometry
anal m.
aneroid m.
anorectal m.
biliary m.
ERCP m.
esophageal m.
rectosigmoid m.
sphincter of Oddi m.
Manson schistosomiasis-pulmonary artery obstruction syndrome
mantle
anechoic m.
m. block
brain m.
cement m.
cerebral m.
m. complex
m. field
hypoechoic m.
m. radiotherapy
manual
m. compression
m. computed method
m. injection
m. pressure over carotid sinus
m. subtraction film
manubria
manubriosternal
m. joint
m. syndrome
manubrium, pl. **manubria**
hypersegmentation of the m.
m. hypersegmentation
manus
digiti m.
Maolate
MAP
mean arterial pressure
map (*See* mapping)
acceleration m.
bladder m.
bull's eye polar m.
cerebral blood volume m.
cylindrical projection m.
decimalized variance m.
end-diastolic polar m.
end-systolic polar m.
sestamibi polar m.
spherical m.
map-guided partial endocardial ventriculotomy
maple
m. bark disease
m. bark stripper's lung
m. bark worker's suberosis
mapping
activation-sequence m.
m. algorithm
body surface potential m.
brain electrical activity m.
cardiac m.
catheter m.
m. of cerebral sulcus
color-flow m.
contour m.
m. of defect
digital road m.
Doppler color-flow m.
2D pulsatility index m.
2D resistance index m.
eddy current m.
electrophysiologic m.
endocardial activation m.
endocardial catheter m.
epicardial m.
homology m.
ice m.
intramural m.
intraoperative electrocortical stimulation m.
IOECS m.
k-space velocity m.
lorentzian field m.
lymphatic m.
magnetic resonance phase velocity m.
MRI m.
pace m.
parallel analog m.
phase difference m.
phase-shift velocity m.
precordial m.
retrograde atrial activation m.
road m.

sinus rhythm m.
spastic m.
spatial m.
straight-line Hough transform m.
susceptibility m.
texture m.
two-dimensional m.
velocity m.

Marable syndrome

marantic
m. clot
m. endocarditis
m. thrombus

marble
m. bone
m. bone disease

marbling
m. of pancreatic parenchyma

Marcacci muscle

march foot

Marchiafava-Bignami disease

Marchi tract

Marex MRI system

Marfan
M. bone syndrome
M. CHD syndrome

marfanoid hypermobility syndrome

margin
m. of apposition
blurring of disk m.'s
cardiac m.
colon m.
convex m.
cortical m.
costal m.
costodiaphragmatic m.
depression of renal m.
disk m.
enhancing ventricular m.
fluffy m.'s
infraorbital m. (IOM)
medial talar m.
m. necrosis
obtuse m.
overhanging m.
periarticular m.
pleural m.
posterior disk m.
psoas m.
m. of scapula
scapular m.
sharp lateral m.
stomach m.
subcostal m.
superomedial m.
supraorbital m. (SOM)
tumor m.

marginal
m. artery of Drummond
m. branch
m. branch of left circumflex coronary artery
m. branch of right coronary artery
m. circumflex artery
m. erosion
m. exostosis
m. fracture
m. gyrus
m. kidney depression
obtuse m. (OM)
m. osteophyte
m. osteophyte formation
m. placenta
m. placenta previa
m. ridge
m. sclerosis
m. serration
m. sinus
m. spur
m. spurring
m. syndesmophyte
m. ulcer
m. vein
m. zone B-cell lymphoma
m. zone lymphoma (MZL)

Marie-Bamberger disease

Marie-Foix sign

Marie-Strumpell disease

Marie-Tooth disease

Marimastat

Marin-Amat phenomenon

Marine-Lenhart syndrome

marked
m. sclerosis
m. shunting of blood

markedly accentuated pulmonic component

marker
implanted imaging opaque m.
lead pellet m.
metallic m.
MicroMark tissue m.
myocardial-specific m.
nipple m.

NOTES

M

marker *(continued)*
radioactive string m.
radiopaque m.
Sitzmarks radiopaque m.
m. transit imaging
m. transit study
marker-channel diagram
marking
accentuation of m.'s
bronchovascular m.'s
bronchovascular m.'s
bronchovesicular m.'s
coarse bronchovascular m.'s
confluence of vascular m.'s
convolutional m.'s
crowding of bronchovascular m.'s
digital m.'s
haustral m.'s
increased interstitial m.'s
increased pulmonary vascular m.'s
interstitial m.'s
linear m.'s
lung m.'s
peribronchial m.'s
perihilar m.'s
pullback arterial m.'s
pulmonary arterial m.'s
pulmonary vascular m.'s
sutural m.'s
vascular m.'s
Markov
M. chain
M. chain Monte Carlo technique
M. random field
Marlex band
Maroteaux-Lamy syndrome
marrow
m. agent bone scintigraphy
bone m.
m. canal
cancellous hematopoietic m.
m. cavity
central nidus of high-intensity m.
m. dosimetry
m. edema pattern
epiphyseal hematopoietic m.
m. fat signal intensity
fatty m.
functional m.
hematopoietically active bone m.
high-signal-intensity yellow m.
hypercellular m.
hypocellular m.
m. infarct
m. infiltrate
peripheral hematopoietic intermediate signal intensity m.
shunting of tracer to the bone m.
sternal m.
m. transplant
uptake in bone m.
Marshall
vein of M.
M. vein
Martin disease
Martinez
M. technique
M. universal interstitial template (MUPIT)
Martorell
M. aortic arch syndrome
M. hypertensive ulcer
M. sign
Martorell-Fabre syndrome
Martz method
Mary Allen Engle ventricle
MAS
Morgagni-Adams-Stokes
MAS syndrome
mAs
milliampere-second
masculine pelvis
masculinizing tumor
mask
convolution m.
ISAH stereotactic immobilizing m.
Orfit m.
particle m.
m. ventilation
mask-based approach
masking
unsharp m.
Mason radial fracture classification
mason's lung
masquerading effect
mass
abdominal cystic fetal m.
abdominopelvic m.
adnexal m.
adrenal cystic m.
air-containing neck m.
airless m.
anechoic m.
anterior mediastinal m.
aortopulmonary window m.
appendiceal m.
apperceptive m.
atomic m.
m. attenuation coefficient
avascular brain m.
avascular kidney m.
avascular renal m.
m. balance
benign m.
bilateral fetal chest m.
bilateral renal m.

bilobed m.
brain m.
calcified brain m.
calcified intracranial m.
calcified kidney m.
calcified renal m.
cardiophrenic right-angle m.
carotid space m.
cavitary m.
cerebellar cystic m.
circumscribed m.
m. collision stopping power
complex m.
congenital nasal m.
conical m.
cord intradural extramedullary m.
cordlike m.
cystic m.
m. defect
dense brain m.
dense cerebral m.
dirty m.
discoid chest m.
discrete m.
doughy m.
dumbbell brain m.
dysplasia with associated lesion or m. (DALM)
echogenic m.
m. effect
elongated m.
encapsulated m.
enhancing m.
epidural m.
expanding intracranial m.
expansile m.
external ear m.
extracardiac m.
extraovarian m.
extrauterine pelvic m.
extravascular m.
fallopian tube m.
fat-containing m.
fetal abdominal cystic m.
fibrin m.
firm m.
fixed m.
fleecy m.
fluctuant m.
fluid-filled kidney m.
focal m.
freely movable m.
friable m.
fusiform m.
glenoid ovoid m.
groin m.
high-signal m.
hilar m.
hyperdense m.
hyperintense m.
hypervascular mediastinal m.
hypodense m.
ill-defined m.
m. imaging
indurated m.
inflammatory polypoid m.
injection m.
inner ear m.
interbronchial m.
intermediate signal m.
intraabdominal m.
intracardiac m.
intracavity m.
intracranial m.
intradural extramedullary m.
intraluminal stomach m.
intrasellar brain m.
intrathoracic fetal m.
intrathoracic low-attenuation m.
intravascular m.
intraventricular m.
irregular m.
isodense m.
isointense m.
jugular foraminal m.
kidney sinus m.
lacrimal m.
large solid adrenal m.
lateral m.
lean m.
left ventricular m. (LVM)
m. lesion
liver m.
lobulated m.
loss of bone m.
low-attenuation mediastinal m.
lower lobe lung m.
low-signal m.
lung m.
lymphomatous m.
mammographic evaluation of breast m.
masticator space m.
mediastinal high-attenuation m.

M

NOTES

mass *(continued)*
mesenteric m.
middle ear m.
middle mediastinal m.
mixed-attenuation m.
mixed-density m.
mixed echogenic solid m.
mixed-signal m.
mobile intraluminal gallbladder m.
molar m.
multilobulated m.
multiloculated m.
mushroom-shaped m.
myocardial m.
nasal vault m.
nasopharyngeal m.
nodular m.
noncalcified nodular m.
nonopaque intraluminal m.
nonpulsatile abdominal m.
omental m.
orbital superolateral quadrant m.
ovarian m.
pancreatic m.
paracardiac m.
paranasal sinus m.
parasagittal intracranial m.
parasellar brain m.
paraspinal soft tissue m.
pelvic cystic m.
perirenal m.
peritoneal m.
perivascular m.
petrous apex dumbbell m.
pharyngeal space m.
phlegmonous m.
pineal m.
pleural m.
polypoid calcified irregular m.
porta hepatis low-density m.
posterior mediastinal m.
prepubertal testicular m.
presacral m.
prevertebral space m.
promontory m.
pulmonary m.
m. radiative stopping power
relativistic m.
renal sinus m.
reniform m.
retrobulbar m.
retrocardiac m.
retroperitoneal m.
retropharyngeal space m.
retrosternal m.
right cardiophrenic angle m.
right ventricular m. (RVM)
saccular m.
scrotal m.
soft tissue m.
solid m.
solitary m.
sonolucent cystic m.
space-occupying m.
spherical m.
spiculated m.
stellate m.
stony m.
subinsular m.
suprasellar m.
suspicious m.
thalamic-hypothalamic m.
thymic m.
m. thymus
tissue m.
tooth m.
tubal m.
tumor m.
umbilical m.
uncinate process m.
unilateral adrenal m.
unilateral fetal chest m.
unilateral kidney m.
urinary bladder extrinsic m.
urinary bladder wall m.
uterine m.
ventricular m.
wedge-shaped m.
well-circumscribed breast m.
well-defined m.
woody m.

Massachusetts (General Hospital) Utility Multiprogramming System
massa intermedia
masseter muscle
Massiot polytome
massive
m. aortic regurgitation
m. ascites
m. atelectasis
m. embolus
m. exsanguinating hemorrhage
m. hepatic necrosis
m. herniated disk
m. infiltrate
m. osteolysis
m. ovarian edema
m. pleural effusion
m. pneumonia
m. pulmonary hemorrhagic edema

massively enlarged heart
masslike configuration
Masson body
MAST
motion artifact suppression technique

MAST suit
MAST technique
mast
m. cell-enhancing activity
mastectomy
extended radical m.
non-skin-sparing m. (non-SSM)
radical m.
segmental m.
skin-sparing m. (SSM)
subcutaneous m.
total m.
Master
M. syndrome
M. two-step exercise stress test
master
m. knot of Henry
masticator
m. muscle
m. space
m. space infection
m. space mass
mastitis
chronic cystic m.
cystic m.
m. fibrosa cystica
fibrous m.
nonpuerperal m.
m. obliterans
periductal m.
puerperal m.
mastocytosis
bone m.
GI tract m.
systemic m.
mastoid
m. antrum
m. bone
m. canal
m. complex
m. fontanelle
m. foramen
m. lymph node
m. polytomography
m. sinus
mastoidectomy
mastoiditis
mastopathy
indurative m.
mastoplasia
cystic m.
match
nontransmural m.
transmural m.
triple m.
matched peripheral dose (MPD)
matching
atlas m.
electron-photon field m.
general pattern m.
impedance m.
matchline
m. technique
m. wedge
mater
dura m.
pia m.
material (*See* agent, contrast, medium)
anthracotic m.
atheromatous m.
ballistic m.
bowel containing opaque m.
byproduct m.
coffee-ground m.
collection of contrast m.
columnization of contrast m.
contrast m.
dental m.
extraneous m.
fecal m.
ferromagnetic m.
flow of contrast m.
hand-instilled contrast m.
inspissated m.
Interpore bone replacement m.
intravenous administration of contrast m.
iodinated contrast m.
layering of contrast m.
lipid-rich m.
low-osmolar contrast m.
magnetic m.
metrizamide contrast m.
metrizoate acid contrast m.
nidus of embolic m.
nonionic contrast m.
^{103}Pd radioactive m.
PET target m.
radioactive m.
residual contrast m.
semisolid fecal m.
silicotic m.
superabsorbent polymer embolic m.

NOTES

material *(continued)*
takeup of radioactive m.
target m.
trophoblastic m.
vessel cutoff of contrast m.
vicarious excretion of contrast m.
maternal
m. lake
m. placenta
Mathews classification of olecranon fractures
matrix, pl. **matrices, matrix**
acquisition m.
bone m.
bone tumor m.
calcific m.
cartilage m.
chondroid m.
decision m.
demineralized bone m. (DBM)
extracellular m.
germinal bleed m.
m. image
image m.
m. injury
k-space m.
osteoid m.
proteoglycan m.
quantization m. (QM)
reduced-acquisition m. (RAM)
solid m.
stromal m.
transformation m.
tumor m.
Matrix LR3300 laser imaging
matter
cortical gray m.
cortical white m.
cytotoxic edema of the gray m.
deep white ischemia m.
gray m.
heterotopic gray m.
particulate m.
periaqueductal gray m.
perilesional white m.
periventricular gray m. (PVG matter, PVG)
periventricular white m.
pulverized plaque particulate m.
PVG m.
periventricular gray matter
scalloped appearance of white m.
shearing of white m.
supratentorial gray m.
supratentorial white m.
white m.
maturation
bone m.
disk m.
m. index
mature
m. bone
m. mediastinum teratoma
m. ovarian cystic teratoma
m. pancreatic pseudocyst
m. pseudocyst of pancreas
skeletally m.
maturity of fetus
Mauchart ligament
Maugeri syndrome
maxilla, pl. **maxillae**
maxillary
m. antrum
m. artery
m. bone
m. canal
m. division
m. fracture
m. nerve anatomy
m. sinus
m. sinus carcinoma
m. sinus hypoplasia
m. sinus opacification
m. sinus radiograph
m. spine
maxillofacial
m. fracture
m. imaging
maxilloturbinal bone
maximal
m. estimated gradient
m. intensity
m. transaortic jet velocity
m. volume of left atrium
m. voluntary ventilation (MVV)
maximum
m. amplitude constant
m. anteroposterior diameter
m. density (D_{max})
m. diameter to minimum diameter ratio
m. entropy processing
full width at half m. (FWHM)
m. inflation pressure
m. inflation time
m. intensity pixel (MIP)
m. intensity projection algorithm
m. intensity projection imaging
m. intensity projection and source image
m. likelihood algorithm
m. midexpiratory flow rate (MMFR)
m. permissible body burden
m. permissible concentration
m. permissible dose (MPD)

m. predicted heart rate (MPHR)
m. slew rate ramp
m. venous outflow (MVO)
m. ventricular elastance
m. walking time (MWT)

maximum-intensity
m.-i. sliding thin slab projection

maximus
gluteus m.

Max Plus MR scanner

Maxwell
M. 3D field simulator
M. pair
M. theory of radiation

Mayer
M. position
M. view

Mayer-Rokitansky-Küster-Hauser syndrome

May-Hegglin anomaly

Mayneord F factor

Mazabraud syndrome

Mazicon

Mazur ankle evaluation classification

MBF
myocardial blood flow

MBq
megabecquerel

mC
microcurie

MCA
multichannel analyzer
multiple congenital anomalies

McArdle
M. disease
M. syndrome

MCAT
myocardial contrast appearance time

McBurney point

McCabe-Fletcher classification

McCallum patch

McCort sign

McCune-Albright syndrome

MCD
mean central dose

MCDK
multicystic dysplastic kidney

MCE
myocardial contrast echocardiography

MCFSR
mean circumferential fiber shortening rate

McGinn-White sign

McGregor line

mCi
millicurie

MCK
multicystic kidney

McKee line

McKusick disease

McKusick-Kaufman syndrome

McKusick-type metaphyseal dysplasia

MCL
midclavicular line

McLain-Weinstein spinal tumor classification

MCLC
medial collateral ligament complex

MCLS
mucocutaneous lymph node syndrome

McMurray sign

McNemar test

MCP
metacarpophalangeal

MCPJ
metacarpophalangeal joint

MCPT
Monte Carlo photon transport
MCPT simulation

McRae line

MCS
middle coronary sinus

MCTC
metrizamide computed tomography cisternography

MCTD
mixed connective tissue disease

McWhirter technique

MDAC
multiplying digital-to-analog converter

MD-Gastroview imaging agent

MDP
methylene diphosphonate

Meadows syndrome

meal
barium m.
Boyden test m.
double-contrast barium m.
Ewald test m.
fatty m.
isotope m.
motor test m.
opaque m.
retention m.

NOTES

M

meal *(continued)*
small bowel m.
test m.
mean
m. ankle-brachial systolic pressure index
m. aortic flow velocity
m. aortic pressure
m. arterial pressure (MAP)
m. atrial pressure
m. blood pressure
m. brachial artery pressure
m. cardiac vector
m. central dose (MCD)
m. circulatory filling pressure
m. circumferential fiber shortening rate (MCFSR)
m. corpuscular volume
m. free path
m. left atrial pressure
m. mitral valve gradient
m. perfusate temperature
m. posterior wall velocity
m. pulmonary artery pressure (MPA pressure, MPAP)
m. pulmonary artery wedge pressure
m. pulmonary capillary pressure (MPCP)
m. pulmonary flow velocity
m. pulmonary transit time (MTT)
m. right atrial pressure
m. systolic gradient
m. vector
m. venous pulsation
m. wall motion score
m. wall motion score index
mean-diameter overframing
mean-square error
Meary metatarsotalar angle
measles pneumonia
measurable endpoint
measure
Hausdorff metric m.
linear m.
measurement
ankle-brachial pressure m.
antegrade perfusion pressure m. (APPM)
attenuation m.
automated cardiac flow m. (ACM)
blood flow m.
bone density m.
breath pentane m.
cardiac output m.
cerebrospinal fluid flow m.
Cerenkov m.
Cobb m.
densitometric m.
diode m.
end-diastolic velocity m.
excitation function m.
fetal foot length m.
fetal long bone m.
flow cytometric DNA m.
gestational sac m.
Hausdorff metric m.
high-sensitivity m.
indicator-dilution method for cardiac output m.
intercomparison m.
International Commission on Radiation Units and M.'s (ICRU)
line-pair m.
low-energy photon attenuation m.
mammographic m.
morphometric m.
National Council on Radiation Protection and M.'s (NCRP)
nutation angle m.
occlusion m.
orbit m.
phase-sensitive flow m.
photon attenuation m.
polarographic needle electrode m.
pressure m.
pulse-echo distance m.
quantitative regional myocardial flow m.
regional washout m.
renal length m.
rocking curve m.
root-mean-squared gradient m.
semiquantitative m.
temperature distribution m.
thermodilution method of cardiac output m.
thyroid uptake m.
time-of-flight flow m.
time-velocity m.
topographic m.
transcutaneous oxygen pressure m. ($tcPO_2$)
true conjugate m.
U1-NA cephalometric m.
m. in vivo
Wits cephalometric m.
xenon CT m.
meatal segment
meatus, pl. **meatus**
acoustic m.
external auditory m.
internal auditory m.
nasal m.
meat wrapper's lung
mebrofenin

mechanical
m. augmentation
m. axis
m. biliary obstruction
m. bowel obstruction
m. counterpulsation
m. dottering effect
m. duct obstruction
m. extrahepatic obstruction
m. ileus
m. insufflation
m. insult
m. intestinal obstruction
m. potential energy
m. respiratory tract obstruction
m. sector scanner
m. small bowel obstruction
m. valve
m. ventilation
mechanically activated implant
mechanics
intramural m.
mechanism
blood-clotting m.
central extensor m. (CEM)
check-valve m.
contrecoup m.
deglutition m.
extensor m.
flap-valve m.
Frank-Starling m.
heart rate reserve m.
homing m.
humeral m.
m. of injury
internal retention m.
iron-transporting protein m.
Laplace m.
osseous pinch m.
pinchcock m.
propulsive m.
sinus m.
sphincteric m.
swallowing m.
Taylor-Blackwood m.
ventricular escape m.
watershed m.
Mecholyl test
Meckel
M. band
M. cavity
M. diverticulitis
M. diverticulum
M. diverticulum rule of 2
M. ligament
M. scan
M. space
M. syndrome
Meckel-Gruber syndrome
meclofenamic acid
Meclomen
meconium
m. aspiration
m. aspiration syndrome
m. ileus
m. ileus equivalent
m. ileus soap-bubble appearance
inspissated m.
m. peristalsis
m. peritonitis
m. plug
m. plug syndrome
m. pseudocyst
MEDDARS cardiac catheterization analysis system
media (*pl. of* medium)
media-adventitia interface
medial
m. angle
m. arch
m. arteriosclerosis
m. aspect
m. basal segmental bronchus
m. border
m. calcific sclerosis
m. carpal capsule
m. collateral ligament
m. collateral ligament calcification
m. collateral ligament complex (MCLC)
m. column calcaneal fracture
m. compartment
m. condyle
m. crus
m. cuneiform bone
m. cystic necrosis
m. dissection
m. eminence
m. end of clavicle osteolysis
m. epicondyle
m. epicondyle fracture
m. epicondylitis
m. extension
m. femoral buttressing

NOTES

M

medial *(continued)*
m. fibroplasia
m. geniculate body
m. geniculate fascia
m. hyperplasia
m. joint line
m. joint space
m. lemniscus
m. longitudinal fasciculus (MLF)
m. longitudinal fasciculus lesion
m. malleolar fracture
m. malleolus
m. malleolus periostitis
m. oblique view
m. occipitotemporal gyrus
m. papillary muscle
m. physis
m. plantar artery
m. plica
m. posterior choroidal (MPCh)
m. pterygoid muscle
m. rotation
m. sesamoid bone
m. shelf
m. supraclavicular node
m. talar margin
m. temporal lobe
m. tibial stress syndrome
m. traction spur

medialis
meniscus m.
vastus m.

medially

median
m. antebrachial vein
m. arcuate ligament
m. arcuate ligament of diaphragm
m. bar
m. cleft lip
m. cruciate ligament
m. facial cleft
m. lethal dose
m. level echo
m. line
m. lip cleft
m. lobe of prostate
multiples of the m. (MOM)
m. nerve
m. nerve entrapment
m. nerve lesion
m. raphe
m. sacral artery
m. sagittal plane
m. septum
m. sternotomy
m. umbilical ligament

mediastinal
m. abscess
m. adenoma
m. adenopathy
m. air
m. border
m. bronchogenic cyst
m. bulk
m. collagenosis
m. cross-sectional imaging
m. deviation
m. dorsal enteric cyst
m. emphysema
m. fat
m. fibrosis
m. fistula
m. germ-cell tumor
m. granuloma
m. hematoma
m. hemorrhage
m. hernia
m. high-attenuation mass
m. invasion
m. lesion
m. lipomatosis
m. lung surface
m. lymph node enlargement
m. lymphoma
m. node
m. pleura
m. pleurisy
m. prominence
m. pseudomass
m. retraction
m. seminoma
m. septum
m. seroma
m. shift
m. structure
m. teratoid tumor
m. thickening
m. tube
m. uptake
m. vein
m. viscera
m. wedge
m. widening
m. window

mediastinitis
chronic m.
fibrosing m.
idiopathic fibrous m.
sclerosing m.

mediastinography
gaseous m.

mediastinum
anterior m.
m. cerebelli
m. cerebri
m. dermoid

deviated m.
m. displacement
m. dysgerminoma
epidermoid m.
m. germinoma
inferior m.
m. lipoma
lipomatosis m.
middle m.
posterior m.
seminoma m.
superior m.
m. teratocarcinoma
teratoid m.
m. teratoma
m. testis
widened m.

medical
m. cyclotron
m. holography
m. internal radiation dose (MIRD)
m. internal radiation dosimetry (MIRD)
m. ultrasound 3D portable, with advanced communication (MUSTPAC)
m. umbilical fold

medicamentosa
thyrotoxicosis m.

medicine
American Institute of Ultrasound in M. (AIUM)
digital imaging and communications in m.
Fellow of the American College of Nuclear M. (FACNM)
nuclear m.
photonic m.
Society of Magnetic Resonance in M.
Society of Nuclear M. (SNM)

Medigraphics analyzer

Medilase angioscope-laser delivery system

MedImage scanner

Medinvent

mediolateral
m. aspect
m. flow direction
m. oblique (MLO)
m. oblique projection
m. oblique view
m. radiocarpal angle
m. stress

medionecrosis
cystic m.
Erdheim cystic m.

medionodular cirrhosis

mediopatellar

Medison scanner

Medi-tech

Mediterranean fever

medium, pl. **media** (*See* agent, contrast, material)
Adenoscan contrast m.
Albunex ultrasound contrast m.
AMI 121 contrast m.
AMI 227 contrast m.
Amipaque contrast m.
Angio-Conray contrast m.
Angiovist contrast m.
Baricon contrast m.
barium sulfate contrast m.
Baro-CAT contrast m.
Baroflave contrast m.
Barosperse contrast m.
Biliscopin contrast m.
Bilivist contrast m.
m. caliber
CO_2 negative contrast m.
contrast m.
Cysto-Conray II contrast m.
Cystografin contrast m.
delayed excretion of contrast m.
diatrizoate meglumine radiopaque m.
Ethiodane contrast m.
Ethiodol contrast m.
extraluminal contrast m.
GastroMARK oral contrast m.
Gastrovist contrast m.
Gd-DOTA contrast m.
Gd oxide contrast m.
hand injection of contrast m.
high-osmolar m. (HOM)
high-osmolarity contrast m. (HOCM)
hot contrast m.
Hypaque contrast m.
Hypaque-76 contrast m.
Hypaque-Cysto contrast m.
Hypaque-M contrast m.
Hypaque Meglumine contrast m.
Hypaque Sodium contrast m.

NOTES

M

medium *(continued)*
hyperconcentration of contrast m.
Imagopaque contrast m.
iocetamic acid contrast m.
iodinated contrast m.
ionic paramagnetic contrast m.
Isopaque contrast m.
isosmolar contrast m. (IOCM)
kinetic energy released in the m. (kerma)
low-osmolar contrast m. (LOCM)
myelographic contrast m.
nephrotoxic contrast m.
nonionic paramagnetic contrast m.
opaque m.
paradoxical hyperconcentration of contrast m.
radiochromic dosimetry m.
radiopaque m.
Tomocat contrast m.
topical water-soluble contrast m.
tunica media
uniphasic contrast m.
water-soluble contrast m.
ZK44012 contrast m.
medium-energy collimator
medium-sized bronchus
medius
digitus m.
gluteus m.
scalenus m.
Medix MF-5500X
Medrad
M. contrast medium injector
M. Mrinnervu endorectal colon probe
M. Mrinnervu endorectal colon probe coil
M. power angiographic injector
medronate
m. scan
technetium-99m m.
medroxyprogesterone acetate
Medsonic plethysmography
Medspec
M. MR imaging system
M. MR imaging system scanner
Medtronic
M. Minix
M. radiofrequency receiver
medulla, pl. **medullae**
adrenal m.
hyperechoic renal m.
lymphatic m.
m. oblongata
ovarian m.
renal m.
rostral m.
spinal m.
medullaris
artery of the conus m.
conus m.
conus arteriosus m.
low conus m.
medullary
m. artery
m. bone
m. bone infarct
m. breast carcinoma
m. calcification
m. canal
m. cavity
m. cone
m. cord
m. cystic disease
m. lamina
m. nephrocalcinosis
m. nephrogram
m. pyramid
m. rod
m. sinus
m. sponge
m. sponge kidney
m. tegmentum
m. thyroid carcinoma
m. vein
m. venous anatomy
medullary-type adenocarcinoma (MTA)
medulloblastoma
m. metastasis
vermian m.
medusae
caput m.
Medweb clinical reporting system
Medx
M. camera
M. scanner
Meese position
Mees line
mefenamic acid
MEG
magnetoencephalography
megabecquerel (MBq)
megabulb
jugular m.
megabulbus
duodenum m.
megacalicosis
megacalix, pl. **megacalices**
mega cisterna magna
megacolon
acquired m.
aganglionic m.
congenital m.
m. dilatation

idiopathic m.
toxic m.
megacystic microcolon
megacystis-microcolon-intestinal hypoperistalsis syndrome
megaduodenum
megaesophagus
m. of achalasia
megahertz (MHz)
megalencephaly
unilateral m.
megalocornea
megalocystis
megalocystis-microcolon-intestinal-hypoperistalsis
megaloencephaly
megalourethra
megarectum
megaureter
congenital primary m.
primary m.
primary congenital m.
megavolt (MV)
megavoltage
m. grid
m. grid therapy
m. radiation
m. radiation therapy
m. treatment beam
m. x-ray therapy
meglumine
m. acetrizoate
diatrizoate m.
iocarmate m.
iodipamide m.
m. iodipamide imaging agent
iodoxamate m.
m. iothalamate
m. iotroxate imaging agent
ioxaglate m.
megophthalmos
meibomian
m. cyst
m. gland carcinoma
Meiboom-Gill sequence
Meige lymphedema
Meigs
M. capillary
M. disease
M. syndrome
Meigs-Cass syndrome
Meigs-Salmon syndrome
Meissner plexus
melanocytoma
meningeal m.
melanocytosis
melanoma
anorectal m.
benign juvenile m.
choroidal m.
intraocular m.
malignant uveal m.
melanotic m.
mucosal m.
node-negative m.
regional m.
spitzoid malignant m.
subungual m.
superficial spreading m.
vulvar m.
melanosarcoma
melanosis
m. coli
neurocutaneous m.
parenchymal neurocutaneous m.
melanotic
m. cancer
m. melanoma
m. neuroectodermal tumor
MELAS
mitochondrial myopathy, encephalopathy, lactic acidosis, and stroke-like episodes
melioidosis
Melnick-Needles syndrome
Melone distal radius fracture classification
melorheostosis
m. of Leri
Melrose solution
melting sign
Meltzer sign
membranacea
placenta m.
membranaceous tendon
membranaceum
membrane
amnionic m.
atlantooccipital m.
Bichat m.
m. of bone
cricothyroid m.
glomerular basement m. (GBM)
hourglass m.
interosseous m. (IOM)

NOTES

membrane *(continued)*
intertwin m.
intraluminal m.
intrauterine m.
Liliequist m.
microporous m.
mucous m.
obturator m.
m. permeability
m. phosphate
premature rupture of m.'s
rolling m.
rupture of m.'s
serous m.
Shrapnell m.
synovial m.
tympanic vascular m.
vascular tympanic m.
vernix m.
membranous
m. bronchiole
m. glomerulonephritis
m. labyrinth
m. obstruction of inferior vena cava
m. pregnancy
m. septum
m. subaortic stenosis
m. subvalvular aortic stenosis
m. urethra
m. ventricular septal defect
Memorial dimension averaging method
memory
Aloka color Doppler real-time 2D blood flow imaging with Cine M.
thermal shape m.
memory-intensive algorithm
MEN
multiple endocrine neoplasms
Mendel-Bekhterev sign
mendelevium
Mendelson syndrome
Ménétrier disease
Mengert index
Menghini
M. biopsy technique
meningeal
m. artery
m. artery groove
m. cell tumor
m. enhancement sign
m. fibroma
m. fibrosis
m. hemangiopericytoma
m. hemorrhage
m. infiltrate
m. inflammation
m. melanocytoma
middle m.
m. sarcoma
m. tuberculosis
m. vein
meninges (*pl. of* meninx)
meningioangiomatosis
meningioma
angioplastic m.
atypical m.
cavernous sinus m.
cerebellopontine angle m.
clival m.
convexity m.
m. of cribriform plate
cystic intraparenchymal m.
ectopic m.
endotheliomatous m.
m. en plaque
falcine m.
falcotentorial m.
fibroblastic m.
fibrous m.
globular m.
intraosseous m.
intraparenchymal m.
intraventricular m.
lipoblastic m.
malignant m.
meningothelial m.
meningotheliomatous m.
multicentric m.
olfactory groove m.
optic nerve sheath m.
parasagittal m.
periauricular m.
perioptic m.
posterior fossa m.
m. of posterior fossa
psammoma body m.
psammomatous m.
sphenoid ridge m.
sphenoid wing m.
spinal m.
subfrontal m.
suprasellar m.
temporal m.
tentorial m.
transitional m.
tuberculum sellae m.
meningiomatosis
meningocele
anterior sacral m.
cervical m.
cranial m.
dorsal m.
lateral lumbar m.
lateral thoracic m.

occipital m.
sacral m.
simple m.
traumatic m.
meningococcemia
meningoencephalitic sign
meningoencephalitis
meningoencephalocele
ethmoidal m.
sphenopharyngeal m.
meningofacial angiomatosis
meningohypophyseal
m. artery
m. trunk
meningomyelocele
meningothelial meningioma
meningotheliomatous meningioma
meninx, pl. **meninges**
meninges of brain
meninges of spinal cord
meniscal
m. cleft
m. fragmentation
m. horn
m. injury
m. ossicle
menisci (*pl. of* meniscus)
meniscocapsular
m. attachment
m. junction
m. separation
meniscocondylar coordination
meniscofemoral
m. attachment
m. ligament
meniscosynovial junction
meniscotibial
m. attachment
m. ligament
m. separation
meniscus, pl. **menisci**
articular m.
m. articularis
discoid m.
discoid lateral m.
diverging m.
dysplastic m.
fibrocartilaginous m.
free-floating m.
m. lateralis
m. lung sign
m. medialis
m. notch sign
radiohumeral m.
m. sign
m. tear
Watanabe classification of discoid m.
Menkes syndrome
Mennell sign
menotropins
menses
menstrual
m. age
menstrualis
mensuration
m. algorithm
fetal m.
mental
m. canal
m. spine
mentoanterior
Mentor prostatic biopsy needle
mentum
Menzel olivopontocerebellar degeneration
meptazinol
meralgia paresthetica
mercaptoacetyltriglycerine (MAG)
mercaptoacetyltriglycine
technetium-99m m.
mercaptoacetythiglycine
^{99m}Tc m.
technetium-99m m.
Mercator projection
Merchant
M. angle
M. view
Mercuhydrin
1-mercuri-2-hydroxypropane (MHP)
mercury
m. artifact
millimeters of m. (mmHg, mm Hg)
Meridian echocardiography
Merkel
M. cell carcinoma
M. cell carcinoma cell line
M. muscle
M. tactile disk
Merland perimedullary arteriovenous fistula classification
mermaid
m. deformity
m. syndrome
meroacrania

NOTES

MERRF
myoclonus epilepsy associated with ragged red fibers
mertiatide
technetium-99m m.
mesalamine enema
mesatipellic pelvis
mesencephalic
m. artery
m. cerebral lymphoma
m. cistern
m. cistern effacement
m. infarct
m. low-density brain lesion
m. reticular formation
m. tract
m. vein
mesencephalitis
mesencephalon
m. aqueduct
mesenchymal
m. chondrosarcoma
m. liver hamartoma
m. neoplasm
m. tissue
m. tumor
mesenchymoma
atrial m.
benign m.
chest wall m.
mesenteric
m. adenitis
m. adenopathy
m. angiography
m. apoplexy
m. arterial thrombosis
m. arteriography
m. artery
m. artery occlusion
m. attachment
m. border
m. calcification
m. cyst
m. fistula
m. infarct
m. ischemia
m. lipodystrophy
m. lymphadenopathy
m. lymphoma
m. mass
m. node
m. panniculitis
m. phlegmon
m. pregnancy
m. rupture
m. sclerosis
m. stranding
superior m.
m. tear
m. tissue
m. triangle
m. vascular insufficiency
m. vascular lesion
m. vein
m. venous thrombosis
m. vessel
m. Weber-Christian disease
mesentericoparietal fossa
mesenteritis
chronic fibrosing m.
fibrosing m.
liposclerotic m.
retractile m.
sclerosing m.
mesenterium commune
mesenteroaxial volvulus
mesentery
fan-shaped m.
fatty m.
intestinal m.
ischemic m.
leaves of m.
lymphangioma m.
root of m.
small intestine m. (SIM)
ventral m.
Weber-Christian m.
mesh
suppressor m.
tantalum m.
tubular wire m.
mesial
m. aspect
m. frontal focus
m. hemisphere
m. hyperperfusion
m. temporal epileptogenic lesion
m. temporal sclerosis
mesial-frontal cortex
mesiodistal plane
mesoappendix
mesoblastic nephroma
mesocardia
mesocephalic head shape
mesocolic
m. band
m. shelf
mesocolon
sigmoid m.
transverse m.
mesocolonic
m. fat
m. vessel
mesocuneiform bone

mesoderm
extraembryonic m.
gastral m.
mesoderma
mesodermal
m. dysplasia
m. sarcoma
mesomelia
mesomelic
m. dwarfism
m. dysplasia
mesometanephric carcinoma
meson
kappa m.
mu m.
pi m.
mesonephric
m. kidney
m. ridge
mesonephros, pl. **mesonephroi**
mesoporphyrine
Bid-Gd m.
mesorectum
mesosigmoid colon
mesosternum
mesothelial cyst
mesothelioma
asbestos-related m.
atrioventricular nodal node m.
benign m.
cystic m.
diffuse malignant peritoneal m.
epithelioid malignant m.
fibrosing m.
localized fibrous m.
malignant pleural m.
peritoneal m.
pleural m.
mesothorium
mesotympanum
mesoversion of heart
mesylate
fenoldopam m.
metabolic
m. bone disease
m. bone disorder
m. bone series
m. calculus
m. cardiomyopathy
m. cirrhosis
m. lesion
m. rate of oxygen
m. response
m. stone
m. tracer uptake
metabolism
carbon m.
cerebral m.
evaluation of glucose m.
fat m.
fatty acid m.
glucose m.
hepatic m.
myocardial m.
oxidative m.
phosphorus m.
metabolite
phosphorus m.
metacarpal
base of m.
m. bone
m. fracture
m. hand sign
m. index
metacarpoglenoidal ligament
metacarpophalangeal (MCP)
m. articulation
m. joint (MCPJ)
m. ligament
metacarpus
metachronous
m. lesion
m. metastasis
m. transitional cell carcinoma
metadiaphyseal
metadiaphysis
metaiodobenzylguanidine (MIBG)
adrenal imaging m.
iodine-131 m.
metal
m. chelate complex
Co-Cr-W-Ni alloy implant m.
cobalt-chromium-tungsten-nickel alloy metal impant
lanthanide m.
m. line-pair phantom
Lipowitz m.
radioactive m.
m. technetium target
transition m.
metallic
m. artifact
m. clip
m. density

M

NOTES

metallic *(continued)*
m. echo
m. foreign body
m. fragment
m. marker
m. needle
m. otologic implant
m. pointer
m. rod fixation
m. screw
m. staple
m. stent
m. suture
m. tip cannula
m. track of bullet
metalloporphyrin
metanephric
m. diverticulum
m. vesicle
metanephros, pl. **metanephroi**
metaphyseal, metaphysial
m. abscess
m. chondrodysplasia
m. dysostosis
m. dysplasia
m. extension
m. flare
m. fracture
m. lucent band
m. metaphysis
metaphyseal-diaphyseal
m.-d. junction
m.-d. low-signal-intensity red marrow inhomogeneity
metaphyseal-epiphyseal angle
metaphysial (*var. of* metaphyseal)
metaphysis, pl. **metaphyses**
agnogenic myeloid m.
autoparenchymatous m.
celomic m.
columnar m.
frayed m.
fundic m.
humeral m.
intestinal m.
metaphyseal m.
myeloid m.
primary myeloid m.
secondary myeloid m.
squamous m.
metaplasia
agnogenic myeloid m.
cartilaginous m.
intestinal m.
keratinizing squamous m.
monarticular synovium-based cartilage m.
myelofibrosis with myeloid m. (MMM)
osteocartilaginous m.
squamous m.
metaplastic
m. carcinoma
m. polyp
metapneumonic
m. empyema
m. pleurisy
metaraminol
metastagenicity
metastasectomy
metastasis, pl. **metastases**
adnexal m.
adrenal m.
air-space m.
aortic node m.
axillary node m.
blastic m.
bone m.
brain m.
breast m.
calcareous m.
calcified m.
calcifying m.
cavitating lung m.
celiac lymph node m.
cerebral m.
clivus m.
cystic m.
diffuse skeletal m.
distant m.
drop m.
echogenic liver m.
echopenic liver m.
endobronchial m.
extracapsular m.
extrahepatic m. (EHM)
extrathoracic m.
gastric m.
hemorrhagic m.
hepatic m.
hypervascular liver m.
inguinal lymph node m.
in-transit m.
intraparenchymal m.
kidney m.
liver m.
local m.
lung m.
lymphangitic m.
lymphatic m.
lymphogenous m.
medulloblastoma m.
metachronous m.
micronodular m.
necrotic m.

neuroendocrine hepatic m.
nodal m.
nonhemorrhagic melanoma m.
occult bone m.
orbital m.
osseous m.
osteoblastic m.
osteolytic m.
ovarian m.
m. of pancreas
pancreatic m.
paracardiac m.
parasellar m.
parenchymal brain m.
peritoneal m.
placental m.
pleura m.
pulmonary m.
pulsating m.
renal m.
satellite m.
skeletal m.
skip m.
small bowel m.
sphenoid sinus m.
spinal cord m.
splenic m.
stomach cancer m.
testicular m.
tumor, node, m. (TNM)
uterine sarcoma m.
Virchow m.
white m.
widespread m.

metastatic
m. abscess
m. adenocarcinoma
m. adenopathy
m. axillary involvement
m. bone survey
m. carcinoid syndrome
m. carcinoma
m. disease
m. lesion
m. lymphoma
m. malignancy
m. myocardial tumor
m. osteosarcoma
m. pneumonia
m. polyp
m. renal neoplasm
m. rhabdomyosarcoma
m. seeding
m. soft tissue calcification
m. testicular lymphoma
m. urothelial cancer

Metastron
M. imaging agent

metasynchronous tumor

metatarsal
angle of declination of m.
m. axis
m. bone
m. fracture
m. head
m. injury
m. joint
m. length ratio
m. parabola
m. synostosis

metatarsocalcaneal angle

metatarsocuneiform
m. joint
m. joint fusion

metatarsophalangeal (MTP)
m. capsule
m. joint (MTPJ)
m. joint arthritis
m. joint fusion

metatarsotalar angle

metatarsus
m. adductocavus deformity
m. adductovarus deformity
m. adductus
m. adductus angle
m. adductus deformity
m. atavicus deformity
m. latus deformity
m. primus angle
m. primus varus deformity
m. valgus
m. varus
m. varus deformity

metatrophic
m. dwarfism
m. dysplasia

metaxalone

metencephalon

meteorism

meter (m)
exposure m.
Gammex RMI DAP (dose-area product) m.
kVp m.

M

NOTES

meter *(continued)*
photovolt pH m.
rate m.
roentgen m. (R meter)
meters per second (mps)
methacholine
methadone lung damage
methicillin-resistant ***Staphylococcus aureus***
methimazole
methiodal
m. sodium
m. sodium imaging agent
methionine
^{11}C m.
methocarbamol
method
Andren m.
Arelin m.
automated airway tree segmentation m.
Bayler-Pinneau m.
Beclere m.
Benassi m.
Benedict-Talbot body surface area m.
Bertel m.
Blackett-Healy m.
border detection m. (BDM)
Born m.
Brasdor m.
Cahoon m.
Caldwell m.
Caldwell-Moloy m.
calibration m.
Cameron m.
Camp-Gianturco m.
Causton m.
Chassard-Lapine m.
Chausse m.
CHESS m.
chemical shift selective
cine-cyclic m.
Cleaves m.
coaxial-needle m.
Colbert m.
Colcher-Sussman m.
column extraction m.
computer m.
Davis m.
2DFT m.
Dooley, Caldwell and Glass m.
double-echo three-point Dixon suppression m.
downstream sampling m.
dual-balloon m.
Duncan-Hoen m.
Dunlap, Swanson and Penner m.
echoplanar imaging m.
empirical m.
Enhance deblurring m.
error diffusion m.
extraction m.
FBP m.
FI m.
full scan with interpolation method
Fick m.
filtered back-projection m.
fixed-grid stereologic m.
forward triangle m.
fractal-based m.
Friedman m.
FS m.
full-scan method
full-scan m. (FS method)
full scan with interpolation m. (FI method)
Garn m.
Gaynor-Hart m.
Gerota m.
gradient-echo m.
gradient-reversal fat suppression m.
Grandy m.
Grashey m.
Graupner m.
Gunson m.
Haas m.
half-scan with extrapolation m.
Harrison-Stubbs m.
Hatt m.
Hawkins m.
Hickey m.
Hirtz m.
incremental passive positioning m.
intrapixel sequential processing neuron evaluation m.
in vivo m.
IPSP neuron evaluation m.
isocenter shift m.
isodose shift m.
Joliot m.
Kandel m.
Kaplan-Meier m.
Kennedy area-length m.
Korotkoff m.
Kouchoukos m.
Kuchendorf m.
KWE m.
Laks m.
Laquerriere-Perquin m.
Lauenstein and Hickey m.
Lawrence m.
Leonard-George m.
Levenberg-Marquardt m.
Lilienfelds m.
long-cannula coaxial m.

Lysholm m.
Mankin m.
manual computed m.
Martz m.
Memorial dimension averaging m.
Meyerding m.
multiple-line scanning m.
multiple-sensitive-point m.
multisection m.
NEUGAT m.
  neutron/gamma transmission method
Owen-Pendergrass m.
parallax m.
Parama m.
Pearson m.
Pfeiffer-Comberg m.
phase-unwrapping m.
Pirie m.
Porcher m.
power law TAR m.
radiotracer foil m.
ray-casting m.
Sansregret m.
m. of Scarpa
segmentation m.
selective excitation m.
selective saturation m.
Settegast m.
Shimazaki area-length m.
shock-monitoring m.
short-cannula coaxial m.
simulated annealing m.
spectroscopic chemical-shift m.
spin-label m.
spin-warp m.
spiral imaging m.
Staunig m.
Steel-Dwaas m.
stereologic m.
Strickler m.
sum-peak m.
surface coil m.
Syed-Neblett brachytherapy m.
tandem-needle m.
Tanner-Whitehouse-Healy m.
Teufel m.
thallium split-dose m.
Thom m.
three-dimensional-FATS (fast adiabetic trajectory in a steady state) m.
thresholding m.
Tilden m.
time-of-flight m.
triangulation m.
trocar drainage m.
two-dye m.
under-scan m.
Valdini m.
Valvassori m.
variable projection m. (VARPRO)
Wehlin m.
Welcker m.
Zimmer m.

methodology
  Gehan m.

methohexital

methotrexate lung damage

methoxystaurosporine
  ^{11}C m.

methyl
  m. methacrylate bead implant
  m. methacrylate beads
  m. methacrylate imaging agent
  m. proton

methyl-ABV

methylene
  m. blue enema
  m. diphosphonate (MDP)
  m. diphosphonate (MDP) concentration

methylglucamine
  m. diatrizoate
  iodipamide m.
  m. iodipamide

methyltransferase
  thiopurine m. (TPMT)

metopic suture

metrizamide
  m. computed tomography cisternography (MCTC)
  m. contrast material
  m. CT cisternogram
  m. imaging agent
  m. myelography
  m. ventriculogram

metrizamide-assisted computed tomography (CTMM)

metrizoate
  m. acid contrast material

NOTES

metrizoate *(continued)*
sodium m.
m. sodium imaging agent
metrizoic
m. acid
m. acid imaging agent
Metrodin
metrology
metronidazole
metroperitoneal fistula
metroplasty
Mevatron 74 linear accelerator
Mexican hat sign
Meyer
M. dysplasia
M. line
M. loop
supratubercular ridge of M.
Meyer-Archambault loop
Meyerding method
Meyer-McKeever tibial fracture classification
Meyers-McKeever classification of tibial fractures
Meyer-Weigert rule
Meynert tract
Meynet node
MF
magnification factor
mf
microfarad
MFG
magnetic field gradient
manofluorography
MFH
malignant fibrous histiocytoma
MFH-B
malignant fibrous histiocytoma of bone
MF-5500X
Medix M.
MHP
1-mercuri-2-hydroxypropane
MHV
middle hepatic vein
MHz
megahertz
MI
mitral insufficiency
myocardial infarct
inferior wall MI
MIBG
metaiodobenzylguanidine
adrenal imaging MIBG
MIBG scintigraphy
MIBG SPECT scan
mica pneumoconiosis
mice
joint m.
micelle
Michaelis
M. complex
rhomboid of M.
Michaelis-Gutmann body
Michel
M. anomaly
M. aplasia
M. deformity
Michels classification
Mickey Mouse ears pelvis
Mick seed applicator
micrencephaly, micrencephalia
microabscess
m. of the spleen
splenic m.
microadenoma
adrenocorticotropin m.
pituitary m.
microampere (μA, mA)
microaneurysm
Charcot-Bouchard intracerebral m.
microangiography
microangiopathy
mineralizing m.
thrombotic m.
microarteriography
microatelectasis
microballoon
Rand m.
microbubble contrast imaging agent
microbubbles
sonicated albumin m.
microcalcification
breast m.
clustered m.
ductal breast m.
lobular breast m.
microcardia
microCase
Micro-Cast collimator
microcatheter
microcavitation
microcephaly
cytomegalovirus with m.
microcirculation
pulmonary m.
microcirculatory blood flow
microcluster
biodegradable magnetic m.
microcoil
Hilal m.
microcolon
megacystic m.
microcolon-megacystis syndrome
microconidia
microcurie (μCi, mC)
m. per milliliter

microcyst
milk-of-calcium m.
microcystic
m. adenoma
m. degeneration
m. encephalomalacia
m. formation
m. lumbar spine
m. pancreatic tumor
m. pilocytic cerebellar astrocytoma
microcystica
microcytosis
microdactylia
microdactyly of big toe
microdistribution
heterogeneous m.
microdosimetry
microembolization
ferromagnetic m.
microembolus, pl. **microemboli**
microenvironment
bone marrow m.
microerosion
microexplosion lithotripsy
microextension
microfarad (mf)
microfixation plate
microfluidization
microfocal spot mammography
microfracture
subchondral m.
trabecular m.
microgallbladder
microgastria
microglandular adenosis
microglioma
microglobulin labeling
micrognathia
Micro-Guide
microimaging
microinfarct
microkymatotherapy
microlithiasis
alveolar m.
pulmonary alveolar m.
testicular m.
microlobular cirrhosis
microlobulation
micromanometer-tip catheter
MicroMark tissue marker
micromelena
micromelia
bowed m.
extreme m.
micromelic
m. dwarfism
m. dysplasia
micrometallic artifact
micrometastasis
systemic m.
micrometastatic disease
micronodular
m. cirrhosis
m. infiltrate
m. lung disease
m. metastasis
m. pattern
micronodule
centrilobular m.
micropapillary
m. carcinoma
m. lesion
Micropaque
microperforation
microporous membrane
microprolactinoma
micropuncture needle
microradiography
microreentrant circuit
microsatellite instability
microscanner
pQCT m.
microscintigraphy
microscope
scanning acoustic m. (SAM)
scanning electron m. (SEM)
x-ray tomographic m. (XTM)
microscopic
m. cortical dysplasia
m. hemorrhage of ligament
m. imaging
m. polyangiitis
microscopy
darkfield m.
DIC m.
differential interference contrast microscopy
3D magnetic resonance m.
electron m.
immune electron m.
light m.
ultrasound backscatter m. (UBM)
in vivo m.

NOTES

M

microsecond pulsed flashlamp pumped dye laser
microsomia
hemifacial m.
microsphere
acrylic m.
degradable starch m.
ferromagnetic m.
m. perfusion scintigraphy
silicone m.
stainless steel m.
superparamagnetic m.
technetium-99m albumin m.
technetium-99m human albumin m.
trisacryl gelatin m.
ytterbium-90 m.
yttrium-90 m.
micro tear
microtomography
view m.
Microtrast
microtrauma
repetitive m.
microtron accelerator
microvascular
m. circulation
m. decompression (MVD)
m. disease
m. retrieval
microvasculature
pulmonary m.
microvenoarteriolar fistula
microvesicular fat
microvolt (μV)
microwave
m. hyperthermia
m. hyperthermia treatment
m. imaging
m. therapy
MID
multiinfarct dementia
midabdominal wall
midaortic
m. arch
m. syndrome
midaxillary line
midazolam
midbody
m. of vertebra
midbrain
m. aqueduct
m. function
m. lesion
m. reticular formation (MRF)
m. tegmentum
tegmentum of pons and m.
midcarpal
m. compartment
m. dislocation
m. instability
m. joint
m. joint cavity
midcircumflex
midclavicular
m. line (MCL)
m. plane
midcolon
midcoronal
m. oblique image
m. plane
mid-diastole
mid-distal
middle
m. aortic syndrome
m. cardiac vein
m. cerebral artery
m. cerebral artery bifurcation
m. cerebral artery infarct
m. coronary sinus (MCS)
m. cranial fossa
m. cuneiform bone
m. ear
m. ear choristoma
m. ear mass
m. ear neoplasm
m. extrahepatic bile duct
m. finger
m. fossa syndrome
m. frontal gyrus
m. hepatic vein (MHV)
m. lobe (ML)
m. lobe bronchus
m. lobe syndrome
m. mediastinal mass
m. mediastinum
m. meningeal
m. meningeal artery
m. meningeal artery groove
m. muscle
m. perforating collagen bundle
m. pole
m. pulmonary lobe atelectasis
m. rectal vein
m. temporal gyrus
m. third shaft
m. third of thoracic esophagus
m. turbinate bone
middle-field-strength MR imaging
middorsal
midepigastrium
midesophageal diverticulum
midesophagus
midexpiratory tidal flow
midface
fetal m.
m. retrusion

midfacial fracture
midfemur
midfoot fracture
midfrontal
m. plane
m. plane coronal section
midget MRI scanner
midgraft stenosis
mid-groove portion of lumina
midgut
m. volvulus
m. volvulus with malrotation
midhumeral line
midinguinal point
midlateral course
midleft sternal border
midline
m. of brain cyst
m. cerebellum
m. cystic structure
m. granuloma
m. herniation of disk
infracolic m.
m. lesion
m. malignant reticulosis
m. mucosa-sparing block
m. parasagittal focus
m. shift
mid-lung
m.-l. field
m.-l. zone
midmarginal
m. branch
m. branch of artery
midpalmar
m. abscess
m. space
midpelvis
midplane
m. depth
m. sagittal image
midpole
midportion
midsagittal
m. diameter (MSD)
m. MR image
m. MR imaging
m. plane
midscapular line
midshaft fracture
midshunt peak velocity (MSPv)
midsigmoid colon
midspinal line
midsternal
m. area
m. line
midsternum
midsystolic
m. buckling of mitral valve
m. notching of velocity spectrum
m. retraction
midtarsal
m. injury
m. joint
midthalamic plane
midthigh amputation
midthoracic spine
midventricular short-axis slice
midwaist scaphoid fracture
midzonal necrosis
mid-zone
Miescher granulomatosis
Mignon granuloma
migraine
migrainous scintillation
migrans
necrolytic erythema m.
visceral brain large m.
visceral larva m.
migration
m. of acetabular cup
catheter m.
embolus m.
gallstone m.
hallux m.
neuronal m.
placenta m.
sesamoid m.
stent m.
tissue m.
migrational
m. abnormality
m. anomaly
migratory
m. patchy infiltrate
m. pneumonia
Mikity-Wilson syndrome
Mikulicz
M. angle
M. disease
M. syndrome

M

NOTES

Milch
M. classification of humeral fractures
M. elbow fracture classification
mild
m. edema
m. head injury
m. subcostal retraction
mildly enlarged heart
miliary
m. aneurysm
m. embolus
m. granuloma
m. lung disease
m. nodule
m. pattern
m. pulmonary tuberculosis
m. tuberculosis
milk
m. of calcium
m. of calcium urinary tract cyst
human m.
m. leg syndrome
m. teeth
milk-alkali syndrome
milkmaid's
m. elbow
m. elbow dislocation
milkman's
m. fracture
m. pseudofracture
Milkman syndrome
milk-of-calcium
m.-o.-c. microcyst
milky
m. effusion
m. way breast
Millar catheter-tip transducer
Miller
M. disease
M. position
Miller-Dieker syndrome
miller's lung
milliampere (ma, mA)
milliampere-second (mAs)
millicurie (mCi)
millijoule (mJ)
Millikan-Siekert syndrome
milliliter (mL)
microcurie per m.
millimeter (mm)
millimeters of mercury (mmHg, mm Hg)
millimole (mmol)
million
parts per m.
millirad (mrad)
milliroentgen (mr)
millisecond (ms, msec)
millivolt (mV)
Milophene
Milroy disease
Milton angioedema disease
Milwaukee
M. brace
M. shoulder syndrome
MIMIC
multivane intensity modulation compensator
mimic
mimicked
mimicker of malignancy
mimicking
mimosa pattern
Minaar classification of coalition
minced rib
mind-body interaction
mineral
m. oil contrast
m. oil imaging agent
mineralization
bone m.
mineralizing microangiopathy
mineralocorticoid secretion
miner's lung
Ming classification of gastric carcinoma
miniature
m. imaging
m. stomach
m. uterine cavity
miniaturized mitral valve
Mini-Balloon system
minicalyx
MINI 6000 C-arm
minicholecystostomy
surgical-radiologic m.
minicoil
minification
minimal
m. luminal diameter (MLD)
m. port diameter (MPD)
m. volume
minimally displaced fracture
minimi
flexor digiti m.
opponens digiti m.
mini-microaggregated albumin colloid (MMAA)
minimum
m. blood pressure
m. intensity projection imaging

m. intensity projection (MIP) image
m. tolerance dose
minimum-intensity sliding thin slab projection
minimus
digitus m.
gluteus m.
scalenus m.
m. scalenus muscle
mining
miniovoid
ministem shaft
Minix
Medtronic M.
minor
m. calix
m. duodenal papilla
m. fissure
globus m.
m. muscle
pectoralis m.
rhomboid m.
teres m.
Minor sign
Minot-von Willebrand syndrome
minus
omentum m.
minusculc
minute
m. bleeding ulcer
blood volume per m.
cycles per m. (cpm)
rotations per m. (rpm)
m. ventilation
m. vessels
m. volume
minute-sequence study
MION
monocrystalline iron oxides
miosis
miotic
MIP
macrophage inflammatory protein
maximum intensity pixel
MIP reconstruction
MIPcor
coronal maximum-intensity projection
coronary maximum-intensity projection
MIR
Mallinckrodt Institute of Radiology
MIR guidclines
MIR intrauterine tandem
MIR system
mirabile
rete m.
miracidia
MIRALVA applicator
MIRD
medical internal radiation dose
medical internal radiation dosimetry
MIRI
myocardial infarction recovery index
Mirizzi syndrome
mirror
beam-splitting m.
m. image aneurysm
m. image reversal
m. imaging
polygon m.
mirror-image
m.-i. artifact
m.-i. brachiocephalic branching
m.-i. interpretation
misalign
miscarriage
misery perfusion
misleading
m. image
m. imaging
mismapping
phase m.
mismatch
FDG-blood flow m.
perfusion-metabolism m.
ventilation-perfusion m.
V/Q m.
misplaced thoracentesis
misregistration
m. artifact
oblique flow m.
missed
m. abortion
m. testicular torsion
missile
m. effect
m. wound
missing pulse steady-state free precession sequence
MIT
monoiodotyrosine
Mitchell classification
mitochondrial
m. encephalomyopathy

NOTES

mitochondrial *(continued)*
m. myopathy, encephalopathy, lactic acidosis, and stroke-like episodes (MELAS)
m. uncoupler
mitosis sign
mitozolomide
mitral
m. apparatus
m. arcade
m. component
m. configuration of cardiac shadow
m. deceleration slope
m. flow velocity index
m. inflow velocity
m. insufficiency (MI)
m. leaflet
m. leak
m. orifice (MO)
posterior m. (PM)
m. regurgitant signal area
m. regurgitation (MR)
m. regurgitation artifact
m. regurgitation-chordal elongation syndrome
m. ring calcification
m. stenosis (MS)
m. valve
m. valve of annulus
m. valve area (MVA)
m. valve atresia
m. valve calcification
m. valve commissure
m. valve cusp
m. valve deformity
m. valve echocardiography
m. valve echogram
m. valve flow
m. valve gradient
m. valve incompetence
m. valve leaflet systolic prolapse
m. valve leaflet tip
m. valve myxomatous degeneration
m. valve opening (MVO)
m. valve orifice (MVO)
m. valve prolapse (MVP)
m. valve regurgitation
m. valve replacement (MVR)
m. valve ring
m. valve septal separation
m. valve stenosis (MVS)
m. valve systolic anterior motion
mitralization
Mitsuyasu staging system
mixed
m. aneurysm
m. bone lesion
m. cell sarcoma
m. connective tissue disease (MCTD)
m. echogenic solid mass
m. fat-water breast lesion density
m. fat-water density lesion
m. germ-cell tumor
m. gonadal dysgenesis
m. IUGR
m. lymphocytic-histiocytic lymphoma
m. petal-fugal flow
m. restrictive-obstructive lung disease
m. rheumatoid and degenerative arthritis
m. sclerotic and lytic bone lesion
m. sclerotic osteolysis
m. small and large cell lymphoma
m. venous blood
m. venous-lymphatic malformation
m. venous saturation
mixed-attenuation mass
mixed-density mass
mixed-signal mass
mixelitine
mixture
barium m.
mJ
millijoule
ML
middle lobe
mL
milliliter
MLC
multileaf collimator
MLD
minimal luminal diameter
MLF
medial longitudinal fasciculus
MLF lesion
MLO
mediolateral oblique
MLS
multiple line scan
mm
millimeter
MMAA
mini-microaggregated albumin colloid
^{99m}Tc MMAA
technetium-99m mini-microaggregated albumin
MMEF
MMFR
maximum midexpiratory flow rate
mmHg, mm Hg
millimeters of mercury
MMM
myelofibrosis with myeloid metaplasia

M-mode
time-motion mode
M-mode display
M-mode echocardiogram imaging
M-mode echocardiography
M-mode echophonocardiography
M-mode sector transducer
M-mode ultrasound
mmol
millimole
Mn
manganese
Mn-TPPS$_4$
manganese tetrasodium-meso-tetra
MO
mitral orifice
Mo
molybdenum
^{99}Mo
molybdenum-99
MoAb
^{131}I-labeled human M.
radiolabeled M.
Moberg-Gedda fracture
Mobetron electron beam system
mobile
cecum m.
cor m.
m. duodenum
m. fluoroscopy
m. gallbladder
m. intraluminal gallbladder mass
m. magnetic resonance
m. radiography
m. thrombus
m. without recapture
m. with recapture
Mobin-Uddin
Mobitz I or II heart block
modality
multislice m.
mode
AAI m.
AAI rate-responsive m.
m. abandonment
active m.
asynchronous transfer m. (ATM)
blink m.
brightness m.
byte m.
cine m.
continuous m.
dispersion m.
dual-demand pacing m.
DVI m.
digital vascular imaging
full-to-empty VAD m.
high-frame-rate m.
high spatial resolution m.
high temporal resolution m.
imaginary m.
inactive m.
magnet m.
motion m.
multiplanar m.
multislice m.
noncommitted m.
pulsed m.
road-mapping m.
semicommitted m.
sequential m.
stimulated-echo acquisition m. (STEAM)
stimulation m.
time-motion m. (M-mode)
triggered pacing m.
underdrive m.
unipolar pacing m.
modeling
3D m.
electromagnetic m.
Monte Carlo m.
thermal m.
three-dimensional m.
ultrasonographic m.
moderately
m. differentiated adenoma
m. dilated ureter
m. well-differentiated carcinoma
moderator band
modest caliber
Modic disk abnormality classification
modification
thiol m.
modified
m. birdcage coil
m. Bruce protocol
m. electron-beam CT scanner
m. Naughton-Balke treadmill protocol
m. projection
m. Simpson rule
m. stage exercise
m. vessel image processor software

NOTES

M

modiolus
modulation
amplitude m.
brightness m.
off-center m.
print reflectance m.
specific m.
m. transfer function (MTF)
module
detecting m.
E-TOF (electron time-of-flight) detecting m.
tube geometry m.
Modulith SL 20
modulus
m. image
Moe and Kettleson distribution of curves in scoliosis
Moenckeberg
M. arteriosclerosis
M. calcification
Mohn-Wriedt brachydactyly
Mohrenheim space
Mohr syndrome
Mohs micrographic surgery
moiety, pl. **moieties**
upper pole m.
moiré
m. fringe
m. fringes artifact
m. pattern
M. photography
molar
m. mass
m. pregnancy
m. teeth
m. tooth configuration
m. tooth fracture
mold
filter m.
molding
atheroma m.
m. of skull
molecular
m. diffusion
m. recognition unit (MRU)
m. weight dependence of relaxation
molecule
accessory adhesion m.
adhesion m.
homing m.
intracellular adhesion m.
molecule-1
vascular cell adhesion m.
moliolus
Moll
adenocarcinoma of M.
molle
fibroma m.
heloma m.
papilloma m.
molluscoid
pseudotumor m.
molluscum, pl. **mollusca**
fibroma m.
m. fibrosum
Molnar disk
molybdenum (Mo)
m. anode
m. target
m. target tube
molybdenum-99 (^{99}Mo)
m. breakthrough test
m. generator
molybdenum-technetium generator
MOM
multiples of the median
moment
macroscopic magnetic m.
magnetic dipole m.
nuclear magnetic m.
quadripole m.
zeroth m.
momentum
angular m.
Monakow tract
monarticular
m. process
m. synovium-based cartilage metaplasia
Mönckeberg
M. arteriosclerosis
M. calcification
M. degeneration
M. medial sclerosis
Mondini
M. anomaly
M. dysplasia
M. malformation
Mondor disease
mongolian spotlike lesion
mongolism
mongoloid features
moniliasis
monitor
beam m.
blood perfusion m. (BPM)
cardiac m.
Doplette m.
Doppler blood flow m.
Doppler ultrasonic fetal heart m.
Life-Pack 5 cardiac m.
radiation m.
radiation beam m.
m. unit

monitoring
electrode m.
m. electrode
photoplethysmographic m.
ultrasound m.
monoarticular
monochorionic
m. diamniotic twin pregnancy
m. monoamniotic twin pregnancy
monochorionic-monoamniotic twin
monochromatic
m. radiation
m. synchrotron
m. synchrotron radiation
Monoclate
monoclonal antibody imaging agent
monocrystalline iron oxides (MION)
monocusp valve
monocyte
monocytopenia
monodactylism
monodermal dermoid
monodisk
monoiodobenzylguanidine (^{131}I-mIB6)
monoiodotyrosine (MIT)
monomalleolar fracture
monomer
ionic m.
nonionic m.
monophasic
Monophen
monophosphate
cyclic adenosine m.
cyclic guanosine m.
monopolar radiofrequency electrocautery
Monopty needle
monorchia
monosodium urate crystals (MSU)
monosomy X
monostotic
m. fibrous dysplasia
monoventricle
monoxide
^{11}C carbon m.
monozygotic twin
Monro
M. aqueduct
M. bursa
mons pubis
monstrocellular sarcoma
Monte
M. Carlo calculation
M. Carlo modeling
M. Carlo photon transport (MCPT)
M. Carlo photon transport simulation
M. Carlo technique
Monteggia
M. dislocation
M. fracture
M. lesion
Montercaux fracture
Montgomery gland
moon sign
Moore fracture
Morand spur
morbid event
morcellation
Robinson-Chung-Farahvar clavicular m.
morcellized bone
Morel syndrome
Morgagni
M. appendix
appendix of M.
column of M.
M. crypt
crypt of M.
foramen of M.
M. foramen
M. hernia
M. hydatid
hyperostosis of M.
M. lacuna
lacuna of M.
M. nodule
sinus of M.
M. syndrome
tubercle of M.
M. ventricle
Morgagni-Adams-Stokes (MAS)
M.-A.-S. syndrome
morgagnian cyst
Morison pouch
morphine
m. sulfate
m. sulfate scintigraphy
morphine-augmented study
morphogen
morphologic
m. criteria
m. growth
m. left ventricle

NOTES

M

morphological
m. correlation
m. and physiological image coregistration
morphologically normal
morphology
bow-tie m.
enhancement m.
joint m.
ovarian m.
residuum m.
turning-point m.
morphometric measurement
morphometry
MRI m.
Morquio
M. sign
M. syndrome
Morris point
mortise
ankle m.
ball-and-socket ankle m.
m. of bone
cuneiform m.
diaphyseal cortical m.
m. joint
m. radiograph
m. view
Morton
M. neuroma
M. toe
Morton-Horwitz nerve crossover sign
morula
MOS
M. capacitator
mosaic
m. artifact
m. attenuation pattern
m. duodenal mucosal pattern
m. pattern
m. perfusion
mosaic-jet signal
Moschcowitz sign
Mose
M. concentric ring
M. technique
MoSearch
Mossbauer spectrometer
moth-eaten
m.-e. appearance
m.-e. bone destruction
m.-e. pattern
mother
infant of diabetic m. (IDM)
mother-in-law phenomenon
motilin
motility
antroduodenal m.
colonic m.
m. disorder
esophageal m.
m. of Golden
ileal m.
jejunal m.
small bowel m.
m. study
motion
akinetic segmental wall m.
anterior wall m.
apical wall m.
m. artifact
m. artifact suppression technique (MAST)
m. blur
bowel m.
brisk wall m.
brownian water m.
cardiac wall m.
catheter tip m.
chest wall paradoxical m.
m. compensation gradient pulse
cusp m.
discernible venous m.
dyskinetic segmental wall m.
forceful parasternal m.
heaving precordial m.
hyperkinetic segmental wall m.
hypokinetic segmental wall m.
incoherent m.
inferior wall m.
intravoxel coherent m.
intravoxel incoherent m.
isotropic m.
leaflet m.
left ventricular function wall m.
left ventricular regional wall m.
limitation of joint m.
linear accelerator isocenter m.
mitral valve systolic anterior m.
m. mode
paradoxical leaflet m.
paradoxical septal m.
parasternal m.
patient m.
photoreceptor m.
posterior wall m.
posterolateral wall m.
precessional m.
random m.
rapid oscillatory m.
regional hypokinetic wall m.
respiratory m.
rocking precordial m.
rotational m.
scapulothoracic m.
segmental wall m.

septal wall m.
stationary zero-order m.
sustained anterior parasternal m.
swirling m.
systolic anterior m. (SAM)
time m. (TM)
translational m.
trifid precordial motion m.
m. unsharpness
venous m.
ventricular wall m.
vibratory m.
visible anterior m.
wall m.
within-view m.

motional
m. averaging
m. narrowing

motion-compensating format converter
motion-induced phase shift
motion-related impingement syndrome
motion-triggered cine kinematic MR image
motoneuron
motor
m. area
m. branch
m. cortex
m. impairment
m. meal barium GI series
m. nucleus
m. paralytic neurogenic bladder
m. reinnervation
m. root
m. sign
m. test meal
m. tract
m. urge incontinence
m. vehicle injury (MVI)
versive m.

motorcyclist's knee
MOTSA
multiple overlapping thin-slab acquisition

mottle
photon m.
quantum m.
radiographic m.

mottled
m. appearance
m. calcification
m. density
m. distribution
m. echotexture
m. gray lung
m. hepatic uptake
m. infiltrate
m. liver uptake
m. pattern
m. thickening

mottling
diffuse m.

Mouchet fracture
moulage sign
mound
infraumbilical m.

Mounier-Kuhn
M.-K. disease
M.-K. syndrome

Mounod sign
mouse
m. bed sign
m. ear erosion
peritoneal m.

mouth (os)
floor of m.
tapir's m.

movable
m. heart
m. kidney

movement
arcuate m.
m. artifact
bowel m.
fetal m. (FM)
fetal breathing m. (FBM)
fiducial m.
m. pattern
pendulum m.
propulsive m.
spontaneous fetal m.
systolic anterior m.

movie sign
moving-slot radiography
moyamoya syndrome
Moyer line
Moynahan syndrome
MPA
main pulmonary artery
MPA pressure

MPAP
mean pulmonary artery pressure
multipurpose access port

MPCh
medial posterior choroidal

NOTES

MPCP
mean pulmonary capillary pressure
MPD
main pancreatic duct
main papillary duct
matched peripheral dose
maximum permissible dose
minimal port diameter
multiplanar display
MPGR
multiplanar gradient recall
MPGR technique
MPHR
maximum predicted heart rate
MPPv
main portal vein peak velocity
MPR
myocardial perfusion reserve
MPR view
MP-RAGE
magnitude preparation-rapid acquisition gradient echo
MP-RAGE protocol
MP-RAGE sequence
MP-RAGE technique
MP-RAGE-WE
magnetization-prepared rapid gradient echo-water excitation
mps
meters per second
MR
magnetic resonance
mitral regurgitation
MR catheter imaging and spectroscopy system scanner
chemical-selective fat-saturation MR
combined multisection diffuse-weighted and hemodynamically weighted echoplanar MR
contrast-enhanced MR
echo FLASH MR
MR echoplanar imaging
first-pass myocardial perfusion MR
MR imaging
lipid-sensitive MR
oxygenation-sensitive functional MR
MR proton spectroscopy
MR simulator
susceptibility weighted MR
mr
milliroentgen
MRA
magnetic resonance angiography
MRA imaging
mrad
millirad
MRC
magnetic resonance cholangiogram
MRCP
magnetic resonance cholangiopancreatography
MRE
magnetic resonance elastography
MRF
midbrain reticular formation
MRI
magnetic resonance imaging
cardiac MRI
chondroitin sulfate iron colloid-enhanced MRI
cine MRI
CSI-enhanced MRI
CSIS-enhanced MRI
dynamic contrast-enhanced MRI
electrocardiogram-gated MRI
extremity MRI (E-MRI)
functional MRI
Gd-DTPA-enhanced turbo FLASH MRI
intravenously enhanced MRI
IV-enhanced MRI
laser-polarized helium MRI
magnetoacoustic MRI
MRI mapping
MRI morphometry
multinuclear MRI
multiplanar MRI
open MRI
opposed-phase MRI
perfusion-weighted MRI
MRI prescan
MRI probe head
MRI probehead
proton-density-weighted MRI
pulsed magnetization transfer contrast MRI
rapid-acquisition relaxation-enhanced MRI
rapid axial MRI
MRI segmentation
T2 quantitative MRI
MRI-guided
M.-g. breast biopsy
M.-g. focused ultrasound transducer
M.-g. laser-induced interstitial imaging
M.-g. laser-induced interstitial thermotherapy
MRM
magnetic resonance mammography
MRN
magnetic resonance neurography
MRS
magnetic resonance spectroscopy
slice-point MRS

MRU
magnetic resonance urography
molecular recognition unit
ThromboScan MRU
MS
mitral stenosis
ms
millisecond
MS-325 contrast agent
MSA
multiple system atrophy
MSA syndrome
MSAD
multiple scan average dose
MSD
midsagittal diameter
msec
millisecond
M-shaped
M.-s. mitral valve pattern
M.-s. pattern of mitral valve
MSI
magnetic source imaging
MSPv
midshunt peak velocity
MSTS
Musculoskeletal Tumor Society
MSTS staging
MSU
monosodium urate crystals
MT
magnetization transfer
MTA
medullary-type adenocarcinoma
MTC
magnetization transfer contrast
99mTc-HMPAO
MTE
main timing event
MTF
modulation transfer function
MTP
metatarsophalangeal
MTP joint
MTPJ
metatarsophalangeal joint
MTR
magnetization transfer ratio
MTT
mean pulmonary transit time
m-tyrosine
^{18}F-labeled derivatives of m.-t.
mu (μ)
m. meson
m. rhythm
mucin-hypersecreting carcinoma
mucinosis
follicular m.
mucinous
m. adenocarcinoma
m. adenoma
m. breast carcinoma
m. cyst
m. cystadenocarcinoma
m. cystadenoma
m. degeneration
m. ductal ectasia of the pancreas
m. ductectatic tumor of pancreas
m. ovarian cystadenocarcinoma
m. ovarian tumor
m. pancreatic cystic neoplasm
mucin-producing
m.-p. adenocarcinoma
m.-p. carcinoma
mucocele
appendix m.
breast m.
bronchial m.
frontal sinus m.
frontoethmoidal m.
orbital m.
paranasal sinus m.
mucocutaneous
m. junction
m. lymph node syndrome (MCLS)
mucoepidermoid
m. carcinoma
m. carcinoma parotis
m. lung carcinoma
mucoid
m. degeneration of umbilical cord
m. impaction
m. impaction of bronchus
m. plugging of airway
m. umbilical cord degeneration
mucopolysaccharidosis cardiomyopathy
mucopyocele
mucormycosis
lung m.
rhinocerebral m.
mucosa, pl. **mucosae**
bronchial m.
buccal m.

NOTES

M

mucosa *(continued)*
burned-out m.
cobblestone m.
colorectal m.
endocervical m.
friable m.
frothy colonic m.
isoeffective bronchial m.
muscularis m.
m. muscularis
nasal m.
outpocketings of m.
polypoid m.
prolapsed antral m.
prolapsed gastric m.
sloughed m.
mucosa-associated
m.-a. lymphoid tissue (MALT)
mucosal
m. abnormality
m. bridge
m. crinkling
m. destruction
m. esophageal stripe sign
m. esophageal tumor
m. fold
m. ganglioneurofibromatosis
m. gland
m. hyperplasia
m. inflammation
m. island
m. lesion
m. lining
m. mass collecting system
m. melanoma
m. necrosis
m. neuroma syndrome
m. pattern
m. pharyngeal space
m. prolapse syndrome
m. relief radiography
m. suspensory ligament
m. thickening
m. ulcer
mucosalesophageal nodule
mucosa-sparing block
mucosum
ligamentum m.
mucous
m. bronchogram
m. carcinoma
m. degeneration
m. fistula
m. lake
m. lake of stomach
m. membrane
m. membrane hyperemia
m. polyp
m. pseudomass
m. retention cyst
mucoviscidosis
mucus
m. hypersecretion
m. plug
m. plugging
m. plug syndrome
mud
biliary m.
Mueller (*var. of* Müller)
MUGA
multiple gated acquisition
MUGA cardiac blood pool imaging
first-pass MUGA
MUGA scan
Muir and Bruce tract
Muir-Torre of hereditary nonpolyposis colon cancer
Mukherjee-Sivaya view
mulberry
m. calculus
m. eye lesion
m. gallstone
m. ovary
m. type classification
mulberry-type calcification
Mulder sign
Müller, Mueller
M. canal
M. fibers
M. humerus fracture classification
M. maneuver
M. muscle
M. sign
M. test
M. tray
M. trigone
müllerian
m. duct
m. duct anomaly
m. duct cyst
multangular
m. bone
m. ridge fracture
multangulum
multiaccess catheter (MAC)
multiarc LINAC radiosurgery
multiaxial classification
multibreath washout study
multicentric
m. angiofollicular lymph node
m. basal cell carcinoma
m. Castleman disease
m. fibromatosis
m. germinoma
m. glioblastoma
m. lytic lesion

m. malignant glioma
m. meningioma
m. osteogenic sarcoma
m. osteosarcoma
multichannel analyzer (MCA)
multicolor flow cytometry
multicompartment clearance
multicoupled loop-gap resonator
multicrystal gamma camera
multicystic
m. acoustic neuroma
m. dysgenetic kidney
m. dysplasia
m. dysplastic kidney (MCDK)
m. kidney (MCK)
multidetector system
multidose vial
multidrug-resistant tuberculosis
multiecho
m. axial
m. axial image
m. coronal image
m. imaging
preinversion m. (PRIME)
m. sequence
standard m.
multielectrode impedance catheter
multielemental neutron activation analysis
multiexponential
m. relaxation
multifield beam
multifocal
m. aggressive infiltrate
m. anaplastic astrocytoma
m. area of hyperintensity
m. brain tumor
m. breast cancer
m. enhancing brain lesion
m. glioblastoma multiforme
m. infarct
m. leukoencephalopathy
m. lymphoma
m. nephroblastomatosis
m. osteosarcoma
m. short stenosis
m. subperitoneal sclerosis
multiformat camera
multiformatted imaging
multiforme
glioblastoma m. (GBM)
multifocal glioblastoma m.
multiform ventricular complex
multigated pulsed Doppler flow system
multigravida
multiilluminant color correction
multiinfarct dementia (MID)
multiinterval
multilamellar periosteal reaction
multilaminar bodies
multileaf
m. collimating system
m. collimator (MLC)
multilevel fusion
multiline scanning technique
multilobular
m. cirrhosis
m. configuration
multilobulated mass
multilocular
m. cystic lesion
m. cystic nephroma
m. renal cyst
multiloculated mass
multilog effect
multimodal image fusion technique
multimodality imaging
multinodular
m. goiter
m. thyroid
multinuclear MRI
multiorgan imaging
multipara
multiparametric color composite display
multiparous
multiparticle cyclotron
multipartite
m. fracture
m. patella
multipennate muscle
multiphasic
m. CT
m. multislice MRI technique
m. multislice spin-echo imaging technique
m. renal computerized tomography
multiplanar
m. compression
m. display (MPD)
m. gradient-echo software
m. gradient recall (MPGR)
m. gradient-recalled echo
m. gradient refocus
m. gradient refocused sequence

NOTES

M

multiplanar *(continued)*
m. mode
m. MRI
m. MR imaging
phase-offset m. (POMP)
phase-ordered m. (POMP)
m. reconstruction
m. reformation
m. reformatted radiographic and digitally reconstructed radiographic imaging
m. reformatting
m. reformatting view (MPR view)
m. scanning
m. transesophageal echocardiography

multiplane dosage calculation

multiple
m. bile duct hamartomas
m. blocks
m. bone myeloma
m. bull's eye lesions bowel wall
m. chords
m. colon filling defects
m. concentric GI rings
m. congenital anomalies (MCA)
m. congenital fibromatosis
m. cortical infarcts
m. emboli
m. enchondromatosis
m. endocrine neoplasia syndrome
m. endocrine neoplasms (MEN)
m. epiphyseal dysplasia
m. fetuses
m. fibroxanthomata
m. focal lesions of spinal cord
m. focus
m. fractures
m. gated acquisition (MUGA)
m. gated acquisition scan
m. gestation
m. gland disease
m. hereditary exostoses
m. idiopathic hemorrhagic sarcoma
m. jointed digitizer
m. jointed digitizer scanner
m. kidney myeloma
m.-lesion osteosclerosis
m. line scan (MLS)
m. loops of small bowel
m. lucent lung lesion
m. lung nodule
m. lytic bone lesions
m. mural dilatation
m. organ failure
m. osteochondromatosis
m. osteolysis
m. osteosclerotic lesions
m. overlapping thin-slab acquisition (MOTSA)
m. parotid gland lesions
m. peripheral papillomas
m. planar gradient-recalled images
m. pleural densities
m. polyposis
m. polyps
m. pregnancy
m. pterygium syndrome
m. pulmonary calcifications
m. pulmonary cysts
m. scan average dose (MSAD)
m. sclerosis
m. sclerosis (MS) plaque
m. sclerosis (MS) plaquing
m. sclerosis plateau
m. sclerotic osteosarcoma
m. sensitive points
m. slice acquisition
m. small bowel filling defects
m. small bowel stenosis
m. small bowel ulcers
m. stenotic lesions
m. stenotic lesions of small bowel
m. stones
m. symmetrical lipomatosis
m. system atrophy (MSA)
m. system atrophy syndrome
m. thin-walled lung cavities
m. thyroid cysts
m. trauma
m. vacuum phenomenon
m. vascular leiomyomas

multiple-beam interface spacing

multiple-echo imaging

multiple-exposure volumetric holography

multiple-gated
m.-g. acquisition scan
m.-g. blood pool imaging

multiple-line
m.-l. scan imaging
m.-l. scanning method

multiple-plane imaging

multiple-sensitive-point method

multiples of the median (MOM)

multiple-suture synostosis

multiplex
dysostosis m.
dysplasia epiphysealis m.

multiplexing

multiplying digital-to-analog converter (MDAC)

Multi-Pro biopsy needle

multipurpose access port (MPAP)

multiray fracture

multirod collimator

multisection
m. diffuse-weighted magnetic resonance imaging
m. method
m. multirepetition acquisition
multisectional dose-volume histogram
multisensor
m. structured light range digitizer
m. structured light-range digitizer scanner
multiseptate appearance
multiseptated gallbladder
multishot echoplanar imaging
multislab magnetic resonance angiography
multislice
m. acquisition
ECG-gated m.
m. first-pass myocardial perfusion imaging
m. FLASH 2D
m. flow-related enhancement
m. modality
m. mode
m. modified KEW direct Fournier imaging
m. spin-echo sequence
m. spin-echo technique
two-dimensional m.
multispectral diffuse transillumination
multispin relaxation
multisweep
high-resolution m. (HRMS)
multitime point imaging
multitracer
m. imaging
m. study
multivane intensity modulation compensator (MIMIC)
multivariant
m. regressional analysis
multizone transmit-receive focus
Münchmeyer disease
MUPIT
Martinez universal interstitial template
mural
m. aneurysm
m. arch
m. architecture
m. clot
m. CNS nodule
m. defect
m. degeneration
m. dilatation
m. endomyocardial fibrosis
m. fibrosing alveolitis
m. hematoma
m. infiltrate
m. kidney
m. leaflet of mitral valve
m. pregnancy
m. stratification
m. thickening
m. thrombus
m. thrombus formation
muramidase
Murphy sign
muscle
abductor digiti quinti m.
abductor hallucis m.
abductor pollicis brevis m.
accessory m.
adductor magnus m.
Aeby m.
Albinus m.
anconeus m.
anterior papillary m. (APM)
antigravity m.
m. artifact
m. atrophy
auricular m.
axillary m.
BBC m.'s
belly of m.
biceps femoris m.
bipennate m.
Bochdalek m.
Bovero m.
Bowman m.
brachioradialis m.
Braune m.
Brücke m.
bulbocavernosus m.
m. bulk
cardiac m.
Casser m.
casserian m.
cervical m.
Chassaignac m.
chin m.
circular m.
Coiter m.
conal papillary m.
m. contracture

NOTES

muscle *(continued)*
Crampton m.
cricopharyngeus m.
dartos m.
deep m.
m. of deglutition
detrusor m.
digastric m.
dorsal m.
Dupré m.
Duverney m.
ECRB m.
ECRL m.
ECU m.
EDB m.
EDC m.
EDL m.
EDQ m.
EHL m.
extensor hallucis longus muscle
EIP m.
EPB m.
EPL m.
extensor carpi radialis brevis m.
extensor carpi radialis longus m.
extensor carpi ulnaris m.
extensor digiti quinti m.
extensor digitorum brevis m.
extensor digitorum communis m.
extensor digitorum longus m.
extensor hallucis longus m. (EHL muscle)
extensor indicis proprius m.
extensor pollicis brevis m.
extensor pollicis longus m.
external oblique m.
extraocular m.
extrinsic foot m.
FCR m.
flexor carpi radialis muscle
FDI m.
first digital interosseous muscle
FDL m.
FDP m.
flexor digitorum profundus muscle
FDQB m.
FDS m.
FHB m.
flexor hallucis brevis muscle
m. fiber
m. fiber wasting
fibrosed m.
first digital interosseous m. (FDI muscle)
fixator m.
flexor carpi radialis m. (FCR muscle)
flexor digiti quinti brevis m.
flexor digitorum longus m.
flexor digitorum profundus m. (FDP muscle)
flexor digitorum superficialis m.
flexor hallucis brevis m. (FHB muscle)
Folius m.
frontotemporal m.
fused papillary m.
Gantzer m.
gastrocnemius m.
Gavard m.
genioglossus m.
Guthrie m.
Hilton m.
Horner m.
Houston m.
hyoglossus m.
hyperintense m.
m. hyperintensity
ileococcygeus m.
iliocostal m.
iliopsoas m.
m. infarct
infarcted heart m.
inferior gemellus m.
infraspinatus m.
innermost intercostal m.
intercostal m.
internal intercostal m.
interosseous m.
interspinal m.
intertransverse m.
intraauricular m.
intrinsic foot m.
m. irritability
ischiocavernosus m.
Jung m.
Klein m.
Lancisi m.
lateral pterygoid m.
lateral rectus m.
latissimus dorsi m.
left ventricular m.
lesser m.
levator m.
longitudinal m.
longus colli m.
Luschka m.
Macalister m.
major m.
Marcacci m.
masseter m.
masticator m.
medial papillary m.
medial pterygoid m.
Merkel m.
middle m.

minimus scalenus m.
minor m.
Müller m.
multipennate m.
mylohyoid m.
myocardial m.
nonstriated m.
oblique m.
obturator internus m.
occipitofrontalis m.
Ochsner m.
Oddi m.
ODQ m.
Oehl m.
omohyoid m.
opponens digiti quinti m.
opposing m.
organic m.
m. ossification
palatal m.
papillary m.
paralaryngeal m.
paraspinal m.
Passavant m.
pectineus m.
pectoralis major m.
pectoralis minor m.
peroneal m.
peroneus quartus m.
pharyngeal m.
Phillips m.
piriform m.
piriformis m.
plantaris m.
platysma m.
posterior papillary m. (PPM)
Pozzi m.
psoas m.
pterygoid m.
pubococcygeus m.
pupillary constrictor m.
pyloric m.
quadrate m.
quadriceps m.
reactive disease of smooth m.
m. recruitment pattern
rectus m.
Reisseisen m.
retronuchal m.
rhomboideus major m.
ribbon m.
rider m.
Riolan m.
rotator cuff m.
Rouget m.
round m.
Ruysch m.
sacrospinalis m.
Santorini m.
sartorius m.
scalenus anterior m.
Sebileau m.
semimembranous m.
semispinal m.
semitendinous m.
septal papillary m.
serratus anterior m.
m. sheath
short m.
shoulder m.
Sibson m.
skeletal m.
smooth m.
Soemmerring m.
soleus m.
somatic m.
m. spasm
sphenomandibularis m.
m. spindle
spindle-shaped m.
sternocleidomastoid m.
sternohyoid m.
sternothyroid m.
m. strain
strap m.
striated m.
styloglossus m.
stylohyoid m.
subaortic m.
subscapularis m.
sucking m.
superficial m.
supraspinatus m.
synergic m.
tailor's m.
temporalis m.
tensor veli palatini m.
Theile m.
thenar m.
thigh m.
m. tissue
Tod m.
Toynbee m.
m. traction-induced periostitis

M

NOTES

muscle *(continued)*
transversus abdominis m.
trapezius m.
Treitz m.
triangular m.
trigonal m.
true back m.
two-bellied m.
unipennate m.
Valsalva m.
vastus medialis m.
ventral m.
vertical m.
visceral m.
vocal m.
vocalis m.
voluntary m.
Wilson m.
wrinkler m.
muscle-fat interface
muscular
m. atrioventricular septum
m. branch
m. bridge
m. crus
m. crus of diaphragm
m. degeneration
m. dystrophy
m. esophageal ring
m. GI tract rim sign
m. hypertrophy
m. insufficiency
m. lesion
m. ring esophagus
m. slip
m. subaortic stenosis
m. tube
m. twig
m. ventricular septal defect
muscularis
mucosa m.
m. mucosa
m. propria
musculature
axial m.
cervical m.
longitudinal taenia m.
paraspinous m.
paravertebral m.
scalene m.
musculoaponeurotic fibromatosis
musculocutaneous
musculofascial pedicle
musculophrenic
m. artery
m. branch
m. vessel
musculoskeletal
m. imaging
m. radiography
m. system
m. tumor
M. Tumor Society (MSTS)
musculotendinous
m. cuff
m. junction
m. retraction
m. unit
musculotendinous-osseous link
musculotubal canal
musculus uvula
mushroom
m. appearance
m. picker's disease
m. sign
m. worker's lung
mushroom-shaped mass
Musset sign
mustache sign
Mustard operation
MUSTPAC
medical ultrasound 3D portable, with advanced communication
MUSTPAC ultrasound imaging
mutant
mutation
point m.
mutational dysostosis
mute toe sign
mutilans
arthritis m.
muzzle velocity
MV
megavolt
mV
millivolt
MVA
mitral valve area
MVD
microvascular decompression
MVI
motor vehicle injury
MVO
maximum venous outflow
mitral valve opening
mitral valve orifice
MVP
mitral valve prolapse
MVR
mitral valve replacement
MVS
mitral valve stenosis
MVV
maximal voluntary ventilation

MWT
maximum walking time
myasthenia gravis
mycalamide A
mycetoma
kidney m.
Mycobacterium tuberculosis
Mycoplasma
Mycoplasma pneumonia
Mycoplasma pneumonitis
mycoplasmal pneumonitis
mycosis, pl. **mycoses**
mycotic
m. aneurysm
m. aortic aneurysm
m. brain aneurysm
m. intracranial aneurysm
m. lung infection
m. pneumonia
m. sinusitis
myelencephalon
myelin
m. ball
m. ball formation
m. sheath
myelination
nerve fiber m.
optic pathway m.
myelinolysis
central pontine m.
extrapontine m.
pontine m.
myelitis
radiation m.
transverse m.
myeloblastoma
myelocele
myelocystocele
myelodysplasia
myelofibrosis
acute m.
m. with myeloid metaplasia (MMM)
myelogenesis
myelogram
myelographic
m. contrast medium
m. imaging agent
myelography
air m.
cervical m.
complete m.
CT m.
extraarachnoid m.
Hypaque m.
m. imaging
lumbar m.
lumbosacral m.
magnetic resonance m.
metrizamide m.
Pantopaque m.
positive contrast m.
thoracic m.
myeloid metaphysis
myelolipoma
adrenal m.
myeloma
amyloidosis of multiple m.
endothelial m.
indolent m.
localized m.
multiple bone m.
multiple kidney m.
sclerosing m.
smoldering multiple m.
solitary bone m.
spinal plasma cell m.
myelomalacia
cystic m.
myelomatosis
myelopathy
carcinomatous m.
cervical m.
cystic m.
necrotizing m.
paracarcinomatous m.
posttraumatic cystic m.
radiation m.
subacute necrotizing m.
myelophthisic splenomegaly
myeloproliferative
m. disorder
m. syndrome
myeloschisis
myelosclerosis
myelotomography
myenteric
m. plexus
m. plexus of Auerbach
Myerson sign
myleran lung damage
mylohyoid
m. muscle
m. ridge

NOTES

myoblastoma
granular breast-cell m.
granular lung-cell m.
granular sella-cell m.
myocardial
m. blood flow (MBF)
m. blush
m. bridge
m. calcification
m. cellular degeneration
m. cellular hypertrophy
m. cold-spot perfusion scintigraphy
m. contractile function
m. contractility
m. contracture
m. contrast appearance time (MCAT)
m. contrast echocardiography (MCE)
m. contusion
m. deposition disease
m. depression
m. dilatation
m. fiber
m. fibrous degeneration
m. function assessment
m. granulomatous disease
m. hibernation
m. image redistribution
m. incompetence
m. infarct (MI)
m. infarct imaging
m. infarction recovery index (MIRI)
m. infiltration
m. inflammation
m. insufficiency
m. insult
m. irritability
m. ischemia
m. jeopardy index
m. mass
m. metabolism
m. muscle
m. necrosis
m. O_2 demand index
m. oxygen consumption
m. perfusion
m. perfusion echocardiography
m. perfusion imaging
m. perfusion reserve (MPR)
m. perfusion scan
m. perfusion tomography
m. preservation
m. protection
m. recovery
m. reperfusion injury
m. revascularization
m. rupture
m. scar
m. stunning
m. tagging
m. thallium imaging
m. thickening
m. tissue viability
m. twist
m. uptake
m. uptake of thallium
m. wall
m. work
myocardial-specific marker
myocardiopathy
myocarditis
fibroid m.
fragmentation m.
myocardium
asynergic m.
calcification of m.
dilated m.
hibernating m.
hypertrophied m.
inferior apical aspect of the m.
ischemic reperfused m.
ischemic viable m.
jeopardized m.
necrotic m.
noninfarcted m.
nonperfused m.
perfused m.
recovery period of m.
refractory period of m.
reperfused m.
rupture of m.
salvage of m.
senile m.
sparkling appearance of m.
stunned m.
ventricular m.
viable m.
myoclonus epilepsy associated with ragged red fibers (MERRF)
myoepithelial sialadenitis
myoepithelioma
myofascial
m. disruption
m. pain
m. pain dysfunction syndrome
myofibrillar disintegration
myofibril volume fraction
myofibroblastoma
intranodal m.
myofibrohistiocytic proliferation
myofibromatosis
infantile m.
myogenesis
myoid hamartoma

myointimal
m. hyperplasia
m. proliferation
myoma
pedunculated subserous m.
submucous m.
uterine m.
myometrium
m. swiss cheese
myonecrosis
myoneural junction
myopathy
carcinomatous m.
myosarcoma
Myoscint
M. imaging
M. imaging agent
myosin
^{111}In murine monoclonal antibody Fab to m.
myosis
endolymphatic stromal m.
myositis
brucellar m.
m. circumscripta ossificans
eye m.
m. ossificans progressiva
m. ossificans traumatica
myostatic contracture
myotendinous
m. junction
m. junction rupture
myotonia atrophica cardiomyopathy
myotonic disorder
myotube
Myoview imaging agent
myxadenoma
myxedema
m. of heart
pretibial m.
myxoglobulosis
myxoid
m. cyst
m. extraskeletal chondrosarcoma
m. malignant fibrous histiocytoma
myxoma, pl. **myxomata, myxomas**
atrial m.
biatrial m.
cardiac m.
complex m.
familial m.
heart m.
m. of heart
left atrial m.
pedunculated uterine m.
vascular m.
ventricular m.
myxomatodes
fibroma m.
myxomatous
m. degeneration
m. liposarcoma
m. proliferation
m. valve leaflet
myxomembranous colitis
myxopapillary ependymoma
MZL
marginal zone lymphoma

NOTES

N
nitrogen
N_{aqs}
^{13}N
nitrogen-13
^{13}N ammonia radioactive tracer
^{13}N ammonia uptake
^{14}N
nitrogen-14
^{15}N
nitrogen-15
^{23}Na
sodium-23
^{24}Na
sodium-24
nabothian
n. cyst
n. follicle
Naclerio
V-sign of N.
nadir
untransformed n.
Naffziger sign
Nägele
N. obliquity
N. pelvis
NaI
sodium iodide
nail
n. bed lesion
hyperconvex n.
intramedullary n.
orthopedic n.
n. plate
n. plate avulsion
spoon-shaped n.
triflanged n.
nailing
elastic stable intramedullary n. (ESIN)
nail-patella syndrome
nail-plate device
Nakata index
naked-facet sign
naked tuberosity sign
naloxone imaging agent
Namaqualand hip dysplasia
nanoparticle
iodinated n.
nanoparticulate imaging agent
napkin-ring
n.-r. annular lesion
n.-r. annular stenosis
n.-r. annular tumor
n.-r. carcinoma
n.-r. trachea
napkin ring defect
Napoleon hat sign
Narco esophageal motility machine
Narcomatic flowmetry
naris, pl. **nares**
narrow
n. anteroposterior diameter
n. caliber
n. chest
n. gating tolerance
narrow-band spectral-selective radiofrequency pulse
narrowed
n. orifice
n. rib space
n. valve
narrowing
airway n.
antral stomach n.
arterial n.
arteriolar n.
n. of artery
n. asymmetry
atherosclerotic n.
bile duct n.
bird-beak configuration or n.
bronchiolar n.
n. of bronchiolar passages
colonic n.
concentric n.
degenerative n.
diffuse n.
disk-space n.
duodenal n.
eccentric n.
esophageal n.
n. exchange
focal esophageal n.
n. of forefoot
gastric n.
glottic n.
high-grade n.
intervertebral disk n.
joint-space n.
n. of joint space
large airway n.
longitudinal n.
long smooth esophageal n.
lower esophageal n.
luminal n.
motional n.
nasopharyngeal n.
neural foraminal n.

N

narrowing *(continued)*
oropharyngeal n.
pancompartmental joint space n.
rectal n.
residual luminal n.
retropharyngeal n.
segmental bronchus n.
smooth esophageal n.
n. of spinal canal
stomach n.
subcritical n.
subglottic n.
supraglottic n.
symmetric n.
n. of thecal sac
tracheal n.
vallecular n.

nasal
n. airway resistance
n. bone
n. bridge
n. canal
n. cavity
n. cavity wall
n. concha
n. fracture
n. intubation
n. meatus
n. mucosa
n. part of pharynx
n. polyp
n. septum
n. septum hematoma
n. sinus
n. spine
n. tip deformity
n. turbinate
n. vault mass

nasal-to-plasma radioactivity ratio
nasion recession
nasociliary nerve
nasofrontal duct
nasogastric
n. intubation
n. (NG) tube

nasojejunal feeding tube
nasolabial
n. cyst
n. lymph node

nasolacrimal
n. canal
n. duct

nasoorbital fracture
nasopalatal fissure
nasopalatine canal
nasopharyngeal
n. atresia
n. blastomycosis
n. cancer
n. carcinoma (NPC)
n. craniopharyngioma
n. hematoma
n. mass
n. mucus retention cyst
n. narrowing
n. reflux
n. squamous cell carcinoma

nasopharynx
nasotracheal
n. intubation
n. tube

natatory ligament
National
N. Biomedical Tracer Facility (NBTF)
N. Bureau of Standards (NBS)
N. Council on Radiation Protection and Measurements (NCRP)
N. Institute of Standards and Technology (NIST)
N. Radiological Protection Board (NRPB)

native
n. aorta
n. aortic valve
n. aortic valve closure
n. atherosclerosis
n. coronary artery
n. image
n. kidney
n. kidney renal artery stenosis
n. kidney renal vein thrombosis
n. tissue harmonic imaging (NTHI)
n. ventricle
n. vessel

natural neon gas
Naumoff
N. disease
N. syndrome

Navarre interventional radiology device
navel string
navicular
n. body
n. body fracture
n. bone
carpal n.
n. to first metatarsal angle
n. hand fracture
ossific nucleus of n.
protrusion of n.
target n.
tarsal n.
n. tuberosity
n. view

naviculare
os n.

navicularis
fossa n.
naviculocapitate
n. fracture
n. syndrome
naviculocuneiform
n. joint
n. ligament
navigable echo signal
navigated spin-echo diffusion-weighted MR imaging
navigation
computer-assisted intracranial n.
navigator
n. echo
n. echo-based real-time respiratory gating and triggering
n. echo motion correction technique
n. pulse
n. shift
NB
neuroblastoma
NBS
National Bureau of Standards
NBTF
National Biomedical Tracer Facility
NCP
noncontrast phase
NCPF
noncirrhotic portal fibrosis
NCRP
National Council on Radiation Protection and Measurements
Nd:YAG
neodymium:yttrium-aluminum-garnet
Nd:YAG laser
near-anatomic
n.-a. position
n.-a. position of joint
nearest neighbor interpolation
near field
near-infrared spectroscopy (NIRS)
near-resonance spin-lock contrast
necessitatis
empyema n.
necessity
fracture of n.
neck
air-containing mass of n.
anatomic n.
n. of aneurysm
aneurysmal n.
n. of bladder
bone n.
n. coil
congenital cystic lesion of n.
dental n.
n. emphysema
femoral n.
n. of femur
n. fracture
n. of gallbladder
n. germ-cell tumor
hyperextension of n.
n. lymphangioma
Madelung n.
n. of pancreas
pancreatic n.
potato tumor of n.
n. of rib
n. shaft angle
surgical n.
n. of talus
n. teratoma
uterine wry n.
vesical n.
webbed n.
necrobiotic nodule
necrolytic
n. erythema migrans
necrosis, pl. **necroses**
acute cortical n.
acute native kidney tubular n.
acute renal transplant tubular n.
acute sclerosing hyaline n. (ASHN)
acute tubular n. (ATN)
alveolar septal n.
aortic idiopathic n.
arteriolar n.
aseptic n.
avascular n. (AVN)
avascular bone n.
avascular cortical infarction n.
avascular femoral head n.
avascular tarsal scaphoid n.
avascular vertebral body n.
bilateral cortical n.
biliary piecemeal n.
bloodless zone of n.
bony n.
bowel n.
bridging n.
caseous n.

NOTES

N

necrosis *(continued)*
central n.
centrilobular n.
coagulation n.
colliquative n.
colonic n.
contraction band n.
cortical kidney n.
cystic medial n.
diffuse n.
dirty n.
embolic n.
epiphyseal ischemic n.
Erdheim cystic medial n.
fascial margin n.
fat breast n.
fatty n.
fibrinoid n.
fibrosing piecemeal n.
Ficat stage of avascular n.
focal fat n.
focal hepatic n.
frank n.
heart muscle n.
hemorrhagic n.
hepatic n.
hyaline n.
indurative n.
intestinal n.
intratumoral n.
ischemic n.
laminar brain n.
liquefaction n.
localized n.
lung n.
margin n.
massive hepatic n.
medial cystic n.
midzonal n.
mucosal n.
myocardial n.
Paget quiet n.
pancreatic n.
papillary n.
peripheral n.
piecemeal n.
postpartum pituitary n.
postsurgical fat n.
posttraumatic aseptic n.
posttraumatic fat n.
pressure n.
progressive emphysematous n.
radiation n.
Ratliff classification of avascular n.
renal allograft n.
renal cortical n.
renal papillary n.
renal tubular n.
septal n.
septic n.
soft tissue n.
strangulation n.
stromal n.
subacute hepatic n.
subcapsular hepatic n.
subcutaneous fat n.
subendocardial n.
submassive hepatic n.
superficial n.
total n.
tracheobronchial mucosal n.
traumatic fat n.
tubular n.
vascular n.
ventricular muscle n.
Zenker n.

necrotic
n. bone
n. bone pseudocyst
n. debris
n. flap
n. inflammation
n. lesion
n. metastasis
n. myocardium
n. renal cell carcinoma
n. sequestrum
n. tissue
n. tumor
n. ulcer

necrotizing
n. angitis
n. emphysema
n. enterocolitis
n. external otitis
n. fasciitis
n. gastritis
n. glomerulonephritis
n. myelopathy
n. pancreatitis
n. papillitis
n. pneumonia
n. respiratory granulomatosis
n. thrombosis
n. ulcerative gingivitis

NECT
nonenhanced computed tomography

NED
no evidence of disease

needle
Abrams biopsy n.
abscission n.
Accucore II biopsy n.
Amplatz angiography n.
Bauer Temno biopsy n.
B-D bone marrow biopsy n.

biopsy n.
n. biopsy
blunt-end sialogram n.
BV2 n.
cesium n.
Conrad-Crosby bone marrow biopsy n.
Cope biopsy n.
core biopsy n.
Cournand arteriography n.
Cournand-Grino angiography n.
Dos Santos aortography n.
dumbbell n.
E-Z-EM cut biopsy n.
flexible biopsy n.
full-intensity n.
half-intensity n.
Hawkins n.
Hawkins-Akins n.
Hawkins breast lesion localization n.
Hawkins one-stick n.
Homerlok n.
Homer Mammalok n.
n. hydrophone
iridium n.
Kormed liver biopsy n.
n. localization
n. localization of breast lesion
Maggi biopsy n.
Mammo-lock n.
Mentor prostatic biopsy n.
metallic n.
micropuncture n.
Monopty n.
Multi-Pro biopsy n.
nonferromagnetic n.
OSTYCUT bone biopsy n.
n. pyelography
Quincke spinal n.
^{226}Ra n.
scalp vein n.
Seldinger n.
self-aspirating cut-biopsy n.
sialography n.
spinal n.
TLA n.
translumbar aortography n.
Tuohy aortography n.
n. visualization
Whitacre spinal n.

needle-hookwire localization
needle-shaped breast calcification
needlestick injury
Neel temperature
Neer
N. impingement sign
N. lateral view
N. transscapular view
Neer-Horowitz
N.-H. classification of humeral fractures
N.-H. humerus fracture classification
NEFA
nonesterified fatty acid
NEFA scintigraphy
negative
n. contrast imaging agent
n. contrast left atriography
n. delta sign
n. image
n. image pulmonary edema
n. predictive value
pulmonary edema photographic n.
true n. (TN)
negative-ion cyclotron
negligible pressure gradient
Negro sign
Nélaton
N. dislocation
N. fold
N. line
N. sphincter
Nelson
N. sign
N. syndrome
NEMD
nonspecific esophageal motility disorder
neoadjuvant
n. hormonal therapy
neoangiogenesis
neoaorta
neoaortic valve
neobladder
ileal n.
neocerebellum
neocholangiole
Neocholex
neodensity
neodymium:YAG laser therapy
neodymium:yttrium-aluminum-garnet (Nd:YAG)
n. laser (Nd:YAG laser)

N

NOTES

neofissure
neogalactosyl albumin
neointima formation
neointimal
- n. hyperplasia
- n. proliferation

Neo-Iopax
neonatal
- n. adrenal ultrasound
- n. ascites
- n. cardiac failure
- n. choroid plexus hemorrhage
- n. cystic pulmonary emphysema
- n. heart failure
- n. hepatitis
- n. intracerebellar hemorrhage
- n. intracranial hemorrhage
- n. intracranial ischemia
- n. intraventricular hemorrhage
- n. omphalitis
- n. pneumonia
- n. wet lung disease

neonate
- n. encephalomalacia
- n. mediastinal shift

neonatorum
- edema n.

neon particle protocol
neopallium
neoplasm, pl. **neoplasia**
- adrenocortical n.
- benign n.
- bone n.
- bronchopulmonary n.
- cavitating n.
- cervical intraepithelial n.
- choroid plexus n.
- colonic n.
- connective tissue n.
- cranial nerve n.
- cystic splenic n.
- ductectatic mucinous cystic n.
- encapsulated n.
- epithelial n.
- esophageal n.
- external ear n.
- firm n.
- focally decreased renal n.
- functioning n.
- gestational trophoblastic n.
- gonadal n.
- hepatic n.
- interdigital n.
- intracranial n.
- intrahepatic biliary n.
- intramedullary compartment n.
- lethal n.
- low-grade n.
- macrocystic n.
- malignant urethral n.
- mesenchymal n.
- metastatic renal n.
- middle ear n.
- mucinous pancreatic cystic n.
- multiple endocrine neoplasms (MEN)
- neuroepithelial n.
- osteocartilaginous parasellar n.
- pancreatic n.
- papillary cystic n.
- papillary epithelial n.
- papillary pancreatic cystic n.
- pearly n.
- pineal gland n.
- primary n.
- radiation-induced n. (RIN)
- second malignant n. (SMN)
- skeletal n.
- soft tissue n.
- spherical n.
- supratentorial n.
- T-cell n.
- thoracic spinal n.
- thymic n.
- transitional cell n.
- trochlear nerve n.
- vaginal intraepithelial n.
- vulvar intraepithelial n.
- well-circumscribed n.

neoplastic
- n. aneurysm
- n. calcification
- n. cyst
- n. destruction of spinal element
- n. fracture
- n. hyperplasia
- n. invasion
- n. lesion
- n. process
- n. stenosis
- n. tissue

Neoprobe radioactivity detector
neopterin
neorectum
NeoTect
neovagina
neovascularity
- tumor n.

neovascularization
neovasculature
- tumor n.

nepheline pneumoconiosis
nephrectomy
nephritic calculus
nephritis, pl. **nephritides**
- acute diffuse bacterial n.

acute focal bacterial n.
acute interstitial n. (AIN)
bacterial n.
Balkan n.
chronic hereditary n.
diffuse bacterial n.
focal bacterial n.
glomerular n.
interstitial n.
nephrocalcinosis n.
radiation n.
salt-losing n.
tubulointerstitial n.

nephroblastoma
cystic partially differentiated n.
polycystic n.

nephroblastomatosis
multifocal n.
superficial diffuse n.

nephrocalcinosis
cortical n.
medullary n.
n. nephritis
renal cortical n.

nephrogenic, nephrogenetic
n. bladder adenoma
n. diabetes insipidus
n. phase

nephroglastomatosis
panlobar n.

nephrogram
cortical rim n.
delayed unilateral n.
increasingly dense n.
medullary n.
obstructive n.
persistent increasing n.
rim n.
n. rim
segmental n.
shell n.
n. shock
spotted n.
striated angiographic n.
sunburst n.
Swiss cheese n.
tubular n.

nephrographic phase (NP)

nephrography

nephrolithiasis

nephrolithotomy

nephroma
congenital mesoblastic n.
cystic n.
mesoblastic n.
multilocular cystic n.

nephronophthisis
juvenile n.

nephropathic cystinosis

nephropathy
analgesic n.
Balkan n.
contrast n.
n. contrast
diabetic n.
HIV n.
obstructive n.
radiation n.
reflux n.
urate n.
uric acid n.

nephroptosis

nephrosclerosis
arterial n.
benign n.
malignant n.
senile n.

nephroscope
Alken-Marberger n.
flexible n.
percutaneous n.
Wickham-Miller n.

nephroscopic fulguration

nephroscopy
percutaneous n.

nephrosis, pl. **nephroses**
congenital Finnish n.

nephrostogram
n. imaging
postprocedure n.

nephrostolithotomy
caliceal n.

nephrostomy
circle wire n.
n. drainage
percutaneous n.
n. puncture

nephrotic
n. edema
n. syndrome

nephrotomogram

nephrotomography
n. imaging

NOTES

N

nephrotoxic contrast medium
nephrotoxicity
contrast media n.
cyclosporin n.
drug-induced n.
nephrotropic MR imaging agent
nephroureteral stent
nephroureterectomy
Neptune trident appearance
neptunium
Neri bowing sign
Nernst equation
nerve
accessory n.
acoustic n.
afferent digital n.
cluneal n.
cochlear n.
cranial n.
dorsal ramus of spinal n.
efferent digital n.
n. entrapment
excrescentic thickening of the optic n.
facial n.
femoral n.
n. fiber myelination
fibrolipomatous hamartoma n.
fifth cranial n.
fourth cranial n.
frontal n.
glossopharyngeal n.
greater superficial petrosal n.
hypoglossal n.
n. injury
intercostal n.
intercostobrachial n.
interosseous n.
lacrimal n.
laryngeal n.
n. of Latarjet
left respiratory n.
lingual n.
mandibular n.
median n.
nasociliary n.
oculomotor n.
ophthalmic n.
optic n.
peripheral n.
periradicular n.
peroneal n.
petrosal n.
pinched n.
n. plexus
posterior interosseous n. (PION)
pseudoneuroma of median n.
recurrent laryngeal n.
recurrent meningeal n.
n. root
n. root axillary pouch
n. root compression
n. root edema
n. root embarrassment
n. root impingement
n. root irritability
rootlet of n.
n. root sheath
n. root sheath effacement
n. root sleeve
n. root tumor
rostral cervical n.
sacral n.
saphenous n.
second cranial n.
n. sheath tumor
spinal accessory n.
subcostal n.
supraspinatus n.
sural n.
trochlear n.
n. trunk
unroofing of n.
vagus n.
vein, artery, n. (VAN)
vestibular division of eighth cranial n.
vestibulocochlear n.
vidian n.
nervosa
dysphagia n.
nervous heart syndrome
nervus intermedius
nesidioblastoma
net
n. magnetization factor
n. magnetization vector
n. shunt
n. tissue magnetization
n. transverse magnetization
network
articular n.
artificial neural n.
hypertrophic duct n.
lymphatic n.
neural n.
vascular n.
venous n.
NEUGAT
neutron/gamma transmission
NEUGAT method
NEUGAT technique
neural
n. arch cleft
n. arch fracture
n. axis vascular malformation

n. canal
n. crest origin
n. evaluation algorithm
n. fibrolipoma
n. foramen
n. foramen remodeling
n. foraminal narrowing
n. groove
n. network
n. origin bone tumor
n. pathway
n. placode
n. sheath
n. tube
n. tube defect (NTD)
n. vertebral arch

neuralgia
sphenopalatine n.

neuraxis
n. radiation therapy
n. staging

neuraxonal dystrophy

neurenteric canal

neurilemoma, neurilemmoma

neurinoma (*var. of* neuroma)

neuritic
n. plaquing
n. senile plaque

neuritis, pl. **neuritides**
axial n.
brachial plexus n.
friction n.
optic n.

Neuro
EasyGuide N.
N. Lobe software
N. SPGR software

neuroangiography

neuroarthropathy

neuroaugmentation

neuroblastoma (NB)
adrenal n.
cerebral n.
chest wall n.
dumbbell-type n.
Hutchinson-type n.
intracranial n.
intraventricular n.
olfactory n.
stage 4S n.
n. staging

neuroblockage

neurocentral synchondrosis

neurocutaneous
n. disorder
n. melanosis
n. syndrome

neurocysticercosis

neurocytoma
intraventricular n.

neurodiagnostic imaging

NeuroEcho software

neuroectoderm

neuroectodermal
n. dysplasia
n. tumor

neuroendocrine
n. hepatic metastasis
n. small-cell carcinoma

neuroenteric cyst

neuroepithelial
n. neoplasm

neuroepithelioma
primitive n.

neurofibrillary tangle

neurofibroma
aryepiglottic fold n.
craniofacial plexiform n.
dumbbell n.
paraspinal n.
plexiform n.

neurofibromatosis
abortive n.
central n.
incomplete n.
kidney n.
peripheral n.
segmental n.
type 1 n.
type 2 n.
n. with bilateral acoustic neuroma

neurofibrosarcoma

neurogenic
n. atrophy
n. bladder dysfunction
n. disorder
n. fracture
n. intestinal obstruction
n. lesion
n. pulmonary edema
n. sarcoma
n. tumor
n. urinary bladder

NOTES

neuroglial
n. tumor
neurography
magnetic resonance n. (MRN)
neuroholography
neuroimaging
functional n.
three-dimensional n.
neurointerventional radiology
Neurolite
N. imaging agent
neurologic
n. bladder lesion
n. soft sign
neuroma, neurinoma
acoustic n.
digital n.
interdigital n.
Morton n.
multicystic acoustic n.
neurofibromatosis with bilateral acoustic n.
postamputation n.
posttraumatic n.
neuromatosa
elephantiasis n.
neuromorphometry
neuromuscular
n. dysfunction
n. junction
n. system electric induction
neuromyopathy
carcinomatous n.
neuron
lower motor n.
pyramidal n.'s
upper motor n.
neuronal
n. cell origin tumor
n. migration
n. proliferation
neuronavigation
Neuropac
neuropathic
n. ankle
n. arthropathy
n. bladder
n. fracture
n. midfoot deformity
n. osteoarthropathy
n. pain
n. tarsometatarsal joint
neuropathicum
papilloma n.
neuropathy
acute n.
compression n.
entrapment n.
neuropore
neuroradiologic
n. examination
n. imaging
neuroradiology
American Society of N.
interventional n.
pediatric n.
neuroreceptor
neurosarcoidosis
neurosarcoma
NeuroScan 3D imager
NeuroSector
N. ultrasound
N. ultrasound system
neurosonogram
neurosonography
neurosonology
neurosyphilis
parenchymatous n.
neuroticum
papilloma n., papilloma neuropathicum
neurotoxic effect
neurotrophic
n. fracture
n. joint
neurotropic imaging agent
neurovascular
n. bundle
n. compression
n. lesion
neurSector scanner
neurulation
neutral
adduction to n.
n. hip position
neutralization plate
neutrino
neutron
n. activation analysis
n. bombardment
fast n.
n. irradiation
n. radiation
slow n.
n. therapy
n. therapy machine
thermal n.
neutron-deficient nucleus
neutron/gamma
n. transmission (NEUGAT)
n. transmission method (NEUGAT method)
n. transmission therapy
neutron-rich biomedical tracer

neutropenic
n. colitis
n. enterocolitis
neutrophil
Nevaiser frozen shoulder classification
nevi (*pl. of* nevus)
Neviaser classification of frozen shoulder
nevoid basal-cell carcinoma
nevus, pl. **nevi**
Becker n.
benign n.
ectopic n.
senile n.
spider n.
stellar n.
n. verrucosus
verrucous n.
new
n. bone formation
newborn renal imaging
newly woven bone
Newman
N. classification of radial neck and head fractures
N. radial fracture classification
Newvicon camera tube
New York Heart Association (NYHA)
NEX
number of excitations
NH_3
anhydrous ammonia
NHL
non-Hodgkin lymphoma
small noncleaved NHL
niche
Barclay n.
Haudek n.
Nicoladoni-Branham sign
Nicolet NMR spectrometer
Nicoll bone
nicotinamide
n. imaging agent
n. radiosensitizer
nidus
n. angle
n. demarcation
n. of embolic material
n. of lesion
thrombus n.
Niemann-Pick disease
Niemeier gallbladder perforation
Nievergelt
N. disease
N. syndrome
Niewenglowski ray
nightstick fracture
nigra
substantia n.
nigricans
acanthosis n.
nigrostriate tract
Nikolsky sign
nimodipine
n. imaging agent
intraarterial superselective n.
nimorazole
niobium/titanium superconductor
Niopam
N. imaging agent
NIP
nonspecific interstitial pneumonia
nipple
adenoma of n.
aortic n.
n. aspiration cytology
deep to the n.
n. discharge
inverted n.
n. marker
out-of-profile n.
Paget disease of n.
n. retraction
n. shadow
nipple-areolar complex
nipplelike
n. common bile duct
n. osteophyte formation
NIPS
noninvasive programmed stimulation
NIRS
near-infrared spectroscopy
Nishimoto Sangyo scanner
Nissen
N. antireflux operation
N. fundoplication
N. fundoplication procedure
NIST
National Institute of Standards and Technology
nitinol
n. filter
n. inferior vena cava filter
niton

NOTES

nitrate
gallium n.
nitriloacetic acid
nitrite
amyl n.
nitrocellulose film
nitrofurantoin lung damage
nitrogen (N)
body n.
n. washout
nitrogen-13 (^{13}N)
n. ammonia imaging agent
nitrogen-14 (^{14}N)
nitrogen-15 (^{15}N)
nitroglycerin
nitrosourea lung damage
nitrous
n. oxide
n. oxide imaging agent
nitroxide-stable free radical
N-methylglucamine
N-methylspiperone
^{11}C N.-m.
^{18}F N.-m.
N-methylspiroperidol (NMS)
^{11}C N.-m.
NMIS
nuclear medicine information system
NMR
nuclear magnetic resonance
continuous-wave NMR
NMR LipoProfile device
magic angle spinning NMR
NMR magnetometer probe
pulsed-electron paramagnetic NMR
NMR quadrature detection array
NMR spectrometer
surface-coil NMR
NMS
N-methylspiroperidol
no
n. discernible finding
n. evidence of disease (NED)
n. frequency wrap
Noble position
nocardial osteomyelitis
nocardiosis
cerebral n.
no-carrier-added ^{18}F imaging agent
nociceptive
nodal
n. conduction
n. disease
n. fibrosis
n. impulse
n. metastasis
n. point
n. premature contraction
n. rhythm
n. rupture
n. tissue
node
abdominal lymph n.
accessory lymph n.
angiofollicular hyperplasia lymph n.
anorectal lymph n.
aortic lymph n.
aortic window n.
apical lymph n.
appendicular lymph n.
Aschoff n.
Aschoff-Tawara n.
atrioventricular n.
auricular lymph n.
AV n.
axillary lymph n. (ALN)
azygos lymph n.
bifurcation lymph n.
brachial lymph n.
brachiocephalic lymph n.
breast lymph n.
bronchopulmonary lymph n.
buccal lymph n.
buccinator lymph n.
n. calcification
cardiac n.
cartilaginous n.
caval lymph n.
celiac lymph n.
central lymph n.
cervical lymph n.
cervical paratracheal lymph n.
Cloquet inguinal lymph n.
common iliac lymph n.
companion lymph n.
coronary n.
cubital lymph n.
cystic lymph n.
Delphian lymph n.
deltopectoral lymph n.
diaphragmatic lymph n.
Dürck n.
eggshell calcification of lymph n.
epicolic lymph n.
epigastric lymph n.
epitrochlear lymph n.
Ewald n.
external iliac lymph n.
fibular lymph n.
Flack sinoatrial n.
foraminal n.
gastric lymph n.
gastroduodenal lymph n.
gastroepiploic lymph n.
gastrohepatic ligament n.
gastroomental lymph n.

Ghon n.
giant hyperplasia lymph n.
gluteal lymph n.
gouty n.
Haygarth n.
Heberden n.
hemal n.
hemolymph n.
Hensen n.
hepatic lymph n.
hilar lymph n.
hot n.
ileocolic lymph n.
iliac circumflex lymph n.
iliac lymph n.
ilioinguinal lymph n.
infraclavicular n.
infrahyoid lymph n.
inguinal lymph n.
intercostal lymph n.
interiliac lymph n.
internal mammary lymph n.
interpectoral lymph n.
intramammary lymph n.
intraparenchymal lymph n.
jugular lymph n.
jugulodigastric n.
juguloomohyoid lymph n.
juxtaintestinal n.
Keith n.
Keith-Flack sinoatrial n.
Koch sinoatrial n.
lacunar n.
lumbar lymph n.
lymph n.
lymphomatous lymph n.
malar lymph n.
mandibular lymph n.
mastoid lymph n.
medial supraclavicular n.
mediastinal n.
mesenteric n.
Meynet n.
multicentric angiofollicular lymph n.
nasolabial lymph n.
obturator lymph n.
occipital lymph n.
Osler n.
pancreatic lymph n.
pancreaticoduodenal lymph n.
pancreaticolienal lymph n.
pancreaticosplenic n.
paraaortic lymph n.
paracardial lymph n.
paracolic lymph n.
paramammary lymph n.
pararectal lymph n.
parasternal lymph n.
paratracheal lymph n.
parauterine lymph n.
paravaginal lymph n.
paravesicular lymph n.
parietal lymph n.
parotid lymph n.
Parrot n.
pectoral lymph n.
pelvic lymph n.
periaortic lymph n.
peribronchial lymph n.
pericardial lymph n.
perisplenic n.
peroneal n.
phrenic lymph n.
popliteal n.
porta hepatis n.
postaortic lymph n.
postcaval lymph n.
posterior mediastinal n.
postvesicular lymph n.
preaortic lymph n.
precaval lymph n.
prececal lymph n.
prelaryngeal n.
prepericardial lymph n.
pretracheal lymph n.
prevertebral lymph n.
prevesicular lymph n.
pulmonary juxtaesophageal lymph n.
pulmonary lymph n.
pyloric lymph n.
Ranvier n.
rectal lymph n.
regional lymph n.
retroaortic lymph n.
retroauricular lymph n.
retrocecal lymph n.
retrocrural n.
retroperitoneal n.
retropharyngeal lymph n.
retropyloric n.
retrorectal lymph n.
Rosenmüller n.
Rotter n.

NOTES

N

node *(continued)*
SA n.
sinoatrial node
sacral lymph n.
satellite n.
scalene n.
Schmorl n.
sentinel lynph n. (SLN)
shotty lymph n.
sick sinus n.
sigmoid lymph n.
signal n.
singer's n.
sinoatrial n. (SA node, SAN)
sinoauricular n.
sinus node
Sister Mary Joseph n.
solitary lymph n.
spinal accessory lymph n.
splenic lymph n.
subcarinal lymph n.
submandibular lymph n.
submental lymph n.
subpyloric n.
subscapular lymph n.
superficial inguinal lymph n.
supraclavicular lymph n.
suprapyloric n.
supratrochlear n.
syphilitic n.
Tawara atrioventricular n.
teacher's n.
thyroid lymph n.
tibial n.
tracheal lymph n.
tracheobronchial lymph n.
Troisier n.
vesicular lymph n.
vestigial left sinoatrial n.
Virchow sentinel n.
Virchow-Troisier n.
visceral lymph n.
node-negative
n.-n. cancer
n.-n. melanoma
node-positive breast cancer
nodohisian bypass tract
nodosa
periarteritis n.
salpingitis isthmica n.
nodosum
nodoventricular
n. bypass fiber
n. bypass tract
n. pathway
n. tachycardia
nodular
n. adrenal hyperplasia
n. aneurysm
n. density
n. enhancement
n. goiter
n. hyperintense focus
n. induration of temporal artery
n. lesion
n. liver
n. liver regeneration
n. lung disease
n. lymphoid hyperplasia
n. mass
n. opacity
n. proliferation
n. regenerative hyperplasia (NRH)
n. sclerosis Hodgkin disease
n. subepidermal fibrosis
n. synovitis
n. thyroid disease
nodularity
calcified n.
coarse n.
lung n.
noncalcified n.
perivenular n.
pulmonary n.
surface n.
vein n.
n. vein
nodule
acinar n.
air-space n.
Albini n.
n.'s of aortic valve
aortic valve n.
Arantius n.
Aschoff n.
autonomous n.
Bianchi n.
calcified lung n.
cartilaginous n.
cavitating lung n.
cerebral n.
cirrhotic n.
cold thyroid n.
cortical n.
Cruveilhier n.
cutaneous n.
Dalen-Fuchs n.
discordant thyroid n.
dysplastic liver n.
echogenic n.
enhancing n.
esophageal mucosal n.
fibrocartilaginous n.
fibrous n.
Fraenkel typhus n.
functioning n.

Gamna n.
Gamna-Gandy n.
Gamna-Gandy n.
glial n.
hemorrhagic lung n.
Hoboken n.
hot thyroid n.
hyperechoic renal n.
hypermetabolic n.
innumerable small enhancing cerebral n.
Kerckring n.
Koeppe n.
laryngeal n.
lingular n.
Lisch n.
lung n.
miliary n.
Morgagni n.
mucosalesophageal n.
multiple lung n.
mural CNS n.
necrobiotic n.
noncavitary n.
nondelineated n.
nonenhancing n.
nonfunctioning thyroid n.
ossific n.
peripheral n.
periumbilical subcutaneous n.
Picker n.
pleura-based lung n.
prostatic hyperplastic n.
pulmonary n.
regenerative liver n.
rheumatoid n.
Rokitansky n.
satellite n.
Scheuermann n.
Schmorl n.
semiautonomous n.
shaggy lung n.
silicotic n.
singer's n.
Sister Mary Joseph n.
solitary lung n.
solitary metastatic lung n.
solitary pulmonary n. (SPN)
subcutaneous n.
surfer's n.
teacher's n.
thyroid adenoma n.
thyroid colloid n.
tobacco n.
toxic n.
tuberculous n.
typhoid n.
typhus n.
warm n.

nodule-in-nodule liver
nodulo-ulcerative basal-cell carcinoma
nodulus Arantius
nodus arcus venae azygos
no-gap technique
noise
acoustic n.
echogenic n.
image n.
lesion-to-cerebrospinal fluid n.
lesion-to-white matter n.
pixel n.
quantum n.
random n.
respiratory n.
n. spike artifact
statistical n.
structured n.
subtractive n.
systematic n.
thermal n.
total image n.
white n.

noise-reduction intercom
Nolke position
nomifensine
^{11}C n.

nominal standard dose (NSD)
nonablative heating
nonaccidental trauma
nonanaplastic glioma
nonaneurysmal perimesencephalic subarachnoid hemorrhage
nonarrhythmic myocardial infarct
nonarticular radial head fracture
nonasbestos pneumoconiosis
nonatherosclerotic disease
nonavid infarct imaging
nonaxial beam technique
nonbacterial
n. gastric emphysema
n. pneumonia

noncalcified
n. coronary stenosis
n. mitral leaflet

N

NOTES

noncalcified *(continued)*
- n. nodularity
- n. nodular mass
- n. ocular process
- n. stone

noncardiac angiography
noncardiogenic
- n. pulmonary edema

noncaseating
- n. granuloma
- n. tubercle

noncavitary nodule
nonchromaffin paraganglioma
noncicatrizing phase
noncircularity degree
noncirrhotic
- n. liver
- n. portal fibrosis (NCPF)

nonclassifiable interstitial pneumonia
noncleaved cell lymphoma
noncoaxial catheter tip position
noncoiled umbilical cord
noncollagenous pneumonoconiosis
noncomedo breast cancer
noncommitted mode
noncommunicating
- n. cyst
- n. hydrocephalus

noncompensatory pause
noncompliant plaque
noncontact imaging technology
noncontained disk
noncontiguous fracture
noncontractile scar tissue
noncontrast phase (NCP)
noncoplanar
- n. arch technique
- n. arc technique
- n. beam technique
- n. therapy beam

noncoronary
- n. cardiomyopathy
- n. cusp
- n. sinus

noncritical
- n. soft tissue
- n. stenosis

nondeciduate placenta
nondecremental
nondelineated nodule
nondependent lung
nondisplaced fracture
nondissociative instability
nondominant
- n. hemisphere lesion
- n. putaminal hemorrhage
- n. vessel

nonechogenic tumor
nonembolic infarct
nonenclosed magnet
nonenhanced
- n. computed tomography (NECT)
- n. CT
- n. CT scan

nonenhancing
- n. lesion
- n. nodule

nonesterified
- n. fatty acid (NEFA)
- n. fatty acid scintigraphy

nonexpansile
- n. multilocular bone lesion
- n. multilocular osteolysis
- n. unilocular bone lesion
- n. unilocular osteolysis
- n. well-demarcated multilocular bone defect
- n. well-demarcated unilocular bone defect

nonfamilial intestinal pseudoobstruction
nonfatal myocardial infarct
nonferromagnetic
- n. needle
- n. positioning device

nonfilarial chylocele
nonfilling venous segment
nonforeshortened angiographic view
nonfunctioning
- n. islet cell tumor
- n. kidney
- n. pituitary adenoma
- n. thyroid nodule

nonfusion of cranial suture
nongestational choriocarcinoma
nonhemorrhagic melanoma metastasis
non-Hodgkin
- n.-H. chest lymphoma
- n.-H. lymphoma (NHL)

nonhomogeneous
- n. consolidation
- n. enhancement

nonhyperfunctioning adrenal adenoma
nonimmune
- n. fetal hydrops
- n. hydrops fetalis

noninducible tachycardia
noninfarcted
- n. myocardium
- n. segment

noninfectious aortitis
noninflammatory joint effusion
noninteger period
noninvasive
- n. aspergillosis
- n. assessment
- n. breast cancer

n. diagnosis
n. imaging
n. imaging study
n. lesion
n. programmed stimulation (NIPS)
n. technique
n. thermometry
n. thymoma
n. ultrasound

nonionic
n. contrast material
n. iodinated contrast
n. monomer
n. paramagnetic contrast imaging agent
n. paramagnetic contrast medium

nonionizing radiation
nonischemic congestive cardiomyopathy
nonislet cell carcinoma
nonisotropic gradient
nonlactating breast
nonlethal
n. dwarfism
n. dysplasia
n. myocardial ischemic injury

nonlinear
n. excitation profile
n. sampling

nonlingular
n. branch
n. branches of upper lobe bronchus

nonlocalized ischemia
nonmagnetization transfer gradient-refocused echo image
nonmeningiomatous malignant lesion
nonmucinous adenocarcinoma
Nonne-Milroy lymphedema
nonneoplastic
n. cyst
n. tumor

nonneurogenic bladder
nonnodular
n. fibrosis
n. silicosis

nonobstructive
n. atelectasis
n. cardiomyopathy
n. hydrocephalus
n. ileus

nonocclusive
n. mesenteric arterial insufficiency
n. mesenteric ischemia

nonolfactory cortex
nonopaque
n. calculus
n. intraluminal mass
n. intraluminal mass in collecting system
n. stone

nonorthogonal plane
nonossifying fibroma
nonosteogenic fibroma
nonpalpable abnormality
nonperfused myocardium
nonphyseal fracture
nonplanar slice
nonpolar crevice
nonpuerperal mastitis
nonpulsatile abdominal mass
non-Q-wave myocardial infarct
nonradiopaque
n. foreign body
n. stone

nonreplantable amputation
nonresonance Raman spectroscopy
nonrheumatic
n. aortic insufficiency
n. valvular aortic stenosis

non-rib-bearing vertebra
nonrotation
nonrotational burst fracture
nonsegmental areas of opacification
nonselective
n. angiography
n. pulse

nonseminomatous
n. germ cell tumor

nonseptic embolic brain infarct
non-skin-sparing mastectomy (non-SSM)
non-small-cell
n.-s.-c. carcinoma
n.-s.-c. lung cancer (NSCLC)

nonspecific
n. accumulation
n. bowel gas pattern
n. changes
n. esophageal motility disorder (NEMD)
n. interstitial pneumonia (NIP, NSIP)
n. phenomenon

NOTES

non-SSM
non-skin-sparing mastectomy
nonstanding lateral oblique view
nonsteroidal antiphlogistics imaging agent
nonstress
n. fetal test
n. test (NST)
nonstriated muscle
nonsubperiosteal cortical defect
nonsubtraction
n. image
n. imaging
nonsuppurative
n. ascending cholangitis
n. destructive cholangitis
nonsyndromic
n. bicoronal synostosis
n. unicoronal synostosis
nontrabeculated atrium
nontransmural
n. match
n. myocardial infarct
nontraumatic epidural hemorrhage
nontriggered phase-contrast MR angiography
nontropical sprue
nonuniform
n. attenuation
n. excitation
n. rotational defect (NURD)
nonunion
atrophic n.
bony n.
fibrous n.
fracture n.
n. of fracture fragments
hypertrophic n.
torsion wedge n.
nonunited fracture
nonvalved conduit
nonviable
n. fetus
n. scar
n. scar from myocardial infarct
n. tissue
nonvisualization
n. of fetal stomach
n. of gallbladder
n. of spleen
nonweightbearing view
Noonan syndrome
noose sign
no-reflow phenomenon
Norland
N. bone densitometry
N. pQCT XCT2000 scanner
N. XR26 bone densitometer
normal
n. anatomic position
n. anatomic variation
n. bladder caliber
borderline n.
n. calcification
n. caliber duct
n. chest film
n. echogenicity
n. fold urethrogram
n. gestation
n. hemodynamic liver parameter
high n.
n. human serum albumin imaging agent
n. lordotic curve
low n.
morphologically n.
n. ovarian surface epithelium (NOSE)
n. perfusion pressure breakthrough
n. planar MR anatomy
n. range
n. renal parenchyma
n. spleen weight
upper limits of n.
n. variant
n. variant of Ga-67 uptake
normal-appearing bronchus
normal-caliber bowel
normalized
n. average glandular dose
n. cross-section
normal-pressure hydrocephalus
normal-region pixel
normoblast
normotensive
n. hydrocephalus
normothermia
normoxia
Norrie disease
North American blastomycosis
NOS
not otherwise specified
NOSE
normal ovarian surface epithelium
nose
beak-shaped n.
nose-chin position
nose-forehead position
nosocomial
n. infection
n. pneumonia
n. tuberculosis transmission
notch
acetabular n.
anacrotic n.
angular n.

antegonial n.
aortic n.
apical n.
auricular n.
cardiac n.
cerebellar n.
n. chest sign
clavicular n.
coracoid n.
costal n.
cotyloid n.
craniofacial n.
dicrotic n.
digastric n.
ethmoidal n.
fibular n.
Frankfort mandibular n.
frontal n.
greater sciatic n.
greater sigmoid n.
interclavicular n.
intercondylar n.
interpeduncular n.
intervertebral n.
kernahorn n.
lesser sciatic n.
ligamentum teres n.
lucent hilar n.
radial sigmoid n.
sacrosciatic n.
scapular n.
sciatic n.
semilunar n.
septal n.
sigmoid n.
spinoglenoid n.
splenic n.
sternal n.
suprasternal n.
trochlear n.
ulnar n.
n. view

notched aortic knob

notching

cortical n.
pelvic n.
n. of pulmonic valve
rib n.
n. ureter
ureteral n.

note

resonant percussion n.

no-therapy zone

Nothnagel syndrome

no-threshold concept

notochord

n. remnant

notochordal

n. canal
n. process

not otherwise specified (NOS)

Novacor left ventricular assist system

novel agent

novo

de n.

Novopaque

N. imaging agent

Novus Medical Image Card

nozzle effect

NP

nephrographic phase

NPC

nasopharyngeal carcinoma

***N*-phosphonoacetyl-*l*-aspartic acid (PALA enhancement)**

n.p.o.

nulla per os

^{59}NP scintigraphy

NRC

Nuclear Regulatory Commission

NRH

nodular regenerative hyperplasia

NRPB

National Radiological Protection Board

NSCLC

non-small-cell lung cancer

NSD

nominal standard dose

N-shaped sigmoid loop

NSIP

nonspecific interstitial pneumonia

NST

nonstress test

NTD

neural tube defect

NTHI

native tissue harmonic imaging

NTP

nucleoside triphosphate

nubbin

n. kidney sign
n. testis sign

nuchae

ligamentum n.

NOTES

nuchal
n. cord
n. cyst
n. cyst syndrome
n. ligament
n. skin thickening
Nuck
canal of N.
N. canal
diverticulum of N.
N. diverticulum
nuclear
n. angiography
n. annular differentiation
n. atom
n. bone imaging
n. cardiovascular imaging
n. chemistry
n. disintegration
n. electric quadripole relaxation
n. enema
n. energy
n. fusion
n. gated blood pool imaging
n. gated blood pool testing
n. hepatobiliary imaging
n. magnetic moment
n. magnetic resonance (NMR)
n. magnetic resonance imaging
n. magnetic resonance (NMR) scan
n. magnetic resonance (NMR) spectography
n. magnetic resonance (NMR) spectroscopy
n. magnetic resonance (NMR) spectrum
n. magnetic resonance tomography
n. magnetism
n. medicine
n. medicine information system (NMIS)
n. Overhauser effect
n. parameter
n. perfusion imaging
n. pleomorphism
n. polarization
n. probe
n. pulse amplifier
N. Regulatory Commission (NRC)
n. renal scintigraphy
n. signal
n. spin
n. spin quantum number
nuclear-tagged red blood cell bleeding study
nucleon
nucleonics
nucleoside
n. phosphonate
n. triphosphate (NTP)
Nucletron
N. applicator
N. MicroSelectron/LDR remote afterloader
nucleus
n. ambiguus lesion
arcuate n.
basal n.
n. basalis lesion
caudate n.
cranial n.
head of the caudate n.
Köllicker n.
lentiform n., lenticular nucleus
motor n.
neutron-deficient n.
oculomotor-trochlear n.
ossific n.
parafascicular n.
pretectal n.
n. pulposus herniation
quadripolar n.
residual n.
sensory n.
sixth n.
ventral cochlear n.
nuclide
n. analysis
n. generator
nulla per os (n.p.o.)
nulling
gradient moment n. (GMN)
null point
number
average gradient n.
Avogadro n. (Λ)
clonogen n.
CT n.
n. of excitations (NEX)
Hounsfield n.
imaginary n.
nuclear spin quantum n.
quantum n.
Reynolds n.
spin quantum n.
numerary renal anomaly
nummular pneumonia
NURD
nonuniform rotational defect
Nurick
N. classification of spondylosis
N. spondylosis classification
nursemaid's elbow

nutation
n. angle
n. angle measurement
nutcracker
n. esophagus
n. fracture
n. phenomenon
n. syndrome
nutrient
n. artery of femur
n. artery of fibula
n. artery growth
n. foramen
nutritional cirrhosis
NX
regional lymph node cannot be addressed
Nycomed
N. contrast
N. imaging agent
Nyegaard
NYHA
New York Heart Association
NYHA congestive heart failure classification
Nyquist
N. criterion
N. frequency
N. limit
N. sampling theorem

NOTES

O
oxygen
O shell
O_2
O_2 consumption index
^{15}O
oxygen-15
^{16}O
oxygen-16
^{17}O
oxygen-17
^{18}O
oxygen-18
OA
osteoarthritis
OAF
off-axis factor
OAR
off-axis ratio
oat-cell carcinoma
OAV
oculoauriculovertebral
OAV dysplasia
OBD
organic brain disease
O'Beirne sphincter
obesity
cardiopulmonary o.
exogenous o.
truncal o.
object
side-by-side o.
object-film distance (OFD)
objective symptoms
object-plane blur
oblique
o. axial MR imaging
o. coronal plane
o. diameter
o. film
o. fissure
o. flow misregistration
left anterior o. (LAO)
left posterior o. (LPO)
o. magnetic resonance imaging
mediolateral o. (MLO)
o. muscle
o. pericardial sinus
o. prescription line
o. projection
o. radiograph
o. ridge
right anterior o. (RAO)
right posterior o. (RPO)
o. sagittal sequence
o. slice
o. spiral fracture
superior o.
trauma o.
T2-weighted fast spin-echo coronal o.
o. vein
o. vein of left atrium
o. view
obliquity
Litzmann o.
magnitude of o.
Nägele o.
pelvic o.
Roederer o.
Solayrès o.
obliquus
vastus medialis o. (VMO)
obliterans
arteriosclerosis o. (ASO)
atherosclerosis o. (ASO)
bronchiolitis o.
bronchiolitis fibrosa o.
endarteritis o.
mastitis o.
thromboangiitis o.
obliterated costophrenic angle
obliteration
subdeltoid fat plane o.
obliterative
o. arteriosclerosis
o. bronchiolitis
o. cardiomyopathy
o. inflammation
oblongata
medulla o.
O'Brien
O. classification of radial fractures
O. radial fracture classification
OBS
organic brain syndrome
obscuration arteriosclerosis
obscure cardiomyopathy
observed maximal uptake
obstetric, obstetrical
o. injury
o. sonography
o. ultrasonography
o. ultrasound
obstipation
obstructed shunt tube
obstructing embolus arteriosclerosis
obstruction
acute abdominal o.
adynamic intestinal o.

obstruction *(continued)*
airway o.
aortic arch o.
aortic outflow o.
aortic valve o.
aortoiliac o.
aqueductal o.
arachnoid villi o.
arterial o.
ball-valve o.
bilateral o.
bile flow o.
biliary tract o.
biliary tree o.
bladder outlet o.
bowel o.
bronchial o.
bronchiolar o.
cardiac o.
catheter o.
cerebrospinal fluid o.
chronic airway o.
closed-loop intestinal o.
colonic o.
common bile duct o.
complete bowel o.
congenital duodenal o.
congenital left-sided outflow o.
congenital subpulmonic o.
cowl-shaped o.
distal common bile duct o.
o. of duct
duct o.
duodenal-gastric outlet o.
embolic o.
endobronchial o.
esophageal o.
extrahepatic binary o.
extrathoracic o.
extrinsic malignant o.
false colonic o.
fecal o.
fetal bowel o.
fetal renal o.
fixed airway o.
fixed coronary o.
flow-dependent o.
food bolus o.
foreign body upper airway o.
functional ureteral o.
gastric outlet o.
gastrointestinal tract o.
hepatic venous outflow o.
high-grade o.
high small bowel o.
hydrocephalic o.
idiopathic o.
ileal o.
incomplete o.
increased pulmonary o.
inferior vena cava o.
infravesical o.
interposed colon segment o.
intestinal o.
intrapancreatic o.
intrathoracic upper airway o.
intraventricular right ventricular o.
intravesical o.
irreversible airways o.
jejunal o.
large bowel o.
left ventricular inflow tract o.
left ventricular outflow tract o. (LVOTO)
low small bowel o.
lymphatic o.
malignant airway o.
mammary duct o.
mechanical biliary o.
mechanical bowel o.
mechanical duct o.
mechanical extrahepatic o.
mechanical intestinal o.
mechanical respiratory tract o.
mechanical small bowel o.
neurogenic intestinal o.
otic o.
outflow o.
outlet o.
pancreatic duct o.
paralytic colonic o.
partial small bowel o.
pelvic venous o.
preocclusive o.
prostatic o.
pulmonary artery o.
pulmonary outflow o.
pulmonary vascular o.
pulmonary venous o.
pyloric outlet o.
pyloroduodenal o.
rectal o.
renal o.
respiratory tract o.
right ventricular outflow o.
Rigler triad of small bowel o.
secondary o.
segmental biliary o.
sequence o.
simple mechanical o.
small bowel o. (SBO)
strangulated o.
subclavian artery o.
subpulmonic o.
subrectus o.
subvalvular aortic o.

subvalvular diffuse muscular o.
superior vena caval o.
suprapancreatic o.
supravesical o.
thrombotic o.
transient shunt o.
tubal o.
upper airway o.
ureteral renal transplant o.
ureteropelvic junction o.
ureterovesical junction o.
urethral o.
urinary o.
vascular o.
venous o.
ventricular o.
vesical outlet o.

obstructive
o. abnormality
o. airway disease
o. atelectasis
o. biliary cirrhosis
o. calculus
o. component
o. dysfunctional ileitis
o. emphysema
o. hydrocephalus
o. hypertrophic cardiomyopathy
o. hypopnea
o. jaundice
o. lesion
o. lung disease
o. nephrogram
o. nephropathy
o. pancreatitis
o. plaque
o. pneumonia
o. pulmonary disease (OPD)
o. pulmonary overinflation
o. renal dysplasia
o. thrombus
o. uropathy
o. ventilatory defect

obtundation

obturating embolus

obturator
o. avulsion fracture
o. externus
o. foramen
o. hernia
o. internus
o. internus fascia
o. internus muscle
o. line
o. lymph node
o. membrane
o. nodal chain
o. sign

obtuse
o. margin
o. marginal (OM)
o. marginal branch (OMB)
o. marginal coronary artery

occipital
o. artery
o. bone
o. bossing
o. cephalocele
o. condyle
o. condyle fracture
o. condyle hypoplasia
o. condyle invasion
o. eminence
o. encephalocele
o. fissure
o. focus
o. fontanelle
o. gyrus
o. horn
o. lesion
o. lobe
o. lobe infarct
o. lymph node
o. meningocele
o. pole
o. protuberance
o. sinus
o. suture
o. tip
o. vessel
o. view
o. view of skull

occipitalization
atlas o.
o. of atlas

occipitoanterior

occipitoatlantoaxial
o. anomaly
o. fusion
o. ligament

occipitoaxial
o. joint
o. ligament

O

NOTES

occipitocervical
o. angle
o. articulation
o. fusion
o. junction
o. plate
occipitofrontal fasciculus
occipitofrontalis muscle
occipitomastoid suture
occipitomental projection
occipitoparietal suture
occipitopontine tract
occipitoposterior
occipitosphenoid suture
occipitotemporal
o. convolution
o. gyrus
o. sulcus
occipitotemporopontine tract
occiput
occlude
occluded
o. graft
o. lumen
occluder
ameroid o.
Flo-Rester vessel o.
radiolucent plastic o.
Rashkind double-disk umbrella o.
occluding
o. spring embolus
occlusal
o. facet
o. film
o. plane
o. radiograph
o. segment
o. surface
occlusion
angiographic o.
o. angiography
aqueductal o.
arterial o.
o. of artery
atrial septal defect o.
balloon test o.
basilar o.
bilateral o.
carotid artery o.
carotid-cavernous fistula o.
cerebral sinovenous o.
complete o.
coronary o.
deep venous o.
diathermic vascular o.
ductus arteriosus o.
dural sinus o.
embolic o.
fallopian tube o.
graft o.
infrapopliteal artery o.
intermittent o.
intracranial vascular o.
late graft o.
o. measurement
mesenteric artery o.
percutaneous thermal o.
pulmonary arterial o.
side-branch o.
snowplow o.
subclavian artery o.
subclavian vein o.
subtotal o.
superficial femoral artery o.
tapering o.
thermal o.
thrombotic o.
total o.
traumatogenic o.
tubal o.
unilateral o.
ureteral o.
vascular brain o.
vein graft o.
venous o.
vertebral artery o.
vertebrobasilar o.
vessel o.
occlusive
o. arterial thrombus
o. cerebrovascular disease
o. cerebrovascular insult
o. ileus
o. impedance phlebography
o. lesion
o. mesenteric infarct
o. vascular brain disease
occult
o. blood
o. bone metastasis
o. carcinoma of the thyroid
o. cerebral vascular malformation (OCVM)
o. detection
o. fracture
o. hydrocephalus
o. lesion
o. papillary carcinoma
o. pericardial constriction
o. primary tumor of testis
o. residual herniated disk
roentgenographically o.
o. spinal dysraphism
o. steal syndrome
o. subluxation
o. vascular brain malformation

occulta
spina bifida o. (SBO)
occultum
cranium bifidum o.
OCG
oral cholecystogram
OCG imaging
ochronosis
Ochsner
O. muscle
O. ring
OCL
oral colonic lavage
OCL bowel preparation
O'Connor finger dexterity test
OCR
off-center ratio
OCT
optical coherence tomography
OctreoScan
O. imaging agent
Octreoscan system
octreotide
o. acetate
O. imaging agent
O. scintigraphy
ocular
o. globe topography
o. implant
o. lesion
o. pneumoplethysmography (OPG)
o. radiation therapy (ORT)
o. rhabdomyosarcoma
o. trauma
oculoauriculovertebral (OAV)
o. dysplasia (OAV dysplasia)
oculomotor
o. apparatus
o. nerve
o. sign
oculomotor-trochlear nucleus
oculopharyngeal dystrophy
oculoplethysmography (OPG)
oculoplethysmography/carotid phonoangiography (OPG/CPA)
oculopneumoplethysmography
oculosubcutaneous syndrome of Yuge
OCVM
occult cerebral vascular malformation
OD
optical density
odd-echo dephasing
Oddi
O. muscle
sphincter of O.
Odelca camera unit
O'Donoghue unhappy triad
odontogenic
o. cyst
o. fibromyxoma
o. keratocyst
o. tumor
odontoid
o. bone
o. condyle fracture
o. dysplasia
o. erosion
o. ligament
pannus deformity of o.
o. process
o. view
odontoideum
os o.
odontoma
ODQ
opponens digiti quinti
ODQ muscle
odynophagia
OEC Series 9600 cardiac system
OEF
oxygen extraction fraction
Oehl muscle
OER
oxygen extraction rate
OFD
object-film distance
off
tapering o.
off-axis
o.-a. dose inhomogeneity
o.-a. factor (OAF)
o.-a. point localization
o.-a. ratio (OAR)
off-center
o.-c. cuts
o.-c. modulation
o.-c. ratio (OCR)
Office of Health Technology Assessment
off-resonance
rotating delivery of excitation o.-r.
o.-r. saturation
o.-r. saturation pulse imaging
o.-r. spin-locking

NOTES

off-resonance *(continued)*
three-dimensional rotating delivery of excitation o.-r.
offset
o. frequency
frequency o.
quarter-detector o.
o. radiofrequency spin echo
Ogden
O. classification of epiphyseal fractures
O. epiphyseal fracture classification
Ogilvie syndrome
Ogston line
Ohio
O. infuser
O. Nuclear Delta 50 FS scanner
O. Nuclear Delta 2000 scanner
ohm
ohmic heating
Ohngren line
OHP
orthogonal-hole test pattern
OI
osteogenesis imperfecta
OIH
iodine-123 orthoiodohippurate
I-123 OIH
iodine-131 OIH
oil
brominized o.
chloriodized o.
o. cyst
o. embolus
o. emulsion imaging agent
ethiodized o.
iodized o.
oil-aspiration pneumonia
oil-water phantom
okadaic acid
Okuda transhepatic obliteration of varices
old
o. hemorrhage
o. myocardial infarct
olecranon
o. bursa
o. bursitis
o. fossa
o. process
o. tip fracture
oleothorax
Olerud and Molander fracture classification
olfactory
o. area
o. bulb
o. canal
o. groove meningioma
o. gyrus
o. neuroblastoma
o. sulcus
o. tract
oligemia
oligoastrocytoma
anaplastic mixed o.
recurrent vermian o.
oligodactylia
oligodendroglioma
bifrontal o.
subependymal o.
oligohydramnios
oligomeganephronia
oligonucleotide probe
olisthesis
olisthetic vertebra
olivary
o. degeneration
o. hypertrophy
olive
posterior o.
o. ring
Oliver-Cardarelli sign
olivopontocerebellar
o. atrophy
o. degeneration (OPCD)
Ollier disease
olsalazine imaging agent
OLT
osteochondral lesion of the talus
olycystic ovarian disease
Olympus
O. endoscopic ultrasound
O. endoscopic ultrasound scanner
O. Gastrocamera GTF-A
O. GF-UM2, GF-UM3 echoendoscope
O. UM-1W transendoscopic ultrasound probe
O. VU-M2 endoscope
O. XIF-UM3 echoendoscope
OM
obtuse marginal
OM artery
OMB
obtuse marginal branch
omega-sella
Omenn syndrome
omental
o. band
o. bursa
o. cake
o. cyst
o. infarct

o. mass
o. tuberosity
omentum, pl. **omenta**
colic o.
gastric o.
gastrocolic o.
gastrohepatic o.
gastrosplenic o.
greater o.
incarcerated o.
lesser o.
o. majus
o. minus
pancreaticosplenic o.
sigmoid o.
splenogastric o.
ominous sign
Omnipaque
O. imaging agent
O. injection
Omniscan
O. imaging agent
omohyoid muscle
omovertebral bone
omphalic
omphalitis
neonatal o.
omphalocele
infraumbilical o.
omphaloma
omphalomesenteric
o. duct
o. duct cyst
o. remnant
omphalopagus
onchocerciasis
oncocalyx
oncocytic thyroid adenoma
oncocytoma
pituitary o.
oncogenesis
radiation o.
oncogenic
o. rickets
oncologist
oncology
American Society for Therapeutic Radiology and O. (ASTRO)
picture archiving and communications systems in radiation o. (PACSRO)
radiation o.
on-column
o.-c. preparation
OncoRad
O. OV103
OncoScint
O. breast imaging agent
O. CR103
O. CR/OV
O. OV103
O. PR
oncosis
OncoSpect imaging agent
oncotaxonomy
OncoTrac
O. imaging agent
oncotropic
one-dimensional
o.-d. chemical-shift imaging (1D-CSI)
o.-d. phase encoding
one-line anion exchange purification
one-part fracture
one-shot echoplanar imaging
one-sided image reconstruction
one-stage amputation
one-step production
"one-stick" system
one-third ejection fraction
one-ventricle heart
onion
o. bulb changes
o. peel appearance
onion-shaped dilatation of duodenum
onionskin
o. appearance
o. configuration of collagenous fiber
o. lesion
o. periosteal reaction
onlay graft
on-line portal imaging
on-off phenomenon
onset
insidious o.
onychoosteodysplasia
familial o.
oocyte
o. retrieval
oogenesis
oophorus
opacification
collecting system o.

NOTES

opacification *(continued)*
contrast o.
extravesical o.
ground-glass o. (GGO)
o. of hemithorax
hemithorax o.
maxillary sinus o.
o. of maxillary sinus
nonsegmental areas of o.
pedal artery o.
o. of posterior longitudinal ligament
opacifying
o. gallstone
o. injection
opacity
air-space o.
bubbly o.
chronic diffuse confluent lung o.
chronic multifocal ill-defined lung o.
diffuse o.
ground-glass o.
homogeneous o.
linear o.
lung o.
nodular o.
parenchymal o.
patchy alveolar o.
pleura-based area of increased o.
reticular o.
opaque
o. calculus
o. meal
o. medium
o. stone
o. synovium
o. wire suture
OPCD
olivopontocerebellar degeneration
OPD
obstructive pulmonary disease
Opdima digital mammography system
open
o. beam
o. bronchus sign
o. dislocation
o. fontanelle
o. fracture
o. magnet
o. MRI
o. neural tube defect
o. pneumothorax
o. reduction
o. reduction and internal fixation (ORIF)
o. tuberculosis
open-architecture system
open-book fracture
open-break fracture
open-configuration magnetic resonance system
open-cord tendon implant
open-ended guide wire
opening (os)
aortic o. (AO, Ao)
aortic valve o.
o. of aortic valve
buttonhole o.
caval o.
esophageal o.
mitral valve o. (MVO)
o. slope
valvular o.
open-mouth odontoid view
OpenPACS system
opera-glass hand
operation
biliary-enteric anastomosis o.
3D connect o.
Mustard o.
Nissen antireflux o.
pulsed-mode o.
three-dimensional-connect o.
Whipple o.
operative
o. cholangiogram
operator exposure
opercula (*pl. of* operculum)
opercular cortex
operculofrontal artery
operculum, pl. **opercula**
cerebral o.
sylvian o.
OPG
ocular pneumoplethysmography
oculoplethysmography
ophthalmoplethysmography
OPG/CPA
oculoplethysmography/carotid phonoangiography
ophenoxic acid
ophthalmic
o. artery
o. biometry by ultrasound echography
o. nerve
o. vein
ophthalmicus
ophthalmopathy
ophthalmoplegia
ophthalmoplethysmography (OPG)
ophthalmoscopy
scanning laser o.
opioid
opisthion

opisthotonic position
Opitz thrombophlebitic splenomegaly
Oppenheim sign
opponens
o. digiti minimi
o. digiti quinti (ODQ)
o. digiti quinti muscle
o. pollicis
opportunistic
o. infection
o. lung cavity infection
opposed
o. GRE image
o. loop-pair quadrature NMR coil
opposed-phase
o.-p. GRE imaging
o.-p. image
o.-p. MRI
o.-p. MR imaging
o.-p. sequence
opposing
o. articular surfaces
o. muscle
o. pleural surfaces
opposite breast cancer
opposition
finger o.
opsoclonus
optic
o. canal
o. chiasm
o. chiasm disease
o. complex tumor
o. excrescentic thickening
o. foramen
o. glioma pathway
o. globe
o. glove
o. nerve
o. nerve compression
o. nerve enlargement
o. nerve fusiform thickening
o. nerve glioma
o. nerve hypoplasia
o. nerve lesion
o. nerve sheath meningioma
o. neuritis
o. pathway myelination
o. radiation
o. recess
o. strut
optical
o. coherence tomography (OCT)
o. density (OD)
o. isomer
o. surface imaging (OSI)
opticochiasmatic cistern
optimal
o. imaging plane
o. visualization
optimally positioned view
optimization
interactive gradient o.
iterative gradient o.
o. parameter
optimum-angle imaging
optimum dose
optional target-to-background ratio
Optiplanimat automated unit
Optiray
O. 320 imaging agent
Optison ultrasound contrast agent
ora (*pl. of* os)
Orabilex
O. sodium imaging agent
Oragrafin
O. Calcium imaging agent
O. Sodium imaging agent
oral
o. bile desaturating agent
o. cavity tumor
o. cephalocele
o. cholecystogram (OCG)
o. cholecystogram imaging
o. colonic lavage (OCL)
o. contrast imaging agent
o. fissure
o. intubation
o. magnetic particle
o. part of pharynx
oral-enhanced CT scan
Oralex ultrasound imaging agent
orange
acridine o.
xylenol o.
Oravue imaging agent
orbicular
o. bone
o. ligament
orbicularis
o. sign
zona o.

NOTES

orbit
angular process of o.
o. artifact
body contour o.
bony o.
egg-shaped o.
electron o.
floor of the o.
o. measurement
Rhese view of o.'s
orbitae
aditus o.
orbital
o. abscess
o. aneurysm
o. apex
o. apex syndrome
o. aspect of frontal lobe
o. base
o. blood cyst
o. blowout fracture
o. bone
o. canal
o. capillary hemangioma
o. cavity
o. cellulitis
o. childhood tumor
o. chocolate cyst
o. coke-bottle sign
o. dermoid cyst
o. edema
o. electrons
o. emphysema
o. fissure
o. floor fracture
o. granulocytic sarcoma
o. gyrus
o. hemangioma
o. infection
o. juvenile pilocytic astrocytoma
o. lymphangioma
o. lymphoma
o. mass compression
o. metastasis
o. mucocele
o. plate
o. pseudotumor
o. rhabdomyosarcoma
o. rim
o. rim stepoff
o. sarcoidosis
o. schwannoma
o. space
o. superolateral quadrant mass
o. teratoma
o. varix
o. varix ophthalmic vein
o. wall
orbitofrontal cortex
orbitography
orbitopathy
thyroid o.
orbitosphenoidal bone
orbitotomy
Krönlein o.
Orbix x-ray unit
Orca C-arm fluoroscopy
orchiectomy
radical o.
orchitis
ordered phase encoding
Orfit mask
organ
accessory o.
annulospiral o.
o. capsule
circumventricular o.
Corti o.
critical o.
extraperitoneal o.
floating o.
hollow o.
o. ischemia
o. piping
poles of o.
retroperitoneal o.
sanctuary o.
secondary retroperitoneal o.
target o.
o. transplant
Zuckerkandl o.
organelle
sphere o.
organic
o. brain disease (OBD)
o. brain syndrome (OBS)
o. free radical
o. granulomatosis
o. lesion
o. muscle
o. sign
organification defect
organized hematoma
organizing
o. focal pneumonia
o. interstitial pneumonia
organoaxial
o. rotation
o. volvulus
organogenesis
organoid structure
organomegaly
organ-specific concentration
organs of Zuckerkandl
Oriental
O. cholangiogram

O. cholangiohepatitis
O. lung fluke
orientation
angle of o.
coronal o.
cruciate o.
disk-to-magnetic field o.
disturbed o.
sagittal o.
slice o.
spatial o.
temporal o.
transverse o.
ORIF
open reduction and internal fixation
orifice
anal o.
aortic o.
atrioventricular nodal o.
cardiac o.
coronary o.
double coronary o.
esophagogastric o.
external urethral o.
gastroduodenal o.
golf-hole ureteral o.
hypoplastic tricuspid o.
ileocecal o.
inferior vena cava o.
internal urethral o.
lingular o.
mitral o. (MO)
mitral valve o. (MVO)
narrowed o.
pharyngeal o.
pulmonary o.
pyloric o.
rectal o.
regurgitant o.
segmental bronchus o.
slitlike o.
tricuspid o.
ureteral o.
urethral o.
vaginal o.
valvular o.
orifice-to-annulus ratio
origin
anomalous o.
o. of artery
histiocytic bone tumor o.
neural crest o.
spatial o.
o. of vessel
Ormond disease
orodigitofacial syndrome
oroendotracheal tube
orofacial fistula
orogastric tube
oropharyngeal
o. airway
o. dysfunction
o. dysphagia
o. emptying
o. narrowing
oropharynx
orotracheal intubation
ORT
ocular radiation therapy
Orthicon
O. camera
O. tube
orthocephalic
orthodeoxia
orthogonal
o. angiographic projection
o. plane
o. projection mammography
o. radiofrequency coil
o. tag line
o. view
o. view on angiography
orthogonal-hole test pattern (OHP)
orthoiodohippurate
iodine-123 o. (OIH)
iodine-131 o.
orthonormal diameter
orthopantogram
o. imaging
orthopedic
o. cement
o. fixation device
o. nail
o. pin
o. plate
o. rod
o. screw
o. staple
orthoroentgenogram
o. imaging
orthosis drop-lock ring
orthostereoscope
orthotic plate

NOTES

orthotopic
o. total heart replacement
o. ureter
o. ureterocele
orthovoltage
o. radiation therapy
Ortner syndrome
Ortolani
O. sign
O. test
Orudis
os, pl. **ora**
mouth
opening
coronary sinus os
external os
internal cervical os
nulla per os (n.p.o.)
per os (p.o.)
os, pl. **ossa**
os acetabulum
os acromiale
os calcis
os calcis bone
os coxae
os cuboides secondarium
os fabella
os infundibulum
os naviculare
os odontoideum
os peroneum
os pubis
os styloidium
os supratrochleare dorsale
os tibiale externum
os trapezium bone
os trapezoideum bone
os trigonum
os trigonum syndrome
Osbil
Osborne ligament
OSCAR ultrasonic bone cement removal system
oscillating
o. electrons
o. gradient
o. grid
o. magnetic field
oscillation
resonant frequency of o.
oscillography
oscilloscope
o. tuning station
oseomyelitis
chronic recurrent multifocal o.
Osgood-Schlatter disease
OSI
optical surface imaging
Osler
O. disease
O. maneuver
O. node
O. sign
O. syndrome
O. triad
Osler-Libman-Sacks syndrome
Osler-Weber-Rendu
O.-W.-R. disease
O.-W.-R. syndrome
O.-W.-R. telangiectasia
Osm
osmole
osmium-194
osmolality
low o.
osmole (Osm)
osmotic
o. demyelination syndrome
o. edema
o. effect
o. load
ossa (*pl. of* os)
ossea
facies o.
leontiasis o.
osseocartilaginous
o. arch
o. thoracic cage
osseoligamentous
o. arch
o. ring
osseous, osteal
o. abnormality
o. bone contusion
o. bridge
o. coalition
o. defect
o. destructive process
o. dysplasia
o. graft
o. hemangioendothelioma
o. hemangioma
o. instability
o. labyrinth
o. lacuna
o. lesion
o. metastasis
o. patellar outgrowth
o. pinch mechanism
o. polyp
o. remodeling
o. spiral lamina
o. structure
o. survey
o. tissue
o. union

ossicle
accessory o.
benign Bergman o.
Kerckring o.
meniscal o.
Riolan o.
ossiferous
ossific
o. nodule
o. nucleus
o. nucleus of navicular
ossificans
fasciitis o.
labyrinthitis o.
myositis circumscripta o.
panniculitis o.
subacute myositis o.
ossification
abnormal o.
Brooker classification of heterotopic o.
o. of cartilaginous structure
o. center
diaphyseal o.
disk o.
ectopic o.
enchondral o.
extraarticular posterior o.
flowing anterior vertebra o.
heterotopic scar o.
intracartilaginous o.
intramembranous o.
irregular enchondral o.
muscle o.
paravertebral o.
periarticular heterotopic o. (PHO)
peripheral o.
o. of the posterior longitudinal ligament
primary center of o.
scar o.
secondary center of o.
soft tissue o.
o. of soft tissue
spine o.
o. variant
vertebral arch ligament o.
ossified
o. body
o. posterior longitudinal ligament
o. scar
ossifying
o. bone fibroma
o. cochleitis
o. epiphysis
o. fibroma of long bone
o. skull fibroma
ossium
fibrogenesis imperfecta o.
fragilitas o.
osteal (*var. of* osseous)
ostealgia
osteitis
o. condensans ilii
o. deformans
o. fibrosa
o. fibrosa cystica
o. pubis
ostemia
ostempyesis
OsteoAnalyzer device
osteoaneurysm
osteoarthritic
o. cartilage
o. change
o. spur
osteoarthritis (OA)
degenerative o.
early o.
erosive o.
generalized o.
o. grade
o. grading classification
hand o.
posttraumatic o.
premature o.
traumatic o.
osteoarthropathy
hypertrophic pulmonary o.
neuropathic o.
primary hypertrophic o.
pulmonary o.
osteoarticular
osteoblastic
o. activity
o. bone regeneration
o. lesion
o. metastasis
o. osteosarcoma
o. presentation
o. tumor
osteoblastoma
expansile o.

NOTES

osteocachexia
osteocartilaginous
o. defect
o. exostosis
o. lesion
o. metaplasia
o. parasellar neoplasm
o. tissue
o. tumor
osteochondral
o. defect
o. fragment
o. lesion
o. lesion of the talus (OLT)
o. loose body
o. slice fracture
osteochondritis
o. dissecans
osteochondrodysplasia
osteochondrodystrophia deformans
osteochondrodystrophy
osteochondrofibroma
osteochondrolysis
osteochondroma
epiphyseal o.
soft tissue o.
osteochondromatosis
bursal o.
multiple o.
synovial o.
tenosynovial o.
osteochondrophyte
osteochondroplastica
tracheobronchopathia o.
tracheopathia o.
osteochondrosis
o. deformans juvenilis
o. dissecans
intervertebral o.
spinal o.
vertebral o.
osteochondrotic
o. loose body
o. separation of epiphysis
osteoclasis
osteoclastic
o. erosion
o. resorption
osteoclastoma
osteocyte
osteocytoma
osteodermopathia hypertrophicans
osteodiastasis
osteodystrophy
Albright hereditary o.
azotemic o.
congenital renal o.
renal o.
osteoenchondroma
osteofibrochondrosarcoma
osteofibromatosis
cystic o.
osteofibrous dysplasia
osteogenesis
distraction o.
o. imperfecta (OI)
o. imperfecta tarda
osteogenic
o. bone fibroma
parosteal o.
o. sarcoma
osteoid
o. carcinoma
malignant o.
o. matrix
o. osteoma
o. seam
tumor o.
osteolipochondroma
osteolipoma
osteolysis
blade-of-grass o.
candle-flame o.
essential o.
expansile multilocular o.
idiopathic o.
lytic o.
malignant acetabular o.
mandible o.
massive o.
medial end of clavicle o.
mixed sclerotic o.
multiple o.
nonexpansile multilocular o.
nonexpansile unilocular o.
o. on both sides of joint
sacral o.
scalloping o.
skull o.
temporomandibular joint o.
trabeculated o.
o. tuft
osteolytic
o. lesion
o. metastasis
osteoma, pl. **osteomas, osteomata**
cancellous osteoid o.
choroidal o.
cortical osteoid o.
costal o.
fibrous o.
giant osteoid o.
intracapsular osteoid o.
juxtaarticular osteoid o.
osteoid o.
parosteal o.

soft tissue o.
spongy o.
subperiosteal osteoid o.
tropical ulcer o.
ulcer o.

osteomalacia
hematogenous o.
hypophosphatemic o.
renal tubular o.
senile o.

osteomalacic pelvis

osteomas (*pl. of* osteoma)

osteomata (*pl. of* osteoma)

osteomatosis

osteomesophyknosis

osteomyelitic sinus

osteomyelitis
Ackerman criteria for o.
active o.
acute hematogenous o. (AHO)
bacterial o.
brucellar o.
childhood o.
early o.
nocardial o.
pyogenic o.
recurrent multifocal o.
sacral o.
o. scintigraphy
sclerosing nonsuppurative o.
spinal o.
synovitis, acne, pustulosis, hyperostosis, o. (SAPHO)
tuberculous o.
vertebral o.

osteomyelofibrosis

osteonal bone

osteonecrosis
radiation o.
spontaneous o.

osteopathia
o. condensans disseminata
o. striata

osteopenia
localized o.

osteopenic bone

osteopetrosis
cranial o.
malignant o.

osteophyte
anterior o.
bony o.
bridging o.
cervical o.
floating o.
o. formation
fringe of o.
horseshoe o.
impinging o.
jagged o.
marginal o.
posterior o.
spinal o.

osteophytic
o. bone lip
o. bridge
o. lipping
o. proliferation
o. spurring

osteophytosis

osteoplastica
tracheopathia o.

osteoplastic flap

osteopoikilosis

osteoporosis
o. of bone
o. circumscripta
corticosteroid-induced o.
disuse o.
ground-glass o.
juvenile o.
localized o.
partial transient o.
periarticular o.
picture-framing o.
postmenopausal o.
posttraumatic o.
regional migratory o.
regional transient o.
senile o.
Singh index of o.
transient regional o.

osteoporotic
o. bone
o. fracture

osteoradiology

osteoradionecrosis

osteosarcoma
cardiac o.
central o.
chondroblastic o.

NOTES

osteosarcoma *(continued)*
classical o.
conventional o.
epithelioid o.
extraosseous o.
extraskeletal o.
extremity o.
fibroblastic o.
gnathic o.
intracortical o.
intraosseous o.
jaw o.
metastatic o.
multicentric o.
multifocal o.
multiple sclerotic o.
osteoblastic o.
parosteal o.
sclerosing o.
secondary o.
surface o.
telangiectatic o.
osteosarcomatosis
osteosclerosis
constitutional o.
diffuse o.
multiple-lesion o.
solitary o.
subchondral o.
o. tuft
o. vertebral sarcoidosis
osteosclerotic lesion
osteosis
osteospongioma
osteosynthesis
biological o.
osteothrombosis
osteotomy
OsteoView
O. desktop hand x-ray system
O. digital bone densitometer
ostial
o. cannulation
o. lesion
o. renal artery stenosis
ostiomeatal
o. complex
o. unit
ostium, pl. **ostia**
o. abdominale tubae uterinae
aortic o.
artery o.
atrioventricular nodal o.
conus branch ostia
coronary artery o.
coronary sinus o.
o. primum
o. primum atrial septal defect
o. secundum
o. secundum atrial septal defect
ostomy bag
Ostreg spinal marker system
Ostwald solubility coefficient (Λ)
OSTYCUT bone biopsy needle
otic
o. capsule
o. ganglion
o. obstruction
oticus
herpes zoster o.
otitis
o. externa
external malignant o.
malignant external o.
necrotizing external o.
otologic implant
otorrhea
otosclerosis
cochlear o.
fenestral o.
retrofenestral o.
stapedial o.
otospongiosis
OTT
overall treatment time
Otto
O. pelvis
O. pelvis dislocation
Otto-Krobak pelvis
out
rule o. (R/O)
silhouetted o.
outcropping of lesion
outer
o. annular/posterior longitudinal ligament complex
o. canthus
o. table
o. table of the skull
Outerbridge
O. degenerative arthritis staging
O. ridge
O. scale
outflow
double o.
o. effect
hepatic venous o.
hypoplastic subpulmonic o.
maximum venous o. (MVO)
o. obstruction
subpulmonic o.
swan neck shape of ventricular o.
o. tract
o. tract gradient
o. of ventricle
outgrowth
osseous patellar o.
outlet
cervical o.

o. impingement
o. obstruction
pelvic o.
pyloric o.
thoracic o.
ventricular o.
o. view
o. view radiograph
widened thoracic o.

outline
absent kidney o.
double o.
gastric o.
renal o.
trabeculated o.

out-of-phase
o.-o.-p. gradient echo
o.-o.-p. GRE imaging

out-of-profile nipple

out-of-slice artifact

outpocketings of mucosa

outpouching
saccular o.

output
adequate cardiac o.
o. amplitude
augmented cardiac o.
cardiac o. (CO, Q)
Douglas back method for determining cardiac o.
Dow method for measuring cardiac o.
Fick method for cardiac o.
Gorlin method for cardiac o.
Hamilton-Stewart formula for measuring cardiac o.
Hetzel forward triangle method for cardiac o.
inadequate cardiac o.
instrument o.
low cardiac o.
o. point
pulmonic o.
reduced systemic cardiac o.
stroke o.
systemic o.
thermodilution cardiac o.
ventricular o.

outrigger arm

outside film

OV
ovarian

OV103
OncoRad O.
OncoScint O.

ova (*pl. of* ovum)

Ovadia-Beals tibial plafond fracture classification

oval
o. shape
o. window

ovalbumin

ovale
centrum o.
foramen o.
patent foramen o. (PFOB)
o. skull base of foramen

ovalis
annulus o.
fossa o.
limbus fossae o.

oval-shaped breast lesion

ovarian (OV)
o. abscess
o. anatomy
o. artery
o. carcinoma
o. choriocarcinoma
o. cortex
o. cystadenofibroma
o. cystadenoma
o. dermoid
o. dermoid cyst
o. Doppler signal
o. dysgenesis
o. dysgerminoma
o. edema
o. fibroma
o. fishnet weave pattern
o. follicular cyst
o. fossa
o. hernia
o. hyperstimulation syndrome
o. image signature cyst
o. mass
o. medulla
o. mesonephroid tumor
o. metastasis
o. morphology
o. polycystic syndrome
o. pregnancy
o. remnant syndrome
o. retention cyst
o. serous cystadenocarcinoma

O

NOTES

ovarian *(continued)*
o. size
o. suspensory ligament
o. systic teratoma
o. torsion
o. vein
o. vein syndrome
o. vein thrombosis
ovarii
struma o.
ovarioabdominal pregnancy
ovary
atrophied o.
clear cell neoplasm of o.
cystic o.
embryonic o.
fibroma-thecoma tumor of o.
o. germ cell tumor
o. gland
hilar cell tumor of o.
hyperstimulation of o.
ligament of o.
mulberry o.
palpable postmenopausal o.
pearly white o.
polycystic o.
postmenopausal o.
sclerocystic o.
stromal carcinoid of o.
suspensory ligament of o.
teratoblastoma of o.
teratocarcinoma of o.
thecoma of o.
transposition of o.
Ovation falloposcopy system
overaeration
overall treatment time (OTT)
overcirculation
pulmonary vessel o.
o. vascularity
overcouch
o. exposure
o. tube
o. view
overdevelopment
bone o.
overdiagnostic bias
overdistention
alveolar o.
pulmonary o.
overdrive suppression
overexpansion
lung o.
pulmonary o.
overframing
horizontal o.
mean-diameter o.
subtotal o.
overgrowth
bony o.
cuticular o.
epiphyseal o.
fibrocartilaginous o.
overhanging margin
Overhauser
O. effect
O. technique
overhead
o. film
o. oblique view
overinflation
lung o.
obstructive pulmonary o.
pulmonary o.
unilateral o.
overlapping
o. finger
o. fracture
o. images
o. suture
overlay plate
overlie
overload
acute hemodynamic o.
cardiac o.
chronic hemodynamic o.
diastolic o.
fluid o.
pressure o.
right ventricular o.
systolic ventricular o.
transfusional iron o.
volume o.
overlying
o. attenuation artifact
o. bowel content
o. bowel gas
o. bowel shadows
o. branching pattern
overpenetrated film
over-read
overrelaxation factor
override
aortic o.
overriding
o. aorta
o. of fracture fragments
o. great artery
o. sutures of fontanelle
o. toes
oversampling
overshooting
conjugate o.
overstaged

overuse
o. injury
o. syndrome
overventilation
alveolar o.
oviductal pregnancy
ovoid
afterloading tandem and o.'s
o. heart
Manchester o.
o. shape
tandem and o.'s
ovulation
o. failure sign
incessant o.
o. induction
ovulatory
o. failure
o. phase
ovum, pl. **ova**
aspiration of ova
Owen-Pendergrass method
Owen view
owl's eye appearance
oxalosis
bone o.
kidney o.
primary o.
Oxford
O. magnet
O. 2-T large-bore imaging system scanner
ox heart
oxidation
Baeyer-Villiger o.
o. state
oxidative metabolism
oxide
deuterium o.
monocrystalline iron o.'s (MION)
nitrous o.
superparamagnetic agent iron o.
superparamagnetic iron o. (SPIO)
oxidized
o. complex
oxidronate
technetium-99m o.
Oxilan
O. imaging agent
oxime
hexamethylpropyleneamine o.
oximeter
oximetry
exercise o.
pulse o.
transcranial cerebral o.
oxine
oxine-indium
lipophilic o.-i.
oxycephaly
oxygen (O)
cerebral metabolic rate of o. ($CMRO_2$)
cistern o.
o. cisternography
o. consumption (QO_2)
o. effect
o. extraction fraction (OEF)
o. extraction rate (OER)
hyperbaric o.
o. imaging agent
inhaled o.
metabolic rate of o.
regional cerebral metabolic rate for o. ($rCMRO_2$)
o. saturation
oxygen-15 (^{15}O)
oxygen-16 (^{16}O)
oxygen-17 (^{17}O)
o. NMR spectroscopy
oxygen-18 (^{18}O)
oxygenated perfluorocarbon blood substitute
oxygenation
extracorporeal membrane o.
tissue o.
oxygenation-sensitive
o.-s. functional MR
o.-s. functional MR imaging
oxygenator
extracorporeal membrane o.
oxygen-dependent emphysema
oxygen-free water
oxyphilic
o. kidney adenoma
o. thyroid adenoma
oyster-pearl breast calcification
Ozonoff-Ogden sign

O

NOTES

π
pi
P
posterior
P loop
P pulmonale pattern
P1-P4 segments of posterior cerebral artery
^{32}P
phosphorus-32
sodium phosphate ^{32}P
9p
trisomy 9p
PA
posteroanterior
pulmonary artery
PA and lateral films
PA projection
Paas disease
PABA
paraaminobenzoic acid
PABP
pulmonary artery balloon pump
pacchionian
p. bodies
p. body
p. depression
p. granulation
pace
p. mapping
pacemaker
p. artifact
bipolar p.
implanted p.
p. lead
p. wire
Pace Plus System scanner
pachydermoperiostosis
pachygyria
pachymeningitis
pachymeninx, pl. **pachymeninges**
pachypleuritis
pacing artifact
packed beads
packing, extraction, and calculation technique
pack-years of cigarette smoking
pack-year smoking history
PACS
picture archiving and communication system
PBT Technologies PACS
PACSRO
picture archiving and communications systems in radiation oncology
PAD
percutaneous abscess drainage
pulmonary artery diastolic pressure
pad
abdominal fat p.
antimesenteric fat p.
Bichat fat p.
p. effect
epicardial fat p.
esophagogastric fat p.
fat p.
fibrocartilaginous p.
fingertip p.
foveal fat p.
haversian fat p.
heel fat p.
Hoffa fat p.
ileocecal fat p.
intracapsular fat p.
intrapatellar fat p.
ischiorectal fat p.
patellar fat p.
pericardial fat p.
pre-Achilles fat p.
Sat P.
scalene fat p.
p. sign
p. sign of aortic insufficiency
thickened heel p.
UltraEase ultrasound p.
ultrasound p.
padding
antral p.
paddle
compression p.
spot-compression p.
PADP-PAWP
pulmonary artery diastolic and wedge pressure
PAEDP
pulmonary artery end-diastolic pressure
Page kidney
Paget
P. abscess
P. carcinoma
P. disease of nipple
P. jaw disease
P. osteitis deformans
P. quiet necrosis
P. temporal bone disease
Paget-associated osteogenic sarcoma
pagetic
pagetoid
p. bone
p. epidermal involvement

Paget-Schroetter venous thrombosis
Paget-von Schroetter syndrome
PAH
paraaminohippurate
pain
abdominal p.
acute flank p.
atypical chest p.
bone p.
congenital absence of p.
congenital insensitivity to p.
flank p.
low back p. (LBP)
myofascial p.
neuropathic p.
perimalleolar p.
phantom limb p.
radicular p.
referred p.
retrosternal chest p.
RUQ p.
pain-free walking time (PFWT)
painful
p. sclerosis
p. scoliosis
painless thyroiditis
paint brush striation
pair
electron-positron p.
line p.
Maxwell p.
p. production
paired
p. inferior vena cava
p. parietal branch
p. visceral branch
Pais fracture
PALA enhancement
palatal muscle
palate
bony p.
Byzantine arch p.
hard p.
high arched p.
soft p.
palatina
uvula p.
palatine
p. bone
p. canal
p. foramen
p. ridge
p. root
p. shelf
p. suture
palatini
levator veli p.
tensor veli p.
palatoglossus
palatomaxillary canal
palatomyograph
palatopharyngeal fold
palatopharyngeus
palatovaginal canal
paleopathologic and radiologic study
palisade formation
palladium (Pd)
p. imaging agent
p. implant
palliative
p. esophagostomy
p. irradiation
p. radiation therapy
pallidus
globus p.
palmar
p. angulation
p. aponeurosis
p. arterial arch
p. cutaneous vein
p. displacement
p. fascia
p. fasciitis
p. fibromatosis
p. ganglion
p. interossei
p. metacarpal ligament
p. plate
p. radiocarpal ligament
p. surface
p. wrist
palmaris
p. brevis
p. longus
palmatae
plicae p.
palmitate
^{11}C p.
retinyl p.
palmoplantar
palpable
p. aortic ejection sound
p. postmenopausal ovary
p. presystolic bulge
p. pulmonic ejection sound
palpatory T-stage prostate cancer
palpebra
levator p.'s
palpebral
p. fissure
p. raphe
palsy
Bell p.
bridegroom's p.
hypoglossal nerve p.

progressive supranuclear p.
waiter's tip p.
PAM
pulmonary artery mean pressure
PAM pressure
pampiniform plexus
panacinar emphysema
panaortic
panbronchiolitis
diffuse p.
pancake
p. appearance
p. kidney
p. MRI magnet
pancarpal destructive arthritis
panchamber
p. enlargement
p. hypertrophy
Pancoast
P. syndrome
P. tumor
pancompartmental joint space narrowing
pancreas, pl. **pancreata**
aberrant p.
accessory p.
annular p.
anterior surface of p.
Aselli p.
body of the p.
p. cystadenoma
degeneration of p.
p. divisum
dorsal p.
ectopic p.
fat-spared area in p.
p. gland
head of the p.
heterotopic p.
interior surface of p.
lesser p.
mature pseudocyst of p.
metastasis of p.
mucinous ductal ectasia of the p.
mucinous ductectatic tumor of p.
neck of p.
posterior surface of p.
p. secretin test
tail of p.
p. transplant
p. ultrasonography imaging
uncinate process of p.
ventral p.
Willis p.
Winslow p.
pancreatic
p. abscess
p. angiography
p. ascites
p. atrophy
p. calcification
p. calculus
p. cancer
p. carcinoma
p. cutaneous fistula
p. cyst
p. cystic fibrosis
p. cystic lymphangioma
p. cystosis
p. degeneration
p. deivisum
p. disease
p. dorsal anlage
p. duct
p. ductal adenocarcinoma
p. duct branch
p. duct dilatation
p. duct obstruction
p. duct sphincter
p. duct stent
p. fluid collection
p. hamartoma
p. head
p. islet cell tumor
p. lipomatosis
p. lymph node
p. lymphoma
p. macrocystic adenoma
p. mass
p. metastasis
p. microcystic adenoma
p. neck
p. necrosis
p. neoplasm
p. phlegmon
p. pseudocyst
p. pseudocyst drainage
p. scan
p. trauma
p. vein
pancreatic-enteric continuity
pancreaticobiliary
p. common channel
p. ductal junction

NOTES

P

pancreaticobiliary *(continued)*
p. function variant
p. sphincter
p. tract
p. ultrasound
pancreaticoblastoma
pancreaticoduodenal
p. artery
p. lymph node
pancreaticoduodenectomy
pancreaticohepatic syndrome
pancreaticolienal lymph node
pancreaticopleural fistula
pancreaticosplenic
p. node
p. omentum
pancreatitis
acute p.
chronic calcifying p.
chronic obstructive p.
diffuse p.
edematous p.
focal p.
necrotizing p.
obstructive p.
phlegmonous p.
p. pseudoaneurysm
Santiani-Stone classification of p.
suppurative p.
tropical p.
pancreatocholangiogram
retrograde p.
pancreatogram
pancreatography
endoscopic retrograde p.
p. imaging
intraoperative p.
percutaneous p.
retrograde p.
pancreatolithiasis
panda
p. appearance
p. sign
Pander island
Pandora pneumonitis
panduriform placenta
panencephalitis
progressive rubella p.
sclerosing p.
subacute sclerosing p. (SSPE)
panfacial fracture
panhypopituitarism
panlobar nephroglastomatosis
panlobular emphysema
panmyelopathy
panmyelosis
Panner disease
panni (*pl. of* pannus)
panniculitis
fasciitis p.
mesenteric p.
p. ossificans
systemic nodular p.
panniculus
pannus, pl. **panni**
p. deformity
p. deformity of odontoid
p. formation
synovial p.
p. of synovium
panoramic
p. CT scan
p. image
p. imaging
p. radiograph
p. rotating machine
p. surface projection
p. x-ray film
Panorex view
pansinusitis
pansystolic mitral regurgitation
pantalar fusion
pantaloon
p. embolus
p. hernia
pantomogram
pantomography
Pantopaque
P. cisternography
P. imaging agent
P. myelography
PAP
pulmonary artery pressure
Papavasiliou classification of olecranon fractures
paper chromatography
paper-doll fetus
Papile classification
papilla, pl. **papillae**
aberrant p.
acoustic p.
bile p.
p. of columnar epithelium
duodenal p.
major duodenal p.
minor duodenal p.
renal p.
Santorini p.
p. of Santorini
sloughed p.
smudged p.
urethral p.
p. of Vater
p. of Vater enlargement
p. of Vater stenosis

papillary
p. adenoma of large intestine
p. apocrine change
p. bile duct stenosis
p. breast carcinoma
p. cystadenoma lymphomatosum
p. cystic adenoma
p. cystic neoplasm
p. duct of Bellini
p. epididymal cystadenoma
p. epithelial neoplasm
p. excrescence
p. fibroelastoma
p. lesion
p. muscle
p. muscle dysfunction (PMD)
p. muscle infarct
p. muscle rupture
p. necrosis
p. pancreatic cystic neoplasm
p. projection
p. proliferation
p. renal cell carcinoma
p. serous adenocarcinoma
p. serous carcinoma
p. thyroid carcinoma
p. tumor
papillitis
necrotizing p.
papillocarcinoma
papillogram
papilloma, pl. **papillomas, papillomata**
p. acuminata
basal cell p.
p. of bladder
breast p.
p. breast
choroid plexus p.
cockscomb p.
p. diffusum
ductal p.
p. durum
fibroepithelial p.
p. of the fourth ventricle
hard p.
Hopmann p.
p. inguinale
intraductal p.
inverted p.
large duct p.
p. molle
multiple peripheral papillomas
p. neuropathicum
p. neuroticum
penile squamous p.
schneiderian p.
soft p.
squamous cell p.
transitional cell p.
transitional urethral cell p.
villous p.
papillomatosis
intraductal breast p.
juvenile breast p.
laryngeal p.
pulmonary p.
recurrent respiratory p.
tracheobronchial p.
papillomatous growth
Papillon-Lefevre syndrome
papillon technique
papillotomy
papova
Pappenheimer body
papular lesion
papulonecrotic lesion
PAPVR
partial anomalous pulmonary venous return
papyracea
lamina p.
papyraceus
fetus p.
p. fetus
PAR
plain abdominal radiography
paraaminobenzoic acid (PABA)
paraaminohippurate (PAH)
paraaminosalicylic acid (PAS)
paraaortic
p. lymphadenectomy
p. lymph node
paraarticular
p. bone remodeling
p. calcification
parabola
digital p.
metatarsal p.
parabolic velocity profile
paracarcinomatous myelopathy
paracardiac
p. mass
p. metastasis
p. tumor

NOTES

P

paracardiac-type total anomalous venous return
paracardial lymph node
paracecal appendix
paracentesis
abdominal p.
paracentral
p. artery
p. gyrus
p. lobule
paracervical lymphatic
parachute
p. deformity of mitral valve
p. mitral valve deformity
paracicatricial emphysema
paracoccidioidal granuloma
paracolic
p. abscess
p. gutter
p. lymph node
paracorporeal
p. heart
paracortical hyperplasia
paracostal
paracystic pouch
paradigm
LENT p.
p. shift
paradoxical
p. bronchospasm
p. cerebral embolus
p. colon dilatation
p. enhancement
p. hyperconcentration of contrast medium
p. leaflet motion
p. middle turbinate
p. septal motion
p. suppression
paradoxicum
paradoxus
pulsus p.
paraduodenal
p. fold
p. fossa
p. hernia
p. recess
paraesophageal
p. hernia
p. varix
paraesophagogastric devascularization
parafascicular nucleus
paraffinoma
paraganglioma
adrenal p.
chromaffin p.
extraadrenal p.
functional p.
gangliocytic p.
nonchromaffin p.
thoracic p.
paragangliomatosis
paraglenoid cyst
paragonimiasis
brain p.
lung p.
paragranuloma
parahiatal hernia
parahilar
parahippocampal gyrus
paraileostomal hernia
paraisopropyliminodiacetic acid (PIPIDA)
paralabral
p. cyst
p. lesion
paralaryngeal
p. muscle
p. space
parallax
p. method
p. view
parallel
p. analog mapping
p. arrays
p. channel sign
p. cine
p. data acquisition coil
p. hole imaging
p. line equal spacing bar pattern
p. M line
p. opposed ports
p. opposed unmodified ports
p. pitch line
p. and spiral flow pattern
p. tag plane
p. virtual machine (PVM)
parallel-hole medium sensitivity collimator
parallelism of articular surface
parallel-line
p.-l. equal spacing (PLES)
p.-l. equal spacing bar
parallel-opposed beams
parallel-tagged MR images
parallel-tag MR imaging
paralysis, pl. **paralyses**
deglutitional p.
p. of diaphragm
diaphragmatic p.
facial nerve p.
hernia p.
Klumpke p.
residual p.
vocal cord p.
paralytic
p. chest

p. colonic obstruction
p. ileus
paralytica
dysphagia p.
paramagnetic
p. artifact
p. cation
p. contrast
p. contrast enhancement
p. effect
p. enhancement accentuation
p. enhancement accentuation by chemical shift imaging
p. imaging agent
p. influence
p. shift
p. shift relaxation
paramagnetism
apparent p.
collective p.
paramalleolar artery
Parama method
paramammary lymph node
paramedian
p. infarct
p. pontine reticular formation
p. position
p. sagittal plane
p. section
p. thalamic artery
p. thalamopeduncular artery
p. triangle
paramediastinal gland
parameningeal rhabdomyosarcoma
parameniscal cyst
paramesonephric
p. duct
p. duct cyst
parameter
clinical p.
extrinsic cellular p.
growth p.
hematologic p.
intrinsic cellular p.
kinetic perfusion p.
normal hemodynamic liver p.
nuclear p.
optimization p.
physiologic p.
scan p.
sonographic p.
thermal treatment p.
timing p.
ventricular function p.
parametrectomy
radical p.
parametric
parametrium, pl. **parametria**
paranasal
p. sinus
p. sinus cancer
p. sinus carcinoma
p. sinusitis
p. sinus mass
p. sinus mucocele
paraneoplastic
p. cerebellar degeneration
p. lung cancer syndrome
p. process
p. thromboembolism
paraorbital
p. lesion
paraosteoarthropathy
paraovarian cyst
paraparesis
parapatellar plica
parapelvic
p. cyst
p. gutter
parapharyngeal
p. abscess
p. space
p. space cyst
paraplegia
parapneumonic effusion
paraprosthetic
p. leak
p. leakage
paraprosthetic-enteric fistula
pararectal
p. abscess
p. fossa
p. lymph node
p. pouch
pararenal
p. abscess
p. aortic aneurysm
p. aortic atherosclerosis
p. space
parasagittal
p. image
p. intracranial mass
p. lesion
p. meningioma

NOTES

P

parasellar
p. brain mass
p. cistern
p. dermoid tumor
p. lesion
p. metastasis
paraseptal
p. emphysema
p. position
parasitic
p. fetus
p. infiltrate
paraspinal
p. abnormality
p. abscess
p. calcification
p. line
p. muscle
p. neurofibroma
p. pleural stripe
p. soft tissue mass
p. soft tissue shadowing
paraspinous musculature
parasternal
p. bulge
p. long-axis view
p. long-axis view echocardiography
p. lymph node
p. motion
p. scanning
p. short-axis view
p. short-axis view echocardiography
p. view of heart
p. window
parastomal hernia
parastriate cortex
parasympathetic
p. fibers
p. ganglia tumor
p. nervous system
paratendinitis
paratenonitis
paraterminal gyrus
paratesticular
p. rhabdomyosarcoma
p. tumor
parathymic syndrome
parathyroid
p. adenoma
p. carcinoma
p. cyst
ectopic p.
p. hyperplasia
p. insufficiency
p. scintigraphy
technetium-99m sestamibi p.
p. tumor
p. ultrasonography imaging
p. vein
P:A ratio
paratracheal
p. adenopathy
p. lymph node
p. soft tissue
p. tissue stripe
paratrooper's fracture
paratubal serous cyst
paraumbilical vein
paraureteral diverticulum
paraurethral
p. canal
p. cyst
p. duct
p. gland
parauterine lymph node
paravaginal
p. lymph node
p. soft tissue
paravalvular
p. leak
p. regurgitation
paraventriculohypophysial tract
paravertebral
p. ganglion
p. groove
p. gutter
p. musculature
p. nerve plexus
p. ossification
p. scanning
p. venous plexus
paravesical
p. fossa
p. pouch
paravesicular lymph node
parchment
p. heart
p. heart syndrome
p. right ventricle
parenchyma
bleeding into brain p.
brain p.
breast p.
cerebral p.
hepatic p.
liver p.
lung p.
mammary p.
marbling of pancreatic p.
normal renal p.
pulmonary p.
renal p.
spinal cord p.
testicular p.

parenchymal
p. blastoma
p. blood
p. brain metastasis
p. breast pattern
p. cone
p. consolidation
p. cysticercosis
p. echogenicity
p. extension
p. fibrous band
p. hematoma
p. hemorrhage
p. infarct
p. laceration
p. lung band
p. lung disease
p. neurocutaneous melanosis
p. opacity
p. peliosis hepatis
p. scarring
p. tissue
p. tracer accumulation
p. transit
parenchymatous
p. atrophy
p. cerebellar degeneration
p. inflammation
p. neurosyphilis
p. phase
p. pneumonia
parenchymography
endoscopic retrograde p. (ERP)
parenchymous goiter
Parenti-Fraccaro disease
parent vein
paresis
Erb-Duchenne p.
hemilingual p.
Klumpke p.
Todd p.
paresthetica
meralgia p.
Parham-Martin band
paricallosal artery
parietal
p. association area
p. band
p. bone
p. boss
p. bossa
p. cephalohematoma
p. convexity
p. cortex
p. cortex lesion
p. eminence
p. encephalocele
p. extension
p. extension of infundibular septum
p. fistula
p. foramen
p. gyrus
p. layer
p. lobe
p. lobe lesion
p. lobe sign
p. lymph node
p. middle cerebral artery
p. pelvic fascia
p. pericardial calcification
p. pericardium
p. peritoneum
p. pleura
p. pleural scarring
p. pregnancy
p. presentation
p. suture
parietography
parietooccipital
p. area
p. branch of posterior cerebellar artery
p. lesion
p. sulcus
p. suture
parietopontine tract
parietotemporal area
Paris system
parity bit
park
p. bench position
P. Medical Systems scanner
Parke
corner sign of P.
P. corner sign
Parkes-Weber syndrome
Parks
P. bidirectional Doppler flowmeter
P. 800 bidirectional Doppler flowmetry
Parona space
paroöphoron
parosteal
p. bone lesion

NOTES

P

parosteal *(continued)*
p. chondrosarcoma
p. osteogenic
p. osteogenic sarcoma
p. osteoma
p. osteosarcoma
parotid
p. abscess
p. duct
p. gland
p. gland sialography
p. lymph node
p. pleomorphic adenoma
p. tumor
parotis
adenoid cystic carcinoma p.
benign mixed tumor p.
cylindroma p.
mucoepidermoid carcinoma p.
pleomorphic adenoma p.
parotitis
parovarian cyst
paroxysmal
p. auricular tachycardia (PAT)
p. AV block
p. change
p. pulmonary edema
Parrot
frontal bossing of P.
P. node
P. sign
parrot-beak
p.-b. labral tear
p.-b. meniscus tear
p.-b. pattern
parry fracture
pars, pl. **partes**
p. flaccida cholesteatoma
p. infravaginalis gubernaculi
p. interarticularis
p. interarticularis defect
p. interarticularis fracture
pedicles and p.
p. tensa cholesteatoma
Parsons
third intercondylar tubercle of P.
P. tubercle
part
fetal small p.'s
presenting p.
partes (*pl. of* pars)
partial
p. anomalous pulmonary venous connection
p. anomalous pulmonary venous return (PAPVR)
p. atrioventricular canal defect
p. brain irradiation
p. bursal surface tear
p. collapse of lung
p. complex seizure
p. corpus callosum agenesis
p. dislocation
p. dislodgement
p. flip-angle fast-scan technique
p. Fourier technique
p. heart block
p. k-space sampling
p. liquid ventilation
p. liquid ventilation with perflubron
p. obliteration of lateral ventricle
p. ossicular replacement prosthesis (PORP)
p. pericardial abscess
p. pericardial absence
p. placenta previa
p. pulmonary venous connection
p. saturation
p. saturation sequence
p. saturation spin echo (PSSE)
p. saturation technique
p. small bowel malrotation
p. small bowel obstruction
p. steal syndrome
p. thickening
p. transient osteoporosis
p. transposition of great arteries
p. ureter duplication
p. volume averaging
p. volume effect
p. volume effect artifact
partial-brain radiation therapy
partially polycystic kidney
partial-thickness split tear
particle
accelerated p.
p. accelerator
alpha p.
beta p.
bone p.
calcium/oxyanion-containing p.
charged p.
heavy charged p.
p. identification
Ivalon p.
large colloidal p.
p. mask
oral magnetic p.
p. size determination
submicron magnetic p.
particle-beam radiation therapy
particulate
p. debris
p. echo
magnetic p.'s
p. matter

partition
atrial p.
p. coefficient
gastric p.
parts per million
parturient canal
parturition
parvus
PAS
paraaminosalicylic acid
pulmonary artery systolic pressure
PASA
proximal articular set angle
pascals of force
PASH
pseudoangiomatous stromal hyperplasia
PASP-SASP
pulmonary to systemic arterial systolic pressure
PASP-SASP ratio
passage
adiabatic fast p.
biliary p.
free air p.
narrowing of bronchiolar p.'s
p. pressure
Passavant
P. bar
P. muscle
P. ridge
passes
interleaved imaging p.
passive
p. atelectasis
p. clot
p. congestive failure
p. edema
p. filling
p. hepatic congestion
p. hyperemia
p. pneumonia
p. shimming
p. smoking
p. track detector
p. vascular congestion
p. venous distention
passively
p. congested lung tissue
p. shimmed superconducting magnet
PASTA
polarity-altered spectral-selective acquisition
PASTA imaging
PASTA technique
paste
ferric ammonium citrate-cellulose p.
pastille, pastil
Sabouraud p.
PAT
paroxysmal auricular tachycardia
Patau syndrome
patch
ash leaf p.
blood p.
p. crinkling
p. electrode
epidural blood p.
Gore-Tex p.
p. graft reconstruction
p. kinking
p. lesion
McCallum p.
pigskin p.
sclerotic calvarial p.
shagreen rough skin p.
subcutaneous p.
patch-graft aortoplasty
patchy
p. air-space consolidation
p. alveolar opacity
p. area of density
p. area of pneumonia
p. atelectasis
p. atrophy of renal cortex
p. colonic ulcer
p. distribution of tracer
p. edema
p. migratory infiltrate
p. zone
patella, pl. **patellae, patellas**
p. alta
apex of head of p.
p. baja
dislocation of p.
floating p.
half-moon p.
high-lying p.
high-riding p.
lower pole of p.
multipartite p.
pebble-shaped p.
skyline view of p.
squared p.

NOTES

patella *(continued)*
subluxing p.
undersurface of p.
patellae
chondromalacia p.
ligamentum p.
patellar
p. bursitis
p. button
p. chondromalacia
p. contour
p. dislocation
p. edge
p. entrapment
p. fat pad
p. fossa
p. groove
p. ligament-patellar ratio
p. malalignment
p. pole
p. retinaculum
p. shaving
p. shelf
p. skyline view
p. sleeve fracture
p. subluxation
p. tendinosis
p. tendon
p. tilt
patellas (*pl. of* patella)
patellectomy
patellofemoral
p. articular cartilage
p. articulation
p. compartment
p. congruence
p. disorder
p. incongruency
p. index
p. joint
p. joint space
p. realignment
patency
arterial p.
p. of artery
coronary artery bypass graft p.
ductus arteriosus p.
ductus venosus p.
graft p.
long-term p.
p. rate
short-term p.
shunt p.
p. trifurcation
p. and valvular reflux of deep vein
vascular p.
vein p.
p. of vein graft
p. of vessel
patent
p. bifurcation
p. bronchus sign
p. ductus arteriosus (PDA)
p. foramen ovale (PFOB)
p. lumen
p. needle tract
p. stent
p. urachus
p. vessel
widely p.
Paterson-Parker
P.-P. rules
P.-P. system
path
free p.
mean free p.
water p.
pathergy test
pathlength
effective p. (EPL)
pathognomonic
p. finding
p. sign
p. signthalamic infiltrating glioma
pathologic, pathological
p. correlation
p. diagnosis
p. dislocation
p. fracture
p. intracranial calcification
p. lid retraction sign
pathology
radiographic p.
pathophysiologic changes
pathway
amygdalofugal p.
anomalous p.
antegrade fast p.
anterior internodal p.
atrio-His p.
cerebellar p.
cerebropontocerebellar p.
cerebrospinal fluid p.
corticospinal motor p.
dentatoolivary p.
dual atrioventricular node p.
hepatobiliary p.
neural p.
nodoventricular p.
optic glioma p.
reticulocortical p.
retrovestibular neural p.
septal accessory p.
synaptic p.
Thorel p.

patient
- Artma Virtual P.
- hypotonic p.
- p. motion
- p. motion artifact
- p. volume

pattern
- abnormal lung p.
- acinar p.
- airspace-filling p.
- airway p.
- alveolar p.
- anhaustral colonic gas p.
- arterial deficiency p.
- atypical vessel colposcopic p.
- ballerina-foot p.
- beam p.
- bigeminal p.
- blood flow p.
- bony trabecular p.
- bowel gas p.
- branching p.
- broken bough p.
- bronchiectatic p.
- bronchovascular p.
- butterfly p.
- cavitating p.
- centrum semiovale p.
- circadian p.
- cobblestone p.
- cobweb p.
- coiled-spring p.
- collimator plugging p.
- colonic urticaria p.
- contractile p.
- convolutional p.
- corduroy cloth p.
- corkscrew p.
- crazy paving p.
- cribriform p.
- degenerative nuclear p.
- p. of destruction
- diffraction p.
- diffuse p.
- dissemination p.
- divergent spiculated p.
- dot-and-dash p.
- ductal p.
- early repolarization p.
- echo p.
- echodense p.
- echolucent p.
- edema p.
- enhancement p.
- esophageal achalasia p.
- extended p.
- fibrotic cavitating p.
- fibrous nodular p.
- filigree p.
- fine reticular p.
- finger-in-glove p.
- fingerprint p.
- fleur-de-lis p.
- flow void p.
- fold p.
- follicular p.
- four-quadrant bar p.
- gas p.
- gastric mucosal p.
- geographic p.
- ground-glass p.
- ground-glass ovary p.
- gyriform p.
- hairbrush p.
- hanging fruit p.
- haustral p.
- helical p.
- hemodynamic p.
- hepatic echo p.
- herringbone p.
- heterogeneous internal echo p.
- heterogeneous perfusion p.
- hierarchical scanning p.
- hole p.
- homogeneous echo p.
- honeycomb p.
- hourglass p.
- infiltration p.
- inhomogeneous echo p.
- interstitial p.
- interstitial lung p.
- interstitial tear p.
- intestinal gas p.
- inverse follicle p.
- juvenile T-wave p.
- kidney mass growth p.
- lacelike trabecular p.
- ladderlike p.
- Laue p.
- left ventricular contraction p.
- left ventricular strain p.
- liver spoke-wheel p.
- lobular p.
- locomotor p.

NOTES

P

pattern *(continued)*
lymphatic drainage p.
M p.
macronodular p.
magnetic resonance enhancement p.
manometric p.
marrow edema p.
micronodular p.
miliary p.
mimosa p.
moiré p.
mosaic p.
mosaic attenuation p.
mosaic duodenal mucosal p.
moth-eaten p.
mottled p.
movement p.
M-shaped mitral valve p.
mucosal p.
muscle recruitment p.
nonspecific bowel gas p.
orthogonal-hole test p. (OHP)
ovarian fishnet weave p.
overlying branching p.
parallel line equal spacing bar p.
parallel and spiral flow p.
parenchymal breast p.
parrot-beak p.
permeative p.
pin p.
PLES bar p.
pneumoencephalographic p.
postembolization angiographic p.
P pulmonale p.
prominent ductal p.
pseudohomogeneous edema p.
pseudoinfarct p.
pseudomantle zone p.
pulmonary flow p.
pulmonary vascular p.
QR p.
railroad track p.
recurrence p.
relief p.
restrictive p.
reticulogranular p.
reticulonodular p.
rheologic p.
right ventricular strain p.
rosary bead p.
rugal p.
seizure p.
sheetlike growth p.
shish kebab p.
sigmoid hair p.
signet ring p.
sinus p.
slice-of-sausage breast p.
small bowel mucosal p.
snowflake p.
snowstorm breast p.
speckled p.
spectral p.
spiral flow p.
spoiler gradient p.
spoke wheel p.
p. of spread
star p.
starry sky p.
start test p.
stellate p.
storiform p.
storiform-pleomorphic p.
strain p.
sulcal p.
sunburst gyral p.
surface convexity p.
Tabar p.
task-rest p.
temporal sawtooth p.
thermal convection p.
three-dimensional physiologic flow p.
TIB p.
tigroid p.
trabecular p.
tram-track p.
transducer beam p.
tree-in-bud p.
trigeminal p.
tubular gas p.
V p.
ventricular contraction p.
vesicular p.
Wolfe mammographic parenchymal p.

patulous
p. cardia
p. hiatus

pauciarticular

pauciostotic

paucity of bowel gas

Pauli exclusion principle

Paul sign

Pauly point

pause
asystolic p.
compensatory p.
noncompensatory p.
postextrasystolic p.
sinus p.

Pauwel
P. angle
P. femoral neck fracture classification

paving-stone degeneration

Pavlik harness
Pavlov stomach
Pawlik
P. triangle
P. trigone
Pawlow
P. position
P. projection
PAWP
pulmonary artery wedge pressure
Payr
P. disease
P. sign
Pb
lead
PBF
pulmonary blood flow
PBI
protein-bound iodine
PBPI
penile-brachial pressure index
PBT Technologies PACS
PBVI
pulmonary blood volume index
PC
posterior commissure
PC imaging
pc, pCi
picocurie
PCA
posterior cerebral artery
posterior communicating artery
PCAVC
persistent complete atrioventricular canal
PCC
peripheral cholangiocarcinoma
pCi
picocurie
pCi (*var. of* pc)
PCICO technique
PCIS
postcardiac injury syndrome
PCL
posterior cruciate ligament
PCLBCL
primary cutaneous large B-cell lymphoma
PCoA
posterior communicating artery
PCOD
polycystic ovarian disease
PCP
pulmonary capillary pressure
PCRA
percutaneous coronary rotational atherectomy
PCS
proximal coronary
PCVD
pulmonary collagen vascular disease
PCWP
pulmonary capillary wedge pressure
Pd
palladium
^{103}Pd
^{103}Pd isotope
^{103}Pd prostatic implant
^{103}Pd radioactive material
PDA
patent ductus arteriosus
poorly differentiated adenocarcinoma
posterior descending artery
PDD
percentage depth dose
pDEXA x-ray peripheral bone densitometer
PDI
power Doppler imaging
PDR
pulsed dose rate
PDT
photodynamic therapy
PE
pericardial effusion
photographic effect
pulmonary embolus
Peacock system
peak
p. airway pressure
airway pressure p.
p. aortic flow velocity
p. area
Bragg ionization p.
carotid pulse p.
p. count density
p. diastolic gradient
diffraction p.
p. dP/dt
p. early diastolic filling velocity
early systolic p.
p. enhancement
p. filling
p. filling rate (PFR)

NOTES

peak *(continued)*
p. fitting
p. flow variability
p. flow velocity
frequency-related p.
p. identification
p. inflation pressure
p. instantaneous gradient
juxtaphrenic p.
p. kilovoltage (pkV)
kilovoltage p. (kVp)
p. late diastolic filling velocity
main glow p.
p. parenchymal activity
photon p.
pressure p.
p. pressure gradient
p. profile
p. pulmonary flow velocity
recirculation p.
p. regurgitant flow velocity
p. regurgitant wave pressure
p. repetition frequency (PRF)
p. right ventricular-right atrial systolic gradient
p. scatter factor
p. shape
single p.
spread Bragg p.
p. systolic aortic pressure (PSAP)
p. systolic and diastolic ratio
p. systolic gradient (PSG)
p. systolic velocity
temporal p. (TP)
p. transmitted velocity
p. velocity of blood flow

peak-to-peak pressure gradient
peak-to-pressure gradient
pearl
keratin p.
p. necklace gallbladder
scrotal p.

pearl-like breast calcification
pearly
p. CNS tumor
p. neoplasm
p. white ovary

pear-shaped
p.-s. defect
p.-s. heart
p.-s. urinary bladder
p.-s. uterus
p.-s. vertebra

Pearson
P. attachment
P. method
P. position

pebble-shaped patella
Pecquet
cistern of P.

pecten pubis
pectinate
p. ligament
p. line

pectineal
pectineus
p. muscle

pectoral
p. girdle
p. heart
p. lymph node
p. ridge

pectoralis
p. major muscle
p. major syndrome
p. minor
p. minor muscle

pectoris
variant angina p.

pectus
p. carinatum deformity
p. excavatum
p. excavatum deformity

pedal
p. artery opacification
p. bone
p. lymphangiography

pedes (*pl. of* pes)
pediatric
p. biplane TEE probe
p. fibroxanthoma
p. hemangioma
p. neuroradiology
p. primary brain tumor
p. radiology
p. solid tumor

pedicle
p. bone graft
p. erosion
p. finger
p. flap
p. fracture
IMA p.
internal mammary artery pedicle
musculofascial p.
p.'s and pars
phrenic p.
p. plate
p. sclerosis
p. signal intensity
spinal p.
splaying of p.'s
vascular p.
p. of vertebra

pedicolaminar fracture-dislocation

pedis
calcar p.
digitus p.
dorsalis p.
dorsum p.
malum perforans p.
pollex p.
pedobarography
dynamic p.
peduncle
cerebellar p.
cerebral p.
inferior cerebellar p.
peduncular
p. loop
p. segment of superior cerebellar artery
p. tract
pedunculated
p. leiomyoma
p. lesion
p. polyp
p. subserous myoma
p. thrombus
p. uterine fibroid
p. uterine myxoma
p. vesical tumor
pedunculation
peel
pleura p.
PEF
PEG
percutaneous endoscopic gastrostomy
pneumoencephalogram
peg
cerebellar p.
rete p.
Pegasys workstation
PEI
postexercise index
Pel-Ebstein disease
peliosis
spleen p.
Pelizaeus-Merzbacher disease
Pelkan spur
Pellegrini-Stieda
P.-S. calcification
P.-S. disease
P.-S. phenomenon
pellet
alanine-silicone p.
p. artifact
radiopaque p.
pellucidum
septum p.
pelvem
aditus ad p.
pelves (*pl. of* pelvis)
pelvic
p. abscess
p. aneurysm
p. arteriography
p. artery
p. bone
p. brim
p. canal
p. chocolate cyst
p. collateral vessel
p. colon
p. cystic mass
p. diameter
p. diaphragm
p. exenteration
p. exostosis
p. fascia
p. femoral angle
p. fibrolipomatosis
p. floor
p. fluid
p. fracture frame
p. girdle
p. infection
p. inflammatory disease (PID)
p. inlet
p. insufficiency fracture
p. ligament
p. lipomatosis
p. lymph node
p. malignancy
p. mass complex
p. mass frequency
p. notching
p. obliquity
p. outlet
p. peritoneum
p. phased-array coil
p. plane
p. plexus
p. rim fracture
p. ring
p. ring fracture
p. sidewall
p. sonography

NOTES

P

pelvic *(continued)*
p. space
p. steal
p. steal test
p. straddle fracture
p. ultrasound
p. ultrasound CT scan
p. unleveling
p. vascular trauma
p. vein thrombosis
p. venous obstruction
p. venous stenosis
p. view
p. viscera
p. wall
pelvicaliceal
p. changes
p. distention
pelvicephalography
pelviectasis
pelvimetry
radiographic p.
pelvis, pl. **pelves**
aditus p.
android p.
anthropoid p.
assimilation p.
beaked p.
bifid p.
bony p.
brachypellic p.
brim of the p.
champagne glass p.
contracted p.
cordate p.
cordiform p.
Deventer p.
dolichopellic p.
dwarf p.
elephant ears p.
extrarenal renal p.
false p.
female p.
flat p.
frozen p.
funnel-shaped p.
goblet-shaped p.
greater p.
gynecoid p.
hardened p.
heart-shaped p.
intrarenal p.
inverted p.
juvenile p.
p. of kidney
Kilian p.
kyphoscoliotic p.
kyphotic p.
lesser p.
longitudinal oval p.
lordotic p.
male p.
masculine p.
mesatipellic p.
Mickey Mouse ears p.
Nägele p.
osteomalacic p.
Otto p.
Otto-Krobak p.
platypelloid p.
portable film of p.
pseudoosteomalacic p.
rachitic p.
renal p.
reniform p.
Rokitansky p.
scoliotic p.
small p.
spider p.
spondylolisthetic p.
tombstone p.
transverse oval p.
trident p.
true p.
ureteral p.
ureteric p.
wineglass p.
pelviureteral junction
pelviureterography
pelvocaliceal
p. effacement
p. system
pelvocephalography
Pena Shokeir syndrome
Pena-Vaandrager metaphyseal dysplasia
pencil
p. bone
p. dosimeter
p. electron beam
pencil-beam
p.-b. approach
p.-b. navigator echoes
pencil-in-cup deformity
penciling
p. deformity
p. of the distal clavicle
p. of rib
p. of terminal tuft
pencil-like deformity
pencil-point metatarsal deformity
pendent positioning
pendetide
indium-111 satumomab p.
Pendred syndrome
pendulous
p. heart

p. pouch
p. urethra
pendulum
cor p.
p. movement
penes (*pl. of* penis)
penetrating
p. aortic ulcer
p. atherosclerotic ulcer
p. fracture
p. lung injury
p. trauma
p. TRD
p. wound
penetration
bowel wall p.
rectal p.
penetrometer
Benoist p.
penile
p. artery
p. fibromatosis
p. implant
p. plaque
p. prosthesis
p. raphe
p. sonography
p. squamous papilloma
p. urethra
p. urethra diverticulum
p. vein
p. vessel
penile-brachial pressure index (PBPI)
penis, pl. **penes**
bulb of p.
bulbospongiosus muscle of p.
clubbed p.
concealed p.
corpora cavernosa p.
corpus spongiosum p.
crus of p.
deep fascia of p.
dorsal artery of p.
dorsal nerve of p.
dorsum of p.
double p.
glans p.
hypoplastic p.
ischiospongiosus muscle of p.
p. lacuna
root of p.
suspensory ligament of p.
webbed p.
peniscopy
penoscrotal
PenRad mammography clinical reporting system
pentacene
pentagastrin
p. imaging agent
pentalogy
p. of Cantrell
p. of Fallot
pentavalent DMSA imaging agent
Pentax EUP-EC124 ultrasound gastroscope
Pentax-Hitachi FG32UA endosonographic system
pentetate
^{111}In imciromab p.
pentetic acid
pentetide
satumomab p.
pentetreotide
p. imaging agent
^{111}In p.
indium-111 p.
pentretreotide scan
penumbra, pl. **penumbrae**
dosimetric p.
hemodynamic p.
p. zone
PEP
preejection period
peppermint oil imaging agent
pepper-pot pitting
Peptavlon
peptic
p. esophagitis
p. stricture
p. ulcer
p. ulcer disease (PUD)
peptide imaging agent
P-ER
pronation-external rotation
P-ER injury
percentage
p. depth dose (PDD)
p. signal intensity loss (PSIL)
Perception scanner
perceptual linearization
Percheron
artery of P.

NOTES

P

perchlorate
potassium p.
p. washout test
Percoll
percreta
placenta p.
percussion
p. sensitivity
p. sign
percutaneous
p. abscess drainage (PAD)
p. antegrade biliary drainage
p. atherectomy device
p. automated diskectomy
p. cecostomy
p. cholangiography
p. coronary rotational atherectomy (PCRA)
p. dilatation of biliary duct
p. endofluoroscopy
p. endoluminal placement
p. endoscopic gastrostomy (PEG)
p. endoscopic gastrostomy (PEG) tube
p. endoscopy
p. ethanol injection
p. femoral arteriography
p. gastroenterostomy
p. interventional radiology
p. intraaortic balloon counterpulsation (PIBC)
p. intracoronary angioscopy imaging
p. nephroscope
p. nephroscopy
p. nephrostomy
p. pancreatography
p. pericardioscopy
p. pin insertion
p. radiofrequency ablation
p. retrograde transfemoral technique
p. stent
p. thermal occlusion
p. transcatheter therapy
p. transhepatic cholangiogram (PTC, PTHC)
p. transhepatic cholangiography (PTHC)
p. transhepatic cholecystostomy
p. transhepatic decompression
p. transhepatic liver biopsy
p. transhepatic portography
p. transluminal balloon dilatation
p. transluminal coronary angiogram
p. transluminal coronary recanalization technique
p. transperineal seed implantation
percutaneously cannulated
Perez sign
perflubron
p. imaging agent
partial liquid ventilation with p.
perfluorocarbon
p. imaging agent
perfluorochemical
perfluorooctyl bromide (PFOB)
perforated
p. aortic cusp
p. carcinoma
p. cholecystitis
p. diverticulum
p. gangrenous appendix
p. hollow viscus
p. ulcer
perforating
p. aneurysm
p. artery
p. artery of foot
p. branch
p. colorectal cancer
p. fracture
p. vein
p. wound
perforation
bladder p.
cardiac p.
central p.
colonic p.
p. of common bile duct
common bile duct spontaneous p.
esophageal p.
gallbladder p.
iatrogenic p.
idiopathic gastric p.
intestinal p.
Niemeier gallbladder p.
renal transplant GI tract p.
septal p.
spontaneous p.
transseptal p.
ulcer p.
ureteral p.
vascular p.
ventricular p.
perforative lesion
perforator
incompetent p.
septal p.
p. vessel
perfusate vessel
perfused
p. myocardium
p. twin
perfusion
p. abnormality
adequate coronary p.
p. agent

antegrade p.
blood p.
brain p.
capillary p.
continuous hyperthermic peritoneal p.
diminished systemic p.
first-pass cardiac p.
p. gradient
homogeneous p.
hypothermic p.
impaired renal p.
increment of p.
intraperitoneal hyperthermic p. (IPHP)
isolated limb p. (ILP)
limb p.
lung p.
p. lung scan
luxury p.
maldistribution of ventilation and p.
p. measurement technique
misery p.
mosaic p.
p. MR imaging
myocardial p.
peripheral p.
poor p.
p. pressure
pulsatile p.
quantitative cardiac p.
regional cerebral p.
regional pulmonary p.
regional vascular p.
renal p.
resting p.
retrograde cardiac p.
p. time
tissue p.
unilateral lung p.
p. and ventilation lung imaging

perfusion-metabolism mismatch

perfusion-weighted
p.-w. imaging
p.-w. MRI

Pergonal

perialveolar fibrosis

periampullary
p. carcinoma
p. diverticulum
p. duodenal tumor

perianal
p. abscess
p. hematoma

periaortic
p. area
p. fibrosis
p. lymph node
p. mediastinal hematoma

periaortitis
chronic p.

periapical
p. cemental dysplasia
p. granuloma
p. lesion
p. radiograph

periappendiceal abscess

periaqueductal
p. gray matter
p. hemorrhage

periarteriolar lymphoid sheath

periarteritis nodosa

periarticular
p. calcification
p. fluid collection
p. fracture
p. heterotopic ossification (PHO)
p. margin
p. osteoporosis
p. tissue

periauricular meningioma

peribronchial
p. alveolar space
p. connective tissue
p. cuffing
p. distribution
p. fibrosis
p. hemorrhage
p. infiltrate
p. lymph node
p. markings
p. thickening

peribronchovascular interstitial compartment

peribursal fat

pericaliceal cyst

pericallosal
p. artery
p. lipoma
p. vein

pericapsular fat infiltrate

pericardia (*pl. of* pericardium)

pericardiacophrenic vein

NOTES

P

pericardiac pleura
pericardial
p. aorta
p. calcification
p. cavity
p. chyle with tamponade
p. cyst
p. defect
p. diaphragmatic adhesion
p. disease
p. effusion (PE)
p. empyema
p. fat pad
p. flap
p. fluid
p. fold
p. hematoma
p. infusion
p. knock sound
p. lymph node
p. reserve volume
p. sac
p. sinus
p. space
p. vein
p. window
pericardiectomy
pericardioperitoneal canal
pericardioscopy
percutaneous p.
pericardiotomy syndrome
pericarditis
bread-and-butter p.
constrictive p.
diffuse p.
hemorrhagic p.
radiation-induced p.
pericardium, pl. **pericardia**
adherent p.
autologous p.
bread-and-butter p.
p. calcareous deposit
calcified p.
congenitally absent p.
crus p.
diaphragmatic p.
p. fibrosum
fibrous p.
inelastic p.
parietal p.
rheumatic adherent p.
roughened state of p.
serous p.
shaggy p.
soldier's patches of p.
veins of p.
visceral p.
pericarinal injury
pericatheter thrombus
pericaval
pericecal abscess
pericentral fibrosis
pericerebral fluid
pericholecystic
p. abscess
p. edema
p. fluid
p. fluid collection
perichondral
p. bone
p. cell seeding
p. ring
perichondrium
pericicatricial emphysema
pericolic abscess
pericolonic
p. abscess
p. fat
pericranii
sinus p.
pericyst
pericystic edema
peridental space
peridiaphragmatic hematoma
peridiploid
peridiverticulitis
periductal
p. calcification
p. fibrosis
p. mastitis
peridural fibrosis
perifascial fluid-like collection
perifocal emphysema
perigastric
p. deformity
p. fat
perigestational hemorrhage
perigraft
p. fluid
p. hematoma
perihepatic space
perihepatitis
gonorrheic p.
perihilar
p. area
p. batwing infiltrate
p. density
p. edema
p. fat
p. fibrosis
p. lung disease
p. markings
p. region
periileal
periinfarction
p. block (PIB)

p. conduction defect (PICD)
p. ischemia
perilabral sulcus
perilesional
p. bone
p. white matter
perilobular
p. connective tissue
p. duct
perilunar
p. dislocation
p. instability
perilunate
p. carpal dislocation
p. fracture-dislocation (PLFD)
p. instability
perimalleolar pain
perimedial
p. dysplasia
p. fibroplasia
p. renal fibroplasia artery
perimedullary
perimembranous ventricular septal defect
perimeniscal capsular plexus
perimesencephalic cistern
perimetry testing
perimuscular
p. fibrosis
p. plexus
perimylolysis
perinatal
p. anoxia
p. asphyxia
p. injury
p. respiratory distress syndrome
perinea (*pl. of* perineum)
perineal
p. descent
p. fascia
p. sinus
p. space
perineogram
p. imaging
perineoplastic edema
perineovaginal fistula
perinephric
p. abscess
p. fat
p. fluid collection
p. hematoma
p. space
p. space hemorrhage
perineum, pl. **perinea**
perineural
p. fat
p. fibroblastoma
p. fibroblastoma tumor
p. fibrosis
p. invasion
p. sacral cyst
p. tumor spread
perinuclear halo
period
antegrade refractory p.
diastasis heart p.
diastolic filling p.
effective refractory p. (ERP)
embryonic p.
fetal p.
functional refractory p. (FRP)
immediate postictal p.
isoelectric p.
isovolumetric p.
last menstrual p. (LMP)
noninteger p.
phase-encoding p.
postbiopsy p.
preejection p. (PEP)
radiofrequency p.
rapid filling p. (RFP)
raster p.
reduced ventricular filling p.
relative refractory p. (RRP)
retrograde refractory p.
roentgen equivalent man p. (REMP)
systolic ejection p. (SEP)
total atrial refractory p. (TARP)
ventricular effective refractory p. (VERP)
ventriculoatrial effective refractory p.
window p.
periodicity
circadian p.
periodontal
p. disease
p. ligament
perioptic meningioma
periorbital
p. bidirectional Doppler

NOTES

P

periorbital *(continued)*
p. directional Doppler ultrasonography
p. Doppler imaging
p. edema
periosteal
p. artery
p. bone
p. bone collar
p. bone ring
p. creep
p. desmoid
p. dysplasia
p. elevation
p. fibroma
p. fibrosarcoma
p. ganglion
p. new bone formation
p. reaction
p. resorption
p. sarcoma
periosteum, pl. **periostea**
p. of rib
periostitis
florid reactive p.
medial malleolus p.
muscle traction-induced p.
periotic bone
peripancreatic
p. artery
p. fluid collection
p. lymphadenopathy
peripartum dilated cardiomyopathy
peripelvic
p. collateral vessel
p. cyst
p. fat proliferation
p. lipomatosis
peripheral
p. air-space disease
p. arterial disease
p. arteriography
p. arteriosclerosis
p. blood
p. blood flow
p. bolus chase
p. carcinoma
p. cholangiocarcinoma (PCC)
p. chondrosarcoma
p. circulation
p. circulatory vasoconstriction
p. consolidation
p. cutaneous vasoconstriction
p. edema
p. embolus
p. enhancement
p. expansion
p. fracture
p. gating
p. hematopoietic intermediate signal intensity marrow
p. hypoperfusion
p. infiltrate
p. intravenous infusion line
p. laser recanalization technique
p. loading
p. lung disease
p. lymphoma
p. meniscocapsular tear
p. necrosis
p. nerve
p. nerve block
p. nerve decompression
p. nerve injury
p. nerve lesion
p. nervous system
p. neuroectodermal tumor
p. neurofibromatosis
p. nodule
p. ossification
p. ossifying fibroma
p. parenchymal atelectasis
p. perfusion
p. perimeniscal capillary ingrowth
p. pneumonia
p. pseudoaneurysm
p. puddling
p. pulmonary artery stenosis (PPAS)
p. quantitative computed tomography (pQCT)
p. quantitative computed tomography technology
p. runoff
p. small airways study
p. vascular disease (PVD)
p. vascular imaging
p. vascular resistance (PVR)
p. vasculature
p. vessel
p. washout liver sign
peripherally
p. inserted central catheter (PICC)
p. inserted central catheter (PICC) line
periphery
echogenic p.
lung p.
periportal
p. area
p. cirrhosis
p. collar
p. fibrosis
p. sinusoidal dilatation
p. tracking
p. tracking of blood

periprosthetic
p. bone resorption
p. fracture
p. leak
periradicular
p. nerve
p. sheath
perirectal fat
perirenal
p. abscess
p. compartment
p. fat
p. hematoma
p. hemorrhage
p. insufflation
p. lymphoma
p. mass
p. septum
p. space
perirolandic parietal cortex
perisellar vascular lesion
perisigmoid colon
perisinusoidal space
perisplenic node
peristalsing bowel
peristalsis
abnormal esophageal p.
absent p.
accelerated p.
anterograde p.
bowel p.
decreased p.
esophageal p.
hyperactive p.
increased p.
meconium p.
primary esophageal p.
retrograde p.
reversed p.
secondary p.
small bowel p.
ureteral seesaw p.
visible p.
yo-yo esophageal p.
yo-yo ureteral p.
peristaltic
p. activity
p. contraction
p. rush
p. wave
peristriate cortex
perisylvian cortex
peritendinitis
peritendinous
p. adhesion
p. calcification
perithyroid vein
peritoneal
p. attachment
p. band
p. carcinomatosis
p. cavity
p. cavity fluid
p. dialysis catheter
p. effusion
p. enhancement
p. fold
p. gutter
p. hernia
p. inclusion cyst
p. ligament
p. lymphopneumatosis
p. mass
p. mesothelioma
p. metastasis
p. mouse
p. recess
p. sac
p. seeding
p. sign
p. space
p. washings
peritoneal-venous shunt patency test
peritonei
carcinomatosis p.
gliomatosis p.
pseudomyxoma p.
peritoneocele
peritoneogram imaging
peritoneography
CT p.
peritoneopericardial diaphragmatic hernia
peritoneovenous shunt (PVS)
peritoneum
p. desmoid tumor
parietal p.
pelvic p.
visceral p.
peritonitis
meconium p.
tuberculous p.
peritrochanteric fracture
peritubular vascular structure

NOTES

peritumoral
p. edema
p. tissue
periumbilical
p. subcutaneous nodule
p. subcutaneous swelling
periungual fibroma
periureteral fibrosis
periureteric venous ring
periurethral
p. gland
p. phlegmon
perivalvular
p. dehiscence
p. disruption
p. leak
p. pseudoaneurysm
perivascular
p. canal
p. cloaking
p. distribution
p. edema
p. fibrosis
p. infiltrate
p. mass
p. plane
p. pseudorosette
p. space
p. space of Virchow-Robin
periventricular
p. border
p. bright signal
p. calcification
p. density
p. echogenicity (PVE)
p. gray matter (PVG matter, PVG)
p. halo
p. hemorrhagic infarct
p. hypodensity
p. lesion
p. leukoencephalopathy
p. leukomalacia (PVL)
p. plaque
p. white matter
perivenular nodularity
perivesical
Perkin line
Perlmann tumor
permanent
p. callus
p. interstitial implant
p. magnet
p. stoma
PermCath
Quinton P.
permeability
capillary p.
membrane p.
pulmonary capillary p.
p. pulmonary edema
tumor capillary p.
permeation
permeative
p. bone destruction
p. lesion
p. neuroectodermal tumor
p. pattern
permutation
pernio lupus
peroneal
p. to anterior compartment ratio (P:A ratio)
p. area
p. artery
p. bone
p. brevis tendon
p. longus tendon
p. muscle
p. muscular atrophy
p. nerve
p. node
p. obliterative thrombus
p. retinaculum
p. sign
p. tendon subluxation
p. tenosynovitis
p. trochlea
p. vein
p. vessel
peroneum
os p.
peroneus
p. longus
p. longus muscle avulsion
p. quartus muscle
p. tertius
peroral
p. cone radiation therapy
p. implantation
per os (p.o.)
peroxyl
Persantine
IV P.
P. thallium stress test
Persantine-thallium imaging
persistent
p. bronchopleural fistula
p. common atrioventricular canal
p. complete atrioventricular canal (PCAVC)
p. cortical kidney lobation
p. ductus arteriosus
p. fetal circulation
p. generalized lymphadenopathy
p. hyperparathyroidism
p. increasing nephrogram

p. left inferior vena cava
p. left superior vena cava
p. metopic suture
p. ossiculum terminale
p. ostium atrioventriculare commune
p. primitive trigeminal artery
p. pulmonary hypertension
p. pylorospasm
p. sciatic artery
p. splenomegaly
p. truncus arteriosus (PTA)

personal ionization chamber
perspective volume rendering (PVR)
pertechnate
technetium p.
Pertechnegas
pertechnetate
free p. (TcO^{4-})
sodium p.
p. sodium
p. sodium imaging agent
^{99m}Tc p.
^{99m}Tc tin colloid/free Tc-99m p.
technetium-99m p.
Perthes
P. disease
P. epiphysis
P. lesion
Perthes-Bankart lesion
Pertofrane
Pertscan 99m
perturbation
magnetic field p.
radiation dose p.
perturbing magnetic field
pertussoid eosinophilic pneumonia
perversus
situs p.
pes, pl. **pedes**
p. abductus
p. adductus
p. anserinus
p. anserinus bursitis
p. arcuatus
p. arcuatus clawfoot deformity
p. calcaneocavus
p. calcaneovalgus
p. calcaneus
p. calvaneovalgus
p. cavovalgus
p. cavovarus
p. cavus
p. cavus clawfoot deformity
p. contortus
p. equinovalgus
p. equinovarus
p. equinus
p. malleus valgus
p. planovalgus
p. planovalgus deformity
p. plantigrade planus
p. planus
p. planus deformity
p. pronation
p. pronatus
p. varus
PET
positron emission tomography
PET balloon
PET balloon Simpson atherectomy device
cardiac PET
^{18}fluoro-deoxy-D-glucose PET
PET imaging
PET lung imaging
PET metabolic imaging
PET myocardial fatty acid imaging
PET perfusion metabolism imaging
PET radioligand
PET target material
petal-fugal flow
petiole
petit
P. disease
P. ligament
p. mal seizure
P. sinus
PETite scanner
Pétrequin ligament
petrobasilar suture
petroclinoid ligament
petromastoid
petrooccipital synchondrosis
petrosal
p. bone
p. cerebellum
p. foramen
p. ganglion
greater p.
lesser p.
p. nerve
p. sinus
p. vein

NOTES

P

petrositis
apical p.
petrosphenobasilar
p. suture
petrosphenoid
petrosphenooccipital
p. suture
petrosquamosal
petrosquamous
p. suture
petrous
p. apex
p. apex dumbbell mass
p. apicitis
p. carotid canal
p. carotid canal stenosis
p. pyramid
p. pyramid scalloping
p. ridge
p. segment of carotid artery
p. temporal bone
PETT
positron emission transaxial tomography
PETT imaging
Peutz-Jeghers
P.-J. gastrointestinal polyposis
P.-J. polyp
Peyronie disease
Pfaundler-Hurler
P.-H. disease
P.-H. gargoylism
Pfeiffer
P. acrocephalosyndactyly
P. disease
P. syndrome
Pfeiffer-Comberg method
PFFD
proximal focal femoral deficiency
PFFD syndrome
Pfizer
P. 200 FS scanner
P. 0450 scanner
PFOB
patent foramen ovale
perfluorooctyl bromide
PFR
peak filling rate
Pfuhl-Jaffé sign
PFWT
pain-free walking time
PGK (Panos G. Koutrouvelis, M.D.) stereotactic device
PGSE
pulsed-gradient spin echo
phagedenic ulcer
phagocytic macrophage
phagocytized fat
phalangeal
p. bone
p. branch
p. diaphyseal fracture
p. glenoidal ligament
p. herniation
p. preponderance
p. shortening
phalanx, pl. **phalanges**
base of p.
drumstick p.
phalanges of foot
phalanges of hand
hourglass p.
ivory p.
rectangular p.
waist of p.
Phalen
P. position
P. sign
phallectomy
phantom
Alderson anthropomorphic p.
p. bone
p. breast tumor
p. dosimetry
gelatin p.
Hine-Duley p.
p. limb pain
p. limb syndrome
p. lung tumor
metal line-pair p.
oil-water p.
p. pregnancy
reference p.
p. study
velocity-evaluation p.
wax p.
pharmacoangiography
pharmacokinetic technique
pharmacologic
p. stress dual-isotope myocardial perfusion SPECT
p. stress echocardiography
p. stress test
pharmacoradiologic disimpaction of esophageal foreign body
pharyngeal
p. abscess
p. area
p. artery
p. canal
p. muscle
p. orifice
p. plexus
p. pouch
p. recess
p. space mass

p. wall cancer
p. wall carcinoma
pharynges (*pl. of* pharynx)
pharyngobasilar fascia
pharyngoesophageal
p. diverticulum
p. function
p. sphincter
pharyngoesophagogram
pharyngotympanic tube
pharynx, pl. **pharynges**
p. cross-section
laryngeal part of p.
nasal part of p.
oral part of p.
postcricoid p.
p. steeple sign
phase
accelerated p.
accumulative p.
p. analysis
p. angle
arterial p.
blastic p.
p. cancellation intensity artifact
chronic p.
cicatrizing p.
p. coherence
p. contrast
corticomedullary p.
p. cycling
p. delay
delayed p.
diastolic depolarization p.
p. difference mapping
p. discontinuity artifact
p. effect
p. encoding
endometrium menstrual p.
equilibrium p.
excretory p. (EP)
expiratory p.
fat-water out of p.
p. filtering
follicular p.
p. gain
hepatic arterial p. (HAP)
p. identification
p. image
inspiratory p.
p. instability
interictal p.
late p.
luteal p.
p. mismapping
nephrogenic p.
nephrographic p. (NP)
noncicatrizing p.
noncontrast p. (NCP)
ovulatory p.
parenchymatous p.
plateau p.
portal venous p. (PVP)
prolonged expiratory p.
prolonged inspiratory p.
rapid early repolarization p.
rapid filling p.
rapid ventricular filling p.
p. relation
p. shift
spent p.
thallium redistribution p.
vascular p.
p. velocity imaging
ventilation scintigraphy equilibrium p.
wash-in p.
washout p.
zero p.
phase-angle display redundancy
phase-contrast
p.-c. angiography
p.-c. imaging (PC imaging)
p.-c. MR angiography
p.-c. (PC) image
phased-array
p.-a. body-coil MR imaging
p.-a. multicoil imaging
p.-a. scanner
p.-a. surface coil
p.-a. surface coil MR imaging
p.-a. torso coil
p.-a. transducer
phase-dependent spectroscopic imaging
phase-encode
p.-e. pulse
p.-e. time-reduced acquisition sequence
p.-e. time-reduced acquisition sequence imaging
phase-encoding
p.-e. direction
p.-e. gradient
p.-e. motion artifact

NOTES

P

phase-encoding *(continued)*
p.-e. period
p.-e. step
phase-offset
p.-o. multiplanar (POMP)
p.-o. multiplanar imaging
phase-ordered
p.-o. multiplanar (POMP)
p.-o. multiplanar imaging
phase-preserving reconstruction
phase-sensitive
p.-s. detector
p.-s. flow measurement
p.-s. gradient-echo MR imaging
phase-shift
p.-s. artifact
p.-s. velocity mapping
phase-shifting interferometry
phase-specific action
phase-unwrapping method
phase-velocity image
phasic
p. contraction
p. pressure
phasicity
phasing-in time
PHCA
profound hypothermic circulatory arrest
Phemister triad
phenazopyridine
phenobarbital
p. biliary atresia
p. imaging agent
phenobutiodil
phenobutiodyl
phenolsulfonphthalein (PSP)
phenomenological effective surface potential
phenomenon, pl. **phenomena**
A p.
aliasing p.
anniversary p.
Aschner p.
Ashman p.
Austin Flint p.
autoimmune p.
baked-brain p.
Bancaud p.
Bell p.
booster p.
Bowditch staircase p.
collapse-related vacuum p.
combined flexion p.
common cavity p.
coronary steal p.
Courvoisier p.
crus p.
Cushing p.
dip p.
dip-and-plateau p.
Doppler p.
Dubin-Johnson p.
embolic p.
entry-slice p.
extinction p.
field p.
first-set p.
flare p.
flow p.
fogging p.
freezing p.
Friedreich p.
Gallavardin p.
gap conduction p.
Gärtner p.
Gibbs p.
glove p.
Goldblatt p.
Gordon knee p.
Gowers p.
Herendeen p.
Hering p.
Hurst p.
iceberg p.
intervertebral disk space vacuum p.
intraluminal flow p.
Jod-Basedow p.
Kasabach-Merritt p.
Katz-Wachtel p.
Kernohan notch p.
kindling p.
Litten diaphragm p.
Luciani-Wenckebach p.
magic-angle p.
Marin-Amat p.
mother-in-law p.
multiple vacuum p.
nonspecific p.
no-reflow p.
nutcracker p.
on-off p.
Pellegrini-Stieda p.
Piltz-Westphal p.
pivot shift p.
Raynaud p.
recall p.
resonance p.
Robin Hood p.
R-on-T p.
Schellong-Strisower p.
Schiff-Sherrington p.
Schramm p.
seizure p.
setting-sun p.
silhouette p.
spin-phase p.

staircase p.
stalactite p.
steal p.
stone heart p.
treppe p.
truncation p.
Uhthoff p.
unilateral Raynaud p.
V p.
vacuum disk p.
vacuum joint p.
vasovagal p.
vertebral steal p.
Wenckebach p.
window-period p.
zone p.

phenoxyacetic acid

Phentetiothalein imaging agent

pheochromocytoma
adrenal p.
bladder p.
p. rule of 10

Philippe-Gombault tract

Philips
P. DVI 1 system
P. Gyroscan ACS scanner
P. Gyroscan NT, NT5, NT15 scanner
P. Gyroscan S5 scanner
P. Gyroscan T5 scanner
P. linear accelerator
P. 1.5-T NT MR scanner
P. Tomoscan 350 CT scanner
P. Tomoscan SR 6000 CT scanner
P. 4.7-T small-bore system scanner
P. T-60 tomoscanner
P. ultrasound machine

Phillips muscle

phlebectasia
malformed p.

phlebectatic peliosis hepatis

phlebitis
postvenography p.

phlebogram
ascending contrast MR p.
direct puncture MR p.
impedance MR p.

phlebography
ascending contrast p.
cervical intervertebral foraminal magnetic resonance p.
cervical magnetic resonance p. (CMRP)
direct puncture p.
impedance p.
magnetic resonance p.
occlusive impedance p.

phlebolith

phlebolith-like calcification

phleborheography (PRG)

phlebosclerosis

phlebostasis

phlebostenosis

phlebothrombosis

phlegmasia
p. cerula dolens
p. dolens alba

phlegmon
Holz p.
mesenteric p.
pancreatic p.
periurethral p.

phlegmonous
p. gastritis
p. mass
p. pancreatitis

PHO
periarticular heterotopic ossification

phocomely, phocomelia

phoenix abscess

phonation

phonatory sign

phonoangiography
carotid p.
oculoplethysmography/carotid p. (OPG/CPA)

phonophotography

phosphate
chromium p.
p. enema
linear p.'s
membrane p.
phosphorus-32 sodium p.
sodium p.
^{99m}Tc p.
technetium-99m phosphate
technetium-99m p. (^{99m}Tc phosphate)

phosphonate
nucleoside p.
tetraazacyclododecanetetraacetic tetramethylene p.

phosphor
cesium iodide input p.

NOTES

phosphor *(continued)*
photostimulable p.
p. plate
phosphorescence
phosphoric acid imaging agent
phosphorus
colloidal chromic p.
p. imaging agent
inorganic p.
p. isotope
p. magnetic resonance spectroscopy (P-MRS)
p. metabolism
p. metabolite
p. poisoning
phosphorus-32 (^{32}P)
p. intracavitary irradiation
p. sodium phosphate
phosphorylase
thymidine p. (TP)
phosphosoda enema
phosphotope oral solution
photic
photoacoustic
p. ultrasonography
p. ultrasound
photoactinic
photoaffinity
photocell plethysmography
photochemotherapy
extracorporeal p.
photochromogen
photocoagulation
interstitial laser p.
intraoperative laser p.
photodeficient region
photodensitometry
photodetector
CCD p.
photodiode
photodisintegration
photodisruption
photodynamic therapy (PDT)
photoechoic effect
photoelasticity
photoelectric
p. absorption
p. effect
p. emission
p. system
photoexcitation
photofluorography
photofrin 2
photographic effect (PE)
photography
CT bone window p.
Moiré p.
photolabel
long wavelength p.
photolysis
flash p.
photometer
HemoCue p.
photomicrograph
cystic hyperplasia p.
photomultiplier (PM)
p. tube (PMT)
photon (hv)
p. attenuation
p. attenuation measurement
Compton scattering p.'s
p. deficiency
degraded p.'s
p. densitometry
p. density
dual p.'s
p. energy
p. flux
p. interaction depth
linear p.'s
p. mottle
p. peak
soft p.'s
p. theory of radiation
p. therapy beam line
photon-deficient
p.-d. bone lesion
p.-d. lesion bone scintigraphy
photonic medicine
photon-neutron
p.-n. mixed-beam radiation therapy
photopeak
photopenia
photopenic
p. area
p. defect
p. region
photoplethysmographic
p. digit
p. monitoring
photoplethysmography (PPG)
photo-plotter film
photoprotein
photoradiation
photoreceptor
p. fractional velocity error
p. motion
photoscan
photostimulable
p. luminescence intensity
p. phosphor
p. phosphor dental radiography (PSP)
p. phosphor digital imaging
phototimer

photo transformation
phototube output circuit
photovolt pH meter
PHP
pseudohypoparathyroidism
phrenic
p. ampulla
p. artery
p. lymph node
p. nerve injury
p. pedicle
phrenicocolic ligament
phrenicoesophageal (*var. of* phrenoesophageal)
phrenicolienal ligament
phrenicosplenic ligament
phrenoesophageal, phrenicoesophageal
p. ligament
phrenogastric
phrenogastric ligament
phrenopericardial angle
phrenosplenic ligament
phrenovertebral junction
phrygian
p. cap
p. cap deformity
phrynoderma
phthinoid chest
phthisis
p. of aneurysm
aneurysmal p.
PHTN
pulmonary hypertension
phyllodes
cystosarcoma p.
p. tumor
physeal
p. bar
p. cartilage
p. closure
p. damage
p. distraction
p. injury
p. plate fracture
physes (*pl. of* physis)
physical
p. half-life
roentgen equivalent p. (REP)
p. stress test
p. trauma
Physicians
Fellow of the American College of Nuclear P. (FACNP)
Physick pouch
physicochemical speciation
physics
American Institute of P. (AIP)
Doppler p.
health p.
radiation p.
physiologic
p. atrophy
p. high activity
p. hypertrophy
p. ovarian cyst
p. parameter
p. regurgitation
p. shunt flow
p. sphincter
physis, pl. **physes**
distal tibial p.
fibular p.
fused p.
medial p.
unfused p.
phytobezoar
PI
pulmonic insufficiency
pi (π)
pia
p. arachnoid
p. mater
pial vessel
piano key sign
PIB
periinfarction block
PIBC
percutaneous intraaortic balloon counterpulsation
PICA
posterior-inferior cerebellar artery
posterior-inferior communicating artery
pica artifact
PICC
peripherally inserted central catheter
PICD
periinfarction conduction defect
Pick
P. body
P. bundle
P. disease
P. tubular adenoma

Picker
P. camera
P. Magnascanner
P. MR scanner
P. nodule
P. PQ 5000 helical CT scanner
P. PQ 2000 spiral CT scanner
P. SPECT attenuation correction
P. Synerview 600 scanner
P. system
picket
p. fence appearance
Picket Fence fiducial localization stereotactic system
pickup tube
picocurie (pc, pCi)
picometer (pm)
picomole (pmol)
picture
p. archival communication system
p. archiving and communications systems in radiation oncology (PACSRO)
p. archiving and communication system (PACS)
p. element
p. frame appearance
p. frame pattern of vertebral bodies
p. frame vertebra
picture-framing osteoporosis
PID
pelvic inflammatory disease
PIE
postinfectious encephalomyelitis
pulmonary interstitial emphysema
piece
chin-occiput p.
piecemeal necrosis
Piedmont fracture
Pierre Robin syndrome
piezoelectric
p. crystals
p. effect
p. transducer
pigeon
p. breeder's pneumonitis
p. chest
p. fancier's lung
pigeon-breast deformity
Pigg-O-Stat
P.-O.-S. immobilization device
P.-O.-S. x-ray chair
pigmented
p. basal cell carcinoma
p. iris hamartoma
p. villonodular bundle (PVB)
p. villonodular synovitis (PVNS)
pigment stone
pigskin patch
pigtail stent
PIH
pseudointimal hyperplasia
pilar
p. sheath
p. tumor of scalp
pilaris
pile
sentinel p.
pillar
faucial p.
p. fracture
p. sign
tonsillar p.
P. view
pill esophagitis
pillion fracture
pillow
p. fracture
p. sign
pilocytic
p. astrocytoma
p. tumor
piloid astrocytoma
pilomatricoma
pilon
p. ankle fracture
pilonidal
p. cyst
p. fistula
p. sinus
p. tract
pilosity
Piltz-Westphal phenomenon
pin
Hagie p.
orthopedic p.
p. pattern
resorbable p.
revolving Ge-68 p.
track of p.
pinchcock mechanism
pinched nerve
pincushion distortion
Pindborg tumor
pineal
p. apoplexy
p. body
p. cyst
p. dysgerminoma
p. germ-cell tumor
p. germinoma
p. gland
p. gland calcification
p. gland neoplasm
p. gland shift

p. gland teratocarcinoma
p. gland tumor
p. gland tumor classification
p. mass
p. parenchymal tumor
p. region
p. region tumor
p. teratocarcinoma
p. teratoma
p. ventricle
pinealcytoma
pinealoblastoma, pineoblastoma
pinealoma
ectopic p.
pineoblastoma, pinealoblastoma
pineocytoma
ping-pong
p.-p. ball deformity
p.-p. fracture
p.-p. heart volume
pinhole
bone p.
p. camera
p. collimator
p. image
p. imaging
pink
hit the p.
p. puffer
p. tetralogy
Pinnacle
P. 3 radiation therapy planning system
pinning
hip p.
in situ p.
Pins sign
PION
posterior interosseous nerve
pion
PIOPED
prospective investigation of pulmonary embolus detection
PIOPED criteria
Piotrowski sign
PIP
proximal interphalangeal joint
PIP articulation
PIP joint
pipe
endoscopic washing p.
pipe smoker's cancer
pipestem
p. artery
p. cirrhosis
p. fibrosis
p. ureter
pipe-stemming of ankle-brachial index
PIPIDA
paraisopropyliminodiacetic acid
PIPIDA hepatobiliary imaging
technetium-99m PIPIDA
piping
organ p.
PIPJ
proximal interphalangeal joint
Pipkin
P. classification of femoral fractures
P. femoral fracture classification
Pirie
P. bone
P. method
piriform, pyriform
p. cortex
p. lobe
p. muscle
p. recess
p. sinus
p. sinus cancer
p. sinus carcinoma
piriformis, pyriformis
p. muscle
p. syndrome
Pirogoff
P. amputation
P. angle
pisiform
p. bone
p. fracture
pisohamate ligament
pisometacarpal ligament
pisotriquetral
p. articulation
p. joint
pisounciform ligament
pisouncinate ligament
pistol-grip femur deformity
pistoning
piston-like reflux
piston sign
pit
anal p.
articular p.

NOTES

P

pit *(continued)*
auditory p.
central p.
colonic p.
costal p.
cutaneous p.
gastric p.
herniation p.
pitch ratio p.
postanal p.
scan pitch p.
spiral CT pitch p.
p. of stomach
synovial herniation p.
pitch
calcaneal p.
p. ratio
p. ratio pit
recon p.
scan p.
spiral CT p.
p. worker's cancer
pitted cartilage
pitting
pepper-pot p.
Pittsburgh pneumonia
pituicytoma
pituilith
pituitary
p. adenoma
p. adenoma chromophobe
p. cyst
p. dwarfism
p. failure
p. fossa
p. gland
p. gland anatomy
p. gland enlargement
p. hyperplasia
p. infarct
p. infundibulum
p. macroadenoma
p. microadenoma
p. oncocytoma
p. stalk
p. stalk distortion (PSD)
p. stone
p. tumor
pivot
p. of calcar
p. joint
p. shift
p. shift phenomenon
pivoting table
pivot-shift sign
pixel
p. block
edge-region p.
maximum intensity p. (MIP)
p. noise
normal-region p.
p. value
pixel-oriented algorithm
Pixsys FlashPoint camera
pizoelectric generator
pkV
peak kilovoltage
placement
annular p.
catheter p.
intracoronary stent p.
intrapericardial patch lead p.
line p.
percutaneous endoluminal p.
radiotherapy field p.
shim p.
shunt p.
subannular p.
subject p.
transcatheter filter p.
transpapillary p.
placenta, pl. **placentae**
abnormal adherence of p.
p. abruptio
accessory p.
p. accreta
adherent p.
annular p.
anterofundal p.
battledore p.
bilobate p.
p. biopsy
chorioallantoic p.
circummarginate p.
cirsoid p.
deciduate p.
Duncan p.
p. enlargement
extrachorial p.
p. extrachorialis
fetal p.
p. of fetus
first-trimester p.
fundal p.
horseshoe p.
incarcerated p.
p. increta
kidney-shaped p.
low-lying p.
marginal p.
maternal p.
p. membranacea
p. migration
nondeciduate p.
panduriform p.
p. percreta

premature senescence p.
p. previa
retained p.
p. rotation
Schultze p.
second-trimester p.
third-trimester p.
p. tumor
vascular space of the p.
velamentous p.
villous p.

placentae
abruptio p.

placental
p. abruption
p. circulation
p. disk
p. edema
p. grade
p. hemorrhage
p. infarct
p. localization
p. metastasis
p. polyp
p. septal cyst
p. septum
p. souffle
p. villus

placentation

placentography

placode
neural p.
unneurulated neural p.

plafond
p. fracture
tibial p.

plagiocephaly

plague pneumonia

plain
p. abdominal radiography (PAR)
p. film
p. film imaging
p. radiograph
p. tomogram
p. view

plain-paper image

plan
isodose p.
posterior transaxial scan p.

plana
coxa p.
vertebra p.

planar
p. circular coil
p. exercise thallium-201 scintigraphy
p. left anterior oblique image
p. plate
p. radionuclide imaging
p. spin imaging
p. thallium imaging
p. thallium scan
p. thallium with quantitative analysis
p. view

Planck quantum theory

plane
AC-PC p.
Addison p.
anatomic p.
areolar p.
auriculoinfraorbital p.
axial p.
axiolabiolingual p.
axiomesiodistal p.
bite p.
buccolingual p.
Calve vertebra p.
capsular p.
circular p.
p. of cleavage
coronal p.
E p.
eye-ear p.
fascial p.
fat p.
first parallel pelvic p.
flexion-extension p.
four-chamber p.
fourth parallel pelvic p.
Frankfort horizontal p.
frontal p.
German horizontal p.
gonion-gnathion p.
Hensen p.
Hodge p.
horizontal p.
imaging p.
p. of intercostal space
internervous p.
interspinous p.
intertubercular p.
ischiorectal fossa p.
Ludwig p.

NOTES

P

plane *(continued)*
median sagittal p.
mesiodistal p.
midclavicular p.
midcoronal p.
midfrontal p.
midsagittal p.
midthalamic p.
nonorthogonal p.
oblique coronal p.
occlusal p.
optimal imaging p.
orthogonal p.
parallel tag p.
paramedian sagittal p.
pelvic p.
perivascular p.
Poschl p.
sagittal p.
scan p.
sella-nasion p.
semicoronal p.
sensitive p.
short-axis p.
p. sign
slicing p.
spinous p.
sternoxiphoid p.
subadventitial p.
subcostal p.
subintimal cleavage p.
supracristal p. (SCP)
suprasternal p.
tag p.
thalamic p.
thoracic p.
transaxial p.
transaxial scan p.
transmedial p.
transpyloric p.
transtrabecular p. (TTP)
transumbilical p. (TUP)
transverse p.
tumor cleavage p.
valve p.
varus-valgus p.
vertical p.
Virchow p.
XY p.
ZY p.

planigram

planigraphic principle

planigraphy

planimeter

planimetry

planning
3D radiation treatment p.
radiation therapy p. (RTP)
radiation treatment p. (RTP)
p. target volume (PTV)

planogram

planography

planovalgus
p. foot
p. foot deformity
pes p.

plantae
quadratus p.

plantar
p. aponeurosis
p. arterial arch
p. aspect
p. axial view
p. bursa
p. calcaneal enthesophyte
p. calcaneal spur
p. capsule
p. compartment
p. compartmental anatomy
p. fasciitis
p. fibromatosis
p. flexion-inversion deformity
p. hyperplasia
p. interossei
p. ligament
p. metatarsal angle
p. metatarsal artery
p. plate
p. shift
p. surface
p. vault

plantarflexion stress view

plantaris
p. muscle
p. rupture
p. tendon
tylosis palmaris et p.

plantarward

planum sphenoidale

planus
pes p.
pes plantigrade p.

plaque
arterial p.
arteriosclerotic p.
asbestos pleural p.
atheromatous p.
atherosclerotic p.
calcified p.
carotid artery p.
p. cleaving
p. compression
concentric atherosclerotic p.
p. constituent
p. cracker
disrupted p.

eccentric atherosclerotic p.
echogenic p.
echolucent p.
endocardial p.
p. erosion
esophageal p.
fatty p.
fibrofatty p.
fibrotic p.
fibrous intima p.
fissured atheromatous p.
focal pleural p.
p. fracture
fungal p.
gastrointestinal p.
hemorrhage p.
p. hemorrhage
heterogeneous carotid p.
homogeneous carotid p.
Hutchinson p.
iliac p.
infiltrating p.
intraluminal p.
lipid-laden p.
luminal p.
meningioma en p.
multiple sclerosis (MS) p.
neuritic senile p.
noncompliant p.
obstructive p.
penile p.
periventricular p.
pleural p.
pleuroparenchymal p.
pulverized p.
Randall p.
p. regression
p. remodeling
residual p.
p. rupture
sclerotic p.
senile p.
sequential paired opposed p. (SPOP)
sessile p.
p. splitting
stenotic p.
talc p.
p. tearing
ulcerated atheromatous p.
ulcerated carotid artery p.
uncalcified pleural p.
p. vaporization

plaque-containing artery

plaquelike
p. lesion
p. linear defect

plaquing
p. calcification
luminal p.
multiple sclerosis (MS) p.
neuritic p.

plasma
p. cell pneumonia
p. emission spectroscopy
p. radioiron disappearance rate
p. radioiron turnover rate
p. volume

plasmablast

plasmablastic lymphoma

plasmacytoma
anaplastic p.
extramedullary leukemic p.
primary pulmonary p.
solitary p.

plasmodium embolus

plaster
p. cast
x-ray in p. (XIP)
x-ray out of p. (XOP)

plastic
p. bowing fracture
carbon fiber-reinforced p.
p. clot
p. pleurisy

plastica
linitis p.

plasticity
brain p.

plate
acetabular reconstruction p.
alar p.
amorphous selenium p.
anal p.
auditory p.
axial p.
basal p.
blade p.
bone flap fixation p.
bony p.
budding p.
buttress p.
cap-and-anchor p.

NOTES

P

plate *(continued)*
cardiogenic p.
cartilaginous growth p.
Casper p.
clinoid p.
cloacal p.
cloverleaf p.
coaptation p.
compression p.
condylar p.
connecting p.
cortical p.
cranial bone fixation p.
cribriform p.
3D p.
dorsal p.
dual p.
end p.
epiphyseal cartilage p.
epiphyseal growth p.
ethmovomerine p.
femoral p.
fenestrated compression p.
fibrocartilaginous volar p.
flat p.
flexor palmar p.
foot p.
Fresnel zone p.
frontal p.
fusion p.
Gallannaugh bone p.
ground p.
growth p.
hilar p.
interfragmentary p.
intertrochanteric p.
localization-compression grid p.
low-contact dynamic compression p. (LC-DCP)
meningioma of cribriform p.
microfixation p.
nail p.
neutralization p.
occipitocervical p.
orbital p.
orthopedic p.
orthotic p.
overlay p.
palmar p.
pedicle p.
phosphor p.
planar p.
plantar p.
prochordal p.
pterygoid p.
quadrigeminal p.
quadrilateral p.
resorbable p.
screw and p.
selenium p.
septal cartilage p.
sinodural p.
skull p.
Spli-Prest p.
stabilization p.
stainless steel p.
stem base p.
subchondral bone p.
supracondylar p.
tarsal p.
tectal p.
tendon p.
tissue p.
titanium p.
vertebral body p.
volar p.
xeroradiographic selenium p.
Y bone p.

plateau
multiple sclerosis p.
p. phase
p. tibia fracture
tibial p.

platelet-rich thrombus

platelets
adhesive p.
radiolabeled p.

platelike
p. atelectasis

platform
Cemax PACS p.
positioning p.

platinocyanoide
barium p.

platinum-based treatment

platinum coil

platinum-resistant
p.-r. disease
p.-r. ovarian cancer

platterlike atelectasis

platycephaly

platypelloid, platypellic
p. pelvis

platypodia

platysma muscle

platyspondylosis

platyspondyly
p. generalisata

play
excessive joint p.
joint p.

pleating
p. of ligamentum flavum
p. of small bowel

pleomorphic
p. adenoma parotis

p. calcification
p. liposarcoma
p. lung adenoma
p. rhabdomyosarcoma
p. T-cell lymphoma
p. type
p. xanthoastrocytoma (PXA)

pleomorphism
nuclear p.

pleonosteosis
Leri p.

PLES
parallel-line-equal spacing
parallel-line equal spacing
PLES bar
PLES bar pattern

plesiocurie therapy

plesiography

plethora

plethoric

plethysmography
air p.
body box p.
digital p.
Doppler ultrasonic velocity detector segmental p.
exercise strain gauge venous p.
impedance p. (IPG)
Medsonic p.
photocell p.
segmental bronchus p.
strain-gauge p.
thermistor p.
venous p.

pleura, pl. **pleurae**
cervical p.
congested p.
costal p.
costodiaphragmatic recess of p.
crus p.
diaphragmatic p.
edematous p.
empyema p.
p. fibrin body
fibromyxoma p.
fibrous tumor p.
hyaloserositis p.
inflamed p.
localized fibrous tumor of p.
mediastinal p.
p. metastasis
parietal p.
p. peel
pericardiac p.
p. pseudotumor
pulmonary p.
scarification of p.
silicotic visceral p.
solitary fibrous tumor of p.
visceral p.
wrinkled p.

pleura-based area of increased opacity

pleura-based lung nodule

pleurae (*pl. of* pleura)

pleural
p. apical hematoma cap
p. calcification
p. canal
p. cavity
p. cupula
p. cyst
p. density
p. disease
p. effusion
p. empyema
p. fibromyxoma
p. fistula
p. flap
p. fluid
p. fluid aspiration
p. fluid collection
p. lines
p. margin
p. mass
p. mesothelioma
p. plaque
p. reaction
p. recess
p. rind
p. ring
p. sac
p. scarring
p. space
p. stripe
p. tail sign
p. thickening
p. tube

pleurectomy

pleurisy
acute p.
Bends asbestos p.
blocked p.
chronic p.
circumscribed p.

NOTES

P

pleurisy *(continued)*
costal p.
diaphragmatic p.
diffuse p.
double p.
dry p.
encysted p.
exudative p.
fibrinopurulent p.
fibrinous p.
hemorrhagic p.
ichorous p.
indurative p.
interlobar p.
latent p.
mediastinal p.
metapneumonic p.
plastic p.
primary p.
proliferation p.
pulmonary p.
pulsating p.
purulent p.
sacculated p.
secondary p.
septic p.
serofibrous p.
serous p.
single p.
suppurative p.
typhoid p.
visceral p.
wet p.
pleuritic pneumonia
pleurocutaneous fistula
pleuroesophageal line
pleurogenic pneumonia
pleurography
pleuroparenchymal plaque
pleuropericardial
p. adhesion
p. canal
p. cyst
p. effusion
pleuroperitoneal
p. canal
p. fold
pleuropulmonary
p. adhesion
p. blastoma
pleuroscopy
plexiform neurofibroma
Plexiglas radiographic ruler
plexogenic pulmonary arteriopathy
plexus, pl. **plexus, plexuses**
abdominal aortic p.
anterior coronary p.
anterior pulmonary p.
aortic p.
Auerbach mesenteric p.
autonomic p.
axillary p.
basilar p.
Batson p.
biliary p.
brachial p.
calcification of choroid p.
cardiac p.
carotid p.
cavernous p.
celiac p.
cervical p.
choroid p.
ciliary ganglionic p.
coccygeal p.
colic p.
colonic myenteric p.
common carotid p.
coronary p.
cystic p.
dangling choroid p.
deep cardiac p.
deferential p.
enteric p.
epidural venous p.
Erb-Duchenne-Klumpke injury to brachial p.
esophageal p.
Exner p.
extradural vertebral p.
facial p.
femoral p.
gastric p.
gastroesophageal variceal p.
glomus of choroid p.
great cardiac p.
hemorrhoidal p.
hepatic nerve p.
hypogastric p.
ileocolic p.
inferior mesenteric p.
p. injury
intermesenteric p.
left coronary p.
lumbar p.
lumbosacral p.
lymph p.
Meissner p.
myenteric p.
nerve p.
pampiniform p.
paravertebral nerve p.
paravertebral venous p.
pelvic p.
perimeniscal capsular p.
perimuscular p.

pharyngeal p.
posterior coronary p.
posterior pulmonary p.
presacral p.
prostatic venous p.
pulmonary p.
rectal p.
retrovertebral p.
right coronary p.
sacral p.
sciatic p.
solar p.
spinal nerve p.
subareolar p.
submucosal venous p.
superficial p.
superior hypogastric p.
superior mesenteric p.
tympanic p.
uterovaginal p.
vaginal p.
vascular p.
venous p.
vertebral venous p.
vesical venous p.

PLFD
perilunate fracture-dislocation

plica, pl. **plicae**
plicae circulares
plicae colliculi
infrapatellar p.
medial p.
plicae palmatae
parapatellar p.
suprapatellar p.
symptomatic lateral synovial p.
p. syndrome
synovial p.

plicated dural sheath

plication
p. defect
disk p.
transmesenteric p.

PLIF
posterior lumbar interbody fusion

P-LINK software

PLL
posterior longitudinal ligament

PLSA
posterolateral spinal artery

plug
bile p.
bone p.
dermoid p.
echogenic p.
finger-in-glove mucous p.
fingerlike mucus p.
p. flow
interbody bone p.
luminal p.
meconium p.
mucus p.
Porstmann Ivalon p.
toothpaste shadows mucus p.

plugging
fingerlike mucus p.
mucus p.

Plumbicon

plumbline
p. sign
p. view

Plumicon camera tube

Plummer sign

plump vessel

plurality of slices

plural pregnancy

pluridirectional tomography (PT)

Plus
Laserprobe-PLR P.
4096 P. PET scanner

plutonism

plutonium
environmental p.

PM
photomultiplier
posterior mitral

Pm
promethium

pm
picometer

PMD
papillary muscle dysfunction

PML
progressive multifocal leukoencephalopathy

pML
posterior mitral leaflet

pmol
picomole

P-MRS
phosphorus magnetic resonance spectroscopy

PMS-Lidocaine Viscous

NOTES

P

PMT
photomultiplier tube
PMT robotic fulcrumless tomographic system
PMV
prolapsed mitral valve
PMVL
posterior mitral valve leaflet
PNC
premature nodal contraction
PNET
primitive neuroectodermal tumor
pneumarthrogram
pneumarthrography
pneumatic bone
pneumatization
pneumatocele
postinfectious p.
traumatic p.
pneumatocyst
pneumatosis
p. coli
p. cystoides intestinalis
epidural p.
gastric p.
p. sphenoidale
stomach p.
pneumencephalography
lumbar p.
pneumoarthrogram
pneumoarthrography
pneumocele
pneumocephalus
intracranial p.
pneumocolon
pneumoconiosis, pl. **pneumoconioses**
aluminum p.
barium p.
bauxite p.
p. classification
coal worker's p.
complicated p.
fiberglass p.
Fuller earth p.
kaolin p.
mica p.
nepheline p.
nonasbestos p.
rheumatoid p.
sericite p.
silicate p.
sillimanite p.
simple coal worker's p.
talc p.
tungsten carbide p.
uncommon p.
zeolite p.
pneumoconstriction
pneumocystic infection
***Pneumocystis carinii* kidney infection**
***Pneumocystis* pneumonia**
pneumocystography
breast p.
pneumocystosis
cutaneous p.
pneumocystotomography
pneumoencephalogram (PEG)
pneumoencephalographic pattern
pneumoencephalography
pneumoencephalomyelogram
pneumoencephalomyelography
pneumogastrography
pneumogram
pneumography
cerebral p.
retroperitoneal p.
pneumogynogram
pneumohemothorax
pneumohydrothorax
pneumointestinalis
pneumolith
pneumomediastinography
pneumomediastinum
postoperative p.
radiolucent p.
spontaneous p.
traumatic p.
pneumomyelography
pneumonectomy
p. chest
pneumonia
accelerated interstitial p.
acute eosinophilic p.
acute interstitial p. (AIP)
adenovirus p.
alcoholic p.
allergic p.
alveolar p.
anthrax p.
apical p.
aspiration p.
asthmatic p.
atypical bronchial p.
atypical interstitial p.
atypical measles p.
atypical primary p.
Bacillus anthracis p.
bacterial p.
bilateral lower lobe p.
bilious bronchial p.
bronchiolitis obliterans with organizing p. (BOOP)
Buhl desquamative p.
capillary p.
caseous p.
catarrhal p.

cavitating p.
central p.
cerebral p.
cheesy p.
chelonian p.
chemical p.
chickenpox p.
cholesterol p.
chronic eosinophilic p.
chronic interstitial p.
classic interstitial p.
community-acquired p.
concomitant p.
consolidative p.
contusion p.
Corrigan p.
cryptogenic organizing p.
cytomegalovirus p.
deglutition p.
delayed resolution of p.
desquamative interstitial p. (DIP)
diffuse p.
double p.
Eaton agent p.
embolic p.
endogenous lipid p.
eosinophilic p.
ephemeral p.
exogenous lipoid p.
extensive bilateral p.
fibrinous p.
fibrous p.
focal organizing p.
Friedländer p.
fungal p.
gangrenous p.
giant cell interstitial p. (GIP)
golden p.
granulomatous p.
gray hepatization stage of p.
Hecht p.
hemorrhagic p.
herpesvirus p.
hypersensitivity p.
hypostatic p.
idiopathic interstitial p.
incomplete resolution of p.
indurative p.
infantile p.
inhalation p.
interstitial organizing p.
interstitial plasma cell p.
irradiation p.
Klebsiella p.
lingular p.
lipoid endogenous p.
lobar p.
lobular p.
Löffler p.
lower lobe p.
lymphocytic interstitial p. (LIP)
lymphoid interstitial p. (LIP)
Macrodantin p.
massive p.
measles p.
metastatic p.
migratory p.
Mycoplasma p.
mycotic p.
necrotizing p.
neonatal p.
nonbacterial p.
nonclassifiable interstitial p.
nonspecific interstitial p. (NIP, NSIP)
nosocomial p.
nummular p.
obstructive p.
oil-aspiration p.
organizing focal p.
organizing interstitial p.
parenchymatous p.
passive p.
patchy area of p.
peripheral p.
pertussoid eosinophilic p.
Pittsburgh p.
plague p.
plasma cell p.
pleuritic p.
pleurogenic p.
Pneumocystis p.
postobstructive p.
posttraumatic p.
progressive tuberculosis (TB) p.
protozoal p.
purulent p.
radiation p.
recurrent p.
red hepatization stage of p.
resolving p.
respiratory syncytial virus p.
rheumatic p.
rickettsial p.

NOTES

P

pneumonia *(continued)*
right-sided p.
round p.
secondary p.
segmental p.
septic p.
subacute allergic p.
superficial p.
suppurative p.
terminal p.
toxemic p.
toxic p.
traumatic p.
tuberculous p.
tularemic p.
typhoid p.
unresolved p.
usual interstitial p. (UIP)
walking p.
wandering p.
Weill sign of p.
white p.
woolsorter's p.
zoster p.
pneumonic infiltrate
pneumonitis
acid aspiration p.
acute interstitial p.
acute radiation p.
aspiration p.
bacterial p.
basilar p.
chemical p.
cholesterol p.
chronic p.
congenital rubella p.
cytomegalovirus interstitial p.
drug-induced p.
early p.
granulomatous p.
hypersensitivity p.
idiopathic interstitial p.
interstitial p.
lipoid p.
lupus p.
lymphocytic interstitial p.
lymphoid interstitial p.
malarial p.
manganese p.
Mycoplasma p.
mycoplasmal p.
Pandora p.
pigeon breeder's p.
radiation p.
staphylococcal p.
trimellitic anhydrotic p.
unusual interstitial p.
uremic p.
usual interstitial p.
ventilation p.
pneumonocirrhosis
pneumonoconiosis
noncollagenous p.
pneumoorbitography
pneumopathy
cobalt p.
pneumoperitoneum
balanced p.
drop test for p.
pneumoplethysmography
ocular p. (OPG)
pneumopyelography
pneumoradiography
pneumoroentgenogram
pneumoroentgenography
pneumoscrotum
pneumothorax, pl. **pneumothoraces**
artificial p.
basilar p.
blowing p.
catamenial p.
closed p.
congenital p.
diagnostic p.
extrapleural p.
induced p.
life-threatening p.
open p.
positive-pressure p.
pressure p.
recurrent p.
simultaneous bilateral spontaneous p. (SBSP)
spontaneous tension p.
sucking p.
tension p.
therapeutic p.
traumatic p.
tuberculous p.
uncomplicated p.
valvular p.
pneumoventriculography
p.o.
per os
pocket
air p.
p. chamber
p. Doppler
p. dosimeter
infraclavicular p.
rectus sheath p.
regurgitant p.
p. shot
subcutaneous p.
subpectoral p.
valve p.

p. of Zahn
Zahn p.
pocketed calculus
pocketing of barium
podagra
point
A p.
Addison p.
alveolar p.
apophyseal p.
auricular p.
bleeding p.
branch p.
breast trigger p.
Cannon p.
Cannon-Boehm p.
cardinal p.
Chauffard p.
choroid p.
Clado p.
coaptation p.
commissural p.
congruent p.
Cope p.
coplanar contour p.
craniometric p.
Crowe pilot p.
D p.
de Mussey p.
dorsal p.
end p.
entry p.
equilibrium p.
Erb p.
frontopolar p.
glenoid p.
Griffith p.
Hartmann p.
ICRU reference p.
p. imaging
Lanz p.
lead p.
p. localization
Mackenzie p.
McBurney p.
midinguinal p.
Morris p.
multiple sensitive p.'s
p. mutation
p. mutation detection using exonuclease amplification couple capture technique (point-EXACCT)
nodal p.
null p.
output p.
Pauly p.
preauricular p.
pressure p.
random p.
reentry p.
Rolando p.
saddle p.
sample p.
p. scanning
seed p.
sensitive p.
Sudeck p.
sylvian p.
target p.
time p.
white p.
pointer
hip p.
metallic p.
shoulder p.
point-EXACCT
point mutation detection using exonuclease amplification couple capture technique
point-in-space stereotactic biopsy
point-resolved
p.-r. spectroscopy (PRESS)
p.-r. spectroscopy sequence (PRESS sequence)
point-spread function (PSR)
point-to-point protocol (PPP)
Poirier space
Poiseuille
P. flow
P. law
P. space
poisoning
lead p.
phosphorus p.
radiation p.
Poisson
P. distributed activity concentration
P. distribution
P. noise fluctuation
P. ratio
poker spine
Poland
P. classification of epiphyseal fractures

NOTES

Poland *(continued)*
P. epiphyseal fracture classification
P. syndrome
polar-bound water
polar coordinate system
polarity-altered
p.-a. spectral-selective acquisition (PASTA)
p.-a. spectral-selective acquisition imaging
polarization
chemically induced dynamic nuclear p.
dynamic nuclear p. (DNP)
linear p.
nuclear p.
polarographic
p. needle electrode
p. needle electrode measurement
Polaroid film
pole
abapical p.
cephalic p.
fetal p.
p. figure texture analysis
frontal p.
germinal p.
inferior p.
kidney p.
lower p.
middle p.
occipital p.
patellar p.
scaphoid p.
p. of scaphoid bone
superior p.
temporal p.
upper p.
p. of vessel
poles of organ
pole-to-pole length of kidney
Polhemus
P. 3 digitizer
P. 3 digitizer scanner
poliomyelitis
polka-dot sclerosis
pollex pedis
pollicis
adductor p.
p. longus tendon
opponens p.
pollicization
Riordan finger p.
pollicized ray
polyadenopathy
angiofollicular and plasmacytic p.
polyalveolar lobe
polyangiitis
microscopic p.
polyarcuate diaphragm
polyarteritis
polyarthropathy
polyarticular symmetric tophaceous joint inflammation
polychemotherapy
polychondritis
relapsing p.
polychromatic radiation
polycystic
p. kidney
p. kidney disease
p. liver
p. liver disease
p. nephroblastoma
p. ovarian disease (PCOD)
p. ovary
p. renal disease
polydactyly
Wassel classification of thumb p.
polyethylene
p. glycol
p. tube
polygelin colloid imaging agent
polyglycolide
self-reinforced p.
polygon mirror
polygyria
polyhydramnios
polylactic acid
polylobar liver
polymastia
polymer
p. dosimetry
p. fume fever
polymethyl methacrylate (PMMA) implant
polymicrogyria
polymorphism
polymyalgia rheumatica
polymyositis
Polynesian bronchiectasis
polyneuropathy
Déjérine-Sottas hypertrophic p.
distal predominantly sensory p.
polynomial stepwise multilinear regression
polyostotic
p. bone lesion
p. fibrous dysplasia
polyp
adenomatous p. (AP)
adenomatous colonic p.
angiomatous nasal p.
antral p.
antrochoanal p.

benign p.
bleeding p.
broad-based p.
bronchial p.
cardiac p.
carpet p.
cervical p.
choanal p.
cholesterol gallbladder p.
colonic adenomatous p.
colonic hamartomatous p.
colorectal p.
cystic p.
dental p.
duodenal p.
endometrial p.
epithelial colonic p.
fibrinous p.
fibroepithelial urethral p.
fibroid p.
fibrous urinary tract p.
fibrovascular p.
filiform p.
gallbladder p.
gastric p.
hamartomatous gastric p.
Hopmann p.
hydatid p.
hyperplastic adenomatous p.
hyperplastic colon p.
hyperplastic gastric p.
hyperplastic stomach p.
inflammatory colonic p.
inflammatory esophagogastric p.
inflammatory fibroid p.
inflammatory stomach p.
juvenile p.
laryngeal p.
lipomatous p.
lymphoid p.
malignant p.
metaplastic p.
metastatic p.
mucous p.
multiple p.'s
nasal p.
osseous p.
pedunculated p.
Peutz-Jeghers p.
placental p.
postinflammatory p.
rectal p.
regenerative gastric p.
retention colon p.
retention stomach p.
sessile p.
sigmoid p.
single p.
stalk of p.
p. stalk
tubular p.
tubulovillous p.
uterine fibroid p.
vascular fibrous p.
villoglandular p.
villous stomach p.

polypectomy
colonoscopic p.

polyphase generator

polyphebus

polyphosphate

polyphosphonate
technetium p.

polypoid
p. adenoma
p. calcified irregular mass
p. carcinoma
p. dysplasia
p. fibroma
p. fibroma collecting system
p. filling defect
p. lesion
p. lymphoid hyperplasia
p. lymphoma
p. mucosa

polyposa
colitis p.

polyposis
adenoma familial p.
diffuse mucosal p.
familial adenomatous p. (FAP)
familial colorectal p.
familial gastrointestinal p.
familial intestinal p.
familial juvenile p.
familial multiple p.
filiform p.
gastric hamartomatous p.
intestinal p.
juvenile p.
multiple p.
Peutz-Jeghers gastrointestinal p.
postinflammatory p.

NOTES

P

polyposis *(continued)*
sinonasal p.
p. syndrome
polyradiculomyelitis
polyradiculoneuropathy
polyradiculopathy
polysplenia syndrome
polystotic
polytetrafluoroethylene
p. (PTFE) graft
polythelia
polytome
Massiot p.
polytomographic radiology
polytomography
mastoid p.
polytrauma
polyurethane
p. foam embolus
p. stent
polyvinyl chloride
POMP
phase-offset multiplanar
phase-ordered multiplanar
POMP imaging
Pompe
P. disease
P. syndrome
pond fracture
Ponfick shadow
Ponomar transjugular clot-trapper device
pons
caudal p.
infarct of p.
rostral p.
tegmentum of p.
ponticulus posticus
pontine, pontile
p. angle
p. angle tumor
p. artery
central p.
p. cistern
p. contusion
p. glioma
p. hemorrhage
p. hydatid cyst
p. infarct
p. isthmus
p. lesion
p. myelinolysis
p. parareticular formation (PPRF)
p. syndrome
p. tegmentum
pontine-medullary level
pontis
brachium p.
pontocerebellar
p. fiber
p. glioma
pontomedullary
p. junction
p. sulcus
pontomesencephalic
p. junction
p. vein
pool
blood p.
focal p.
gastric p.
vascular blood p.
white-appearing blood p.
pooling
venous p.
poor
p. perfusion
p. screen/film contact
p. sensitivity
p. shimming of MRI magnet
p. visualization
poorly
p. circumscribed tumor
p. concentrated isotope
p. differentiated adenocarcinoma (PDA)
p. differentiated adenoma
p. differentiated tumor
popcorn calcification
popcornlike appearance
Popeye arm
popliteal
p. artery
p. artery aneurysm
p. artery entrapment syndrome
p. artery occlusive disease
p. artery pulsation artifact
p. artery trifurcation
p. cavity
p. cyst
p. fossa
p. hiatus
p. ligament
p. line
p. node
p. recess
p. space
p. tendon
p. tendonitis
p. trifurcation
p. vein
popliteus bursa
Poppel sign
poppet
barium-impregnated p.
disk p.

poppy seedlike calcification
porcelain
p. aorta
p. gallbladder
Porcher method
porcine
p. gallbladder
p. heart xenograft
pore
Kohn and Lambert p.'s
skin p.
porencephalic cyst
porencephaly
acquired p.
agenetic p.
encephaloclastic p.
true p.
porokeratosis plantaris discreta
porosis
cerebral p.
porous
p. bone
p. ingrowth
p. kidney
p. metallic stent
PORP
partial ossicular replacement prosthesis
Porstmann Ivalon plug
port
Cordis multipurpose access p.
p. film
implantable infusion p.
injection p.
multipurpose access p. (MPAP)
parallel opposed p.'s
parallel opposed unmodified p.'s
radiation p.
radiotherapy p.
simulation of converging p.'s
single p.
subcutaneous implanted injection p.
tangential p.
treatment p.
porta
p. cirrhosis
p. hepatis
p. hepatis defect
p. hepatis low-density mass
p. hepatis node
portable
p. C-arm image intensifier fluoroscopy
p. C-arm intensifier
p. chest film
p. film of pelvis
p. radiography
p. view
p. x-ray
Port-A-Cath
portacaval
p. shunt
p. space
portal
p. canal
p. decompression
p. fibrosis
p. fissure
fixed-beam p.
p. flow
radiocarpal p.
simulation of tangential p.'s
p. space
superomedial p.
p. triad
p. vascular bed
p. vein
p. vein aneurysm
p. vein cavernoma
p. vein congestion index
p. vein system
p. vein thrombosis
p. vein velocity
p. venography
p. venous gas
p. venous phase (PVP)
p. venous pressure (PVP)
portalization
hepatic vein p.
portal-phased spiral CT scan
portal-to-portal
p.-t.-p. bridge
p.-t.-p. fibrosis
PortalVision radiation oncology system
portion
intrapericardial p.
supraclinoid p.
portio vaginalis
portoenterostomy
portogram
portography
arterial p.
computed tomography angiographic p. (CTAP)

NOTES

P

portography *(continued)*
computed tomography arterial p. (CTAP)
double-spiral CT arterial p.
percutaneous transhepatic p.
splenic p.
portohepatic
portopulmonary shunt
portosplenic thrombosis
portosystemic
p. collateral circulation
p. collateral vessel
p. gradient
p. shunt
portovenography
portovenous
Posada fracture
Posadas-Wernicke coccidioidomycosis
Poschl plane
Posicam HZ PET scanner
position
Albers-Schönberg p.
Albert p.
anatomic p.
anterior oblique p.
barber chair p.
bayonet fracture p.
beachchair p.
Beclere p.
Benassi p.
Bertel p.
Blackett-Healy p.
Broden p.
Caldwell p.
Camp-Coventry p.
cardiac p.
catheter p.
catheter tip p.
central venous line p.
Chassard-Lapine p.
Cleaves p.
Clements-Nakayama p.
cock-robin p.
conus medullaris p.
Coyle trauma p.
decubitus p.
dorsal decubitus p.
dorsal recumbent p.
dorsosacral p.
dwell p.
p. encoding
erect p.
Feist-Mankin p.
Fick p.
Fleischner p.
Fowler p.
Friedman p.
frogleg p.
Fuchs p.
full lateral p.
Gaynor-Hart p.
Grashey p.
Haas p.
heart p.
Hickey p.
horizontal p.
infragenicular p.
infrapulmonary p.
Isherwood p.
jackknife p.
Johnson p.
Kurzbauer p.
LAO p.
Larkin p.
lateral decubitus p.
lateral left anterior oblique p.
Law p.
Lawrence p.
left anterior oblique p.
left posterior oblique p.
left-side-down decubitus p.
Leonard-George p.
Lilienfelds p.
lordotic p.
lotus p.
Low-Beers p.
LPO p.
Mayer p.
Meese p.
Miller p.
near-anatomic p.
neutral hip p.
Noble p.
Nolke p.
noncoaxial catheter tip p.
normal anatomic p.
nose-chin p.
nose-forehead p.
opisthotonic p.
paramedian p.
paraseptal p.
park bench p.
Pawlow p.
Pearson p.
Phalen p.
prone p.
pulmonary capillary wedge p.
reclining p.
rectus p.
recumbent p.
reverse Trendelenburg p.
right anterior oblique (RAO) p.
right posterior oblique (RPO) p.
right-side-down p.
right-side-down decubitus p.
Schüller p.

semilateral p.
semiupright p.
Settegast p.
side-lying p.
Sims p.
spatial p.
squatting p.
Staunig p.
Stecher p.
steep Trendelenburg p.
stepping-source p.
supine p.
swimmer's p.
Tarrant p.
Taylor p.
three-quarters prone p.
Titterington p.
Towne p.
Trendelenburg p.
tripod p.
upright p.
ventral decubitus p.
Walcher p.
Waters p.
Wigby-Taylor p.
Zanelli p.

positional
p. dysfunction
p. variation

positioning
p. error
pendent p.
p. platform

positive
p. bottle sign
p. contrast myelography
p. electron
p. end-expiratory pressure
p. predictive value (PPV)
p. ray
p. tilt test
true p. (TP)

positive-ion cyclotron

positive-pressure pneumothorax

positron
p. emission tomography (PET)
p. emission tomography balloon (PET balloon)
p. emission tomography compound
p. emission tomography imaging
p. emission tomography (PET) radiopharmaceutical
p. emission tomography (PET) scan
p. emission transaxial tomography (PETT)
p. emission transaxial tomography imaging
p. emitting radionucleotide
p. imaging
labeled p.
p. matter-antimatter annihilation reaction
p. scanning
p. scintillation camera

post
status p. (S/P)

postablation

postamputation neuroma

postanal pit

postangioplasty
p. angiography
p. aortography
p. intimal flap
p. mural thrombosis
p. restenosis
p. stenosis

postaortic lymph node

postaugmentation

postbeat filtration

postbiopsy
p. change
p. period
p. renal AV fistula

postbulbar
p. ulcer

postbypass spasm

postcapillary venule

postcardiac injury syndrome (PCIS)

postcardiotomy lymphocytic splenomegaly

postcaval
p. lymph node
p. ureter

postcentral
p. gyrus
p. sulcus

postcholecystectomy syndrome

postcontrast
p. echocardiography
p. MR imaging

postcricoid
p. area

NOTES

P

postcricoid *(continued)*
p. carcinoma
p. defect
p. pharyngeal cancer
p. pharynx
p. web
postcubital
postdilatation arteriography
postdrainage
p. cystogram
p. imaging
p. projection
postductal
p. aortic coarctation
p. coarctation of aorta
Postel destructive coxarthropathy
postembolization
p. angiographic pattern
p. angiography
p. syndrome
postenhancement sequence
posterior (P)
p. abdominal wall
p. acoustic shadowing
p. aorta transposition of great arteries
p. apical segment
p. arch fracture
p. aspect
p. auricular vein
p. axillary line
p. basal segmental bronchus
p. border
p. border of heart
p. calcaneal bursitis
p. cardinal vein
p. central gyrus
p. cerebral artery (PCA)
p. cerebral territory infarct
p. cervical space
p. cervical triangle
p. choroidal artery
p. circumflex humeral artery
p. cistern
p. colliculus
p. column deficit
p. column demyelination
p. column lesion
p. column of spine
p. column syndrome
p. commissure (PC)
p. communicating artery (PCA, PCoA)
p. communicating artery aneurysm
p. compartment
p. compartment lesion
p. coronary plexus
p. cruciate ligament (PCL)
p. cruciate ligament injury
p. cusp
p. descending artery (PDA)
p. descending branch
p. disk margin
p. element fracture
p. epidural fat
p. fascicular block
p. fontanelle
p. fossa-atrial shunt
p. fossa circulation
p. fossa cyst
p. fossa-foramen magnum lesion
p. fossa hematoma
p. fossa meningioma
p. fossa tumor
p. fracture dislocation
p. free wall
p. gray column of cord
p. gray horn
p. iliac crest
p. impingement
p. inferior tibiofibular ligament
p. intercostal artery
p. intercostal branch
p. interosseous nerve (PION)
p. interosseous nerve (PIN) entrapment
p. interventricular groove
p. interventricular sulcus
p. interventricular vein
p. joint syndrome
p. junction line
p. language area lesion
p. leaflet prolapse
p. lie
p. lip
p. longitudinal ligament (PLL)
p. lumbar interbody fusion (PLIF)
p. lumbar vessel
p. median septum
p. mediastinal mass
p. mediastinal node
p. mediastinum
p. membrane articulation
p. metatarsal arch
p. mitral (PM)
p. mitral leaflet (pML)
p. mitral valve leaflet (PMVL)
p. neck surface coil
p. oblique ligament
p. olive
p. osteophyte
p. papillary muscle (PPM)
p. parietal artery
p. patch aortoplasty
p. pharyngeal wall carcinoma
p. pituitary fossa

p. pituitary gland ectopia
p. pleural recess
p. predominance
p. probability
p. projection
p. pulmonary plexus
p. rectus sheath
p. ring fracture
p. root entry zone (PREZ)
p. root ganglion
p. scalloping of vertebra
p. semicircular canal
p. septal space
p. skull view
p. spinal artery
p. spinal cord horn
p. spine fusion (PSF)
p. spinocerebellar tract
p. spur
p. subluxation
superior labral anterior to p. (SLAP)
p. surface
p. surface of pancreas
p. surface of prostate
p. talofibular ligament (PTF ligament)
p. temporal artery
p. terminal vein (PTV)
p. tibial artery
tibialis p.
p. tibial tendon
p. tibiotalar ligament
p. transaxial scan plan
p. tricuspid leaflet (PTL, pTL)
p. urethra
p. urethral injury (PUI)
p. urethral valve (PUV)
p. urethrovesical angle
p. vagal trunk
p. ventricular branch
p. vertebral elements blowout lesion
p. vertebral scalloping
p. wall (PW)
p. wall fracture
p. wall motion
p. wall myocardial infarct
p. wall thickness (PWT)

posterior-inferior
p.-i. cerebellar artery (PICA)
p.-i. cerebellar artery aneurysm
p.-i. communicating artery (PICA)
p.-i. spine

posteroanterior (PA)
p. chest film
p. projection
p. view

posteroapical defect

posterobasal
p. segment
p. wall myocardial infarct

posteroinferior
p. myocardial infarct

posterolateral
p. aspect
p. capsule
p. compartment
p. corner injury
p. corner (PLC) of knee
p. disk herniation
p. fontanelle
p. rotatory instability
p. rotatory subluxation
p. sclerosis
p. segment
p. spinal artery (PLSA)
p. wall
p. wall motion
p. wall myocardial infarct

posteromedial
p. compartment
p. tibia

posterooblique view

posterosuperior glenoid impingement

postevacuation
p. film
p. view

postexercise
p. echocardiography
p. image
p. imaging
p. index (PEI)

postextrasystolic pause

postgadolinium scan

postganglionic
p. gray fibers
p. sympathetic fibers

postglomerular arteriolar constriction

postglucose loading examination

posthemorrhagic hydrocephalus

posthepatic cirrhosis

postictal cerebral blood flow scan

NOTES

posticus
 ponticulus p.
postinfarction
 p. ventricular aneurysm
 p. ventriculoseptal defect
postinfectious
 p. bronchiectasis
 p. demyelination
 p. encephalitis
 p. encephalomyelitis (PIE)
 p. hydrocephalus
 p. pneumatocele
postinflammatory
 p. adenopathy
 p. polyp
 p. polyposis
 p. pulmonary fibrosis
 p. renal atrophy
 p. scarring
postinjection
 p. echocardiography
 p. imaging
postintraarticular paramagnetic contrast injection T1-weighted image
postirradiation
 p. fracture
 p. osteogenic sarcoma
 p. vascular insufficiency
postischemic recovery
postlaminectomy
 p. instability
 p. kyphosis
postlumpectomy
 p. skin thickening
postlymphangiography
postmastectomy
 p. lymphedema
 p. lymphedema syndrome
postmaturity syndrome
postmenopausal
 p. adnexal cyst
 p. bleeding
 p. endometrial thickness
 p. endometrium
 p. estrogen therapy
 p. osteoporosis
 p. ovary
 p. uterine atrophy
 p. uterine bleeding
postmetrizamide
 p. CT imaging
 p. CT scan
postmyocardial
 p. infarct
 p. infarction echocardiography
 p. infarction syndrome
postmyocardiotomy infarct
postmyocarditis dilated cardiomyopathy
postnatal injury
postnecrotic
 p. cirrhosis
 p. scarring
postneuritic atrophy
postobstructive
 p. pneumonia
 p. renal atrophy
postoperative
 p. angiography
 p. breast hematoma
 p. breast scar
 p. cholangiography imaging
 p. chylothorax
 p. diagnosis
 p. emphysema
 p. ileus
 p. mediastinal hemorrhage
 p. pneumomediastinum
 p. seroma
 p. skull defect
 p. thoracic deformity
 p. view
postorchiectomy paraaortic radiation therapy
postpartum
 p. cardiomyopathy
 p. pituitary apoplexy
 p. pituitary necrosis
postperfusion lung syndrome
postpericardiotomy syndrome
postphlebitic
 p. leg
 p. valvular incompetence
postpolio syndrome
postprimary pulmonary tuberculosis
postprocedure nephrostogram
post-PTCA residual stenosis
postpyelonephritis cortical scarring
postradiation fibrosis
postreduction
 p. mammoplasty
 p. view
 p. x-ray
postrheumatic cusp retraction
postrolandic parietal cortex
postrubella syndrome
postsphenoid bone
poststenotic dilatation
poststress
 p. ankle/arm Doppler index
 p. image
 p. imaging
postsurgical
 p. emphysema
 p. fat necrosis
 p. lumbosacral syndrome

p. pseudoaneurysm
p. recurrent ulcer
posttemporal middle cerebral artery
postterm
p. fetus
p. pregnancy
posttherapy change
postthoracotomy change
postthrombolytic coronary reocclusion
posttourniquet occlusion angiography
posttransplant
p. acute renal failure
p. coronary artery disease
posttraumatic
p. angulation
p. aseptic necrosis
p. atrophy of bone
p. cavus
p. chondrolysis
p. cystic myelopathy
p. fat necrosis
p. fibrosis
p. hemorrhage
p. hydrocephalus
p. intradiploic pseudomeningocele
p. neuroma
p. oil cyst
p. osteoarthritis
p. osteoporosis
p. pneumonia
p. pulmonary insufficiency
p. spinal cord cyst
p. subcapsular hepatic fluid collection
p. syringomyelia
postulnar bone
postural
p. motor sign
p. reduction
posture
benediction p.
postvagotomy dysphagia
postvasectomy change in epididymis
postvenography phlebitis
postvesicular lymph node
postviral leukoencephalopathy
postvoid
p. residual
p. residual urine
p. residual urine volume
p. view
postvoiding
p. cystogram
p. film
Potain sign
potassium (K)
p. bromide
p. imaging agent
p. iodide
ionic p.
p. perchlorate
total exchangeable p. (TEK)
potassium-39 (^{39}K)
potassium-40 (^{40}K)
potassium-42 (^{42}K)
potassium-43 (^{43}K)
potato
p. liver
p. tumor of neck
potential
electrostatic p.
ionization p.
low metastatic p.
phenomenological effective surface p.
recruitment p.
resting phase of cardiac action p.
sorption p.
upstroke phase of cardiac action p.
variable tube p.
potentiator
potentiometer
Pott
P. abscess
P. aneurysm
P. ankle fracture
P. disease
P. puffy tumor
P. shunt
P. sign
Pottenger sign
Potter
P. classification
P. dysplasia
P. sequence
P. syndrome
P. type IV kidney
Potter-Bucky diaphragm
pouce flottant (floating thumb)
pouch
antral p.
apophyseal p.
arachnoid retrocerebellar p.

NOTES

pouch *(continued)*
axillary p.
blind upper esophageal p.
branchial p.
Broca pudendal p.
celomic p.
deep perineal p.
p. of Douglas
Douglas rectouterine p.
dural root p.
endodermal p.
endorectal ileal p.
fourth branchial cleft p.
gastric p.
Hartmann p.
haustral p.
Heidenhain p.
hepatorenal p.
hernia p.
hypophysial p.
ileal S p.
ileoanal p.
ileocecal p.
Indiana p.
jejunal p.
Morison p.
nerve root axillary p.
paracystic p.
pararectal p.
paravesical p.
pendulous p.
pharyngeal p.
Physick p.
Prussak p.
Rathke p.
rectal p.
rectouterine p.
rectovaginal p.
rectovaginouterine p.
rectovesical p.
renal p.
Seessel p.
S-shaped p.
superficial inguinal p.
superficial perineal p.
suprapatellar p.
two-loop ileal J p.
ultimobranchial p.
uterovesical p.
vesicouterine p.
Willis p.
W-shaped ileal p.
Zenker p.
pouchogram
pouchography
evacuation p.
Poupart inguinal ligament
Pourcelot index
powder
bone p.
p. pseudocalcification
tantalum p.
power
p. Doppler
p. Doppler imaging (PDI)
p. Doppler sonography
p. Doppler ultrasound
p. gain
p. injection
p. injector
p. law TAR method
mass collision stopping p.
mass radiative stopping p.
p. ratio
resolving p.
scanning p.
p. spectral analysis (PSA)
stopping p.
stroke p.
PowerVision ultrasound
Pozzi muscle
PPAF
progressive perivenular alcoholic fibrosis
PPAS
peripheral pulmonary artery stenosis
PPG
photoplethysmography
PPH
primary pulmonary hypertension
PPM
posterior papillary muscle
PPO
2,5-diphenyloxazole
PPP
point-to-point protocol
PPPMA
progressive postpolio muscle atrophy
PPRF
pontine parareticular formation
PPV
positive predictive value
pQCT
peripheral quantitative computed tomography
pQCT microscanner
PQCT microscanner scanner
P:QRS ratio
PR
pulmonic regurgitation
OncoScint PR
PRA
proximal reference axis
praecox
Praestholm
preablation
pre-Achilles fat pad

preacinar arterial wall thickness
preampullary portion of bile duct
preangioplasty stenosis
preaortic lymph node
preauricular point
precancerous
p. change
p. disease
precapillary lung hypertension
precatheterization
precaval lymph node
prececal lymph node
precentral
p. artery
p. cerebellar vein
p. gyrus
p. sulcus
precentroblast
precessing proton
precession
p. angle
fast imaging with steady-state free p. (FISP)
free p.
Larmor p.
reverse fast imaging with steady-state free p. (PSIF)
steady state free p. (SSFP)
precessional
p. frequency
p. motion
precharred fiber
prechiasmal optic nerve lesion
precipitated contrast
precipitate evacuation
precipitating event
precipitation
contrast p.
precirrhosis
precision
test-retest p.
precocious puberty
precommunicating segment of anterior cerebral artery
precontrast
p. echocardiography
p. imaging
p. scan
precordial
p. bulge
p. lead
p. mapping
precordium, pl. **precordia**
active p.
anterior p.
bulging p.
lateral p.
precoronal sagittal sinus
precuneus
precursor
bone marrow myeloid p.
p. sign
p. sign to rupture of aneurysm
predental space
predicted
p. cardiac index
p. maximal uptake
p. target heart rate
predictor
predisposition
hereditary p.
prediverticular
p. change
p. disease
predominance
anterior p.
posterior p.
predominant p.
temporal p.
predominant
p. flow load
p. predominance
preductal
p. aortic coarctation
p. coarctation of aorta
preejection
p. interval
p. period (PEP)
preemphasis
preenhancement sequence
preepiglottic
p. soft tissue
p. space
preesophageal dysphagia
preexcitation
ventricular p.
preexposure prophylaxis
preformed clot
prefrontal
p. artery
p. bone of von Bardeleben

NOTES

P

pregnancy
abdominal ectopic p.
ampullar p.
anembryonic p.
bigeminal p.
broad ligament p.
cervical p.
combined p.
compound p.
cornual ectopic p.
diamniotic p.
dichorionic diamniotic twin p.
ectopic p. (EP)
extrauterine p.
failed p.
failing p.
fallopian p.
false p.
gemellary p.
heterotopic p.
hydatid p.
hypervolemia of p.
interstitial ectopic p.
intraligamentary p.
intraperitoneal p.
intrauterine p.
membranous p.
mesenteric p.
molar p.
monochorionic diamniotic twin p.
monochorionic monoamniotic twin p.
multiple p.
mural p.
ovarian p.
ovarioabdominal p.
oviductal p.
parietal p.
phantom p.
plural p.
postterm p.
prevalence ectopic p.
prolonged p.
pseudointraligamentary p.
sarcofetal p.
sarcohysteric p.
selective reduction of p.
sextuplet p.
spurious p.
stump p.
p. test
toxemia of p.
tubal p.
tuboabdominal p.
tuboligamentary p.
tuboovarian p.
tubouterine p.
p. tumor
twin ectopic p.
uteroabdominal p.
uterotubal p.
p. wastage

pregnant
p. uterus
p. uterus rupture

Pregnyl

preinjection echocardiography

preinsular gyrus

preintegration complex

preinterparietal bone

preinvasive
p. carcinoma
p. disease of cervix, vagina, and vulva

preinversion multiecho (PRIME)

Preiser disease

prelaryngeal node

preliminary
p. film
p. view

preload
left ventricular p.
p. reserve

premammillary artery

premasseteric
p. space
p. space abscess

premature
p. atherosclerosis
p. calcification
p. closure of ductus arteriosus
p. closure of valve
p. isolated adrenarche
p. isolated thelarche
p. labor
p. middiastolic closure of mitral valve
p. nodal contraction (PNC)
p. osteoarthritis
p. placental senescence
p. rupture of membranes
p. senescence placenta
p. suture synostosis
p. uterine membrane rupture
p. valve closure
p. ventricular contraction (PVC)

prematurely closed suture

prematurity
retinopathy of p.

premaxillary bone

premedication

premedullary arteriovenous fistula

premolar teeth

premonitory sign

premotor
p. area
p. cortex
premyocardial infarction echocardiography
prenatal injury
preocclusive obstruction
preoperative
p. angiography
p. assessment
p. diagnosis
p. imaging
p. localization
p. resting MUGA scan
p. view
preosteonecrosis marrow edema
prepapillary bile duct
preparation
bowel p.
Colonlite bowel p.
CoLyte bowel p.
crush p.
dry bowel p.
Dulcolax bowel p.
Emulsoil bowel p.
p. error
Evac-Q-Kwik bowel p.
faulty p.
Fleet bowel p.
flow cytometry sample p.
GoLYTELY bowel p.
inadequate bowel p.
international reference p.
Ioban p.
kit p.
OCL bowel p.
on-column p.
touch p.
Tridrate bowel p.
wet bowel p.
X-Prep bowel p.
prepatellar
p. bursa
p. bursitis
prepectoral fascia
prepectorally
prepericardial lymph node
preperitoneal fat
preplacental hemorrhage
preponderance
phalangeal p.
prepontine
p. cistern
p. white epidermoidoma
prepubertal testicular mass
prepulse
spin-lock p.
prepyloric
p. antrum
p. atresia
p. fold
p. sphincter
p. ulcer
p. vein
prereduction
p. view
p. x-ray
prerenal
p. aortic aneurysm
p. failure
p. fat
prerupture of aneurysm
presacral
p. anomaly
p. cystic lesion
p. mass
p. plexus
p. space
presaturation
fat-selective p.
p. projection
p. pulse
spatial p.
p. technique
presbyesophagus
presbyophrenia
prescan
MRI p.
prescapula
presenile arteriosclerosis
presentation
aleukemic p.
breech p.
brow p.
cephalic p.
compound p.
cord p.
face p.
footling p.
frank breech p.
osteoblastic p.
parietal p.
shoulder p.

NOTES

presentation *(continued)*
transverse p.
vertex p.
presenting part
preservation
breast p.
myocardial p.
p. of native aortic valve
sphincter p.
presinusoidal
pre-slip
p.-s. change
p.-s. staging
presphenoid bone
PRESS
point-resolved spectroscopy
PRESS sequence
pressure
acoustic p.
airway p.
alveolar p.
p. amplitude
ankle-arm p.
ankle systolic p.
aortic root p.
arterial peak systolic p.
atmospheric p.
A-wave p.
bile duct p.
blood p.
bone marrow p. (BMP)
brachial artery cuff p.
brachial artery end-diastolic p.
brachial artery peak systolic p.
brachial artery pulse p.
capillary hydrostatic p.
capillary wedge p.
cardiac filling p.
central aortic p.
central venous p. (CVP)
colloid oncotic p. (COP)
continuous positive airway p. (CPAP)
coronary perfusion p.
coronary wedge p.
p. cuff
C-wave p.
damping of catheter tip p.
diastolic blood p.
diastolic filling p. (DFP)
diastolic perfusion p.
distal coronary perfusion p.
Doppler ankle systolic p.
Doppler blood p.
draining with venous p.
drifting wedge p.
elevated p.
end-diastolic p.
end-expiratory p.
end-inspiratory p.
endocardial p.
end-systolic p. (ESP)
p. epiphysis
equalization of p.
p. equalization
equalized diastolic p.
esophageal peristaltic p.
extravascular p.
feeding mean arterial p. (FMAP)
filling p.
p. fracture
p. gradient on pullback
p. half-time
p. half-time technique
hepatic wedge p. (HWP)
high filling p.
high interstitial p.
high wedge p.
increased central venous p.
increased intracranial p.
increased intrapericardial p.
increased pulmonary arterial p.
p. injector
inspiratory increase in venous p.
interstitial fluid hydrostatic p.
intracardiac p.
intracranial p. (ICP)
intracranial epidural p. (ECIDP)
intraductal p.
intraluminal esophageal p.
intramuscular fluid p.
intrapericardial p.
intrapleural p.
intrapulmonary p.
intrathoracic p.
jugular venous p.
labile blood p.
left atrial p. (LAP)
left atrial end-diastolic p.
left-sided heart p.
left subclavian central venous p. (LSCVP)
left ventricular p. (LVP)
left ventricular cavity p.
left ventricular end-diastolic p. (LVEDP)
left ventricular filling p.
left ventricular function p.
left ventricular peak systolic p.
left ventricular systolic p. (LVs pressure)
lower esophageal sphincter p. (LESP)
low urethral p. (LUP)
LVs p.
left ventricular systolic pressure

maximum inflation p.
mean aortic p.
mean arterial p. (MAP)
mean atrial p.
mean blood p.
mean brachial artery p.
mean circulatory filling p.
mean left atrial p.
mean pulmonary artery p. (MPA pressure, MPAP)
mean pulmonary artery wedge p.
mean pulmonary capillary p. (MPCP)
mean right atrial p.
p. measurement
minimum blood p.
MPA p.
mean pulmonary artery pressure
p. necrosis
p. overload
PAM p.
passage p.
p. peak
peak airway p.
peak inflation p.
peak regurgitant wave p.
peak systolic aortic p. (PSAP)
perfusion p.
p. perfusion imaging
p. perfusion study
phasic p.
p. pneumothorax
p. point
portal venous p. (PVP)
positive end-expiratory p.
pulmonary arterial wedge p.
pulmonary artery p. (PAP)
pulmonary artery diastolic p. (PAD)
pulmonary artery diastolic and wedge p. (PADP-PAWP)
pulmonary artery end-diastolic p. (PAEDP)
pulmonary artery mean p. (PAM)
pulmonary artery peak systolic p.
pulmonary artery/pulmonary capillary wedge p.
pulmonary artery systolic p. (PAS)
pulmonary artery wedge p. (PAWP)
pulmonary capillary p. (PCP)
pulmonary capillary venous wedge p.
pulmonary capillary wedge p. (PCWP)
pulmonary to systemic arterial systolic p. (PASP-SASP)
pulmonary venous capillary p.
pulmonary venous wedge p.
pulmonary wedge p. (PWP)
pulse p.
raised intracranial p.
p. reading
recoil p.
regional cerebral perfusion p. (rCPP)
right atrial p. (RAP)
right-sided heart p.
right ventricular p. (RVP)
right ventricular diastolic p.
right ventricular end-diastolic p.
right ventricular peak systolic p.
right ventricular volume p.
Rolleston rule for systolic blood p.
segmental bronchus lower extremity Doppler p.
shockwave p.
stump p.
subatmospheric p.
superior vena cava p.
supersystemic pulmonary artery p.
systemic diastolic blood p.
systemic mean arterial p. (SMAP)
systolic blood p. (SBP)
systolic-diastolic blood p.
toe systolic p.
torr p.
transmyocardial perfusion p.
transpulmonary p. (PTP)
venous p.
ventricular p.
ventricularization of p.
in vivo balloon p.
V-wave p.
p. wave
p. waveform
wedge p.
wedge hepatic venous p. (WHVP)
withdrawal p.
X′-wave p.
Y-wave p.
Z-point p.

NOTES

pressure-controlled intermittent coronary occlusion technique (PCICO technique)
pressure-flow gradient
pressure-volume loop
pressurized fluid jet
Pressurometer
prestenotic dilatation
prestomal ileitis
prestyloid recess
presumptive diagnosis
pretectal
p. lesion
p. nucleus
pretendinous
p. band
p. cord
pretherapy imaging
pretibial
p. dimple
p. myxedema
pretracheal lymph node
prevalence ectopic pregnancy
Prevel sign
prevertebral
p. fascia
p. ganglion
p. lymph node
p. soft tissue (PVST)
p. space
p. space mass
p. width
prevesicular lymph node
previa
central placenta p.
complete placenta p.
incomplete placenta p.
lateral placenta p.
marginal placenta p.
partial placenta p.
placenta p.
total placenta p.
vasa p.
previable fetus
Prévost sign
PREZ
posterior root entry zone
PRF
peak repetition frequency
PRG
phleborheography
prickle cell carcinoma
primary
p. achalasia
p. acquired cholesteatoma
p. adrenal insufficiency
p. amyloidosis
p. aspergillosis
p. atelectasis
p. auditory cortex
p. beam
p. benign liver tumor
p. biliary cirrhosis
p. bone lymphoma
p. brain lymphoma
p. cancer
cancer of unknown p. (CUP)
p. cardiomyopathy
p. cartilage joint
p. center of ossification
p. CNS cholesteatoma
p. CNS lymphoma
p. CNS tumor classification
p. coccidioidomycosis
p. complex
p. congenital megaureter
p. cutaneous large B-cell lymphoma (PCLBCL)
p. cyst of spleen
p. digital acquisition
p. esophageal peristalsis
p. familial xanthomatosis
p. glaucoma
p. hepatocellular carcinoma
p. hydrocele
p. hydrocephalus
p. hyperparathyroidism
p. hypertrophic osteoarthropathy
p. hypothyroidism
p. implanted tumor
p. intracerebral hematoma
p. intracranial germ cell tumor
p. intraosseous carcinoma
p. left bronchus
p. lesion
p. lymphomasonography
p. malignant liver tumor
p. megaureter
p. motor strip
p. myeloid metaphysis
p. neoplasm
p. neuroendocrine small cell carcinoma
p. optic atrophy
p. ovarian choriocarcinoma
p. oxalosis
p. peristaltic wave
p. pleurisy
p. progressive cerebellar degeneration
p. pulmonary hypertension (PPH)
p. pulmonary lobule
p. pulmonary lymphangiectasia
p. pulmonary malignancy
p. pulmonary malignant fibrous histiocytoma
p. pulmonary plasmacytoma

p. pulmonary tuberculosis
p. radiation
p. ray
p. refractory Burkitt lymphoma
p. renal tumor
p. retroperitoneal fibrosis
p. rhabdomyosarcoma
p. right bronchus
p. sarcoma
p. sclerosing cholangitis
p. sclerosis
p. sequestrum
p. teeth
p. temporal bone cholesteatoma
p. thrombus
p. tumor bed
unknown p.
p. vasospasm
p. vesical calculus
p. visual cortex
p. vitreous
p. yolk sac

PRIME
preinversion multiecho
PRIME pulse sequence

Primicon

priming effect

primitive
p. acoustic artery
p. bone
p. dislocation
p. gut
p. hindgut
p. hypoglossal artery
p. neuroectodermal tumor (PNET)
p. neuroepithelial tumor
p. neuroepithelioma
p. streak
p. trigeminal artery (PTA)
p. ventricle
p. yolk sac

primordial
p. follicle
p. tooth cyst

primum
ostium p.
septum p.

primus
digitus p.

principal
p. artery of pterygoid canal
p. bronchus
p. eigenvector

principle
Dodge p.
Doppler shift p.
Fick p.
Fuchs p.
Grossman p.
Huygens p.
indicator fractionation p.
line focus p.
Pauli exclusion p.
planigraphic p.
submicron magnetic p.
tracer p.
uncertainty p.

print reflectance modulation

Priodax
P. imaging agent

prior probability

Priscoline

prism
p. interpolation
p. method for ventricular volume

proactinium

probability
absolute emission p.
emission p.
posterior p.
prior p.

probe
AngeLase combined mapping-laser p.
P. balloon dilatation system
biplane sector p.
p. dilatation
Doppler flow echocardiographic p.
EFF p.
electromagnetic focusing field probe
electromagnetic flow p.
electromagnetic focusing field p. (EFF probe)
gamma p.
gamma-detection p.
hand-held exploring electrode p.
hand-held mapping p.
high-frequency miniature p.
hot-tipped laser p.
hybrid p.
hybridization p.

NOTES

P

probe *(continued)*
hyperthermia p.
interstitial p.
intraoperative gamma p.
laparoscopic Doppler p.
laser-Doppler flowmetry p. (LDF probe)
Laserflow Doppler p.
LDF p.
laser-Doppler flowmetry probe
localizing p.
magnetometer p.
Medrad Mrinnervu endorectal colon p.
NMR magnetometer p.
nuclear p.
oligonucleotide p.
Olympus UM-1W transendoscopic ultrasound p.
pediatric biplane TEE p.
relaxation p.
shift p.
side-hole cannulated p.
Teflon p.
transesophageal echocardiography (TEE) p.
truncated NMR p.
ultrasound p.
USCI p.

probehead
MRI p.

PROBE-SV spectrometer

problematic abdominal activity

proboscis

Probst
P. callosal bundle

procarbazine lung damage

procedure
catheter-directed interventional p.
Chamberlain p.
diagnostic p.
endoscopic p.
gastric pull-through p.
interventional p.
intestinal bypass p.
invasive radiological vascular p.
limb-lengthening p.
magnetic resonance angiography-directed bypass p.
Nissen fundoplication p.
psoas hitch p.
revascularization p.
Roux-en-Y p.
spatial localization p.
stereotactic p.
Swenson pull-through p.
two-step p.
Whipple p.

process
accessory p.
acromion p.
alar p.
alveolar consolidative p.
apical p.
articular p.
ascending p.
auditory p.
basilar p.
bony p.
calcaneal p.
carrier-free separation p.
caudate p.
clinoid p.
cochleariform p.
condyloid p.
conoid p.
consolidative p.
coracoacromial p.
coracoid p.
coronoid p.
costal p.
cribriform p.
cystic p.
destructive p.
energy transfer p.
ensiform p.
ethmoidal p.
falciform p.
fibroplastic p.
frontal p.
frontonasal p.
frontosphenoidal p.
glenoid p.
inflammatory synovial p.
interspinous p.
intravascular clotting p.
jugular p.
knobby p.
left ventricular posterior superior p.
lumbar transverse p.
monarticular p.
neoplastic p.
noncalcified ocular p.
notochordal p.
odontoid p.
olecranon p.
osseous destructive p.
paraneoplastic p.
prominent xiphoid p.
pterygoid p.
radial styloid p.
radiostyloid p.
sacral p.
sacralized transverse p.
space-occupying p.
spinous p.

SSFP p.
styloid p.
supracondylar p.
supracondyloid p.
temporal p.
transverse p.
trochlear p.
ulnar styloid p.
uncinate p.
vermiform p.
vertebral p.
vertebrospinous p.
xiphoid p.
zygomatic p.

processing
digital imaging p. (DIP)
intrapixel sequential p. (IPSP)
maximum entropy p.
signal p.

processor
fast-array p.
sequence p.

processus vaginalis

prochordal plate

proctogram
balloon p.
video p.

proctographic features

proctography
evacuation p.

proctostat

procurvature deformity

product
brightness area p. (BAP)
Committee of Radiation from Radioactive Medicinal P.'s (CRRMP)
fibrin-split p.
fission p.
iodine-labeled p.
real-time dose area p. (DAP)
respiratory burst p.
spallation p.

production
Cerenkov radiation p.
fast routine p.
lactoferrin p.
one-step p.
pair p.
radionuclide p.
radiopharmaceutical p.
remote-controlled p.
secondary electron p.

Profasi HP

profile
3D dose p.
excitation p.
flat time-intensity p.
flow velocity p.
fluence p.
P. mammography system
nonlinear excitation p.
parabolic velocity p.
peak p.
projection p.
rectangular section p.
section-sensitivity p.
slice sensitivity p. (SSP)
three-dimensional dose p.
ultra-low p. (ULP)
velocity p.

profilogram

profluens
hydrops tubae p.

profound hypothermic circulatory arrest (PHCA)

profoundly obtunded infant

profunda
colitis cystica p.
p. femoris artery

profundal popliteal collateral index

profundus
flexor digitorum p. (FDP)

profusion

progeny
radon p.

progeria
adult p.

prognathic dilatation

prognathism

programmer wand

progress
abortion in p.

progression
inexorable p.
inflow disease p.
insidious p.
interval p.
steady-state free p. (SSFP)

progression-free

progressiva
encephalopathia subcorticalis p.
fibrodysplasia ossificans p.

NOTES

P

progressiva *(continued)*
fibrous dysplasia ossificans p.
myositis ossificans p.
rhinitis gangrenosa p.
progressive
p. coccidioidomycosis
p. degeneration
p. diaphyseal dysplasia
p. disease
p. dysphagia
p. emphysematous necrosis
p. familial cirrhosis
p. hydrocephalus
p. interstitial pulmonary fibrosis
p. massive fibrosis
p. multifocal leukoencephalopathy (PML)
p. neuropathic muscle atrophy
p. nodular pulmonary fibrosis
p. perivenular alcoholic fibrosis (PPAF)
p. postpolio muscle atrophy (PPPMA)
p. primary tuberculosis
p. rubella panencephalitis
p. spin saturation
p. stroke
p. subcortical gliosis
p. suppurative cholangitis
p. supranuclear palsy
p. systemic sclerosis
p. tuberculosis (TB) pneumonia
p. uptake
ProHance
P. imaging agent
projectile horn
projection
p. angiogram
anterior p.
anteroposterior (AP) p.
apical lordotic p.
average pixel p. (APP)
axial p.
back p.
base p.
Berteil p.
p. binning
Blineau p.
bony vertebra p.
Caldwell p.
carpal tunnel p.
cartographic p.
caudad p., caudal p.
caudocranial p.
Chassard-Lapine p.
Chaussier p.
coronal maximum-intensity p. (MIPcor)
coronary maximum-intensity p. (MIPcor)
crosstable lateral p.
cylindrical map p.
Didiee p.
divergent ray p.
3D stereotactic surface p.
fan-beam p.
FI p.
full scan with interpolation projection
p. fiber damage
fingerlike p.
frogleg lateral p.
FS p.
full-scan projection
full-scan p. (FS projection)
full scan with interpolation p. (FI projection)
Granger p.
half-axial p.
half-scan with extrapolation p.
Hermodsson tangential p.
Lambert p.
LAO p.
Laquerriere-Perquin p.
lateral p.
lateromedial p.
Lauenstein and Hickey p.
left anterior oblique p.
left lateral p.
left posterior oblique p.
Loepp p.
Low-Beers p.
maximum-intensity sliding thin slab p.
mediolateral oblique p.
Mercator p.
minimum-intensity sliding thin slab p.
modified p.
oblique p.
occipitomental p.
orthogonal angiographic p.
PA p.
panoramic surface p.
papillary p.
Pawlow p.
postdrainage p.
posterior p.
posteroanterior p.
presaturation p.
p. profile
ray-sum p.
Rhese p.
right anterior oblique (RAO) p.
right posterior oblique (RPO) p.
rotating tomographic p.

Rumstrom p.
saturation inversion p. (SIP)
simulated annealing method p.
steep left anterior oblique p.
steep Towne p.
Stenvers p.
stereographic p.
stereotactic surface p. (SSP)
straight lateral p.
submental vertex p.
submentovertical p.
surface p.
Templeton and Zim carpal tunnel p.
three-dimensional stereotactic surface p.
Towne p.
p. tract imaging
transaxial maximum-intensity p.
under-scan method p.
Vogt bone free p.
Waters p.

projection-reconstruction
p.-r. imaging
p.-r. technique

projector
cine p.
white light pattern p.

prolactin-secreting pituitary macroadenoma

prolapse
anterior leaflet p.
p. of aortic valve
aortic valve leaflet p.
billowing mitral valve p.
cord p.
gastroduodenal mucosal p.
gastrojejunal mucosal p.
holosystolic mitral valve p.
intestinal p.
intracranial fat p.
mitral valve p. (MVP)
mitral valve leaflet systolic p.
posterior leaflet p.
rectal p.
p. of rectum
p. of right aortic valve cusp
p. of spleen
systolic p.
tricuspid valve p.
p. of umbilical cord
valve p.

prolapsed
p. antral mucosa
p. gastric mucosa
p. mitral valve (PMV)
p. stoma
p. tumor

prolapsing scallop

proliferation
angiofibroblastic p.
p. area
benign sclerosing ductal p.
bile duct p.
p. of bone
bony p.
collagen tissue p.
connective tissue p.
extranodal p.
fibroplastic p.
p. of fibrous tissue
glandular p.
intimal p.
myofibrohistiocytic p.
myointimal p.
myxomatous p.
neointimal p.
neuronal p.
nodular p.
osteophytic p.
papillary p.
peripelvic fat p.
p. pleurisy
p. rate
synovial p.
villous p.

proliferative
p. bronchiolitis
p. glomerulonephritis
p. index
p. inflammation
p. phase endometrium

prolonged
p. ejection time
p. expiratory phase
p. inspiratory phase
p. interval
p. left ventricular impulse
p. pregnancy

promethium (Pm)

prominence
aortic p.
p. of bone
bony p.

NOTES

P

prominence *(continued)*
hilar p.
interstitial p.
mediastinal p.
tibial tubercle p.
upper lobe vein p.
prominent
p. ductal pattern
p. ductal vascular structure
p. liver
p. pyramidal thyroid lobe
p. rim of radiolucency
p. septal lymphatics
p. spur
p. tubercle
p. uptake
p. xiphoid process
promontory
p. mass
sacral p.
p. of sacrum
pronation
hallucal p.
pes p.
pronation-abduction
p.-a. fracture
p.-a. injury
pronation-eversion fracture
pronation-external
p.-e. rotation (P-ER)
p.-e. rotation injury
pronator
p. fat pad sign
p. quadratus
p. quadratus line
round p.
p. teres
pronatus
pes p.
prone
p. film
p. lateral view
p. position
pronephron
rudimentary p.
pronephros, pl. **pronephroi**
propagation speed artifact
proper digital nerve branch
properitoneal
p. fat
p. fat line
p. flank stripe
p. hernia
prophylaxis
preexposure p.
propidium iodide
proportion
aneurysmal p.
proportional
p. counter
p. ratio
proportionality
cephalofacial p.
propoxyphene lung damage
propria
lamina p.
muscularis p.
substantia p.
tunica p.
proprius
extensor indicis p. (EIP)
extensor quinti p. (EQP)
proptosis
propulsive
p. mechanism
p. movement
propyliodone
p. imaging agent
prosencephalon
prospective
p. analysis
p. investigation of pulmonary embolus detection (PIOPED)
ProSpeed CT scanner
ProstaScint
P. monoclonal antibody imaging agent
P. system
prostate
p. abscess
p. anatomy
apex of p.
p. cancer
p. capsule
carcinoma of p.
floating p.
p. gland
p. hypoechoic lesion
p. implant
inferolateral surface of p.
lateral lobe of p.
lymph vessel of p.
median lobe of p.
posterior surface of p.
p. seeding
transurethral incision of the p.
transurethral resection of p. (TURP)
prostatectomy
transurethral ultrasound-guided laser-induced p.
prostatic
p. adenoma
p. bed
p. calculus
p. carcinoma

p. cyst
p. duct
p. fluid
p. hyperplasia
p. hyperplastic nodule
p. obstruction
p. sinus
p. stent
p. transition zone
p. urethra
p. urethroplasty
p. uterus
p. venous plexus
prostaticovesical junction
prostatism
prostatitis
cavitary p.
diverticular p.
prosthesis, pl. **prostheses**
p. dehiscence
iridium p.
partial ossicular replacement p. (PORP)
penile p.
unicompartmental knee p.
prosthetic
p. cup
p. device
p. femoral distal graft
p. heart valve
p. implant
p. mitral valve
p. replacement
p. valve embolus
protection
p. factor
International Commission on Radiation P. (ICRP)
myocardial p.
radiation p.
region of p.
protein
macrophage inflammatory p. (MIP)
protein-bound iodine (PBI)
proteoglycan matrix
proteolysis
protium
protocol
Balke-Ware treadmill exercise stress testing p.
Bruce p.
chronotropic assessment exercise p.
Cornell p.
2D GRE dynamic p.
Ellestad p.
modified Bruce p.
modified Naughton-Balke treadmill p.
MP-RAGE p.
neon particle p.
point-to-point p. (PPP)
Sheffield modification of Bruce treadmill p.
standard Bruce p.
telomere repeat amplification p.
treadmill exercise Bruce p.
UCLA imaging p.
protodensity MR imaging
protodiastole
protodiastolic reversal of blood flow
proton
p. chemical shift imaging
p. density
p. density-weighted imaging
high-energy p.
p. irradiation
lactate p.
p. magnetic resonance
p. magnetic resonance signal
methyl p.
p. nuclear magnetic resonance spectroscopy
p. nuclear magnetic resonance spectrum
precessing p.
p. relaxation
p. relaxation enhancement
p. spin-lattice relaxation time
proton-density axial MR scan
proton-density-weighted MRI
proton-electron dipole-dipole interaction
proton-proton magnetization exchange
protoplasmic astrocytoma
protopulmonary bilharziasis
protozoal pneumonia
protracted
p. exposure sensitization
p. venous infusion (PVI)
protrude
protruded disk
protruding
p. atheroma
p. fat

NOTES

P

protrusio
p. acetabuli
p. shill
protrusion
acetabular p.
anal p.
p. of cystocele
disk p.
hip p.
p. of navicular
spicular p.
spoonlike p.
vascular p.
protuberance
bony p.
occipital p.
provisional callus
provocable ischemia
provocative testing
Provocholine
Prowazek body
Prowazek-Greeff body
proximal
p. acinar emphysema
p. anterior descending artery
p. anterior tibial artery
p. articular set angle (PASA)
p. aspect
p. brain shift
p. carpal row
p. circumflex artery
p. coil
p. colon
p. convoluted tubule
p. coronary (PCS)
p. digital artery
p. and distal portion of vessel
p. femoral focal deficiency syndrome (PFFD syndrome)
p. femoral fracture
p. femur
p. fibula
p. focal femoral deficiency (PFFD)
p. humeral fracture
p. interphalangeal joint (PIP, PIPJ)
p. interphalangeal joint articulation
p. left anterior descending artery
p. loop syndrome
p. part of dorsal duct
p. popliteal artery
p. radioulnar joint
p. reference axis (PRA)
p. segment
p. small bowel
p. third shaft
p. tibia
p. tibial metaphyseal fracture
p. tubular adenoma
proximally
proximal-to-distal ring
proximity injury
pruned
p. appearance of pulmonary vasculature
pruned-tree
p.-t. appearance
p.-t. arteriography
pruned-tree-appearance bile duct
pruning
p. of pancreatic duct branch
pulmonary artery p.
p. sign
Prussak
P. pouch
P. space
Prussian helmet sign
PS
pulmonary sequestration
pulmonary stenosis
pulmonic stenosis
PSA
power spectral analysis
psammoma
p. body
p. body meningioma
Virchow p.
psammomatoid ossifying fibroma
psammomatous
p. calcification
p. meningioma
PSAP
peak systolic aortic pressure
psathyrosis
PSD
pituitary stalk distortion
pseudarthrosis (*var. of* pseudoarthrosis)
pseudoacardia
pseudoachondroplasia
pseudoaneurysm
anastomotic p.
aortic p.
chronic posttraumatic aortic p.
heart p.
hepatic artery p.
pancreatitis p.
peripheral p.
perivalvular p.
postsurgical p.
renal transplant p.
splenic artery p.
traumatic aortic p.
pseudoangiomatous stromal hyperplasia (PASH)
pseudoangiosarcoma
pseudoarthritis

pseudoarthrosis, pseudarthrosis
long bone p.
pseudoarticulation
pseudoascites
pseudo-AV block
pseudoblind loop syndrome
pseudobulbar sign
pseudocalcification
powder p.
pseudocalculus
p. bile duct
pseudocapsule
pseudocarcinoma
pseudocarcinomatous
pseudocavitation
lung p.
pseudochylous effusion
pseudocirrhosis
cholangiodysplastic p.
pseudocoarctation
p. of aorta
pseudocolor
p. B mode
p. B-mode display
pseudocryptorchidism
pseudocyst
adrenal p.
gelatinous brain p.
mature pancreatic p.
meconium p.
necrotic bone p.
pancreatic p.
pulmonary p.
splenic p.
subarticular p.
umbilical cord p.
pseudocystic hygroma
pseudo-Dandy-Walker malformation
pseudodextrocardia
pseudodiffusion
pseudodislocation
pseudodissection
pseudodiverticula
small bowel p.
pseudodiverticulosis
intramural esophageal p.
pseudodiverticulum
retrograde ureteral p.
pseudodynamic MR imaging
pseudoepiphysis
pseudoexstrophy
pseudofollicle
pseudofollicular
p. salpingitis
pseudo-Foster-Kennedy sign
pseudofracture
p. artifact
milkman's p.
pseudogap signal
pseudogating
diastolic p.
pseudogestational sac
pseudoglioma
pseudogout
pseudogynecomastia
pseudohaustration
pseudohermaphroditism
female p.
pseudohomogeneous edema pattern
pseudo-Hurler deformity
pseudohypertrophy
pseudohypoparathyroidism (PHP)
pseudoinfarct pattern
pseudointestinal wall sign
pseudointimal
p. formation
p. hyperplasia (PIH)
pseudointraligamentary pregnancy
pseudointussusception
pseudo-Jefferson fracture
pseudojoint
pseudokidney sign
pseudoluxation
pseudolymphoma
breast p.
gastric p.
lung p.
p. syndrome
pseudomalignant tumor
pseudomantle zone pattern
pseudomass
mediastinal p.
mucous p.
pseudomembrane
fetal neck p.
pseudomembranous
p. colitis
p. inflammation
p. radiation gastritis
pseudomeningocele
posttraumatic intradiploic p.
pseudomitral leaflet
pseudomucinous cystadenocarcinoma
pseudomyxoma peritonei

NOTES

pseudoneoplasm
pseudonephritis
athlete's p.
pseudoneuroma
p. of median nerve
pseudoobstruction
bowel p.
chronic idiopathic intestinal p. (CIIP)
colonic p.
familial intestinal p.
idiopathic intestinal p.
nonfamilial intestinal p.
pseudoomphalocele
pseudoorbital tumor
pseudoosteomalacic pelvis
pseudopalsy
pseudopancreatitis
pseudo-Pelger-Huet change
pseudoperiostitis
pseudopneumoperitoneum
pseudopod formation
pseudopodia
pseudopolyp
p. definition
pseudopolyposis lymphatica
pseudoporencephaly
pseudo-post Billroth I appearance
pseudoprecocious puberty
pseudopregnancy
pseudo-pseudohypoparathyroidism
pseudopyogenic granuloma
pseudorosette
perivascular p.
pseudosac
pseudosacculation
pseudosarcoma
esophageal p.
pseudosarcomatous fasciitis
pseudosclerosis
spastic p.
pseudosheath
pseudospondylolisthesis
Junghans p.
pseudostone
pseudostricture
colon p.
pseudosubluxation
C-spine p.
pseudotear
pseudothickening
pseudothrombophlebitis syndrome
pseudothrombosis
pseudotrabecula
pseudotrochanteric bursitis
pseudotruncus arteriosus
pseudotumor
abdominal p.
atelectatic asbestos p.
p. cerebri (PTC)
fibrosing inflammatory p.
hemophilic p.
inflammatory idiopathic orbital p.
inflammatory intestinal p.
kidney p.
p. molluscoid
orbital p.
pleura p.
renal p.
p. sign
small bowel p.
vermian p.
xanthomatous p.
pseudo-Turner syndrome
pseudoulceration
pseudoureterocele
pseudovagina
pseudo-Whipple disease
pseudowidening
joint space p.
pseudoxanthoma elasticum
pseudo-Z-E syndrome
PSF
posterior spine fusion
P-S flow ratio
PSG
peak systolic gradient
PSH-25GT transcranial imaging transducer
PSIF
reverse fast imaging with steady-state free precession
PSIL
percentage signal intensity loss
psoas
p. abscess
p. absence
p. fascia
p. hitch procedure
p. line
p. major
p. margin
p. muscle
p. shadow
p. shadow angle
p. sign
p. stripe
psoralen plus ultraviolet light of A wavelength (PUVA)
psoriatic arthritis
PSP
phenolsulfonphthalein
photostimulable phosphor dental radiography
^{31}P spectroscopy

PSR
  point-spread function
PSSE
  partial saturation spin echo
    PSSE technique
psychogenic water intoxication
PT
  pluridirectional tomography
PTA
  persistent truncus arteriosus
  primitive trigeminal artery
PTAB
  pterygoalar bar
PTC
  percutaneous transhepatic cholangiogram
  pseudotumor cerebri
PTCA
    PTCA angiogram
    PTCA coronary angiography
pterion
p-terphenyl
pterygium colli
pterygoalar bar (PTAB)
pterygoid
    p. artery
    p. bone
    p. canal
    p. chest
    p. fossa
    p. muscle
    p. plate
    p. process
pterygoideus hamulus
pterygomandibular
    p. ligament
    p. raphe
pterygopalatine
    p. canal
    p. fossa
    p. ganglion
pterygospinous ligament
PTF ligament
PTHC
  percutaneous transhepatic cholangiogram
  percutaneous transhepatic
   cholangiography
PTL, pTL
  posterior tricuspid leaflet
ptosis, pl. **ptoses**
ptotic
    p. kidney
PTP
  transpulmonary pressure
PTT
  pulmonary transit time
PTV
  planning target volume
  posterior terminal vein
ptyalography
pubertal development
puberty
    precocious p.
    pseudoprecocious p.
    true precocious p.
pubescent uterus
pubic
    p. arch
    p. bone
    p. bone maldevelopment
    p. crest
    p. ramus
    p. symphysis
    p. tubercle
pubis
    mons p.
    os p.
    osteitis p.
    pecten p.
    ramus of p.
    symphysis p.
    widened symphysis p.
pubocapsular ligament
pubocervical ligament
pubococcygeal line
pubococcygeus muscle
pubofemoral ligament
puboischial area
puboprostatic ligament
puborectalis loop
pubovesical ligament
Puck
    P. cutfilm changer
    P. film changer
PUD
  peptic ulcer disease
puddle sign
puddling
    p. of contrast
    peripheral p.
pudenda
    ulcerating granuloma of p.
pudendal
    p. blood supply

NOTES

pudendal *(continued)*
p. branch
p. canal
p. cleft
p. vein
puerperal
p. mastitis
p. ovarian vein thrombophlebitis
puffer
pink p.
puff-of-smoke
p.-o.-s. brain
p.-o.-s. vessels
Pugh Child grading system for bleeding esophageal varices
PUI
posterior urethral injury
Pulec and Freedman classification of congenital aural atresia
pullback
p. across aortic valve
aortic p.
p. arterial markings
p. imaging
p. pressure gradient
pressure gradient on p.
p. pressure recording
p. study
pulled elbow
pulley of finger
pull maneuver
pulmoaortic canal
pulmogram
pulmolith
pulmolithiasis
pulmonale
atrium p.
cor p.
pulmonary
p. abscess
p. adenopathy
p. alveolar microlithiasis
p. alveolus
p. angioma
p. aplasia
p. arc
p. arterial circulation
p. arterial flow insufficiency
p. arterial hypertension
p. arterial input impedance
p. arterial malformation
p. arterial markings
p. arterial occlusion
p. arterial resistance index
p. arterial vent
p. arterial wedge pressure
p. arteriography
p. arteriolar resistance
p. arteriolar vasoconstriction
p. arteriosclerosis
p. arteriovenous aneurysm
p. arteriovenous fistula
p. arteriovenous malformation
p. artery (PA)
p. artery agenesis
p. artery aneurysm
p. artery apoplexy
p. artery atresia
p. artery balloon pump (PABP)
p. artery bifurcation
p. artery blockage
p. artery-bronchus ratio
p. artery compression ascending aortic aneurysm
p. artery diastolic pressure (PAD)
p. artery diastolic and wedge pressure (PADP-PAWP)
p. artery dilatation
p. artery end-diastolic pressure (PAEDP)
p. artery hemorrhage
p. artery interruption
p. artery intima
p. artery mean pressure (PAM)
p. artery obstruction
p. artery peak systolic pressure
p. artery pressure (PAP)
p. artery pruning
p. artery/pulmonary capillary wedge pressure
p. artery to right ventricle diastolic gradient
p. artery sarcoma
p. artery stenosis
p. artery systolic pressure (PAS)
p. artery wedge angiography
p. artery wedge pressure (PAWP)
p. asbestosis
p. aspiration
p. atrium
p. barotrauma
p. blood flow (PBF)
p. blood flow redistribution
p. blood volume
p. blood volume index (PBVI)
p. capillary endothelium
p. capillary hemangiomatosis
p. capillary permeability
p. capillary pressure (PCP)
p. capillary venous wedge pressure
p. capillary wedge position
p. capillary wedge pressure (PCWP)
p. capillary wedge tracing
p. carcinoma
p. and cardiac sclerosis

p. cartilage
p. cavitation
p. cavity
p. cirrhosis
p. collagen vascular disease (PCVD)
p. conduit outflow tract
p. confluence
p. consolidation
p. contusion
p. cyst
p. cystic lymphangiectasis
p. density
p. dysmaturity
p. edema
p. edema photographic negative
p. embolic septic disease
p. embolus (PE)
p. failure
p. flow pattern
p. function test
p. gas
p. gas exchange
p. hamartoma
p. heart
p. hilum
p. histoplasmosis
p. hyalinizing granuloma
p. hyperinflation
p. hypertension (PHTN)
p. hypoperfusion
p. hypoplasia
p. idiopathic fibrosis
p. incompetence
p. infarct
p. interstitial disease
p. interstitial emphysema (PIE)
p. interstitial idiopathic fibrosis
p. interstitium
p. juxtaesophageal lymph node
p. Kaposi sarcoma
p. lesion
p. ligament
p. linearity
p. lobe
p. lymphangiectasia
p. lymphangiomatosis
p. lymph node
p. lymphoid disorder
p. lymphoma
p. mainline granulomatosis
p. mass
p. metastasis
p. microcirculation
p. microvasculature
p. nodularity
p. nodule
p. nodule enhancement
p. orifice
p. osteoarthropathy
p. outflow gradient
p. outflow obstruction
p. overdistention
p. overexpansion
p. overinflation
p. papillomatosis
p. parenchyma
p. parenchymal changes
p. parenchymal infection
p. parenchymal infiltrate
p. parenchymal injury
p. parenchymal window
p. perfusion imaging
p. perfusion and ventilation
p. pleura
p. pleurisy
p. plexus
p. pseudocyst
p. quantitative differential function study
p. resection
p. sarcoidosis
p. scar
p. scintigraphy
p. segment
p. sequestration (PS)
p. sequestration spectrum
p. sinus
p. sling
p. sling complex
p. stenosis (PS)
p. subcutaneous encephalitis emphysema
p. sulcus
p. to systemic arterial systolic pressure (PASP-SASP)
p. talcosis
p. telangiectasia
p. thromboembolic disease
p. thromboembolism
p. thromboembolization
p. thrombosis
p. time activity curve
p. transit time (PTT)

NOTES

P

pulmonary *(continued)*
p. trunk
p. trunk bifurcation
p. trunk idiopathic dilatation
p. tuberculosis
p. tumor
p. valve
p. valve annulus
p. valve atresia
p. valve cusp
p. valve deformity
p. valve dysplasia (PVD)
p. valve insufficiency
p. valve stenosis
p. valve stenosis dilatation
p. varix
p. vascular bed
p. vascular bed impedance
p. vascular congestion
p. vascularity
p. vascular markings
p. vascular obstruction
p. vascular pattern
p. vascular redistribution
p. vascular reserve
p. vascular resistance (PVR)
p. vascular resistance index (PVRI)
p. vasculature
p. vasoreactivity
p. vein
p. vein apoplexy
p. vein atresia
p. vein fibrosis
p. vein stenosis
p. vein wedge angiography
p. venolobar syndrome
p. venous capillary pressure
p. venous congestion (PVC)
p. venous drainage
p. venous hypertension
p. venous obstruction
p. venous return
p. venous system
p. venous-systemic air embolus
p. venous wedge pressure
p. ventilation imaging
p. vesicle
p. vessel
p. vessel overcirculation
p. wedge pressure (PWP)

pulmonic
p. area
p. atresia
p. infiltrate
p. insufficiency (PI)
p. output
p. output flow
p. output index
p. regurgitation (PR)
p. stenosis (PS)
p. valve (PV)
p. valve gradient
p. valve regurgitation
p. valvular stenosis
p. versus systemic flow

pulmonic-systemic flow ratio (P-S flow ratio)

pulmonis
lingula p.

pulp
p. canal
p. of finger
p. space
p. stone

pulposus
herniated nucleus p. (HNP)

pulsate

pulsatile perfusion

pulsatility
arterial p.
p. index

pulsating
p. empyema
p. metastasis
p. pleurisy
p. vein

pulsation
p. artifact
capillary p.
mean venous p.

pulse
adiabatic slice-selective radiofrequency p.
compensated composite spin-lock p.
composite p.
dampened obstructive p.
DANTE-selective p.
depth p.
p. design
diastolic depolarization p.
Doppler p.
p. Doppler interrogation
2D spatially selective radiofrequency p.
E point of cardiac apex p.
p. fashion pulse spray
fat suppression p.
p. flip angle
frequency-selective p.
gradient p.
p. height analyzer
p. height spectral analysis
inversion p.
p. labeling
p. length
motion compensation gradient p.

narrow-band spectral-selective radiofrequency p.
navigator p.
nonselective p.
p. oximetry
phase-encode p.
6-p., 3-phase generator
12-p., 3-phase generator
presaturation p.
p. pressure
radiofrequency p.
radiofrequency excitation p.
p. reappearance time
p. repetition frequency
p. repetition time
resting p.
section-select p.
selective p.
sequence p.
p. sequence
p. sequence echoplanar imaging
p. shape
small water-hammer p.
spatially selective inversion p.
steady-state field p.
synchronous carotid arterial p.
tidal wave of carotid arterial p.
trough of venous p.
twin-peaked p.
velocity-compensating gradient p.
vertical synchronization p. (V SYNC)
p. voltage
p. volume recorder
p. volume recording (PVR)
p. volume waveform
V peak of jugular venous p.
p. width (PW)
p. width variation

pulsed
p. Doppler flowmetry
p. Doppler transesophageal echocardiography
p. Doppler ultrasound
p. Doppler waveform
p. dose rate (PDR)
p. electron paramagnetic imaging
p. gradient
p. infrared laser
p. L-band ESR spectrometry
p. magnetization transfer contrast MRI
p. magnetization transfer MR imaging
p. metal vapor laser
p. mode
p. wave

pulsed-electron paramagnetic NMR

pulsed-gradient
p.-g. spin echo (PGSE)
p.-g. spin-echo technique

pulsed-mode operation

pulsed-wave
p.-w. Doppler
p.-w. Doppler recording
p.-w. (PW) Doppler echocardiography

pulse-echo distance measurement

PulseSpray
P. injector
P. pulsed infusion system

pulsing current

pulsion diverticulum

pulsus
p. alternans
p. paradoxus

pulverized
p. plaque
p. plaque particulate matter

pulvinar
p. hip joint

pump
balloon p.
implantable infusion p.
intraaortic balloon p. (IABP)
ion p.
p. lung
pulmonary artery balloon p. (PABP)

punch
Sweet sternal p.

punched-out
p.-o. appearance
p.-o. area
p.-o. bony defect
p.-o. lytic bone lesion

punched-pout ulcer

punch-through

puncta (*pl. of* punctum)

punctata
chondrodysplasia p.
rhizomelic chondrodysplasia p.

punctate
p. calcification

NOTES

P

punctate *(continued)*
p. enhancement
p. hyperintense focus
p. infiltrate
p. ulcer
p. white matter hyperintensity
punctation
punctum, pl. **puncta**
puncture
antegrade p.
cisternal p.
direct needle p.
fine-needle p.
p. fracture
lumbar p.
nephrostomy p.
retrograde nephrostomy p.
stereotactic p.
p. transducer
p. ulcer
ultrasound-guided nephrostomy p.
pupillary
p. constrictor muscle
p. sign
purging
bone marrow p.
immunomagnetic p.
purification
one-line anion exchange p.
purified
p. water
p. water contrast
purity
radiochemical p.
radioisotopic p.
radionuclide p.
radiopharmaceutical p.
Purkinje fibers
purse-stringing effect
purulent
p. lesion
p. pleurisy
p. pneumonia
p. salpingitis
p. synovitis
push maneuver
push-pull
p.-p. ankle stress view
p.-p. hip view
pustulotic arthrosteitis
putamen
putaminal hemorrhage
putty kidney
PUV
posterior urethral valve
PUVA
psoralen plus ultraviolet light of A wavelength
PUVA radiation
PV
pulmonic valve
PVB
pigmented villonodular bundle
PVC
premature ventricular contraction
pulmonary venous congestion
PVD
peripheral vascular disease
pulmonary valve dysplasia
PVE
periventricular echogenicity
PVG
periventricular gray matter
PVG matter
PVI
protracted venous infusion
PVL
periventricular leukomalacia
PVM
parallel virtual machine
PVNS
pigmented villonodular synovitis
PVP
portal venous phase
portal venous pressure
PVR
peripheral vascular resistance
perspective volume rendering
pulmonary vascular resistance
pulse volume recording
PVR fly-through viewing
PVRI
pulmonary vascular resistance index
PVS
peritoneovenous shunt
PVST
prevertebral soft tissue
PVST shadow
PVST swelling
PW
posterior wall
pulse width
PWP
pulmonary wedge pressure
PWT
posterior wall thickness
PXA
pleomorphic xanthoastrocytoma
pyarthrosis, pl. **pyarthroses**
pycnodysostosis
pyelectasia
pyelectasis
fetal p.

pyelitis
p. cystica
emphysematous p.
pyelocaliceal, pyelocalyceal
p. diverticulum
p. system
pyelocaliectasis
pyelofluoroscopy
pyelogenic cyst
pyelogram
pyelographic appearance time
pyelography
antegrade p.
excretory intravenous p.
p. imaging
intravenous p. (IVP)
needle p.
rapid-sequence intravenous p.
retrograde p.
pyelolymphatic backflow
pyelolysis
pyelonephritis
acute suppurative p.
atrophic p.
chronic atrophic p.
emphysematous p. (EPN)
suppurative p.
xanthogranulomatous p.
pyeloplasty
pyelorenal backflow
pyeloscopy
pyelostogram
pyclotubular backflow
pyelotumoral backflow
pyeloureteritis cystica
pyeloureterography
pyeloureterostomy
pyelovenous backflow
pyemic embolus
Pyle disease
pylori (*pl. of* pylorus)
pyloric
p. antrum
p. canal
p. cap
p. channel
p. channel ulcer
p. hypertrophy
p. insufficiency
p. lymph node
p. muscle
p. orifice
p. outlet
p. outlet obstruction
p. ring
p. sphincter
p. stenosis
p. stricture
p. string sign
p. teat
p. valve
pyloroduodenal
p. junction
p. obstruction
pyloroplasty
pylorospasm
infantile p.
persistent p.
pylorus, pl. **pylori**
p. cervix sign
hypertrophic p.
torus p.
pyocele
pyocephalus
pyoderma granulosa
pyogenic
p. brain abscess
p. cholangitis
p. liver
p. liver abscess
p. osteomyelitis
pyogenicum
pyometra
pyomyositis
pyonephrosis
pyopneumothorax
pyosalpinx
pyothorax
pyothorax-associated pleural lymphoma
pyoureter ectopic ureterocele
PYP
pyrophosphate
PYP imaging
PYP technetium myocardial scan
pyramid
medullary p.
p. method for ventricular volume
petrous p.
renal medullary p.
pyramidal
p. bone
p. eminence
p. fracture
p. hemorrhagic zone

NOTES

pyramidal *(continued)*
p. layer of cerebral cortex
p. lobe
p. neurons
p. sign
p. system
p. tract
pyriform (*var. of* piriform)
pyriformis (*var. of* piriformis)
pyrimidine
p. analog
halogenated p.
pyrogen testing
Pyrolite
pyrophosphate (PYP)
p. crystals
p. imaging
p. scintigraphy
stannous p.
^{99m}Tc p.
technetium-99m pyrophosphate
^{99m}Tc p.
technetium-99m p. (^{99m}Tc pyrophosphate)
p. technetium myocardial scan

Q
cardiac output
quotient
Q angle
Q space
Q-angle
QC
Mammo Q.
QCA
quantitative coronary arteriography
Q-catheter catheterization recording system
QCT
quantitative computed tomography
QCT imaging
QDE
quantum detection efficiency
QDR-1500 bone densitometer
QDR-2000 bone densitometer
QEEG
quantitative electroencephalography
QF
quality factor
QGS
quantitative gated SPECT
QHS
quantitative hepatobiliary scintigraphy
QM
quantization matrix
QO_2
oxygen consumption
QPC
quadrigeminal plate cistern
QPD
quadrature phase detector
QR pattern
QRS
Q. interval
Q. score
Q. synchronized shock
Q. vector
Q-switching
QUAD
Q. 12000 high-field open MRI scanner
Quad-Lumen drain with radiopaque stripe
quadrangle cartilage
quadrangulation of Frouin
quadrant
q. of death
left lower q. (LLQ)
left upper q. (LUQ)
right lower q. (RLQ)
right upper q.
upper outer q.
quadrantectomy
quadrate
q. gyrus
q. ligament
q. lobe of liver
q. muscle
quadratic
q. dependence
q. phase gain
quadrature
q. cervical spine coil
q. detection
q. excitation
q. phase detector (QPD)
q. phase detector artifact
q. radiofrequency receiver coil
q. setting
q. surface coil MRI system
q. T/L (terminal latency) surface coil
quadratus
q. femoris
q. femoris fascia
q. lumborum
q. plantae
pronator q.
quad resonance NMR probe circuit
quadriceps
q. apron
q. atrophy
q. femoris
q. femoris tendon reflex test
q. muscle
q. tendon
q. tendon tear
quadricuspid pulmonary valve
quadrigeminal
q. plate
q. plate cistern (QPC)
q. vein
quadrigeminy
quadrilateral
q. bone
q. brim
q. plate
q. retinoblastoma
q. space syndrome
quadripartite sesamoid bone
quadriplegia
quadriplegic
quadripolar
q. nucleus
q. signal broadening

quadripole
q. moment
Quain fatty degeneration of heart
qualitative study
quality factor (QF)
quanta (*pl. of* quantum)
quantification
acoustic q.
automated q.
flow q.
shunt q.
quantify
quantitative
q. amniotic fluid volume
q. analysis
q. cardiac perfusion
q. computed tomography (QCT)
q. coronary arteriography (QCA)
q. CT during expiration
q. digital radiography
q. Doppler assessment
q. electroencephalography (QEEG)
q. exercise thallium-201 variable
q. fluorescence imaging
q. gated SPECT (QGS)
q. hepatobiliary scintigraphy (QHS)
q. lung perfusion imaging
q. magnetization transfer
q. regional myocardial flow measurement
q. scan
q. spirometrically controlled CT
q. spirometrically controlled CT imaging
q. track etch autoradiography
quantity
spectrophotometric q.
quantization
q. error
q. matrix (QM)
q. matrix scaling
sequential scalar q. (SSQ)
wavelet scalar q. (WSQ)
quantizer-design algorithm
quantum, pl. **quanta**
q. detection efficiency (QDE)
q. energy
q. limit
q. mottle
q. mottle index
q. noise
q. number
q. sink
q. theory
quarter-detector offset
quartz glass
quasi-accelerated fractionation
quasiradiographic image
Queckenstedt sign
quellung reaction
Quénu-Muret sign
questionable lesion
Quick CT9800 scanner
quiescence
Quik-Prep
Quinton Q.-P.
Quimby implant system
Quinby classification of pelvic fractures
Quincke
Q. angioedema disease
Q. sign
Q. spinal needle
quinti
abductor digiti q. (ADQ)
extensor digiti q. (EDQ)
opponens digiti q. (ODQ)
Quinton
Q. PermCath
Q. Quik-Prep
quotient (Q)
Rayleigh q.
QUS-2 calcaneal ultrasonometer
Q-wave myocardial infarct

R
radius
resistance
roentgen
root
R meter
R1
longitudinal relaxivity
R2
transverse relaxivity
r
roentgen
RA
right atrium
Ra
radium
^{226}Ra
radium-226
^{226}Ra needle
RAA
right atrial appendage
Raaf Cath vascular catheter
RAAPI
resting ankle-arm pressure index
rabbit
r. ear sign
r. ear strands
RACAT
rapid acquisition computed axial tomography
raccoon eye
racemose
r. aneurysm
r. cyst
racemosum
angioma venosum r.
racetrack microtron accelerator
rachioscoliosis
rachischisis of atlas
rachitic
r. pelvis
r. rosary
r. rosary sign
raclopride
^{11}C r.
Racobalamin-57 radioactive imaging agent
RAD
radiation-absorbed dose
reactive airways disease
right axis deviation
rad
radian
Gy rad
gray radiation absorbed dose
rad surface dose (RSD)
radarkymography
radiability
radiable
radial
r. aplasia
r. artery to cephalic vein fistula
r. bone
r. breast scar
r. bursa
r. collateral ligament
r. deviation
r. digital artery
r. drift
r. epiphyseal displacement
r. facing of metacarpal heads
r. fossa
r. head
r. head fracture
r. head subluxation (RHS)
r. metacarpal ligament
r. neck fracture
r. neck groove
r. ray anomaly
r. ray defect
r. ridge
r. sclerosing lesion
r. sigmoid notch
r. split tear
r. styloid fracture
r. styloid process
r. tuberosity
r. vascular thermal injury
radialis
flexor carpi r. (FCR)
r. sign
radialized
radian (rad)
radiant
r. energy
radiata
corona r.
radiate sternocostal ligament
radiation
adjuvant r.
afterloading r.
alpha r.
r. anemia
annihilation r.
background r.
r. beam
r. beam monitor
beta r.
r. biology

radiation *(continued)*
bone injury r.
braking r.
r. carcinogenesis
r. caries
r. cataract
Cerenkov r.
r. chimera
corpuscular r.
r. cystitis
diagnostic r.
r. dose perturbation
r. dosimetry
r. dosimetry calculation
r. effect
r. effect unit (reu)
electromagnetic r.
r. energy
r. enhancement
r. enteritis
r. exposure
external beam r.
fatal dose of r.
r. fistula
gamma r.
gastritis r.
r. hepatitis
heterogeneous r.
high linear energy transfer r.
homogeneous r.
hyperfractionated r.
hypofractionated r.
r. intensity
r. interrogation
involved-field r.
ionizing r.
Maxwell theory of r.
megavoltage r.
r. monitor
monochromatic r.
monochromatic synchrotron r.
r. myelitis
r. myelopathy
r. necrosis
r. nephritis
r. nephropathy
neutron r.
nonionizing r.
r. oncogenesis
r. oncology
optic r.
r. osteonecrosis
r. pericardial disease
photon theory of r.
r. physics
r. pneumonia
r. pneumonitis
r. poisoning
polychromatic r.
r. port
primary r.
r. protection
PUVA r.
radiofrequency r.
rectum r.
r. response (RR)
r. risk
scatter r.
scattered r.
secondary r.
r. seed
r. sensitivity testing
r. sensitizer
r. sickness
solar r.
superficial r.
synchrotron r.
therapeutic external r. (TER)
r. therapy
R. Therapy Oncology Group (RTOG)
r. therapy planning (RTP)
r. therapy planning system
thorny bone r.
tissue tolerance to r.
r. toxicity syndrome
r. treatment planning (RTP)
r. weighting factor

radiation-absorbed dose (RAD)

radiation-attenuating surgical gloves

radiation-induced
r.-i. cancer
r.-i. change
r.-i. colitis
r.-i. fibrosis (RIF)
r.-i. ischemia
r.-i. leukoencephalopathy
r.-i. liver disease (RILD)
r.-i. neoplasm (RIN)
r.-i. pericarditis
r.-i. peripheral nerve tumor
r.-i. pulmonary toxicity
r.-i. sarcoma
r.-i. skin injury
r.-i. ulcer
r.-i. upregulation

radiation-related
r.-r. ischemia
r.-r. ischemic change

radiative hyperthermia device

radical
r. abdominal hysterectomy
r. cystectomy
free r.
heterocyclic free r.
leucine r.

r. mastectomy
nitroxide-stable free r.
r. orchiectomy
organic free r.
r. parametrectomy
stable free r.
r. vaginal hysterectomy
r. vulvectomy
radices (*pl. of* radix)
radicular
r. artery
r. compression
r. cyst
r. pain
r. vessels
radiculomedullary artery
radiculopathy
radiculospinal artery
radiferous
radii (*pl. of* radius)
radii
capitulum r.
Radinyl
radioactive
r. aerosol
r. atom
r. bolus
r. cancer-specific targeting agent
r. cobalt
r. colloid
r. constant (Λ)
r. cow
^{11}C palmitic acid r.
r. cyanocobalamin
r. decay
r. disintegration
r. emission
r. equilibrium
r. fibrinogen imaging
r. fibrinogen scan
r. gold
r. half-life
r. iodide (RAI)
r. iodine (RAI)
r. iodine uptake imaging
r. iodine uptake test (RAIU)
r. isotope
r. isotope imaging agent
r. label
r. labeling
r. material
r. metal
r. radon
r. seeding
r. source
r. string marker
r. thallium
r. thyroxine
r. tracer
r. xenon clearance
r. xenon gas inhalation
radioactively tagged
radioactivity
artificial r.
r. detection
r. distribution
induced r.
r. per volume
unit of r.
radioaerosol
r. clearance
r. imaging study
radioassay
radioautogram
radioautography
radiobiologic, radiobiological
radiobiology
radiocalcium
radiocapitellar
r. articulation
r. joint
r. joint ganglion
r. line
radiocarbon
radiocarcinogenesis
radiocardiogram
radiocardiography
radiocarpal
r. angle
r. articulation
r. compartment
r. dislocation
r. joint
r. ligament
r. portal
radioccipital
radiocephalic
radiocephalpelvimetry
radiocesium
radiochemical
r. purity
r. study
radiochemistry
radiochlorine

NOTES

radiocholangiography
radiocholecystography
radiochromic
r. dosimetry medium
r. film
radiocineangiocardiography
radiocineangiography
radiocinematography
radiocobalt
radiocolloid
r. lymphoscintigraphy
radiocontaminant
radiocontrast-associated
radiocurable
radiode
radiodense
r. lesion
radiodensity
r. area
radiodermatitis
radiodiagnosis
radiodiagnostics
radiodigital
radioelement
r. solution
surface application of r.
radioenzyme
radioepithelitis
radiofibrinogen uptake scan
radiofluorinated
Radiofocus Glidewire
radiofreqency radiogenic leukopenia
radiofrequency (RF)
r. ablation (RFA)
r. ablation therapy
r. absorption
r. catheter ablation (RFCA)
r. coil (RFC)
r. energy
r. excitation pulse
r. gangliolysis
r. hyperthermia
r. lesion
r. magnetic shield
r. modification transcatheter
r. overflow artifact
r. period
r. pulse
r. radiation
r. radiogold
r. radiographic control
r. radiographic hallmark
r. (RF) electromagnetic field
r. (RF) spoiling
r. saturation band
r. screen
r. spatial distribution problem reconstruction artifact
r. spin echo
r. transmitter-receiver coil
radiofrequency-generated thermal balloon catheter
radiogallium
radiogammetry
radiogenesis
radiogenic
r. leukopenia
radiogold
r. colloid
radiofrequency r.
radiogram
radiograph (*See* radiography)
axial r.
bitewing r.
cephalometric r.
decubitus r.
digitally reconstructed r. (DRR)
double-contrast r.
dual-energy r. (DER)
erect r.
frontal cephalometric r.
internal oblique r.
lateral cephalometric r.
lateral decubitus r.
lateral oblique r.
lateral skull r.
maxillary sinus r.
mortise r.
oblique r.
occlusal r.
outlet view r.
panoramic r.
periapical r.
plain r.
scout r.
soft tissue r.
spot r.
submental vertex r.
submentovertex r.
supine r.
Trendelenburg r.
tunnel r.
radiographer
radiographic
r. baseline (RBL)
r. blurring
r. contrast
r. control
r. criteria
r. density
r. mottle
r. parallel line shadow
r. pathology
r. pelvimetry
r. pincushion distortion
r. stability of lesion

radiographically
r. firm synostosis
r. normal imaging
r. occult fracture
radiography
advanced multiple-beam equalization r. (AMBER)
air-gap r.
bedside r.
bedside chest r.
body section r.
cardiac r.
computed r. (CR)
dental r.
digital r. (DR)
digital video gastrointestinal r.
electron r.
filmless r.
high-resolution, low-speed r.
interventional r.
intraoperative r.
intraoral periapical r.
magnification r.
mobile r.
moving-slot r.
mucosal relief r.
musculoskeletal r.
photostimulable phosphor dental r. (PSP)
plain abdominal r. (PAR)
portable r.
quantitative digital r.
rapid serial r.
scanned projection r. (SPR)
scanning equalization r.
sectional r.
serial r.
slit r.
soft-copy computed r.
spot-film r.
stress r.
video digital gastrointestinal r.
radiohumeral
r. articulation
r. bursitis
r. meniscus
radioimmunity
radioimmunoassay (RIA)
scintillation proximity r.
radioimmunodetection (RAID)
radioimmunodiffusion
radioimmunoelectrophoresis
radioimmunoglobulin scintigraphy (RIS)
radioimmunoguided surgery
radioimmunoimaging
radioimmunolocalization
radioimmunoprecipitation
radioimmunoscintigraphy
radioimmunoscintimetry
radioimmunosorbent
radioimmunotherapy
radioinduced sarcoma
radioiodide
radioiodinated
r. serum albumin (RISA)
radioiodination
direct r.
electrophilic r.
radioiodine
r. uptake
radioiron
r. oral absorption
r. red cell utilization
radioisotope
r. camera
carrier-free r.
cistern r.
r. cisternography
r. cisternography imaging
r. gallium imaging
Gd-DTPA r.
r. indium-labeled white blood cell imaging
r. labeling
r. lung scan
r. scanner
r. scintigraphy
r. stent
r. technetium imaging
transplutonium r.
trapping of r.
r. uptake
r. voiding cystogram
radioisotopic purity
radiolabeled
r. compound
r. estrogen analog
r. fibrinogen
r. MoAb
r. MoAb imaging agent
r. platelets
r. thyroxine

NOTES

radiolabeled *(continued)*
r. water study
r. WBCs
radiolabeling
area of increased r.
radiolead
radiolesion
radioligand
PET r.
radiologic
r. anatomy
r. diagnosis
r. guidance
r. percutaneous gastrostomy
r. sphincter
radiologic-anatomic correlation
radiologic-histopathologic study
radiologic-pathologic correlation
radiologist
American Club of Therapeutic R.'s (ACTR)
Association of University R.'s (AUR)
Fellow of the American College of R.'s (FACR)
Fellow of the Faculty of R.'s (FFR)
radiology
American Board of R. (ABR)
American College of R. (ACR)
cardiovascular r.
chest r.
computed r. (CR)
diagnostic r.
forensic r.
interventional r.
Mallinckrodt Institute of R. (MIR)
neurointerventional r.
r. outcomes data
pediatric r.
percutaneous interventional r.
polytomographic r.
skeletal r.
storage phosphor r.
r. telephone access system (RTAS)
therapeutic r.
radiolucency
linear band of maximal r.
prominent rim of r.
relative r.
soap-bubble r.
radiolucent
r. area
r. cleft
r. crescent line
r. crescent sign
r. density
r. fat
r. focus
r. gallstone
r. joint space
r. lesion
r. linear filling defect
r. liver sign
r. operating room table extension
r. plastic occluder
r. pneumomediastinum
r. roll
r. spine frame
r. stone
radiolunate articulation
radiolunotriquetral ligament
radiolymphoscintigraphy
radiolysis
radiomedullary artery
radiometer
radiomicrometer
radiomimetic
radiomuscular
radiomutation
radionecrosis
cerebral r.
radioneuritis
Radionics CRW stereotactic head frame
radionitrogen
radionuclear venography
radionucleotide
positron emitting r.
radionuclide
absorption of r.
r. angiocardiography
r. angiogram (RNA)
r. blood flow study
r. bone scan
r. bone scintigraphy
r. carrier
r. carrier system
r. cineangiography
r. cisternography
concentration of r.
r. cystogram
r. ejection fraction
r. esophageal dead time
r. esophagogram
r. flow scan
r. gated blood pool imaging
r. gated blood pool scan
r. generator
gold-195m r.
r. inflammation
inhaled r.
r. injection
injection of r.
r. label
r. liver scan
lung perfusion r.

r. mammography
r. milk imaging
r. milk scan
r. production
r. purity
renal r.
r. renal imaging
r. renography imaging
r. shuntogram
r. signal
r. stenosis
r. stroke volume
r. table
r. testicular scintigraphy
r. thyroid imaging
uptake of r.
r. venography
ventilation r.
r. ventriculogram (RNV, RVG, RVN)
r. voiding study

radiopacity
linear r.

radiopaque
r. bone cement
r. density
r. distal tip
r. drain
r. fluid extravasation
r. foreign body
r. imaging agent
r. lesion
r. marker
r. medium
r. pellet
Shiner r.
r. suture
r. urine
r. vesical calculus
r. wire of counteroccluder buttonhole
r. xenon gas

radiopathology

radiopelvimetry

radiopharmaceutical
r. ablation
r. chemistry
r. dacryocystography
diagnostic r.
r. localization
positron emission tomography (PET) r.
r. production
r. purity
r. quality control
r. synovectomy
r. therapy
trace amount of r.
r. tracer
r. uptake
r. voiding cystogram
r. volume-dilution technique

radiophobia

radiophosphate

radiophosphorus

radiophotography

radiophylaxis

radiopotassium

radiopotentiation

radioprotectant

radioprotective agent

radiopulmonography

radioreaction

radioreceptor

radioresistance

radioresponsiveness

radioscaphocapitate ligament

radioscaphoid
r. articulation
r. joint
r. ligament

radioscapholunate ligament

radioscintigraphy

radioscopy

radiosensitive tumor

radiosensitivity
fibroblast r.

radiosensitization

radiosensitizer
carbogen r.
halogenated thymidine analog r.
nicotinamide r.

radiosodium

radiostereoscopy

radiostrontium

radiostyloid process

radiosulfur

radiosurgery
Bragg peak r.
charged-particle r.
dynamic stereotactic r.
gamma knife r.
heavy-charged particle Bragg peak r.

NOTES

radiosurgery *(continued)*
image-guided r.
interstitial r.
LINAC r.
multiarc LINAC r.
stereotactic r.
Winston-Lutz for LINAC-based r.
radiotherapeutic agent
radiotherapist
radiotherapy
abdominal strip r.
AVM r.
continuous hyperfractionated accelerated r. (CHAR)
dynamic r.
electron-beam intraoperative r. (EBIORT)
r. field placement
high-dose r.
iceberg r.
interstitial r.
intracavitary r.
intraoperative r.
involved-field r.
large-field r.
r. localization
locoregional field r.
mantle r.
r. port
rotational r.
short-distance r.
split-course accelerated r.
stereotactic r.
teletherapy r.
three-dimensional conformal r.
whole-brain r.
r. with hyperthermia
r. without hyperthermia
radiothermy
radiothyroidectomy
radiothyroxin
radiotoxemia
radiotoxicity
radiotracer
r. activity
decreased uptake of r.
r. foil method
increased uptake of r.
r. technique
r. uptake
radiotransparency
radiotransparent
radiotropic
radioulnar
r. articulation
r. joint
r. subluxation
r. surface
radioulnarproximodistal translation
radium (Ra)
r. beam therapy
r. emanation
intracavitary r.
r. radioactive source
radium-226 (^{226}Ra)
radius, pl. **radii (R)**
Bohr r.
r. of curvature
r. hypoplasia
sigmoid cavity of r.
radix, pl. **radices**
radix-two algorithm
RadNet
R. radiology information system
radon (Rn)
r.-222 (^{222}Rn)
r. progeny
radioactive r.
r. seed implantation
RadStat
RADstation radiology workstation
radwaste radioactivity detection
RAE
right atrial enlargement
Raeder-Arbitz syndrome
Raeder paratrigeminal syndrome
ragged urethra
ragpicker's disease
RAI
radioactive iodide
radioactive iodine
RAI uptake
RAID
radioimmunodetection
railroad
r. track appearance
r. track ductus arteriosus
r. track heart calcification
r. track pattern
r. track sign
Raimiste sign
raised intracranial pressure
raiser
stress r.
RAIU
radioactive iodine uptake test
RAIU imaging
rake ulcer
RAM
reduced-acquisition matrix
Raman spectroscopy
Ramesh and Pramod algorithm
rami (*pl. of* ramus)
ramp
folded step r.
maximum slew rate r.

ramping
Ramsay
R. Hunt cerebellar myoclonic dyssynergia
R. Hunt syndrome
ram's horn sign
ramus, pl. **rami**
dorsal primary r.
inferior pubic r.
r. intermedius artery
r. intermedius artery branch
ischiopubic r.
r. of ischium
r. of lateral sulcus
mandibular r.
r. medialis artery
r. medialis artery branch
pubic r.
r. of pubis
superior pubic r.
ventral primary r.
Randall plaque
Rand microballoon
random
r. motion
r. noise
r. point
randomized
r. controlled trial
r. trial
range
absorbed dose r.
dynamic r.
emission r.
frequency r.
gray-scale r.
normal r.
reference r.
therapeutic r.
water r.
range-gated
r.-g. Doppler spectral flow analysis
r.-g. pulsed Doppler
ranine tumor
rank
Spearman r.
Ranke angle
ranula
Ranvier
R. groove
R. node
RAO
right anterior oblique
RAP
right atrial pressure
raphe
abdominal r.
amnionic r.
anococcygeal r.
anogenital r.
longitudinal r.
median r.
palpebral r.
penile r.
pterygomandibular r.
scrotal r.
tendinous r.
unicusp with central r.
rapid
r. acquisition computed axial tomography (RACAT)
r. acquisition with relaxation enhancement (RARE)
r. axial MRI
r. axial MR imaging
r. deceleration injury
r. dephasing
r. dissolution formula (RDF)
r. distribution
r. early repolarization phase
r. filling (RF)
r. filling period (RFP)
r. filling phase
r. filling wave (RFW)
r. film changer
r. fluid expansion
r. image transfer
r. inspiratory flow rate
r. oscillatory motion
r. pull-through technique (RPT)
r. scan fluoroscopy
R. Scan spectrometery
r. scan technique
r. sequential CT scan
r. serial radiography
r. thoracic compression technique
r. ventricular filling phase
r. ventricular rate
r. ventricular response
rapid-acquisition relaxation-enhanced MRI
Rapido
Rapido-mat

NOTES

rapid-sequence
r.-s. imaging
r.-s. intravenous pyelography
r.-s. IVP
raptus of attention
RARE
rapid acquisition with relaxation enhancement
RARE-derived pulse sequence
rare-earth screen
rarefaction
bony r.
r. of cortex
fluffy r.
rarefied area
RAS
renal artery stenosis
Rokitansky-Aschoff sinus
rotational atherectomy system
Rashkind
R. double-disk umbrella occluder
R. double umbrella device
R. umbrella
Rasmussen mycotic aneurysm
Rastelli type A, B, C atrioventricular canal defect
raster
r. frequency
r. line
r. period
r. spacing error
rat-bite erosion
rate
ACR r.
r. analysis
atrial r. (AR)
digital sampling r.
dipole-dipole relaxation r.
flow r.
glomerular filtration r.
high-dose r. (HDR)
inspiratory flow r.
instantaneous enhancement r.
intraoperative high dose r. (IOHDR)
lipid fraction relaxation r.
magnet r.
maximum midexpiratory flow r. (MMFR)
maximum predicted heart r. (MPHR)
mean circumferential fiber shortening r. (MCFSR)
r. meter
oxygen extraction r. (OER)
patency r.
peak filling r. (PFR)
plasma radioiron disappearance r.
plasma radioiron turnover r.
predicted target heart r.
proliferation r.
pulsed dose r. (PDR)
rapid inspiratory flow r.
rapid ventricular r.
relaxation r.
shear strain r.
Solomon-Bloembergen theory of dipole-dipole relaxation r.
specific absorption r. (SAR)
spirometer flow r.
standby r.
stroke ejection r.
time to peak filling r. (TPFR)
transverse relaxation r.
ultra-low dose r. (ULDR)
valley-to-peak dose r.
variable response r.
ventricular r.
ratemeter
Rathke
R. cleft cyst
R. duct
R. pouch
R. pouch tumor
rating scale
ratio
adrenal-to-spleen r. (ASR)
ankle-brachial pressure r.
AO:AC r.
aortic valve opening to aortic valve closing ratio
aortic root r.
aortic valve opening to aortic valve closing r. (AO:AC ratio)
apnea/bradycardia r.
artery/aortic velocity r.
bone age r.
brain-to-background r.
bronchus-pulmonary artery r.
cardiothoracic r. (CT, CTR)
r. of caudate to right hepatic lobe
CBV/CBF r.
cerebral blood volume/cerebral blood flow ratio
cerebral blood volume/cerebral blood flow r. (CBV/CBF ratio)
chemical-shift r.
C/N r.
compression r.
conduction r.
contrast-to-noise r. (C/N)
conversion r.
CT r.
diastolic velocity r.
dose nonuniformity r. (DNR)
E:A wave r.

end-systolic wall index/end-systolic volume r. (ESWI-ESVI ratio)
escape-peak r.
ESP/ESV r.
ESWI-ESVI r.
 end-systolic wall index/end-systolic volume ratio
false negative r.
false positive r.
FL/AC r.
 femur length to abdominal circumference
gray to white matter activity r.
gray-white matter contrast r.
gray to white matter utilization r.
grid r.
gyromagnetic r.
HC/AC r.
 head circumference to abdominal circumference ratio
head circumference to abdominal circumference r. (HC/AC ratio)
heart-to-background r.
heart-to-lung r. (HLR)
Holdaway r.
I:E r.
inferior-anterior count r.
Insall r.
Insall Salvati r.
inspiratory to expiratory r.
inverse inspiratory-expiratory time r.
iodine-to-particle r.
isotopic r.
kidney-to-background r.
LA/AR r.
L/A peak r.
L/B r.
 lesion-to-brain ratio
left atrium/aortic root r.
left ventricular systolic time interval r.
lesion-to-background r.
lesion-to-brain r. (L/B ratio)
lesion-to-muscle r.
lesion-to-nonlesion count r.
liver/aorta peak r.
liver/liver peak r. (L/LP ratio)
L/LP r.
 liver/liver peak ratio
LQ r.
magnetization transfer r. (MTR)
magnetogyric r.
maximum diameter to minimum diameter r.
metatarsal length r.
nasal-to-plasma radioactivity r.
off-axis r. (OAR)
off-center r. (OCR)
optional target-to-background r.
orifice-to-annulus r.
P:A r.
 peroneal to anterior compartment ratio
PASP-SASP r.
patellar ligament-patellar r.
peak systolic and diastolic r.
peroneal to anterior compartment r. (P:A ratio)
pitch r.
Poisson r.
power r.
P:QRS r.
proportional r.
P-S flow r.
 pulmonic-systemic flow ratio
pulmonary artery-bronchus r.
pulmonic-systemic flow r. (P-S flow ratio)
right ventricular to left ventricular systolic pressure r. (RVP-LVP pressure ratio)
RVP-LVP pressure r.
 right ventricular to left ventricular systolic pressure ratio
scatter-air r. (SAR)
scatter-maximum r. (SMR)
scatter-to-primary r.
S/D r.
 systolic/diastolic ratio
sensitizer enhancement r.
septal to free wall r.
signal intensity r.
signal-to-clutter r.
signal-to-noise r. (S/N ratio, SNR)
SI joint to sacrum r.
S/N r.
 signal-to-noise ratio
spleen-to-liver r.
stroke count r.
stroke volume r.
systolic/diastolic r. (S/D ratio)
systolic velocity r.
target-to-background r.
T-D r.

NOTES

ratio *(continued)*
thickness to diameter of ventricle ratio
thallium-to-scalp r.
thermal enhancement r. (TER)
thickness to diameter of ventricle r. (T-D ratio)
tissue-air r. (TAR)
tissue-maximum r. (TMR)
tissue-phantom r. (TPR)
TME r.
trapezium-metacarpal eburnation ratio
r. transformer
trapezium-metacarpal eburnation r. (TME ratio)
tumor to normal brain r.
tumor-to-normal brain r.
ventilation-perfusion r.

Ratliff
R. avascular necrosis classification
R. classification of avascular necrosis

rat-tail
r.-t. common bile duct
r.-t. esophagus
r.-t. sign

Rau
apophysis of R.

Rauchfuss triangle

rave
fracture en r.

RAW
resistance airway

ray
actinic r.
alpha r.
r. amputation
anode r.
beta r.
cathode r.
central r. (CR)
chemical r.
digital r.
direct r.
gamma r.
glass r.
grenz r.
H r.'s
hard r.
hypermobile first r.
incident r.
indirect r.
infrared r.
intermediate r.
keV gamma r.
long axis r.
Niewenglowski r.
pollicized r.
positive r.
primary r.
reflected r.
roentgen r.
secondary r.
soft r.
r. sum
r. therapeutics
r. tracing
ultraviolet r.
W r.

Raybar 75

ray-casting method

Rayleigh
R. quotient
R. scattering
R. scattering law

Raymond-Cestan syndrome

Raynaud
R. disease
R. phenomenon
R. syndrome

Rayopak

rays

ray-sum
r.-s. projection
r.-s. view

Ray-Tec x-ray detectable surgical sponge

Rayvist

Rb
rubidium

^{82}Rb-based cardiac imaging

RBBB
right bundle-branch block

RBC
red blood cell
Cr-heated RBC
labeled RBC
Tc-99m-tagged RBC
technetium-99m-labeled RBC
technetium-99m-tagged RBC

RBE
relative biologic effectiveness

RB-ILD
respiratory bronchiolitis-associated interstitial lung disease

RBL
radiographic baseline
Reid baseline

RCA
retained cortical activity
right coronary angiography
right coronary artery
rotational coronary atherectomy

rCBF
regional cerebral blood flow

rCBF PET (regional cerebral blood flow positron emission tomography) scan

rCBV
regional cerebral blood volume

$rCMRO_2$
regional cerebral metabolic rate for oxygen

rCPP
regional cerebral perfusion pressure

rd
rutherford

RDF
rapid dissolution formula

RDG
retrograde duodenogastroscopy

RDPA
right descending pulmonary artery

RDS
respiratory distress syndrome

RE
reflux esophagitis

Re
rhenium
^{186}Re
rhenium-186
^{188}Re
rhenium-188
generator-produced ^{188}Re

reabsorption
r. atelectasis
bony r.
sodium r.

reaccumulation

reactance
inductive r. (XL)

reaction
allergic r.
alloxan-Schiff r.
anaphylactic r.
annihilation r.
arrest r.
choriodecidual r.
complex periosteal r.
Crohn-like lymphoid r.
dystonic r.
Eisenmenger r.
endoergic r.
exoergic r.
extrapyramidal r.
first-order r.
fluffy periosteal r.
hair-on-end periosteal r.
hilar r.
hypersensitivity r. (HSR)
inflammatory r.
interrupted periosteal r.
Jones-Mote r.
lamellar periosteal r.
multilamellar periosteal r.
onionskin periosteal r.
periosteal r.
pleural r.
positron matter-antimatter annihilation r.
quellung r.
r. recovery time
sarcoid-like r.
scar tissue r.
Schultz r.
shell type of periosteal r.
soft tissue r.
solid periosteal r.
sunburst periosteal r.
symmetric periosteal r.
r. vial

reactivation tuberculosis

reactive
r. airways disease (RAD)
r. airways dysfunction syndrome
r. arteriole
r. bone sclerosis
r. cyst cord
r. disease of smooth muscle
r. follicular hyperplasia
r. gliosis
r. hyperemia
r. interface
r. lymphadenopathy
r. lymphoid hyperplasia
r. lymphoid lesion
r. marrow edema
r. proliferating angioendotheliomatosis
r. remodeling
r. spinal cyst
r. woven bone

reactivity
bronchial r.

reactor
fast-breeder r.

Reader paratrigeminal syndrome

reading
batch r.

NOTES

reading *(continued)*
pressure r.
wet x-ray r.
readout
r. delay
r. gradient
r. wavelength
REAL
Revised European-American Lymphoma
REAL classification
realignment
patellofemoral r.
real-time
r.-t. assessment
r.-t. biplanar needle tracking
r.-t. chirp Z transformer
r.-t. color Doppler imaging
r.-t. CT fluoroscopy
r.-t. 2D blood flow imaging
r.-t. display
r.-t. Doppler
r.-t. dose area product (DAP)
r.-t. echocardiogram imaging
r.-t. echocardiography
r.-t. echoplanar image
r.-t. enhancement
r.-t. format converter
r.-t. magnetic resonance imaging tracking
r.-t. respiratory feedback
r.-t. scan ultrasound
r.-t. sector scanning
r.-t. sonogram
r.-t. two-dimensional Doppler flow-imaging system
r.-t. ultrasonography
r.-t. volume rendering
rearfoot varus
rebleeding of aneurysm
rebound
r. excitation
r. sign
rebreathing ventilation scan
Rebuck skin window technique
recalcitrant
recall
multiplanar gradient r. (MPGR)
r. phenomenon
recanalization technique
recanalized
r. artery
r. ductus
recapture
mobile with r.
mobile without r.
stuck with r.
stuck without r.
receive-only circular surface coil
receiver
r. coil
r. dead time
Medtronic radiofrequency r.
r. operating characteristic curve (ROC curve)
r. operating characteristics
recent
r. dislocation
r. lymphangiographic contrast
receptor binding
recess
attic r.
azygoesophageal r.
cecal r.
cerebellopontine r.
cochlear r.
costodiaphragmatic r.
costomediastinal r.
costophrenic r.
duodenojejunal r.
epitympanic r. (EPR)
hepatorenal r.
ileocecal r.
inferior duodenal r.
infraglenoid r.
intersigmoid r.
lacrimal r.
lateral r.
optic r.
paraduodenal r.
peritoneal r.
pharyngeal r.
piriform r.
pleural r.
popliteal r.
posterior pleural r.
prestyloid r.
rectouterine r.
rectovesical r.
retrocecal r.
retroduodenal r.
sacciform r.
sphenoethmoidal r.
splenorenal r.
sublabral r.
subphrenic r.
subscapularis r.
superior azygoesophageal r.
superior duodenal r.
twining r.
recession
nasion r.
rib r.
reciprocal
r. agonist-antagonist relaxation
r. changes

r. depression
r. rhythm
reciprocating conduction
recirculation peak
Recklinghausen
R. disease of bone
R. tumor
reclining position
recoarctation
r. of aorta
recoil
r. atom
r. electrons
r. pressure
recon pitch
reconstitution
r. of blood flow in artery
r. via profunda artery
reconstructed radiographic imaging
reconstruction
r. algorithm
analytic r.
r. of aorta
aortic r.
r. artifact
breast r.
coronal r.
3D image r.
Dor r.
external gamma dose r.
fan-beam r.
Fourier transformation r.
Fourier two-dimensional projection r.
gated 3D r.
image r.
iterative r.
magnitude r.
MIP r.
multiplanar r.
one-sided image r.
patch graft r.
phase-preserving r.
renovascular r.
respiration gated 3D r.
sagittal r.
spatial r.
r. study
three-dimensional r.
transannular patch r.
r. view
zygomaticomalar r.
reconstructive imaging
reconstructor
dynamic planar r. (DPR)
dynamic spatial r. (DSR)
recorder
circadian event r.
event r.
pulse volume r.
recording
color Doppler r.
continuous-wave Doppler r.
pullback pressure r.
pulsed-wave Doppler r.
pulse volume r. (PVR)
segmental limb pressure r.
simultaneous r.
recovery
arrhythmia-insensitive flow-sensitive alternating inversion r. (A-FAIR)
cardiac r.
3D turbo fluid-attentuated inversion r.
fast short tau inversion r.
fluid-attenuated inversion r. (FLAIR)
inversion r.
myocardial r.
r. period of myocardium
postischemic r.
saturation r.
selective saturation r.
shape r.
short tau inversion r. (STIR)
short TI inversion r. (STIR)
silver r.
r. time (RT, TR)
r. time image
uneventful r.
recrudescence
recrudescent tuberculosis
recruitment potential
recta
vasa r.
rectal
r. balloon
r. cancer
r. carcinoma
r. dilatation
r. distention
r. duplication cyst
r. endoscopic ultrasonography (REU)

NOTES

rectal *(continued)*
r. endosonography
r. fascia
r. fisting
r. fistula
r. fold
r. halo sign
r. intussusception
r. lesion
r. lymph node
r. multiplane transducer
r. muscle cuff
r. narrowing
r. obstruction
r. orifice
r. penetration
r. plexus
r. polyp
r. pouch
r. prolapse
r. radiation injury
r. sheath hematoma
r. shelf
r. stenosis
r. stump
r. target sign
r. tear
r. tip
r. valve
r. vault
rectangular
r. field of view
r. phalanx
r. section profile
recti (*pl. of* rectus)
rectification
full-wave r.
rectifier
full-wave r.
silicon-controlled r. (SCR)
r. subblock
r. tube
rectilinear
r. bone scan
r. bone scan imaging
r. scanner
r. thyroid scan
rectocele
rectogenital septum
rectosigmoid
r. cancer
r. carcinoma
r. function
r. junction
r. manometry
r. polypoid lesion
rectouterine
r. fold
r. fossa
r. pouch
r. recess
rectovaginal
r. fistula
r. pouch
r. septum
rectovaginouterine pouch
rectovesical
r. fistula
r. pouch
r. recess
r. septum
rectum
benign lymphoma of r.
Hartmann closure of r.
prolapse of r.
r. radiation
rectus, pl. **recti**
r. abdominis
r. femoris
gyrus recti
r. muscle
r. position
r. sheath
r. sheath pocket
recumbent
r. position
r. view
recurrence
ipsilateral breast tumor r. (IBTR)
local r. (LR)
r. pattern
tumor r.
recurrent
r. artery of Heubner
r. bronchiectasis
r. canal
r. cancer
r. carcinoma
r. digital fibroma
r. dislocation
r. embolus
r. fleeting infiltrate
r. high-grade malignant glioma
r. hyperparathyroidism
r. laryngeal nerve
r. lateral patellar subluxation
r. lesion
r. lymphoma
r. meningeal nerve
r. multifocal osteomyelitis
r. pneumonia
r. pneumothorax
r. pyogenic cholangiogram (RPC)
r. pyogenic cholangitis
r. pyogenic hepatitis
r. respiratory papillomatosis

r. sialadenitis
r. stricture
r. ulcer
r. vermian oligoastrocytoma
recursive partitioning analysis
recurvatum
r. deformity
genu r.
red
r. blood cell (RBC)
r. blood cell scintigraphy
r. cell ghost
congo r.
r. hepatization stage of pneumonia
r. infarct
Texas R.
redirection of inferior vena cava
redistributed thallium scan
redistribution
blood flow r.
flow r.
r. image
myocardial image r.
r. myocardial imaging
pulmonary blood flow r.
pulmonary vascular r.
r. of pulmonary vascular flow
r. study
r. thallium-201 imaging
vascular r.
Redi-Vu teleradiology system
red-out
reduced
r. acquisition
r. alveolar ventilation
r. circulation
r. compliance of chamber
r. filling
r. plasma volume
r. prominence of pulmonary vessels
r. pulmonary compliance
r. signal intensity
r. stroke volume
r. subluxation
r. systemic cardiac output
r. ventricular filling period
reduced-acquisition
r.-a. matrix (RAM)
r.-a. matrix FAST
reduction
anatomic r.
blood viscosity r.
Burwell-Charnley classification of fracture r.
closed r.
concentric r.
congruent r.
r. deformity
electrolytic r.
fracture r.
gradient moment r. (GMR)
limb r.
r. mammoplasty
r. mammoplasty tissue
open r.
postural r.
stable r.
redundancy
r. of interposed colon segment
phase-angle display r.
redundant
r. aortic valve leaflet
r. capsule
r. carotid artery
r. mitral valve leaflet
r. scallop of posterior annulus
reefing
capsular r.
r. of medial retinaculum of knee
reentrant
r. loop
r. well chamber
reentry
bundle-branch r. (BBR)
r. circuit
functional r.
intraatrial r.
r. point
sinus nodal r.
reexpansion
lung r.
r. of lung
r. pulmonary edema
reexploration
reference
r. coordinate system
r. dose
frame of r.
r. line
r. phantom
r. range
rotating frame of r.
r. site

NOTES

reference *(continued)*
sternospinal r.
r. wave
referred pain
REFI
regional ejection fraction imaging
refill
capillary r.
reflected
r. edge of Poupart ligament
r. inguinal ligament
r. ray
reflection coefficient
reflectivity
echo r.
high r.
reflectometer tuning unit
reflector
diffuse r.
specular r.
reflex
r. arc
conditioned r. (CR)
genitourinary r.
r. ileus
r. sympathetic dystrophy
refluoromyelography
reflux
acid r.
r. activity
r. atrophy
r. of barium
bile r.
congenital vesicoureteral r.
duodenobiliary r.
duodenogastric r. (DGR)
duodenogastroesophageal r.
duodenopancreatic r.
esophageal r.
r. esophagitis (RE)
free r.
r. gastritis
gastroesophageal r. (GER)
r. grades I–V
intrarenal r.
nasopharyngeal r.
r. nephropathy
piston-like r.
r. regurgitation
uretero-ureteral r.
vesicoureteral r. (VUR)
refluxing spastic neurogenic bladder
refocus
multiplanar gradient r.
reformat
reformation
DentaScan multiplanar r.
multiplanar r.
reformatting
multiplanar r.
refraction
refractive shadowing
refractory
r. anemia
r. congestive heart failure
r. hypertension
r. period of myocardium
r. to treatment
r. tumor
refractured bone
regeneration
imperfect r.
nodular liver r.
osteoblastic bone r.
r. of tissue
regenerative
r. chondrocyte
r. gastric polyp
r. liver nodule
region
dark r.
hyperechoic r.
hypermetabolic r.
hypervariable r.
insular r.
r. of interest (ROI)
perihilar r.
photodeficient r.
photopenic r.
pineal r.
r. of protection
regional
r. asynergy
r. cerebral blood flow (rCBF)
r. cerebral blood flow response
r. cerebral blood volume (rCBV)
r. cerebral metabolic rate for oxygen (rCMRO$_2$)
r. cerebral oxygen saturation
r. cerebral perfusion
r. cerebral perfusion pressure (rCPP)
r. colitis
r. contractile reserve
r. dyskinesia
r. dyssynergia
r. ejection fraction
r. ejection fraction image
r. ejection fraction imaging (REFI)
r. enteritis
r. granulomatous lymphadenitis
r. hypokinesis
r. hypokinetic wall motion
r. ileitis
r. left ventricular function
r. lymph node

r. lymph node cannot be addressed (NX)
r. melanoma
r. migratory osteoporosis
r. myocardial blood flow
r. myocardial ischemia
r. myocardial uptake of thallium
r. neurolytic block
r. pulmonary perfusion
r. spread
r. tracer uptake
r. transient osteoporosis
r. transmural ischemia
r. tumor confinement
r. vascular perfusion
r. ventilation
r. wall motion assessment
r. washout measurement

region-of-interest
r.-o.-i. fluoroscopy
r.-o.-i. imaging technique

registration
r. and alignment of 3D images
2D portal image r.
landmark r.
robust r.
spastic r.
spatial r.
surface r.

Regnauld degeneration of MTP joint

Regnauld-type great toe degeneration

regression
caudal r.
plaque r.
polynomial stepwise multilinear r.
spontaneous r.
stepwise r.

regressive remodeling

regrowth delay

regular
r. connective tissue
r. wedge delay

regulation
volume r.

regurgitant
r. flow delay
r. fraction
r. jet
r. lesion
r. lesion delay
r. orifice
r. orifice area (ROA)
r. pandiastolic flow
r. pocket
r. stream
r. stroke volume (RSV)
r. systolic flow
r. velocity

regurgitation
aortic r. (AR)
congenital aortic r.
congenital mitral r. (CMR)
Dexter-Grossman classification of mitral r.
Doppler tricuspid r.
factitious r.
Grossman scale for r.
ischemically mediated mitral r.
massive aortic r.
mitral r. (MR)
mitral valve r.
pansystolic mitral r.
paravalvular r.
physiologic r.
pulmonic r. (PR)
pulmonic valve r.
reflux r.
semilunar aortic valve r.
semilunar pulmonic valve r.
silent r.
sour fluid r.
syphilitic aortic r.
transient tricuspid r.
tricuspid orifice r.
tricuspid valve r.
r. of valve
valvular r. (VR)

Reichek method of calculating end-systolic wall stress

Reichert
R. canal
R. flexible sigmoidoscope

Reichert-Mundinger-Fischer stereotactic frame

Reid
R. baseline (RBL)
R. lobule

Reil
R. band
island of R.
R. island

Reilly body

NOTES

reimplantation
r. lung response
r. technique
reinfarction
Reinhardt syndrome
reinjection thallium stress examination
Reinke space
reinnervation
motor r.
reintimalization
reirradiation
Reisseisen muscle
Reiter
R. disease
R. syndrome
R. syndrome arthritis
rejection
accelerated acute kidney r.
acute renal transplant r.
allograft r.
borderline severe r.
chronic humoral r.
chronic lung transplant r.
chronic renal transplant r.
end-stage r.
first-set r.
focal moderate r.
graft r.
hyperacute lung transplant r.
hyperacute renal transplant r.
low moderate r.
lung transplant r.
renal transplant r.
resolving r.
second-set r.
severe acute r.
transplant r.
vasculitic r.
relapse
bone marrow r.
solitary r.
testicular r.
relapse-free survival (RFS)
relapsing
r. course
r. polychondritis
relation
end-diastolic pressure-volume r.
end-systolic pressure-volume r.
force-frequency r.
force-length r.
force-velocity r.
Frank-Starling r.
phase r.
relationship
dentoskeletal r.
dose-time r.
dose-volume r.
globe-orbit r.
Karplus r.
Reynolds r.
tumor cell-host bone r.
relative
r. biologic effectiveness (RBE)
r. conversion factor
r. error
r. hypoxia
r. mitral stenosis
r. radiolucency
r. refractory period (RRP)
r. shunt flow
r. value scale
relativistic mass
relaxation
r. atelectasis
ferromagnetic r.
isovolumetric r.
longitudinal r.
molecular weight dependence of r.
multiexponential r.
multispin r.
nuclear electric quadripole r.
paramagnetic shift r.
r. probe
proton r.
r. rate
r. rate frequency dependence
reciprocal agonist-antagonist r.
sinusoidal r.
spin-lattice r.
spin-spin r.
r. technique
r. time
tissue-based T2 r.
transverse r.
T2 star r.
relaxivity
longitudinal r. (R1)
transverse r. (R2)
relaxometer
Bruker PC-10 r.
Bruker TC-10 r.
IBM field-cycling research r.
relaxometry
releasing factor
relief pattern
reloading
anode tube r.
REM
roentgen equivalent man
remasking
remineralization
remitting course
remnant
cystic duct r.
ductal r.

gastric r.
heart r.
notochord r.
omphalomesenteric r.
thyroglossal duct r.

remodeling
bone r.
craniofacial r.
intimal r.
neural foramen r.
osseous r.
paraarticular bone r.
plaque r.
reactive r.
regressive r.
stress-induced r.
thrombus r.

remote
r. control afterloading machine
r. diagnosis
r. history
r. ischemia
r. lower motor neuron lesion

remote-controlled
r.-c. implantation of radioactive source
r.-c. production

REMP
roentgen equivalent man period

remyelinization

renal
r. r.
r. abscess
r. adenocarcinoma
r. agenesis
r. allograft
r. allograft necrosis
r. anatomy
r. angiography
r. angiography imaging
r. angiomyolipoma
r. arteriography
r. arteriosclerosis
r. artery
r. artery aneurysm
r. artery fibromuscular dysplasia
r. artery stenosis (RAS)
r. artery string-of-beads sign
r. artery transplant thrombosis
r. axis
r. calcification
r. calculus
r. calix
r. cancer
r. capsule
r. carbuncle
r. carcinosarcoma
r. cholesterol embolus
r. choristoma
r. clearance
r. colic
r. collecting structure
r. collecting system
r. collecting system atony
r. column
r. cortex
r. cortical adenoma
r. cortical carcinoma
r. cortical isotope scanning agent
r. cortical necrosis
r. cortical nephrocalcinosis
r. CT imaging
r. cyst beak sign
r. cyst claw sign
r. cystic disease
r. cyst imaging
r. cyst study
r. Doppler
r. duplex imaging
r. duplex scan
r. duplication
r. dwarfism
r. dysfunction
r. edema
r. failure
r. fascia
r. flow curve
r. function differential
r. function impairment
r. fungal infection
r. fungus ball
r. gallium scintigraphy
r. halo sign
r. hamartoma
r. hemangiopericytoma
r. hilar vessel
r. hilum
r. impression
r. infarct
r. inflammation
r. injury
r. insufficiency
r. isthmus
r. labyrinth

NOTES

renal *(continued)*
r. leiomyoma
r. length measurement
r. lithiasis
r. lymphoma
r. malrotation
r. mass lesion
r. medulla
r. medullary pyramid
r. metastasis
r. obstruction
r. osteodystrophy
r. outline
r. papilla
r. papillary necrosis
r. parenchyma
r. parenchymal blush
r. parenchymal disease
r. parenchymal malakoplakia
r. pelvic fibrolipomatosis
r. pelvic urothelial carcinoma
r. pelvis
r. perfusion
r. pouch
r. pseudotumor
r. radionuclide
r. reflux atrophy
r. resistive index
r. scarring
r. sclerosis
r. shadow
r. shutdown
r. sinus
r. sinus complex
r. sinus cyst
r. sinus disease
r. sinus echo
r. sinus fat
r. sinus lipomatosis
r. sinus mass
r. size
r. stone
r. stone mineral composition
r. transplant
r. transplant GI tract perforation
r. transplant hypertension
r. transplant lymphocele
r. transplant pseudoaneurysm
r. transplant rejection
r. transplant urine extravasation
r. trauma
r. tuberculosis
r. tubular degeneration
r. tubular dysgenesis
r. tubular ectasia
r. tubular necrosis
r. tubular osteomalacia
r. tubule
r. tumor
r. ultrasonography imaging
r. ultrasound
r. vascular anatomy
r. vascular damage
r. vascular hypertension (RVH)
r. vein
r. vein thrombosis (RVT)
r. vein transplant thrombosis
r. venography imaging
vertebral, anal, tracheal, esophageal, r. (VATER)

rendering
3D r.
perspective volume r. (PVR)
real-time volume r.
surface r.
surface projection r.
three-dimensional r.
transparent r.
volume r.
voxel gradient r.

Rendu-Osler-Weber disease

Renee creak sign

reniform
r. contour
r. mass
r. pelvis

renin-angiotensin-dependent outer cortex

reninculus

reninoma

renin-secreting tumor

ren lobatus

Renografin

Renografin-60
R. imaging agent

Renografin-76
R. microbubbles imaging agent

renogram
r. curve
imaging r.
r. imaging

renography
ACE inhibition r.
DTPA r.
enalaprilat-enhanced r.
Lasix r.

Reno-M-30
R.-M. imaging agent

Reno-M-60
R.-M. imaging agent

Reno-M-Dip
R.-M.-D. imaging agent

Renotec
R. imaging agent

renovascular
r. disease

r. reconstruction
r. stent
Renovist
R. II
R. II imaging agent
R. II injector
R. imaging agent
Renovue
Renovue-65 imaging agent
Renovue-Dip imaging agent
rent
fascial r.
reocclusion
postthrombolytic coronary r.
reordering
r. of phase encoding
reoxygenation
tumor r.
REP
roentgen equivalent physical
reparative giant cell granuloma
repeated free-induction decay
reperfused
r. artery
r. myocardium
reperfusion
r. injury of postischemic lung
r. lung edema
r. therapy
repetition time (RT, TR)
repetitive
r. microtrauma
r. pulse sequence
r. seizures
r. strain injury (RSI)
r. stress injury (RSI)
rephased transverse magnetization
rephasing
echo r.
even-echo r.
field-echo sequence with even-echo r. (FEER)
r. gradient
gradient moment r. (GMR)
gradient motion r. (GMR)
replacement
aortic root r.
aortic valve r. (AVR)
bipolar hip r.
r. bone
r. fibrosis
hip r.
low-signal-intensity r.
mitral valve r. (MVR)
orthotopic total heart r.
prosthetic r.
SAF hip r.
self-articulating femoral hip replacement
self-articulating femoral hip r. (SAF hip replacement)
valve r.
replantable amputation
replantation of finger
replanted digit
repolarization
ventricular r.
reproducibility
reproducible baseline
reproduction
colorimetric color r.
reproductive tract embryology
reprogramming therapy
Repronex
requirement
increased myocardial oxygen r.
rerotation
varus r.
reroute
rerupture of aneurysm
resampling
volumetric r.
rescue
autologous bone marrow r.
bone marrow r.
resectability
resectable
r. colorectal cancer
r. lesion
resecting fracture
resection
absolute curative r.
absolute noncurative r.
atrial septal r.
r. cavity
colosigmoid r.
computer-assisted stereotactic r.
en bloc r.
extraarticular r.
pulmonary r.
rim r.
subtotal gastric r.
transurethral r. (TUR)
wedge r.

NOTES

reserve
blood flow r.
brain perfusion r.
cardiac r.
r. cardiac function
contractile r.
coronary flow r. (CFR)
diastolic r.
r. force
left ventricular systolic functional r.
myocardial perfusion r. (MPR)
preload r.
pulmonary vascular r.
regional contractile r.
stenotic flow r. (SFR)
systolic r.
vascular r.
ventricular r.

reservoir
r. effect
ICV r.
shunt r.

residual
r. barium
r. carcinoma
r. cement
r. contrast material
r. disease
r. ductal tissue
fibrocalcific r.
fibrocystic r.
fibrotic r.
gastric r.
r. gradient
r. hemiparesis
r. imaging agent
r. interstitial changes
r. limb-shaped change
r. luminal narrowing
r. magnetization
r. metal fragment shavings
r. nucleus
r. paralysis
r. plaque
postvoid r.
r. stone
r. stress analysis
r. urine
r. urine accumulation
r. volume (RV)
r. volume/total lung capacity (RV/TLC)

residue
fecal r.

residuum morphology

resilient artery

resin
IRA-400 r.
r. sphere

resistance (R)
airway r.
r. airway (RAW)
arteriolar r.
r. blood flow
calculated r.
coronary vascular r.
decreased peripheral vascular r.
decreased systemic r.
drug-induced drug r.
efferent arteriolar r.
end organ r.
expiratory r.
fixed pulmonary valvular r.
increased cerebrovascular r.
increased outflow r.
increased peripheral r.
increased pulmonary vascular r.
index of runoff r.
nasal airway r.
peripheral vascular r. (PVR)
pulmonary arteriolar r.
pulmonary vascular r. (PVR)
systemic vascular r. (SVR)
total peripheral r. (TPR)
total pulmonary r. (TPR)
vascular systemic r.
r. wire heater
Wood units index of r.

resistive
r. exercise table
r. index (RI)
r. index angiography
r. magnet

resistivity
conductor r.

resistor

resolution
angle variation r.
anisotropic r.
axial r.
contrast r.
energy r.
high temporal r.
image spatial r.
interval r.
intrinsic energy r.
isotropic r.
lateral r.
spatial r.
r. stage

resolving
r. ischemic neurologic defect
r. pneumonia
r. power

r. rejection
r. time
resonance
bandbox r.
cough r.
cracked-pot r.
electron paramagnetic r. (EPR)
electron spin r. (ESR)
fast-scan magnetic r.
focused nuclear magnetic r. (Fonar)
r. frequency
gated inflow magnetic r.
r. generator
r. line
localized magnetic r. (LMR)
low-field magnetic r.
magnetic r. (MR)
mobile magnetic r.
nuclear magnetic r. (NMR)
r. phenomenon
proton magnetic r.
rotating delivery of excitation off r. (RODEO)
skodaic r.
tagging cine magnetic r.
topical magnetic r. (TMR)
T1-weighted magnetic r.
resonant
r. frequency
r. frequency of oscillation
r. percussion note
resonator
birdcage r.
bridged loop-gap r.
Faraday shielded r.
flexible surface-coil-type r. (FSCR)
multicoupled loop-gap r.
resorbable
r. pin
r. plate
r. rod
r. screw
resorcinol spray
resorption
bone r.
cortical bone r.
dependent edema fluid r.
fluid r.
r. lacuna
osteoclastic r.
periosteal r.
periprosthetic bone r.
r. phase of healing
subarticular bone r.
subchondral bone r.
subperiosteal bone r.
terminal tuft r.
r. of terminal tuft
trabecular bone r.
resorptive atelectasis
respiration
cardiac gated r.
r. gated 3D reconstruction
respiratory
r. atrium
r. bronchiolar dilatation
r. bronchiole
r. bronchiolitis
r. bronchiolitis-associated interstitial lung disease (RB-ILD)
r. burst
r. burst product
r. capacity
r. compensation
r. compromise
r. decompensation
r. diaphragm
r. distress syndrome (RDS)
r. disturbance of acid base
r. effort
r. embarrassment
r. failure
r. frequency
r. gating
r. insufficiency
r. modulation of vascular impedance
r. motion
r. motion artifact
r. muscle weakness
r. noise
r. ordered phase encoding (ROPE)
r. sorted phase encoding
r. spasm
r. stridor
r. syncytial virus pneumonia
r. system
r. tract
r. tract infection
r. tract obstruction
r. volume
respiratory-esophageal fistula
response
abnormal ejection fraction r.

NOTES

response *(continued)*
autoimmune r.
blood flow r.
blood pressure r.
cardioinhibitory r.
clinical complete r.
clinical partial r.
controlled ventricular r.
deconditioned exercise r.
effective direct radiation electrodermal r. (EDR)
end-organ r.
healing flare r.
hemodynamic r.
high-rate ventricular r.
immune r.
magnet r.
metabolic r.
radiation r. (RR)
rapid ventricular r.
regional cerebral blood flow r.
reimplantation lung r.
slow ventricular r.
synovial inflammatory r.
therapeutic r.
vasoactive r.
vasoconstrictor r.
vasodepressor r.
vasodilatory r.
ventricular r.
whole-body inflammatory r.

responsiveness
airway r.

rest
r. and exercise gated nuclear angiography
r. injection
r. left ventricular function
r. magnetization
r. myocardial perfusion imaging
r. right ventricular function
r. thallium-201 myocardial imaging

restenosis
postangioplasty r.

restiform body

restiformia
corpora r.

resting
r. ankle-arm pressure index (RAAPI)
r. echocardiography
r. electrocardiogram
r. end-systolic wall stress
r. energy expenditure
r. forefoot supination angle
r. heart
r. left ventricular ejection fraction
r. MUGA imaging
r. perfusion
r. phase of cardiac action potential
r. pulse
r. regional myocardial blood flow
r. regional myocardial hypoperfusion

resting-redistribution thallium-201 scintigraphy

restoration
r. algorithm
r. of flow

rest-redistribution
r.-r. examination
r.-r. imaging

restricted diffusion

restriction
intrauterine growth r.
unilateral flow r.

restrictive
r. abnormality
r. bulboventricular foramen
r. cardiac syndrome
r. cardiomyopathy
r. hemodynamic syndrome
r. lung disease
r. myocardial disease
r. pattern
r. pulmonary emphysema
r. ventilatory defect

restrictor
beam r.

restructuring

result
concordant r.
false-negative r.
false-positive r.
suboptimal r.

resurrection bone

retained
r. barium
r. cortical activity (RCA)
r. dead fetus
r. fetal lung fluid
r. foreign body
r. gallstone
r. gastric antrum
r. placenta
r. products of conception
r. root
r. secretion
r. urine

retardation (*See* IUGR)
asymmetric intrauterine growth r.
deafness, onychodystrophy, osteodystrophy, mental r. (DOOR)
fetal growth r.

growth r.
intrauterine growth r. (IUGR)
rete, pl. **retia**
r. mirabile
r. peg
r. ridge
r. testis
retention
r. of barium
CO_2 r.
r. colon polyp
r. cyst
r. enema
fluid r.
r. meal
r. stomach polyp
r. of stool
uptake and r.
water r.
reticula (*pl. of* reticulum)
reticular
r. activating formation
r. activating substance
r. connective tissue
r. formation (RF)
r. formation of the brainstem
gray r.
r. infiltrate
r. opacity
r. type
reticularis
zona r.
reticulated bone
reticulation
r. artifact
chronic diffuse r.
coarse lung r.
diffuse, fine lung r.
lower lobe r.
r. with hilar adenopathy
reticule
reticulocortical pathway
reticuloendothelial
r. imaging
r. imaging agent
r. system
r. tumor
reticulogranular
r. appearance
r. pattern
r. pulmonary density
reticulohistiocytic granuloma
reticuloid
actinic r.
reticulonodular
r. infiltrate
r. lung disease
r. pattern
reticulosis
midline malignant r.
reticulospinal tract
reticulum, pl. **reticula**
r. bone cell sarcoma
r. brain cell sarcoma
hematopoietic r.
retina
angiomatosis of r.
retinacular
r. disruption
r. ligament
retinaculum, pl. **retinacula**
avulsed r.
cubital tunnel r.
retinacula cutis
extensor r.
flexor r.
free-floating r.
inferior extensor r.
inferior quadriceps r.
patellar r.
peroneal r.
superior extensor r.
superior peroneal r. (SPR)
retinal
r. angiomatosis
r. anlage tumor
r. artery
r. astrocytoma
r. degeneration
r. dysplasia
r. embolus
retinalis
retinoblastoma
r. hereditary human carcinoma
quadrilateral r.
trilateral r.
retinocerebellar angiomatosis
retinochoroiditis
retinocortical time
retinocytoma
retinoma
retinopathy
r. of prematurity
retinyl palmitate

NOTES

retracted
r. rib
r. stoma
retractile
r. mesenteritis
r. testis
retracting clot sign
retraction
chest wall r.
clot r.
costa r.
inspiratory r.
intercostal r.
late systolic r.
leaflet r.
mediastinal r.
midsystolic r.
mild subcostal r.
musculotendinous r.
nipple r.
postrheumatic cusp r.
r. ring
sternocleidomastoid r.
sternum r.
substernal r.
superior r.
suprasternal r.
systolic r.
upward r.
retrieval
microvascular r.
oocyte r.
transvaginal oocyte r.
transvesical oocyte r.
retroaortic
r. lymph node
r. renal vein
retroappendiceal fossa
retroareolar
r. density
r. dysplasia
retroauricular lymph node
retrobulbar
r. hemorrhage
r. mass
retrocalcaneal
r. bursa
r. bursitis
r. exostosis
r. spur
retrocardiac
r. area
r. density
r. infiltrate
r. mass
r. space
retrocaval ureter
retrocecal
r. appendix
r. lymph node
r. recess
retrocerebellar arachnoid cyst
retrochiasmal
r. lesion
r. optic tract
retroclavicular
retrocochlear hearing loss
Retro-Conray
retrocrural
r. adenopathy
r. air
r. lymphadenopathy
r. node
r. space
retrodiskal
r. temporomandibular joint pad inflammation
r. tissue
retrodisplaced fracture
retroduodenal recess
retroesophageal
r. aorta
r. arch
r. right subclavian artery
retrofenestral otosclerosis
retroflexed
r. uterus
r. view
retroflexion
retrogastric space
retrograde
r. aortography
r. arteriography
r. atherectomy
r. atrial activation mapping
r. block
r. blood flow across valve
r. blood velocity
r. cannulation
r. cardiac perfusion
r. coronary sinus infusion
r. cystogram
r. cystography imaging
r. degeneration
r. duodenogastroscopy (RDG)
r. embolus
r. femoral aortography
r. femoral arterial approach
r. filling
r. injection
r. jejunoduodenogastric intussusception
r. left ventriculogram
r. nephrostomy puncture
r. pancreatocholangiogram

r. pancreatography
r. peristalsis
r. pyelography
r. refractory period
r. systolic flow
r. transaxillary aortography
r. transfemoral aortography
r. translumbar aortography
r. transurethral prostatic urethroplasty
r. ureteral pseudodiverticulum
r. ureterogram
r. ureterography
r. ureteropyelogram
r. ureteropyelography imaging
r. urethrocystography
r. urethrogram (RUG)
r. urography
r. ventriculoatrial conduction

retrohepatic vena cava
retroileal appendix
retroiliac ureter
retrolental fibroplasia
retrolisthesis
vertebral body r.
retromalleolar sulcus
retromammary
r. fascia
r. fat
r. space
r. space view
retromandibular
retromedullary arteriovenous malformation
retromembranous hematoma
retromolar trigone cancer
retronuchal muscle
retroorbital space
retropancreatic
r. preaortic space
r. tunnel
retroparotid space
retropectoral mammary implant
retroperfusion
coronary sinus r.
synchronized r.
retroperitoneal
r. actinomycosis
r. adenopathy
r. area
r. calcification
r. cavity
r. cyst
r. drain
r. fat stripe displacement
r. fibrosis (RPF)
r. fistula
r. hematoma
r. hemorrhage
r. infection
r. leiomyosarcoma
r. liposarcoma
r. lymphadenopathy
r. lymphangioma
r. lymphoma
r. mass
r. node
r. organ
r. pneumography
r. space
r. tumor
r. tunnel
r. viscera
retroperitoneum
retropharyngeal
r. abscess
r. hematoma
r. hemorrhage
r. lymph node
r. narrowing
r. soft tissue
r. space
r. space mass
retroplacental hematoma
retropneumoperitoneum
retropulsed fracture fragment
retropulsion
retropyloric node
retrorectal
r. cystic hamartoma
r. lymph node
retrosomatic cleft
retrospective gating
retrosphenoidal space
retrosternal
r. air space
r. area
r. chest pain
r. mass
r. space
r. thyroid
retrotorsion
femoral r.

NOTES

retrotracheal
r. adenoma
r. goiter
retrovascular goiter
retroversion
r. of acetabular cup
femoral r.
retrovertebral plexus
retroverted uterus
retrovesical
r. septum
r. space
retrovestibular neural pathway
retrusion
midface r.
Rett syndrome
return
anomalous pulmonary venous r.
arterial r.
r. to baseline
central r.
impaired venous r.
infracardiac-type total anomalous venous r.
interatrial transposition of venous r.
paracardiac-type total anomalous venous r.
partial anomalous pulmonary venous r. (PAPVR)
pulmonary venous r.
supracardiac total anomalous venous r.
systemic venous r.
total anomalous pulmonary venous r. (TAPVR)
venous r.
Retzius
R. foramen
ligament of R.
R. ligament
line of R.
space of R.
R. stripe
system of R.
R. system
R. vein
vein of R.
REU
rectal endoscopic ultrasonography
reu
radiation effect unit
REV
room's eye view
revascularization
cerebral r.
coronary ostial r.
endosteal r.
foot r.
graft r.
infrainguinal r.
myocardial r.
r. procedure
revascularized tissue
reverberation
r. artifact
echo r.
r. echo
reversal
r. of cervical lordosis
end-systolic r.
gradient r.
mirror image r.
shunt r.
r. sign
reverse
r. augmentation
r. Barton fracture
r. Colles fracture
r. 3 configuration
r. distribution
r. fast imaging with steady-state free precession (PSIF)
r. figure-3 sign
r. Hill-Sachs defect
r. Hill-Sachs lesion
r. Monteggia fracture
r. peripheral bat-wing infiltrate
r. pivot shift (RPS)
r. S sign
r. tennis elbow
r. transport
r. Trendelenburg position
reversed
r. coarctation
r. coarctation of aorta
r. ductus arteriosus
r. greater saphenous vein
r. Mercedes-Benz sign
r. peristalsis
r. shunt
r. vein graft
r. vertebral blood flow (RVBF)
reversible
r. airways disease
r. bronchiectasis
r. ischemic defect
r. ischemic neurologic deficit (RIND)
r. myocardial ischemia
r. organic brain syndrome
Revised
R. European-American Lymphoma (REAL)
R. European-American Lymphoma classification
revolving Ge-68 pin

Reynolds
R. number
R. relationship
Reynold sign
REZ
root exit zone
RF
radiofrequency
rapid filling
reticular formation
RFA
radiofrequency ablation
RFC
radiofrequency coil
RFCA
radiofrequency catheter ablation
R&F camera
RFP
rapid filling period
RFS
relapse-free survival
RF-spoiled FAST
RFW
rapid filling wave
Rh
rhodium
rhabdoid
r. suture
r. tumor
rhabdomyoblast
rhabdomyolysis
exertional r.
rhabdomyoma
cardiac r.
heart r.
r. of heart
rhabdomyosarcoma (RMS)
alveolar r.
bladder-prostate r.
cardiac r.
chest wall r.
childhood r.
embryonal r.
extremity r.
female genital tract r.
genitourinary r.
metastatic r.
ocular r.
orbital r.
parameningeal r.
paratesticular r.
pleomorphic r.
primary r.
truncal r.
rhabdosarcoma
rhebosis
rhenium (Re)
r.-186 (^{186}Re)
r.-186 etidronate
r.-188 (^{188}Re)
r. 186-HEDP
r. imaging agent
r. isotope
rheologic pattern
Rhese
R. projection
R. view
R. view of orbits
rheumatic
r. adherent pericardium
r. aortic insufficiency
r. aortic valvular stenosis
r. arthritis-associated interstitial lung disease
r. chorea
r. fever
r. granuloma
r. heart disease
r. heart valve
r. lesion
r. mitral stenosis
r. pneumonia
r. tricuspid stenosis
r. valvular disease
rheumatica
polymyalgia r.
rheumatism
articular r.
desert r.
hydroxyapatite r.
rheumatoid
r. arthritis
r. lung
r. nodule
r. pneumoconiosis
r. spondylitis
rheumatologist
rhinencephalic mamillary body
rhinitis gangrenosa progressiva
rhinocerebral mucormycosis
rhinoplasty
rhinoscleroma
rhizomelia

NOTES

rhizomelic
r. brachymelia
r. chondrodysplasia punctata
r. dwarfism
r. dysplasia
rhizotomy
rhodium (Rh)
r. anode
r. filter
r. isoimmunization
rhombencephalitis
rhombencephalon
rhombencephalosynapsis
rhomboid
r. fossa
r. ligament
r. major
r. of Michaelis
r. minor
rhomboideus major muscle
RHS
radial head subluxation
RHV
right hepatic vein
rhythm
atrial bigeminal r.
atrioventricular nodal r.
bisferious pulse r.
escape-capture r.
idioventricular r. (IVR)
mu r.
nodal r.
reciprocal r.
sinus r.
transitional r.
ventricular r.
rhythmic
r. paradoxical eruption
r. segmentation
RI
resistive index
RIA
radioimmunoassay
rib
angle of r.
beaded r.
bed of r.
bicipital r.
bifid r.
bone lesion of the r.
cervical r.
r. contusion
cough fracture of r.
dense r.
r. detail
double-exposed r.
false r.
fifth r.
first r.
floating r.
r. fracture
fused r.
guillotine r.
gumma of r.
head of r.
hyperlucent r.
hypoplastic horizontal r.
inferior margin of superior r.
jail-bar r.
r. lesion
lumbar r.
minced r.
neck of r.
r. notching
penciling of r.
periosteum of r.
r. recession
retracted r.
ribbon r.
rudimentary r.
r. shadowing
shaft of r.
short r.
slipping r.
sternal r.
Stiller r.
superior border of r.
superior margin of inferior r.
true r.
r. tubercle
tubercle of r.
twisted ribbonlike r.
vertebral r.
vertebrocostal r.
vertebrosternal r.
r. view
wide r.
rib-bearing vertebra
Ribbert thrombosis
ribbing disease
ribbon
r. application
r. bowel
hollow r.
^{192}Ir r.
r. muscle
r. rib
seed r.
r. uterus
rice joint body
rice-like muscle calcification
Richet
tibioastragalocalcaneal canal of R.
R. tibioastragalocalcaneal canal
Richter hernia
Richter-Monroe line

rickets
r. classification
dietary r.
familial hypophosphatemic r.
gastroenterogenous r.
hypophosphatemic vitamin D refractory r.
oncogenic r.
vitamin D-dependent r.
vitamin D-resistant r.
rickettsial pneumonia
rider muscle
rider's
r. bone
r. tendon
ridge
alveodental r.
alveolar r.
apical ectodermal r. (AER)
basal r.
bicipital r.
bisagittal r.
bony r.
broad maxillary r.
buccocervical r.
buccogingival r.
bulbar r.
cerebral r.
cranial r.
cutaneous r.
dental r.
dorsal r.
epicondylar r.
epidermal r.
epipericardial r.
fibrocartilaginous r.
fibromuscular r.
ganglion r.
gastrocnemial r.
genital r.
gluteal r.
greater multangular r.
humeral r.
interarticular r.
interosseous r.
intertrochanteric r.
interureteric r.
keel-like r.
longitudinal r.
marginal r.
mesonephric r.
mylohyoid r.
oblique r.
Outerbridge r.
palatine r.
Passavant r.
pectoral r.
petrous r.
radial r.
rete r.
ridging r.
sagittal r.
semicircular r.
septal r.
sphenoid r.
supraaortic r.
supracondylar r.
supracoronary r.
supraorbital r.
tentorial r.
transverse r.
triangular r.
ulnar r.
urethral r.
vastus lateralis r.
wolffian r.
ridged-convoluted villus
ridging ridge
riding
r. embolus
r. stomach
Ridley
R. sinus
R. syndrome
Riechert-Mundinger technique
Riedel
R. lobe
R. struma
R. thyroiditis
Riemann classification
Rieux hernia
RIF
radiation-induced fibrosis
right
r. anterior oblique (RAO)
r. anterior oblique position ventriculogram
r. anterior oblique (RAO) position
r. anterior oblique (RAO) projection
r. anterior oblique view
r. aortic arch
r. aortic arch with mirror image branching

NOTES

right *(continued)*
- r. atrial appendage (RAA)
- r. atrial chamber
- r. atrial cuff
- r. atrial enlargement (RAE)
- r. atrial extension of uterine leiomyosarcoma
- r. atrial function
- r. atrial hypertrophy
- r. atrial patch positioned over right atrioventricular sulcus
- r. atrial pressure (RAP)
- r. atrial sarcoma
- r. atrium (RA)
- r. atrium oxygen saturation
- r. auricle
- r. axis deviation (RAD)
- r. border of heart
- r. bundle branch
- r. bundle-branch block (RBBB)
- r. cardiophrenic angle mass
- r. colon
- r. colonic flexure
- r. coronary angiography (RCA)
- r. coronary artery (RCA)
- r. coronary cusp
- r. coronary plexus
- r. crus
- r. descending pulmonary artery (RDPA)
- r. dominant coronary anatomy
- r. femoral artery
- r. gutter
- r. heart
- r. hemisphere
- r. hepatic duct
- r. hepatic vein (RHV)
- r. inferior epigastric artery
- r. internal iliac artery
- r. internal jugular artery
- r. lateral decubitus view
- r. and left ankle index
- r. and left atrial phasic volumetric function
- r. or left lateral decubitus film
- r. lobe bronchus
- r. lobe of liver
- r. lower lobe (RLL)
- r. lower lobe lesion
- r. lower quadrant (RLQ)
- r. lung
- r. mainstem bronchus
- r. middle lobe (RML)
- r. middle lobe lingula
- r. posterior oblique (RPO)
- r. posterior oblique (RPO) position
- r. posterior oblique (RPO) projection
- r. primary bronchus
- r. pulmonary artery (RPA)
- r. pulmonary vein (RPV)
- r. subclavian central venous (RSCVP)
- r. triangular ligament
- r. upper lobe (RUL)
- r. upper lobe lesion
- r. upper quadrant
- r. ventricle
- r. ventricle of heart
- r. ventricle-pulmonary artery conduit
- r. ventricle-to-ear time
- r. ventricular
- r. ventricular apex (RVA)
- r. ventricular assist device (RVAD)
- r. ventricular branch of right coronary artery
- r. ventricular bypass tract
- r. ventricular cardiomyopathy
- r. ventricular chamber
- r. ventricular coil
- r. ventricular conduction defect
- r. ventricular diastolic pressure
- r. ventricular dilatation
- r. ventricular dimension (RVD)
- r. ventricular dysplasia
- r. ventricular ejection fraction (RVEF)
- r. ventricular end-diastolic pressure
- r. ventricular end-diastolic volume (RVEDV)
- r. ventricular end-systolic volume (RVESV)
- r. ventricular enlargement (RVE)
- r. ventricular failure
- r. ventricular hypertrophy (RVH)
- r. ventricular infarct
- r. ventricular inflow view
- r. ventricular infundibulum
- r. ventricular internal diameter (RVID)
- r. ventricular to left ventricular systolic pressure ratio (RVP-LVP pressure ratio)
- r. ventricular to main pulmonary artery pressure gradient
- r. ventricular mass (RVM)
- r. ventricular outflow obstruction
- r. ventricular outflow tract (RVOT)
- r. ventricular overload
- r. ventricular peak systolic pressure
- r. ventricular pressure (RVP)
- r. ventricular strain pattern
- r. ventricular stroke volume
- r. ventricular stroke work (RVSW)

r. ventricular stroke work index (RVSWI)
r. ventricular systolic/diastolic function
r. ventricular volume pressure
right-angle chest tube
right-angled telescopic lens
right-handedness
ventricular r.-h.
right-left
r.-l. disorder
r.-l. disorientation
right-sided
r.-s. arch
r.-s. cardiomyopathy
r.-s. empyema
r.-s. heart failure
r.-s. heart pressure
r.-s. pneumonia
right-sidedness
bilateral r.-s.
right-side-down
r.-s.-d. decubitus position
r.-s.-d. position
right-to-left
r.-t.-l. shift
r.-t.-l. shunting of blood
rightward
juxtaposed r.
rigid
r. endofluoroscopy
r. ureter
rigidity
lead-pipe r.
rigidus
hallux r.
Rigler
R. sign
R. triad
R. triad of small bowel obstruction
RIGScan CR49 imaging agent
RILD
radiation-induced liver disease
Riley-Day
R.-D. disease
R.-D. syndrome
rim
r. apophysis
bony glenoid r.
r. of capsule
dark signal intensity r.
r. degeneration
dorsal r.
r. enhancement
r. of fascia
glenoid r.
high-density r.
hypoechoic r.
low-density r.
nephrogram r.
r. nephrogram
orbital r.
r. resection
sclerotic r.
r. sign
signal intensity r.
volar r.
rim-enhancing lesion
rimlike calcium distribution
RIN
radiation-induced neoplasm
RIND
reversible ischemic neurologic deficit
rind
pleural r.
Rindfleisch
fold of R.
ring
abdominal r.
Ace-Colles half r.
amnion r.
annular r.
anorectal r.
aortic subvalvular r.
apex of external r.
r. apophysis
arc r.
atrial r.
atrioventricular nodal r.
r. badge
Bickel r.
r. blush on cerebral arteriography
brain lesion r.
Cannon r.
Carpentier r.
cartilaginous r.
CBI stereotactic r.
centering r.
Charnley centering r.
choroidal r.
ciliary r.
common tendinous r.
congenital r.
constriction r.

NOTES

ring *(continued)*
Crawford suture r.
crural r.
distal esophageal r.
double-flanged valve sewing r.
double-populated detector r.
doughnut r.
drop-lock r.
r. of enhancement
r. enhancement
enhancement r.
r. epiphysis
esophageal A r.
esophageal B r.
esophageal contractile r.
esophageal mucosal r.
esophageal muscular r.
external inguinal r.
femoral r.
fibrocartilaginous r.
fibrous r.
r. finger
r. of fire sign
Fischer r.
r. fracture
half r.
halo r.
ilioinguinal r.
iliopsoas r.
Ilizarov r.
inguinal r.
internal abdominal r.
internal inguinal r.
intrahaustral contraction r.
ischial weightbearing r.
isometric contractile force r.
Kayser-Fleischer r.
r. lesion
r. ligament
low-density r.
lower esophageal mucosal r.
lymphoid r.
r. man shoulder
mitral valve r.
Mose concentric r.
multiple concentric GI r.'s
muscular esophageal r.
Ochsner r.
olive r.
orthosis drop-lock r.
osseoligamentous r.
pelvic r.
perichondral r.
periosteal bone r.
periureteric venous r.
pleural r.
proximal-to-distal r.
pyloric r.
retraction r.
Schatzki r.
r. shadow
r. sign
Silastic r.
silicone elastomer r.
sizing r.
sodium iodide r.
sphincter contraction r.
stereotactic r.
superficial inguinal r.
supraannular suture r.
supravalvular r.
symptomatic vascular r.
tracheal r.
tricuspid valve r.
tubal r.
umbilical r.
valve r.
vascular r.
vertebral epiphysis r.
r. of Vieussens
Vieussens r.
Waldeyer r.
Wimberger r.
Zinn r.

ring-and-arc calcification

ring-disrupting fracture

ring-down
r.-d. artifact
r.-d. echo

ring-enhancing brain lesion

ringing
edge r.

ringlike
r. configuration
r. contraction
r. structure

Ring-MacLean sump

ring-shaped form

ring-type
r.-t. imaging
r.-t. imaging system

Riolan
arch of R.
R. arch
R. artery
R. bone
R. muscle
R. ossicle

Riordan
R. club hand classification
R. finger pollicization
R. sign

ripple
triple r.

RIS
radioimmunoglobulin scintigraphy

RISA
radioiodinated serum albumin
Riseborough-Radin
R.-R. classification of intercondylar fracture
R.-R. intercondylar fracture classification
rise time
risk
radiation r.
Risser sign
Ritchie index
Riva-Rocci manometer
Rivero-Carvallo
R.-C. maneuver
R.-C. sign
Riviere sign
Rivinus
R. canal
R. duct
RLL
right lower lobe
RLQ
right lower quadrant
RML
right middle lobe
RMS
rhabdomyosarcoma
Rn
radon
^{222}Rn
radon-222
RNA
radionuclide angiogram
Epstein-Barr-encoded RNA (EBER)
gated RNA
RNV
radionuclide ventriculogram
R/O
rule out
ROA
regurgitant orifice area
road-mapping
r.-m. mode
r.-m. technique
road mapping
Robengatope radioactive imaging agent
Robert
R. ligament
R. syndrome
Robertson
giant limb of R.
R. sign
robertsonian translocation
Robin
R. anomalad
R. Hood phenomenon
R. sequence
Robinow syndrome
Robinson-Chung-Farahvar clavicular morcellation
robot
Lausanne stereotactic r.
Long Beach stereotactic r.
robotics
robotics-controlled stereotactic frame
Robson
R. modification of Flocks-Kadesky system
R. staging classification
robust
r. registration
r. registration technique
ROC
ROC curve
rocker-bottom foot
rockerbottom foot deformity
rocking
r. curve measurement
r. precordial motion
Rockwood
R. acromioclavicular injury classification
R. classification of clavicular fracture
rod
r. eyelet
Harrington r.
Hopkins r.
IM r.
Isolar r.
Luque r.
medullary r.
orthopedic r.
resorbable r.
thermoluminescent dosimeter r. (TLD rod)
TLD r.
thermoluminescent dosimeter rod
rodding
IM r.
intramedullary r.

NOTES

rodent ulcer
RODEO
rotating delivery of excitation off resonance
3D RODEO
rod-shaped calcification
Roederer obliquity
rOEF
roentgen (R, r)
r. equivalent man (REM)
r. equivalent man period (REMP)
r. equivalent physical (REP)
r. knife
r. meter (R meter)
r. ray
r. stereophotogrammetric analysis (RSA)
r. unit
roentgen-equivalent-physical
roentgenkymogram
roentgenkymograph
roentgenkymography
roentgenogram
Knuttsen bending r.
roentgenographic
r. change
r. control
r. diagnosis
r. finding
r. silhouette
roentgenographically occult
roentgenography
abdominal r.
roentgenologist
roentgenology
roentgenometer
roentgenoscope
roentgenotherapy
Rogan teleradiology system
Roger
maladie de R.
R. system
R. ventricular septal defect
ROI
region of interest
Rokitansky
R. diverticulum
R. lobe
R. nodule
R. pelvis
Rokitansky-Aschoff sinus (RAS)
Rokitansky-Cushing ulcer
Rokitansky-Mayer-Küster-Hauser syndrome
Rokus view
rolandic
r. artery
r. cortex
r. fissure
r. sulcus
Rolando
R. angle
R. area
fissure of R.
R. fracture
R. line
R. point
R. tubercle
R. zone
rolandoparietal glioma
roll
radiolucent r.
rolled
r. edge deformity
r. view
Rolleston rule for systolic blood pressure
Rollet stroma
rolling
r. hiatal hernia
r. membrane
Rolloscope
R. II
Romano-Ward syndrome
Romberg-Wood syndrome
Romer test
Romhilt-Estes score for left ventricular hypertrophy
ROMI
rule out myocardial infarct
R-on-T phenomenon
roof
acetabular r.
r. of insula
intercondylar r.
r. of ventricle
roofless fourth ventricle diverticulum
room
gantry r.
room's eye view (REV)
root (R)
anatomic r.
r. of aorta
aortic r.
r. canal
cervical nerve r.
cochlear r.
r. compression
coronary sinus r.
cranial r.
dental r.
dilated aortic r.
r. end granuloma
r. entry zone
r. entry-zone lesion
r. exit zone (REZ)

extrathecal nerve r.
facial r.
insula r.
intradural nerve r.
intrathecal r.
lateral r.
left atrium/aortic r. (LA/AR)
lingual r.
lumbar nerve r.
lung r.
r. of lung
r. of mesentery
motor r.
nerve r.
palatine r.
r. of penis
retained r.
sensory r.
spinal r.
ventral r.
ventricle r.

rootlet of nerve

root-mean-squared
r.-m.-s. gradient measurement

ROPE
respiratory ordered phase encoding

ropelike cord

ropy
r. density

Roques syndrome

rosary
r. bead configuration
r. beading
r. beading bone scintigraphy
r. beading esophagus
r. bead pattern
rachitic r.

Rösch technique

rose
r. bengal sodium I-131 biliary imaging
r. bengal sodium ^{131}I radioactive biliary agent

Rose-Bradford kidney

Rosenbach
R. sign
R. syndrome

Rosen-Castleman-Liebow syndrome

Rosenmüller
fossa of R.
R. node

Rosenthal
basal vein of R. (BVR)
R. basal vein
R. canal

rosette
acinar r.
Homer-Wright r.

Ross body

rostral
r. brainstem ischemia
r. cervical nerve
r. connection
r. hypothalamus
r. medulla
r. pons
r. spinal cord
r. terminus

rostrally

rostrocaudal extent signal abnormality

rostrum
r. of corpus callosum
r. sphenoidale

Rotablator thrombectomy system

rotary
r. ankle instability
r. deviation
r. subluxation of scaphoid
r. thoracolumbar scoliosis

rotated
abducted and externally r. (ABER)

rotating
r. anode
r. anode tube
r. delivery of excitation off resonance (RODEO)
r. delivery of excitation off-resonance
r. delivery of excitation off-resonance (RODEO) MR imaging
r. frame imaging
r. frame of reference
r. gamma camera
r. tomographic projection

rotating frame

rotating-frame zeugmatography

rotation
360° r.
anisotropic r.
gantry r.
internal femoral r.
medial r.
organoaxial r.

NOTES

rotation *(continued)*
r.'s per minute (rpm)
placenta r.
pronation-external r. (P-ER)
short-T2 in anisotropic r.
SPECT center of r.
r. therapy
tibiotalar r.
tube position r.

rotational
r. alignment
r. atherectomy system (RAS)
r. burst fracture
r. contact lithotripsy
r. coronary atherectomy (RCA)
r. correlation time
r. deformity
r. dislocation
r. displacement
r. field
r. force
r. frequency
r. instability
r. malalignment
r. motion
r. radiation therapy
r. radiotherapy
r. scanography
r. therapy technique

rotator
r. cuff
r. cuff arthropathy
r. cuff lesion
r. cuff muscle
r. cuff tear
r. interval

rotatory
r. instability
r. load
r. load on spine

Rotch sign
Rothschild sign
Roth spot
Rotor syndrome
rotoscoliosis
rotoscoliotic deformity
Rotter node
rotundum
foramen r.

Rouget muscle
roughened
r. articular surface
r. cartilage
r. state of pericardium

rough zone
round
r. back deformity
r. bone-cell tumor
r. cell sarcoma
r. heart
r. ligament
r. ligament of uterus
r. lucent lesion
r. muscle
r. pneumonia
r. pronator
r. shift
r. shoulder deformity
r. ulcer

roundback stem
round-cell tumor
rounded
r. atelectasis
r. border of lung
r. convex border

Rous
R. sarcoma
R. tumor

route
thoracic duct r.

routine magnification view
Rouviere
ligament of R.
R. ligament

Roux-en-Y
R.-e.-Y. limb
R.-e.-Y. procedure

Rovighi sign
Rovsing sign
row
carpal r.
distal carpal r.
first carpal r.
proximal carpal r.

Rowasa enema
Rowe calcaneal fracture classification
Rowe-Lowell
R.-L. fracture-dislocation classification
R.-L. fracture-dislocation classification system

row-mode sinogram imaging
Royer-Wilson syndrome
RPA
right pulmonary artery

RPC
recurrent pyogenic cholangiogram

RPF
retroperitoneal fibrosis

rpm
rotations per minute

RPO
right posterior oblique

RPS
reverse pivot shift

RPT
rapid pull-through technique
RPV
right pulmonary vein
RR
radiation response
RRP
relative refractory period
RSA
roentgen stereophotogrammetric analysis
RSCVP
right subclavian central venous
RSD
rad surface dose
RSI
repetitive strain injury
repetitive stress injury
RSV
regurgitant stroke volume
RT
recovery time
repetition time
RT 3200 Advantage ultrasound
RT 3200 Advantage ultrasound scanner
RT 6800 ultrasound
RT 6800 ultrasound scanner
RTA
RTAS
radiology telephone access system
RTOG
Radiation Therapy Oncology Group
R-to-R imaging
RTP
radiation therapy planning
radiation treatment planning
3D RTP
RTP system
^{82}Ru
rubidium-82
rubber
r. drain
r. vessel loop
rubeola
rubidium (Rb)
r.-82 (^{82}Ru)
r. chloride imaging agent
Rubin test
Rubratope-57 imaging agent
rubrobulbar tract
rubrospinal tract
rubrous
Rudick red flag
rudimentary
r. bone
r. lung
r. outlet chamber
r. pronephron
r. rib
r. sinus
r. ventricle
r. ventricular chamber
Ruedi-Allgower
R.-A. tibial plafond fracture
R.-A. tibial plafond fracture classification
ruffled border formation
RUG
retrograde urethrogram
ruga, pl. **rugae**
gastric rugae
rugal
r. fold
r. pattern
Ruge-Simon syndrome
rugger
r. jersey appearance
r. jersey vertebra
rugger-jersey spine
RUL
right upper lobe
rule
1-7-11 r.
carcinoid r. of 1/3
fuzzy r.'s
hydrostatic reduction r. of 3
Meckel diverticulum r. of 2
Meyer-Weigert r.
modified Simpson r.
r. of 3
r. out (R/O)
r. out myocardial infarct (ROMI)
Paterson-Parker r.'s
rule-based scheme
ruler
endocatheter r.
Plexiglas radiographic r.
Rumstrom
R. projection
R. view
runner's
r. bump
r. knee

R

NOTES

runoff
absent r.
aortic r.
aortofemoral r.
arterial r.
r. arteriography
digital r.
distal r.
inadequate r.
peripheral r.
r. resistance index
single-vessel r.
suboptimal r.
three-vessel r.
two-vessel r.
vessel r.
r. vessel
Runyon classification
rupture
abdominal aortic aneurysm r.
Achilles tendon r.
amnion r.
aneurysmal r.
aortic r.
appendix r.
arch r.
arterial dilatation and r.
Berry aneurysm r.
bladder r.
breast prosthesis r.
bronchial r.
buttonhole r.
capsular ligament r.
cardiac r.
chordae tendineae r.
chordal r.
complete Achilles tendon r.
complex extraperitoneal r.
contained aneurysmal r.
contained aortic r.
delayed splenic r.
diaphragmatic r.
esophageal r.
extraperitoneal bladder r.
forniceal r.
frank r.
hemidiaphragm r.
hernia r.
interventricular septal r.
intramural esophageal r.
intraperitoneal r.
intratendinous r.
r. of membranes
mesenteric r.
myocardial r.
r. of myocardium
myotendinous junction r.
nodal r.
papillary muscle r.
plantaris r.
plaque r.
pregnant uterus r.
premature uterine membrane r.
silicone implant r.
simple extraperitoneal r.
splenic r.
tendon r.
testicular r.
tracheobronchial r.
traumatic aortic r.
urinary bladder r.
ventricular free wall r.
ventricular septal r.
vessel r.
ruptured
r. aneurysm
r. aortic cusp
r. capillary
r. chordae tendineae
r. disk
r. emphysematous bleb
r. follicle
r. hollow viscus
r. intracranial aneurysm
r. spleen
r. thoracic duct
r. ulcer
RUQ pain
rush
peristaltic r.
Russell
R. body
R. effect
Russell-Rubinstein
R.-R. cerebrovascular malformation classification
R.-R. classification of cerebrovascular malformation
Russell-Silver
R.-S. dwarfism
R.-S. syndrome
Rust sign
rutherford (rd)
r. unit
Rutner
R. balloon dilatation helical stone extractor set
Ruvalcaba-Myhre-Smith syndrome
Ruysch
R. disease
R. muscle
RV
residual volume
RVA
right ventricular apex
RVA electrogram

RVAD
right ventricular assist device
RVBF
reversed vertebral blood flow
RVD
right ventricular dimension
RVE
right ventricular enlargement
RVEDV
right ventricular end-diastolic volume
RVEF
right ventricular ejection fraction
RVESV
right ventricular end-systolic volume
RVG
radionuclide ventriculogram
RVH
renal vascular hypertension
right ventricular hypertrophy
RVID
right ventricular internal diameter
RVM
right ventricular mass
RVN
radionuclide ventriculogram
RVOT
right ventricular outflow tract
RVP
right ventricular pressure
RVP-LVP pressure ratio
RVSW
right ventricular stroke work
RVSWI
right ventricular stroke work index
RVT
renal vein thrombosis
RV/TLC
residual volume/total lung capacity
RX400
Apogee R.

NOTES

S
S. contour
S. distortion
S. shape
S. sign of Golden
^{35}S
sulfur-35
SA
sarcoma
serratus anterior
sinoatrial
splenic artery
SA node
SAB
sinoatrial block
Sabathie sign
saber-sheath
s.-s. trachea
saber-shin
s.-s. appearance
s.-s. deformity
s.-s. tibia
sabot
coeur en s.
s. heart
Sabouraud-Noiré instrument
Sabouraud pastille
sac
abdominal s.
air s.
alveolar s.
amnionic s.
s. of aneurysm
aneurysmal s.
aortic s.
bursal s.
chorionic s.
common dural s.
cystic s.
decidual s.
dental s.
double decidual s.
double-walled fibroserous s.
drop metastasis in thecal s.
dural s.
embryonic s.
empty gestational s.
endolymphatic s.
enterocele s.
false s.
fibroserous pericardial s.
fluid-filled s.
gestational s. (GS)
greater peritoneal s.
heart s.
hernial s.
indirect hernia s.
intrauterine s.
lacrimal s.
lesser peritoneal s.
lymphatic s.
main s.
narrowing of thecal s.
pericardial s.
peritoneal s.
pleural s.
primary yolk s.
primitive yolk s.
pseudogestational s.
secondary yolk s.
spinal s.
terminal air s.
thecal s.
tight dural s.
wide-mouth s.
wrapped aneurysmal s.
yolk s.
sacciform
s. aneurysm
s. kidney
s. recess
saccular
s. aneurysm
s. bronchiectasis
s. collection
s. dilatation
s. formation
s. malformation
s. mass
s. outpouching
sacculated pleurisy
sacculation
saccule
sacculocochlear canal
sacculoutricular canal
sacculus ventricularis
Sack-Barabas syndrome
saclike
s. cavity
s. space
sacral
s. agenesis
s. ala
s. aneurysm
s. bone
s. bone tumor
s. canal
s. chordoma
s. crest
s. cyst

S

sacral *(continued)*
s. foramen
s. gutter
s. hyperintensity
s. insufficiency fracture (SIF)
s. lymph node
s. meningocele
s. nerve
s. osteolysis
s. osteomyelitis
s. plexus
s. process
s. promontory
s. spine
s. vertebra
sacralization
sacralized transverse process
sacrococcygeal
s. chordoma
s. joint
s. remnant tumor
sacrococcyx
sacrodural ligament
sacrogenital fold
sacrohorizontal angle
sacroiliac (SI)
s. articulation
s. disease
s. fracture
s. infection
s. joint
s. joint fusion
s. joint widening
s. sprain
s. subluxation
sacroiliitis
infectious s.
septic s.
sacropubic diameter
sacrosciatic
s. foramen
s. notch
sacrospinalis muscle
sacrospinous ligament
sacrotuberous
s. ligament
sacrouterine
sacrovertebral angle
sacrum
ala of s.
chordoma of s.
cornu of s.
promontory of s.
scimitar s.
tilted s.
SACT
sinoatrial conduction time
saddle
s. coil
s. embolus
s. joint
s. lesion
s. peristalsis ureter
s. point
saddlebag sign
saddle-shaped
s.-s. uterine fundus
s.-s. uterus
SADIA
small-angle double-incidence angiogram
Sadowsky breast marking system
SaECG
signal-averaged electrocardiogram
Saemisch ulcer
Saethre-Chotzen acrocephalosyndactyly
SAF
self-articulating femoral
SAF hip replacement
SAFHS
sonic-accelerated fracture-healing system
Saf-T-coil
Sage-Salvatore
S.-S. acromioclavicular joint injury classification
S.-S. classification of acromioclavicular joint injury
sagittal
s. and coronal reconstruction view
s. cranial suture
s. fontanelle
s. gradient-echo imaging
s. groove
s. oblique imaging
s. orientation
s. plane
s. plane fault
s. plane loop
s. plane vectorcardiography
s. porta hepatis
s. reconstruction
s. ridge
s. roll spondylolisthesis
s. scan
s. section
s. sinus
s. slice
s. synostosis
s. thrombosis
s. T1 imaging
s. tomogram
s. transabdominal imaging
s. ultrasound
s. view
SAH
subarachnoid hemorrhage

Sahara
S. clinical bone sonometer
S. portable bone densitometer
sail-like tricuspid valve
sail sign
Saint triad
Sakellarides
S. calcaneal fracture classification
S. classification of calcaneal fractures
Saldino-Noonan syndrome
salicylate
s. lung damage
sodium s.
salient physical finding
saline
s. implant
s. solution
s. torch
saline-enhanced
s.-e. MR arthrography
s.-e. MR imaging
s.-e. RF tissue ablation
salivary
s. calculus
s. gland
s. gland cancer
s. gland carcinoma
s. gland dysfunction
s. gland function study
s. gland infection
s. gland lymphoepithelioma
s. stone
Salkowski test
salmon-patch hemorrhage
salpinges (*pl. of* salpinx)
salpingitis
chronic interstitial s.
follicular s.
hemorrhagic s.
interstitial s.
s. isthmica nodosa
pseudofollicular s.
purulent s.
tuberculous s.
salpingogram
salpingography
selective osteal s.
salpingo-oophorectomy
bilateral s.-o.
total abdominal hysterectomy and bilateral s.-o. (TAHBSO)
unilateral s.-o. (USO)
salpingopharyngeus
salpinx, pl. **salpinges**
Salpix
S. imaging agent
salt-and-pepper duodenal erosion
saltans
coxa s.
hallux s.
Salter
S. I–IV fracture
Salter-Harris
S.-H. classification of epiphyseal fractures
S.-H. fracture classification
Salter-Harris-Rang epiphyseal fracture classification
salt-losing nephritis
Saltzman anatomy
salvage of myocardium
salvo of echoes
Salyrgan
SAM
scanning acoustic microscope
systolic anterior motion
samarium (Sm)
s. imaging agent
samarium-153
same-day microsurgical arthroscopic lateral-approach laser-assisted (SMALL) fluoroscopic diskectomy
sample
decalcified bone marrow s.
s. point
sampling
angular s.
asymmetric data s.
s. error
Gibbs s.
length-biased s.
nonlinear s.
partial k-space s.
zonal s.
SAN
sinoatrial node
San
S. Joaquin fever
S. Joaquin Valley fever
SANA
sinoatrial node artery

NOTES

Sanchez-Perez
S.-P. automatic film changer
S.-P. cassette changer
sanctuary
s. organ
s. site
sandal-gap deformity
sandbagging
s. fracture
s. fracture of long bone
sandbag hazard
Sanders sign
sandlike lucency
Sandrock test for thrombosis
sand tumor
sandwich
s. appearance
s. configuration
s. configuration adenopathy
s. patch closure
s. sign
s. vertebra
Sanfilippo
S. disease
S. syndrome
Sansom sign
Sansregret method
Santiani-Stone classification of pancreatitis
Santorini
accessory duct of S.
S. canal
S. duct
duct of S.
S. labyrinth
S. ligament
S. muscle
papilla of S.
S. papilla
SAPA
spatial average-pulse average
saphenofemoral junction
saphenous
s. nerve
s. system
s. varix
s. vein
s. vein bypass graft
s. vein graft
s. vein incompetence
s. vein stenosis
SAPHO
synovitis, acne, pustulosis, hyperostosis, osteomyelitis
SAPHO syndrome
Sappey
S. ligament
S. line
saprophytic aspergillosis
SAR
scatter-air ratio
specific absorption rate
Sarbo sign
sarcofetal pregnancy
sarcohysteric pregnancy
sarcoid
Boeck lung s.
s. granuloma
sarcoid-like reaction
sarcoidosis
acinar s.
alveolar s.
bone s.
hepatic s.
orbital s.
osteosclerosis vertebral s.
pulmonary s.
spinal cord s.
spleen s.
sarcoma, pl. **sarcomata, sarcomas (SA)**
Abernethy s.
African Kaposi s.
alveolar soft part s.
ameloblastic s.
angiolithic s.
bone-forming s.
breast s.
cardiac s.
cerebellar s.
cervical s.
clear cell s.
clear kidney cell s.
embryonal liver s.
endobronchial Kaposi s.
endometrial stromal s.
epicardial Kaposi s.
epithelioid s.
Ewing s.
extraosseous Ewing s.
fascicular s.
giant cell s.
giant cell monstrocellular s.
hemangioendothelial bone s.
hemangioendothelial liver s.
hepatic anaplastic s.
high-grade surface osteogenic s.
intracolonic Kaposi s.
intracortical osteogenic s.
intrathoracic Kaposi s.
Ito cell s.
juxtacortical osteogenic s.
Kaposi s. (KS)
Kaposi epicardial s.
Kupffer cell s.
lipoblastic s.
low-grade central osteogenic s.

lymphatic s.
malignant myeloid s.
meningeal s.
mesodermal s.
mixed cell s.
monstrocellular s.
multicentric osteogenic s.
multiple idiopathic hemorrhagic s.
neurogenic s.
orbital granulocytic s.
osteogenic s.
Paget-associated osteogenic s.
parosteal osteogenic s.
periosteal s.
postirradiation osteogenic s.
primary s.
pulmonary artery s.
pulmonary Kaposi s.
radiation-induced s.
radioinduced s.
reticulum bone cell s.
reticulum brain cell s.
right atrial s.
round cell s.
Rous s.
sclerotic osteogenic s.
small cell osteogenic s.
soft tissue s.
Sternberg s.
synovial s.
telangiectatic osteogenic s.
tendosynovial s.
undifferentiated liver s.
vascular s.
vasoablative endothelial s. (VABES)

sarcomatode

sarcomatosis
diffuse s.
sclerosing osteogenic s.

sarcomatous

sarcomere

sartorius
s. muscle

SAS
supravalvular aortic stenosis

Sassouni analysis

SATA
spatial average-temporal average

satellite
s. cartilaginous focus
s. lesion
s. metastasis
s. node
s. nodule
s. structure

Saticon

Sat Pad

satumomab
s. pendetide imaging agent
s. pentetide

saturated potassium iodide solution (SSKI)

saturation
aortic oxygen s.
arterial oxygen s.
frequency-selective fat s.
gaussian line s.
s. index (SI)
s. inversion projection (SIP)
jugular venous oxygen s.
line s.
lorentzian line s.
mixed venous s.
off-resonance s.
oxygen s.
partial s.
progressive spin s.
s. recovery
s. recovery sequence
s. recovery technique
regional cerebral oxygen s.
right atrium oxygen s.
selective s.
spatial-spectral prepulses for fat s.
s. stripe
systemic oxygen s.
s. transfer

Satvioni cryptoscope

saucerization of vertebra

saucer-shaped excavation

sausage
s. digit
s. finger
s. segment effect

sausaging of vein

Sauvage filamentous velour graft

sawtooth
s. appearance
s. configuration
s. edge
s. irregularity of bowel contour
s. sign
s. ureter

NOTES

SBDX
scanning-beam digital x-ray
SBE
self-breast examination
small bowel enteroscopy
subacute bacterial endocarditis
SBF
systemic blood flow
SBFT
small bowel followthrough
SBO
small bowel obstruction
spina bifida occulta
SBP
systolic blood pressure
SBS
shaken baby syndrome
SBSP
simultaneous bilateral spontaneous pneumothorax
^{47}Sc
scandium-47
SCA
superior cerebellar artery
scabbard trachea
SCAD
spontaneous coronary artery dissection
scalar
s. coupling
s. effect
scale
Abbreviated Injury S.
digital gray s.
false color s.
Flint Colon Injury S.
gray s.
Hunt-Hess subarachnoid hemorrhage s.
Injury Severity S. (ISS)
Outerbridge s.
rating s.
relative value s.
SOMA s.
subjective, objective, management, and analytic
scalene
s. fat pad
s. maneuver
s. musculature
s. node
s. triangle
s. tubercle
scalenus
s. anterior
s. anterior muscle
s. anticus muscle hypertrophy
s. anticus syndrome
s. medius
s. minimus
s. tunnel syndrome
scaling
quantization matrix s.
scallop
prolapsing s.
scalloped
s. appearance
s. appearance of white matter
s. bowel lumen
s. commissure
s. luminal configuration
scalloping
s. contour
s. of margin of vertebral body
s. osteolysis
petrous pyramid s.
posterior vertebral s.
s. of vertebra
vertebral s.
scalp
s. branch of external carotid artery
s. hematoma
s. hypothermia
pilar tumor of s.
s. vein needle
scalpel
interactive electronic s.
ultrasonically activated s.
scan (*See* scanning)
aerosol ventilation s.
attenuation s.
axial s.
Becton Dickinson FAC s.
bile duct s.
biphasic helical CT s.
blood pool radionuclide s.
bone s.
brain s.
bremsstrahlung s.
Captopril renal s.
cardiac s.
Cardiolite heart imaging s.
CE-FAST s.
cerebral perfusion SPECT s.
clearance phase ventilation s.
colloid shift on s.
color-flow duplex s.
computed tomography s. (CT scan)
s. converter
coronal s.
coronary artery s. (CAS)
CT s.
computed tomography scan
s. decrement
s. defect
dental s.
DEXA s.

diuretic renal s.
double helical CT s.
2D sector s.
dual-phase s.
elbow coronal s.
electromagnetic interference s.
EMI s.
enhanced CT s.
s. equalization
equilibrium MUGA s.
^{18}FDG PET s.
flow portion of bone s.
^{67}Ga bone s.
gadolinium s.
gallium s.
gastric emptying s.
helical thin-section CT s.
hepatobiliary s.
hepatoiminodiacetic acid s.
HIDA s.
^{125}I fibrinogen s.
indium-111-labeled white blood cell s.
intravenously enhanced CT s.
iodine-131 whole-body s.
isotope bone s.
isotopic lung s.
kidney s.
labeled leukocyte s.
left ventricular gated blood pool s.
liver s.
liver-lung s.
liver-spleen s.
longitudinal s.
lung s.
Meckel s.
medronate s.
MIBG SPECT s.
MUGA s.
multiple-gated acquisition s.
multiple gated acquisition s.
multiple line s. (MLS)
myocardial perfusion s.
nonenhanced CT s.
nuclear magnetic resonance (NMR) s.
oral-enhanced CT s.
pancreatic s.
panoramic CT s.
s. parameter
pelvic ultrasound CT s.
pentretreotide s.
perfusion lung s.
s. pitch
s. pitch pit
planar thallium s.
s. plane
portal-phased spiral CT s.
positron emission tomography (PET) s.
postgadolinium s.
postictal cerebral blood flow s.
postmetrizamide CT s.
precontrast s.
preoperative resting MUGA s.
proton-density axial MR s.
PYP technetium myocardial s.
pyrophosphate technetium myocardial s.
quantitative s.
radioactive fibrinogen s.
radiofibrinogen uptake s.
radioisotope lung s.
radionuclide bone s.
radionuclide flow s.
radionuclide gated blood pool s.
radionuclide liver s.
radionuclide milk s.
rapid sequential CT s.
rCBF PET (regional cerebral blood flow positron emission tomography) s.
rebreathing ventilation s.
rectilinear bone s.
rectilinear thyroid s.
redistributed thallium s.
renal duplex s.
sagittal s.
scintillation s.
sector s.
segmental lung defect s.
segmenting dual-echo MR head s.
serial duplex s.
single-photon emission computed tomography (SPECT) technetium sestamibi s.
spin-echo s.
stacked s.
stereotactic CT s.
stimulation s.
stress thallium s.
strip s.
sulfur colloid s.
suppression s.

S

NOTES

scan *(continued)*
survey s.
teboroxime cardiac s.
technetium-99m hepatoiminodiacetic acid s.
thallium single-photon emission computed tomography (SPECT) s.
three-head s.
thyroid stimulation s.
thyroid suppression s.
thyroid whole-body s.
s. time
transaxial CT s.
transaxial joint s.
transmission s.
triple-phase bone s.
T2-weighted s.
unenhanced magnetic resonance imaging s.
venous s.
ventilation-perfusion s.
ventilation-perfusion lung s.
s. volume
volumetric s.
V/Q lung segment s.
washout phase ventilation s.
water signal on magnetic resonance imaging s.
whole-body PET s.
s. with contrast enhancement

Scanditronix
S. MLC system
S. PET scanner

scandium-47 (^{47}Sc)

Scanmaster
S. DX system
S. DX x-ray film digitizer
S. DX x-ray film digitizer scanner

scannable tumor

scanned projection radiography (SPR)

scanned-slot detector system

scanner
Acoma s.
Acuson 128EP s.
Acuson ultrasound s.
Advanced NMR Systems s.
Agfa Medical s.
All-Tronics s.
Aloka ultrasound linear s.
Aloka ultrasound sector s.
American Shared-CuraCare s.
ANMR Insta-scan MR s.
Aquilion CT s.
Artoscan MRI s.
ATL Mark 600 real-time sector s.
ATL Neurosector real-time s.
Aurora MR breast imaging system s.
Biospec MR imaging system s.
biplane sector s.
Bruel-Kjaer ultrasound s.
Bruker s.
Canon s.
Cardio Data MK3 Holter s.
cardiovascular computed tomographic s. (CVCT)
Cemax/Icon s.
Cencit surface s.
charge-coupled device s.
cine CT s.
CT9000 s.
CT9800 s.
CTI 933/04 ECAT s.
CTI PET s.
CT Max 640 s.
Delarnette s.
Diasonics ultrasound s.
Dornier s.
DSR s.
3D surface digitizer s.
duplex s.
DuPont s.
Eastman Kodak s.
electron-beam CT s.
Elscint Excel 905 s.
Elscint MR s.
Elscint Twin CT s.
EMED s.
EMI 7070 s.
EMI CT 500 s.
Evolution XP s.
Fonar Stand-Up MRI s.
Galen Scan s.
Gammex RMI s.
GE Advance PET s.
GE CT Advantage s.
GE CT Max s.
GE CT Pace s.
GE 8800 CT/T s.
GE Genesis CT s.
GE GN 500-MHz s.
GE 9800 high-resolution CT s.
GE HiSpeed Advantage helical CT s.
GE MR Max s.
GE MR Signa s.
GE MR Vectra s.
GE Omega 500-MHz s.
GE Pace CT s.
GE QE 300-MHz s.
GE Signa 5.2 s.
GE Signa 4.7 MRI s.
GE Signa 1.5-T s.
GE Signa 5.2 with SR-230 three-axis EPI gradient upgrade s.

GE single-axis SR-230 echoplanar s.
GE Spiral CT s.
GE Vectra MR s.
Gyroscan S15 s.
helical CT s.
Hewlett-Packard s.
high-field open MRI s.
high-field-strength s.
Hilight Advantage System CT s.
Hispeed CT s.
Hitachi CT s.
Hitachi MR s.
Hitachi Open MRI System s.
Hitachi 0.3-T unit s.
Hologic 2000 s.
Hologic QDR 1000W dual-energy x-ray absorptiometry s.
Howtek Scanmaster DX s.
IDSI s.
Imatron C-150L EBCT s.
Imatron C-1000 UFCT s.
Imatron C-100 Ultrafast CT s.
Imatron C-100XL CT s.
Imatron Fastrac C-100 cine x-ray CT s.
Indomitable s.
Innervision MR s.
InstaScan s.
Integris 3000 s.
intensified radiographic imaging system s.
Irex Exemplar ultrasound s.
IRIS s.
Konica s.
large-bore 0.6-T imaging system s.
large-bore 1.5-T imaging system s.
Lumiscan s.
Lunar s.
LymphoScan nuclear imaging system s.
3M s.
Magna-SL s.
Magnes 2500 whole-blood s.
Magnetom SP63 s.
Magnetom 1.5-T s.
Magnex MR s.
Mallinckrodt s.
Max Plus MR s.
mechanical sector s.
MedImage s.
Medison s.
Medspec MR imaging system s.
Medx s.
midget MRI s.
modified electron-beam CT s.
MR catheter imaging and spectroscopy system s.
multiple jointed digitizer s.
multisensor structured light-range digitizer s.
neurSector s.
Nishimoto Sangyo s.
Norland pQCT XCT2000 s.
Ohio Nuclear Delta 2000 s.
Ohio Nuclear Delta 50 FS s.
Olympus endoscopic ultrasound s.
Oxford 2-T large-bore imaging system s.
Pace Plus System s.
Park Medical Systems s.
Perception s.
PETite s.
Pfizer 0450 s.
Pfizer 200 FS s.
phased-array s.
Philips Gyroscan ACS s.
Philips Gyroscan NT, NT5, NT15 s.
Philips Gyroscan S5 s.
Philips Gyroscan T5 s.
Philips 1.5-T NT MR s.
Philips Tomoscan 350 CT s.
Philips Tomoscan SR 6000 CT s.
Philips 4.7-T small-bore system s.
Picker MR s.
Picker PQ 5000 helical CT s.
Picker PQ 2000 spiral CT s.
Picker Synerview 600 s.
4096 Plus PET s.
Polhemus 3 digitizer s.
Posicam HZ PET s.
PQCT microscanner s.
ProSpeed CT s.
QUAD 12000 high-field open MRI s.
Quick CT9800 s.
radioisotope s.
rectilinear s.
RT 3200 Advantage ultrasound s.
RT 6800 ultrasound s.
Scanditronix PET s.
Scanmaster DX x-ray film digitizer s.

S

NOTES

scanner *(continued)*
scintillation s.
scintiscanner s.
sector s.
Shimadzu CT s.
Shimadzu MR s.
Siemens DRH CT s.
Siemens Magnetom GBS II s.
Siemens Magnetom SP 4000 s.
Siemens Magnetom 1.5-T s.
Siemens Magnetom Vision s.
Siemens One Tesla s.
Siemens Somaform 512 CT s.
Siemens Somatom DR2 and DR3 whole-body s.
Siemens Sonoline Elegra ultrasound s.
Siemens SP 4000 s.
SieScape ultrasound s.
Signa Horizon s.
Signa 1.5-T s.
SmartPrep s.
Somatom DR CT s.
spiral CT s.
spiral XCT s.
supercam scintillation s.
Swissray s.
TCT900S helical CT s.
Technicare Delta 2020 s.
Tecmag Libra-S16 system s.
Toshiba MR s.
Toshiba 900S helical CT s.
Toshiba 900S/XII s.
Toshiba TCT-80 CT s.
Toshiba Xpress SX helical CT s.
Toshiba Xvision s.
Trionix s.
ultrafast computed tomography s.
Ultramark s.
Ultramark 9 s.
UM 4 real-time sector s.
Varian CT s.
Vidar s.
Vision MRI s.
Vision Ten V-scan s.
whole-body 3T MRI system s.
whole-body 1.5-T Siemens Vision s.
Xpress/SW helical CT s.
Xpress/SX helical CT s.

scanning
s. acoustic microscope (SAM)
s. beam digital system
body s.
collimation s.
combined ^{99m}Tc-DMSA and ^{99m}Tc-DTPA s.
diffusion-weighted s.
dual isotope s.
s. electron microscope (SEM)
s. equalization radiography
external s.
full-line s.
gated equilibrium blood pool s.
high-resolution ultrasound s.
IDA (iminodiacetic acid) s.
isotopic bone s.
s. laser ophthalmoscopy
light s.
linear s.
s. locus
multiplanar s.
parasternal s.
paravertebral s.
point s.
positron s.
s. power
real-time sector s.
sensitive point s.
spiral CT s.
spot s.
suprasternal s.
s. technique
three-phase bone s.
total body s.
transabdominal s.
whole-body ^{29}FDG s.
wide-beam s.
xenon CT s.

scanning-beam digital x-ray (SBDX)

scanogram
s. imaging

scanography
rotational s.

scanty finding

scaphocapitate
s. joint
s. syndrome

scaphocephalic head shape

scaphocephaly

scaphoid
s. abdomen
s. bone
congenital bipartite s.
s. facet
s. fat stripe
s. hand fracture
s. pole
rotary subluxation of s.
s. shape
s. stomach

scapholunate (SL)
s. advanced collapse (SLAC)
s. arthritic collapse (SLAC)
s. arthritic collapse wrist
s. dislocation

s. dissociation
s. joint
s. ligament (LSS)
s. space
s. widening
scaphotrapeziotrapezoid (STT)
s. joint
scaphotriquetral ligament
scapula, pl. **scapulae**
body of s.
high-riding s.
inferior tip of s.
margin of s.
swallowtail malformation of s.
winged s.
scapulae
incisura s.
levator s.
scapular
s. angle
s. body
s. bone
dorsal s.
s. flap
s. margin
s. notch
s. winging
scapuloclavicular
s. articulation
scapulocostal syndrome
scapuloperoneal muscular atrophy
scapulothoracic
s. joint
s. motion
scapulovertebral border
scar (*See* scarring)
s. band
s. cancer
s. carcinoma
central pancreatic lesion s.
s. contracture
dense s.
s. emphysema
femoral physeal s.
fibrocartilaginous s.
s. formation
infarcted s.
lung starfish s.
myocardial s.
nonviable s.
s. ossification
ossified s.
postoperative breast s.
pulmonary s.
radial breast s.
s. tissue
s. tissue reaction
tumor of liver s.
well-demarcated s.
scarification of pleura
scarified duodenum
Scarpa
canal of S.
fascia of S.
S. fascia
S. ganglion
ganglion of S.
ligament of S.
method of S.
triangle of S.
S. triangle
scarred
s. duodenum
s. kidney
scarring (*See* scar)
apical s.
basilar pleural s.
fibrotic s.
glial s.
interstitial s.
parenchymal s.
parietal pleural s.
pleural s.
postinflammatory s.
postnecrotic s.
postpyelonephritis cortical s.
renal s.
selective s.
valvular s.
scatter
s. compensation
s. correction
s. degradation factor
s. dose
s. radiation
s. and veiling glare (SVG)
scatter-air ratio (SAR)
scattered
s. air bronchogram
s. radiation
scatterer depth
scattering
coherent s.
collimator s.

NOTES

S

scattering *(continued)*
Compton s.
s. foil
s. foil compensator
forward-angle light s.
image-degrading s.
low-angle s.
Rayleigh s.
side s.
small-angle multiple s.
s. system
Thomson s.
scatter-maximum ratio (SMR)
scatterplot
scatter-to-primary ratio
scavenging system
Sceratti goniometer
SCFE
slipped capital femoral epiphysis
Scharff-Bloom-Richardson grade
Schatzker fracture classification
Schatzki
S. ring
S. view
Schaumann
S. body
S. lymphogranuloma
Scheibe dysplasia
Scheie
S. disease
S. syndrome
Schellong-Strisower phenomenon
scheme
computer-aided diagnosis s.
decay s.
encryption s.
Fibonacci search s.
gradient s.
rule-based s.
Schepelmann sign
Scheuermann
S. disease
S. juvenile kyphosis
S. nodule
Schick
S. sign
S. sign of tuberculosis
Schiefferdecker disk
Schiff-Sherrington phenomenon
Schilder disease
Schiller-Duval body
schistosomal bladder carcinoma
schizencephaly
Schlemm
canal of S.
S. canal
S. ligament
Schlesinger
S. sign
vein of S.
S. vein
Schmid disease
Schmid-like
S.-l. metaphyseal chondrodysplasia
Schmidt optics system
Schmid-type metaphyseal dysplasia
Schmincke tumor
Schmitt disease
Schmorl
S. disease
S. node
S. nodule
schneiderian
s. carcinoma
s. papilloma
Schoeber sign
Schoemaker line
Schonander film changer
Schramm phenomenon
Schroedinger equation
Schüller
S. position
S. view
Schultze
S. bundle
comma tract of S.
S. comma tract
S. placenta
Schultz reaction
Schumacher criteria
Schütz tract
Schwalbe space
Schwann
S. cell of myelin sheath
S. tumor
schwannoma
acoustic s.
facial s.
geniculate ganglion s.
jugular foramen s.
orbital s.
s. trigeminal
vestibular s.
Schwartz
S. criteria
S. test for patency of deep saphenous veins
Schwartze sign
Schwartz-Jampel syndrome (SJS)
SCI
spinal cord injury
sciatic
s. endometriosis
s. nerve irritation

s. notch
s. plexus
sciatica
scimitar
s. deformity
s. sacrum
s. sign
s. syndrome
s. vein
scimitar-shaped
s.-s. flap
s.-s. shadow
scinticisternography
Scinticore multicrystal scintillation camera
scintigram
spatial resolution s.
SPECT thallium s.
scintigraphic
s. angiography
s. balloon
s. balloon topography
s. evidence
s. perfusion defect
s. scan imaging
s. study
scintigraphy
ACE inhibition s.
adrenal s.
AMA-Fab s.
antimyosin antibody-Fab scintigraphy
antifibrin s.
s. artifact
blood pool s.
bone s.
bone marrow s.
brain perfusion s.
cardiac s.
cold defect renal s.
cortical s.
dipyridamole thallium-201 s.
dual intracoronary s.
early bone s.
exercise stress-redistribution s.
exercise thallium s.
gallium bone s.
gallium lung s.
gallium tumor s.
gastrointestinal s.
gated blood pool s.
GI tract s.
heart s.
hepatobiliary s.
indium-111 antimyosin s.
infarct-avid hot-spot s.
In-pentetreotide s.
iodine s.
iodomethyl-norcholesterol-59 s. (^{59}NP scintigraphy)
isotope s.
labeled free fatty acid s.
liver s.
long segmental diaphyseal uptake bone s.
lung s.
lymphoma gallium s.
marrow agent bone s.
MIBG s.
microsphere perfusion s.
morphine sulfate s.
myocardial cold-spot perfusion s.
NEFA s.
^{59}NP s.
iodomethyl-norcholesterol-59 scintigraphy
nuclear renal s.
Octreotide s.
osteomyelitis s.
parathyroid s.
photon-deficient lesion bone s.
planar exercise thallium-201 s.
pulmonary s.
pyrophosphate s.
s. quality control
quantitative hepatobiliary s. (QHS)
radioimmunoglobulin s. (RIS)
radioisotope s.
radionuclide bone s.
radionuclide testicular s.
red blood cell s.
renal gallium s.
resting-redistribution thallium-201 s.
rosary beading bone s.
single-photon planar s. (SPPS)
soft tissue uptake bone s.
source of artifact s.
SPECT brain perfusion s.
SPECT thallium s.
splenic s.
split-function s.
sulfur colloid s.
^{99m}Tc-DMSA s.
technetium ^{99m}Tc-PYP s.

NOTES

S

scintigraphy *(continued)*
thallium-201 myocardial s.
thallium perfusion s.
three-phase bone s. (TPBS)
thyroid s.
time course fracture s.
transit s.
vesicoureteral s.
white blood cell with indium-111 s.
scintillascope
scintillation
s. camera
s. camera field uniformity
s. camera geometry
s. camera linearity
s. camera linearity differential
s. camera uniformity differential
s. counter
s. counting technique
s. crystal
s. detector
s. imaging
migrainous s.
s. proximity radioimmunoassay
s. scan
s. scanner
s. spectrometry
scintillometer
scintimammography (SMM)
scintiphotograph
scintiphotography
liver s.
scintirenography
scintiscan
scintiscanner
s. scanner
Scintiview nuclear computer system
Scintron IV nuclear computer system
scirrhous
s. breast carcinoma
s. infiltrating adenocarcinoma
s. lesion
s. tumor
scission
double-strand s.
single-strand s.
scissoring of legs
SCIWORA
spinal cord injury without radiographic abnormality
SCL
sinus cycle length
SCLBCL
secondary cutaneous large B-cell lymphoma
SCLC
small-cell lung carcinoma
scleral canal
sclerocystic ovary
sclerodactyly
scleroderma
diffuse s.
s. of esophagus
hand arthritis s.
scleroma R
scleromyxedema R
sclerosed temporal bone
sclerosing
s. adenitis
s. adenosis
s. agent
s. basal cell carcinoma
s. cholangitis
s. duct hyperplasia
s. hepatic carcinoma (SHC)
s. inflammation
s. injection
s. lesion
s. mediastinitis
s. mesenteritis
s. myeloma
s. nonsuppurative osteomyelitis
s. osteogenic sarcomatosis
s. osteomyelitis of Garré
s. osteosarcoma
s. panencephalitis
sclerosis, pl. **scleroses**
Ammon horn s.
amyotrophic lateral s. (ALS)
s. of aorta
aortic s.
arterial s.
arteriocapillary s.
arteriolar s.
Baló concentric s.
bony s.
calcified s.
chronic subperitoneal s.
congenital hippocampal s.
coronary s.
diaphyseal s.
diffuse CNS s.
diffuse myelinoclastic s.
disseminated s.
endocardial s.
endplate s.
esophageal variceal s.
familial amyotrophic lateral s.
focal bone s.
gastric s.
hepatic s.
hepatoportal s.
hippocampal s.
idiopathic hypertrophic subaortic s. (IHSS)

incisural s.
Krabbe diffuse s.
laser s.
lobar s.
marginal s.
marked s.
medial calcific s.
mesenteric s.
mesial temporal s.
Mönckeberg medial s.
multifocal subperitoneal s.
multiple s.
painful s.
pedicle s.
polka-dot s.
posterolateral s.
primary s.
progressive systemic s.
pulmonary and cardiac s.
reactive bone s.
renal s.
segmental vein s.
subchondral low-signal-intensity s.
subendocardial s.
systemic s.
temporal bone s.
tuberous s. (TS)
tumefactive multiple s.
valvular s.
variceal s.
vascular s.
venous s.

sclerostenosis

sclerotic

s. area
s. calvarial patch
s. calvarium bone island
s. coronary artery
s. degeneration
s. kidney
s. lesion
s. osteogenic sarcoma
s. plaque
s. rim
s. stomach

scoliosis

adolescent idiopathic s. (AIS)
Aussies-Isseis unstable s.
Cobb measurement of s.
dextrorotary s.
Dwyer correction of s.
Fergusson method for measuring s.
fixation of s.
functional s.
idiopathic s.
King classification of thoracic s.
King-Moe s.
levorotary s.
lumbar s.
Moe and Kettleson distribution of curves in s.
painful s.
rotary thoracolumbar s.
S-shaped s.
thoracic s.
thoracolumbar s.
uncompensated rotary s.
Winter-King-Moe s.

scoliotic

s. pelvis
s. spine

score

biophysical profile s. (BPS)
fetal biophysical profile s.
Injury Severity S. (ISS)
late effects toxicity s.
LENT s.
late effects of normal tissues score
mean wall motion s.
QRS s.
stroke scale s.
thallium SPECT s.
wall motion s.

scored cartilage

scorings on bone

scotograph

scotometry

scotomization

scottie, scotty

s. dog appearance
s. dog fracture
s. dog sign
s. dog view

scout

s. film
s. image
s. imaging
s. radiograph
s. view

ScoutView targeting

SCP

supracristal plane

SCR

silicon-controlled rectifier

NOTES

scrambled
s. image
s. imaging
scrape cytology
screen
s. craze artifact
fluorescent s.
guilt s.
intensifying s.
Lanex medium s.
radiofrequency s.
rare-earth s.
s. type film
screen-film
s.-f. contact
s.-f. mammography
screening
breast cancer s.
s. mammography
screening-detected abnormality
screen-intensifying factor (IF)
screw
bicortical s.
bone s.
cancellous s.
compression plate and s.
s. fixation
interference s.
lag s.
metallic s.
orthopedic s.
s. and plate
resorbable s.
transfixing s.
unicortical s.
scriptorius
calamus s.
scroll bone
scrotal
s. abscess
s. anatomy
s. area
s. calcification
s. fasciitis
s. fibroma
s. gas
s. hematocele
s. hernia
s. histiocytoma
s. mass
s. pearl
s. raphe
s. vein
s. wall thickening
scrotum, pl. **scrota, scrotums**
acutely symptomatic s.
SCT
allogeneic stem-cell transplantation
star-cancellation test
SCTA
spiral computed tomography arteriography
spiral CT angiography
Scully tumor
scutum, pl. **scuta**
scybalum
scyphoid
SD
SDH
subdural hemorrhage
S/D ratio
SDRI
small, deep, recent infarct
^{75}Se
selenium-75
^{75}Se selenomethionine radioactive agent
SEA
spinal epidural abscess
sea
s. anemone ulcer
s. urchin granuloma
seagull
s. joint
s. sign
seal-fin deformity
seam
osteoid s.
seatbelt
s. fracture
s. injury
sebaceous
s. adenoma
s. carcinoma
s. cyst
s. gland calcification
sebaceum
adenoma s.
SEBI
stereotactic external-beam irradiation
Sebileau muscle
second
s. branchial arch
s. branchial cleft cyst
counts per s.
s. cranial nerve
s. cuneiform bone
cycles per s. (cps)
s. diagonal branch
s. malignant neoplasm (SMN)
meters per s. (mps)
s. portion of duodenum
s. ventricle of cerebrum

secondarium
os cuboides s.
secondary
s. achalasia
s. acquired cholesteatoma
s. amyloidosis
s. archnoid cyst
s. atelectasis
s. axillary adenopathy
s. axillary lymphadenopathy
s. biliary cirrhosis
s. brain lymphoma
s. bronchus
s. calcification
s. cardiomyopathy
s. cartilaginous joint
s. center of ossification
s. chondromatosis
s. coccidioidomycosis
s. collimation
s. contracture
s. cutaneous large B-cell lymphoma (SCLBCL)
s. degeneration
s. electron production
s. electrons
s. extravasation
s. fracture
s. hydrocele
s. hydrocephalus
s. hyperparathyroidism
s. hypertension
s. hypoparathyroidism
s. hypothyroidism
s. lesion
s. lymphangiectasia
s. malignancy
s. myeloid metaphysis
s. obstruction
s. osteosarcoma
s. ovarian tumor
s. peristalsis
s. pleurisy
s. pneumonia
s. pulmonary lobule
s. radiation
s. ray
s. retroperitoneal fibrosis
s. retroperitoneal organ
s. sclerosing cholangitis
s. sequestrum
s. sign
s. sonographic finding
s. teeth
s. ulcer
s. union
s. venous insufficiency
s. wave
s. yolk sac
second-degree
s.-d. AV block
s.-d. heart block
second-echo image
second-order
s.-o. chorda
s.-o. compensation
second-set rejection
second-trimester
s.-t. gestational dating
s.-t. placenta
secretin
secretion
adrenocortical s.
bowel s.
gastric s.
hyperdense sinus s.
mineralocorticoid s.
retained s.
sinonasal s.
tubular kidney s.
secretion-filled bronchus
secretory
s. adenocarcinoma
s. breast disease
s. capacity
s. carcinoma
s. component
s. phase endometrium
section
axial s.
cesarean s.
coronal s.
distal leg cross s.
flood s.
hip muscle cross s.
midfrontal plane coronal s.
paramedian s.
sagittal s.
serial s.
serpiginous s.
step s.
tomographic s.
transverse s.

S

NOTES

sectional
s. radiography
s. segmental anatomy
section-select
s.-s. flow compensation
s.-s. pulse
section-sensitivity profile
sector
s. echocardiography
lower field visual s.
s. scan
s. scan echocardiography
s. scanner
Sommer s.
s. transducer
sector-scan echocardiography imaging
secular equilibrium
secundum
s. atrial septal defect
ostium s.
septum s.
secundus
digitus s.
sedimented calcium
seed
encapsulated radioactive s.
gold s.'s
s. point
radiation s.
s. ribbon
s. voxel
seeding
intracranial s.
metastatic s.
perichondral cell s.
peritoneal s.
prostate s.
radioactive s.
subarachnoid s.
subependymal s.
TheraSeed s.
tumor s.
s. of tumor
seen on end
seesaw peristalsis ureter
Seessel pouch
segment
aganglionic s.
akinetic s.
angulated s.
anterobasal s.
anterolateral s.
aortic s.
aperistaltic distal ureteral s.
apical s.
apicoposterior s.
arterial s.
atretic s.
blind s.
bronchopulmonary s.
cardiac s.
coarcted s.
contiguous s.
diaphragmatic s.
distal s.
s. distraction
diversity s.
duodenal s.
endarterectomized s.
expansile aortic s.
hypokinetic s.
infarcted lung s.
inferoapical s.
inferobasal s.
inferoposterior s.
intercalated s.
interleaved inversion-readout s.
interposed colon s.
intradiaphragmatic aortic s.
intramuscular aortic s.
ischemic s.
joint s.
liver s.
meatal s.
nonfilling venous s.
noninfarcted s.
occlusal s.
posterior apical s.
posterobasal s.
posterolateral s.
proximal s.
pulmonary s.
redundancy of interposed colon s.
septal wall s.
superior s.
taillike s.
variable s.
vaterian s.
venous s.
segmental
s. asynergy
s. atelectasis
s. biliary obstruction
s. bone defect
s. bone loss
s. bowel infarct
s. branch
s. branch of artery
s. bronchus
s. bronchus consolidation
s. bronchus defect
s. bronchus fracture
s. bronchus ischemia
s. bronchus lesion
s. bronchus lower extremity Doppler pressure

s. bronchus narrowing
s. bronchus orifice
s. bronchus perfusion abnormality
s. bronchus plethysmography
s. bronchus renal artery waveform
s. bronchus sign
s. bronchus symptom
s. demyelination
s. dyssynergia
s. k-space turbo gradient-echo breath-hold sequence imaging
s. limb pressure recording
s. liver anatomy
s. lung defect scan
s. lung density
s. mastectomy
s. necrotizing glomerulonephritis
s. nephrogram
s. neurofibromatosis
s. omental infarct
s. pneumonia
s. portal hypertension
s. stenosis
s. vein sclerosis
s. wall motion

segmentation
s. anomaly
automatic lumen edge s.
barium s.
Cannon s.
lung s.
s. method
s. method for real-time display
MRI s.
rhythmic s.
time-resolved imaging by automatic data s. (TRIADS)
vascular s.

segmentectomy

segmented
s. k-space acquisition
s. k-space cardiac tagging
s. k-space time-of-flight MR angiography
s. k-space turbo gradient echo breath-hold sequence

segmenting
s. dual-echo MR head scan
s. dual-echo MR imaging

Segond fracture

Segre chart

Seguin sign

SEH
spinal epidural hemorrhage

SEI
subendocardial infarct

Seidelin body

Seidlitz powder test

Seinsheimer
S. classification of femoral fractures
S. femoral fracture classification

Seitz sign

seizure
absence s.
generalized s.
grand mal s.
s. localization
partial complex s.
s. pattern
petit mal s.
s. phenomenon
repetitive s.'s
s. threshold

Seldinger
S. angiography
S. needle
S. percutaneous technique

selection
s. bias
coil s.
delay time s.
gradient s.
guidance system s.
slice s.

selective
s. angiography
s. arterial injection
s. arterial magnetic resonance angiography
s. cannulation
s. cerebral arteriography
chemical shift s. (CHESS method, CHESS)
s. coronary arteriography
s. coronary arteriography view
s. coronary cineangiography
s. excitation
s. excitation method
s. excitation projection reconstruction imaging
s. hole burning
s. injection
s. irradiation

NOTES

S

selective *(continued)*
s. laser sintering
s. osteal salpingography
s. presaturation MR angiography
s. pulse
s. reduction of pregnancy
s. saturation
s. saturation method
s. saturation recovery
s. scarring
s. separation
S. Tubal Assessment to Refine Reproductive Therapy (STARRT)
s. venography
s. venous magnetic resonance angiography
s. visceral aortography
s. visceral arteriography
s. visualization
selectivity
spatial s.
Selectron system
selenium
s.-75 (^{75}Se)
s. imaging agent
s. plate
selenium-based digital detector
selenium-labeled
s.-l. bile acid imaging
self-articulating
s.-a. femoral (SAF)
s.-a. femoral hip replacement (SAF hip replacement)
self-aspirating cut-biopsy needle
self-breast examination (SBE)
self-expanding
s.-e. metallic endoprosthesis
s.-e. tulip sheath
self-reinforced polyglycolide
self-selection bias
sella, pl. **sellae**
atrophy of dorsum s.
ballooned s.
decalcified dorsum s.
diaphragma s.
dorsum sellae
empty s.
enlargement of s.
s. enlargement
J-shaped s.
tuberculum s.
s. turcica
s. turcica calcification
s. turcica diaphragm
s. turcica tubercle
sella-nasion plane
sellar
s. destruction
s. floor
s. tomography
SEM
scanning electron microscope
semiautonomous nodule
semicircular
s. canal
s. canal hydrops
s. ridge
semicommitted mode
semiconductor
complementary metal oxide s. (CMOS)
semicoronal plane
semidynamic splint
semihorizontal heart
semiinvasive aspergillosis
semilateral position
semiliquid feces
semilobar holoprosencephaly
semilunar
s. aortic valve regurgitation
s. bone
s. bone formation
s. calcification
s. cartilage
s. fold
s. indentation
s. line
s. notch
s. pulmonic valve regurgitation
s. tract
s. valve
s. valve cusp
semilunaris
hiatus s.
linea s.
semimembranosus
s. bursa
s. tendon
semimembranous muscle
seminal
s. colliculus
s. tract
s. vesicle
s. vesicle atrophy
s. vesicle cyst
s. vesicle hypoplasia
s. vesicle invasion (SVI)
seminiferous
s. tubular damage
s. tubule
seminoma
extragonadal s.
mediastinal s.
s. mediastinum
testicular s.
seminomatous tumor

semiopaque
semiovale
centrum s.
semiquantitative measurement
semisolid fecal material
semispinal muscle
semitendinosus tendon
semitendinous muscle
semiupright
s. position
s. view
semivertical heart
^{77}Se MRI spectroscopy
senescence
premature placental s.
senescent
s. aortic stenosis
s. change
senile
s. amyloidosis
s. ankylosing hyperostosis
s. arteriosclerosis
s. change
s. degeneration
s. emphysema
s. fibroma
s. myocardium
s. nephrosclerosis
s. nevus
s. osteomalacia
s. osteoporosis
s. plaque
s. subcapital fracture
senilis
coxa s.
Senographe 500-T mammography
SenoScan mammography system
sensing
s. coil
s. error
sensitive
s. bladder
s. plane
s. plane projection reconstruction imaging
s. point
s. point scanning
s. volume
sensitivity
s. analysis
contrast s.
line-shape s.
percussion s.
poor s.
spectral s.
uniform s.
sensitization
protracted exposure s.
sensitizer
s. enhancement ratio
radiation s.
sensitizing gradient
sensitometric
s. curve
s. strip
sensitometry
sensor
temperature s.
sensorimotor cortex
sensorineural hearing loss
sensory
s. ganglion
s. impairment
s. neurogenic bladder
s. nucleus
s. paralytic bladder
s. root
s. strip
s. tract
s. urgency
sentinel
s. clot sign
s. fold
s. fracture
s. loop
s. loop sign
s. lymphadenectomy
s. lynph node (SLN)
s. node dissection
s. pile
s. transoral hemorrhage
SEP
separation of ghosts
systolic ejection period
separation
acromioclavicular joint s.
aortic cusp s.
atlantoaxial s.
atlantooccipital s.
s. of bowel loop
carrier-free s.
chorioamnionic s.
chromatographic s.
collagen fiber s.

NOTES

S

separation *(continued)*
costochondral junction s.
E point to septal s. (EPSS)
fat/water signal s.
fracture fragment s.
frequency s.
s. of ghosts (SEP)
leaflet s.
meniscocapsular s.
meniscotibial s.
mitral valve septal s.
selective s.
septal s.
shoulder s.

separator tube

Sephadex beads

septal
s. accessory pathway
s. amplitude
s. arcade
s. area
s. asymmetry
s. band
s. bone
s. cartilage plate
s. cirrhosis
s. cusp
s. cusp of calve
s. defect
s. deviation
s. dip
s. to free wall ratio
s. hyperperfusion
s. hypertrophy
s. hypokinesis
s. hypoperfusion
s. leaflet
s. line
s. malformation
s. myocardial infarct
s. necrosis
s. notch
s. papillary muscle
s. perforating branch
s. perforation
s. perforator
s. perforator artery
s. placenta cyst
s. ridge
s. separation
s. tricuspid annulus
s. vein
s. wall
s. wall motion
s. wall motion on echocardiography
s. wall segment
s. wall thickness

septate
s. hypertrophy

septation
gallbladder s.
s. septal defect

septic
s. arthritis
s. bursitis
s. cholangitis
s. diskitis
s. embolus
s. lung
s. lung syndrome
s. necrosis
s. pleurisy
s. pneumonia
s. pulmonary embolus
s. pulmonary infarct
s. sacroiliitis
s. thrombosis

septomarginal
s. band
s. trabecula
s. tract

septostomy
atrial s.
balloon atrial s.

septum
alveolar s.
anal intermuscular s.
anteroapical trabecular s.
aortic s.
aortopulmonary s.
atrial s.
atrioventricular nodal s.
s. band
s. of Bertin
bronchial s.
bulbar s.
canal s.
cartilaginous s.
s. cavum vergae
conal s., conus s.
connective tissue s.
crural s.
distal bulbar s.
dyskinetic s.
epirenal s.
femoral s.
fibrous s.
gingival s.
infundibular s.
intact ventricular s.
interatrial s. (IAS)
interhaustral s.
interlobar s.
interlobular s.
interlobular lung s.

intermuscular s.
internal intermuscular s.
intraventricular s.
Kürner s.
low-signal-intensity fibrous s.
median s.
mediastinal s.
membranous s.
muscular atrioventricular s.
nasal s.
parietal extension of infundibular s.
s. pellucidum
s. pellucidum cavity
perirenal s.
placental s.
posterior median s.
s. primum
rectogenital s.
rectovaginal s.
rectovesical s.
retrovesical s.
s. secundum
sinus s.
subarachnoid s.
thickened s.
s. transversum
s. transversum defect
ventricular s. (VS)

sequela, pl. **sequelae**
late normal tissue s.
significant s.
tissue s.

sequence
amnion rupture s.
breath-hold gradient-recalled echo (GRE) s.
s. bypass graft
cardiac gated PGSE (pulsed-gradient spin-echo) s.
Carr-Purcell s.
Carr-Purcell-Meiboom-Gill s.
cine gradient-echo s.
conventional pulse s.
CP s.
CPMG s.
DANTE s.
diffusion pulse s.
diffusion-sensitive s.
diffusion-weighted pulse s.
double inversion recovery s.
3D spoiled gradient-recalled echo (GRE) s.
3D time-of-flight magnetic resonance angiographic s.
3D transesophageal echocardiographic s.
dual-echo s.
dual gradient-recalled echo (GRE) pulse s.
s. echoplanar imaging
echoplanar pulse s.
fast gradient-echo (GE) s.
FAST pulse s.
Fourier-acquired steady-state technique pulse sequence
fat-suppressed T2-weighted fast spin-echo s.
FISP pulse s.
FLASH 3D pulse s.
flow-compensated gradient-echo s.
gradient-echo imaging s.
gradient-echo pulse s.
GRASS pulse s.
hypervariable s.
in-phase s.
interleaved GRE s.
IRSE s.
Klippel-Feil s.
long TR/TE s.
magnetization-prepared 3D gradient-echo s.
magnetization-prepared rapid acquisition gradient-echo s.
Meiboom-Gill s.
missing pulse steady-state free precession s.
s. monophasic shock
MP-RAGE s.
multiecho s.
multiplanar gradient refocused s.
multislice spin-echo s.
oblique sagittal s.
s. obstruction
opposed-phase s.
partial saturation s.
phase-encode time-reduced acquisition s.
point-resolved spectroscopy s. (PRESS sequence)
postenhancement s.
Potter s.
preenhancement s.
PRESS s.

NOTES

S

sequence *(continued)*
point-resolved spectroscopy sequence
PRIME pulse s.
s. processor
s. pulse
pulse s.
s. quantitative MR imaging
RARE-derived pulse s.
repetitive pulse s.
Robin s.
saturation recovery s.
segmented k-space turbo gradient echo breath-hold s.
Shine-Dalgamo s.
short repetition time s.
short TI inversion recovery pulse s.
simulated-echo s.
single-echo versus multiple-echo s.
single-shot adiabatic localization pulse s.
spin-echo imaging s.
spin-echo pulse s.
spin-echo pulse s.
spin-warp pulse s.
spiral-pulse s.
steady-state free precession s.
STIR s.
susceptibility-sensitive s.
Szumowski s.
three-dimensional time-of-flight MR angiographic s.
s. time
TONE s.
turbo FLASH s.
turbo inversion recovery s.
turbo IR s.
turbo pulse s.
turbo SE s.
T1-weighted coronal fat-suppressed fast spin-echo s.
T2-weighted pulse s.
T2-weighted spin-echo (SE) s.
twin-reversed arterial perfusion s.
velocity-encoded s.
voiding s.
water-selective SE imaging s.

sequential
s. balloon inflation
s. circulator
s. determinant
s. extraction-radiotracer technique
s. films
s. first-pass imaging
s. image acquisition
s. line imaging
s. mode
s. paired opposed plaque (SPOP)
s. plane imaging
s. point imaging
s. postcontrast MR image
s. quantitative MR imaging
s. scalar quantization (SSQ)

sequestered
s. disk
s. lobe
s. lobe of lung

sequestration
bronchopulmonary s.
disk s.
extralobar s.
extrapulmonary s.
fluid s.
intralobar s.
labeled red blood cell s.
pulmonary s. (PS)
s. system
third-space s.

sequestrum, pl. **sequestra**
associated s.
bony s.
kissing sequestra
necrotic s.
primary s.
secondary s.
tertiary s.

sequoiosis

Serax

serendipity view

serial
s. changes
s. cholangiogram
s. contrast MR imaging
s. CT slice
s. cut film technique
s. duplex imaging
s. duplex scan
s. film changer
s. injection
s. lesion
s. radiographic survey
s. radiography
s. section
s. splinting
s. static image
s. static imaging
s. subtraction films

serialography
s. imaging

sericite pneumoconiosis

series, pl. **series**
abdominal s.
acute abdominal s.
cardiac s.
decay s.

dynamic s.
FCS s.
full cervical spine series
gallbladder s. (GBS)
gastrointestinal s.
intubated small bowel s.
lumbosacral s.
metabolic bone s.
motor meal barium GI s.
sinus s.
small bowel s.
upper gastrointestinal s.
seriograph
seriography
serioscopy
SER-IV
supination-external rotation IV
SER-IV fracture
serofibrinous pericardial effusion
serofibrous pleurisy
seroma
mediastinal s.
postoperative s.
seromuscular layer
Serophene
serosa
cecal s.
serosal
s. surface
s. tear
serosanguineous fluid
serous
s. adenocarcinoma
s. carcinoma
s. cyst
s. cystadenocarcinoma
s. cystadenoma
s. effusion
s. intestine
s. ligament
s. membrane
s. ovarian tumor
s. pericardium
s. pleurisy
serpentine
s. aneurysm
s. structure
serpiginosum
angioma s.
serpiginous
s. band
s. low signal intensity border
s. section
s. ulcer
serrated appearance
serration
marginal s.
serratus
s. anterior (SA)
s. anterior muscle
Sertoli
S. syncytium
Sertoli-cell testis tumor
Sertoli-Leydig
S.-L. cell tumor
S.-L. ovarian cell tumor
Servelle vein
Servox amplifier
sesamoid
bipartite s.
s. bone
s. complex
s. injury
s. ligament
s. migration
sesamoidometatarsal joint
sesamophalangeal ligament
sessile
s. adenoma
s. filling defect
s. hydatid
s. lesion
s. nodular carcinoma
s. plaque
s. polyp
s. tumor
sestamibi
s. imaging agent
s. polar map
s. stress scan imaging
s. stress test
technetium-99m s.
s. technetium-99m
set
Amplatz dilator s.
s. angle
s. angle of toes
data s.
3D MRI data s.
Greene biopsy s.
Hawkins inside-out nephrostomy s.
Rutner balloon dilatation helical stone extractor s.
volumetric data s.

NOTES

S

Sethotope radioactive imaging agent
Settegast
S. method
S. position
setting
quadrature s.
simulation-aided field s.
wide window s.
window/level s.'s
setting-sun
s.-s. phenomenon
s.-s. sign
Sever disease
severe
s. acute liver disease
s. acute rejection
s. head injury
s. infarct
s. stenosis
SEW
slice excitation wave
sextuplet pregnancy
sexual differentiation disorder
SFA
superficial femoral artery
SFD
source-film distance
SFR
stenotic flow reserve
shaded-surface
s.-s. display (SSD)
s.-s. display algorithm (SSD algorithm)
s.-s. display CT angiography
s.-s. display imaging (SSD imaging)
shading
s. artifact
image s.
shadow (*See* shadowing)
bandlike s.
bat's wing s.
s. box
breast s.
butterfly breast s.
cardiac s.
cardiothymic s.
cardiovascular s.
centrilobular s.
clean s.
companion s.
concatenation of s.'s
cortical signet ring s.
discoid s.
double-arc gallbladder s.
double-bubble s.
dumbbell-shaped s.
effusion s.
fusiform s.
hilar s.
iliopsoas muscle s.
kidney s.
large thymus s.
line s.
linear s.
mitral configuration of cardiac s.
nipple s.
overlying bowel s.'s
Ponfick s.
psoas s.
PVST s.
radiographic parallel line s.
renal s.
ring s.
scimitar-shaped s.
snowstorm s.
soft tissue s.
spindle-shaped s.
summation of s.'s
superimposition of bowel s.
toothpaste lung s.
tramline s.
tumorlike s.
wall-echo s. (WES)
widened heart s.
shadowing
acoustic s.
dirty acoustic s.
interstitial s.
lateral wall refractive s.
paraspinal soft tissue s.
posterior acoustic s.
refractive s.
rib s.
s. stone
shaft
bone s.
femoral s.
s. flange
s. fracture
middle third s.
ministem s.
proximal third s.
s. of rib
shag
aortic s.
shagging of cardiac border
shaggy
s. aorta syndrome
s. esophagus
s. heart border
s. lung nodule
s. pericardium
shagreen rough skin patch
shaken baby syndrome (SBS)

shallow
s. inspiration
s. inspiratory effort
shank bone
Shape
S. Maker system
shape
baseball bat s.
brachycephalic head s.
cardiac s.
cricket bat s.
dumbbell s.
exponential s.
gooseneck s.
half-moon s.
head s.
horseshoe s.
hourglass s.
line s.
mesocephalic head s.
oval s.
ovoid s.
peak s.
pulse s.
s. recovery
S s.
scaphocephalic head s.
scaphoid s.
sickle s.
spherical s.
spheroid s.
wineglass s.
shaper
beam s.
Shapiro sign
shared coronary artery
sharp
s. border of lung
s. carina
s. dissection
s. lateral margin
Sharpey fibers
sharply demarcated circumferential lesion
Sharp-Purser test
shattered
s. kidney
s. spleen
Shaver disease
shaving
femoral condylar s.
patellar s.
residual metal fragment s.'s
SHC
sclerosing hepatic carcinoma
shear
s. fracture
s. interface
s. strain
s. strain rate
s. stress
shearing
axonal s.
s. force
s. of white matter
s. white matter injury
sheath
angioplasty s.
anterior rectus s.
ArrowFlex s.
arterial s.
axillary s.
bicipital synovial s.
bicipital tendon s.
carotid s.
catheter s.
caudal s.
Check-Flo s.
check-valve s.
Colapinto s.
common synovial flexor s.
Cordis s.
crural s.
dentinal s.
dural s.
extensor carpi ulnaris s.
fascial s.
femoral s.
fenestrated s.
fibrous s.
flexor tendon s.
giant cell tumor of the tendon s. (GCTTS)
guiding s.
Henle s.
intratendon s.
s. ligament
muscle s.
myelin s.
nerve root s.
neural s.
periarteriolar lymphoid s.
periradicular s.

NOTES

S

sheath *(continued)*
pilar s.
plicated dural s.
posterior rectus s.
rectus s.
Schwann cell of myelin s.
self-expanding tulip s.
s. and side-arm
synovial s.
tendon s.
transseptal s.
tulip s.
unplicated s.
vascular s.
venous s.
working s.
sheathing canal
Shebele physician reporting workstation
Sheehan syndrome
sheet
amnionic s.
s. sign
sheetlike
s. dysplasia
s. growth pattern
Sheffield
S. gamma unit
S. modification of Bruce treadmill protocol
Shekelton aneurysm
shelf, pl. **shelves**
Blumer rectal s.
buccal s.
dental s.
lateral s.
medial s.
mesocolic s.
palatine s.
patellar s.
rectal s.
synovial s.
shell
acetabular s.
K s.
L s.
M s.
s. nephrogram
O s.
s. type of periosteal reaction
shelling off of cartilage
shell-of-bone appearance
Shelton femur fracture classification
shelves (*pl. of* shelf)
shelving edge of Poupart ligament
Shenton line
Shepherd fracture
shepherd's
s. crook configuration
s. crook deformity
Shepp-Logan filter function
SHG
sonohysterography
Shibley sign
shibuol
shield
apron s.
Faraday s.
lead apron s.
lead eye s.
radiofrequency magnetic s.
tungsten eye s.
shielding
s. block
faulty radiofrequency s.
magnetic s.
shift
anterior capsular s.
chemical s.
colloid s.
diamagnetic s.
distal s.
Doppler frequency s.
intracranial s.
lanthanide-induced s.
left-to-right s.
mediastinal s.
midline s.
motion-induced phase s.
navigator s.
neonate mediastinal s.
paradigm s.
paramagnetic s.
phase s.
pineal gland s.
pivot s.
plantar s.
s. probe
proximal brain s.
reverse pivot s. (RPS)
right-to-left s.
round s.
simple s.
square brain s.
ST-segment s.
superior frontal axis s.
tracheal s.
velocity-induced phase s.
s. of ventricle
ventricular s.
shill
protrusio s.
shim
s. coil
s. placement

Shimada histopathologic classification
Shimadzu
S. CT scanner
S. MR scanner
S. system
Shimazaki area-length method
shimmed magnet
shimmering
visual s.
shimming
localized s.
passive s.
shin
s. bone
s. splint
Shine-Dalgamo sequence
Shiner radiopaque
Shinnar-LeRoux algorithm
Shirodkar cerclage
shish
s. kebab esophagus
s. kebab pattern
Shmoo sign
shock
s. block
bowel s.
s. bowel
cardiac s.
circulation s.
distributive s.
hypovolemic s.
joule s.
lung s.
s. lung
nephrogram s.
QRS synchronized s.
sequence monophasic s.
shocklike syndrome
shock-monitoring method
shockwave pressure
shoemaker's breast
Shone
S. anomaly
S. syndrome
Shope
S. fibroma
short
s. bone
s. esophagus-type hiatal hernia
s. gut syndrome
s. half-life
s. head
s. head of biceps
s. insular gyrus
s. inversion recovery imaging
s. limb dysplasia
s. muscle
s. oblique fracture
s. radiolunate ligament
s. repetition time sequence
s. rib
s. rib-polydactyly syndrome
s. scale contrast
s. tau inversion recovery (STIR)
s. tau inversion recovery (STIR) image
s. TI inversion recovery (STIR)
s. TI inversion recovery imaging
s. TI inversion recovery pulse sequence
s. T1 inversion recovery (STIR) image
s. T1 relaxation time
short-axis
s.-a. acquisition
s.-a. image
s.-a. parasternal view
s.-a. plane
s.-a. slice
s.-a. view echocardiography
short-bore magnet
short-cannula coaxial method
short-distance
s.-d. radiation therapy
s.-d. radiotherapy
short-echo time
short-echo-time proton spectroscopy
shortening
Achilles tendon s.
circumferential s.
fractional s. (FS)
fractional myocardial s.
left ventricular functional s. (LVFS)
leg s.
phalangeal s.
skeleton s.
suboccipital s.
systolic fractional s.
T1 s.
T2 s.
tendon s.
short-increment sensitivity index
short-range isotope

NOTES

short-T2 in anisotropic rotation
short-term patency
shot
cusp s.
fast low-angle s. (FLASH)
fluid-attenuated inversion recovery-fast low-angle s. (FLAIR-FLASH)
guiding s.
pocket s.
shotgun sign
shotty lymph node
shoulder
s. ankylosis
arthrotomography of s.
baseball s.
curvilinear threshold s.
s. dislocation
s. dome
double-contrast arthrotomography of s.
drooping s.
drop s.
dynamic ultrasound of s. (DUS)
s. dystocia
flail s.
frozen s.
s. girdle
s. of heart
s. immobilizer
s. impingement
s. impingement syndrome
intrathoracic dislocation of s.
s. isocenter
s. joint
s. joint instability
knocked-down s.
s. labral capsular complex
Little Leaguer s.
loose s.
s. muscle
Neviaser classification of frozen s.
s. pad sign
s. pointer
s. presentation
ring man s.
s. separation
sprained s.
step-down deformity of s.
subcoracoid dislocation of s.
subglenoid dislocation of s.
s. surface coil
swimmer's s.
tennis s.
shoulder-hand syndrome
shoulder-upper extremity-thoracic outlet syndrome
shower
s. of echoes
embolic s.
Shprintzen velocardiofacial syndrome
shrapnel
Shrapnell membrane
shrinkage
graft s.
tumor s.
shriveled kidney
shrugging sign
shrunken
s. bladder
s. gallbladder
s. liver
s. lung
shudder
carotid s.
shunt
barium-sulfate impregnated s.
bidirectional s.
biliopancreatic s.
Blalock s.
Blalock-Taussig s.
cardiac atrial s.
cardiovascular s.
cerebral s.
cystoatrial s.
Davidson s.
Denver ascites s.
dialysis s.
distal splenorenal s.
esophageal s.
s. evaluation
s. fraction
Glenn s.
indwelling nonvascular s.
jejunoileal s.
net s.
s. patency
peritoneovenous s. (PVS)
s. placement
portacaval s.
portopulmonary s.
portosystemic s.
posterior fossa-atrial s.
Pott s.
s. quantification
s. reservoir
s. reversal
reversed s.
small bowel s.
transjugular intrahepatic portosystemic s. (TIPS)
s. tube
s. tubing
s. valve
s. with normal left atrium

shunted
s. blood
s. tracer
shunting
s. circuit
s. of tracer to the bone marrow
shuntogram
s. imaging
radionuclide s.
shuntography
shutdown
renal s.
SI
sacroiliac
saturation index
signal intensity
sinus irregularity
stroke index
SI joint
SI joint to sacrum ratio
S/I
superior/inferior
Si
S. (Li) detector
sialadenitis
acute suppurative s.
autoimmune s.
chronic recurrent s.
myoepithelial s.
recurrent s.
sialectasis
sialoadenitis, sialadenitis
sialogram
sialography
CT s.
s. imaging
magnetic resonance s.
s. needle
parotid gland s.
submaxillary s.
sialolithiasis
sialometaplasia
sialometry
sialosis
siboroxime
technetium-99m s.
Sibson
S. fascia
S. groove
S. muscle
sickle shape
sickle-shaped fold
sickling
intravascular s.
sickness
decompression s.
radiation s.
sick sinus node
SID
source-to-image receptor distance
side
s. branch
s. lobe artifact
s. scattering
side-arm
sheath and s.-a.
side-branch occlusion
side-by-side
s.-b.-s. object
s.-b.-s. transposition of great arteries
side-hole cannulated probe
side-lying position
Sideris buttoned double-disk device
sideropenic dysphagia
siderotic splenomegaly
sideswipe fracture
sidewall
s. impingement
pelvic s.
Siemens
S. AG system
S. DRH CT scanner
S. gamma camera
S. Lithostar lithotripter
S. Magnetom GBS II scanner
S. Magnetom SP 4000 scanner
S. Magnetom 1.5-T scanner
S. Magnetom Vision scanner
S. Mevatron 74 linear accelerator
S. One Tesla scanner
S. Satellite CT evaluation console
S. Somaform 512 CT scanner
S. Somatom DR2 and DR3 whole-body scanner
S. Somatom nonhelical unit
S. Sonoline Elegra ultrasound
S. Sonoline Elegra ultrasound scanner
S. SP 4000 scanner
S. 1.5-T system
SieScape
S. ultrasound

S

NOTES

SieScape *(continued)*
S. ultrasound imaging
S. ultrasound scanner
sieve bone
sievert (Sv)
SIF
sacral insufficiency fracture
sigma
s. filter
sigmoid
s. carcinoma
s. cavity
s. cavity of radius
s. cavity of ulna
s. colon
s. colon volvulus
s. curve
s. diverticulitis
s. diverticulum
s. flexure
s. fold
s. hair pattern
s. kidney
s. loop
s. lymph node
s. mesocolon
s. notch
s. omentum
s. polyp
s. sinus
s. valve
s. volvulus
sigmoidoscope
Reichert flexible s.
sigmoidoscopy
sigmoid-shaped configuration
sign
Aaron s.
abdominal aorta crescent s.
abdominal football s.
abdominal string-of-beads s.
Abrahams s.
absent diaphragm s.
absent kidney s.
ace of spades s.
Achilles bulge s.
acute interstitial lung disease s.
Adson s.
air-crescent lung s.
Allen s.
Allis s.
alveolar disease s.
Amoss s.
amputation s.
aneurysmal bone cyst doughnut s.
angel-wing s.
Anghelescu s.
antecedent s.
anterior drawer s.
anterior tibial s.
antler s.
antral nipple s.
anvil s.
aortic arch aneurysm s.
aortic calcification s.
aortic nipple s.
aortic nitrogen-nipple s.
apical cap s.
Apley s.
applesauce s.
Ashhurst s.
Auenbrugger s.
Baart de las Faille s.
Baccelli s.
bagpipe s.
Balance s.
ball-bearing eye s.
Bamberger s.
Bancroft s.
barber pole s.
barber's chair s.
barium snake-head s.
Barlow s.
Battle s.
bayonet s.
B6 bronchus s.
beading s.
beak s.
bear paw s.
Becker s.
Beevor s.
Bergman s.
Bethea s.
beveled edge s.
Biermer s.
bilateral pyramidal s.
Biot s.
Bird s.
bite s.
black pleura s.
bladder-within-bladder s.
Blumberg s.
bottle s.
Bouillaud s.
bowstring s.
bow-tie s.
Boyce s.
Bozzolo s.
Bragard s.
brain aneurysm target s.
brain cord s.
brainstem s.
Braunwald s.
brim s.
Broadbent inverted s.
Brockenbrough-Braunwald s.

bronchial cuff s.
bronchus s.
Brudzinski s.
Bryant s.
bubble s.
bull's eye s.
s. of the burnuous
s. of the burnuous appearance
Burton s.
buttock s.
C s.
calcification s.
calcium s.
camelback s.
Cantelli s.
Carabello s.
Cardarelli s.
cardinal s.
cardiorespiratory s.
Carman s.
Carman-Kirklin meniscus s.
Carman meniscal s.
Carnett s.
carotid dissection string s.
carpal s.
Carvallo s.
Castellino s.
catheter coiling s.
cecal bar s.
Cegka s.
celery stalk s.
cerebral cortical vein s.
Chaddock s.
chain of lakes s.
chest sail s.
chest wave s.
Chilaiditi s.
choppy sea s.
Christmas tree s.
chronic interstitial lung disease s.
Chvostek-Weiss s.
Claybrook s.
Cleeman s.
clockwise whirlpool s.
cobblestoning s.
Codman s.
Cogan lid twitch s.
cogwheel s.
Cole s.
collapsed cava s.
collapsing cord s.
collar s.
Collier s.
colon cutoff s.
colon saw tooth s.
colon whirl s.
comb s.
comet-tail s.
comet-tail lung lesion s.
commemorative s.
common bile duct target s.
Comolli s.
computed tomographic bubble s.
continuous diaphragm s.
contralateral s.
Coopernail s.
cord s.
Corrigan s.
cortical rim s.
cortical vein s.
corticospinal tract s.
coughing s.
Courvoisier s.
cranial nerve s.
crescent s.
crescent hip s.
crescent-in-doughnut s.
crescent lung s.
Crohn disease string s.
Crohn disease target s.
cross-chest impingement s.
crossed sciatica s.
crow's foot gallstone s.
crow's foot lung s.
Cruveilhier s.
CT angiogram lung s.
CT bubble s.
CT halo lung s.
cuff s.
Cullen s.
cupola s.
cutoff colon s.
cyst rebound s.
dagger s.
D'Amato s.
Dance s.
Dawbarn s.
deep sulcus s.
Déjérine s.
de la Camp s.
Delbet s.
Delmege s.
Demianoff s.
de Musset s.

NOTES

sign *(continued)*
de Mussey s.
dense sigmoid sinus s.
dense vein s.
Desault s.
d'Espine s.
detour s.
Deyerle s.
diamond s.
diaphragm collar s.
differential heart density s.
dirty fat s.
displaced crus s.
displaced fat pad s.
Doge cap s.
doorbell s.
Dorendorf s.
dorsal column s.
double-arc lung shadow s.
double-ball s.
double-barrel shotgun s.
double-bleb s.
double-bubble s.
double-bubble duodenal s.
double-camelback s.
double-channel s.
double-cortex s.
double-delta s.
double-density s.
double-duct s.
double-fragment s.
double-fungus-ball wall s.
double-halo s.
double-lesion s.
double-line hip s.
double-target liver s.
double track s.
double-track pylorus s.
double-vessel s.
double wall s.
doughnut s.
drooping lily s.
drooping lily kidney s.
Drummond s.
Duchenne s.
Dupuytren s.
dural trail s.
Duroziez s.
E s.
Ebstein s.
echogenic ring s.
Egawa s.
Ellis s.
Erb s.
Erichsen s.
erosive gastritis target s.
Ewart s.
extrapyramidal tract s.
Fajersztajn crossed sciatic s.
falciform ligament s.
fallen lung s.
false localizing s.
fan s.
fat heart-pad s.
fat-pad s.
fawn-tail s.
Federici s.
feeding-vessel s.
figure-3 s.
figure-of-eight s.
finger-in-glove s.
fingertip s.
Finkelstein s.
Fischer s.
fishnet s.
fissure s.
flank stripe s.
Fleck s.
Fleischner s.
flip-flop s.
floppy-thumb s.
focal neurologic s.
football s.
Forestier bowstring s.
four-artery s.
Fox s.
Frank s.
Fränkel s.
Franz s.
Friedreich s.
Froment paper s.
frontal lobe s.
Frostberg-3 s.
Frostberg inverted-3 s.
Fürbringer s., Fuerbringer
Gaenslen s.
Galant s.
Galeazzi s.
gallbladder halo s.
gallbladder rim s.
garland s.
Garland brain s.
Gerhardt s.
geyser s.
giant cell tumor doughnut s.
Gilbert s.
Glasgow s.
gloved-finger s.
Goldthwait s.
gooseneck s.
Gordon s.
Gottron s.
Gowers s.
Grancher s.
gray-bone-cortex s.
Greene s.

Green-Joynt s.
Grey Turner s.
Griesinger s.
Grocco s.
Grossman s.
guarding s.
Guilland s.
Gunn crossing s.
Hale-Denver s.
Hall s.
halo s.
Hamman pneumopericardium s.
harlequin eye s.
Hart s.
hatchet s.
hay-fork s.
head cheese s.
Heberden s.
Heim-Kreysig s.
Helbing s.
Henning s.
hepatic angle s.
hilar comma s.
hilar waterfall s.
Hildreth s.
Hill s.
hip doughnut s.
hip equator s.
Hirschberg s.
Hoffmann s.
Holman carotid slim s.
Honda s.
Hoover s.
Hope s.
Horn s.
hot-nose s.
Howship-Romberg s.
Huchard s.
Hueter fracture s.
hump and dip breast s.
Huntington s.
hyperdense middle cerebral artery s.
hyperintense ring s.
iliopsoas s.
indistinct liver s.
inferior triangle s.
infundibulum s.
insular ribbon s.
interrupted duct s.
interstitial OB line s.
intestinal doughnut s.
intussusception target s.
inverted pancreatic 3 s.
inverted teardrop s.
inverted-V s.
ipsilateral cerebellar s.
ipsilateral corticospinal tract s.
irregular infrapatellar fat-pad s.
IVP rim s.
J s.
Jaccoud s.
Jackson s.
Jenet s.
jugular s.
jump s.
Jürgensen s.
Kanavel s.
Kantor s.
Kaplan s.
Karplus s.
Katz-Wachtel s.
Keen s.
Kehr s.
Kellgren s.
Kellock s.
Kernig s.
Kerr s.
Kirklin s.
kissing-cousin heart s.
Klemm s.
knuckle lung s.
Kocher-Cushing s.
Korányi-Grocco s.
Kussmaul s.
Lachman s.
Laënnec s.
Lancisi s.
Landolfi s.
Langoria s.
lariat s.
Lasègue s.
lasso s.
lateralizing s.
Laugier s.
Lazarus s.
Leichtenstern s.
lemon s.
Lennhoff s.
Leri s.
Levine s.
ligamentum teres s.
lily-pad s.
Linder s.

NOTES

S

sign *(continued)*
linguine breast s.
liver flap s.
liver-jugular s.
liver ring s.
liver target s.
Livierato abdominocardiac s.
localizing s.
lollipop tree s.
long tract s.
Lorenz s.
Löwenberg s.
Ludloff s.
1-2-3 lung s.
Macewen s.
Mahler s.
Maisonneuve s.
malignant melanoma target s.
Mannkopf s.
Marie-Foix s.
Martorell s.
McCort s.
McGinn-White s.
McMurray s.
melting s.
Meltzer s.
Mendel-Bekhterev s.
meningeal enhancement s.
meningoencephalitic s.
meniscus s.
meniscus lung s.
meniscus notch s.
Mennell s.
metacarpal hand s.
Mexican hat s.
Minor s.
mitosis s.
moon s.
Morquio s.
Morton-Horwitz nerve crossover s.
Moschcowitz s.
motor s.
moulage s.
Mounod s.
mouse bed s.
movie s.
mucosal esophageal stripe s.
Mulder s.
Müller s.
Murphy s.
muscular GI tract rim s.
mushroom s.
Musset s.
mustache s.
mute toe s.
Myerson s.
Naffziger s.
naked-facet s.
naked tuberosity s.
Napoleon hat s.
Neer impingement s.
negative delta s.
Negro s.
Nelson s.
Neri bowing s.
neurologic soft s.
Nicoladoni-Branham s.
Nikolsky s.
noose s.
notch chest s.
nubbin kidney s.
nubbin testis s.
obturator s.
oculomotor s.
Oliver-Cardarelli s.
ominous s.
open bronchus s.
Oppenheim s.
orbicularis s.
orbital coke-bottle s.
organic s.
Ortolani s.
Osler s.
ovulation failure s.
Ozonoff-Ogden s.
pad s.
panda s.
parallel channel s.
parietal lobe s.
Parke corner s.
Parrot s.
patent bronchus s.
pathognomonic s.
pathologic lid retraction s.
Paul s.
Payr s.
percussion s.
Perez s.
peripheral washout liver s.
peritoneal s.
peroneal s.
Pfuhl-Jaffé s.
Phalen s.
pharynx steeple s.
phonatory s.
piano key s.
pillar s.
pillow s.
Pins s.
Piotrowski s.
piston s.
pivot-shift s.
plane s.
pleural tail s.
plumbline s.
Plummer s.

Poppel s.
positive bottle s.
postural motor s.
Potain s.
Pott s.
Pottenger s.
precursor s.
premonitory s.
Prevel s.
Prévost s.
pronator fat pad s.
pruning s.
Prussian helmet s.
pseudobulbar s.
pseudo-Foster-Kennedy s.
pseudointestinal wall s.
pseudokidney s.
pseudotumor s.
psoas s.
puddle s.
pupillary s.
pyloric string s.
pylorus cervix s.
pyramidal s.
Queckenstedt s.
Quénu-Muret s.
Quincke s.
rabbit ear s.
rachitic rosary s.
radialis s.
radiolucent crescent s.
radiolucent liver s.
railroad track s.
Raimiste s.
ram's horn s.
rat-tail s.
rebound s.
rectal halo s.
rectal target s.
renal artery string-of-beads s.
renal cyst beak s.
renal cyst claw s.
renal halo s.
Renee creak s.
retracting clot s.
reversal s.
reversed Mercedes-Benz s.
reverse figure-3 s.
reverse S s.
Reynold s.
Rigler s.
rim s.
ring s.
ring of fire s.
Riordan s.
Risser s.
Rivero-Carvallo s.
Riviere s.
Robertson s.
Rosenbach s.
Rotch s.
Rothschild s.
Rovighi s.
Rovsing s.
Rust s.
Sabathie s.
saddlebag s.
sail s.
Sanders s.
sandwich s.
Sansom s.
Sarbo s.
sawtooth s.
Schepelmann s.
Schick s.
Schlesinger s.
Schoeber s.
Schwartze s.
scimitar s.
scottie dog s.
seagull s.
secondary s.
segmental bronchus s.
Seguin s.
Seitz s.
sentinel clot s.
sentinel loop s.
setting-sun s.
Shapiro s.
sheet s.
Shibley s.
Shmoo s.
shotgun s.
shoulder pad s.
shrugging s.
signet ring s.
silhouette s.
Sister Mary Joseph s.
Skoda s.
slim carotid artery s.
small bowel beak s.
small bowel string-of-beads s.
small bowel whirl s.
Smith s.

S

NOTES

sign *(continued)*
soft neurologic s.
somatic s.
sonographic Murphy s.
sonographic whirlpool s.
Soto-Hall s.
Spalding s.
Speed s.
spinal s.
Spinnaker-sail s.
spread suture s.
spring onion s.
Spurling s.
square-root s.
squeeze s.
stairs s.
steeple s.
Steinberg s.
Steinmann s.
stellate s.
stepladder s.
Sterles s.
Sterling-Okuniewski s.
Sternberg s.
Stewart-Holmes s.
Stierlin s.
Strauss s.
stretch s.
string s.
string-and-double-track s.
string-of-beads s.
string-of-pearls s.
stripe s.
Strümpell s., Struempell
Strunsky s.
subglottic inverted V s.
Sumner s.
superior triangle s.
Swiss cheese liver s.
tail s.
target brain s.
TCC stipple s.
telangiectatic osteosarcoma doughnut s.
telltale triangle s.
Terry fingernail s.
Terry Thomas s.
testis doughnut s.
tethered-bowel s.
theater s.
Thomas s.
thorn s.
thread-and-streaks tumor thrombus s.
thumbprinting s.
Thurston Holland s.
thyroid halo s.
tibialis s.
Tinel percussion s.
toe spread s.
transverse colon stripe s.
trapezius ridge s.
Traube aortic regurgitation s.
Trimadeau s.
triple-bubble s.
triple-pylorus track s.
triple-track s.
tripod s.
Troisier s.
trolley-track s.
Trömner s., Troemner
trough s.
Trousseau s.
trumpet nerve root s.
Turner s.
Turyn s.
twin peak s.
Uhthoff s.
upper motor neuron s.
urachal GI tract s.
ureter Bergman s.
ureter catheter coiling s.
ureter goblet s.
ureteric rim s.
vacuum cleaner s.
Vanzetti s.
vein s.
vital s.
Voshell s.
Waddell s.
wall s.
Walter-Murdoch wrist s.
Wartenberg s.
washout liver s.
waterfall right hilum s.
water lily lung s.
wave s.
Weill s.
Weiss s.
Westermark s.
wet leather s.
whirl s.
whirlpool s.
white cerebellum s.
white matter s.
Williams s.
Williamson s.
Wilson s.
Wimberger s.
windshield wiper s.
windsock s.
winking owl spinal s.
Wintrich s.
wooden shoe s.

Signa
S. Advantage system

S. GEMS MR imaging system
S. Horizon scanner
S. 1.5-T scanner

signal
abnormal bright s.
s. acquisition
s. attenuation
s. average
s. blooming
bright s.
s. change
color Doppler s.
composite s.
D s.
s. dephasing
s. depth
differential s.
disk water s.
Doppler blood flow velocity s.
Doppler ovary s.
s. drop-out artifact
s. enhancement
s. fallout
flow velocity s.
free-induction s.
gamma s.
high-intensity s.
high-pitched s.
hyperintense s.
hypointense s.
increased echo s.
s. intensity (SI)
s. intensity inhomogeneity
s. intensity ratio
s. intensity rim
s. intensity time curve
s. joint
lipid s.
s. loss
magnetic resonance s.
s. magnification
mosaic-jet s.
navigable echo s.
s. node
nuclear s.
ovarian Doppler s.
periventricular bright s.
s. processing
proton magnetic resonance s.
pseudogap s.
radionuclide s.
s. sonographic feature analysis
s. source
SSFP s.
stimulus-correlated s.
stimulus-correlated water s.
superimposition of s.'s
s. time course
s. transducer
s. transduction
turbulent s.
s. void
weak s.

signal-averaged
s.-a. electrocardiogram (SaECG)

signal-to-clutter ratio

signal-to-noise
s.-t.-n. calculation
s.-t.-n. ratio (S/N ratio, SNR)
s.-t.-n. threshold

signature
echo s.
gut s.

signet
s. ring appearance
s. ring cell carcinoma
s. ring pattern
s. ring sign

significance level

significant
s. axis deviation
s. residual deficit
s. sequela

Silastic
S. collar-reinforced stoma
S. finger joint
S. ring

silence
electrocerebral s. (ECS)

silent
s. area of brain
s. cerebral embolus
s. gallstone
s. ischemic episode
s. mitral stenosis
s. myocardial infarct
s. myocardial ischemia
s. patent ductus arteriosus
s. regurgitation

silhouette
cardiac s.
cardiovascular s.
enlarged cardiac s.

S

NOTES

silhouette *(continued)*
figure-of-eight cardiac configuration s.
heart s.
s. image
s. imaging
luminal s.
s. phenomenon
roentgenographic s.
s. sign
s. sign of Felson
s. technique
widened cardiac s.
silhouetted out
silicate pneumoconiosis
silicon
amorphous s.
s. diode array
s. diode dosimeter
silicon-controlled rectifier (SCR)
silicone
s. elastomer band
s. elastomer ring
s. elastomer rubber ball implant
s. fluid
s. implant leakage
s. implant rupture
s. injection
s. microsphere
s. wrist implant
Silicon Graphics Reality Engine system
silicosis
chronic simple s.
complicated s.
Liverpool s.
nonnodular s.
simple s.
silicotic
s. fibrosis of lung
s. granuloma
s. material
s. nodule
s. visceral pleura
silicotuberculosis
silk
s. suture
s. tuft
sillimanite pneumoconiosis
silo
s. filler's disease
s. filler's lung
s. filler's lung
silver
s. bromide
s. finisher's lung
s. fork fracture
Grocott methenamine s.
s. halide film
s. polisher's lung
s. recovery
s. wire effect
SIM
small intestine mesentery
simian griffe
Simmond disease
Simon
S. focus
Simonart
S. band
S. ligament
SIM/Plant
simple
s. block
s. bolus
s. bone cyst
s. breast cyst
s. capillary lymphangioma
s. coal worker's pneumoconiosis
s. cortical renal cyst
s. dislocation
s. extraperitoneal rupture
s. goiter
s. mechanical obstruction
s. meningocele
s. shift
s. silicosis
s. skull fracture
s. ureterocele
simplex
xanthoma tuberosum s.
Simpson
S. atherectomy
S. atherectomy device
S. AtheroCath
S. Coronary AtheroCath (SCA) system
S. rule method for ventricular volume
white line of S.
S. white line
Sims position
simulated
s. annealing
s. annealing method
s. annealing method projection
s. echo
s. echo artifact
s. equilibrium factor study
simulated-echo sequence
simulation
s. of converging ports
s. film
laboratory s.
MCPT s.
Monte Carlo photon transport s.

s. of tangential portals
s. of treatment arena
simulation-aided field setting
simulator
AcQsim CT s.
magnetic resonance s.
Maxwell 3D field s.
MR s.
virtual reality s.
Ximatron s.
simultaneous
s. balloon inflation
s. bilateral spontaneous pneumothorax (SBSP)
s. fluoroscopy
s. recording
s. thermoradiotherapy (STRT)
s. volume imaging
sincalide
sincipital cephalocele
Sinding-Larsen-Johansson disease (SLJD)
sine wave
singer's
s. node
s. nodule
Singh
S. index of osteoporosis
S. osteoporosis index
single
s. atrium
s. axis
s. breath-hold
s. colonic filling defect
s. fill/void technique
s. isocenter
s. label
s. peak
s. plane left ventriculogram
s. pleurisy
s. polyp
s. port
s. suture synostosis
s. umbilical artery
s. ventricle
s. x-ray dosimetry
single-breath view
single-cannula atrial cannulation
single-cavity cochlea
single-contrast
s.-c. arthrography
s.-c. barium enema
single-dose gadolinium imaging
single-echo
s.-e. diffusion imaging
s.-e. versus multiple-echo sequence
single-energy x-ray absorptiometer (SXA)
single-field hyperthermia technique
single-head rotating gamma camera
single-lumen silicone breast implant
single-lung transplantation
single-outlet heart
single-photon
s.-p. absorptiometry (SPA)
s.-p. counting system (SPC system)
s.-p. densitometer
s.-p. emission computed tomography (SPECT)
s.-p. emission computed tomography (SPECT) technetium sestamibi scan
s.-p. emission CT
s.-p. emission tomography (SPET)
s.-p. planar scintigraphy (SPPS)
single-plane angiography
single-pole double-throw (SPDT)
single-shot
s.-s. adiabatic localization pulse sequence
s.-s. imaging technique
s.-s. MR cholangiogram
single-slice
s.-s. gradient-echo image
s.-s. long-axis tomogram
s.-s. modified KEW direct Fournier imaging
"single-stick" system
single-strand scission
single-stripe colitis (SSC)
single-vessel
s.-v. disease
s.-v. runoff
single-view oblique mammography
single-voxel
s.-v. proton brain spectroscopy imaging
s.-v. proton spectroscopy
sinistral portal hypertension
sinistrum
atrium s.
sink
s. effect
quantum s.

NOTES

sink-trap malformation
sinoatrial (SA)
s. block (SAB)
s. branch
s. bundle
s. conduction time (SACT)
s. exit block
s. nodal reentry tachycardia
s. node (SA node, SAN)
s. node artery (SANA)
s. node dysfunction
s. node infarct
sinoauricular node
sinodural plate
Sinografin
S. imaging agent
sinogram
sinography
sinonasal
s. carcinoma
s. cavity
s. lesion
s. lymphoma
s. polyposis
s. psammomatoid ossifying fibroma
s. secretion
s. tumor
sinotubular junction
sinovaginal bulb
sintering
selective laser s.
sinus
accessory s.
alternating s.
aortic valve s.
s. arrest
artery of inferior cavernous s. (AICS)
atlas articular s.
barber's pilonidal s.
basilar s.
branchial s.
Breschet s.
bronchial s.
carotid s.
cavernous s.
s. cavity
cerebral venous s.
cervical s.
circular s.
coccygeal s.
coronary s. (CS)
costomediastinal s.
cranial s.
s. cycle length (SCL)
dilated intercavernous s.
distal coronary s. (DCS)
dorsal dermal s.
dorsal enteric s.
draining s.
dural venous s.
dura mater venous s.
endodermal s.
s. of epididymis
ethmoid s.
frontal s.
granulomatous lesion of s.
Guérin s.
s. histiocytosis
s. hyperplasia
hypoechoic renal s.
s. hypoplasia
inferior sagittal s. (ISS)
intercavernous s.
s. irregularity (SI)
lactiferous s.
lateral s.
s. lateralis
left coronary s.
s. lipomatosis
lumbosacral dermal s.
lymph node s.
manual pressure over carotid s.
marginal s.
mastoid s.
maxillary s.
s. mechanism
medullary s.
middle coronary s. (MCS)
s. of Morgagni
nasal s.
s. nodal artery
s. nodal reentry
s. node
s. node automaticity
s. node depression
s. node dysfunction
s. node exit block
s. node recovery time (SNRT)
noncoronary s.
oblique pericardial s.
occipital s.
opacification of maxillary s.
osteomyelitic s.
paranasal s.
s. pattern
s. pause
pericardial s.
s. pericranii
perineal s.
Petit s.
petrosal s.
pilonidal s.
piriform s.
precoronal sagittal s.
prostatic s.

pulmonary s.
s. of pulmonary trunk
renal s.
s. rhythm
s. rhythm mapping
Ridley s.
Rokitansky-Aschoff s. (RAS)
rudimentary s.
sagittal s.
s. septum
s. series
sigmoid s.
s. slowing
sphenoid s.
sphenoparietal s.
subeustachian s.
superior sagittal s. (SSS)
tarsal s.
s. tarsi syndrome
thickened s.
s. thrombosis
s. tract
s. tract imaging
s. tract study
transverse pericardial s.
urachal s.
urogenital s.
s. of Valsalva
s. of Valsalva aneurysm
valve of coronary s.
s. of vena cava
s. venosus
s. venosus atrial septal defect
venous s.
vertebral articular s.

sinusitis
acute s.
allergic s.
bacterial s.
bronchiectasis-ethmoid s.
s. cerebritis
chronic s.
mycotic s.
paranasal s.
sphenoidal s.

sinusoid
hepatic s.
s. reference function

sinusoidal
s. capillary
s. histiocyte
s. lesion
s. relaxation
s. vascular space
s. waveform

sinuum
confluens s.

sinuvertebral nerve of Luschka

SIP
saturation inversion projection

siphon
carotid s.

Sipple
S. disease
S. syndrome

sirenomelia

SISCO spectrometer

Sister
S. Mary Joseph node
S. Mary Joseph nodule
S. Mary Joseph sign

site
anastomotic s.
binding s.
bleeding s.
cellular binding s.
donor s.
extraadrenal s.
extranodal s.
fracture s.
ipsilateral antegrade s.
s. of maximal intensity
reference s.
sanctuary s.
unknown primary s.

site-specific labeling

sitting-up
s.-u. view
s.-u. view angiography

situ
adenocarcinoma in s.
carcinoma in s.
ductal carcinoma in s. (DCIS)
in s.
intracystic breast papillary carcinoma in s.
lobular carcinoma in s. (LCIS)

situs
atrial s.
s. atrialis solitus
s. concordance
D-loop ventricular s.
s. inversus totalis
s. inversus viscerum

NOTES

situs *(continued)*
L-loop ventricular s.
s. perversus
s. transversus
s. viscerum inversus
Sitzmarks radiopaque marker
sixth
s. compartment
s. nucleus
s. ventricle
size
abnormal placental s.
borderline heart s.
decreased placenta s.
embryo s.
s. estimation error
gallbladder s.
kernel s.
kidney s.
ovarian s.
renal s.
s. of spinal cord
top normal limits of s.
uterine s.
ventricular s.
voxel s.
x-ray beam s.
sizing ring
Sjögren
S. orbital syndrome
S. syndrome
SJS
Schwartz-Jampel syndrome
skeletal
s. amyloidosis
s. bed
s. biopsy
s. disruption
s. dysplasia
s. dysplasia in fetus
s. emphysema
s. hyperostosis
s. hypoplasia
s. lesion
s. lymphoma
s. metastasis
s. muscle
s. muscle fiber
s. neoplasm
s. radiology
s. survey
s. system
skeletally
s. immature
s. mature
skeleton
appendicular s.
articulated s.
axial s.
bony s.
cardiac s.
fibrous s.
gill arch s.
laryngeal s.
s. shortening
spidering s.
spiky s.
sulcal s.
visceral s.
skeletonizing
skier's
s. fracture
s. injury
s. thumb
skijump view
Skillern fracture
skimming of magnetic field
skin
s. bridge
s. calcification
s. cancer
s. collimation
s. crease artifact
s. depth
s. dose
s. effect
s. fold
s. fold artifact
s. lesion
s. lesion artifact
s. line
s. pore
s. staple
s. thickening
skin-rolling scapular tenderness
skin-sparing
s.-s. effect
s.-s. mastectomy (SSM)
Skiodan
S. Acacia
S. imaging agent
skip
s. aganglionosis
s. area
s. lesion
s. metastasis
skodaic resonance
Skoda sign
skull
abnormally thin s.
s. asymmetry
base of s. (BOS)
s. base
beaten brass s.
beaten silver appearance of s.
button sequestrum s.

cloverleaf s.
dentate suture of s.
s. film
s. fracture
geographic s.
hair-on-end of s.
hammered silver s.
hammer-marked s.
hot-cross-bun s.
s. hyperostosis
indented fracture of s.
inner table of the s.
lacunar s.
lytic lesion of s.
molding of s.
occipital view of s.
s. osteolysis
outer table of the s.
s. plate
sonolucent s.
thin s.

skull-base tumor

skyline
s. view
s. view of patella

SL
scapholunate
SL joint
SL technique

slab
coronal s.
interleaved axial s.

SLAC
scapholunate advanced collapse
scapholunate arthritic collapse
SLAC wrist

slant hole collimator

slanting
tibiotalar joint s.
s. tibiotalar joint

SLAP
superior labral anterior to posterior
SLAP lesion
SLAP tear

sleeve
s. fracture
s. lobectomy
nerve root s.
thoracic root s.

slice
angled s.
apical short-axis s.
axial s.
basal short-axis s.
contiguous s.'s
coronal s.
digitized s.'s
digitized CT s.
s. excitation wave (SEW)
s. format
s. fracture
s. geometry
horizontal long axis s.
s. interference
intermediate CT s.
long-axis s.
midventricular short-axis s.
nonplanar s.
oblique s.
s. orientation
s. overlap artifact
plurality of s.'s
s. profile artifact
sagittal s.
s. selection
s. selection gradient
s. sensitivity profile (SSP)
serial CT s.
short-axis s.
texture s.
s. thickness
tissue s.
tomographic s.
transaxial s.
transverse s.
two-dimensional sequential s.
vertical long-axis s.
s. volume

slice-of-sausage breast pattern

slice-point MRS

slice-selective excitation

slicing plane

slider crank theory

sliding
s. hiatal hernia
s. thin-slab maximum intensity projection CT imaging
s. thin-slab, minimum intensity projection technique

slim
s. carotid artery sign
s. disease

sling
cardiac s.

NOTES

sling *(continued)*
s. muscle fiber
pulmonary s.
s. ring complex
tendon s.
vascular s.
slip
s. angle
diaphragmatic s.
muscular s.
slip-angle spondylolisthesis
slip-in connection
slippage
epiphyseal s.
film s.
slipped
s. capital femoral
s. capital femoral epiphysis (SCFE)
s. intervertebral disk
s. tendon
s. upper femoral epiphysis (SUFE)
slipping
s. rib
s. rib syndrome
slip-ring
s.-r. camera
s.-r. CT
s.-r. gantry system
s.-r. imaging
s.-r. technology
slit
s. hemorrhage
s. radiography
s. ventricle
slitlike
s. lumen
s. orifice
slit-shaped vessel lumen
slit-ventricle syndrome
sliver
bone s.
SLJD
Sinding-Larsen-Johansson disease
SLN
sentinel lynph node
slope
s. blot analysis
closing s.
decreased E-to-F s.
disappearance s.
downward s.
D-to-E s.
E-to-F s.
flat diastolic s.
flattened E-to-F s.
mitral deceleration s.
opening s.
ST/HR s.
ST segment/heart rate slope
treadmill s.
triquetrohamate helicoid s.
valve opening s.
sloughed
s. mucosa
s. papilla
s. urethra syndrome
slow
s. exchange soft tissue
s. filling wave
s. neutron
s. stroke
s. ventricular response
slow-channel blocking drug
slow-flow
s.-f. lesion
s.-f. vascular anomaly
s.-f. vascular malformation
slowing
sinus s.
slowly
s. developing atelectasis
s. developing lesion
SLP
sludge
s. ball
biliary s.
blood s.
gallbladder s.
tumefactive s.
tumefactive biliary s.
sludge-like intraluminal echo
sludging of retinal vein
sluggish flow
sluggishly flowing blood
Sly disease
Sm
samarium
SMA
spinal muscular atrophy
small
s. airway
s. airway dysfunction
s. angle double incidence
s. B-cell lymphoma
s. bowel
s. bowel adenocarcinoma
s. bowel adenoma
s. bowel atresia
s. bowel beak sign
s. bowel benign tumor
s. bowel cancer
s. bowel cavitary lesion
s. bowel contents
s. bowel delayed transit
s. bowel diverticulum
s. bowel duplication cyst

s. bowel enema
s. bowel enteroscopy (SBE)
s. bowel filling defect
s. bowel fold anatomy
s. bowel folds atrophy
s. bowel followthrough (SBFT)
s. bowel gas
s. bowel hemangioma
s. bowel hemorrhage
s. bowel infarct
s. bowel leiomyoma
s. bowel leiomyosarcoma
s. bowel loop
s. bowel malignant tumor
s. bowel malrotation
s. bowel meal
s. bowel metastasis
s. bowel motility
s. bowel mucosal pattern
s. bowel multiple ulcer
s. bowel obstruction (SBO)
s. bowel peristalsis
s. bowel pseudodiverticula
s. bowel pseudotumor
s. bowel series
s. bowel shunt
s. bowel string-of-beads sign
s. bowel transit time
s. bowel volvulus
s. bowel whirl sign
s. cardiac vein
s. cell carcinoma of lung
s. cell osteogenic sarcoma
s. cleaved-cell lymphoma
s., deep, recent infarct (SDRI)
s. feminine aorta
s. field-of-view MR imaging
s. gallbladder
s. gut
s. internal auditory canal
s. intestine
s. intestine cancer
s. intestine mesentery (SIM)
s. left colon syndrome
s. lymphocytic T-cell lymphoma
s. noncleaved NHL
s. parts of fetus
s. pelvis
s. round cell carcinoma
s. saphenous vein
s. spleen
s. unilateral adrenal tumor
s. urinary bladder capacity
s. vertebral body
s. water-hammer pulse

small-angle
s.-a. double-incidence angiogram (SADIA)
s.-a. multiple scattering

small-aorta syndrome

small-cell
s.-c. cribriform cancer
s.-c. lung carcinoma (SCLC)
s.-c. undifferentiated carcinoma

small-cuff syndrome

small-droplet fatty liver

small-for-gestational-age fetus

small-lunged emphysema

small-step distraction

small-vessel stroke

SMAP
systemic mean arterial pressure

SmartPrep
S. imaging agent

SmartPrep scanner

SmartSpot
S. high-resolution digital imaging
S. high-resolution digital imaging system

SMAS
superior mesenteric artery syndrome

smear fragment

Smith
S. dislocation
S. fracture
S. orthogonal hole test
S. sesamoid position classification
S. sign

Smith-Lemli-Opitz syndrome

SMM
scintimammography

SMN
second malignant neoplasm

smokelike echo

smoker's
s. bronchiolitis
s. lung

smoking
passive s.

smoldering multiple myeloma

smooth
s. border
s. brain
s. esophageal narrowing

NOTES

smooth *(continued)*
s. hyperplasia
s. muscle
s. muscle tumor
smooth-bordered
smoothed curve fit
smoothing
gaussian s.
smooth-muscle hypertrophy
SMR
scatter-maximum ratio
smudged papilla
SMV
superior mesenteric vein
Smythe syndrome
Sn
stannum
^{113}Sn
tin-113
snake graft
snake's head appearance
snapping
s. fascia lata
s. hip
s. hip syndrome
snapshot
contrast-enhanced dynamic s.
dynamic s.
Sneppen fracture of talus
sniff test
SNM
Society of Nuclear Medicine
snowflake pattern
snowman
s. abnormality
s. appearance of heart
s. deformity
s. heart configuration
snowplow
s. effect
s. occlusion
snowstorm
s. breast pattern
s. shadow
SNR
signal-to-noise ratio
S/N ratio
SNRT
sinus node recovery time
snuffbox
anatomic s.
snufftaker's pituitary disease
Snyder classification
soap
calcium bile s.
soap-bubble radiolucency
Society
American Roentgen Ray S.
S. of Magnetic Resonance in Medicine
Musculoskeletal Tumor S. (MSTS)
S. of Nuclear Medicine (SNM)
Southeastern Neuroradiological S.
Western Neuroradiological S.
World Federation of Neuroradiological S.'s
socket/residuum interface
socket-stump interface
sodium
s.-23 (^{23}Na)
s.-2-mercaptoethane sulfonate
acetrizoate s.
s. bicarbonate solution imaging agent
s. chloride imaging agent
s. chromate
s. detector
s. diatrizoate imaging agent
s. diatrizoate with Menoquinon imaging agent
fluorescein s.
s. imaging
s. iodide (NaI)
s. iodide crystal
s. iodide iodine-131
s. iodide ring
s. iodide ring imaging agent
s. iodipamide imaging agent
iodohippurate s.
s. iodohippurate imaging agent
iodomethamate s.
s. iodomethamate imaging agent
iothalamate s.
s. iothalamate imaging agent
ioxaglate s.
ipodate s.
s. ipodate imaging agent
liothyronine s.
methiodal s.
s. methiodal imaging agent
s. metrizoate
s. pertechnetate
pertechnetate s.
s. pertechnetate imaging agent
s. phosphate
s. phosphate ^{32}P
s. reabsorption
s. salicylate
technetium-99m pertechnetate s.
tetrabromophenolphthalein s.
s. tetradecyl sulfate
tetraiodophenolphthalein s.
s. thiosulfate
s. thorium tartrate imaging agent
total exchangeable s. (TENa)

tyropanoate s.
s. tyropanoate imaging agent

sodium-24 (^{24}Na)

Soemmerring
S. ligament
S. muscle

soft
s. disk
s. disk herniation
s. food dysphagia
s. infiltrate
s. neurologic sign
s. palate
s. palate cancer
s. papilloma
s. photons
s. pigment stone
s. ray
s. tissue
s. tissue abnormality
s. tissue abscess
s. tissue attenuation value
s. tissue canal encroachment
s. tissue chondroma
s. tissue contracture
s. tissue contusion
s. tissue defect
s. tissue density
s. tissue density structure
s. tissue distraction
s. tissue entrapment
s. tissue envelope
s. tissue fibroma
s. tissue ganglion
s. tissue gas
s. tissue hemangioma
s. tissue injury
s. tissue interposition
s. tissue lesion classification
s. tissue lipoma
s. tissue lipomatosis
s. tissue mass
s. tissue necrosis
s. tissue neoplasm
s. tissue ossification
s. tissue osteochondroma
s. tissue osteoma
s. tissue radiograph
s. tissue reaction
s. tissue sarcoma
s. tissue shadow
s. tissue stranding
s. tissue swelling
s. tissue uptake bone scintigraphy
s. tissue window

softball sliding injury

soft-copy computed radiography

softening
s. of brain
s. of cartilage

software
DecThreads s.
Kodak s.
modified vessel image processor s.
multiplanar gradient-echo s.
NeuroEcho s.
Neuro Lobe s.
Neuro SPGR s.
P-LINK s.
SPARC s.
Starlink s.
VERT s.
Viewmax s.
Viewnex s.
Voxel-Man s.
VoxelView s.

SOG
supraorbital groove

sojourn time

solar
s. plexus
s. radiation

Solayrès obliquity

soldier's
s. heart
s. heart syndrome
s. patches of pericardium
s. spot

soleal
s. line
s. vein

solenoid
s. surface coil

soleus
s. muscle

Soleus syndrome

solid
s. bolus challenge
s. bone
s. bony union
s. circumscribed breast carcinoma
s. and cystic pancreatic tumor
s. echo
s. edema

NOTES

solid *(continued)*
s. edema of lung
s. food dysphagia
s. lesion spleen
s. lesion thymus
s. mass
s. matrix
s. ovarian teratoma
s. ovarian tumor
s. and papillary pancreatic carcinoma
s. periosteal reaction
s. phase extraction
s. pilocytic astrocytoma
s. splenic lesion
s. thymic lesion
s. viscus injury
solid-phase extraction tube
solid-state
s.-s. detector
s.-s. manometry catheter
s.-s. nuclear track detector
solitary
s. bone cyst
s. bone myeloma
s. cold lesion
s. dilated duct
s. fibrous tumor of pleura
s. gallstone
s. left IVC
s. lung nodule
s. lymph node
s. mass
s. metastatic lung nodule
s. osteochondroma
s. osteosclerosis
s. osteosclerotic lesion
s. plasmacytoma
s. pleura tumor
s. pulmonary nodule (SPN)
s. rectal ulcer
s. rectal ulcer syndrome
s. relapse
s. small bowel filling defect
solitus
abdominal situs s.
atrial situs s.
cardiac situs s.
situs atrialis s.
visceral situs s.
Solomon-Bloembergen
S.-B. equation
S.-B. theory of dipole-dipole relaxation rate
Solomon syndrome
Solu-Biloptin
S.-B. imaging agent
solute
solution
aqueous s.
Carnoy s.
hyperosmotic s.
Melrose s.
phosphotope oral s.
radioelement s.
saline s.
saturated potassium iodide s. (SSKI)
Solutrast
solvent
s. suppression
s. water TI frequency dependence
SOM
supraorbital margin
SOMA
subjective, objective, management, and analytic
SOMA classification
SOMA scale
somatic
s. muscle
s. sign
Somatom DR CT scanner
somatosensory cortex
Somatostatin imaging agent
Sommer sector
Sondermann canal
Sones
S. cineangiography technique
S. coronary arteriography imaging
S. selective coronary arteriography
S. technique for cineangiography
sonic-accelerated fracture-healing system (SAFHS)
sonicated
s. albumin microbubbles
s. meglumine sodium imaging agent
s. Renografin-76 imaging agent
sonication
Sonicator portable ultrasound
sonic effect
Sonifer sonicating system
SONK
spontaneous osteonecrosis of knee
Sonnenberg classification of erosive esophagitis
sonoangiogram
Sonocut ultrasonic aspirator
sonogram
dual transverse linear-array s.
fatty meal s. (FMS)
real-time s.
transabdominal s.

Sonographers
American Registry of Diagnostic Medical S. (ARDMS)
sonographic
s. assessment
s. diagnosis
s. echo
s. feature analysis
s. guidance
s. hip type
s. Murphy sign
s. parameter
s. whirlpool sign
sonography
abdominal s.
Acuson computed s.
Acuson transvaginal s.
breast s.
carotid s.
color-coded duplex s.
color-coded real-time s.
color-flow Doppler s.
color power transcranial Doppler s.
compression s.
Doppler s.
duplex pulsed Doppler s.
endoanal s.
endoluminal s.
endoscopic s.
endovaginal s.
fatty meal s. (FMS sonography)
fetal s.
FMS s.
fatty meal sonography
freehand interventional s.
gray-scale s.
hysterosalpingo-contrast s.
intraoperative s. (IOS)
obstetric s.
pelvic s.
penile s.
power Doppler s.
thoracic s.
transabdominal color Doppler s.
transcranial real-time color-flow Doppler s.
transrectal s.
transvaginal s. (TVS)
sonohysterography (SHG)
Sonoline
S. Elegra ultrasound system
S. Sierra ultrasound imaging system
sonologist
sonolucent
s. area
s. cystic lesion
s. cystic mass
s. doughnut
s. halo
s. layer
s. skull
s. zone
sonometer
Sahara clinical bone s.
SoundScan 2000 bone s.
SoundScan Compact bone s.
SonoRx
Sonos ultrasonographic transducer
Sorbie
S. calcaneal fracture classification
S. classification of calcaneal fracture
sorbitol 70% imaging agent
Sorbol heel
sorption
s. kinetics
s. potential
sorter
FACSVantage cell s.
fluorescence-activated cell s. (FACScan)
Soto-Hall sign
Sotos syndrome
souffle
funic s.
funicular s.
placental s.
systolic mammary s.
sound
s. beam
bowel s.'s
heart s.'s
palpable aortic ejection s.
palpable pulmonic ejection s.
pericardial knock s.
s. transmission
s. wave
SoundScan
S. 2000 bone sonometer
S. Compact bone sonometer

NOTES

sour
s. fluid regurgitation
s. stomach
source
americium radioactive s.
s. of artifact scintigraphy
cobalt radioactive s.
discrete bleeding s.
dummy s.
external heat generating s.
fiberoptic light s.
gold radioactive s.
heat-generating s.
Heyman-Simon s.
s. imaging
interstitial heat-generating s.
intracavitary radiation s.
intrastitial radiation s.
iodine radioactive s.
radioactive s.
radium radioactive s.
remote-controlled implantation of radioactive s.
signal s.
yttrium radioactive s.
source-film distance (SFD)
source-skin distance (SSD)
source-surface distance (SSD)
source-to-image receptor distance (SID)
source-tray distance (STD)
Southeastern Neuroradiological Society
S/P
status post
SP6 camera
SPA
single-photon absorptiometry
space (*See* spacing)
abdominal s.
acromioclavicular s.
air s.
alveolar dead s.
anatomic dead s.
antecubital s.
anterior clear s.
anterior pararenal s. (APS)
apical air s.
arachnoid s.
axillary s.
Baros s.
Berger s.
Bogros s.
Bowman s.
buccal s.
Burns s.
capsular s.
carotid s.
cartilage joint s.
Chassaignac s.
Cloquet s.
Colles s.
coracoclavicular s.
Cotunnius s.
C-Y color s.
dead s.
s. deficit
disk s.
Disse s.
dorsal subaponeurotic s.
dorsal subcutaneous s.
echo s.
echo-free s.
enlarged presacral s.
epicardial s.
epidural s.
episcleral s.
epitympanic s.
extraaxial s.
extracellular s.
extradural s.
extrapleural s.
fibulocalcaneal s.
fifth intercostal s.
fluid s.
focal dilatation of air s.
foraminal s.
fourth intercostal s.
free pericardial s.
gingival s.
Henke s.
His perivascular s.
Holzknecht s.
hyperintense marrow s.
increased lateral joint s.
infraglottic s.
inframesocolic s.
intercellular s.
intercondylar joint s.
intercostal s.
interlobar s.
intermetatarsal s.
interosseous s.
interpeduncular s.
interpleural s.
interstitial fluid s.
intervertebral disk s.
intrathecal s.
intravascular s.
joint s.
Kiernan s.
Kretschmann s.
Kuhnt s.
lateral joint s.
left intercostal s. (LICS)
Lesgaft s.
Lesshaft s.
lung air s.

Magendie s.
Malacarne s.
masticator s.
Meckel s.
medial joint s.
midpalmar s.
Mohrenheim s.
mucosal pharyngeal s.
narrowed rib s.
narrowing of joint s.
orbital s.
paralaryngeal s.
parapharyngeal s.
pararenal s.
Parona s.
patellofemoral joint s.
pelvic s.
peribronchial alveolar s.
pericardial s.
peridental s.
perihepatic s.
perineal s.
perinephric s.
perirenal s.
perisinusoidal s.
peritoneal s.
perivascular s.
plane of intercostal s.
pleural s.
Poirier s.
Poiseuille s.
popliteal s.
portacaval s.
portal s.
posterior cervical s.
posterior septal s.
predental s.
preepiglottic s.
premasseteric s.
presacral s.
prevertebral s.
Prussak s.
pulp s.
Q s.
radiolucent joint s.
Reinke s.
retrocardiac s.
retrocrural s.
retrogastric s.
retromammary s.
retroorbital s.
retropancreatic preaortic s.
retroparotid s.
retroperitoneal s.
retropharyngeal s.
retrosphenoidal s.
retrosternal s.
retrosternal air s.
retrovesical s.
s. of Retzius
s. of Retzius abscess
saclike s.
scapholunate s.
Schwalbe s.
sinusoidal vascular s.
subacromial s.
subarachnoid s.
subdural s.
subhepatic s.
subperitoneal s.
subphrenic s.
subpulmonic pleural s.
subtalar joint s.
subtendinous s.
subtrapezial s. (STS)
subumbilical s.
supracolic s.
suprahepatic s.
supralevator s.
supratentorial s.
syndesmotic clear s.
Talairach s.
target tarsometatarsal joint s.
Tarin s.
terminal air s.
thenar s.
tibiocalcaneal s.
tissue s.
trapezium-trapezoid joint s.
Traube semilunar s.
Trautmann triangular s.
vascular placenta s.
ventricular s.
vesicovaginal s.
Virchow perivascular s.
Virchow-Robin s.
Waldeyer s.
web s.
Westberg s.
widened joint s.
widened retrogastric s.
Zang s.
zonular s.

S

NOTES

space-occupying
s.-o. lesion
s.-o. mass
s.-o. process
spacing
gray-level s.
multiple-beam interface s.
parallel-line-equal s. (PLES)
spade
s. field
s. finger
spadelike
s. appearance
s. hand
spade-shaped valvotome
Spalding sign
spall
spallation
s. product
SPAMM
spatial modulation of magnetization
SPAMM technique
span
levator s.
liver s.
ventricular s.
SPARC software
sparing
arytenoid s.
spark gap generator
sparkling appearance of myocardium
SPARS
spatially resolved spectroscopy
sparsity of bone formation
spasm
arterial s.
bowel s.
bronchial smooth muscle s.
catheter-induced coronary artery s.
colonic s.
coronary artery s. (CAS)
coughing s.
diffuse arteriolar s.
diffuse esophageal s. (DES)
esophageal s.
hemifacial s.
inspiratory s.
intermittent diffuse esophageal s.
muscle s.
postbypass s.
respiratory s.
vascular s.
venous s.
spasmodic stricture
spastic
s. bowel syndrome
s. colitis
s. colon
s. electron paramagnetic resonance (EPR) imaging
s. equinovarus deformity
s. esophagus
s. heart
s. hindfoot valgus deformity
s. ileus
s. mapping
s. pseudosclerosis
s. registration
s. urinary bladder
spastica
dysphagia s.
spatial
s. average-pulse average (SAPA)
s. average-pulse average (SAPA) intensity
s. average-temporal average (SATA)
s. average-temporal average (SATA) intensity
s. encoding
s. filter
s. frequency
s. frequency domain
s. frequency error
s. localization procedure
s. mapping
s. misregistration artifact
s. modulation of magnetization (SPAMM)
s. modulation of magnetization (SPAMM) image
s. offset image artifact
s. orientation
s. origin
s. peak-temporal average (SPTA)
s. peak-temporal average (SPTA) intensity
s. position
s. presaturation
s. reconstruction
s. registration
s. resolution
s. resolution scintigram
s. selectivity
s. vectorcardiography
spatially
s. resolved spectroscopy (SPARS)
s. selective inversion pulse
spatial-spectral prepulses for fat saturation
SPC system
SPDT
single-pole double-throw
Spearman rank
special bolus
speciation
physicochemical s.

specific
s. absorption rate (SAR)
s. activity
s. modulation
specified
not otherwise s. (NOS)
specimen
breast core biopsy s.
specious finding
speck finger
speckle
blood s.
speckled pattern
SPECT
single-photon emission computed tomography
acetazolamide-enhanced SPECT
brain perfusion SPECT
SPECT brain perfusion scintigraphy
SPECT center of rotation
cerebral SPECT
dual-head SPECT
dual-isotope SPECT
dynamic volumetric SPECT
electrocardiogram-gated SPECT
FDG SPECT
GE SPECT
gradient-echo
ictal technetium Tc-99m HMPAO (hexamethylpropyleneamine oxime) brain SPECT
SPECT imaging
interictal SPECT
pharmacologic stress dual-isotope myocardial perfusion SPECT
SPECT quality control
quantitative gated SPECT (QGS)
^{99m}Tc red blood cell SPECT
SPECT thallium scintigram
SPECT thallium scintigraphy
Trionix SPECT
SPECT uniformity
spectamine
s. brain imaging
iodine-123 brain imaging s.
spectography
nuclear magnetic resonance (NMR) s.
spectra (*pl. of* spectrum)
spectral
s. analysis
s. broadening
s. diffusion
s. Doppler
s. Doppler imaging
s. emission
s. line
s. noise distribution
s. pattern
s. sensitivity
s. ultrasound
s. waveform
s. width
s. window
spectral-spatial
s.-s. fat suppression
s.-s. image
Spectranetics excimer laser
spectrin
spectrofluorometry
spectrometer
beta-ray s.
Bragg s.
Bruker AMX 300 NMR s.
Compton suppression s.
EDXRF s.
gamma-ray s.
GE GN300 7.05-T/89-mm bore multinuclear s.
GE NMR s.
IBM NMR s.
liquid scintillation s.
Mossbauer s.
Nicolet NMR s.
NMR s.
PROBE-SV s.
Rapid Scan s.
SISCO s.
Varian Associates 11.7-T, 51-mm bore s.
Varian NMR s.
VT multinuclear s.
x-ray s.
spectrometry
accelerator mass s. (AMS)
Compton suppression s.
Fourier transform NMR s.
liquid scintillation s.
pulsed L-band ESR s.
scintillation s.
spectrophotometer
F-1200 fluorescence s.
F-2000 fluorescence s.

NOTES

spectrophotometer *(continued)*
F-4500 fluorescence s.
U-1100 UV-Vis s.
spectrophotometric
s. calculation
s. quantity
spectrophotometry
atomic absorption s.
ultraviolet s.
spectroscopic chemical-shift method
spectroscopy
atomic absorption s.
carbon-13 s.
circular dichroism s.
COSY H-1 MR s.
CSI s.
depth-resolved surface coil s. (DRESS)
diffusion s.
2D J-resolved 1H MR s.
double-spin echo proton s.
electrospray ionization mass s.
flame emission s. (FES)
fluorescence s.
fluorine-19 s.
Fourier transform infrared s.
Fourier transform Raman s.
glutamate s.
H-1 MR s.
image-selected in vivo s.
INVOS 2100 optical s.
ISIS s.
localized H1 s.
magnetic resonance s. (MRS)
MR proton s.
near-infrared s. (NIRS)
nonresonance Raman s.
nuclear magnetic resonance (NMR) s.
oxygen-17 NMR s.
^{31}P s.
phosphorus magnetic resonance s. (P-MRS)
plasma emission s.
point-resolved s. (PRESS)
proton nuclear magnetic resonance s.
Raman s.
^{77}Se MRI s.
short-echo-time proton s.
single-voxel proton s.
spatially resolved s. (SPARS)
surface-coil rotating-frame s.
in vivo proton MR s.
spectrum, pl. **spectra, spectrums**
absorption x-ray s.
S. DG-P pediatric cradle
electromagnetic s.
energy s.
frequency s.
gamma-ray s.
infinitesimal Z s.
infrared s.
invisible s.
lissencephaly-pachygyria s.
midsystolic notching of velocity s.
nuclear magnetic resonance (NMR) s.
proton nuclear magnetic resonance s.
pulmonary sequestration s.
thermal s.
ultraviolet s.
Wiener s.
x-ray s.
SPECTurn chair
specular
s. echo
s. reflector
speech area
speed
film s.
incremental increases in treadmill s.
Speed sign
Spence
axillary tail of S.
tail of S.
Spengler fragment
Spens syndrome
spent phase
spermatic
s. artery
s. calculus
s. cord
s. cord torsion
s. vein
s. venography
spermatocele
spermatogonia
sperm granuloma
SPET
single-photon emission tomography
SPGR
spoiled GRASS
S-phase
S.-p. analysis
S.-p. fraction
S.-p. fractionation
sphenocephaly
sphenoethmoidal
s. encephalocele
s. recess
s. suture
sphenoid
s. angle

s. bone
s. bone fracture
s. fontanelle
s. ridge
s. ridge meningioma
s. ridge tumor
s. sinus
s. sinus metastasis
s. wing
s. wing meningioma

sphenoidal
s. encephalocele
s. fissure syndrome
s. fossa
s. sinusitis
s. turbinated bone

sphenoidale
planum s.
pneumatosis s.
rostrum s.

sphenomandibularis muscle

sphenomandibular ligament

sphenomaxillary encephalocele

sphenooccipital
s. chordoma
s. suture
s. synchondrosis

sphenoorbital
s. encephalocele
s. suture

sphenopalatine
s. canal
s. ganglion
s. neuralgia

sphenoparietal
s. sinus
s. sulcus
s. suture

sphenopetrosal suture

sphenopharyngeal
s. canal
s. encephalocele
s. meningoencephalocele

sphenosquamous suture

sphenotemporal suture

sphenovomerine suture

sphere
s. organelle
resin s.

spherical
s. lesion
s. map
s. mass
s. neoplasm
s. shape
s. structure

spheroid
s. shape
tumor s.

spherule

sphincter
antral s.
s. atony
basal s.
bicanalicular s.
s. of bile duct
Boyden s.
canalicular s.
cecal s.
choledochal s.
colic s.
s. contraction ring
cricopharyngeal s.
duodenal s.
duodenojejunal s.
external anal s.
external urethral s.
extrinsic s.
first duodenal s.
functional s.
hypertensive lower esophageal s.
Hyrtl s.
s. incompetence
inferior esophageal s. (IES)
lower esophageal s. (LES)
Lutkens s.
Nélaton s.
O'Beirne s.
s. of Oddi
s. of Oddi manometry
pancreatic duct s.
pancreaticobiliary s.
pharyngoesophageal s.
physiologic s.
prepyloric s.
s. preservation
pyloric s.
radiologic s.
upper esophageal s. (UES)

sphincteric mechanism

sphygmography

spicular
s. density
s. protrusion

NOTES

spiculated
s. carcinoma
s. distortion
s. mass
s. scirrhous lesion
spicule
bony s.
thorny s.
spider
s. angioma
s. finger
s. nevus
s. pelvis
stainless steel s.
s. x-ray view
spidering skeleton
spiderlike
s. calix
s. pelvocaliceal system
spiderweb
s. appearance
s. circulation
spigelian
s. fascia
s. hernia
s. lobe
spike
s. averaging
s. loading
s. staple
spiking
interictal s.
spiky skeleton
spill
ileal s.
spin
s. coupling
s. density
s. density weighted
s. dephasing
s. diffusion
s. echo
electron s.
s. exchange
s. flip
flowing s.
high s.
J-coupled s.
nuclear s.
s. quantum number
stationary s.
s. tagging
uncoupled s.
s. vector
spina, pl. **spinae**
s. bifida
s. bifida aperta
s. bifida occulta (SBO)
erector spinae
s. ventosa
spinal
s. accessory lymph node
s. accessory nerve
s. angiogram
s. angulation
s. artery
s. axis
s. axis tumor
s. chordoma
s. column stabilization
s. concussion
s. cord
s. cord atrophy
s. cord caliber
s. cord canal
s. cord cleft
s. cord compression
s. cord decompression
s. cord depression
s. cord diameter
s. cord ependymoma
s. cord glioma
s. cord hemisection
s. cord infarct
s. cord injury (SCI)
s. cord injury without radiographic abnormality (SCIWORA)
s. cord laceration
s. cord lesion
s. cord metastasis
s. cord parenchyma
s. cord sarcoidosis
s. cord stroke
s. cord transsection
s. cord tumor
s. degeneration
s. dermal sinus tract
s. dermoid
s. diastematomyelia
s. dorsal horn
s. dural arteriovenous fistula
s. empyema
s. endplate change
s. epidural abscess (SEA)
s. epidural hemorrhage (SEH)
s. epidural lymphoma
s. fixation
s. fixation device
s. fluid
s. fracture
s. fusion
s. ganglion
s. growth
s. hemiplegia
s. hydatid cyst
s. infection

s. inflammation
s. instability
s. integrity
s. lordosis
s. medulla
s. meningioma
s. muscular atrophy (SMA)
s. needle
s. nerve plexus
s. nerve root avulsion
s. osteochondrosis
s. osteomyelitis
s. osteophyte
s. pedicle
s. plasma cell myeloma
s. root
s. sac
s. sign
s. stenosis
s. subarachnoid hemorrhage
s. subdural hemorrhage (SSH)
s. syndesmophyte
s. teratoma
s. tuberculosis
s. vascular malformation
ventral derotating s. (VDS)
s. videofluoroscopy

spinalis
funiculus medullae s.

spindle
aortic s.
s. colonic groove
His s.
muscle s.
ureteral s.

spindle-shaped
s.-s. aneurysm
s.-s. muscle
s.-s. shadow

spine
alar s.
s. angioreticuloma
angulation of s.
anterior column of s.
anterior-inferior iliac s.
anterior maxillary s.
anterior-superior iliac s. (ASIS)
anteroposterior iliac s.
arachnoid loculation of the s.
bamboo s.
caroticojugular s.
cervical s.
cervical fusion of s.
Charcot s.
coccygeal s.
dendritic s.
dens view of cervical s.
dorsal s.
epidermoid s.
extension injury of s.
fetal s.
functional units of s.
iliac s.
instability of s.
intermaxillary s.
ischial s.
kinetic cervical s.
kissing s.
lateral bending views of s.
s. lipoma
lumbar s.
lumbarized s.
lumbosacral s. (LS)
maxillary s.
mental s.
microcystic lumbar s.
midthoracic s.
nasal s.
s. ossification
poker s.
posterior column of s.
posterior-inferior s.
rotatory load on s.
rugger-jersey s.
sacral s.
scoliotic s.
static cervical s.
thin-plate s.
thoracic s.
thoracolumbar s.
trochanteric s.

spin-echo
s.-e. cardiac imaging
s.-e. image
s.-e. imaging sequence
inversion recovery s.-e. (IRSE)
s.-e. magnetic resonance imaging
s.-e. pulse sequence
s.-e. pulse sequence
s.-e. scan
s.-e. technique
s.-e. using repeated gradient echoes

NOTES

S

spin-label
s.-l. method
s.-l. technique
spin-lattice
s.-l. relaxation
s.-l. relaxation time
spin-lock
s.-l. imaging technique (SL technique)
s.-l. and magnetization transfer imaging
s.-l. prepulse
spin-lock-induced T1-rho weighted image
spin-locking
off-resonance s.-l.
Spinnaker-sail sign
spinning-top
s.-t. test
s.-t. urethra
spinocerebellar
s. ataxia
s. degeneration
s. tract
spinocervical tract
spinocervicothalamic tract
spinoglenoid
s. ligament
s. notch
spinographic
s. angle
s. line
spinography
digitized s.
spinoreticular tract
spinosum
foramen s.
spinotectal tract
spinothalamic tract
spinous
s. foramen
s. plane
s. process
s. process avulsion
s. process fracture
spin-phase
s.-p. graph
s.-p. phenomenon
spin-spin
s.-s. coupling
s.-s. relaxation
s.-s. relaxation time
spintharicon
spinthariscope
spin-warp
s.-w. imaging
s.-w. method
s.-w. pulse sequence
SPIO
superparamagnetic iron oxide
SPIO imaging
SPIO imaging agent
spiperone
^{18}F s.
spiral
s. appearance
s. arthrosis
s. band of Gosset
s. computed tomography
s. computed tomography arteriography (SCTA)
s. CT angiography (SCTA)
s. CT pitch
s. CT pitch pit
s. CT scanner
s. CT scanning
s. dissection
s. flow pattern
s. fold
s. imaging method
s. ligament
s. oblique fracture
s. scanning technique
s. valve
s. volumetric CT
s. XCT scanner
s. x-ray computed tomography (SVCT)
spiral-pulse sequence
spirometer flow rate
spirometric acquisition
spirometrically
s. controlled CT
s. controlled CT imaging
spirometry
full-volume loop s.
Spitzka-Lissauer tract
spitzoid malignant melanoma
splanchnic
s. aneurysm
s. AV fistula
s. blood
s. vascular imaging
s. vasculature
s. venous system
s. vessel
splash
succussion s.
splayed cranial suture
splayfoot deformity
splaying
s. of frontal horn
s. of pedicles
spleen
aberrant s.
absence of s.

accessory s.
s. angiosarcoma
delayed rupture s.
s. dimension
ectopic s.
epithelial s.
floating s.
hamartoma s.
hyperdense s.
increased density s.
s. inflammation
inflammatory s.
large s.
s. lesion
liver, kidneys, and s. (LKS)
long axis of s.
microabscess of the s.
nonvisualization of s.
s. peliosis
primary cyst of s.
prolapse of s.
ruptured s.
s. sarcoidosis
shattered s.
small s.
solid lesion s.
tip of s.
s. ultrasonography imaging
wandering s.

spleen-to-liver ratio
splenectomy
splenia (*pl. of* splenium)
splenial branch of posterior cerebral artery
splenic

s. abscess
s. angle
s. arteriography
s. artery (SA)
s. artery aneurysm
s. artery pseudoaneurysm
s. AV fistula
s. B-cell lymphoma
s. bleeding
s. bump
s. calcification
s. capsule
s. cleft
s. congestion
s. epidermoid cyst
s. flexure
s. flexure cancer
s. hamartoma
s. hemangioma
s. hilum
s. hyperplasia
s. infarct
s. lesion
s. lobule
s. lymph node
s. metastasis
s. microabscess
s. notch
s. portal venography
s. portography
s. pseudocyst
s. rupture
s. scintigraphy
s. torsion
s. trauma
s. vein
s. vein thrombosis
s. venography
s. vessel

spleniculus, pl. **spleniculi**
splenium, pl. **splenia**

s. of corpus callosum

splenization
splenobronchial fistula
splenocaval
splenocolic ligament
splenogastric omentum
splenography
splenoma
splenomegaly

congenital s.
congestive s.
Egyptian s.
fibrocongestive s.
Gaucher s.
hemolytic s.
infectious s.
myelophthisic s.
Opitz thrombophlebitic s.
persistent s.
postcardiotomy lymphocytic s.
siderotic s.

splenomyelomalacia
splenoportal junction
splenoportogram
splenoportography

s. imaging

splenorenal

s. anastomosis

NOTES

splenorenal *(continued)*
s. angle
s. arterial bypass graft
s. ligament
s. recess
splenosis
abdominal s.
thoracic s.
splenunculus, pl. **splenunculi**
splicing
spline curve
splint
birdcage s.
semidynamic s.
shin s.
thigh s.
splintered
s. bone
s. fracture
splinter hemorrhage
splinting
serial s.
Spli-Prest
S.-P. buffer
S.-P. latex
S.-P. negative control
S.-P. plate
S.-P. positive control
split
s. atlas
s. brain
s. compression fracture
s. cranium
s. foot deformity
s. image artifact
s. renal function decrease
s. spinal cord
split-brain
s.-b. imaging
s.-b. study
split-cord syndrome
split-course
s.-c. accelerated radiation therapy
s.-c. accelerated radiotherapy
s.-c. hyperfractionated radiation therapy
s.-c. technique
split-function scintigraphy
split-heel fracture
split-notochord syndrome
splitter
beam s.
splitting
s. fracture
plaque s.
sternal s.
zero-field s.
Spli-Tube
SPN
solitary pulmonary nodule
SPOCS
Surgical Planning and Orientation Computer System
spoiled
s. gradient-echo imaging
s. gradient-recalled acquisition
s. GRASS (SPGR)
spoiler
s. gradient
s. gradient pattern
lucite beam s.
spoiling
radiofrequency (RF) s.
surface s.
spoke
s. bone
s. wheel pattern
Sponastrine dysplasia
spondylarthritis
spondylitic
s. change
s. deformity
spondylitis
ankylosing s.
cryptococcal s.
s. deformans
lung ankylosis s.
rheumatoid s.
tuberculous s.
spondyloarthritis, pl. **spondyloarthritides**
spondyloarthropathy
destructive s.
spondyloepiphyseal dysplasia
spondylolisthesis
degenerative s.
isthmic s.
sagittal roll s.
slip-angle s.
spondylolytic s.
traumatic s.
spondylolisthetic pelvis
spondylolysis
traumatic s.
spondylolytic spondylolisthesis
spondylomalacia
spondylosis
cervical spine s.
s. deformans
degenerative s.
diffuse s.
Nurick classification of s.
spondylosyndesis
sponge
blood-filled bone s.
Ivalon s.
s. kidney

medullary s.
Ray-Tec x-ray detectable surgical s.
surgical s.
Vistec x-ray detectable s.

spongiform
s. change
s. degeneration
s. leukoencephalopathy

spongioblastoma

spongiocytoma

spongiosa of mitral valve

spongiosis

spongiosum
corpus s.

spongy
s. appearance
s. bone
s. osteoma
s. white matter degeneration

spontaneous
s. abortion
s. carotid dissection
s. closure of defect
s. conversion
s. coronary artery dissection (SCAD)
s. detorsion
s. disintegration
s. drainage
s. echo contrast
s. fetal movement
s. fracture
s. hematoma
s. infantile ductal aneurysm
s. intracranial hypotension
s. involution
s. lesion
s. osteonecrosis
s. osteonecrosis of knee (SONK)
s. perforation
s. perforation of common bile duct
s. pneumomediastinum
s. regression
s. renal hemorrhage
s. subsidence
s. tension pneumothorax
s. transient vasoconstriction
s. urinary extravasation

spoonlike
s. protrusion
s. protrusion of leaflet

spoon-shaped nail

SPOP
sequential paired opposed plaque
SPOP technique

sporadic
s. Burkitt lymphoma
s. colorectal carcinoma
s. tumor

sporotrichosis

spot
blooming focal s.
capitate soft s.
Carleton s.
coast of California café-au-lait s.
coast of Maine café-au-lait s.
cold s.
s. compression
s. compression magnification mammography
s. compression view
cotton-wool s.
s. film
focal s. (FS)
hematocystic s. (HCS)
hot s.
hyperechoic splenic s.
s. image
s. magnification
s. radiograph
Roth s.
s. scanning
soldier's s.
thermal hot s.
tree-shaped s.

spot-compression paddle

spot-film
s.-f. fluorography
s.-f. imaging
s.-f. radiography

spotted nephrogram

SPPS
single-photon planar scintigraphy

SPR
scanned projection radiography
superior peroneal retinaculum

sprain
acute s.
chronic s.
eversion s.
s. fracture
inversion s.

NOTES

S

sprain *(continued)*
sacroiliac s.
syndesmosis s.
sprained
s. ankle
s. shoulder
sprain-strain
spray
pulse fashion pulse s.
resorcinol s.
spread
s. Bragg peak
distant s.
intraocular s.
pattern of s.
perineural tumor s.
regional s.
subependymal s.
s. suture
s. suture sign
transfascial s.
s. of tumor
Sprengel deformity
spring
s. ligament
s. onion sign
s. onion ureter
spring-driven system
Springer fracture
sprinter's fracture
sprodiamide imaging agent
sprue
celiac s.
nontropical s.
tropical s.
SPTA
spatial peak-temporal average
spur
acromial s.
anterior s.
bone s.
bronchial s.
calcaneal s.
calcific s.
degenerative s.
drum s.
s. formation
heel s.
hypertrophic marginal s.
impingement s.
inferior s.
marginal s.
medial traction s.
Morand s.
osteoarthritic s.
Pelkan s.
plantar calcaneal s.
posterior s.
prominent s.
retrocalcaneal s.
traction s.
uncovertebral s.
spuriae
costae s.
spurious
s. aneurysm
s. ankylosis
s. finding
s. pregnancy
Spurling sign
spurring
bony s.
degenerative s.
hypertrophic marginal s.
marginal s.
osteophytic s.
ulnar traction s.
uncovertebral s.
squamocolumnar junction
squamooccipital bone
squamosal suture
squamosomastoid suture
squamosoparietal suture
squamososphenoid suture
squamous
s. bone
s. cell carcinoma
s. cell papilloma
s. endothelium
s. intraepithelial lesion
s. metaphysis
s. metaplasia
s. metaplasia white epithelium
s. odontogenic tumor
s. suture
s. urinary bladder
square
s. brain shift
s. wave
squared
s. patella
s. vertebral body
squared-off
s.-o. heart
s.-o. thorax
square-root sign
squares
least s. (LS)
squatting
s. facet
s. maneuver
s. position
squeeze sign
Squibb system

SQUID
superconducting quantum interference device
Sr
strontium
^{89}Sr
strontium-89
^{89}Sr (strontium) bracelet
^{90}Sr
strontium-90
^{90}Sr-loaded eye applicator
SSC
single-stripe colitis
SSD
shaded-surface display
source-skin distance
source-surface distance
SSD algorithm
SSD imaging
SSFP
steady-state free precession
steady-state free progression
SSFP magnetization
SSFP process
SSFP signal
SSH
spinal subdural hemorrhage
S-shaped
S.-s. pouch
S.-s. scoliosis
SSKI
saturated potassium iodide solution
SSM
skin-sparing mastectomy
SSP
slice sensitivity profile
stereotactic surface projection
subclavian steal syndrome
SSPE
subacute sclerosing panencephalitis
SSQ
sequential scalar quantization
SSS
superior sagittal sinus
stability
bony s.
s. of fracture
stabilization
s. plate
spinal column s.
stabilizer
dynamic s.
static s.
stabilizing bullet
stable
s. cavitation
s. disease
s. fracture
s. free radical
s. isotope
s. reduction
s. xenon CT
stable-state tuberculosis
stacked
s. ovoid lesion
s. scan
s. tomogram
stacked-coin appearance
stacked-foil technique
stacked-metaphor workstation
stacked-scan imaging
STAG
striped tag myocardial tagging system
stage
exudative s.
resolution s.
s. 4S neuroblastoma
staghorn
s. calculus
s. stone
staging
Berndt-Hardy talar lesion s.
Chang s.
distraction-flexion s. (DFS)
Ficat avascular necrosis s.
Gottschalk s.
Greulich and Pyle skeletal maturation s.
invasive surgical s. (ISS)
Jackson s.
Jewitt-Whitmore s.
Kadish s.
lymphoma s.
s. of malignancy
malignant melanoma s.
MSTS s.
neuraxis s.
neuroblastoma s.
Outerbridge degenerative arthritis s.
pre-slip s.
stagnant-loop syndrome
stag wound

NOTES

stainless
s. steel coil
s. steel mesh stent
s. steel microsphere
s. steel plate
s. steel spider
staircase phenomenon
stairs sign
stairstep
s. air-fluid level
s. artifact
s. fracture
stalactite phenomenon
stalk
body s.
fibrovascular s.
infundibular s.
pituitary s.
polyp s.
s. of polyp
tumor s.
standard
ACR teleradiology s.
s. Bruce protocol
s. deviation
gold s.
Greulich and Pyle bone age s.
international s. (IS)
s. multiecho
National Bureau of S.'s (NBS)
s. single echo
s. uptake value (SUV)
Wilmad reference s.
standby rate
standing
s. dorsoplantar view
s. lateral view
s. postvoid view
s. wave
s. weightbearing view
standoff
standstill
atrial s.
cardiac s.
ventricular s.
Stanford
S. aortic dissection classification
S. type B aortic dissection
S. and Wheatstone stereoscope
Stanley cervical ligament
stannous
s. chloride
s. pyrophosphate
stannum (Sn)
stapedes (*pl. of* stapes)
stapedial
s. artery
s. nerve anatomy
s. otosclerosis
stapedius
stapes, pl. **stapedes**
staphylococcal pneumonitis
staphyloma
staple
metallic s.
orthopedic s.
skin s.
spike s.
stone s.
surgical s.
star
s. artifact
s. effect
s. pattern
Starcam camera
star-cancellation test (SCT)
Starling curve
Starlink software
Starr-Edwards valve
STARRT
Selective Tubal Assessment to Refine Reproductive Therapy
STARRT falloposcopy system
starry sky pattern
star-shaped vessel lumen
start test pattern
stasis, pl. **stases**
antral s.
bile s.
bladder s.
s. of blood flow
chronic venous s.
circulation s.
s. cirrhosis
s. edema
s. gallbladder
s. liver
s. ulcer
ureteral s.
venous s.
state
cardiac steady s.
chronic constrictive s.
contrast-enhanced fast-acquisition in a steady s. (CE-FAST)
s. equilibrium
fast adiabatic trajectory in steady s. (FATS)
gradient-recalled acquisition in a steady s. (GRASS)
ground s.
high-output s.
hypoperfused s.
inducibility basal s.
oxidation s.

Statham electromagnetic flowmetry
static
s. cervical spine
s. coupling
s. 3D FLASH imaging
s. foot deformity
s. image
s. image display
s. lung
s. magnetic field
s. stabilizer
s. view
station
MacSpect real-time NMR s.
oscilloscope tuning s.
stationary
s. field
s. spin
s. zero-order motion
statistical noise
status
compromised respiratory s.
intravascular volume s.
Karnofsky performance s. (KPS)
s. post (S/P)
ventricular s.
Staunig
S. method
S. position
STD
source-tray distance
SteadFAS
steady-state
s.-s. field pulse
s.-s. free precession (SSFP)
s.-s. free-precession imaging
s.-s. free precession sequence
s.-s. free progression (SSFP)
s.-s. gradient-echo imaging
steal
arterial s.
coronary artery s.
false s.
pelvic s.
s. phenomenon
subclavian s.
s. syndrome
transmural s.
STEAM
stimulated-echo acquisition mode
steatosis
hepatic s.
liver s.
Stecher position
steel coil
Steel-Dwaas
S.-D. analysis
S.-D. method
steep
s. left anterior oblique projection
s. left anterior oblique view
s. Towne projection
s. Trendelenburg position
steeple sign
steering
beam s.
coaxial s.
electronic independent beam s.
steganography
Steinberg
S. classification
S. sign
Steinbrocker rheumatoid arthritis classification
Steinert epiphyseal fracture classification
Stein-Leventhal syndrome
Steinmann sign
Steinstrasse calculus
Stejskal and Tanner pulsed-gradient spin-echo technique
stellar nevus
stellate
s. border breast lesion
s. configuration
s. confluence
s. crease
s. defect
s. granuloma
s. ligament
s. mass
s. pattern
s. sign
s. skull fracture
s. tear
s. undepressed fracture
stem
s. base plate
bronchus s.
roundback s.
straight s.
stem-loop structure
Stener lesion

NOTES

S

stenocardia
stenogyria
stenosed aortic valve
stenosing ring of left atrium
stenosis, pl. **stenoses**
acquired aortic valve s.
acquired mitral s.
acquired spinal s.
ampullary s.
anal s.
anastomotic s.
antral s.
s. of aorta
aortic s. (AS)
aortoiliac s.
aqueductal s.
s. area
arterial s.
atheromatous s.
atherosclerotic s.
atypical aortic valve s.
benign papillary s.
bicuspid valvular aortic s.
bilateral carotid s.
bowel s.
branch pulmonary artery s.
bronchial s.
buttonhole mitral s.
calcific bicuspid valvular s.
calcific senile aortic valvular s.
canal s.
carotid artery s.
central canal s.
central spinal s.
cerebral artery s.
cervical s.
choledochoduodenal junctional s.
circumferential venous s.
common pulmonary vein s.
concentric hourglass s.
congenital aortic valve s.
congenital esophageal s.
congenital mitral s.
congenital subglottic s.
congenital subvalvular s.
congenital valvular s.
coronary artery s.
coronary luminal s.
coronary ostial s.
critical coronary s.
critical valvular s.
cross-sectional area s.
culprit s.
s. diameter
diffuse s.
discrete subaortic s.
discrete subvalvular aortic s. (DSAS)
duodenal hourglass s.
dynamic subaortic s.
eccentric s.
esophageal s.
external iliac s.
femoropopliteal atheromatous s.
fibromuscular subaortic s.
fishmouth mitral s.
fixed-orifice aortic s.
flow-limiting s.
focal eccentric s.
foraminal s.
graft s.
granulation s.
hemodynamically significant s.
hepatic artery s.
high-grade proximal s.
hourglass s.
hypercalcemic supravalvular aortic s.
hypertrophic infundibular subpulmonic s.
hypertrophic pyloric string sign s.
hypertrophic pyloric target sign s.
hypertrophic subaortic s.
idiopathic hypertrophic subaortic s.
ileal s.
iliac artery s.
iliofemoral venous s.
infrainguinal bypass s.
infrarenal s.
infundibular pulmonary s.
infundibular subpulmonic s.
innominate artery s.
intrarenal s.
intrinsic vein graft s.
iris-like s.
juxtaanastomotic s.
lateral recess s.
linear s.
lumbar spinal s.
luminal s.
membranous subaortic s.
membranous subvalvular aortic s.
midgraft s.
mitral s. (MS)
mitral valve s. (MVS)
multifocal short s.
multiple small bowel s.
muscular subaortic s.
napkin-ring annular s.
native kidney renal artery s.
neoplastic s.
noncalcified coronary s.
noncritical s.
nonrheumatic valvular aortic s.
ostial renal artery s.
papillary bile duct s.

papilla of Vater s.
pelvic venous s.
peripheral pulmonary artery s. (PPAS)
petrous carotid canal s.
postangioplasty s.
post-PTCA residual s.
preangioplasty s.
pulmonary s. (PS)
pulmonary artery s.
pulmonary valve s.
pulmonary vein s.
pulmonic s. (PS)
pulmonic valvular s.
pyloric s.
radionuclide s.
rectal s.
relative mitral s.
renal artery s. (RAS)
rheumatic aortic valvular s.
rheumatic mitral s.
rheumatic tricuspid s.
saphenous vein s.
segmental s.
senescent aortic s.
severe s.
silent mitral s.
spinal s.
stomal s.
string-sign s.
subaortic s.
subclavian artery s.
subglottic s.
subinfundibular pulmonary s.
subpulmonic infundibular s.
subsonic s.
subvalvular aortic s.
subvalvular pulmonary s.
supraaortic s.
supraclavicular aortic s.
suprarenal s.
supravalvular aortic s. (SAS, SVAS)
supravalvular mitral s.
supravalvular pulmonary s.
tapering s.
tight s.
tracheal s.
tricuspid s.
true mitral s.
truncal renal artery s.
tubular s.
tunnel subaortic s.
tunnel subvalvular aortic s.
uncomplicated supraclavicular s.
unicuspid aortic valve s.
unilateral carotid s.
ureteral s.
valvular aortic s.
valvular pulmonic s.
vein graft s.
vertebral artery s.

stenotic
s. coronary artery
s. esophagogastric anastomosis
s. flow reserve (SFR)
s. gradient
s. isthmus
s. lesion
s. plaque
s. tricuspid valve

Stensen
S. canal
S. duct
S. foramen
S. gland

stent
biliary s.
biodegradable s.
coil vascular s.
double-helix prostatic s.
double-J ureteral s.
esophageal s.
s. expansion
indwelling s.
intravascular s.
^{192}Ir-loaded s.
metallic s.
s. migration
nephroureteral s.
pancreatic duct s.
patent s.
percutaneous s.
pigtail s.
polyurethane s.
porous metallic s.
prostatic s.
radioisotope s.
renovascular s.
stainless steel mesh s.
straight s.
tandem s.
tantalum s.
s. thrombosis

NOTES

stent *(continued)*
transhepatic biliary s.
T-tube s.
ureteral s.
urethral metallic s.
urinary s.
U-tube s.
vascular s.
zig-zag s.
stent-graft
endovascular s.-g.
stenting
intracoronary s.
intravascular s.
stentless porcine aortic valve
stent-mounted
s.-m. allograft valve
s.-m. heterograft valve
stent-vessel wall contact
Stenvers
S. projection
S. view
step
phase-encoding s.
s. section
s. wedge
step-down
s.-d. deformity of shoulder
s.-d. shoulder deformity
s.-d. transformer
stepdown unit
stepladder
s. appearance
s. sign
stepoff
s. of fracture
orbital rim s.
stepping-source position
step-up
s.-u. transformer
stepwise
s. regression
s. regression analysis
stercoral
s. ulcer
stercoroma
stereocinefluorography
stereofluoroscopy
stereogram
stereographic projection
stereography
StereoGuide
LORAD S.
S. prone breast biopsy system
stereolithography
StereoLoc upright biopsy system
stereologic
s. method
s. method of volume estimation
stereomammography
stereoradiography
stereoroentgenogram
stereoroentgenography
stereoscope
binocular s.
Stanford and Wheatstone s.
stereoscopic
s. view
s. vision
stereoscopy
stereotactic, stereotaxic
s. ablation
s. add-on device
s. automated technique
s. cerebral angiography
s. CT scan
s. data
s. external-beam irradiation (SEBI)
s. head frame
s. localization
s. localization frame
s. mammography
s. percutaneous needle biopsy
s. procedure
s. proton irradiation
s. puncture
s. radiation therapy
s. radiosurgery
s. radiotherapy
s. ring
s. surface projection (SSP)
s. surgery
stereotaxis
computer-assisted volumetric s.
imaging-based s.
volumetric minimally invasive s.
stereotaxy
frameless s.
Steripaque-BR
Steripaque-V
Sterles sign
Sterling imaging agent
Sterling-Okuniewski sign
sterna (*pl. of* sternum)
sternal
s. abscess
s. angle
s. angle of Louis
s. apex
s. border
s. cartilage
s. clip

s. edge
s. joint
s. lift
s. marrow
s. notch
s. rib
s. splitting
s. suture
s. view
Sternberg
S. myocardial insufficiency
S. sarcoma
S. sign
sterni
corpus s.
sternochondral junction
sternoclavicular
s. angle
s. hyperostosis
s. joint
s. joint disk
s. ligament
sternocleidomastoid
clavicular head of s.
s. muscle
s. muscle border
s. retraction
sternocostal
s. joint
s. surface of heart
sternohyoid muscle
sternomanubrial joint
sternopericardial ligament
sternospinal reference
sternothyroid muscle
sternotomy
median s.
s. wire
sternoxiphoid plane
sternum, pl. **sterna**
anterior bowing of s.
s. retraction
tie s.
Steward-Milford fracture classification
Stewart-Hamilton equation
Stewart-Holmes sign
Stewart-Treves syndrome
ST/HR slope
Stickler disease
Stieda fracture
Stierlin sign
stiff-lung syndrome
stiff-man syndrome
stiffness
aortic s.
s. coefficient
lung s.
ventricular s.
stiff noncompliant lung
Still disease
Stiller rib
Stilling canal
stimulated
s. echo
s. echo-tagging technique
stimulated-echo acquisition mode (STEAM)
stimulation
alternating hemifield s.
electric s.
high-voltage pulsed galvanic s. (HVPGS)
intraoperative electrocortical s. (IOECS)
s. mode
noninvasive programmed s. (NIPS)
s. scan
stimulator
bone growth s.
transcutaneous electrical nerve s. (TENS)
stimulus-correlated
s.-c. signal
s.-c. water signal
stippled
s. appearance
s. calcification
s. soft tissue
stippling of lung field
STIR
short tau inversion recovery
short TI inversion recovery
fast STIR
STIR imaging
STIR sequence
STIR technique
stirrup bone
stocking-glove distribution
Stoerck loop
Stokes theorem
stoma
abdominal s.
anastomotic s.
bowel s.

NOTES

stoma *(continued)*
diverting s.
gastroenterostomy s.
gastrointestinal s.
permanent s.
prolapsed s.
retracted s.
Silastic collar-reinforced s.

stomach
aberrant umbilical s.
s. adenocarcinoma
angulus of s.
antrum of s.
s. atony
s. bed
bilocular s.
body of the s.
s. bubble
s. bull's eye lesion
s. calculus
canal of s.
s. cancer metastasis
cardiac s.
cascade s.
cobblestone appearance s.
contrast-filled s.
convex border of s.
coronary artery of s.
cup-and-spill s.
s. curvature
s. defect incisura
distal blind s.
distended s.
s. diverticulum
dumping s.
s. filling defect
s. fundus
greater curvature of s.
Holzknecht s.
hourglass s.
intrathoracic s.
J-shaped s.
leatherbottle s.
s. leiomyoma
s. leiomyosarcoma
lesser curvature of s.
s. margin
miniature s.
mucous lake of s.
s. narrowing
nonvisualization of fetal s.
Pavlov s.
pit of s.
s. pneumatosis
riding s.
scaphoid s.
sclerotic s.
sour s.
thoracic s.
trifid s.
s. tube
s. ulcer
upset s.
upside-down s.
s. varioliform erosion
s. varix
s. volvulus
s. wall
waterfall s.
water-trap s.
wet s.

stomal
s. bag
s. edema
s. intussusception
s. stenosis

stone
barrel-shaped s.
bile duct s.
biliary tract s.
bilirubinate s.
black faceted s.
bladder s.
bosselated s.
calcium bilirubinate s.
cholesterol s.
common bile duct s.
cystic duct remnant s.
s. extraction
extrahepatic s.
fecal s.
floating gallbladder s.
gallbladder s.
gas-containing s.
s. heart
s. heart phenomenon
high-attenuation s.
impacted urethral s.
s. impaction
intrahepatic s.
intraluminal s.
intravesical s.
kidney s.
lung s.
metabolic s.
multiple s.'s
noncalcified s.
nonopaque s.
nonradiopaque s.
opaque s.
pigment s.
pituitary s.
pulp s.
radiolucent s.
renal s.
residual s.

salivary s.
shadowing s.
soft pigment s.
staghorn s.
s. staple
ureteral s.
urinary bladder s.
vein s.
vesical s.
womb s.

stonelike calculus
stony mass
stool
retention of s.
stool-tagging agent
stop-action
s.-a. image
s.-a. imaging
stopcock
three-way s.
stopping power
storage
digital s.
magnetic tape s.
s. phosphor radiology
s. phosphor system
storiform pattern
storiform-pleomorphic pattern
Storm Von Leeuwen chamber
Stortz thoracoscope
Stouffer syndrome
stoved finger
straddle
s. fracture
s. injury
straddling embolus
straight
s. anterior vertebral border
s. AP pelvic injection
s. chest tube
s. cord
s. interposition graft
s. lateral projection
s. stem
s. stent
s. tubule
s. ureter
straightening of anterior vertebral border
straight-line Hough transform mapping
strain
adductor muscle s.
s. fracture
left ventricular hypertrophy with s.
ligamentous s.
lumbosacral spine s.
muscle s.
s. pattern
shear s.
strain-gauge plethysmography
strain-rate MR imaging
strain-sprain injury
strand
s.'s of increased density
rabbit ear s.'s
stranding
fascial s.
glial s.
mesenteric s.
soft tissue s.
strandy
s. density
s. infiltrate
strangulated
s. bowel
s. inguinal hernia
s. obstruction
s. viscus
strangulation necrosis
stranguria
strap muscle
stratification
mural s.
stratigraphy
Stratis II MRI system
Strauss sign
strawberry gallbladder
strawberry-shaped head
stray neutron field
streak
s.'s of atelectasis
atherosclerotic fatty s.
fatty intima s.
s.'s of increased density
primitive s.
streak-like configuration
streaky density
stream
regurgitant s.
Streeter dysplasia
strength
air-kerma s.
field s.

S

NOTES

streptavidin peroxidase technique
stress
adduction s.
biomechanical s.
s. Broden view
s. cystogram
s. echocardiography
s. endpoint
s. eversion view
s. film
s. fracture
s. gated blood pool cardiac examination
hoop s.
s. incontinence
s. injury
s. inversion view
mediolateral s.
s. perfusion and rest function
s. radiography
s. raiser
Reichek method of calculating end-systolic wall s.
resting end-systolic wall s.
shear s.
s. test
s. thallium image
s. thallium-201 myocardial imaging
s. thallium scan
torque s.
torsional s.
s. ulcer
valgus s.
varus s.
wall shear s.
stress-and-rest image
stress-induced
s.-i. ischemia
s.-i. left ventricular dilatation
s.-i. remodeling
stress-redistribution
s.-r. examination
s.-r. imaging
stress-rest-reinjection examination
stress-strain curve
stretched
s. lung
s. out ligament
stretch sign
striata
osteopathia s.
striatal lesion
striate
s. cortex
s. hemorrhage
s. vein
striated
s. angiographic nephrogram
s. muscle
striation
S. across image
fiber-bundle s.
paint brush s.
urothelial s.
striatum
corpus s.
Strickler method
stricture
anal s.
anastomotic s.
annular esophageal s.
antral s.
benign biliary s.
bile duct s.
biliary s.
Bismuth classification of benign bile duct s.
bronchial s.
choledochojejunostomy s.
cicatricial s.
colonic s.
common bile duct s.
congenital urethral s.
contractile s.
duodenal s.
enteric s.
esophageal s.
gastroesophageal junction s.
irritable s.
longitudinal esophageal s.
Makar s.
peptic s.
pyloric s.
recurrent s.
spasmodic s.
tracheal s.
ureteral s.
urethral s.
stridor
inspiratory s.
laryngeal s.
respiratory s.
string
s. cell carcinoma
s. guideline
navel s.
s. sign
string-and-double-track sign
stringlike bands of fibrous tissue
string-of-beads
s.-o.-b. appearance
s.-o.-b. sign
string-of-pearls
s.-o.-p. appearance

s.-o.-p. nuclear arrangement
s.-o.-p. sign
string-sign stenosis
strionigral tract
strip
Fluorets ophthalmic s.
Ful-Glo ophthalmic s.
primary motor s.
s. scan
sensitometric s.
sensory s.
stripe
Baillarger s.
central high-signal intensity s.
central intraluminal saturation s.
flank s.
Gennari s.
s. of Gennari
paraspinal pleural s.
paratracheal tissue s.
pleural s.
properitoneal flank s.
psoas s.
Quad-Lumen drain with radiopaque s.
Retzius s.
saturation s.
scaphoid fat s.
s. sign
tracheal wall s.
vertebral s.
Vicq d'Azyr s.
striped tag myocardial tagging system (STAG)
striping
horizontal s.
stripped atom
stripping
fibrin sleeve s.
stroke
cardiogenic embolic s.
cerebrovascular s.
completed s.
s. count image
s. count ratio
s. ejection rate
embolic s.
s. in evolution
evolving s.
s. force
hemisphere s.
hemorrhagic s.
hyperacute s.
hypertensive s.
incomplete s.
s. index (SI)
lacunar s.
s. output
s. power
progressive s.
s. scale score
slow s.
small-vessel s.
spinal cord s.
thromboembolic s.
vertebrobasilar distribution s.
s. volume (SV)
s. volume image
s. volume imaging
s. volume index (SVI)
s. volume ratio
stroke-work index (SWI)
stroma, pl. **stromata**
bone marrow s.
cartilage s.
cervical s.
extralobular s.
gonadal s.
Rollet s.
stromal
s. carcinoid of ovary
s. cell tumor
s. matrix
s. necrosis
strongyloidiasis
strontium (Sr)
s. imaging agent
s. isotope
strontium-89 (^{89}Sr)
s. chloride
strontium-90 (^{90}Sr)
STRT
simultaneous thermoradiotherapy
structural
s. anomaly
s. epilepsy
s. lesion
s. weakness
structure
biliary s.
bony s.
branching linear s.
branching tubular s.
calcified density s.

NOTES

structure *(continued)*
central hilar s.
cervical s.
collagenous s.
cord s.
cystic s.
demineralized bony s.
denture-supporting s.
elongated s.
high-density s.
hilar s.
hollow s.
intratumoral s.
labyrinthine s.
low-contrast s.
low-density s.
mediastinal s.
midline cystic s.
organoid s.
osseous s.
ossification of cartilaginous s.
peritubular vascular s.
prominent ductal vascular s.
renal collecting s.
ringlike s.
satellite s.
serpentine s.
soft tissue density s.
spherical s.
stem-loop s.
submillimeter s.
superior mediastinal s.
supraglottic s.
test tube s.
tree-like airway s.
tuboreticular s.
tubular s.
vascular s.

structured
s. coil electromagnet
s. noise
s. water

struma, pl. **strumae**
s. ovarii
Riedel s.

Strümpell-Lorrain disease

Strümpell-Marie disease

Strümpell sign

Strunsky sign

strut
bone s.
s. chorda
corticocancellous s.
s. fracture
optic s.
tricuspid valve s.
valve outflow s.

Struthers
S. arcade
ligament of S.
S. ligament

struvite

Stryker
S. frame
S. notch view

STS
subtrapezial space

ST segment/heart rate slope (ST/HR slope)

ST-segment shift

STT
scaphotrapeziotrapezoid
STT joint

stuck
s. twin
s. without recapture
s. with recapture

studded fissure

studding of endometriosis

study
aerosol ventilation s.
anisotropic volume s.
barium s.
biplane pelvic oblique s.
bladder contractility s.
blood flow s.
bone density s.
bone length s.
bone mineral content s.
cardiac gated s.
carotid duplex s.
cerebral perfusion s.
cerebrospinal fluid leak s.
conventional s.
cornflake esophageal motility s.
correlative Doppler s.
Doppler flow probe s.
double-contrast barium s.
dual-contrast s.
dynamic contrast-enhanced subtraction s.
efficacy s.
electromagnetic blood flow s.
endovascular flow wire s.
first-pass s.
fistula tract s.
flow s.
gallbladder s.
gas ventilation s.
gated imaging s.
gated planar s.
Gd-DOTA-enhanced subtraction dynamic s.
ictal phase s.

imaging s.
inhalation s.
interictal PET FDG s.
interictal SPECT s.
intervention s.
isotopic 3D s.
isotopic volume s.
Joliot sorption s.
kidney function s.
kinematic MRI s.
marker transit s.
minute-sequence s.
morphine-augmented s.
motility s.
multibreath washout s.
multitracer s.
noninvasive imaging s.
nuclear-tagged red blood cell bleeding s.
paleopathologic and radiologic s.
peripheral small airways s.
phantom s.
pressure perfusion s.
pullback s.
pulmonary quantitative differential function s.
qualitative s.
radioaerosol imaging s.
radiochemical s.
radiolabeled water s.
radiologic-histopathologic s.
radionuclide blood flow s.
radionuclide voiding s.
reconstruction s.
redistribution s.
renal cyst s.
salivary gland function s.
scintigraphic s.
simulated equilibrium factor s.
sinus tract s.
split-brain s.
TECA s.
  technetium albumin study
technetium albumin s. (TECA study)
three-phase technetium s.
thymidine suicide s.
ureteral reflux s.
urodynamic s.
in vivo disposition s.
voiding s.
wall motion s.
xenon washout s.

stump
  appendiceal s.
  bulbous s.
  s. cancer
  cystic duct s.
  duodenal s.
  gastric s.
  s. pregnancy
  s. pressure
  rectal s.

stunned myocardium

stunning
  myocardial s.
  thyroid s.

stunted fetus

Sturge-Weber
  S.-W. disease
  S.-W. syndrome
  S.-W. telangiectasia

Sturge-Weber-Dimitri syndrome

stylet
  Inrad HiLiter ultrasound-enhanced s.

styloglossus muscle

stylohyoid
  s. ligament
  s. muscle

styloid
  s. process
  ulnar s.

styloidium
  os s.

stylomandibular ligament

stylomastoid
  s. foramen

stylomaxillary ligament

stylopharyngeus

subacromial
  s. bursa
  s. bursal adhesion
  s. bursitis
  s. enthesophyte
  s. pain syndrome
  s. space

subacromial-subdeltoid
  s.-s. bursa
  s.-s. bursitis

subacute
  s. allergic pneumonia
  s. bacterial endocarditis (SBE)
  s. bronchopneumonia

NOTES

subacute *(continued)*
s. cardiac tamponade
s. combined spinal cord degeneration
s. denervation atrophy
s. encephalitis
s. extrinsic allergic alveolitis
s. granulomatous
s. hemorrhage
s. hepatic necrosis
s. inflammation
s. ischemic brain infarct
s. myocardial infarct
s. myositis ossificans
s. necrotizing myelopathy
s. renal vein thrombosis
s. sclerosing panencephalitis (SSPE)
s. subdural hematoma
s. testicular torsion
s. thyroiditis
subadditivity
subadventitial
s. fibrosis
s. hyperplasia
s. plane
s. tissue
subannular
s. calcification
s. placement
subaortic
s. curtain
s. gland
s. muscle
s. stenosis
subapical
s. bronchus
subaponeurotic abscess
subarachnoid
s. cavity
s. cistern
s. clot
s. cyst
s. cysticercosis
s. hemorrhage (SAH)
s. injection
s. instillation
s. metastatic disease
s. nerve block
s. phenol block
s. seeding
s. septum
s. space
subareolar
s. cancer
s. plexus
subarticular
s. bone resorption
s. cyst
s. pseudocyst
subastragalar dislocation
subastrocytic tumor
subatheromatous ulcer
subatmospheric pressure
subband
wavelet s.
subblock
rectifier s.
subcallosal gyrus
subcapital
s. fracture
subcapsular
s. hepatic necrosis
s. renal hematoma
subcardinal vein
subcarina
subcarinal
s. angle
s. lymph node
subcecal appendix
subchondral
s. bone
s. bone plate
s. bone resorption
s. collapse
s. cyst
s. cystic cavity
s. fracture
s. fracture line
s. lesion
s. low-signal-intensity sclerosis
s. marrow edema
s. marrow hyperemia
s. microfracture
s. osteosclerosis
s. trabecular compression
subchorionic
s. hematoma
s. hemorrhage
subclavian
s. aneurysm
s. arteriography
s. artery
s. artery obstruction
s. artery occlusion
s. artery stenosis
s. flap
s. flap aortoplasty
s. line
s. loop
s. steal
s. steal syndrome (SSP)
s. turndown technique
s. vein
s. vein occlusion
s. vein thrombosis

s. vessel
s. vessel thrombosis
subclavicular
subclavius
subcollateral gyrus
subcoracoid dislocation of shoulder
subcortical
s. arteriosclerotic encephalopathy
s. atherosclerotic encephalopathy
s. CNS hamartoma
s. defect
s. infarct
s. intracerebral hemorrhage
s. intracranial lesion
s. ischemic vascular dementia
s. Sudeck osteoporotic atrophy
s. tumor
subcostal
s. artery
s. branch
s. four-chamber view
s. long-axis view
s. margin
s. nerve
s. plane
s. short-axis view
s. short-axis view echocardiography
s. window
subcritical narrowing
subcutaneous
s. air
s. array electrode
s. arterial bypass graft
s. connective tissue
s. edema
s. emphysema
s. fascia
s. fat
s. fat line
s. fat necrosis
s. fibroma
s. fracture
s. hemangioma
s. implanted injection port
s. infiltrate
s. infusion
s. injection of contrast artifact
s. mastectomy
s. nodule
s. patch
s. pocket
s. sacrococcygeal myxopapillary ependymoma
s. tissue gas
s. tumor
s. tunnel
s. vein
subcuticular layer
subdeltoid
s. bursa
s. bursal adhesion
s. bursal effusion
s. bursitis
s. fat plane obliteration
subdiaphragmatic abscess
subdivision
subdural
s. abscess
s. blood
s. button
s. cavity
s. clot
s. contrast injection
s. effusion
s. empyema
s. hemorrhage (SDH)
s. hygroma
s. interhemispheric hematoma
s. space
s. window
subendocardial
s. infarct (SEI)
s. injury
s. ischemia
s. myocardial infarct
s. necrosis
s. sclerosis
subendometrial halo
subependymal
s. cyst
s. germinolysis
s. giant cell astrocytoma
s. hamartoma
s. hemorrhage
s. oligodendroglioma
s. seeding
s. spread
s. vein
subependymoma
suberosis
maple bark worker's s.
subeustachian sinus
subfalcine herniation

S

NOTES

subfascial
s. hematoma
s. transposition
subfascially
subfrontal meningioma
subgaleal
s. abscess
s. cerebrospinal fluid
s. hematoma
s. hemorrhage
subglenoid dislocation of shoulder
subglottic
s. area
s. carcinoma
s. edema
s. hemangioma
s. inverted V sign
s. narrowing
s. stenosis
subglottis
subhepatic
s. abscess
s. area
s. cecum
s. space
subinfundibular pulmonary stenosis
subinsular mass
subintimal
s. cleavage plane
s. dissection
s. fibrosis
s. filling
subject
s. contrast
s. placement
subjective
s., objective, management, and analytic (SOMA, SOMA scale)
s., objective, management and analytic classification
subjective,
sublabral
s. foramen
s. recess
subligamentous
s. disk herniation
s. extension
Sublimaze
sublingual
s. gland
s. varix
sublux
subluxation
anterior tibial s.
s. articulation
atlantoaxial s.
s. complex
distal radioulnar s.
element s.
forward s.
lateral s.
occult s.
patellar s.
peroneal tendon s.
posterior s.
posterolateral rotatory s.
radial head s. (RHS)
radioulnar s.
recurrent lateral patellar s.
reduced s.
sacroiliac s.
tendon s.
Volkmann s.
subluxed, subluxated
s. vertebra
subluxing patella
submandibular
s. duct
s. ganglion
s. gland
s. lymph node
s. triangle
submassive
s. hepatic necrosis
s. pulmonary embolus
submaxillary
s. gland
s. sialography
s. view
submembranous placental hematoma
submental
s. lymph node
s. vertex projection
s. vertex radiograph
s. vertex view
submentovertex
s. radiograph
submentovertical projection
submicron
s. magnetic particle
s. magnetic principle
submillimeter structure
submucosal
s. circular fold
s. colon tumor
s. esophageal tumor
s. fibroid
s. hemorrhage
s. lesion
s. thickening
s. venous plexus
submucous myoma
suboccipital shortening
suboptimal
s. detail
s. effort

s. examination
s. film
s. result
s. runoff
s. visualization
suboptimally visualized
subpectoral
s. implant
s. pocket
subperiosteal
s. abscess
s. bone resorption
s. cortical abrasion
s. cortical defect
s. desmoid
s. fracture
s. hematoma
s. hemorrhage
s. infection
s. new bone
s. new bone formation
s. osteoid osteoma
subperitoneal space
subphrenic
s. abscess
s. biloma
s. fluid
s. recess
s. space
subpleural
s. bleb
s. curvilinear line
s. dot
s. effusion
s. lymphatic
s. pulmonary arcade
subpubic arch
subpulmonic
s. effusion
s. fluid
s. infundibular stenosis
s. obstruction
s. outflow
s. pleural space
subpyloric node
subrectus obstruction
subsartorial
s. canal
s. tunnel
subscapular
s. artery
s. bursa
s. fossa
s. lymph node
s. notch syndrome
subscapularis
s. muscle
s. recess
s. tendon
subsecond FLASH imaging
subsegmental
s. atelectasis
s. bibasilar atelectasis
s. bronchus
s. lower lobe atelectasis
s. perfusion abnormality
s. perfusion defect
subsegment of lung
subselective cannulation
subseptate uterus
subseptus
uterus s., subseptate uterus
subserosal
s. fibroid
s. fibrosis
s. hemorrhage
s. layer
s. tumor
subsidence
spontaneous s.
subsonic stenosis
subspinous dislocation
substance
bone s.
brain s.
diamagnetic s.
reticular activating s.
substantia
s. nigra
s. propria
substantial emphysema
substernal
s. angle
s. goiter
s. retraction
s. thyroid
s. thyroid gland
substitute
bone s.
oxygenated perfluorocarbon blood s.
substituted benzamide
substitution bone
substrate
main energy s.

NOTES

subtalar
s. angle
s. articulation
s. axis
s. instability
s. joint
s. joint space
s. varus
s. view
subtendinous space
subtentorial lesion
subthalamus
subtotal
s. gastric exclusion
s. gastric resection
s. lesion
s. occlusion
s. overframing
subtraction
s. cloning
computer-assisted blood background s. (CABBS)
digital s.
dual-energy s.
energy s.
Epistar s.
film s.
s. film
s. image
s. imaging
s. technique
subtractive noise
subtrapezial space (STS)
subtrochanteric
s. fracture
s. varus deformity
subumbilical space
subungual
s. abscess
s. glomus tumor
s. melanoma
subunit
functional s. (FSU)
subvalvular
s. aneurysm
s. aortic obstruction
s. aortic stenosis
s. diffuse muscular obstruction
s. gradient
s. pulmonary stenosis
subvesical duct
subxiphoid
s. echocardiography view
s. implantation
s. view echocardiography
succenturiate placental lobe
succimer
technetium-99m s.
succussion splash
sucking
s. muscle
s. pneumothorax
Sucquet-Hoyer
S.-H. anastomosis
S.-H. canal
sucralfate
gadolinium s.
sucrose
s. dosimeter
s. polyester contrast
s. polyester imaging agent
suction
s. device
s. drainage
s. tube
Sudbury system
sudden
s. blockage of coronary artery
s. cardiac death
Sudeck
S. atrophy
S. dystrophy
S. point
SUFE
slipped upper femoral epiphysis
suffocative goiter
sugar-icing liver
sugar tumor
suit
MAST s.
suite
angiography s.
sulcal
s. atrophy
s. enhancement
s. enlargement
s. pattern
s. skeleton
sulcation
sulcomarginal tract
sulcus, pl. **sulci**
s. angle
angularis s.
atrioventricular s.
basilar s.
blunted posterior s.
s. calcanei
s. of calcaneus
calcarine s.
callosal s.
central s.
cerebral s.
cingulate s.
collateral s.
coronary s.
cortical s.

costal s.
costophrenic s.
dilatation of s.
s. dilatation
s. effacement
effacement of s.
frontal s.
Harrison s.
hippocampal s.
hypothalamic s.
lateral occipital s.
lips of lateral s.
mapping of cerebral s.
occipitotemporal s.
olfactory s.
parietooccipital s.
perilabral s.
pontomedullary s.
postcentral s.
posterior interventricular s.
precentral s.
pulmonary s.
ramus of lateral s.
retromalleolar s.
right atrial patch positioned over right atrioventricular s.
rolandic s.
sphenoparietal s.
superior frontal s.
superior pulmonary s.
superior temporal s.
supracallosal s.
s. talus
temporal s.
ulnar s.
widened s.

sulfasalazine-induced pulmonary infiltrate

sulfate
barium s. ($BaSO_4$)
barium lead s.
barium strontium s.
manganese s.
morphine s.
sodium tetradecyl s.

sulfobromophthalein imaging agent

sulfonate
sodium-2-mercaptoethane s.

sulfur
s. colloid
s. colloid imaging agent
s. colloid scan
s. colloid scintigraphy

sulfur-35 (^{35}S)

sum
field-echo s.
ray s.

summation
s. shadow artifact
s. of shadows

summing correction

Summit
S. LoDose collimator

summit
ventricular septal s.

Sumner sign

sump
s. drain
Ring-MacLean s.

sum-peak method

sun
Brett s.
S. SPARCstation system
S. workstation

sunburst
s. appearance
s. brain vascularity
s. gyral pattern
s. nephrogram
s. periosteal reaction

sunrise view

sunset view

superabsorbent polymer embolic material

superbound water

supercam scintillation scanner

superciliary arch

superconducting
s. magnet
s. quantum interference device (SQUID)

superconductor
niobium/titanium s.

superdominant left anterior descending artery

superfecundation

superfemale syndrome

superfetation

superficial
s. angioma
s. basal cell carcinoma
s. depressed carcinoma
s. diffuse nephroblastomatosis

NOTES

superficial *(continued)*
s. dorsal sacrococcygeal ligament
s. external pudendal artery
s. femoral artery (SFA)
s. femoral artery occlusion
s. femoral vein
s. hyperthermia treatment
s. inguinal lymph node
s. inguinal pouch
s. inguinal ring
s. lesion
s. lymphadenopathy
s. lymph vessel
s. muscle
s. necrosis
s. palmar arterial arch
s. palmaris longus tendon
s. perineal pouch
s. plexus
s. pneumonia
s. posterior compartment
s. posterior sacrococcygeal ligament
s. radiation
s. spreading esophageal carcinoma
s. spreading melanoma
s. spreading stomach carcinoma
s. temporal artery
s. temporalis fascia
s. temporoparietal fascia
s. transverse metacarpal ligament
s. transverse metatarsal ligament
superficialis
s. arcade
flexor digitorum s. (FDS)
superimposed
s. acute partial tear
s. bowel gas
superimposition
s. artifact
s. of bowel shadow
s. of signals
superincumbent
s. spinal curve
superior
s. articular facet
s. aspect
s. azygoesophageal recess
s. bilateral vena cava
s. border
s. border of heart
s. border of rib
s. caval defect
s. cerebellar artery (SCA)
s. cervical ganglion
s. colliculus
s. costal facet
s. costotransverse ligament
s. duodenal fold
s. duodenal recess
s. epigastric artery
s. extensor retinaculum
s. frontal axis shift
s. frontal gyrus
s. frontal sulcus
s. genicular artery
s. gluteal vessel
s. hypogastric plexus
s. intercostal artery
s. intercostal vein
s. jugular vein bulb
s. labral anterior to posterior (SLAP)
s. labral anterior to posterior tear
s. labral anteroposterior
s. labral anteroposterior (SLAP) injury
s. labral anteroposterior (SLAP) lesion
s. lobe
s. lobe bronchus
s. lobe of lung
s. longitudinal fasciculus
s. marginal defect
s. margin of inferior rib
s. maxillary foramen
s. mediastinal structure
s. mediastinum
s. mesenteric
s. mesenteric arteriography
s. mesenteric artery
s. mesenteric artery syndrome (SMAS)
s. mesenteric ganglion
s. mesenteric plexus
s. mesenteric vein (SMV)
s. oblique
s. occipitofrontal fasciculus
s. olivary complex
s. ophthalmic vein
s. ophthalmic vein thrombosis
s. orbital fissure
s. orbital fissure anatomy
s. parietal lobule gyrus
s. peroneal retinaculum (SPR)
s. phrenic branch
s. pole
s. pubic ligament
s. pubic ramus
s. pulmonary artery
s. pulmonary sulcus
s. pulmonary sulcus tumor
s. pulmonary vein
s. rectal vein
s. retraction
s. sagittal sinus (SSS)
s. sagittal sinus thrombosis

s. segment
s. segmental bronchus
s. sulcus tumor
s. temporal gyrus
s. temporal sulcus
s. thoracic aperture
s. thyroid artery
s. transverse rectal fold
s. transverse scapular ligament
s. triangle sign
s. turbinated bone
s. vena cava (SVC)
s. vena caval obstruction
s. vena cava pressure
s. vena cava syndrome

superior/inferior (S/I)
superior-inferior flow direction
superioris
levator palpebrae s.
supernormal
s. artery
s. excitation
supernumerary
s. digit
s. kidney
s. parathyroid gland
s. sesamoid bone
superoinferior heart
superolateral
s. aspect
s. displacement
superolaterally
superomedial
s. margin
s. portal
s. surface
superoxide dismutase
superparamagnetic
s. agent iron oxide
s. iron oxide (SPIO)
s. iron oxide imaging
s. iron oxide imaging agent (SPIO imaging agent)
s. microsphere
Superscan
superselective
s. angio-CT
s. angiography
supersystemic pulmonary artery pressure
supervoltage
s. generator
supination
s. deformity
supination-adduction
s.-a. fracture
s.-a. injury
supination-eversion fracture
supination-external
s.-e. rotation injury
s.-e. rotation IV (SER-IV)
supination, external rotation type IV fracture (SER-IV fracture)
supination-outward rotation injury
supinator
supine
s. bicycle stress echocardiography
s. film
s. full view
s. position
s. radiograph
supplemental beam filtration
supply
accessory blood s.
arterial s.
arterial scrotum s.
collateral blood s.
dual blood s.
indirect blood s.
longitudinal blood s.
pudendal blood s.
thrcc-phase voltage s.
tumor blood s.
vascular s.
support
advanced life s. (ALS)
autologous bone marrow s.
ligamentous s.
wedge-shaped s.
supportive therapy
suppression
bone marrow s.
chemotherapy-related myeloid s.
chemsat fat s.
Cytomel s.
DIET method of fat s.
double-echo three-point Dixon method fat s.
drug-induced bone marrow s.
fat s.
overdrive s.
paradoxical s.
s. scan

NOTES

suppression *(continued)*
solvent s.
spectral-spatial fat s.
suppressor mesh
suppuration
suppurative
s. ascending cholangitis
s. inflammation
s. pancreatitis
s. pleurisy
s. pneumonia
s. pyelonephritis
s. thyroiditis
supraanal fascia
supraannular
s. constriction
s. suture ring
supraaortic
s. ridge
s. stenosis
supracallosal
s. gyrus
s. sulcus
supracardiac total anomalous venous return
supracardinal vein
supraceliac aorta
supracervical hysterectomy
supraclavicular
s. aortic stenosis
s. fossa
s. lymph node
s. node involvement
s. triangle
supraclinoid
s. carotid aneurysm
s. carotid artery
s. portion
supracolic
s. compartment
s. space
supracollicular spike of cortical bone
supracondylar
s. femoral fracture
s. humeral fracture
s. plate
s. process
s. ridge
s. Y-shaped fracture
supracondyloid process
supracoronary ridge
supracricoid interval
supracristal
s. plane (SCP)
s. ventricular septal defect
supradditivity
supradiaphragmatic aorta
supraepicondylar
supraepitrochlear
supraglenoid tubercle
supraglottic
s. carcinoma
s. edema
s. laryngectomy
s. larynx
s. narrowing
s. structure
supraglottis
suprahepatic
s. caval cuff
s. hypertension
s. space
s. vena cava
suprahisian block
suprahyoid
suprailiac aortic mesenteric graft
suprainterparietal bone
supralevator space
supraligamentous disk herniation
supramalleolar open amputation
supramarginal gyrus
supramesocolic compartment
supranuclear lesion
supraoccipital bone
supraorbital
s. artery
s. canal
s. fissure
s. foramen
s. groove (SOG)
s. margin (SOM)
s. ridge
suprapancreatic obstruction
suprapatellar
s. bursa
s. plica
s. pouch
suprapharyngeal bone
suprapubic area
suprapyloric node
suprarenal
s. aortic aneurysm
s. extension of aneurysm
s. gland
s. impression
s. stenosis
suprascapular
s. ligament
s. nerve entrapment
s. notch syndrome
suprasellar
s. adenoma
s. aneurysm
s. atypical teratoma
s. capsule
s. extension

s. extension of tumor
s. hemorrhagic germinoma
s. low-density lesion
s. mass
s. mass calcification
s. meningioma
s. subarachnoid cistern
suprasinatus tendinosis
suprasphincteric fistula
supraspinatus
s. muscle
s. musculotendinous junction
s. nerve
s. tendon
supraspinous
s. ligament
s. ligament disruption
suprasternal
s. bone
s. bulge
s. notch
s. notch view
s. plane
s. retraction
s. scanning
s. window
suprasyndesmotic fixation
supratentorial
s. astrocytoma
s. brain tumor
s. cerebral blood flow
s. flow compensation
s. glioma
s. gray matter
s. lesion
s. neoplasm
s. primitive neuroectodermal tumor
s. space
s. white matter
suprathreshold
supratip nasal tip deformity
supratrochlear
s. artery
s. node
supratubercular ridge of Meyer
supravalvular
s. aortic stenosis (SAS, SVAS)
s. aortography
s. mitral stenosis
s. pulmonary stenosis
s. ring
supravaterian duodenum
supraventricular
s. crest (SVC)
s. level
s. tachyarrhythmia
s. tachycardia
s. venous echo
supraventricularis
crista s.
supravesical obstruction
supreme turbinate bone
suralis
tensor fasciae s.
sural nerve
SureStart
S. feature of Aspire continuous imaging
S. imaging system
surface
acromial articular s.
anterolateral s.
anteromedial s.
s. application of radioelement
apposing articular s.
articular s.
articulating s.
arytenoidal articular s.
attenuated cortical s.
auricular s.
axial s.
basal s.
bone s.
bosselated s.
buccal s.
calcaneal articular s.
carpal articular s.
cartilaginous joint s.
cerebral s.
s. coil
s. coil localization
s. coil method
colic s.
s. configuration
contiguous articular s.'s
s. convexity pattern
corrugated fat-pad s.
costal s.
cuboidal articular s.
diaphragmatic s.
distal s.
s. distance
endosteal s.
endothelial s.

NOTES

S

surface *(continued)*
epicardial s.
s. epithelium
s. epithelium vascular channel
erosion of articular s.
fibular articular s.
gastric s.
glenoid s.
grooving of articular s.
immunostained s.
joint articular s.
s. matching technique
mediastinal lung s.
s. nodularity
occlusal s.
opposing articular s.'s
opposing pleural s.'s
s. osteosarcoma
s. ovarian epithelium tumor
palmar s.
parallelism of articular s.
plantar s.
posterior s.
s. projection
s. projection rendering
s. radioelement application
radioulnar s.
s. registration
s. rendering
roughened articular s.
serosal s.
s. spoiling
superomedial s.
synovial s.
s. tension of lung
s. variable-attenuation correction
ventral s.
weightbearing s.

surface-coil
s.-c. NMR
s.-c. rotating-frame spectroscopy

surface-dose application

surface-projection rendering image

surfer's
s. knot
s. nodule

surgeon's tarsal joint

surgery
conservation s.
CT-guided stereotactic s.
gastric bypass s. (GBS)
image-guided s.
Mohs micrographic s.
radioimmunoguided s.
stereotactic s.

surgical
s. angle
s. artifact
s. clip
s. decompression
s. emphysema
s. endarterectomy
s. neck
s. neck fracture
s. neck of humerus
s. neurangiographic technique
S. Planning and Orientation Computer System (SPOCS)
s. simulation CT
s. sponge
s. staple
s. venous interruption
s. wound

surgically created resection cavity

surgical-radiologic minicholecystostomy

surveillance

survey
bone s.
s. film
four-view wrist s.
isotopic skeletal s.
joint s.
metastatic bone s.
osseous s.
s. scan
serial radiographic s.
skeletal s.

survey-view
s.-v. image
s.-v. imaging

survival
cause-specific s. (CSS)
disease-free s. (DFS)
failure-free s. (FFS)
relapse-free s. (RFS)

susceptibility
s. artifact
diamagnetic s.
s. effect
magnetic s.
s. mapping
s. weighted MR

susceptibility-sensitive sequence

susceptibility-weighted MR imaging

suspended
s. heart
s. heart syndrome
s. inspiration

suspension
barium s.
s. characteristics
chromic phosphate ^{32}P colloidal s.
colloidal s.
E-Z-Paque barium s.
fast exchange-cellular s.
s. of kidney

suspensory
s. ligament
s. ligament of ovary
s. ligament of penis
s. muscle of duodenum
suspicious
s. lesion
s. mass
sustained
s. anterior parasternal motion
s. apical impulse
s. left ventricular heave
sustentacular trauma
sustentaculum
s. lienis
s. tali
sutural
s. bone
s. calcification
s. diastasis
s. ligament
s. markings
suture
apical s.
basilar s.
biparietal s.
bregmatomastoid s.
coronal s.
cranial s.
delayed closure of s.
dentate s.
diastasis of s.
diastatic lambdoid s.
ethmoidolacrimal s.
ethmoidomaxillary s.
frontal s.
frontoethmoidal s.
frontolacrimal s.
frontomaxillary s.
frontonasal s.
frontoparietal s.
frontosphenoid s.
frontozygomatic s.
Gillies s.
Gruber s.
infiltration s.
interparietal s.
jugal s.
lambdoidal cranial s.
s. line
s. line cancer
mamillary s.
metallic s.
metopic s.
nonfusion of cranial s.
occipital s.
occipitomastoid s.
occipitoparietal s.
occipitosphenoid s.
opaque wire s.
overlapping s.
palatine s.
parietal s.
parietooccipital s.
persistent metopic s.
petrobasilar s.
petrosphenobasilar s.
petrosphenooccipital s.
petrosquamous s.
prematurely closed s.
radiopaque s.
rhabdoid s.
sagittal cranial s.
silk s.
sphenoethmoidal s.
sphenooccipital s.
sphenoorbital s.
sphenoparietal s.
sphenopetrosal s.
sphenosquamous s.
sphenotemporal s.
sphenovomerine s.
splayed cranial s.
spread s.
squamosal s.
squamosomastoid s.
squamosoparietal s.
squamososphenoid s.
squamous s.
sternal s.
temporal s.
wide s.
zygomaticofrontal s.
zygomaticotemporal s.
SUV
standard uptake value
SV
stroke volume
Sv
sievert
SVAS
supravalvular aortic stenosis

NOTES

SVC
superior vena cava
supraventricular crest
SVCT
spiral x-ray computed tomography
SVG
scatter and veiling glare
SVI
seminal vesicle invasion
stroke volume index
SvO_2
systemic vascular resistance index
SVR
systemic vascular resistance
SVRI
systemic vascular resistance index
swallow
barium s.
dry s.
Gastrografin s.
Hypaque s.
ice-water s.
water-soluble contrast esophageal s.
wet s.
swallowing
s. artifact
s. center
s. dysfunction
fetal s.
s. function
s. mechanism
s. syncope
swallow-tail configuration
swallowtail malformation of scapula
swamp-static artifact
swan-neck finger deformity
swan neck shape of ventricular outflow
Swanson finger joint
sweat
s. duct adenoma
s. gland carcinoma
s. test
Swediaur disease
sweep
duodenal s.
widened duodenal s.
Sweet sternal punch
swelling
ankle s.
blennorrhagic s.
brain s.
s. of cartilage
congestive brain s.
fusiform s.
joint s.
periumbilical subcutaneous s.
PVST s.
soft tissue s.
Swenson pull-through procedure
swept gain
SWI
stroke-work index
swimmer's
s. position
s. shoulder
s. view
swimming pool granuloma
swinging
s. flashlight test
s. heart
swirling
s. motion
s. smokelike echoes
Swiss
S. Alps appearance
S. cheese air bronchogram
S. cheese appearance
S. cheese liver sign
S. cheese nephrogram
S. cheese ventricular septal defect
S. roll technique
Swissray scanner
switched B-gradient technique
swivel dislocation
swollen
s. brain hemisphere
s. tissue
Swyer-James
S.-J. syndrome
S.-J. unilateral hyperlucency of lung
Swyer-James-MacLeod syndrome
Swyer syndrome
SXA
single-energy x-ray absorptiometer
Syed-Neblett
S.-N. brachytherapy method
S.-N. template
Syed-Puthawala-Hedger esophageal applicator
Syed template
sylvian
s. aqueduct
s. aqueduct syndrome
s. candelabra
s. cistern
s. fissure
s. operculum
s. point
s. triangle
sylvian-rolandic junction
Sylvius
aqueduct of S.
cistern of S.
fissure of S., sylvian fissure
fossa of S.

S. fossa
S. ventricle
Syme ankle disarticulation amputation
Symmers fibrosis
symmetric, symmetrical
bilaterally s.
s. chest
s. distribution
s. echo
s. heart hypertrophy
s. IUGR
s. narrowing
s. periosteal reaction
s. phased array
s. pulmonary congestion
s. thorax
sympathectomy
sympathetic
s. block
s. chain
s. denervation
s. discharge
s. dystrophy
s. ganglia tumor
s. ganglion
s. innervation
s. nervous tissue
s. vascular instability
sympathogonia
symphysis
s. cartilage joint
pubic s.
s. pubis
symptom
constellation of s.'s
constitutional s.'s
objective s.'s
segmental bronchus s.
Tar s.
vasomotor s.
symptomatic
s. coarctation of aorta
s. gallstone
s. hydrocephalus
s. lateral synovial plica
s. metastatic spinal cord compression
s. vascular ring
symptomatology
synaptic
s. cleft
s. dopamine concentration
s. pathway
s. vesicle
SYNC
V S.
vertical synchronization pulse
syncephalus
synchondrosis
cartilaginous s.
low signal intensity s.
neurocentral s.
petrooccipital s.
sphenooccipital s.
synchronicity
synchronization device
synchronized retroperfusion
synchronous
s. carotid arterial pulse
s. disease
s. lesion
s. transitional cell carcinoma
synchrony
ventricular s.
synchrotron
monochromatic s.
s. radiation
syncope
carotid sinus s.
deglutition s.
swallowing s.
syncytium
circular s.
Sertoli s.
syndactylization of digit
syndactyly
s. in fetus
syndesmophyte
marginal s.
spinal s.
syndesmosis, pl. **syndesmoses**
s. sprain
s. sprain of ankle
tibiofibular s.
syndesmotic
s. clear space
s. diastasis
s. impingement
s. ligament
s. ligament complex
syndrome
acquired immunodeficiency s. (AIDS)
acute central cord s.

NOTES

S

syndrome *(continued)*
acute compartment s.
acute radiation s.
acute radiation bone marrow s.
acute respiratory distress s. (ARDS)
acute retroviral s.
Adams-Stokes s.
Addison s.
adenomatous polyposis s.
adrenal feminizing s.
adrenal virilizing s.
adrenogenital s.
adult respiratory distress s. (ARDS)
afferent loop s.
Aicardi s.
Alagille s.
Albright s.
Albright-McCune-Sternberg s.
Aldrich s.
AMBRI s.
amnionic band s.
angiomatous s.
angioosteohypertrophy s.
anomalous innominate artery compression s.
anomalous vein of scimitar s.
anterior cerebellar artery s.
anterior compartment s.
anterior cord s.
anterior spinal artery s.
Anton s.
aortic arch hypoplasia s.
aortitis s.
apallic s.
Archer s.
Arnold-Chiari s.
arrhythmogenic right ventricular dysplasia s.
Asherman s.
Asherson s.
ataxia-hemiparesis s.
atherosclerotic occlusive s.
Avellis s.
axonopathic neurogenic thoracic outlet s.
Balint s.
ballooning mitral valve prolapse s.
Bannayan-Riley-Ruvalcaba s.
Banti s.
bare lymphocyte s.
Barlow s.
Barré-Lieou s.
Bartter s.
basal cell nevus s.
basilar artery s.
battered child s.
beat-knee s.
Beckwith-Wiedemann s.
Behçet chest s.
Behr s.
Bernard-Horner s.
Beuren s.
biliary obstruction s.
Bing-Horton s.
Blackfan-Diamond s.
blind loop s.
blind pouch s.
Bloom s.
blueberry muffin s.
blue-digit s.
blue rubber-bleb nevus s.
blue-toe s.
Boerhaave s.
Bouveret s.
Bouveret-Hoffmann s.
Bradbury-Eggleston s.
Brett s.
Brissaud s.
broad thumb s.
Brock meddle lobe s.
bronchiectasis-bronchomalacia s.
Brown-Séquard s.
bubbly lung s.
buckled innominate artery s.
Budd-Chiari s., Budd syndrome
Burke s.
Buschke-Ollendorff s.
Cacchione s.
Caffey-Kempe s.
capillary leak s.
Caplan s.
carcinoid s.
cardiac radiation s.
cardiocutaneous s.
cardiofacial s.
cardiosplenic s.
carotid blowout s.
carotid cavernous s.
carotid sinus s. (CSS)
carpal tunnel s.
cauda equina s. (CES)
cavernous sinus s.
cavitary mesenteric lymph node s.
Cayler s.
Ceelen-Gellerstedt s.
celiac artery compression s.
celiac axis s.
cerebellar s.
cerebral steal s.
cerebrohepatorenal s. (CHRS)
cervical aorta s.
cervical disk s.
cervical dorsal outlet s.
cervical kink s.
cervical pain s.

cervical rib s.
Céstan-Chenais s.
Chandra-Khetarpal s.
Chédiak-Steinbrinck-Higashi s.
Chiari-Budd s.
Chiari-Foix-Nicolesco s.
Chilaiditi s.
chronic overuse s.
chronic venous statis s.
Churg-Strauss s.
circulation hyperkinetic s.
Clarke-Hadefield s.
Claude s.
cleft face s.
Clerc-Levy-Cristeco s. (CLC)
clumsy-hand s.
coarctation s.
Cobb s.
cobbler's chest s.
Cockayne s.
Cogan s.
Colinet-Caplan s.
Collet-Sicard s.
compartment s.
compression s.
congenital adrenogenital s.
congenital heart disease s.
congenital pulmonary venolobar s.
congenital vascular-bone s. (CVBS)
Conn s.
Conradi-Hünermann s.
constriction band s.
coronary artery steal s.
coronary-subclavian steal s.
cortical renal cyst s.
Corvisart s.
costal margin s.
costoclavicular s.
Cotton-Berg s.
Cowley s.
craniofacial pain s.
craniomandibular s.
CREST s.
cri-du-chat s.
Cronkhite-Canada s.
crush s.
cubital tunnel s.
Curracino-Silverman s.
Cushing s.
Cyriax s.
Dandy-Walker s.
Davies-Colley s.
deafness, onychodystrophy, osteodystrophy, mental retardation s.
de Lange s.
De Martini-Balestra s.
Demons-Meigs s.
de Morsier s.
Determann s.
DiGeorge s.
DiGimard s.
distal intestinal obstruction s.
disuse s.
DOOR s.
double outlet right ventricle s.
Down s.
Drash s.
Dressler postmyocardial infarction s.
drowned newborn s.
Dubin-Johnson s.
dumping s.
Dusard s.
Dyke-Davidoff-Masson s.
dysarthria s.
dysgenetic s.
dysmyelopoietic s.
Eagle-Barrett s.
ectopic ACTH s.
ectopic parathyroid s.
ectrodactyly-ectodermal dysplasia-clefting s.
Edward s.
EEC s.
Eisenmenger s.
elbow-patella s.
Ellis-van Creveld s.
Elsner s.
empty sella s.
encephalotrigeminal s.
enlarged vestibular aqueduct s.
entrapment s.
Erdheim I s.
euthyroid sick s.
excessive lateral pressure s. (ELPS)
external carotid steal s.
extrinsic sick sinus s.
facet s.
facioauriculovertebral s.
failed back s. (FBS)
failed back surgery s. (FBSS)
failing ovary s.
Fallot s.
familial adenomatous polyposis s.

S

NOTES

syndrome *(continued)*
familial dysplastic nevus s.
familial polyposis s.
Fanconi-Hegglin s.
Farber s.
fasciitis panniculitis s.
fat embolism s. (FES)
fat pad impingement s.
Feldaker s.
Felty s.
feminizing testes s.
fetal cardiosplenic s.
fibrocystic breast s.
Fiessinger-Leroy s.
Fiessinger-Leroy-Reiter s.
Fissinger-Rendu s.
Fitz-Hugh and Curtis s.
Fleischner s.
floppy valve s.
Fluckiger s.
focal cerebral s.
Foix-Alajouanine s.
Foix-Chavany-Marie s.
Forney s.
Forrester s.
Frey s.
Friedel Pick s.
Frimodt-Moller s.
functional bowel s.
Gaisbock s.
Garcin s.
Gardner bone s.
Gardner-Diamond s.
Gardner GI tract s.
Garland s.
gas-bloat s.
gastrocardiac s.
gastrointestinal s.
generalized lymphadenopathy s.
Goldenhar s.
Goodpasture s.
Gorham s.
Gorham-Stout s.
Gouley s.
Gowers s.
Graham-Burford-Mayer s.
Grisel s.
Gsell-Erdheim s.
Guillain-Barré s.
Hajdu-Cheney s.
Hale s.
Hallermann-Streiff-François s.
Hamman-Rich s.
hand-foot s.
Harbitz-Mueller s.
Harkavy s.
Hayem-Widal s.
Heerfordt s.
Hegglin s.
hemisensory s.
hemopleuropneumonia s.
hemorrhagic lung s.
hepatorenal s. (HRS)
Heryln-Werner-Wunderlich s.
heterotaxia s.
hindgut s.
Hippel-Lindau s.
holiday heart s.
Holmes s.
Holt-Oram s.
Hood s.
Hughes-Stovin s.
Hutchinson s.
Hutchinson-Gilford s.
Hutinel-Pick s.
hyperabduction s.
hyperviscosity s.
hypogenetic lung s.
hypoperistalsis s.
hypoplastic aorta s.
hypoplastic heart s.
hypoplastic left heart s. (HLHS)
hypoplastic left ventricle s.
hypoplastic right heart s.
hyposensitive carotid sinus s.
ileocecal s.
iliocaval compression s.
ilioinguinal s.
iliotibial band friction s.
s. of impending thrombosis
impingement s.
incomplete Kartagener s.
infantile s.
inferior vena cava s.
inflammatory response s.
inframammary s.
infrapatellar contracture s. (IPCS)
infratentorial s.
inguinal ligament s.
innominate artery compression s.
intercoronary steal s.
intermediate coronary s.
internal snapping hip s.
intestinal Behçet s.
intestinal hypoperistalsis s.
intestinal pseudoobstruction s.
intrauterine parabiotic s.
intrinsic sick sinus s.
irritable bowel s.
isolated tethered cord s.
Ivemark CHD s.
Jaffe-Campanacci s.
Janus s.
Jarcho-Levin s.
Jeune s.
Jeune-Tommasi s.

Joubert s.
jugular foramen s.
Kartagener s.
Kasabach-Merritt s.
Kast s.
Katayama s.
Kawasaki s.
Kearns-Sayre s.
Kemp-Elliot-Gorlin s.
Kimmelstiel-Wilson s.
kinky-hair s.
Kinsbourne s.
Klauder s.
Kleffner-Landau s.
Klein-Waardenburg s.
Klinefelter s. (KS)
Klippel-Feil s.
Klippel-Trenaunay s.
Klippel-Trenaunay-Weber s.
Klippel-Trenaunay-Weber-Rubashov s.
Koerber-Salus-Elschnig s.
Korsakoff s.
Kurtz-Sprague-White s.
Lady Windermere s.
Laslett-Short s.
Laubry-Pezzi s.
Laurence-Moon-Biedl s.
Laurence-Moon-Biedl-Bardet s.
left heart s.
left parietal s.
Leitner s.
Leriche s.
Leri-Layani-Weill s.
Lesch-Nyhan s.
lethal wasting s.
Lhermitte s.
Lian-Siguier-Welti venous thrombosis s.
Lightwood s.
Loehr-Kindberg s.
Löffler s.
Looser-Milkman s.
Louis-Bar s.
low back s.
Low-Beers s.
low cardiac output s.
low-flow s.
Lown-Ganong-Levine s. (LGL)
lumbar thecoperitoneal shunt s.
Lutembacher s.
luxury perfusion s.
Lyell s.
lymphadenopathy s.
lymph node s.
Macleod s.
Maffucci s.
Majewski s.
malabsorption s.
mal de Meleda s.
male Turner s.
Mallory-Weiss s.
Manson schistosomiasis-pulmonary artery obstruction s.
manubriosternal s.
Marable s.
Marfan bone s.
Marfan CHD s.
marfanoid hypermobility s.
Marine-Lenhart s.
Maroteaux-Lamy s.
Martorell aortic arch s.
Martorell-Fabre s.
MAS s.
Master s.
Maugeri s.
Mayer-Rokitansky-Küster-Hauser s.
Mazabraud s.
McArdle s.
McCune-Albright s.
McKusick-Kaufman s.
Meadows s.
Meckel s.
Meckel-Gruber s.
meconium aspiration s.
meconium plug s.
medial tibial stress s.
megacystis-microcolon-intestinal hypoperistalsis s.
Meigs s.
Meigs-Cass s.
Meigs-Salmon s.
Melnick-Needles s.
Mendelson s.
Menkes s.
mermaid s.
metastatic carcinoid s.
microcolon-megacystis s.
midaortic s.
middle aortic s.
middle fossa s.
middle lobe s.
Mikity-Wilson s.
Mikulicz s.

NOTES

syndrome *(continued)*
milk-alkali s.
milk leg s.
Milkman s.
Miller-Dieker s.
Millikan-Siekert s.
Milwaukee shoulder s.
Minot-von Willebrand s.
Mirizzi s.
mitral regurgitation-chordal elongation s.
Mohr s.
Morel s.
Morgagni s.
Morgagni-Adams-Stokes s.
Morquio s.
motion-related impingement s.
Mounier-Kuhn s.
moyamoya s.
Moynahan s.
MSA s.
mucocutaneous lymph node s. (MCLS)
mucosal neuroma s.
mucosal prolapse s.
mucus plug s.
multiple endocrine neoplasia s.
multiple pterygium s.
multiple system atrophy s.
myeloproliferative s.
myofascial pain dysfunction s.
nail-patella s.
Naumoff s.
naviculocapitate s.
Nelson s.
nephrotic s.
nervous heart s.
neurocutaneous s.
Nievergelt s.
Noonan s.
Nothnagel s.
nuchal cyst s.
nutcracker s.
occult steal s.
Ogilvie s.
Omenn s.
orbital apex s.
organic brain s. (OBS)
orodigitofacial s.
Ortner s.
Osler s.
Osler-Libman-Sacks s.
Osler-Weber-Rendu s.
osmotic demyelination s.
os trigonum s.
ovarian hyperstimulation s.
ovarian polycystic s.
ovarian remnant s.
ovarian vein s.
overuse s.
Paget-von Schroetter s.
Pancoast s.
pancreaticohepatic s.
Papillon-Lefevre s.
paraneoplastic lung cancer s.
parathymic s.
parchment heart s.
Parkes-Weber s.
partial steal s.
Patau s.
pectoralis major s.
Pena Shokeir s.
Pendred s.
pericardiotomy s.
perinatal respiratory distress s.
Pfeiffer s.
PFFD s.
proximal femoral focal deficiency syndrome
phantom limb s.
Pierre Robin s.
piriformis s.
plica s.
Poland s.
polyposis s.
polysplenia s.
Pompe s.
pontine s.
popliteal artery entrapment s.
postcardiac injury s. (PCIS)
postcholecystectomy s.
postembolization s.
posterior column s.
posterior joint s.
postmastectomy lymphedema s.
postmaturity s.
postmyocardial infarction s.
postperfusion lung s.
postpericardiotomy s.
postpolio s.
postrubella s.
postsurgical lumbosacral s.
Potter s.
proximal femoral focal deficiency s. (PFFD syndrome)
proximal loop s.
pseudoblind loop s.
pseudolymphoma s.
pseudothrombophlebitis s.
pseudo-Turner s.
pseudo-Z-E s.
pulmonary venolobar s.
quadrilateral space s.
radiation toxicity s.
Raeder-Arbitz s.
Raeder paratrigeminal s.

Ramsay Hunt s.
Raymond-Cestan s.
Raynaud s.
reactive airways dysfunction s.
Reader paratrigeminal s.
Reinhardt s.
Reiter s.
respiratory distress s. (RDS)
restrictive cardiac s.
restrictive hemodynamic s.
Rett s.
reversible organic brain s.
Ridley s.
Riley-Day s.
Robert s.
Robinow s.
Rokitansky-Mayer-Küster-Hauser s.
Romano-Ward s.
Romberg-Wood s.
Roques s.
Rosenbach s.
Rosen-Castleman-Liebow s.
Rotor s.
Royer-Wilson s.
Ruge-Simon s.
Russell-Silver s.
Ruvalcaba-Myhre-Smith s.
Sack-Barabas s.
Saldino-Noonan s.
Sanfilippo s.
SAPHO s.
scalenus anticus s.
scalenus tunnel s.
scaphocapitate s.
scapulocostal s.
Scheie s.
Schwartz-Jampel s. (SJS)
scimitar s.
septic lung s.
shaggy aorta s.
shaken baby s. (SBS)
Sheehan s.
shocklike s.
Shone s.
short gut s.
short rib-polydactyly s.
shoulder-hand s.
shoulder impingement s.
shoulder-upper extremity-thoracic outlet s.
Shprintzen velocardiofacial s.
sinus tarsi s.
Sipple s.
Sjögren s.
Sjögren orbital s.
slipping rib s.
slit-ventricle s.
sloughed urethra s.
small-aorta s.
small-cuff s.
small left colon s.
Smith-Lemli-Opitz s.
Smythe s.
snapping hip s.
soldier's heart s.
Soleus s.
solitary rectal ulcer s.
Solomon s.
Sotos s.
spastic bowel s.
Spens s.
sphenoidal fissure s.
split-cord s.
split-notochord s.
stagnant-loop s.
steal s.
Stein-Leventhal s.
Stewart-Treves s.
stiff-lung s.
stiff-man s.
Stouffer s.
Sturge-Weber s.
Sturge-Weber-Dimitri s.
subacromial pain s.
subclavian steal s. (SSP)
subscapular notch s.
superfemale s.
superior mesenteric artery s. (SMAS)
superior vena cava s.
suprascapular notch s.
suspended heart s.
Swyer s.
Swyer-James s.
Swyer-James-MacLeod s.
sylvian aqueduct s.
systemic inflammatory response s.
TAR s.
target tunnel s.
tarsal tunnel s. (TTS)
Taussig-Snellen-Alberts s.
terminal reservoir s.
tethered cord s. (TCS)
thoracic inlet s.

NOTES

syndrome *(continued)*
thoracic outlet s. (TOS)
Tietze s.
tight filum terminal s.
Tolosa-Hunt s.
transient bone marrow edema s.
trashfoot s.
Treacher Collins s.
trisomy D s.
trisomy E s.
trisomy 8 mosaicism s.
Trousseau s.
tumor lysis s. (TLS)
Turcot s.
Turkish sabre s.
Turner s.
Turner s.
twiddler's s.
twin embolization s.
twin-to-twin transfusion s. (TTTS)
ugly foot s.
Uhl s.
ulnar abutment s.
ulnar impaction s.
ulnar tunnel s.
ulnolunate impaction s.
uncal herniation s.
unroofed coronary sinus s.
upper limb-cardiac s.
Upshaw-Schulman s.
urethral s.
VACTERL s.
van Buchem s.
Van der Hoeve s.
vanishing bone s.
vanishing lung s.
vanishing testes s.
vascular leak s.
vasodepressor s.
vasovagal s.
vena cava s.
venolobar s.
vertebral artery s.
vertebrobasilar artery s.
vestibular aqueduct s. (VAS)
Villaret-Mackenzie s.
visceral cholesterol embolization s.
von Hippel-Lindau s.
von Recklinghausen s.
Von Rokitansky s.
Waardenburg s.
Wallenberg lateral medullary s.
Weil s.
Weill-Marchesani s.
Weinberg-Himelfarb s.
Weisenburg s.
Weiss-Baker s.
Werner s.
Wernicke-Korsakoff s.
wet-lung s.
white-lung s.
Wiedemann-Beckwith s.
Wilkie s.
Wilkinson s.
Williams s.
Williams-Beuren s.
Williams-Campbell s.
Williams elfin facies s.
Wilson-Mikity s.
s. with multiple cortical renal cyst
Wolff-Parkinson-White s.
Wolf-Hirschhorn s.
Wyburn-Mason s.
xiphoid process s.
XXY s.
XY s.
Yunis-Varon s.
Zeek s.
Zellweger s.
Ziegler s.
Zieve s.
Zinner s.
Zollinger-Ellison s.

synechia, pl. **synechiae**
uterine s.
s. vulvae

synergic muscle

synergism

synergy
S. ultrasound
S. ultrasound system

syngeneic
s. bone marrow transplant
s. tissue

syngraft

synkinesis

synostosis, pl. **synostoses**
bicoronal s.
cervical s.
congenital radioulnar s.
coronal s.
craniofacial s.
lambdoid s.
metatarsal s.
multiple-suture s.
nonsyndromic bicoronal s.
nonsyndromic unicoronal s.
premature suture s.
radiographically firm s.
sagittal s.
single suture s.
terminal s.
tibiofibular s.
unicoronal s.

synovectomy
radiopharmaceutical s.

synovial
s. bursa
s. cavity
s. chondromatosis
s. cyst
s. diarthroidal joint
s. diffuse lipoma
s. envelope
s. fluid
s. fringe
s. gutter
s. hemangioma
s. herniation pit
s. inflammatory response
s. ligament
s. membrane
s. osteochondromatosis
s. pannus
s. plica
s. proliferation
s. sarcoma
s. sheath
s. shelf
s. surface
s. thickening
s. tissue
synoviogram
synovioma
synovitis
boggy s.
brucellar s.
intraarticular localized nodular s.
nodular s.
pigmented villonodular s. (PVNS)
purulent s.
toxic s.
transient s.
transitory s.
s. tumor
synovitis, acne, pustulosis, hyperostosis, osteomyelitis (SAPHO)
synovium
boggy s.
exuberant s.
hyperplastic s.
opaque s.
pannus of s.
synovium-filled degenerative cyst
synovium-lined fascicle
synpneumonic empyema
synthesis
automated s.
facile s.
synthesizer
frequency s.
synthetic
s. bone implant
s. graft bypass to ankle
s. valve
s. vascular bypass graft
syphilis
bone s.
tertiary s.
syphilitic
s. aortic aneurysm
s. aortic regurgitation
s. aortitis
s. node
syringe
electric s.
Ultraject pre-filled s.
syringes (*pl. of* syrinx)
syringobulbia
syringocarcinoma
syringocele
syringoencephalia
syringoencephalomyelia
syringohydromyelia
holocord s.
syringohydromyelic cavity
syringoma
chondroid s.
syringomeningocele
syringomyelia
ape hand of s.
cervical s.
communicating s.
posttraumatic s.
syringopontia
syrinx, pl. **syringes**
s. cavity
traumatic s.
system
Acuson 128XP ultrasound s.
AEGIS sonography management s.
Agfa CR s.
Agfa PACS s.
AI 5200 diagnostic ultrasound s.
air-filtration s.
Airis II MRI s.
Aloka SSD ultrasound s.
ALT ultrasound s.

S

NOTES

system *(continued)*
American Medical Association Ligament Injury Classification S.
Angiomat 6000 contrast delivery s.
AngioRad radiation s.
AngioVista angiographic s.
anterolateral s.
aortoiliac inflow s.
Apogee CX 200 echo s.
Apollo DXA bone densitometry s.
AquaSens FMS 1000 fluid monitoring s.
Arcitumomab diagnostic imaging s.
Artoscan MRI s.
Ashhurst fracture classification s.
Aspen digital ultrasound s.
Aspire continuous imaging s.
Atlas 2.0 diagnostic ultrasound s.
ATL HDI 3000 ultrasound s.
Aurora dedicated breast MRI s.
automated angle-encoder s.
autonomic nervous s.
Aviva mammography s.
axial spinal s.
BAK-1 interbody fusion s.
Bard CPS s.
Bard percutaneous cardiopulmonary support s.
Bard rotary atherectomy s. (BRAS)
Batson vertebral brain s.
Bevalac s.
Biad SPECT imaging s.
biliary s.
Biosound AU (Advanced Ultrasonography) s.
Biospec MR imaging s.
biphasic s.
biventricular support s. (BVS)
Bracco s.
Breast Imaging Reporting and Data S. (BIRADS)
Bristol-Myers s.
British engineering s. (BES)
Bruker CSI MR s.
caliceal s.
CardioCamera imaging s.
Cardio3DScope imaging s.
cardiopulmonary support s.
cardiovascular s.
carrier-mediated transport s.
cartesian reference coordinate s.
CathTrack catheter locator s.
CDRPan digital x-ray s.
central nervous s. (CNS)
CGR biplane angiographic s.
Chachoua staging s.
Chemo-Port perivena catheter s.
circumflex coronary s.
codominant s.
collateral s.
collecting s.
collimating s.
Compass stereotactic frame s.
Compton-suppression s.
Computerized Thermal Imaging s.
continuous-wave, high-frequency Doppler ultrasound s.
continuous-wave laser s.
Contour mammography s.
contour tilting compression mammography s.
Cordis endovascular s.
Coroskop C cardiac imaging s.
Cotrel-Dubousset s.
CrystalEYES video s.
Curix Capacity Plus film processing s.
Cyberware s.
data-acquisition s. (DAS)
dedicated breast biopsy s.
DELTAmanager MedImage s.
Desilets introducer s.
Diastonics s.
Dictaphone Digital Express clinical reporting s.
digestive s.
Digital Add-On Bucky image acquisition s.
Digital Equipment s.
digital holography s.
digital mammographic s.
Digital Traumex s.
Digitron digital subtraction imaging s.
DIMAQ integrated ultrasound s.
directly coupled sample changer s.
display s.
dominant left coronary artery s.
dominant right coronary artery s.
dryer s.
DryView laser imaging s.
dual-head gamma camera s.
dual screen/dual emulsion s.
duplicated renal collecting s.
DuPont Rare Earth imaging s.
dye laser s.
Dynarad portable imaging s.
E.CAM dual-head emission imaging s.
Echovar Doppler s.
effaced collecting s.
electrostatic imaging s.
Elscint s.
Elston-Scharff-Bloom-Richardson histologic grade s.
endocavitary applicator s.

engorged collecting s.
Evans-D'Angio staging s.
Evans fracture classification s.
excimer laser s.
external jugular s.
extracranial carotid s.
extrapyramidal s.
femoropopliteal outflow s.
fetal musculoskeletal s.
fibroepithelial polyp collecting s.
Ficat-Marcus grading s.
fiducial alignment s.
filling defect collecting s.
FlimFax teleradiology s.
Flocks-Kadesky s.
FluoroPlus angiography s.
FluoroPlus Roadmapper digital fluoroscopy s.
fluoroptic thermometry s.
Fonar s.
Fränkel classification s.
Fuji AC2 storage phosphor computed radiology s.
Fuji FCR9000 computed radiology s.
full-field digital mammography s.
Galen teleradiology s.
GE CT Hi-Speed Advantage s.
GE Signa MR s.
GE single-axis SR-230 echoplanar s.
GE 1.5-T s.
gradient s.
greater saphenous s.
Greenfield vena cava filter s.
guided coaxial balloon catheter s.
Hardy-Vezine classification s.
HDI 1000 ultrasound s.
HDI 3000 ultrasound s.
HDI 5000 ultrasound imaging s.
Helios laser s.
Helix multihead nuclear imaging s.
hepatic ductal s.
hepatic venous s.
Hewlett-Packard phased-array imaging s.
high-field s.
HIMAC s.
Hi-Star midfield MRI s.
Hitachi Open MRI s.
homonuclear spin s.
House grading s.
HP SONOS 5500 ultrasound imaging s.
Hunt-Hess aneurysm grading s.
HyperPACS s.
IBM Speech Server clinical reporting s.
IDIS angiography s.
iiRAD DR1000C digital radiographic s.
image analysis s.
image recording s.
imaging center information s. (ICIS)
Imatron s.
Immunomedics s.
Impax PACS s.
implantable drug delivery s.
Innovator Holter s.
Instrumentation Laboratory s.
intensified radiographic imaging s. (IRIS)
internal carotid s.
Intra-Op autotransfusion s.
intrarenal collecting s.
Isocam scintillation imaging s.
Isocam SPECT imaging s.
Jackson staging s.
Kadish staging s.
Kelley-Goerss Compass stereotactic s.
Krigel staging s.
Lagios classification s.
Laitinen CT guidance s.
Lanier clinical reporting s.
laser s.
left iliac s.
left ventricular support s.
Leksell stereotactic s.
LENT scoring s.
lesser saphenous s.
Liebel-Flarsheim CT 9000 contrast delivery s.
lipophilic sequestration s.
lower pole collecting s.
Luxtec fiberoptic s.
LVs s.
LymphoScan nuclear imaging s.
Magnes biomagnetometer s.
Magnetom Open s.
Magnetom Vision MR s.
Magnex Alpha MR s.
mamillary s.

S

NOTES

system *(continued)*
Mammotest breast biopsy s.
Manchester LDR implant s.
Marex MRI s.
Massachusetts (General Hospital) Utility Multiprogramming S.
MEDDARS cardiac catheterization analysis s.
Medilase angioscope-laser delivery s.
Medspec MR imaging s.
Medweb clinical reporting s.
Mini-Balloon s.
MIR s.
Mitsuyasu staging s.
Mobetron electron beam s.
mucosal mass collecting s.
multidetector s.
multigated pulsed Doppler flow s.
multileaf collimating s.
musculoskeletal s.
NeuroSector ultrasound s.
nonopaque intraluminal mass in collecting s.
Novacor left ventricular assist s.
nuclear medicine information s. (NMIS)
Octreoscan s.
OEC Series 9600 cardiac s.
"one-stick" s.
Opdima digital mammography s.
open-architecture s.
open-configuration magnetic resonance s.
OpenPACS s.
OSCAR ultrasonic bone cement removal s.
OsteoView desktop hand x-ray s.
Ostreg spinal marker s.
Ovation falloposcopy s.
parasympathetic nervous s.
Paris s.
Paterson-Parker s.
Peacock s.
pelvocaliceal s.
PenRad mammography clinical reporting s.
Pentax-Hitachi FG32UA endosonographic s.
peripheral nervous s.
Philips DVI 1 s.
photoelectric s.
Picker s.
Picket Fence fiducial localization stereotactic s.
picture archival communication s.
picture archiving and communication s. (PACS)
Pinnacle 3 radiation therapy planning s.
PMT robotic fulcrumless tomographic s.
polar coordinate s.
polypoid fibroma collecting s.
portal vein s.
PortalVision radiation oncology s.
Probe balloon dilatation s.
Profile mammography s.
ProstaScint s.
pulmonary venous s.
PulseSpray pulsed infusion s.
pyelocaliceal s.
pyramidal s.
Q-catheter catheterization recording s.
quadrature surface coil MRI s.
Quimby implant s.
radiation therapy planning s.
radiology telephone access s. (RTAS)
radionuclide carrier s.
RadNet radiology information s.
real-time two-dimensional Doppler flow-imaging s.
Redi-Vu teleradiology s.
reference coordinate s.
renal collecting s.
respiratory s.
reticuloendothelial s.
s. of Retzius
Retzius s.
ring-type imaging s.
Robson modification of Flocks-Kadesky s.
Rogan teleradiology s.
Roger s.
Rotablator thrombectomy s.
rotational atherectomy s. (RAS)
Rowe-Lowell fracture-dislocation classification s.
RTP s.
Sadowsky breast marking s.
saphenous s.
Scanditronix MLC s.
Scanmaster DX s.
scanned-slot detector s.
scanning beam digital s.
scattering s.
scavenging s.
Schmidt optics s.
Scintiview nuclear computer s.
Scintron IV nuclear computer s.
Selectron s.
SenoScan mammography s.
sequestration s.
Shape Maker s.

Shimadzu s.
Siemens AG s.
Siemens 1.5-T s.
Signa Advantage s.
Signa GEMS MR imaging s.
Silicon Graphics Reality Engine s.
Simpson Coronary AtheroCath (SCA) s.
single-photon counting s. (SPC system)
"single-stick" s.
skeletal s.
slip-ring gantry s.
SmartSpot high-resolution digital imaging s.
sonic-accelerated fracture-healing s. (SAFHS)
Sonifer sonicating s.
Sonoline Elegra ultrasound s.
Sonoline Sierra ultrasound imaging s.
SPC s.
  single-photon counting system
spiderlike pelvocaliceal s.
splanchnic venous s.
spring-driven s.
Squibb s.
STARRT falloposcopy s.
StereoGuide prone breast biopsy s.
StereoLoc upright biopsy s.
storage phosphor s.
Stratis II MRI s.
striped tag myocardial tagging s. (STAG)
Sudbury s.
Sun SPARCstation s.
SureStart imaging s.
Surgical Planning and Orientation Computer S. (SPOCS)
Synergy ultrasound s.
Tecmag Libra-S16 s.
TEGwire ST s.
thermal dosimetry s.
tibioperoneal runoff s.
time-of-flight PET imaging s.
TMS three-dimensional radiation therapy planning s.
TNM staging s.
Tomolex tomographic s.
Trex digital mammography s. (TDMS)
Triad SPECT imaging s.
TRON 3 VACI cardiac imaging s.
trumpet-like pelvocaliceal s.
Trunkey fracture classification s.
two-channel phased-array RF receiver coil s.
UltraPACS diagnostic imaging s.
ultrasound s.
UltraSTAR computer-based ultrasound reporting s.
University of Florida staging s.
s. unsharpness
uPACS picture archiving s.
upper pole collecting s.
USCI Probe balloon-on-a-wire dilatation s.
Vac-Lok patient immobilization s.
vacuum cassette s.
Varian brachytherapy s.
Varian MLC s.
VARIS radiation oncology s.
VasoView balloon dissection s.
VAX 4100 s.
ventricular s.
VentTrak monitoring s.
vertebral artery s.
vertebrobasilar s.
VEST s.
view shadow projection microtomographic s.
Vingmed Sound CFM ultrasound s.
Virtuoso portable three-dimensional imaging s.
VISION high-performance gradient s.
Vitrea 3D s.
VoiceRAD clinical reporting s.
VoxelView s.
widened collecting s.
xenon trap s.
Xillix LIFE-GI fluorescence endoscopy s.
XKnife stereotactic radiosurgery s.
x-ray shadow projection microtomographic s.
Zickel fracture classification s.
Zlatkin grading s.

systematic
  s. noise
  s. relaxation effect
  s. ultrasound-guided biopsy

systemic
  s. adjuvant therapy

NOTES

systemic *(continued)*
s. arterial circulation
s. arterial hypertension
s. arterial vasoconstriction
s. arteriolar resistance index
s. blood flow (SBF)
s. brain lymphoma
s. diastolic blood pressure
s. disorder
s. erythematosus lupus
s. heart
s. heparinization
s. hypoperfusion
s. inflammatory response syndrome
s. lesion
s. mastocytosis
s. mean arterial pressure (SMAP)
s. mercury intoxication
s. micrometastasis
s. nodular panniculitis
s. output
s. output flow
s. output index
s. oxygen saturation
s. sclerosis
s. vascular resistance (SVR)
s. vascular resistance index (SvO_2, SVRI)
s. vein
s. venous
s. venous hypertension
s. venous return

systole
atrial s.
end s. (ES)
end of atrial s.
left ventricular internal dimension at end s. (LVIDs)
left ventricular internal end s.
ventricular s.

systolic
s. acceleration time
s. anterior motion (SAM)
s. anterior motion of mitral valve
s. anterior movement
s. atrial volume
s. blood pressure (SBP)
s. ejection fraction
s. ejection period (SEP)
s. fractional shortening
s. function
s. gating
s. gradient
s. heart failure
s. hypertension
s. impulse
s. mammary souffle
s. pressure-time index
s. prolapse
s. prolapse of mitral valve leaflet
s. reserve
s. retraction
s. retraction of apex
s. S wave
s. toe/brachial index
s. upstroke time
s. velocity ratio
s. velocity-time integral
s. ventricular overload

systolic-diastolic blood pressure

systolic/diastolic ratio (S/D ratio)

Szumowski sequence

γ-T
γ-tocopherol
T
temporal
tesla
thoracic
T artifact
T condylar fracture
T fracture
T loop
T tubogram
T vector
T1
T. relaxation time
T. shortening
T2
T. quantitative MRI
T. relaxation time
T. shortening
T. star relaxation
T. time constant
T_4
thyroxinc
t
transformer
T2-gradient refocused image
T3 resin uptake test
T4 uptake
Ta
tantalum
^{178}Ta
tantalum-178
^{182}Ta
tantalum-182
Tabar pattern
tabes
burned-out t.
t. dorsalis
table
critical dose t.
dual lookup t.
Hadlock t.
Hydradjust IV t.
inner t.
outer t.
pivoting t.
t. of radiation dose
radionuclide t.
resistive exercise t.
tilt t.
tachyarrhythmia
supraventricular t.
tachycardia
atrial ectopic automatic t.
nodoventricular t.
nonincudible t.
paroxysmal auricular t. (PAT)
sinoatrial nodal reentry t.
supraventricular t.
ventricular paroxysmal t.
tachycardia-induced cardiomyopathy
tachykinin
tachypnea
transient t.
tackler's exostosis
tactile disk
taenia tissue
tag
t. of cartilage
t. plane
Tagarno 3SD cine projector for angiography
tagged
t. atom
radioactively t.
tagging
bolus t.
cine magnetic resonance t.
t. cine magnetic resonance
t. cine MR imaging
myocardial t.
segmented k-space cardiac t.
spin t.
TAH
total artificial heart
TAHBSO
total abdominal hysterectomy and bilateral salpingo-oophorectomy
tail
axillary t.
t. bone
t. of breast
comet t.
common bile duct rat t.
dural t.
t. of epididymis
t. of pancreas
t. sign
t. of Spence
wool t.
tailgut cyst
taillike segment
tailored
t. excitation
tailor's
t. ankle
t. muscle
Takayasu
T. aortitis
T. arteritis

takeoff
t. of artery
high t.
t. of vessel
takeup of radioactive material
Talairach space
talar
t. avulsion fracture
t. beaking
t. body fusion
t. dome
t. dome cyst
t. dome fracture
t. dome ischemia
t. impingement
t. neck fracture
t. osteochondral fracture
t. tilt angle
talc
t. plaque
t. pneumoconiosis
talcosis
lung t.
pulmonary t.
tali (*gen. and pl. of* talus)
talipes
t. arcuatus
t. calcaneus
t. calcaneus calcaneocavus
t. cavovalgus
t. cavus
t. cavus calcaneocavus
t. equinovarus
t. valgus
t. varus
T-ALL
T-cell acute lymphoblastic leukemia
talocalcaneal
t. angle
anteroposterior t. (APTC)
t. articulation
t. coalition
t. index
t. index classification
t. joint
lateral t. (LATC)
t. ligament
talocalcaneonavicular
t. articulation
t. joint
talocrural
t. angle
t. fusion
t. joint
talofibular
t. impingement
t. joint
t. ligament
t. ligament injury
talometatarsal angle
talonavicular
t. angle
t. articulation
t. beaking
t. capsule
t. joint
t. ligament
talus, gen. and pl. **tali**
beaking of head of t.
t. bone
Cedell fracture of t.
congenital vertical t.
flat-top t.
t. foot deformity
neck of t.
osteochondral lesion of the t. (OLT)
Sneppen fracture of t.
sulcus t.
sustentaculum tali
vertical t.
tam-o-shanter appearance
tampon
vaginal t.
tamponade
balloon t.
cardiac t.
chronic t.
esophagogastric t.
florid cardiac t.
full-blown cardiac t.
heart t.
low-pressure cardiac t.
pericardial chyle with t.
subacute cardiac t.
tandem
t. applicator
external beam with t.
Fletcher-Suit-Delclos t.
t. lesion
MIR intrauterine t.
t. and ovoids
t. stent
t. technique
t. transplant
tandem-needle method
tangential
t. breast field
t. constriction
t. cuts
t. layer of hand
t. port
t. scapular view
tangentially

tangle
intraneuronal neurofibrillary t.
neurofibrillary t.
Tanner-Whitehouse-Healy method
tannex
bisacodyl t.
tantalate
lutetium t.
tantalum (Ta)
t. bronchogram
t. imaging agent
t. mesh
t. powder
t. stent
tantalum-178 (^{178}Ta)
tantalum-182 (^{182}Ta)
taper
fiberoptic t.
tapered finger
tapering
t. dose
t. occlusion
t. off
t. stenosis
tapeworm
tapir
bouche de t.
tapir's mouth
TAPVD
total anomalous pulmonary venous drainage
TAPVR
total anomalous pulmonary venous return
TAR
tissue-air ratio
TAR syndrome
Tar
T. symptom
tarda
osteogenesis imperfecta t.
tardive
forme t.
tardus-parvus waveform
target
angiographic t.
t. appearance
t. arch
t. bone
t. brain sign
t. calcification
t. canal
t. coalition
t. depth
gas t.
internal cyclotron t.
t. lung lesion
t. material
metal technetium t.
molybdenum t.
t. navicular
t. organ
t. point
t. sign appendicitis
t. tarsometatarsal joint space
three-dimensional reconstructed t.
t. tissue
tungsten t.
t. tunnel syndrome
targeted imaging
target-film distance (TFD)
targeting
angiographic t.
t. beads
ScoutView t.
targetoid growth
target-skin distance (TSD)
target-to-background ratio
Tarin space
Tarlov cyst
TARP
total atrial refractory period
Tarrant position
tarsal
t. arch
t. bone
t. canal
t. coalition
t. cyst
t. joint
t. ligament
t. navicular
t. plate
t. sinus
t. tunnel
t. tunnel syndrome (TTS)
tarsoepiphyseal aclasis
tarsometatarsal
t. angle
t. articulation
t. joint
t. ligament
tartrate
thorium t.
task-rest pattern

NOTES

Taussig-Bing
T.-B. anomaly
T.-B. congenital malformation of heart
T.-B. disease
Taussig-Snellen-Alberts syndrome
taut pericardial effusion
TAV
transcutaneous aortovelography
Taveras injector
Tawara atrioventricular node
Taybi
T. type I–III
Taylor-Blackwood mechanism
Taylor position
TB
toluidine blue
tuberculosis
TBI
total body irradiation
tracheobronchial injury
traumatic brain injury
TBNA
transbronchial needle aspiration
TBT
transcervical balloon tuboplasty
TBW
total body water
Tc
technetium
Tc bond
^{99m}Tc
^{99m}Tc albumin aggregated imaging agent
^{99m}Tc albumin colloid imaging agent
^{99m}Tc albumin microaggregated imaging agent
^{99m}Tc albumin microspheres imaging agent
^{99m}Tc biciromab imaging agent
^{99m}Tc bicisate imaging agent
^{99m}Tc Ceretec
^{99m}Tc Ceretec bind
^{99m}Tc colloid imaging agent
^{99m}Tc dimercaptosuccinic acid imaging agent
^{99m}Tc disofenin imaging agent
^{99m}Tc DTPA
^{99m}Tc etidronate imaging agent
^{99m}Tc exametazime imaging agent
^{99m}Tc ferpentetate imaging agent
^{99m}Tc furifosmin imaging agent
^{99m}Tc Glucarate hot spot imaging agent
^{99m}Tc gluceptate imaging agent
^{99m}Tc glucoheptanoate
^{99m}Tc human serum albumin imaging agent
^{99m}Tc lidofenin imaging agent
^{99m}Tc MAA
^{99m}Tc MDP uptake
^{99m}Tc mebrofenin imaging agent
^{99m}Tc medronate disodium imaging agent
^{99m}Tc mercaptoacetythiglycine
^{99m}Tc mertiatide imaging agent
^{99m}Tc MMAA
^{99m}Tc oxidronate imaging agent
^{99m}Tc pentetate calcium trisodium imaging agent
^{99m}Tc pentetate sodium imaging agent
^{99m}Tc pentetic acid imaging agent
^{99m}Tc pertechnetate
^{99m}Tc phosphate
^{99m}Tc polyphosphate imaging agent
^{99m}Tc pyrophosphate
^{99m}Tc pyrophosphate
^{99m}Tc red blood cell SPECT
^{99m}Tc riisocyanide imaging agent
^{99m}Tc rimetaphosphates imaging agent
^{99m}Tc sestamibi imaging agent
^{99m}Tc siboroxime imaging agent
^{99m}Tc sodium gluceptate imaging agent
^{99m}Tc sodium pertechnetate imaging agent
^{99m}Tc succimer imaging agent
^{99m}Tc sulfur colloid
^{99m}Tc sulfur colloid imaging agent
^{99m}Tc sulfur microcolloid imaging agent
^{99m}Tc macroaggregated albumin
^{99m}Tc teboroxime imaging agent
^{99m}Tc tetrofosmin imaging agent
^{99m}Tc tin colloid/free Tc-99m pertechnetate
Tc-99 DISIDA
Tc-99m-tagged RBC
TCA
tentorium cerebelli attachment
transcondylar axis
TCAT
transmission computer-assisted tomography
TCBF
total cerebral blood flow
^{99m}Tc-bicisate
^{99m}Tc-bis-dimethylphosphonoethane (DMPE)
TCC
transitional cell carcinoma
TCC stipple sign

TCD
transcranial Doppler
TCD ultrasound
^{99m}Tc-DMSA scintigraphy
T-cell
T.-c. acute lymphoblastic leukemia (T-ALL)
T.-c. lymphoblastic lymphoma
T.-c. malignancy
T.-c. neoplasm
T4-cell
^{99m}Tc-glucoheptonate
TcHIDA
^{99m}Tc-HMPAO cerebral perfusion SPECT imaging
Tc-99m
TcO^{4-}
free pertechnetate
T-configuration
$tcPO_2$
transcutaneous oxygen pressure measurement
Tc-PYP
aerosolized T.-P.
Tc-RBC
denatured T.-R.
heat-damaged T.-R.
TCS
tethered cord syndrome
TCT900S helical CT scanner
TDLU
terminal ductal lobular unit
TDMS
Trex digital mammography system
T-D ratio
TE, T-E
echo delay time
echo time
thromboembolic
tracheoesophageal
TE fistula
teacher's
t. node
t. nodule
teacup
t. breast calcification
t. fracture
Teale amputation
tear
annulus fibrosus t.
attritional t.
bowstring t.
bucket-handle meniscus t.
buttonhole t.
cleavage t.
degenerative horizontal cleavage t.
dural t.
entry t.
esophageal t.
fishtail t.
flap t.
full-thickness t.
high-grade partial t.
iatrogenic dural t.
interstitial meniscal t.
intimal t.
intrasubstance cleavage t.
Johnson-Jahss classification of posterior tibial tendon t.
ligament t.
Mallory-Weiss esophageal t.
Mallory-Weiss mucosal t.
meniscus t.
mesenteric t.
micro t.
parrot-beak labral t.
parrot-beak meniscus t.
partial bursal surface t.
partial-thickness split t.
peripheral meniscocapsular t.
quadriceps tendon t.
radial split t.
rectal t.
rotator cuff t.
serosal t.
SLAP t.
stellate t.
superimposed acute partial t.
superior labral anterior to posterior t.
tendon t. (types I–IV)
tibial tendon t.
traumatic aortic t.
tricorn bucket-handle t.
vertical split nondetached t.
teardrop
t. appearance
t. bladder
t. burst fracture
t. heart
t. pelvic anatomy
t. ventriculomegaly
teardrop-shaped flexion-compression fracture

NOTES

T

tearing
plaque t.
teat
pyloric t.
teboroxime
t. cardiac scan
t. imaging agent
t. resting washout (TRW)
technetium-99m t.
TEC-2100 postioning laser
TECA study
Technegas
Techneplex
T. imaging agent
TechneScan
T. MAG3 imaging
T. MAG3 imaging agent
T. Q-12 imaging agent
technetated aggregated human albumin imaging agent
technetium (Tc)
t. albumin study (TECA study)
t. bond (Tc bond)
t. human serum albumin labeling
hydrolyzed t.
t. imaging agent
t. labeled fibrinogen
t. pertechnate
t. polyphosphonate
t. stannous pyrophosphate (TSPP)
t. stannous pyrophosphate imaging
t. Tc99m venography
t. ^{99m}Tc-PYP scintigraphy
technetium-99m-tagged RBC
technetium-labeled phosphate analog
technetium-99m
t. acetanilide iminodiacetic acid
t. albumin colloid
t. albumin microsphere
t. antibody labeling
t. antimyosin Fab fragment
t. bicisate
t. Ceretec (^{99m}Tc Ceretec)
t. Ceretec bind (^{99m}Tc Ceretec bind)
t. diethylenetriamine penta-acetic acid
t. dimercaptosuccinic acid
t. DISIDA (Tc-99 DISIDA)
t. disofenin
t. DMSA
t. DTPA (^{99m}Tc DTPA)
t. DTPA aerosol
t. etidronate
t. ferpentetate
t. furifosmin
t. gluceptate
t. glucoheptanoate (^{99m}Tc glucoheptanoate)
t. heat-denatured erythrocyte
t. hepatoiminodiacetic acid scan
t. human albumin microsphere
t. human serum albumin
t. IDA analog
t. iron-ascorbate-DTPA
t. lidofenin
t. MAA (^{99m}Tc MAA)
t. macroaggregated albumin
t. MDP uptake (^{99m}Tc MDP uptake)
t. medronate
t. mercaptoacetyltriglycine
t. mercaptoacetythiglycine
t. mertiatide
t. mini-microaggregated albumin (^{99m}Tc MMAA)
t. mini-microaggregated albumin colloid
t. oxidronate
t. pertechnetate
t. pertechnetate GI bleed
t. pertechnetate sodium
t. pertechnetate thyroid
t. phosphate (^{99m}Tc phosphate)
t. PIPIDA
t. pyrophosphate (^{99m}Tc pyrophosphate)
sestamibi t.
t. sestamibi
t. sestamibi parathyroid
t. siboroxime
t. succimer
t. sulfur colloid
t. sulfur colloid GI bleed
t. teboroxime
t. tetrofosmin
technetium-99m-labeled
t.-l. RBC
t.-l. WBC
technetium-tagged
t.-t. Cardiolite
t.-t. RBC labeling
t.-t. red blood cell
technetium-thallium subtraction imaging
technical charge
Technicare
T. camera
T. Delta 2020 scanner
Technicians
Association of University Radiologic T. (AURT)
technique
acquisition t.
adiabatic fast scanning t.
afterloading t.
air-gap t.

algebraic reconstruction t. (ART)
antialiasing t.
background subtraction t.
bayesian t.
Beckenbaugh t.
blended beam t.
Bolton-Hunter t.
bougienage t.
brain surface matching t.
bread-loaf t.
breast mammographic t.
Brown-Roberts-Wells t.
bull's eye t.
cardiovascular imaging t.
catheter-securing t.
chemical shift imaging t.
chemical shift selective suppression t.
computer subtraction t.
Corbin t.
coronal oblique t.
Cr-chromate-labeled red cell t.
cress-correlation t.
Cr-labeled red cell t.
cross-correlation t.
cuboid squeeze t.
cuboid whip t.
cut-film t.
3D t.
deblurring t.
Debye-Scherrer photographic t.
deconvolution t.
dephase-rephase magnitude subtraction t.
depth-pulse t.
destructive interference t.
DNA microinjection t.
double-contrast t.
double-freeze t.
double-umbrella t.
double-wire atherectomy t.
driven equilibrium Fourier transform t.
2D time-of-flight t.
dye injection t.
dynamic bolus tracking t.
echo-tagging t.
Egan t.
ejection fraction by first-pass t.
Eklund t.
electron arc t.
endofluoroscopic t.
endovascular t.
enzyme-multiplied immunoassay t.
Epistar perfusion t.
equilibrium radionuclide angiocardiography t.
esophageal balloon t.
exclusion-HPLC t.
external looping t.
fast-FLAIR t.
fat-suppressed T2-weighted FSE t.
field-fitting t.
first-pass t.
FLAK t.
flow cytometry t.
flow mapping t.
fluoroscopic pushing t.
fluoroscopic road-mapping t.
four-field t.
Fourier-acquired steady-state t.
Fourier imaging t.
Fraunfelder t.
FRODO t.
full-bladder ultrasound t.
gated inflow t.
graded compression sonography t.
gradient-echo cine t.
gradient-echo recall t.
grasping t.
grid t.
Grüntzig PTCA t.
guide wire exchange t.
Hahnemann University Hospital t.
hairpin t.
half-Fourier three-dimensional t.
half-Fourier transformation t.
half-wedged field t.
Hampton t.
hanging-block t.
HARC-C wavelet compression t.
Hawkins inside-out nephrostomy t.
Hawkins single-stick t.
high-kV t.
high-resolution bone algorithm t.
hybridization-subtraction t.
hybrid subtraction t.
immersion t.
inhalation t.
intercomparison measurement t.
interleaved phase contrast t.
intraoperative scanning t.
intraoral swage t.
intravascular MRI catheter-based t.

NOTES

T

technique *(continued)*
inverse radiotherapy t.
inversion-recovery t.
isolation-perfusion t.
Judkins t.
jugular t.
Kennedy ligament t.
kinematic MR t.
kissing atherectomy t.
kissing-balloon t.
Klein t.
large-core t.
Laue photographic t.
Leksell t.
loading t.
localization t.
low-angle shot t.
low-dose film mammographic t.
low-dose screen-film t.
magnetization transfer t.
mammography t.
Markov chain Monte Carlo t.
Martinez t.
MAST t.
matchline t.
McWhirter t.
Menghini biopsy t.
Monte Carlo t.
Mose t.
motion artifact suppression t. (MAST)
MPGR t.
MP-RAGE t.
multiline scanning t.
multimodal image fusion t.
multiphasic multislice MRI t.
multiphasic multislice spin-echo imaging t.
multislice spin-echo t.
navigator echo motion correction t.
NEUGAT t.
no-gap t.
nonaxial beam t.
noncoplanar arc t.
noncoplanar arch t.
noncoplanar beam t.
noninvasive t.
Overhauser t.
packing, extraction, and calculation t.
papillon t.
partial flip-angle fast-scan t.
partial Fourier t.
partial saturation t.
PASTA t.
PCICO t.
pressure-controlled intermittent coronary occlusion technique
percutaneous retrograde transfemoral t.
percutaneous transluminal coronary recanalization t.
perfusion measurement t.
peripheral laser recanalization t.
pharmacokinetic t.
point mutation detection using exonuclease amplification couple capture t. (point-EXACCT)
presaturation t.
pressure-controlled intermittent coronary occlusion t. (PCICO technique)
pressure half-time t.
projection-reconstruction t.
PSSE t.
pulsed-gradient spin-echo t.
radiopharmaceutical volume-dilution t.
radiotracer t.
rapid pull-through t. (RPT)
rapid scan t.
rapid thoracic compression t.
Rebuck skin window t.
recanalization t.
region-of-interest imaging t.
reimplantation t.
relaxation t.
Riechert-Mundinger t.
road-mapping t.
robust registration t.
Rösch t.
rotational therapy t.
saturation recovery t.
scanning t.
scintillation counting t.
Seldinger percutaneous t.
sequential extraction-radiotracer t.
serial cut film t.
silhouette t.
single-field hyperthermia t.
single fill/void t.
single-shot imaging t.
SL t.
spin-lock imaging technique
sliding thin-slab, minimum intensity projection t.
Sones cineangiography t.
SPAMM t.
spin-echo t.
spin-label t.
spin-lock imaging t. (SL technique)
spiral scanning t.
split-course t.
SPOP t.
stacked-foil t.

Stejskal and Tanner pulsed-gradient spin-echo t.
stereotactic automated t.
stimulated echo-tagging t.
STIR t.
streptavidin peroxidase t.
subclavian turndown t.
subtraction t.
surface matching t.
surgical neurangiographic t.
Swiss roll t.
switched B-gradient t.
tandem t.
tetrahedral interpolation t.
thallium booster reinjection t.
three-dimensional gradient echo acquisition t.
three-dimensional volume t.
three-point Dixon t.
time-of-flight t.
tissue characterization t.
Todd-Wells t.
tourniquet t.
transcatheter t.
transgluteal CT-guided t.
trephine t.
trocar-cannula t.
two-dimensional t.
two-needle t.
two-step t.
upgated t.
ureteral compression t.
in vivo t.
volumetric mapping t.
water-suppression t.
wedged-pair t.
Welin t.
xeroradiographic t.

Technologists
American Registry of Radiologic T.
American Society of Radiologic T. (ASRT)
American Society of Registered T. (ASRT)

technology
acoustic response t. (ART)
automated cardiac flow measurement ultrasound t.
CellSeek t.
National Institute of Standards and T. (NIST)
noncontact imaging t.
peripheral quantitative computed tomography t.
slip-ring t.
ultrasound imaging t.

Techtides

Tecmag
T. Libra-S16 system
T. Libra-S16 system scanner

tecta (*pl. of* tectum)

tectal
t. beaking
t. lesion
t. plate

tectobulbar tract

tectocerebellar tract

tectoral ligament

tectospinal tract

tectum, pl. **tecta**
t. commissure

TED
thromboembolic disease

Tedlar bag

TEE
transesophageal echocardiography

teeth
carious t.
floating t.
Hutchinson t.
incisor t.
milk t.
molar t.
premolar t.
primary t.
secondary t.
wisdom t.

TEF
tracheoesophageal fistula

Teflon probe

tegmental tract

tegmentospinal tract

tegmentum
t. of brainstem
medullary t.
midbrain t.
t. of pons
t. of pons and midbrain
pontine t.

tegmen tympani

TEGwire
T. ST system

NOTES

Teichholz
T. ejection fraction
T. equation
T. equation for left ventricular volume
TEK
total exchangeable potassium
tela choroidea
telangiectasia, pl. **telangiectases**
ataxia t.
t. brain capillary
capillary t.
Osler-Weber-Rendu t.
pulmonary t.
Sturge-Weber t.
telangiectatic
t. angioma
t. cancer
t. fibroma
t. lesion
t. osteogenic sarcoma
t. osteosarcoma
t. osteosarcoma doughnut sign
t. vessel
telangiectaticum
Telebrix
telecobalt
t. therapy
telecurietherapy
telemammography
TeleMax
telencephalic
t. malformation
t. ventriculofugal artery
telencephalon
TelePACS
Telepaque
T. imaging agent
telephone handle bone
teleradiography
teleradiology
t. videoconferencing
teleradium
t. therapy
teleroentgenography
teleroentgentherapy
teletherapy
C-60 t.
t. radiotherapy
telltale triangle sign
telognosis
telomere repeat amplification protocol
Telos radiographic stress device
Temodal
temperature
t. distribution measurement
firing t.
mean perfusate t.
Neel t.
t. sensor
template
t. irradiation
Martinez universal interstitial t. (MUPIT)
Syed t.
Syed-Neblett t.
Templeton and Zim carpal tunnel projection
temporal (T)
t. aliasing
t. artery
t. artery tap maneuver
t. average intensity
t. bone
t. bone anatomy
t. bone fracture
t. bone sclerosis
t. bone tomogram
t. bone tumor
t. canal
t. filter
t. fossa
t. granulomatous arteritis
t. gyrus
t. horn
t. horn atrophy
t. horn of lateral ventricle
t. instability artifact
t. isthmus
t. lobe
t. lobe epilepsy
t. lobe herniation
t. lobe infarct
t. lobe lesion
t. lobe tumor
t. meningioma
t. orientation
t. peak (TP)
t. peak intensity
t. phase delay
t. pole
t. predominance
t. process
t. sawtooth pattern
t. space infection
t. sulcus
t. suture
temporalis muscle
temporally
temporary
t. aortic shunt bypass
t. atrial pacing wire
t. interstitial implant
t. pacing catheter
temporoinsular astrocytoma

temporomandibular
t. joint (TMJ)
t. joint arthrography
t. joint disk
t. joint osteolysis
t. ligament
temporomandibular joint destruction
temporooccipital
t. artery
t. glioma
t. junction
temporoparietooccipital junction
temporopontine tract
TENa
total exchangeable sodium
tenderness
skin-rolling scapular t.
tendineae
ruptured chordae t.
tendines (*pl. of* tendo)
tendinitis (*var. of* tendonitis)
tendinopathy
tendinosis
angiofibroblastic t.
common extensor t.
patellar t.
suprasinatus t.
tendinous
t. attachment
t. band
t. insertion
t. raphe
tendo, pl. **tendines**
t. Achillis
t. calcaneus
tendon
Achilles t.
anterior tibial t.
t. aponeurosis
t. attenuation
attrition rupture of t.
biceps brachii t.
bifid biceps t.
boomerang t.
bowing of t.
calcaneal t.
central perineal t.
common t.
conjoined t.
coronary t.
cricoesophageal t.
extensor t.
flexor t.
goose foot t.
gracilis t.
hamstring t.
t. of Hector
heel t.
iliopsoas t.
infrapatellar t.
infraspinatus t.
longitudinal split biceps t.
membranaceous t.
patellar t.
peroneal brevis t.
peroneal longus t.
plantaris t.
t. plate
pollicis longus t.
popliteal t.
posterior tibial t.
quadriceps t.
rider's t.
t. rupture
semimembranosus t.
semitendinosus t.
t. sheath
t. sheath giant cell tumor
t. sheath space infection
t. shortening
t. sling
slipped t.
t. subluxation
subscapularis t.
superficial palmaris longus t.
supraspinatus t.
t. tear (types I–IV)
t. tissue
Todaro t.
t. of Zinn
Zinn t.
tendonitis, tendinitis
calcific t.
popliteal t.
tendonosis
tendosynovial sarcoma
tenesmus
tennis
t. elbow
t. leg
t. shoulder
t. toe
tenocyte hyperplasia

NOTES

tenodesis
band t.
tenography
tenonavicular
tenosynovial osteochondromatosis
tenosynovitis
flexor t.
peroneal t.
tibialis posterior t.
tuberculous t.
TENS
transcutaneous electrical nerve stimulator
tense fontanelle
tensile
t. force
t. injury
Tensilon
tension
t. cyst
t. endothorax
epicardial t.
t. fracture
intraventricular systolic t.
t. pneumothorax
tension-time index (TTI)
tensor
t. fasciae femoris
t. fasciae latae
t. fasciae suralis
t. tympani
t. veli palatini
t. veli palatini muscle
tentative diagnosis
tented up
tenth-value layer
tenting
baseline t.
t. of diaphragm
t. of hemidiaphragm
tentorial
t. edge
t. meningioma
t. notch herniation
t. ridge
t. traversal
tentorium
t. cerebelli
t. cerebelli attachment (TCA)
t. keyhole configuration
TER
therapeutic external radiation
thermal enhancement ratio
teratoblastoma of ovary
teratocarcinoma
mediastinum t.
t. of ovary
pineal t.
pineal gland t.
teratogen
teratogenesis
teratogenic effect
teratogenicity
t. of contrast agent
teratoid
t. mediastinum
t. tumor
teratoma, pl. **teratomata**
atypical brain t.
cardiac t.
CNS t.
cystic t.
embryonal ovary t.
immature ovarian t.
malignant t.
mature mediastinum t.
mature ovarian cystic t.
mediastinum t.
neck t.
orbital t.
ovarian systic t.
pineal t.
solid ovarian t.
spinal t.
suprasellar atypical t.
testicular t.
testis t.
teres
ligamentum t.
t. major
t. minor
pronator t.
Teridax
terminal
t. air sac
t. air space
t. aorta
t. bile duct
t. bronchiole
t. carcinoma
t. crest
t. ductal lobular unit (TDLU)
t. edema
t. head
t. ileitis
t. ileum
t. inversion
t. pneumonia
t. reservoir syndrome
t. synostosis
t. thrombosis
t. tuft
t. tuft autoamputation
t. tuft resorption
t. ventricle
t. web
t. zone of the Yakolev

terminale
fatty filum t.
filum t.
persistent ossiculum t.
tight filum t.
terminalis
cistern of lamina t.
ventriculus t.
termination
early-phase t.
late-phase t.
underdrive t.
terminus
duodenal t.
intrapapillary t.
rostral t.
Terry
T. fingernail sign
T. Thomas sign
tertiary
t. collimation
t. hyperparathyroidism (tHPT)
t. hypothyroidism
t. sequestrum
t. syphilis
t. wave
tertius
condylus t.
peroneus t.
Terumo guide wire
tesla (T)
t. (T) field
Tesla magnetic resonance imager
Teslascan
test (*See* testing)
abduction stress t.
acid t.
aluminum ion breakthrough t.
Ames t.
axial manual traction t.
Barlow hip instability t.
Bayer Immuno 1 Dpd assay automated bone-resorption t.
bolus challenge t.
capillary resistance t.
cardiac stress t.
^{14}C lactose breath t.
colorimetric t.
compounding sterility t.
conglutinating complement absorption t.
congo red t.
contraction stress t. (CST)
Coombs t.
costoclavicular t.
Cytomel suppression t.
Dehio t.
Dicopac t.
dipyridamole echocardiography t.
dipyridamole handgrip t.
dipyridamole infusion t.
dipyridamole tomographic thallium stress t.
duplex screening t.
dye reduction spot t.
ergonovine t.
exercise thallium-201 stress t.
exercise tolerance t. (ETT)
fetal stress t.
film screen contact t.
Fisher exact t.
flat-hand t.
Graham-Cole t.
Heaf t.
heart stress t.
Immuno 1 Dpd assay automated bone-resorption t.
t. injection
internal carotid balloon t.
intrinsic field uniformity t.
isometric exercise stress t.
Kolmogorov-Smirnov normality t.
Kveim-Stilzbach t.
Leclercq t.
Linsman water t.
liver enzyme t.
liver function t.
log-rank t.
love t.
Master two-step exercise stress t.
McNemar t.
t. meal
Mecholyl t.
molybdenum-99 breakthrough t.
Müller t.
nonstress t. (NST)
nonstress fetal t.
O'Connor finger dexterity t.
Ortolani t.
pancreas secretin t.
pathergy t.
pelvic steal t.
perchlorate washout t.
peritoneal-venous shunt patency t.

NOTES

T

test *(continued)*
Persantine thallium stress t.
pharmacologic stress t.
physical stress t.
positive tilt t.
pregnancy t.
pulmonary function t.
quadriceps femoris tendon reflex t.
radioactive iodine uptake t. (RAIU)
Romer t.
Rubin t.
Salkowski t.
Seidlitz powder t.
sestamibi stress t.
Sharp-Purser t.
Smith orthogonal hole t.
sniff t.
spinning-top t.
star-cancellation t. (SCT)
stress t.
sweat t.
swinging flashlight t.
thyroid perchlorate washout t.
thyroid suppression t.
tilt t.
treadmill exercise t. (TET)
treadmill exercise stress t.
Trendelenburg t.
T3 resin uptake t.
Triboulet t.
triple-marker screening t.
t. tube structure
ureteral perfusion t.
USP XX t.
vessel t.
water-siphon t.
Wetzel t.
Whitaker t.
Whitfield t.
Wilcoxon signed-rank t.
Yergason t.

testes (*pl. of* testis)

testicle
undescended t.

testicular
t. abscess
t. adrenal rest tissue
t. appendage torsion
t. artery
t. artery avulsion
t. atrophy
t. cancer
t. choriocarcinoma
t. cyst
t. cystic lesion
t. degeneration
t. ectopia
t. feminization
t. gland
t. infarct
t. ischemia
t. metastasis
t. microlithiasis
t. parenchyma
t. posttraumatic edema
t. relapse
t. rupture
t. seminoma
t. stromal cell tumor
t. teratoma
t. torsion appendage
t. trauma
t. tubular adenoma
t. vein

testing (*See* test)
Balke protocol for cardiac exercise stress t.
bronchial provocation t.
Doppler ultrasound segmental blood pressure t.
nuclear gated blood pool t.
perimetry t.
provocative t.
pyrogen t.
radiation sensitivity t.

testis, pl. **testes**
appendix t.
burned-out tumor of t.
t. cancer
descended t.
dilated rete t.
t. doughnut sign
t. dysfunction
t. dysplasia
ectopic t.
efferent ductules of t.
t. fracture
t. germ cell tumor
infarcted t.
maldescended t.
malpositioned t.
mediastinum t.
occult primary tumor of t.
rete t.
retractile t.
t. teratoma
torsion of t.
tubular ectasia of rete t.
undescended t.

testobulbar tract

test-retest precision

Tesuloid
T. imaging agent

TET
treadmill exercise test

tethered
- t. cord syndrome (TCS)
- t. small bowel fold
- t. spinal cord

tethered-bowel sign
tetraazacyclododecanetetraacetic
- t. acid
- t. tetramethylene phosphonate

tetrabromophenolphthalein
- t. sodium

tetrad
- Fallot t.

tetradentate thioiminato
tetradiploid tumor
tetrahedral interpolation technique
tetrahedron chest
tetrahydrouridine
tetraiodophenolphthalein
- t. sodium

tetralogy
- t. of Fallot (TOF)
- pink t.

tetraphocomelia
tetraploid tumor
tetrasodium-meso-tetra
- manganese t.-m.-t. (Mn-$TPPS_4$)

tetrofosmin
- technetium-99m t.

Teufel method
Teutleben ligament
texaphyrin
- gadolinium t.

texaphyrins
Texas Red
texture
- echo t.
- inhomogeneous echo t.
- t. mapping
- t. slice

TFA
- thigh-foot angle
- tibiofemoral angle

T1-FAST
TFC
- threaded fusion cage
- triangular fibrocartilage

TFCC
- triangular fibrocartilaginous complex

TFD
- target-film distance

T1FS
- T1-weighted fat-suppressed image

TGA
- transposition of great arteries

TGC
- time-gain compensation

TGF
- therapeutic gain factor

thalami (*pl. of* thalamus)
thalamic
- t. edema
- t. fracture
- t. fracture of calcaneus
- t. glioma
- t. hemorrhage
- t. infarct
- t. lesion
- t. plane
- t. vein

thalamic-hypothalamic mass
thalamocaudate artery
thalamogeniculate artery
thalamoolivary tract
thalamoperforating artery
thalamostriate vein
thalamotegmental involvement
thalamus, pl. **thalami**
- intralaminar t.

thalidomide
thallium (Tl)
- t. booster reinjection technique
- t. debris
- t. imaging agent
- t. myocardial perfusion imaging
- t. myocardial scan with SPECT imaging
- myocardial uptake of t.
- t. perfusion scintigraphy
- radioactive t.
- t. redistribution phase
- regional myocardial uptake of t.
- t. rest-redistribution imaging
- t. scintography imaging
- t. single-photon emission computed tomography (SPECT) scan
- t. SPECT score
- t. split-dose method
- t. stress imaging

thallium-201 (**^{201}Tl**)
- t. chloride
- dipyridamole t.
- t. imaging
- t. myocardial scintigraphy

NOTES

thallium-201 *(continued)*
t. single-photon emission CT
t. uptake and distribution
thallium-to-scalp ratio
thallous chloride imaging agent
Thal-Quick chest tube
thanatophoric
t. dwarfism
t. dysplasia
thatched-roof worker's lung
Thayer-Doisy unit
THC
transhepatic cholangiogram
THE
transhiatal esophagectomy
theater sign
thebesian
t. circulation
t. foramen
t. valve
t. vein
theca, pl. **thecae**
t. externa
t. interna
theca-cell ovarian tumor
thecal
t. abscess
t. sac
theca-lutein ovarian cyst
thecoma
t. of ovary
Theile
T. canal
T. muscle
thelarche
premature isolated t.
thenar
t. eminence
t. muscle
t. space
t. space abscess
theophylline attenuation
theorem
Bayes t.
Nyquist sampling t.
Stokes t.
theory
Bohr t.
crystal field t. (CFT)
Culiner t.
density matrix t.
electron t.
Fourier optical t.
fuzzy set t.
Kubelka-Munk t.
Planck quantum t.
quantum t.
slider crank t.
therapeutic
t. amniocentesis
t. angiography
t. barium enema
t. chemoembolization
t. cordocentesis
t. embolus
t. external radiation (TER)
t. gain factor (TGF)
t. index
t. pneumothorax
t. radiology
t. range
t. response
t. thrombosis
therapeutics
ray t.
therapy
ablative laser t.
accelerated hyperfractionated radiation t.
adjunctive t.
adjuvant t.
antiestrogen radiologic t.
antitubercular t.
arc t.
beam t.
beta-ray ophthalmic plaque t.
boost t.
Bragg peak photon-beam t.
brisement t.
cesium t.
chemoradiation t.
combined modality radiation t.
compartmental radioimmunoglobulin t.
computer-controlled conformal radiation t. (CCRT)
concomitant boost radiation t.
conformal neutron and photon radiation t.
conformal radiation t. (CRT)
continuous hyperfractionated accelerated radiation t. (CHART)
conventionally fractionated stereotactic radiation t.
craniospinal axis radiation t.
3D conformal radiation t.
directly observed t.
dynamic conformal t.
dynamic radiation t.
electron arc t.
electron beam t.
embolization transcatheter t.
extended-field irradiation t.
external beam radiation t. (EBRT)
external x-ray t.
eye-view 3D conformal radiation t.

eye-view 3D-CRT radiation t.
fast neutron radiation t.
fast-neutron radiation t.
Fletcher-Suit system for radium t.
fluoroscopy-guided subarachnoid phenol block t.
four-fiber t.
fractionated external beam radiation t.
fractionated stereotactic radiation t.
fragmentation t.
grid t.
hadron t.
half-body radiation t.
high-dose t.
high-dose-rate (HDR) intracavitary radiation t.
hyperfractionated accelerated radiation t. (HART)
hypofractionated radiation t.
I-B1 radiolabeled antibody injection radiation t.
ICRU 50 radiation t.
image-guided t.
indicator dilution t.
infusion transcatheter t.
intensity-modulated radiation t. (IMRT)
internal radiation t.
interstitial t.
interstitial radioactive colloid t.
intraarticular radiopharmaceutical t.
intracavitary radiation t.
intracavitary radioactive colloid t.
intracoronary radiation t. (ICRT)
intracoronary thrombolytic t.
intraoperative radiation t. (IORT)
intravascular radiopharmaceutical t.
^{192}Ir seed t.
large-field radiation t.
megavoltage grid t.
megavoltage radiation t.
megavoltage x-ray t.
microwave t.
neoadjuvant hormonal t.
neodymium:YAG laser t.
neuraxis radiation t.
neutron t.
neutron/gamma transmission t.
ocular radiation t. (ORT)
orthovoltage radiation t.
palliative radiation t.
partial-brain radiation t.
particle-beam radiation t.
percutaneous transcatheter t.
peroral cone radiation t.
photodynamic t. (PDT)
photon-neutron mixed-beam radiation t.
plesiocurie t.
postmenopausal estrogen t.
postorchiectomy paraaortic radiation t.
radiation t.
radiofrequency ablation t.
radiopharmaceutical t.
radium beam t.
reperfusion t.
reprogramming t.
rotation t.
rotational radiation t.
Selective Tubal Assessment to Refine Reproductive T. (STARRT)
short-distance radiation t.
split-course accelerated radiation t.
split-course hyperfractionated radiation t.
stereotactic radiation t.
supportive t.
systemic adjuvant t.
telecobalt t.
teleradium t.
three-dimensional conformal radiation t.
thrombolytic t.
tiered t.
timed-sequential t.
total androgen suppression t.
transcatheter t.
triple t. (TT)
ultra-early thrombolytic t.
updraft t.
upper mantle radiation t.
whole-brain radiation t. (WBRT)
wide-field radiation t. (WFRT)
x-ray t.
t. zone

TheraSeed
T. imaging agent
T. seeding

Theratides

thermal
t. bioeffect

NOTES

thermal *(continued)*
t. compression
t. convection pattern
t. diffusion
t. dosimetry system
t. effect
t. energy
t. enhancement ratio (TER)
t. equilibrium
t. hot spot
t. modeling
t. neutron
t. noise
t. occlusion
t. shape memory
t. spectrum
t. treatment parameter
Thermex
Direx T.
thermistor plethysmography
thermoactinomyces vulgaris
thermodilution
t. cardiac output
t. ejection fraction
t. method of cardiac output measurement
t. stroke volume
thermogram
liquid crystal t.
thermography
blood vessel t.
infrared t.
laser-induced t. (LITT)
liquid crystal t. (LCT)
liquid crystal contact t.
thermoluminescence
t. dosimetry
thermoluminescent
t. dosimeter (TLD)
t. dosimeter rod (TLD rod)
thermometry
invasive t.
noninvasive t.
thermonic emission
thermonuclear
thermophilic actinomycetes
thermoplacentography
thermoradiosensitization
thermoradiotherapy
interstitial t.
simultaneous t. (STRT)
thermotherapy
laser-induced t. (LITT)
MRI-guided laser-induced interstitial t.
thermotolerance
thesaurosis
thick
t. bone
t. echo
thickened
t. aortic valve
t. bladder
t. bladder wall
t. duodenal fold
t. gallbladder wall
t. gastric fold
t. heel pad
t. irregular endometrium
t. irregular small bowel fold dilatation
t. nodular irregular small bowel fold
t. septum
t. sinus
t. smooth small bowel fold dilatation
t. stomach fold
t. straight small bowel fold
thickening
antral mucosal t.
aortic valve t.
aortic wall t.
apical pleural t.
beaded t.
bladder wall t.
breast skin t.
bronchial wall t.
capsular t.
circumferential t.
diffuse gallbladder wall t.
diffuse intimal t.
diffuse pleural t.
disproportionate upper septal t.
facial t.
fissural t.
focal gallbladder wall t.
focal intimal t.
fusiform t.
heel pad t.
interlobular septal t.
intimal t.
irregular gallbladder wall t.
ligamentous t.
ligamentum flavum t.
mediastinal t.
mottled t.
mucosal t.
mural t.
myocardial t.
nuchal skin t.
optic excrescentic t.
optic nerve fusiform t.
partial t.
peribronchial t.

pleural t.
postlumpectomy skin t.
scrotal wall t.
skin t.
submucosal t.
synovial t.
trabecular t.
urinary bladder wall t.
valve t.
wall t.

thickness
arterial wall t.
bladder wall t.
t. to diameter of ventricle ratio (T-D ratio)
endometrial t.
full t.
increased skull t.
interventricular septal t. (IVST)
intimomedial t.
posterior wall t. (PWT)
postmenopausal endometrial t.
preacinar arterial wall t.
septal wall t.
slice t.
ventricular free wall t.
wall t.

thick-slice
t.-s. image
t.-s. imaging

thick-walled
t.-w. gallbladder
t.-w. ventricle

Thiemann disease

thigh
t. bone
t. muscle
t. muscle cross-section
t. splint

thigh-foot angle (TFA)

thin
t. border
t. cylindrical uniform field volume
t. fibrous cap
t. film analysis
t. skull

thin-collimation
t.-c. image
t.-c. imaging

thin-film transistor array

thinned cartilage

thinning
apical t.
cortical t.
white matter t.

thin-plate spine

thin-section
t.-s. axial image
t.-s. CT

thin-slice
t.-s. CT
t.-s. image
t.-s. imaging

thin-walled
t.-w. atrium
t.-w. cyst
t.-w. gallbladder
t.-w. lung cavity

thioiminato
tetradentate t.

thiol
t. augmentation
t. modification

thionamide

thiopental

thiopurine methyltransferase (TPMT)

thiosulfate
sodium t.

third
t. branchial arch
t. intercondylar tubercle of Parsons
t. portion of duodenum
t. ventricle
t. ventricle of cerebrum
t. ventricle tumor
t. ventricular hemangioblastoma

third-degree
t.-d. AV block
t.-d. heart block

third-order chorda

third-space sequestration

third-trimester
t.-t. gestational dating
t.-t. placenta

Thixokon
T. imaging agent

Thomas sign

Thom method

Thompson-Epstein
T.-E. classification of femoral fractures
T.-E. femoral fracture classification

Thompson ligament

NOTES

T

Thomson scattering
thoracentesis
misplaced t.
thoraces (*pl. of* thorax)
thoracic (T)
t. adenopathy
t. angiography
t. aorta
t. aortic aneurysm
t. arch aortography
t. asymmetry
t. bone
t. cage configuration
t. cavity
t. circumference
t. crush
t. deformity
t. disk
t. disk herniation
t. duct
t. duct cyst
t. duct route
t. dysplasia
t. empyema
t. esophagus
t. fistula
t. gas volume
t. gibbus
t. index
t. inlet
t. inlet lesion
t. inlet soft tissue
t. inlet syndrome
t. joint
t. kidney
t. kyphosis
t. lordosis
t. myelography
t. outlet
t. outlet syndrome (TOS)
t. paraganglioma
t. plane
t. pulsion diverticulum
t. root sleeve
t. root sleeve diverticulum
t. scoliosis
t. sonography
t. spinal cord
t. spinal neoplasm
t. spine
t. spine anatomy
t. spine curve
t. spine fracture
t. splenosis
t. stomach
t. vent
t. vertebra
t. view
t. wall
thoracoabdominal
t. aorta
t. aortic aneurysm
t. diaphragm
t. duplication
t. gradient
t. wall
thoracoacromial artery
thoracodorsal artery
thoracoepigastric vein
thoracofemoral conversion
thoracolumbar
t. fascia
t. junction fracture
t. kyphosis
t. scoliosis
t. spine
t. spine column
t. vertebral disk
thoracoomphalopagus
thoracopagus
Thoracoport
thoracoscope
Stortz t.
thoracoscopy
video-assisted t. (VAT)
thoracotomy
Thoramat
thorax, pl. **thoraces**
t. articulation
asymmetric t.
bony t.
cylindrical t.
squared-off t.
symmetric t.
Thorel
T. bundle
T. pathway
thorium
t. compound
t. dioxide
t. dioxide granuloma
t. dioxide imaging agent
t. emanation
t. tartrate
t. X
thorn
t. sign
t. ulcer
thorny
t. bone radiation
t. spicule
Thorotrast
T. accumulation
T. imaging agent
thorotrastosis

Thorpe plastic lens
tHPT
tertiary hyperparathyroidism
thread-and-streaks
t.-a.-s. tumor thrombus sign
t.-a.-s. vascular channels
threaded fusion cage (TFC)
threatened
t. vessel closure
three-axis gradient coil
three-chambered heart
three-column injury
three-compartment
t.-c. arthrography
t.-c. wrist angiography
three-cornered bone
three-dimensional
t.-d. conformal radiation therapy
t.-d. conformal radiotherapy
t.-d. dose profile
t.-d. fast low-angle shot imaging
t.-d. fast spin-echo magnetic resonance imaging
t.-d. format
t.-d. Fourier imaging
t.-d. Fourier transform (3DFT)
t.-d. Fourier transform volume image
t.-d. freehand ultrasound
t.-d. gadolinium-enhanced MR angiography
t.-d. gradient echo acquisition technique
t.-d. helical CT angiography
t.-d. holography
t.-d. inflow MR angiography
t.-d. modeling
t.-d. neuroimaging
t.-d. phase-contrast MR angiography
t.-d. physiologic flow pattern
t.-d. processed ultrafast CT
t.-d. projection reconstruction imaging
t.-d. reconstructed target
t.-d. reconstruction
t.-d. rendering
t.-d. rotating delivery of excitation off-resonance
t.-d. stereotactic surface projection
t.-d. time-of-flight MR angiographic sequence
t.-d. transesophageal echocardiography
t.-d. volume
t.-d. volume technique
three-dimensional-connect operation
three-dimensional-FATS (fast adiabetic trajectory in a steady state) method
three-head scan
three-level Haar wavelet decomposition
three-part fracture
three-phase
t.-p. bone scanning
t.-p. bone scintigraphy (TPBS)
t.-p. imaging
t.-p. technetium study
t.-p. voltage supply
three-point Dixon technique
three-quarters prone position
three-stopcock manifold
three-vessel
t.-v. coronary disease
t.-v. runoff
t.-v. umbilical cord
three-way stopcock
thresher's lung
threshold
above selected t. (AST)
attenuation t.
cell-dose t.
erythema t.
t. of Firooznia
fracture t.
malignancy t.
seizure t.
signal-to-noise t.
ultrasound t.
thresholding
gray-level t.
t. method
thrombi (*pl. of* thrombus)
thromboangiitis obliterans
thromboembolic (TE, T-E)
t. disease (TED)
t. lung disease
t. stroke
thromboembolism
aortic t.
chronic lung t.
paraneoplastic t.
pulmonary t.
thromboembolization
catheter-induced t.

NOTES

T

thromboembolization *(continued)*
deep venous t.
pulmonary t.
venous t.
thromboembolus
thrombogenic coil
thrombolysis in myocardial infarct (TIMI)
thrombolytic
t. therapy
thrombophlebitis
breast t.
cerebral t.
puerperal ovarian vein t.
thromboresistance
ThromboScan
T. imaging
T. imaging agent
T. molecular recognition unit
T. MRU
thrombosed giant vertebral artery aneurysm
thrombosis, pl. **thromboses**
abdominal aorta t.
acute renal vein t.
aortic t.
aortoiliac t.
arterial t.
ascending medullary vein t.
atrial t.
atrophic t.
axillary vein traumatic t.
axillosubclavian vein t.
calf vein t.
capsular t.
cardiac t.
catheter-induced subclavian vein t.
central splanchnic venous t. (CSVT)
chronic renal vein t.
coronary t. (CT)
cortical vein t.
deep venous t. (DVT)
dural sinus t.
dural venous sinus t.
effort t.
femoropopliteal t.
hepatic artery t.
hepatic vein t.
iliofemoral t.
infective t.
intentional reversible t.
intervillous placental t.
intraarterial t.
intracranial sinus t.
intravascular t.
jugular vein t.
large-vessel t.
luminal t.
mesenteric arterial t.
mesenteric venous t.
native kidney renal vein t.
necrotizing t.
ovarian vein t.
Paget-Schroetter venous t.
pelvic vein t.
portal vein t.
portosplenic t.
postangioplasty mural t.
pulmonary t.
renal artery transplant t.
renal vein t. (RVT)
renal vein transplant t.
Ribbert t.
sagittal t.
Sandrock test for t.
septic t.
sinus t.
splenic vein t.
stent t.
subacute renal vein t.
subclavian vein t.
subclavian vessel t.
superior ophthalmic vein t.
superior sagittal sinus t.
syndrome of impending t.
terminal t.
therapeutic t.
transverse sinus t.
vein graft t.
venous sinus t.
thrombostasis
thrombotic
t. aneurysm
t. endocarditis
t. infarct
t. microangiopathy
t. obstruction
t. occlusion
t. pulmonary artery (TPA)
thrombus, pl. **thrombi**
adherent t.
anechoic t.
ball-valve t.
blood plate t.
t. calcification
calcified t.
coral t.
t. embolus
t. extension
t. formation
iliocaval t.
intraaneurysmal t.
intraarterial t.
intraatrial t.
intracardiac t.

intraluminal t.
intramural t.
intravascular tumor t.
laminated intraluminal t.
laser desiccation of t.
marantic t.
mobile t.
mural t.
t. nidus
obstructive t.
occlusive arterial t.
pedunculated t.
pericatheter t.
peroneal obliterative t.
platelet-rich t.
primary t.
t. remodeling
tibial obliterative t.
traumatic t.
tumor t.
through-and-through
t.-a.-t. fracture
t.-a.-t. guide wire
t.-a.-t. injury
through-sound transmission
through-the-scope (TTS)
through-transfer imaging
through-transmission
thrower's
t. elbow
t. fracture
throwing arm injury
thrush breast heart
thrusting ventricle
thumb
adducted t.
adductor sweep of t.
basal joint of t.
base of t.
bowler's t.
cortical t.
fingerized hypoplastic t.
floating t.
gamekeeper's t.
hitchhiker's t.
hypoplastic t.
pouce t. (floating thumb)
skier's t.
triphalangeal t.
t. web
thumb-in-palm deformity
thumbprinting
t. appearance of the colon
t. sign
Thurston
T. Holland fracture
T. Holland sign
thymectomy
thymic
t. agenesis
t. carcinoid
t. carcinoma
t. cyst
t. dysplasia
t. enlargement
t. hyperplasia
t. lymphoma
t. mass
t. neoplasm
thymidine
^{11}C t.
t. labeling index (TLI)
t. phosphorylase (TP)
t. suicide study
tritiated t. (TT)
thymolipoma
thymoma
benign t.
t. of heart
malignant t.
noninvasive t.
thymus
congenital absence of t.
diffuse enlargement of the t.
ectopic t.
t. gland
hyperplasia t.
mass t.
solid lesion t.
t. weight
thyroarytenoid
thyrocardiac disease
thyrocervical
t. trunk
t. trunk of subclavian artery
thyroepiglottic ligament
Thyrogen
thyroglossal
t. duct
t. duct cyst
t. duct remnant
thyrohyoid ligament

NOTES

thyroid
t. abscess
t. acropachy
t. adenoma
t. adenoma calcification
t. adenoma nodule
t. artery
t. cancer
t. capsule
t. carcinoma
t. cartilage
cold nodule t.
t. colloid nodule
t. cyst
t. cystadenoma
cystic area t.
t. degeneration
discordant nodule t.
t. disease
t. dysgenesis
t. eminence
t. follicle
t. gland
t. gland inflammation
t. goiter
t. halo sign
t. hyperplasia
t. insufficiency
intrathoracic t.
iodine-123 t.
iodine-131 t.
t. isthmus
lingual t.
t. lobe
t. lymph node
t. lymphoma
multinodular t.
occult carcinoma of the t.
t. orbitopathy
t. organification defect
t. perchlorate washout test
t. psammoma body
t. radioiodine treatment
t. radioiodine uptake
retrosternal t.
t. scintigraphy
t. stimulation scan
t. stunning
substernal t.
t. suppression scan
t. suppression test
technetium-99m pertechnetate t.
t. trapping defect
t. ultrasonography imaging
t. uptake measurement
t. whole-body scan

thyroidectomy

thyroiditis
acute suppurative t.
chronic lymphocytic t.
de Quervain t.
painless t.
Riedel t.
subacute t.
suppurative t.

thyrotoxicosis
t. medicamentosa

thyrotoxicotic cardiomyopathy

thyrotroph cell adenoma

thyrotropin alpha

thyroxine (T_4)
labeled t.
radioactive t.
radiolabeled t.

Thyrx timer

TI
inversion time
thallium
tricuspid incompetence
tricuspid insufficiency

Ti
titanium

TIA
transient ischemic attack
carotid distribution TIA
crescendo TIA
ipsilateral hemispheric carotid TIA

TIB
tree-in-bud
TIB pattern

tibarius
torsus t.

tibia, pl. **tibiae**
anterior bowing t.
t. bone
focal fibrocartilaginous dysplasia of t.
posteromedial t.
proximal t.
saber-shin t.
t. vara

tibiae
malleolus t.

tibial
t. artery
t. artery disease
t. bending fracture
t. collateral ligament
t. condyle
t. condyle fracture
t. crest
t. diaphyseal fracture
t. epiphysis
t. flare
t. intercondylar eminence

t. medullary canal
t. node
t. obliterative thrombus
t. open fracture
t. pilon fracture
t. plafond
t. plafond fracture
t. plateau
t. plateau fracture
t. sesamoid bone
t. sesamoid ligament
t. shaft fracture
t. tendon tear
t. torsion
t. triplane fracture
t. tubercle
t. tubercle ossification center
t. tubercle prominence
t. tuberosity
t. tuberosity fracture
t. varus
t. vein

tibialis
t. anterior
t. posterior
t. posterior tenosynovitis
t. sign

tibioastragalocalcaneal canal of Richet

tibiocalcaneal
t. fusion
t. joint complex
t. ligament
t. space

tibiofemoral angle (TFA)

tibiofibular
t. articulation
t. diastasis
t. fracture
t. joint
t. ligament
t. syndesmosis
t. synostosis

tibioligamentous fascicle

tibionavicular ligament

tibioperoneal
t. occlusive disease
t. runoff system
t. trunk

tibiotalar
t. angle
t. joint
t. joint slanting
t. rotation

tibiotalocalcaneal fusion

tibiotarsal dislocation

TICA
traumatic intracranial aneurysm

tidal
t. inspiratory flow volume
t. wave of carotid arterial pulse

tiered therapy

tie sternum

Tietze syndrome

tiger
t. heart
t. lily heart

tight
t. dural sac
t. filum terminale
t. filum terminal syndrome
t. lesion
t. spinal canal
t. stenosis

tigroid pattern

Tilden method

Tillaux-Chaput fracture

Tillaux fracture

Tillaux-Kleiger fracture

tilt
bent-knee pelvic t.
caudal t.
gantry t.
lunate t.
patellar t.
t. table
t. test
valgus t.
varus t.

tilted
t. optimized nonsaturating excitation (TONE)
t. sacrum

tilting-disk valve

time
acceleration t.
acquisition t.
activated partial thromboplastin t.
t. activity function
asymmetric appearance t.
atrial activation t.
atrioventricular t.
background equivalent radiation t.
bleeding t.

NOTES

time *(continued)*
calculated clearance t.
capillary filling t.
carotid ejection t.
cerebral circulation t.
circulation t. (CT)
t. compensation gain
concentration times t. (C x T)
t. constant
corrected sinus node recovery t.
t. course fracture scintigraphy
cycle t.
data acquisition t.
decay t.
deceleration t.
delayed transit t.
diastolic perfusion t.
diffusion t.
t. to distant failure (TTDF)
t. domain
echo t. (TE, T-E)
echo delay t. (TE, T-E)
effective transverse relation t.
efficient relaxation t.
ejection t. (ET)
emptying t.
esophageal transit t.
t. of flight (TOF)
gastric transit t.
image-acquisition t.
image-reconstruction t.
imaging t.
increased left ventricular ejection t.
interpulse t.
inversion t. (TI)
ischemic t.
isovolumetric contraction t.
isovolumic relaxation t. (IVRT)
lattice relaxation t.
left ventricular ejection t. (LVET)
left ventricular fast filling t.
left ventricular slow filling t. ($LVFT_2$)
t. to local failure (TTLF)
longitudinal recovery t.
longitudinal relaxation t.
maximum inflation t.
maximum walking t. (MWT)
mean pulmonary transit t. (MTT)
t. motion (TM)
myocardial contrast appearance t. (MCAT)
overall treatment t. (OTT)
pain-free walking t. (PFWT)
t. to peak activity
t. to peak contrast (TPC)
t. to peak filling rate (TPFR)
perfusion t.
phasing-in t.
t. point
prolonged ejection t.
proton spin-lattice relaxation t.
pulmonary transit t. (PTT)
pulse reappearance t.
pulse repetition t.
pyelographic appearance t.
radionuclide esophageal dead t.
reaction recovery t.
receiver dead t.
recovery t. (RT, TR)
relaxation t.
repetition t. (RT, TR)
resolving t.
retinocortical t.
right ventricle-to-ear t.
rise t.
rotational correlation t.
scan t.
sequence t.
short-echo t.
short T1 relaxation t.
sinoatrial conduction t. (SACT)
sinus node recovery t. (SNRT)
small bowel transit t.
sojourn t.
spin-lattice relaxation t.
spin-spin relaxation t.
systolic acceleration t.
systolic upstroke t.
transit t.
transverse relaxation t.
T1 relaxation t.
T2 relaxation t.
t. trend
venous filling t. (VFT)
venous refill t. (VRT)
venous return t. (VRT)
ventricular activation t. (VAT)
ventricular isovolumic relaxation t.

time-activity curve

time-attenuation curve

time-averaged flow

time-compensated gain

timed
t. bolus delivery
t. imaging

time-density curve

timed-sequential therapy

time-gain compensation (TGC)

time-insensitive

time-intensity curve

time-lapse quantitative computed tomography lymphography

time-motion mode (M-mode)

time-of-flight (TOF)
t.-o.-f. echoplanar imaging

t.-o.-f. effect
t.-o.-f. enhancement
t.-o.-f. flow measurement
t.-o.-f. imaging
t.-o.-f. magnetic resonance angiography
t.-o.-f. method
t.-o.-f. PET imaging system
t.-o.-f. signal loss
t.-o.-f. technique
two-dimensional t.-o.-f. (2D TOF)

time-out
ventriculoatrial t.-o.

timer
Thyrx t.

time-resolved imaging by automatic data segmentation (TRIADS)

time-sensitive

time-to-treatment
t.-t.-t. bias
t.-t.-t. failure

time-varied
t.-v. gain (TVG)
t.-v. gain control

time-varying magnetic field

time-velocity measurement

TIMI
thrombolysis in myocardial infarct

timing
gradient t.
t. parameter

tin-113 (^{113}Sn)

Tinel percussion sign

tiny ventricle

tip
t. angle
catheter t.
t. deflector
t. dispersion characteristic
hockey-stick appearance of catheter t.
mitral valve leaflet t.
occipital t.
radiopaque distal t.
rectal t.
t. of spleen
valve t.

tip-deflecting guide wire

TIPS
transjugular intrahepatic portosystemic shunt
TIPS failure
TIPS imaging

tissue
aberrant t.
abnormal t.
adipose t.
adventitial t.
aerated t.
anisotropic t.
apical t.
areolar connective t.
bony t.
breast t.
bronchus-associated lymphoid t. (BALT)
cancellous t.
t. capsule
cartilaginous t.
cavernous t.
t. characterization
t. characterization technique
chondroid t.
chorionic t.
collagenous t.
t. conductivity
connective t.
t. contrast
cortical t.
crushed t.
dartoic t.
dead t.
t. deficit compensator
degenerated t.
dense connective t.
t. density
destruction of t.
devitalized t.
t. Doppler imaging
ectopic thyroid t.
edematous t.
engorged t.
escape of air into lung connective t.
extraadrenal chromaffin t.
extralobular connective t.
exuberant granulation t.
fast exchange-soft t.
fatty prostatic t.
fetal lymphoid t.
t. of fetus
fibroadipose t.
fibroareolar t.

NOTES

tissue *(continued)*
fibrocartilaginous t.
fibrocollagenous connective t.
fibrofatty breast t.
fibroglandular t.
fibromuscular t.
fibrosing t.
fibrotic t.
fibrous connective t.
fibrous scar t.
fibrovascular t.
t. flow
gangrenous t.
gastrointestinal-associated lymphoid t.
gelatinous t.
granulation t.
grumous t.
gut-associated lymphoid t. (GALT)
herniation of brain t.
hyperplastic t.
hypertrophic t.
hypervascular granulation t.
t. imaging agent
t. imprint
indurated t.
t. inhomogeneity factor
interlobular t.
interstitial t.
intertrabecular soft t.
intralobular connective t.
island of t.
t. island
isointense soft t.
isotropic t.
joint t.
late effects of normal t. (LENT)
lipomatous t.
lymphatic t.
lymph node t.
lymphoid t.
lymphoreticular t.
mammary t.
t. mass
mesenchymal t.
mesenteric t.
t. migration
mucosa-associated lymphoid t. (MALT)
muscle t.
necrotic t.
neoplastic t.
nodal t.
noncontractile scar t.
noncritical soft t.
nonviable t.
osseous t.
ossification of soft t.
osteocartilaginous t.
t. outflow valve
t. oxygenation
paratracheal soft t.
paravaginal soft t.
parenchymal t.
passively congested lung t.
t. perfusion
periarticular t.
peribronchial connective t.
perilobular connective t.
peritumoral t.
t. plate
preepiglottic soft t.
prevertebral soft t. (PVST)
proliferation of fibrous t.
reduction mammoplasty t.
regeneration of t.
regular connective t.
residual ductal t.
reticular connective t.
retrodiskal t.
retropharyngeal soft t.
revascularized t.
scar t.
t. sequela
t. slice
slow exchange soft t.
soft t.
t. space
stippled soft t.
stringlike bands of fibrous t.
subadventitial t.
subcutaneous connective t.
swollen t.
sympathetic nervous t.
syngeneic t.
synovial t.
taenia t.
target t.
tendon t.
testicular adrenal rest t.
thoracic inlet soft t.
t. tolerance dose (TTD)
t. tolerance to radiation
tongue of t.
tuberculosis granulation t.
underlying t.
vascular t.
t. veil
t. viability
t. water content
t. weighting factor

tissue-air ratio (TAR)
tissue-based T2 relaxation
tissue-maximum ratio (TMR)
tissue-phantom ratio (TPR)
titanium (Ti)

t. compound
t. plate
Titterington position
Tl-201
Cardiolite T.
^{201}Tl
thallium-201
TLA
translumbar aortography
TLA needle
TLD
thermoluminescent dosimeter
tumor lethal dose
TLD rod
TLI
thymidine labeling index
TLS
tumor lysis syndrome
TM
time motion
TMA
transmetatarsal amputation
true metatarsus adductus
TME
trapezium-metacarpal eburnation
TME ratio
TMJ
temporomandibular joint
TMR
tissue-maximum ratio
topical magnetic resonance
TMS three-dimensional radiation therapy planning system
TN
true negative
TNM
tumor, node, metastasis
TNM staging system
tobacco
t. heart
t. nodule
tocolysis
tocopherol
alpha t.
gamma t. (γ-T)
Todani
T. classification
T. type cyst
Todaro
T. tendon
triangle of T.
T. triangle
Todd
T. cirrhosis
T. paresis
toddler's fracture
Todd-Wells technique
Tod muscle
toe
base of t.
cock-up deformity of t.
dynamic hammer t.
fixed hammer t.
interphalangeal joint arthritis of great t.
microdactyly of big t.
Morton t.
overriding t.'s
set angle of t.'s
t. spread sign
t. systolic pressure
tennis t.
TOF
tetralogy of Fallot
time of flight
time-of-flight
2D TOF
two-dimensional time-of-flight
TOF imaging
tolerance
drug t.
Fletcher rule of irradiation t.
irradiation t.
narrow gating t.
Tolosa-Hunt syndrome
toluidine blue (TB)
tomato tumor
tombstone
t. pelvis
t. pelvis configuration
Tomocat
T. contrast medium
T. imaging agent
tomogram
blurred-image t.
plain t.
sagittal t.
single-slice long-axis t.
stacked t.
temporal bone t.
tomograph
tomographic
t. cuts
t. imaging

T

NOTES

tomographic *(continued)*
t. section
t. slice
t. view
tomography
automated computed axial t. (ACAT)
computed t. (CT)
computed transmission t.
computerized axial t. (CAT)
computerized cranial t.
computerized transverse axial t. (CTAT, CTAT imaging)
contrast-enhanced computed t. (CECT)
conventional t.
cranial computed t. (CCT)
dynamic computed t.
electrical impedance t. (EIT)
electron beam t. (EBT)
electron-beam computed t. (EBCT)
emission computed t. (ECT)
emission computer-assisted t. (ECAT)
exercise thallium-201 t.
expiratory computed t.
FDG positron emission t.
flow mode ultrafast computed t.
fluoride ion-positron emission t. (F-18-PET)
^{18}fluoro-deoxy-D-glucose positron emission t. (^{18}FDP PET)
focused appendix computed t. (FACT)
gated single-photon emission computed t. (GSPECT)
helical biphasic computed t. (HBCT imaging)
helical computed t.
high-resolution computed t. (HRCT)
high-spatial-resolution cine computed t. (HSRCCT)
high-temporal-resolution cine computed t. (HTRCCT)
hypocycloidal t.
hypocycloidal ankle t.
indirect computed t.
kidney t.
lateral t.
limited-slice computed t.
linear t.
metrizamide-assisted computed t. (CTMM)
multiphasic renal computerized t.
myocardial perfusion t.
nonenhanced computed t. (NECT)
nuclear magnetic resonance t.
optical coherence t. (OCT)
peripheral quantitative computed t. (pQCT)
pluridirectional t. (PT)
positron emission t. (PET)
positron emission transaxial t. (PETT)
quantitative computed t. (QCT)
rapid acquisition computed axial t. (RACAT)
sellar t.
single-photon emission t. (SPET)
single-photon emission computed t. (SPECT)
spiral computed t.
spiral x-ray computed t. (SVCT)
transmission computed t.
transmission computer-assisted t. (TCAT)
trispiral t.
two-phase helical computed t.
ultrafast computed t. (UFCT)
ultrafast CT electron beam t.
ultrasound computed t. (UCT)
ultrasound diffraction t.
volumetric computed t.
water-contrast computed t.
xenon computed t. (XeCT)
xenon-enhanced computed t.
x-ray computed t. (XCT)
Z-dependent computed t.
tomolevel
Tomolex tomographic system
tomomyelography
tomoscanner
Philips T-60 t.
tomoscintigraphy
tomosynthesis
digital t.
TomTec
TONE
tilted optimized nonsaturating excitation
TONE sequence
tone
fetal t.
vascular t.
tongue
t. cancer
t. fasciculation
t. fracture
t. of tissue
t. and trough bone
tongue-shaped villus
tongue-type intraarticular fracture
tonsil
t. cancer
cerebellar t.
herniated cerebellar t.
lingual t.

tonsillar
t. carcinoma
t. ectopia
t. herniation
t. pillar
tonus
arterial t.
tooth
fibroosteoma of the t.
t. mass
toothpaste
t. lung shadow
t. shadows mucus plug
tophaceous gout
tophus, pl. **tophi**
t. formation
gouty t.
topical
t. magnetic resonance (TMR)
t. water-soluble contrast medium
top normal limits of size
Topo
T. II
topoisomerase II
topodermatography
topogram
topographic
t. identification
t. measurement
topography
arterial t.
balloon t.
ocular globe t.
scintigraphic balloon t.
vessel t.
x-ray t.
topoisomerase
t. II (Topo II)
torch
saline t.
torcula
torcular Herophili
torcular-lambdoid inversion
tori (*pl. of* torus)
torn meniscotibial ligament
Tornwaldt
T. bursitis
T. cyst
torque
t. control guide wire
high t.
t. stress
torr pressure
torsed appendage
torsion
acute testicular t.
adnexal t.
chronic testicular t.
extravaginal testicular t.
t. of fracture fragment
gallbladder t.
internal tibial t. (ITT)
internal tibiofibular t.
intravaginal t.
lung t.
missed testicular t.
ovarian t.
spermatic cord t.
splenic t.
subacute testicular t.
testicular appendage t.
t. of testis
tibial t.
t. wedge nonunion
torsional
t. abnormality
t. alignment
t. attenuating diameter guide wire
t. deformity
t. fracture
t. impaction force
t. stress
torso phased-array coil (TPAC)
torsus tibarius
torticollis
tortuosity
elongation and t.
t. of ureter
tortuous
t. aorta
t. aortic arch
t. emptying
t. esophagus
t. tubule
t. vein
t. vein dilatation
t. vessel
toruloma
torus, pl. **tori**
t. fracture
t. hyperplasia
t. mandibularis
t. pylorus
t. tubarius

NOTES

TOS
thoracic outlet syndrome
Toshiba
T. Aspire continuous imaging
T. echocardiograph machine
T. MR scanner
T. 900S helical CT scanner
T. 900S/XII scanner
T. TCT-80 CT scanner
T. Xpress SX helical CT scanner
T. Xvision scanner
total
t. abdominal hysterectomy
t. abdominal hysterectomy and bilateral salpingo-oophorectomy (TAHBSO)
t. ablation
t. androgen suppression therapy
t. anomalous pulmonary venous connection
t. anomalous pulmonary venous drainage (TAPVD)
t. anomalous pulmonary venous return (TAPVR)
t. artificial heart (TAH)
t. atrial refractory period (TARP)
t. body irradiation (TBI)
t. body scan imaging
t. body scanning
t. body water (TBW)
t. cerebral blood flow (TCBF)
t. condylar depression fracture
t. exchangeable potassium (TEK)
t. exchangeable sodium (TENa)
t. fracture
t. glossectomy
t. hip arthroplasty
t. image noise
t. knee implant
t. lesion
t. lung capacity
t. mastectomy
t. necrosis
t. occlusion
t. peripheral resistance (TPR)
t. placenta previa
t. pulmonary resistance (TPR)
t. pulmonary venous connection
t. reference air-kerma (TRAK)
t. stroke volume (TSV)
totalis
situs inversus t.
toto
in t.
touch preparation
Touraine-Solente-Gole disease
tourniquet
caval t.
t. technique
Tourtual canal
towering cerebellum
Towne
T. position
T. projection
T. view
Townsend avalanche
toxemia of pregnancy
toxemic pneumonia
toxic
t. adenoma
t. cardiomyopathy
t. cirrhosis
t. megacolon
t. multinodular goiter
t. nodular goiter
t. nodule
t. pneumonia
t. synovitis
toxicity
bone marrow t.
dose-limiting t. (DLT)
radiation-induced pulmonary t.
toxin
bacterial t.
toxoabscess
Toynbee muscle
TP
temporal peak
thymidine phosphorylase
true positive
TPA
thrombotic pulmonary artery
TPAC
torso phased-array coil
TPBS
three-phase bone scintigraphy
TPC
time to peak contrast
TPFR
time to peak filling rate
TPMT
thiopurine methyltransferase
T-portagram
TPR
tissue-phantom ratio
total peripheral resistance
total pulmonary resistance
TR
recovery time
repetition time
ultralong TR
trabecula, pl. **trabeculae**
septomarginal t.

trabecular
t. bone
t. bone resorption
t. carcinoma
t. degeneration
t. destruction
t. disruption
t. fracture
t. microfracture
t. pattern
t. thickening
trabeculated
t. atrium
t. bone
t. bone lesion
t. osteolysis
t. outline
trabeculation
endocardial t.
trace
t. amount of radiopharmaceutical
t. edema
t. element distribution
tracer
t. abnormality
t. accumulation
t. activity
t. bolus
delayed transport of t.
deposition of t.
t. dose
focal pooling of t.
^{13}N ammonia radioactive t.
neutron-rich biomedical t.
patchy distribution of t.
t. principle
radioactive t.
radiopharmaceutical t.
shunted t.
transependymal uptake of t.
uptake of t.
t. uptake
trachea, pl. **tracheae**
annular ligament of t.
carina of t.
carrot-shaped t.
intrathoracic t.
lunate-shaped t.
napkin-ring t.
saber-sheath t.
scabbard t.
tracheal
t. anastomosis
t. aspiration
t. "B" button
t. bifurcation
t. bifurcation angle
t. bronchus
t. caliber
t. cartilage
t. deviation
t. displacement
t. diverticulosis
t. fracture
t. lumen
t. lymph node
t. narrowing
t. ring
t. shift
t. stenosis
t. stricture
t. tube
t. tumor
t. wall stripe
tracheobiliary fistula
tracheobronchial
t. fistula
t. foreign body
t. hypersensitivity
t. injury (TBI)
t. lymph node
t. mucosal necrosis
t. papillomatosis
t. rupture
t. tree
tracheobronchoesophageal fistula
tracheobronchomalacia
acquired t.
tracheobronchomegaly
tracheobronchopathia osteochondroplastica
tracheocele
tracheoesophageal (TE, T-E)
t. fistula (TEF)
t. junction
tracheomalacia
congenital t.
tracheopathia
t. osteochondroplastica
t. osteoplastica
tracheostomy
t. tube

NOTES

tracing
carotid pulse t.
electrocardiogram t.
pulmonary capillary wedge t.
ray t.
vessel t.
track
t. cone length
deep white matter t.
t. etching
t. of pin
t. valve
tracking
abnormal t.
anterior t.
automatic peak t. (APT)
bolus t.
t. limit
magnetic bolus t.
magnetic resonance needle t.
periportal t.
real-time biplanar needle t.
real-time magnetic resonance imaging t.
tract
aerodigestive t.
alimentary t.
anterior corticospinal t.
anterior spinocerebellar t.
anterior spinothalamic t.
apple-peel appearance of the GI t.
ascending t.
association t.
atriofascicular t.
atrio-His bypass t.
atrioventricular nodal bypass t.
Behçet GI t.
Bekhterev t.
biliary t.
blind tibial outflow t.
brainstem pyramidal t.
bronchial t.
Bruce and Muir t.
bulbar t.
Burdach t.
candy-cane appearance of GI t.
carcinoid GI t.
central tegmental t. (CTT)
cerebellar t.
cerebellorubral t.
cerebellorubrospinal t.
cerebellospinal t.
cerebellotegmental t.
cerebellothalamic t.
concealed bypass t.
corticobulbar t. (CBT)
corticopontine t.
corticorubral t.
corticospinal t. (CST)
corticotectal t.
crossed pyramidal t.
cuneocerebellar t.
Deiters t.
dentatothalamic t.
dermal sinus t.
descending t.
digestive t.
direct pyramidal t.
dorsal spinocerebellar t.
dorsolateral t.
extracorticospinal t.
extrapyramidal t.
fascial t.
fasiculoventricular bypass t.
fastigiobulbar t.
fetal urogenital t.
fistulous t.
Flechsig t.
flow t.
free wall t.
frontopontine t.
frontotemporal t.
gastrointestinal t. (GI tract)
geniculocalcarine t.
geniculostriate t.
genital t.
genitourinary t.
GI t.
gastrointestinal tract
Goll t.
Gombault-Philippe t.
Gowers t.
habenulopeduncular t.
Helweg t.
hepatic outflow t.
hypothalamohypophysial t.
ileal inflow t.
iliotibial t.
intermediolateral t.
intersegmental t.
interstitiospinal t.
intestinal t.
intrahepatic biliary t.
lateral corticospinal t.
lateral lemniscus t.
lateral spinothalamic t.
left ventricular outflow t. (LVOT)
Lissauer t.
long t.
Lowenthal t.
lower t.
Maissiat t.
mamillopeduncular t.
mamillotegmental t.
mamillothalamic t.
Marchi t.

mesencephalic t.
Meynert t.
Monakow t.
motor t.
Muir and Bruce t.
nigrostriate t.
nodohisian bypass t.
nodoventricular bypass t.
occipitopontine t.
occipitotemporopontine t.
olfactory t.
outflow t.
pancreaticobiliary t.
paraventriculohypophysial t.
parietopontine t.
patent needle t.
peduncular t.
Philippe-Gombault t.
pilonidal t.
posterior spinocerebellar t.
pulmonary conduit outflow t.
pyramidal t.
respiratory t.
reticulospinal t.
retrochiasmal optic t.
right ventricular bypass t.
right ventricular outflow t. (RVOT)
rubrobulbar t.
rubrospinal t.
Schultze comma t.
Schütz t.
semilunar t.
seminal t.
sensory t.
septomarginal t.
sinus t.
spinal dermal sinus t.
spinocerebellar t.
spinocervical t.
spinocervicothalamic t.
spinoreticular t.
spinotectal t.
spinothalamic t.
Spitzka-Lissauer t.
strionigral t.
sulcomarginal t.
tectobulbar t.
tectocerebellar t.
tectospinal t.
tegmental t.
tegmentospinal t.
temporopontine t.
testobulbar t.
thalamoolivary t.
transverse t.
tree-barking urinary t.
triangular t.
trigeminal nerve t.
trigeminothalamic t.
tuberohypophysial t.
upper aerodigestive t.
upper gastrointestinal (UGI) t.
urinary t.
urogenital t.
ventral amygdalofugal t.
ventral spinocerebellar t.
ventral spinothalamic t.
ventricular outflow t.
vestibulocerebellar t.
vestibulospinal t.
Vicq d'Azyr t.

traction
breast t.
bronchiectasis t.
t. diverticulum
t. epiphysis
t. exostosis
t. fracture
t. spur

tragus

trailing edge

train
Carr-Purcell-Meiboom-Gill echo t.
echo t.
fast spin-echo (SE) t.

TRAK
total reference air-kerma

tramline
t. cortical calcification
t. shadow

trampoline fracture

tram-track
t.-t. cortical calcification
t.-t. ductus arteriosus calcification
t.-t. gyral calcification
t.-t. pattern
t.-t. renal cortical necrosis calcification

transabdominal
t. color Doppler sonography
t. imaging
t. left lateral retroperitoneal maneuver

NOTES

transabdominal *(continued)*
t. scanning
t. sonogram
transannular
t. patch reconstruction
transaortic
t. radiofrequency ablation
t. systolic gradient
transapical endocardial ablation
transaxial
t. CT scan
t. image
t. imaging
t. joint scan
t. maximum-intensity projection
t. plane
t. scan plane
t. slice
t. thoracic inlet
transaxillary lateral view
transbronchial needle aspiration (TBNA)
transcaphoid fracture
transcapitate fracture
transcarpal amputation
transcatheter
t. ablation
t. arterial chemoembolization
t. filter placement
t. oily chemoembolization
radiofrequency modification t.
t. technique
t. therapy
transceiver
transcerebral medullary vein
transcervical
t. balloon tuboplasty (TBT)
t. catheterization of fallopian tube imaging
t. femoral fracture
transchondral talar fracture
transcondylar
t. amputation
t. axis (TCA)
t. fracture
t. line
transcoronal STIR image
transcranial
t. alteral view
t. cerebral oximetry
t. color-coded duplex ultrasound
t. Doppler (TCD)
t. Doppler ultrasound (TCD ultrasound)
t. real-time color Doppler imaging
t. real-time color-flow Doppler sonography
transcutaneous
t. aortovelography (TAV)
t. broadband sector transducer
t. crush injury
t. electrical nerve stimulator (TENS)
t. extraction catheter atherectomy
t. oxygen pressure measurement ($tcPO_2$)
transducer
Acuson linear array t.
ART t.
t. beam pattern
biopsy t.
broadband t.
catheter-borne sector t.
end-viewing t.
epicardial Doppler flow sector t.
Gaeltec catheter-tip pressure t.
Gould Statham pressure t.
high-frequency t.
high-resolution linear array t.
linear array t.
magnetic resonance imaging-guided focused ultrasound sector t.
Millar catheter-tip t.
M-mode sector t.
MRI-guided focused ultrasound t.
phased-array t.
piezoelectric t.
PSH-25GT transcranial imaging t.
puncture t.
rectal multiplane t.
sector t.
signal t.
Sonos ultrasonographic t.
transcutaneous broadband sector t.
transesophageal t.
Ultramark 8 t.
ultrasound t.
V5M Multiplane t.
transducer-skin interface
transduction
signal t.
transduodenal
t. endoscopic decompression
t. endosonography
transdural fistula
transection (*var. of* transsection)
transependymal uptake of tracer
transepiphyseal fracture
transesophageal
t. Doppler color flow imaging
t. echocardiography (TEE)
t. echocardiography (TEE) probe
t. transducer
transethmoidal encephalocele
transfascial spread
transfemoral arteriography

transfer
energy t.
Fourier t.
gradient echo MR with magnetization t.
His-Haas muscle t.
t. imaging
inversion t.
t. lesion
linear energy t. (LET)
magnetization t. (MT)
quantitative magnetization t.
rapid image t.
saturation t.
ultrafast video t.
transferase
chloramphenicol acetyl t. (CAT)
hypoxantine-guanosine phosphoribosyl t. (HGPT)
transfibular fusion
transfixing screw
transform
cosine t.
discrete Fourier t. (DFT)
driven equilibrium Fourier t.
fast Fourier t. (FFT)
Fourier t.
Hough t. (HT)
inverse Fourier t. (IFT)
three-dimensional Fourier t. (3DFT)
two-dimensional Fourier t. (2DFT)
wavelet t.
transformation
blastic t.
cavernous portal vein t.
t. constant
enthesopathic t.
fast Fourier t.
Fourier discrete t.
t. matrix
photo t.
vascular t.
t. zone
transformer (t)
closed core t.
Coolidge t.
distribution t.
doughnut t.
t. equation
filament t.
high-voltage t.
t. law
t. loss
ratio t.
real-time chirp Z t.
step-down t.
step-up t.
transfusional iron overload
transgastric endosonography
transgluteal CT-guided technique
transgression
cortical t.
transhamate fracture
transhepatic
t. biliary disease
t. biliary stent
t. cholangiogram (THC)
t. drainage
transhiatal esophagectomy (THE)
transient
t. AV block
t. bone marrow edema syndrome
t. cavitation
t. cerebral ischemia
t. chyle leak
t. equilibrium
t. gallbladder hydrops
t. hemispheric attack
t. hiatal hernia
t. infiltrate
t. ischemic attack (TIA)
t. ischemic carotid insufficiency
t. left ventricular dilatation
t. myocardial ischemia
t. osteoporosis of hip
t. perfusion defect
t. pleural effusion
t. regional osteoporosis
t. shunt obstruction
t. sinus arrest
t. synovitis
t. synovitis of hip
t. tachypnea
t. tricuspid regurgitation
transiliac fracture
transillumination
t. of head
multispectral diffuse t.
transit
biliary-to-bowel t.
bolus t.
delayed small bowel t.
impaired tubular t.
parenchymal t.

NOTES

transit *(continued)*
t. scintigraphy
small bowel delayed t.
t. time
tubular t.
t. volume
transition
allowed beta t.
beta t.
t. electrons
isomeric t.
isometric t.
t. metal
t. ureteral cell cancer
t. zone
transitional
t. cell cancer
t. cell carcinoma (TCC)
t. cell neoplasm
t. cell papilloma
t. kidney cell cancer
t. meningioma
t. rhythm
t. urethral cell papilloma
t. urinary bladder cell cancer
t. vertebra
t. zone fissure
transitory synovitis
transjugular
t. cholangiogram
t. intrahepatic portosystemic shunt (TIPS)
t. intrahepatic portosystemic shunt imaging
t. venography
translation
condylar t.
radioulnarproximodistal t.
translational
t. diffusion
t. motion
translation-invariant filter
translesional gradient
translocation
t. of coronary artery
robertsonian t.
translucency
first-trimester nuchal t.
translucent depression
translumbar
t. amputation
t. aortography (TLA)
t. aortography needle
transluminal
t. atherectomy
t. atherectomy imaging
t. balloon angioplasty imaging
t. coronary artery angioplasty complex
t. dilatation
t. endarterectomy
transluminally placed stented graft
transmalleolar
t. ankle
t. axis-thigh angle
transmedial plane
transmesenteric plication
transmetatarsal amputation (TMA)
transmetatarsal-thigh angle
transmissible venereal tumor
transmission
airborne t.
t. block
t. computed tomography
t. computer-assisted tomography (TCAT)
t. data
t. dosimetry
nosocomial tuberculosis t.
t. scan
sound t.
through-sound t.
transmitral
t. flow
t. gradient
transmit-receive coil
transmitter coil
transmural
t. colitis
t. fibrosis
t. inflammation
t. invasion
t. match
t. myocardial infarct
t. steal
transmyocardial perfusion pressure
transnasal
t. endoluminal ultrasonography
t. endoluminal ultrasound
transnasally
transonic
transoral
transorally
transosseous venography
transpapillary placement
transparent rendering
transpedicular decompression
transperineal implant
transphyseal
t. bone bridge
transplant
allogeneic bone marrow t.
allogeneic peripheral cell t.
arteriovenous fistula t.
autologous bone marrow t.

bone marrow t.
cadaveric renal t.
heart t.
heart-lung t.
hepatic t.
kidney t.
kidney-pancreas t.
liver t.
lung t.
marrow t.
organ t.
pancreas t.
t. rejection
renal t.
syngeneic bone marrow t.
tandem t.

transplantation
allogeneic stem-cell t. (SCT)
autologous stem-cell t.
bone marrow t.
heart and lung t.
single-lung t.

transplutonium radioisotope

transporionic axis

transport
forward t.
iodide t.
Monte Carlo photon t. (MCPT)
reverse t.

transposed
t. adnexa
t. aorta

transposition
atrial t.
carotid-subclavian t.
t. cipher
t. complex
congenitally corrected t.
gastric t.
t. of great arteries (TGA)
great vessel t.
t. of great vessels
t. of inferior vena cava
inferior vena cava t.
Jatene t.
t. of ovary
subfascial t.
ventricular t.

transpulmonary pressure (PTP)

transpulmonic gradient

transpyloric plane

transradial styloid perilunate dislocation

transradiancy

transradiant
t. air
t. zone

transrectal
t. echography
t. sonography
t. ultrasound (TRUS)

transsacral fracture

transscaphoid
t. dislocation fracture
t. perilunate dislocation

transscapular view

transsection, transection
aortic t.
spinal cord t.
t. of spinal cord
traumatic aortic t.

transseptal
t. angiocardiography
t. angiography
t. perforation
t. radiofrequency ablation
t. sheath

transsexual

transsphincteric anal fistula

transstenotic gradient

transsyndesmotic screw fixation

transtelephonic ICD interrogation

transtentorial
t. herniation

transtentorially

transthoracic
t. echocardiography (TTE)
t. esophagectomy
t. imaging
t. needle aspiration biopsy (TTNAB)
t. three-dimensional echocardiography
t. ultrasound

transthoracic-three-dimensional echocardiography

transtrabecular plane (TTP)

transtracheal aspiration

transtricuspid valve diastolic gradient

transtriquetral fracture

transudate

transudation

NOTES

transudative
t. pericardial fluid
t. pleural effusion
transumbilical plane (TUP)
transurethral
t. incision of the prostate
t. resection (TUR)
t. resection of bladder
t. resection of prostate (TURP)
t. ultrasound-guided laser-induced prostatectomy
transvaginal
t. cone
t. echography
t. hysterosonography (TVHS)
t. implant
t. oocyte retrieval
t. sonography (TVS)
t. ultrasonography
t. ultrasound-guided drainage
transvalvular pressure gradient
transvenous
t. digital subtraction angiography
t. implantation
transversalis fascia
transversarium
foramen t.
transverse
t. acoustic wave
t. aortic arch
t. atlantal ligament
t. band
t. carpal ligament
t. cervical ligament
t. colon
t. colon carcinoma
t. colon loop
t. colon stripe sign
t. comminuted fracture
t. cord lesion
t. costal facet
t. crural ligament
t. diameter between ischia
t. esophageal fold
t. genicular ligament
t. heart
t. humeral ligament
t. hypoplasia
t. intertarsal ligament
t. lie
t. ligaments of atlas
t. lucent metaphyseal line
t. magnetization
t. maxillary fracture
t. mesocolon
t. metacarpal ligament
t. metatarsal ligament
t. myelitis
t. orientation
t. oval pelvis
t. pelvic diameter
t. pericardial sinus
t. perineal ligament
t. plane
t. plane alignment
t. plane force
t. plane vectorcardiography
t. presentation
t. process
t. process fracture
t. process of vertebra
t. relaxation
t. relaxation rate
t. relaxation time
t. relaxivity (R2)
t. ridge
t. section
t. section imaging
t. sinus thrombosis
t. slice
t. tarsal joint
t. temporal gyrus
t. tibiofibular ligament
t. tract
t. ultrasound
t. view
transversely oriented endplate compression fracture
transverse/neutral view
transversum
septum t.
transversus
t. abdominis muscle
situs t.
transvesical oocyte retrieval
trapezia (*pl. of* trapezium)
trapeziometacarpal joint
trapezioscaphoid joint
trapeziotrapezoid joint
trapezium, pl. **trapezia**
t. bone
t. fracture
trapezium-metacarpal
t.-m. eburnation (TME)
t.-m. eburnation ratio (TME ratio)
trapezium-trapezoid joint space
trapezius
t. muscle
t. ridge sign
trapezoid
t. body
t. bone
t. bone of Henle
t. bone of Lyser
t. of Henle bone
t. ligament

trapping
air t.
t. of aneurysm
t. of radioisotope
t. thyroid defect
trashfoot syndrome
Traube
T. aortic regurgitation sign
T. heart
T. semilunar space
trauma
abdominal blunt t.
acoustic t.
bladder contusion t.
bladder rupture t.
blunt chest t.
blunt gastrointestinal t.
blunt pancreatic t.
cardiothoracic t.
carotid artery dissection t.
eye t.
gallbladder t.
genitourinary tract t.
GI tract t.
head t.
hepatic t.
high-energy t.
hypovolemia t.
intracerebral hemorrhage t.
kidney t.
liver t.
multiple t.
nonaccidental t.
t. oblique
ocular t.
pancreatic t.
pelvic vascular t.
penetrating t.
physical t.
renal t.
splenic t.
sustentacular t.
testicular t.
urethral t.
urinary bladder t.
vascular t.
vessel t.
traumatic
t. amputation
t. aortic disruption
t. aortic injury
t. aortic pseudoaneurysm
t. aortic rupture
t. aortic tear
t. aortic transsection
t. arthritis
t. avulsion
t. bone cyst
t. brain injury (TBI)
t. degeneration
t. diaphragmatic hernia
t. dislocation
t. emphysema
t. fat necrosis
t. head injury
t. infarct
t. intracranial aneurysm (TICA)
t. lipid cyst
t. lung cyst
t. meningeal hemorrhage
t. meningocele
t. osteoarthritis
t. pneumatocele
t. pneumomediastinum
t. pneumonia
t. pneumothorax
t. rupture of the diaphragm (TRD)
t. spondylolisthesis
t. spondylolysis
t. syrinx
t. thrombus
t. tricuspid incompetence
traumatica
diplegia spinalis brachialis t.
myositis ossificans t.
traumatogenic occlusion
Trautmann triangular space
traversal
tentorial t.
traverse
traversing the fracture
tray
Bucky view t.
Müller t.
TRD
traumatic rupture of the diaphragm
penetrating TRD
Treacher Collins syndrome
treadmill
t. exercise Bruce protocol
t. exercise stress test
t. exercise test (TET)
inclination of t.
t. slope

NOTES

treatment
allocation of t.
cobalt-60 gamma knife radiosurgical t.
t. energy
ferromagnetic microembolization t.
fibrinolytic t.
interstitial hyperthermia t.
intracavitary hyperthermia t.
iodine-131 antiferritin t.
low-energy radiofrequency conduction hyperthermia t.
microwave hyperthermia t.
platinum-based t.
t. port
refractory to t.
superficial hyperthermia t.
thyroid radioiodine t.
ultrasound hyperthermia t.
tree
airway t.
arterial t.
t. artifact
biliary t.
bronchial t.
coronary artery t.
hepatobiliary t.
iliocaval t.
intrahepatic biliary t.
lower extremity arterial t.
tracheobronchial t.
tree-barking
t.-b. kidney
t.-b. urinary tract
tree-in-bud (TIB)
t.-i.-b. bronchiole
t.-i.-b. pattern
tree-in-winter bile duct appearance
tree-like airway structure
tree-shaped spot
trefoil
t. appearance
t. deformity
Treitz
T. fossa
T. hernia
ligament of T.
T. muscle
tremolite
trend
t. correction
time t.
Trendelenburg
T. position
T. radiograph
T. test
trephine technique
treppe phenomenon
Trevor disease
Trex digital mammography system (TDMS)
triad
acute compression t.
Beck t.
Bergqvist t.
Bradbury-Eggleston t.
Charcot t.
Currarino t.
Cushing t.
Dieulafoy t.
Garland t.
Grancher t.
hepatic t.
Kartagener t.
O'Donoghue unhappy t.
Osler t.
portal t.
Rigler t.
Saint t.
T. SPECT imaging system
Virchow thrombosis t.
wall-echo shadow (WES) t.
Whipple t.
TRIADS
time-resolved imaging by automatic data segmentation
triamine
triangle
apex of Koch t.
aponeurotic t.
auricular t.
axillary t.
Burger scalene t.
Calot t.
t. of Capener
cardiohepatic t.
carotid t.
cephalic t.
cervical t.
clavipectoral t.
Codman t.
crural t.
cysticohepatic t.
deltoideopectoral t.
digastric t.
Einthoven t.
facial t.
femoral t.
Garland t.
Gerhardt t.
Grynfeltt t.
Henke t.
Hesselbach t.
iliofemoral t.
inguinal t.
insular t.

internal jugular t.
Kager t.
Koch t.
Korányi-Grocco t.
Labbé t.
t. of Laimer
Langenbeck t.
Lesgaft t.
Livingston t.
lumbocostoabdominal t.
mesenteric t.
paramedian t.
Pawlik t.
posterior cervical t.
Rauchfuss t.
scalene t.
Scarpa t.
t. of Scarpa
submandibular t.
supraclavicular t.
sylvian t.
Todaro t.
t. of Todaro
urogenital t.
vertebrocostal t.
Ward t.

triangular
t. area of dullness
t. bone
t. defect
t. disk
t. external ankle fixation
t. fibrocartilage (TFC)
t. fibrocartilaginous complex (TFCC)
t. fontanelle
t. ligament
t. muscle
t. ridge
t. tract

triangulation
t. of Carrel
t. method

triatrial heart

triatriatum
cor t.

Triboulet test

tributary
extrahepatic portal vein t.
large venous t.

triceps brachii

trichinous embolus

trichobezoar

trichoptysis

trichorhinophalangeal (TRP)

tricorn bucket-handle tear

tricuspid
t. aortic valve
t. area
t. incompetence (TI)
t. insufficiency (TI)
t. orifice
t. orifice regurgitation
t. stenosis
t. valve (TV)
t. valve annulus
t. valve anomaly
t. valve atresia
t. valve closure
t. valve cusp
t. valve deformity
t. valve dysplasia
t. valve flow
t. valve gradient
t. valve prolapse
t. valve regurgitation
t. valve ring
t. valve strut

trident
t. hand
t. pelvis

Tridrate bowel preparation

trifascicular block

trifid
t. precordial motion motion
t. stomach

triflanged nail

trifurcation
t. of artery
patency t.
popliteal t.
popliteal artery t.

trigeminal
t. cavernous fistula
t. cavity
t. cistern
t. ganglion
t. hemangioma
t. nerve anatomy
t. nerve tract
t. pattern
schwannoma t.
t. trigeminy
t. trigonal hypertrophy

NOTES

trigeminothalamic tract
trigeminy
  trigeminal t.
trigger
  ECG t.
  electrocardiogram t.
  t. finger
  t. finger deformity
triggered pacing mode
triggering
  navigator echo-based real-time respiratory gating and t.
trigona (*pl. of* trigonum)
trigonal
  t. hypertrophy
  t. muscle
trigone
  angles of t.
  t. of bladder
  collateral t.
  deltoideopectoral t.
  fibrous t.
  Henke t.
  hypertrophied t.
  hypoglossal t.
  inguinal t.
  lateral ventricle t.
  Lieutaud t.
  Müller t.
  Pawlik t.
  t. of ventricle
  vertebrocostal t.
trigonocephaly
trigonum, pl. **trigona**
  t. calcis
  os t.
triiodinated imaging agent
triiodobenzoic acid
triiodothyronine
triisocyanide ^{99m}Tc imaging agent
trilaminar appearance
trilateral retinoblastoma
trilayer appearance
trileaflet
  t. aortic valve
trilinear interpolation
Trilisate
trilocular heart
trilogy of Fallot
Trimadeau sign
trimalleolar
  t. ankle fracture
trimellitic anhydrotic pneumonitis
trimester
triode tube
Trionix
  T. camera
  T. scanner
  T. SPECT
Triosil
tripartite
  t. duodenal carcinoma
  t. sesamoid bone
triphalangeal
  t. thumb
  t. thumb deformity
triphasic
  t. spiral CT
  t. waveform
Triphasix generator
triphenyltetrazolium chloride (TTC)
triphosphate
  adenosine t.
  arabinsylguanosine t.
  cyclic guanosine t.
  nucleoside t. (NTP)
triplane fracture
triple
  t. label
  t. match
  t.-resonance NMR probe circuit
  t. ripple
  t. therapy (TT)
triple-bubble sign
triple-dose gadolinium imaging
triple-head camera
triple-leaf collimator
triple-marker screening test
triple-peak cerebellum configuration
triple-phase
  t.-p. bone scan
  t.-p. bone scan imaging
triple-pylorus track sign
triplet
  t. gestation
triple-track sign
triple-voiding cystogram
tripod
  t. fracture
  t. position
  t. sign
tri-point bullet
Tripter
  Direx T.
triquetral
  t. bone
  t. fracture
  t. impingement
triquetrohamate
  t. helicoid slope
  t. joint
  t. ligament
triquetrolunate dislocation
triquetropisiform articulation

triquetroscaphoid
t. fascicle
t. ligament
triquetrotrapezoid fascicle
triquetrum
triradial cartilage
triradiate cartilage
trisacryl gelatin microsphere
trisegmentectomy
trismus
trisodium
mangafodipir t.
trisomic fetus
trisomy
t. 8 mosaicism syndrome
t. 9p
t. 13
t. 18
t. 21
t. 22
t. D syndrome
E t.
t. E syndrome
t. G
trispiral tomography
tristimulus
t. value
t. value flip
tritiated
t. thymidine (TT)
t. thymidine labeling index
tritium
triton tumor
trocar
t. drainage method
trocar-cannula technique
trochanter
greater t.
lesser t.
trochanteric
t. bursa
t. bursitis
t. flare
t. spine
trochlea, pl. **trochleae**
peroneal t.
trochlear
t. defect
t. groove
t. nerve
t. nerve neoplasm
t. notch
t. process
trochleocapitellar groove
troika
aponeurotic t.
Troisier
T. node
T. sign
troland
Trolard
vein of T.
trolley-track sign
Trömner sign
TRON 3 VACI cardiac imaging system
Tronzo
T. classification of intertrochanteric fractures
T. intertrochanteric fracture classification
trophedema
trophic
t. fracture
t. lesion
trophoblastic material
tropical
t. pancreatitis
t. sprue
t. ulcer osteoma
tropic ulcer
tropism
facet t.
tropolone
tropomyosin
trough
t. line
t. sign
t. of venous pulse
X t.
Y t.
Trousseau
T. sign
T. syndrome
TRP
trichorhinophalangeal
true
t. aortic aneurysm
t. back muscle
t. channel
t. conjugate measurement
t. dynamic joint imaging
t. event
t. heart aneurysm

NOTES

true *(continued)*
t. hermaphroditism
t. histiocytic lymphoma
t. intersex
t. lateral view
t. lumen
t. metatarsus adductus (TMA)
t. mitral stenosis
t. negative (TN)
t. pelvis
t. porencephaly
t. positive (TP)
t. precocious puberty
t. rib
t. umbilical cord knot
t. ventricular aneurysm
t. vertebra
t. vocal cord
Trümmerfeld zone
trumpet
t. bone
t. nerve root sign
trumpet-like pelvocaliceal system
truncal
t. artery
t. instability
t. obesity
t. renal artery stenosis
t. rhabdomyosarcoma
t. valve
truncated
t. arch index
t. atrial appendage
t. NMR probe
truncation
t. band artifact
t. phenomenon
truncus arteriosus
trunk
aortopulmonary t.
arterial brachiocephalic t.
atrioventricular t.
bifurcation of t.
brachiocephalic t.
bronchomediastinal lymph t.
celiac t.
cordlike t.
costocervical t.
dilated pulmonary t.
joints of t.
lumbosacral t.
lymphatic t.
meningohypophyseal t.
nerve t.
posterior vagal t.
pulmonary t.
sinus of pulmonary t.
thyrocervical t.
tibioperoneal t.
twin t.
vagal t.
Trunkey
T. fracture classification
T. fracture classification system
TRUS
transrectal ultrasound
Tru-Scint imaging agent
TRW
teboroxime resting washout
TS
tuberous sclerosis
TSC
T-Scan 2000
TSD
target-skin distance
TSE
turbo-spin echo
T-shaped
T.-s. fracture
T.-s. uterus
TSPP
technetium stannous pyrophosphate
TSPP imaging
TS2000 TransScan 2000
TSV
total stroke volume
TT
triple therapy
tritiated thymidine
TTC
triphenyltetrazolium chloride
T-tube cholangiogram
TTD
tissue tolerance dose
TTDF
time to distant failure
TTE
transthoracic echocardiography
TTI
tension-time index
TTL
TTLF
time to local failure
TTNAB
transthoracic needle aspiration biopsy
TTP
transtrabecular plane
TTS
tarsal tunnel syndrome
through-the-scope
TTTS
twin-to-twin transfusion syndrome
T-tube
T.-t. cholangiogram (TTC)
French T.-t.
T.-t. stent

tubal
t. canal
t. insufflation
t. mass
t. obstruction
t. occlusion
t. pregnancy
t. ring
tubarius
torus t.
tube (*See* tubing)
angled pleural t.
anode t.
apically directed chest t.
auditory t.
bilateral pleural t.
blocked shunt t.
bronchial t.
calix t.
capillary t.
cathode-ray t. (CRT)
Chaoul voltage x-ray t.
chest t.
collecting t.
corneal t.
cuffed endotracheal t.
t. current
decompression t.
t. decompression
digestive t.
Dobbhoff feeding t.
t. drainage
electron multiplier t.
endobronchial t.
endotracheal t.
eustachian t.
fallopian t.
fenestrated t.
field emission t.
Frederick-Miller t.
gastrostomy t.
Geiger-Müller t.
t. geometry module
hot cathode x-ray t.
image Orthicon t.
interstitial afterloading nylon t.
intestinal t.
J-shaped t.
large-caliber t.
Lenard ray t.
mediastinal t.
molybdenum target t.
muscular t.
nasogastric (NG) t.
nasojejunal feeding t.
nasotracheal t.
neural t.
Newvicon camera t.
obstructed shunt t.
oroendotracheal t.
orogastric t.
Orthicon t.
overcouch t.
percutaneous endoscopic gastrostomy (PEG) t.
pharyngotympanic t.
photomultiplier t. (PMT)
pickup t.
pleural t.
Plumicon camera t.
polyethylene t.
t. position rotation
rectifier t.
right-angle chest t.
rotating anode t.
separator t.
shunt t.
solid-phase extraction t.
stomach t.
straight chest t.
suction t.
Thal-Quick chest t.
tracheal t.
tracheostomy t.
triode t.
uterine t.
vacuum t.
valve t.
Vidicon camera t.
t. voltage waveform
x-ray t.
tuber
brain t.
t. cinereum
t. cinereum hamartoma
cortical t.
tubercle
accessory t.
acoustic t.
adductor t.
amygdaloid t.
articular t.
auricular t.
calcaneal t.

NOTES

tubercle *(continued)*
carotid t.
Chaput t.
conoid t.
corniculate t.
costal t.
crown t.
cuneiform t.
darwinian t.
dental t.
dissection t.
dorsal t.
epiglottic t.
fibrous t.
genial t.
Gerdy t.
Ghon t.
greater t.
iliac t.
intercondylar t.
jugular t.
lesser t.
Lister t.
Lower t.
t. of Morgagni
noncaseating t.
Parsons t.
prominent t.
pubic t.
t. of rib
rib t.
Rolando t.
scalene t.
sella turcica t.
supraglenoid t.
tibial t.
ulnar t.
tuberculoma
brain t.
intracranial t.
lung t.
tuberculosis (TB)
acinar t.
adrenal t.
airways t.
anorectal t.
anthrocotic t.
atypical t.
basal t.
bone t.
cavitary t.
cestodic t.
covitary t.
cystic t.
Delmege sign of t.
disseminated t.
endobronchial t.
extrapulmonary t.
exudative t.
fibroproductive t.
fulminant t.
genitourinary t.
GI tract t.
t. granulation tissue
GU tract t.
hematogenous t.
inhalation t.
meningeal t.
miliary t.
miliary pulmonary t.
multidrug-resistant t.
Mycobacterium t.
open t.
postprimary pulmonary t.
primary pulmonary t.
progressive primary t.
pulmonary t.
reactivation t.
recrudescent t.
renal t.
Schick sign of t.
spinal t.
stable-state t.
tuberculous
t. arthritis
t. bone
t. bronchiectasis
t. bronchopneumonia
t. cystitis
t. effusion
t. empyema
t. granuloma
t. infiltrate
t. lesion
t. mediastinal adenopathy
t. nodule
t. osteomyelitis
t. peritonitis
t. pneumonia
t. pneumothorax
t. salpingitis
t. spondylitis
t. tenosynovitis
tuberculum
t. sella
t. sellae meningioma
tuberohypophysial tract
tuberosity
bicipital t.
calcaneal t.
coracoid t.
costal t.
deltoid t.
femoral t.
greater t.
iliac t.

infraglenoid t.
ischial t.
lesser t.
navicular t.
omental t.
radial t.
tibial t.
ulnar t.
unguicular t.

tuberous sclerosis (TS)

tubing
dialysis t.
shunt t.

tuboabdominal pregnancy

tubogram
T t.

tuboligamentary pregnancy

tuboovarian
t. abscess
t. pregnancy

tuboplasty
balloon t.
transcervical balloon t. (TBT)

tuboreticular structure

tubotympanic canal

tubouterine pregnancy

tubular
t. aneurysm
t. aortic hypoplasia
t. bone
t. breast carcinoma
t. bronchiectasis
t. cancer
t. cavity
t. dysgenesis
t. ectasia
t. ectasia of rete testis
t. fertility index
t. function
t. gas pattern
t. kidney secretion
t. lesion
t. lung density
t. magnet
t. necrosis
t. nephrogram
t. polyp
t. stenosis
t. structure
t. transit
t. ventricle
t. wire mesh

tubule
collecting t.
connecting t.
convoluted t.
dental t.
dentinal t.
discharging t.
distal convoluted t.
proximal convoluted t.
renal t.
seminiferous t.
straight t.
tortuous t.

tubulointerstitial nephritis

tubulovillous
t. colon adenoma
t. polyp

Tuffier inferior ligament

tuft
finger resorption of terminal t.
t. fracture
osteolysis t.
osteosclerosis t.
penciling of terminal t.
resorption of terminal t.
silk t.
terminal t.
ungual t.
vascular t.

tularemic pneumonia

tulip
t. bulb aorta
t. sheath

tumefactive
t. biliary sludge
t. multiple sclerosis
t. sludge

tumor
abdominal wall desmoid t.
Abrikosov t.
acidophilic pituitary t.
acinic cell t.
acoustic nerve sheath t.
ACTH-producing t.
acute splenic t.
adenoid t.
adenomatoid odontogenic t.
adipose t.
adrenal t.
adrenocortical rest cell t.
amelanotic t.
ameloblastic adenomatoid t.

NOTES

tumor *(continued)*
ampulla t.
amyloid t.
androgen-producing t.
angiomatoid t.
aortic body t.
apple-core t.
astrocytic t.
astroglial t.
Azzopardi t.
ball-valve t.
basiocciput t.
B-cell t.
t. bed
Bednar t.
benign congential Wilms t.
benign duodenal t.
benign fibrous bone t.
benign lung t.
benign lymphoepithelial parotid t.
benign ovarian t.
benign small bowel t.
benign teratoid mediastinum t.
benign urethral t.
bladder t.
t. blood supply
blood vessel t.
t. blush
t. blush on angiography
bone t.
bone-forming bone t.
t. boundary
brain t.
Braun t.
breast phyllode t.
Brenner t.
bright-signal-intensity t.
bronchial carcinoid t.
Brooke t.
brown t.
bulky t.
t. burden
burned-out t.
Buschke-Löwenstein t.
t. capillary permeability
t. capsule
carcinoid t.
cardiac t.
carotid body t.
cartilage-containing giant cell t.
cartilage-forming bone t.
cartilaginous soft-tissue t.
cavernous t.
cell t.
t. cell-host bone relationship
cellular t.
central nervous system t.
cerebellopontine angle t.
cervical t.
chemoreceptor t.
chemoresistant t.
chondrogenic t.
chromaffin t.
t. cleavage plane
clivus meningioma t.
CNS ghost t.
CNS multifocal t.
Codman t.
collision t.
colloid cystic t.
congenital cardiac t.
connective tissue fibrous t.
cystic t.
deep t.
deep-seated t.
t. defect
t. d'emblee mycosis fungoides
Denys-Drash t.
dermal duct t.
dermoid t.
desmoid t.
desmoplastic small round-cell t. (DSRCT)
destructive t.
discrete t.
t. dormancy
drug-resistant t.
ductectatic mucinous t.
dumbbell t.
duodenum malignant t.
dysembryoplastic neuroepithelial t. (DNET)
echogenic t.
eighth nerve t.
t. embolus
embryonic t., embryonal tumor
endobronchial t.
endocrine t.
endodermal sinus ovarian t.
endodermal sinus testis t.
endometrioid t.
epidermoid t.
epithelial t.
Erdheim t.
t. erosion
esophageal t.
estrogen-producing t.
Ewing t.
t. extension
extension of t.
t. extirpation
extraaxial t.
extracompartmental t.
extradural t.
extrahepatic primary malignant t.
extramedullary t.

extratesticular t.
fatty soft tissue t.
fecal t.
feign t.
feminizing adrenal t.
fetal mesenchymal t.
fibroid t.
fibrous connective tissue t.
finger of t.
flocculonodular t.
focal t.
focus of t.
fourth ventricle t.
friable t.
frontal lobe t.
fungating t.
galeal extension of t.
ganglion cell t.
gasserian ganglion t.
gastrointestinal stromal t. (GIST)
germ-cell t. (GCT)
gestational trophoblastic t.
giant cell t.
Glazunov t.
glial brain t.
globular t.
glomus body t.
glomus jugulare t.
glomus neck t.
Godwin t.
gonadal stromal t.
granulosa-theca cell t.
Grawitz t.
gross t.
Gubler t.
heart t.
hepatic t.
high-grade t.
highly vascular t.
hilar t.
Hodgkin t.
hourglass t.
HPV16-associated t.
HPV18-associated t.
hypervascular pancreatic t.
hypodiploid t.
hypoechogenic t.
hypopharyngeal t.
hypothalamus t.
t. hypoxia
t. implant
incomplete t.
inflammatory myofibroblastic t.
infratentorial Lindau t.
infundibular t.
t. of infundibulum
inoperable brain t.
intestinal carcinoid t.
intraaxial brain t.
intracavitary extension of t.
intracerebral t.
intracompartmental t.
intracranial t.
intraductal mucin-producing t.
intradural t.
intramedullary spinal cord t.
intramural t.
intraosseous desmoid t.
intrasellar t.
intraspinal t.
intraventricular brain t.
invasive malignant sheath t.
islet pancreatic cell t.
juxtaglomerular t.
Klatskin t.
t. lethal dose (TLD)
Leydig cell t.
lipogenic t.
lipomatous t.
t. of liver scar
lobulated t.
localized pleura t.
locally invasive t.
lung t.
lymphoepithelial parotid t.
lymphoid t.
t. lysis syndrome (TLS)
main t.
malignant duodenal t.
malignant mediastinum teratoid t.
malignant ovarian germ-cell t.
malignant ovarian teratoma t.
malignant small bowel t.
t. margin
masculinizing t.
t. mass
t. matrix
mediastinal germ-cell t.
mediastinal teratoid t.
melanotic neuroectodermal t.
meningeal cell t.
mesenchymal t.
metastatic myocardial t.
metasynchronous t.

NOTES

tumor *(continued)*
microcystic pancreatic t.
mixed germ-cell t.
mucinous ovarian t.
mucosal esophageal t.
multifocal brain t.
musculoskeletal t.
napkin-ring annular t.
neck germ-cell t.
necrotic t.
t. neovascularity
t. neovasculature
nerve root t.
nerve sheath t.
neural origin bone t.
neuroectodermal t.
neurogenic t.
neuroglial t.
neuronal cell origin t.
t., node, metastasis (TNM)
nonechogenic t.
nonfunctioning islet cell t.
nonneoplastic t.
nonseminomatous germ cell t.
t. to normal brain ratio
odontogenic t.
optic complex t.
oral cavity t.
orbital childhood t.
osteoblastic t.
osteocartilaginous t.
t. osteoid
ovarian mesonephroid t.
ovary germ cell t.
Pancoast t.
pancreatic islet cell t.
papillary t.
paracardiac t.
parasellar dermoid t.
parasympathetic ganglia t.
paratesticular t.
parathyroid t.
parotid t.
pearly CNS t.
pediatric primary brain t.
pediatric solid t.
pedunculated vesical t.
periampullary duodenal t.
perineural fibroblastoma t.
peripheral neuroectodermal t.
peritoneum desmoid t.
Perlmann t.
permeative neuroectodermal t.
phantom breast t.
phantom lung t.
phyllodes t.
pilocytic t.
Pindborg t.
pineal germ-cell t.
pineal gland t.
pineal parenchymal t.
pineal region t.
pituitary t.
placenta t.
pontine angle t.
poorly circumscribed t.
poorly differentiated t.
posterior fossa t.
Pott puffy t.
pregnancy t.
primary benign liver t.
primary implanted t.
primary intracranial germ cell t.
primary malignant liver t.
primary renal t.
primitive neuroectodermal t. (PNET)
primitive neuroepithelial t.
prolapsed t.
pseudomalignant t.
pseudoorbital t.
pulmonary t.
radiation-induced peripheral nerve t.
radiosensitive t.
ranine t.
Rathke pouch t.
Recklinghausen t.
t. recurrence
refractory t.
renal t.
renin-secreting t.
t. reoxygenation
reticuloendothelial t.
retinal anlage t.
retroperitoneal t.
rhabdoid t.
round bone-cell t.
round-cell t.
Rous t.
sacral bone t.
sacrococcygeal remnant t.
sand t.
scannable t.
Schmincke t.
Schwann t.
scirrhous t.
Scully t.
secondary ovarian t.
t. seeding
seeding of t.
seminomatous t.
serous ovarian t.
Sertoli-cell testis t.
Sertoli-Leydig cell t.
Sertoli-Leydig ovarian cell t.
sessile t.

t. shrinkage
sinonasal t.
skull-base t.
small bowel benign t.
small bowel malignant t.
small unilateral adrenal t.
smooth muscle t.
solid and cystic pancreatic t.
solid ovarian t.
solitary pleura t.
sphenoid ridge t.
t. spheroid
spinal axis t.
spinal cord t.
sporadic t.
spread of t.
squamous odontogenic t.
t. stalk
stromal cell t.
subastrocytic t.
subcortical t.
subcutaneous t.
submucosal colon t.
submucosal esophageal t.
subserosal t.
subungual glomus t.
sugar t.
superior pulmonary sulcus t.
superior sulcus t.
suprasellar extension of t.
supratentorial brain t.
supratentorial primitive neuroectodermal t.
t. of surface epithelium
surface ovarian epithelium t.
sympathetic ganglia t.
synovitis t.
temporal bone t.
temporal lobe t.
tendon sheath giant cell t.
teratoid t.
testicular stromal cell t.
testis germ cell t.
tetradiploid t.
tetraploid t.
theca-cell ovarian t.
third ventricle t.
t. thrombus
tomato t.
tracheal t.
transmissible venereal t.
triton t.
turban t.
ulcerative t.
umbilical t.
urethral t.
urinary bladder t.
uroepithelial t.
vaginal t.
vanishing lung t.
t. vascularity
vascular origin bone t.
vasoactive intestinal peptide-secreting t.
ventricular t.
vertebral body bone t.
villous t.
t. volume
t. volumetry
von Hippel retina t.
Warthin t.
well-circumscribed t.
well-differentiated polycystic Wilms t.
Wharton t.
Wilms benign congenital t.
Yaba t.
yolk sac ovary t.
Zollinger-Ellison t.

tumoral
t. calcification
t. calcinosis
t. callus
t. fat
t. invasion

tumor-bearing bone
tumorectomy
tumorigenesis
mammary t.

tumorlike
t. bone lesion
t. shadow

tumor-mimicking breast lesion
tumorostatic agent
tumor-to-normal brain ratio
tungstate
calcium t.

tungsten
t. anode
t. carbide pneumoconiosis
t. eye shield
t. target

tungsten-188 (^{188}**W**)
tunica, pl. **tunicae**

NOTES

tunica *(continued)*
t. adventitia
t. albuginea
t. albuginea cyst
t. intima
t. media
t. propria
t. vaginalis
tunnel
aortic-left ventricular t.
baffled t.
carpal t.
cubital t.
fibroosseous t.
intramural t.
t. radiograph
retropancreatic t.
retroperitoneal t.
t. subaortic stenosis
subcutaneous t.
subsartorial t.
t. subvalvular aortic stenosis
tarsal t.
t. view
Tuohy aortography needle
Tuohy-Borst introducer
TUP
transumbilical plane
TUR
transurethral resection
turban tumor
turbid effusion
turbinate
t. bone
nasal t.
paradoxical middle t.
turbo
t. FLAIR imaging
t. FLASH imaging
t. FLASH sequence
t. inversion recovery sequence
t. IR sequence
t. pulse sequence
t. SE sequence
turbo-spin echo (TSE)
turbulence
turbulent
t. blood flow
t. intraluminal flow
t. signal
turcica
sella t.
Turcot syndrome
turf-toe
Turkish sabre syndrome
turn
insufficient cochlear t.
turned-up pulp deformity
Turner
T. marginal gyrus
T. sign
T. syndrome
turning-point morphology
TURP
transurethral resection of prostate
turret exostosis
turricephaly
Turyn sign
TV
tricuspid valve
TVG
time-varied gain
TVHS
transvaginal hysterosonography
TVS
transvaginal sonography
T1-weighted
T.-w. axial localizer
T.-w. coronal fat-suppressed fast spin-echo sequence
T.-w. coronal image
T.-w. coronal imaging
T.-w. FAST
T.-w. fat-suppressed image (T1FS)
T.-w. image (T1WI)
T.-w. magnetic resonance
T.-w. sagittal imaging
T.-w. spin echo
T.-w. spin-echo examination
T2-weighted
T.-w. fast spin-echo coronal oblique
T.-w. image (T2WI)
T.-w. pulse sequence
T.-w. sagittal oblique image
T.-w. scan
T.-w. spin-echo examination
T.-w. spin-echo image
T.-w. spin-echo (SE) sequence
T1WI
T1-weighted image
T2WI
T2-weighted image
twiddler's syndrome
twig
t. of artery
cutaneous t.
muscular t.
twin
conjoined t.'s
dichorionic-diamniotic t.
discordant t.
dizygotic t.
donor t.
t. ectopic pregnancy
t. embolization syndrome

fraternal t.
monochorionic-monoamniotic t.
monozygotic t.
t. peak sign
perfused t.
t. pregnancy discordant growth
stuck t.
t. trunk
vanishing t.

twin-beam CT

twining
t. line
t. recess

twinkling artifact

twin-peaked pulse

twin-reversed arterial perfusion sequence

twin-to-twin transfusion syndrome (TTTS)

twist
myocardial t.

twisted
t. ankle
t. body habitus
t. ribbonlike rib
t. small bowel ribbon appearance

two-bellied muscle

two-chamber echocardiography

two-channel phased-array RF receiver coil system

two-column injury

two-dimensional
t.-d. B-mode ultrasound
t.-d. echocardiography
t.-d. format
t.-d. Fourier transform (2DFT)
t.-d. Fourier transformation imaging
t.-d. gradient-encoded image
t.-d. mapping
t.-d. multislice
t.-d. portal image
t.-d. sequential slice
t.-d. technique
t.-d. time-of-flight (2D TOF)

two-dye method

two-frame gated imaging

two-loop ileal J pouch

two-needle technique

two-part fracture

two-phase
t.-p. computed tomographic imaging
t.-p. CT imaging
t.-p. helical computed tomography
t.-p. helical CT

two-plane
t.-p. fluorometry
t.-p. view

two-stage
t.-s. amputation
t.-s. fusion
t.-s. venous cannulation

two-step
t.-s. procedure
t.-s. technique

two-vessel
t.-v. runoff
t.-v. umbilical cord

two-view
t.-v. chest x-ray
t.-v. film-screen mammography

tylectomy

tylosis, pl. **tyloses**
t. palmaris et plantaris

tympani
tegmen t.
tensor t.

tympanic
t. bone
t. cavity
t. plexus
t. vascular membrane

tympanicum
glomus t.

tympanohyal bone

tympanosclerosis

type
t. A–C right ventricular hypertrophy
centrocyte-like t.
diffuse fibrosis t.
t. II (infracristal) ventricular septal defect
t. I (supracristal) ventricular septal defect
t. IV (muscular) ventricular septal defect
t. 1 neurofibromatosis
t. 2 neurofibromatosis
pleomorphic t.
reticular t.
sonographic hip t.
Wiberg classification of patellar t.'s

typhlitis

NOTES

T

typhoid
- t. nodule
- t. pleurisy
- t. pneumonia

typhus nodule
tyropanoate
- t. sodium
- t. sodium imaging agent

tyropanoic acid
Tyropaque imaging agent
tyrosinase
T-zone lymphoma

U
unit
uranium
U fiber
U-1100 UV-Vis spectrophotometer
U1-NA cephalometric measurement
UBM
ultrasound backscatter microscopy
UBM imaging
UC
ulcerative colitis
undifferentiated carcinoma
UCG
ultrasonic cardiogram
UCL
ulnar collateral ligament
UCLA imaging protocol
UCT
ultrasound computed tomography
UE
upper extremity
UES
upper esophageal sphincter
UFCT
ultrafast computed tomography
U-fiber damage
UGI
upper gastrointestinal
ugly foot syndrome
Uhl
U. anomaly
U. syndrome
UHMM
ultra-high magnification mammography
Uhthoff
U. phenomenon
U. sign
UIP
usual interstitial pneumonia
usual interstitial pneumonia of Liebow
UJ joint
UL
upper lobe
ulcer, ulceration
acid peptic u.
active duodenal u.
acute peptic u.
anastomotic u.
anterior wall antral u.
antral u.
aortic penetrating u.
aphthous stomach u.
apical duodenal u.
arteriolar ischemic u.
atheromatous u.
atherosclerotic aortic u.
Barrett u.
u. base
bear claw u.
benign gastric u.
bleeding u.
bulbar peptic u.
channel pyloric u.
chronic peptic u.
collar-button u.
colonic u.
u. crater
craterlike u.
Cruveilhier u.
Curling u.
Cushing u.
Cushing-Rokitansky u.
decubitus u.
u. disease
duodenal u.
esophageal u.
flask-shaped u.
focal u.
frontier u.
gastric u. (GU)
gastrointestinal u.
giant duodenal u.
giant peptic u.
greater curvature u.
healing u.
Hunner u.
hypertensive ischemic u.
indolent radiation-induced rectal u.
intestinal u.
intractable u.
ischemic u.
jejunal u.
juxtapyloric u.
kissing u.
Kocher dilatation u.
lesser curvature u.
linear u.
malignant gastric u.
marginal u.
Martorell hypertensive u.
minute bleeding u.
mucosal u.
multiple small bowel u.'s
necrotic u.
u. osteoma
patchy colonic u.
penetrating aortic u.
penetrating atherosclerotic u.
peptic u.
perforated u.

U

ulcer *(continued)*
u. perforation
phagedenic u.
postbulbar u.
postsurgical recurrent u.
prepyloric u.
punched-pout u.
punctate u.
puncture u.
pyloric channel u.
radiation-induced u.
rake u.
recurrent u.
rodent u.
Rokitansky-Cushing u.
round u.
ruptured u.
Saemisch u.
sea anemone u.
secondary u.
serpiginous u.
small bowel multiple u.
solitary rectal u.
stasis u.
stercoral u.
stomach u.
stress u.
subatheromatous u.
thorn u.
tropic u.
urinary u.
venous u.
V-shaped u.
u. with heaped-up edges
ulcerated
u. atheromatous plaque
u. carotid artery plaque
ulcerating
u. adenocarcinoma
u. granuloma of pudenda
ulceration (*var. of* ulcer)
ulcerative
u. colitis (UC)
u. jejunitis
u. jejunoileitis
u. lesion
u. lymphoma
u. tumor
ULDR
ultra-low dose rate
Ullmann line
ulna, pl. **ulnae**
capitulum ulnae
sigmoid cavity of u.
ulnar
u. abutment syndrome
u. bone
u. bursa
u. chondromalacia
u. collateral ligament (UCL)
u. deviation
u. deviation view
u. digital artery
u. drift deformity
u. extensor
u. facing of metacarpal heads
u. fracture
u. groove
u. hand
u. head
u. impaction syndrome
u. nerve entrapment
u. nerve lesion
u. notch
u. ridge
u. sesamoid bone
u. styloid
u. styloid process
u. sulcus
u. traction spurring
u. translocation of the carpus
u. tubercle
u. tuberosity
u. tunnel syndrome
u. variance
ulnaris
extensor carpi u. (ECU)
flexor carpi u.
ulnocarpal ligament
ulnolunate
u. impaction syndrome
u. impingement
u. ligament
ulnotriquetral ligament
ULP
ultra-low profile
ultimobranchial pouch
UltraCision ultrasonic knife
Ultracranio T
ultra-early thrombolytic therapy
UltraEase ultrasound pad
ultrafast
u. computed tomography (UFCT)
u. computed tomography scanner
u. CT
u. CT electron beam tomography
u. CT imaging
u. video transfer
ultrafiltration
ultra-high
u.-h. magnification
u.-h. magnification mammography (UHMM)
Ultraject pre-filled syringe
ultralong TR

ultra-low
u.-l. dose rate (ULDR)
u.-l. profile (ULP)
Ultramark
U. scanner
U. 9 scanner
U. 8 transducer
U. 4 ultrasound
UltraPACS diagnostic imaging system
ultrasmall-particle superparamagnetic iron oxide imaging agent (USPIO imaging agent)
ultrasonic
u. aortography
u. assessment
u. assessment of injury
u. atherolysis
u. attenuation
u. cardiogram (UCG)
u. cephalometry
u. guidance
u. lithotripsy
u. lithotripter cannula
u. tomographic image
u. tomographic imaging
u. wave
ultrasonically activated scalpel
ultrasonogram
ultrasonographic
u. echo
u. modeling
ultrasonographically guided injection
ultrasonography (US) (*See* ultrasound)
axillary u.
B-mode u.
carotid duplex u.
compression u.
continuous-wave (CW) Doppler u.
Doppler u.
duplex u.
endorectal u.
endoscopic u.
endovaginal u.
endovascular u.
fetal u.
gray-scale u.
intracaval endovascular u.
intracavitary prostate u.
intraductal u.
intraportal endovascular u. (IPEUS)
intravascular u.
laparoscopic contact u. (LCU)
obstetric u.
periorbital directional Doppler u.
photoacoustic u.
real-time u.
rectal endoscopic u. (REU)
transnasal endoluminal u.
transvaginal u.
ultrasonometer
QUS-2 calcaneal u.
ultrasound (US)
abdominal u.
ACM u.
automated cardiac flow measurement ultrasound
Acuson u.
ADR Ultramark 4 u.
AI 5200 diagnostic u.
Aloka linear u.
Aloka sector u.
A-mode u.
A-scan u.
Aspen digital u.
ATL real-time u.
u. augmented mammography
automated cardiac flow measurement u. (ACM ultrasound)
u. backscatter microscopy (UBM)
u. backscatter microscopy imaging
BladderManager u.
BladderScan u.
breast u.
Bruel-Kjaer u.
carotid duplex u.
color-coded duplex u.
color-coded real-time u.
color Doppler u.
color duplex u.
color power transcranial Doppler u.
u. computed tomography (UCT)
contact B-scan u.
contrast-enhanced u.
cranial u.
CT-guided u.
3D freehand u.
u. diagnosis
diagnostic u.
diagnostic range u.
Diasonics u.
diathermy u.
u. diffraction tomography
Doppler u.
duplex B-mode u.

NOTES

U

ultrasound *(continued)*
duplex carotid u.
duplex pulsed Doppler u.
u. echocardiography
EchoGen-enhanced u.
endoanal u.
endoscopic u. (EUS)
endovascular u.
FDI u.
frequency domain imaging
fetal u.
FloWire Doppler u.
freehand interventional u.
full bladder u.
gallbladder u.
gastrointestinal endoscopic u.
u. gel
graded compression u.
gray-scale u.
Hewlett-Packard u.
high-frequency Doppler (HFD) u.
high-frequency therapeutic u.
high-intensity focused u. (HIFU)
high-resolution u.
Hitachi u.
u. hyperthermia treatment
hypoechoic area of u.
u. imaging technology
immersion B-scan u.
intracaval endovascular u. (ICEUS)
intracavitary prostate u.
intracoronary u. (ICUS)
intraluminal u. (ILUS)
intrarectal u.
intravascular u. (IVUS)
Irex Exemplar u.
laparoscopic u. (LUS)
laparoscopic contact u.
laparoscopic intracorporeal u. (LICU)
level I obstetric u.
low-intensity pulsed u.
M-mode u.
u. monitoring
neonatal adrenal u.
NeuroSector u.
noninvasive u.
obstetric u.
Olympus endoscopic u.
u. pad
pancreaticobiliary u.
pelvic u.
photoacoustic u.
power Doppler u.
PowerVision u.
u. probe
pulsed Doppler u.
real-time scan u.
renal u.
RT 6800 u.
RT 3200 Advantage u.
sagittal u.
Siemens Sonoline Elegra u.
SieScape u.
Sonicator portable u.
spectral u.
Synergy u.
u. system
TCD u.
transcranial Doppler ultrasound
three-dimensional freehand u.
u. threshold
transcranial color-coded duplex u.
transcranial Doppler u. (TCD ultrasound)
u. transducer
transnasal endoluminal u.
transrectal u. (TRUS)
transthoracic u.
transverse u.
two-dimensional B-mode u.
Ultramark 4 u.
u. venography
Vingmed u.

ultrasound-guided
u.-g. nephrostomy puncture
u.-g. percutaneous cholecystostomy
u.-g. percutaneous interstitial laser ablation
u.-g. stereotactic biopsy
u.-g. transthoracic needle aspiration

UltraSTAR computer-based ultrasound reporting system

ultrastructural abnormality

ultratherm

ultraviolet
extravital u.
u. fluorescent dosimeter
intravital u.
u. ray
u. spectrophotometry
u. spectrum
u. (UV) irradiation

Ultravist imaging agent

umbilical
u. artery
u. canal
u. cord
u. cord anatomy
u. cord angiomyxoma
u. cord cyst
u. cord edema
u. cord hemangioma
u. cord hematoma
u. cord lesion
u. cord pseudocyst

u. fissure
u. granuloma
u. hernia
u. ligament
u. mass
u. ring
u. tumor
u. vein
u. vein varix
umbilicalis
annulus u.
umbilicovesical fascia
umbilicus
umbrella
Rashkind u.
UM 4 real-time sector scanner
unattached
u. fractions
unbalanced hemivertebra
unbuttoning of device
uncal
u. gyrus
u. herniation
u. herniation syndrome
uncalcified pleural plaque
uncertainty principle
unciform bone
uncinate
u. aura
u. gyrus
u. process
u. process fracture
u. process mass
u. process of pancreas
uncommitted metaphyseal lesion
uncommon pneumoconiosis
uncompensated rotary scoliosis
uncomplicated
u. myocardial infarct
u. pneumothorax
u. supraclavicular stenosis
uncontrolled bronchospasm
uncoupled spin
uncoupler
mitochondrial u.
uncovertebral
u. joint (UJ joint)
u. spur
u. spurring
uncus
arachnoid of u.
u. corporis
u. of temporal lobe
undefined lymphoma
undepressed skull fracture
undercorrection
underdetection
underdrive
u. mode
u. termination
underinflation
lung u.
u. of lung
underloading
ventricular u.
underlying tissue
underperfusion
under-scan
u.-s. method
u.-s. method projection
undersurface
u. of liver
u. of patella
underventilated lung
underventilation
undescended
u. testicle
u. testis
undifferentiated
u. carcinoma (UC)
u. liver sarcoma
u. lymphoma
u. nasopharyngeal carcinoma
u. non-Hodgkin lymphoma
undisplaced fracture
undiversion
Undritz anomaly
undulant impulse
undulating
u. contour
u. course
unenhanced
u. magnetic resonance imaging scan
u. MR imaging
unequal pulmonary blood flow
uneventful recovery
uneven ventilation
unfused physis
ungual
u. fibroma
u. tuft
unguicular tuberosity

U

NOTES

unicaliceal kidney
unicameral
u. bone cyst
u. brain
unicentric angiofollicular lymph node hyperplasia
unicollis
unicommissural aortic valve
unicompartmental knee prosthesis
unicondylar fracture
unicornis
u. unicollis uterus
uterus u.
unicornuate uterus
unicoronal synostosis
unicortical screw
unicuspid
u. aortic valve stenosis
u. with aortic valve
unicusp with central raphe
unidirectional block
unidurectional lead configuration
unifascicular block
unifocal
unifocalization
uniform
u. attenuation coefficient
u. distribution
u. loading
u. sensitivity
u. TR (repetition time) excitation
u. uptake
uniformity
differential u.
extrinsic field u.
field u.
intrinsic field u.
scintillation camera field u.
SPECT u.
unigravida
unilateral
u. adrenal mass
u. bronchogram
u. carotid stenosis
u. consolidation
u. diaphragmatic elevation
u. fetal chest mass
u. flow restriction
u. fracture
u. fragmentation
u. hallux valgus
u. hydrocephalus
u. hyperlucent lung
u. hypertrophy
u. interfacetal dislocation
u. intrafacetal dislocation
u. kidney mass
u. large smooth kidney
u. lesion
u. lobar emphysema
u. locked facet injury
u. lung perfusion
u. megalencephaly
u. occlusion
u. overinflation
u. pleural effusion
u. pulmonary agenesis
u. pulmonary edema
u. Raynaud phenomenon
u. salpingo-oophorectomy (USO)
u. small kidney
unilobular cirrhosis
unilocular
u. cyst
u. cystic lesion
u. well-demarcated bone defect expansile lesion
unimalleolar fracture
uninfected infarct
uninhibited bladder
union
bony u.
delayed fracture u.
faulty u.
fibrous u.
u. of fracture fragments
osseous u.
secondary u.
solid bony u.
unipapillary kidney
unipara
unipennate muscle
uniphasic
u. contrast medium
u. imaging agent
unipolar pacing mode
unit (U)
adapted standard mammography u.
Ångström u.
atomic mass u. (amu)
Bart abdominoperipheral angiography u.
BICAP u.
British thermal u. (BTU)
burst-forming u.
C-arm portable x-ray u.
CT u.
electromagnetic u. (emu)
EMI u.
gamma u.
gray u.
heat u. (H.U.)
Hewlett-Packard ultrasound u.
Holzknecht u. (H)
Hounsfield u. (HU)

Hounsfield calcium density measurement u.
intensive care u.
intensive therapy u. (ITU)
International Commission on Radiological U.'s
Kienböck u. (X)
Leksell gamma u.
linear accelerator u.
Mammotest u.
molecular recognition u. (MRU)
monitor u.
musculotendinous u.
Odelca camera u.
Optiplanimat automated u.
Orbix x-ray u.
ostiomeatal u.
radiation effect u. (reu)
u. of radioactivity
reflectometer tuning u.
roentgen u.
rutherford u.
Sheffield gamma u.
Siemens Somatom nonhelical u.
stepdown u.
terminal ductal lobular u. (TDLU)
Thayer-Doisy u.
ThromboScan molecular recognition u.
video display u. (VDU)
u. of wavelength
Wood u.

uniting canal
UniTone
univentricular heart
universalis
calcinosis u.
University
U. of Florida linear accelerator
U. of Florida staging system
Unix/X11 workstation
unknown
u. primary
u. primary site
unleveling
pelvic u.
unmitigated
unmodulated radiofrequency current
unmyelinated nerve fiber
unneurulated neural placode
unopacified
unopposed image
unossified cartilage
unpaired
u. parietal branch
u. visceral branch
unplicated sheath
unraveling
digital u.
unresectable
u. colorectal cancer
u. lesion
unresolved pneumonia
unroofed coronary sinus syndrome
unroofing of nerve
unruptured follicle
unsegmented vertebral bar
unsharp masking
unsharpness
absorption u.
u. of the costophrenic angles
geometric u.
motion u.
system u.
unshunted hydrocephalus
unstable
u. bladder
u. fracture
u. joint
u. lesion
unsuppressed
u. examination
u. imaging
untethered
untransformed nadir
ununited fracture
unused colon
unusual
u. interstitial pneumonitis
u. marrow distribution
unwinding of aorta
unwrapping
Dixon method of phase u.
up
tented u.
UP7 film
uPACS picture archiving system
updraft therapy
upgated technique
uphill varix
UPJ
ureteropelvic junction
upper
u. aerodigestive tract

NOTES

upper *(continued)*
u. airway obstruction
u. esophageal sphincter (UES)
u. extremity (UE)
u. gastrointestinal (UGI)
u. gastrointestinal endoscopy
u. gastrointestinal hemorrhage
u. gastrointestinal series
u. gastrointestinal (UGI) tract
u. GI with small bowel followthrough
u. jaw bone
u. limb-cardiac syndrome
u. limits of normal
u. lobe (UL)
u. lobe vein prominence
u. lung disease
u. lung field
u. mantle radiation therapy
u. moiety ureter
u. motor neuron
u. motor neuron lesion
u. motor neuron sign
u. outer quadrant
u. pole
u. pole collecting system
u. pole moiety
u. pole of ureter
u. pulmonary lobe atelectasis
u. rate interval
u. respiratory tract disease
u. sternal border
u. thoracic esophagus
u. thoracic spine fracture

upregulation
radiation-induced u.

upright
u. chest film
u. position
u. postvoid view

UPSC
uterine papillary serous carcinoma

upscanning

upset stomach

Upshaw-Schulman syndrome

upside-down stomach

upstairs-downstairs heart

upstream blood

upstroke
carotid pulse u.
u. phase of cardiac action potential
weak carotid u.

uptake
absence of u.
bilateral diffuse increased u.
u. in bone marrow
cell preparation bone marrow u.
contrast u.
decreased thyroid radiotracer u.
diffuse lung u.
dye u.
u. and excretion
^{18}F u.
^{18}F 2-deoxyglucose u.
FDG u.
fluorescein u.
focal u.
gallium u.
heterogeneous u.
increased isotope u.
increased thyroid u.
increased tracer u.
intense u.
isotope u.
localized u.
long segmental diaphyseal u.
mediastinal u.
metabolic tracer u.
mottled hepatic u.
mottled liver u.
myocardial u.
^{13}N ammonia u.
normal variant of Ga-67 u.
observed maximal u.
predicted maximal u.
progressive u.
prominent u.
radioiodine u.
radioisotope u.
u. of radionuclide
radiopharmaceutical u.
radiotracer u.
RAI u.
regional tracer u.
u. and retention
T4 u.
^{99m}Tc MDP u.
technetium-99m MDP uptake
thyroid radioiodine u.
tracer u.
u. of tracer
uniform u.

uptilted cardiac apex

upward
u. and backward dislocation
u. lens dislocation
u. retraction

urachal
u. abnormality
u. anomaly
u. carcinoma
u. cyst
u. diverticulum
u. GI tract sign
u. ligament
u. sinus

urachus
patent u.
uracil
uranium (U)
^{235}u., u.-235
u. imaging agent
urate nephropathy
uremia
acquired cystic disease of u.
uremic
u. amaurosis
u. pneumonitis
ureter
atonic u.
beaded u.
u. Bergman sign
u. catheter coiling sign
champagne glass u.
circumcaval u.
cobra-head u.
u. cobra head
corkscrew u.
curlicue u.
u. deviation
dilatation of u.
dilated u.
ectopic u.
extravesical infrasphincteric ectopic u.
u. goblet sign
hockey-stick appearance of the u.'s
hood-shaped u.
intestinal u.
intramural portion of distal u.
intravesical u.
J-hook deformity of distal u.
J-shaped u.
kinked u.
lower moiety u.
lower pole u.
moderately dilated u.
notching u.
orthotopic u.
pipestem u.
postcaval u.
retrocaval u.
retroiliac u.
rigid u.
saddle peristalsis u.
sawtooth u.
seesaw peristalsis u.
spring onion u.
straight u.
tortuosity of u.
upper moiety u.
upper pole of u.
ureteral
u. achalasia
u. adenomyosis
u. bud
u. bud bifurcation
u. calculus
u. carcinoma
u. compression technique
u. dilatation
u. distention
u. division
u. duplication
u. endometriosis
u. filling
u. filling defect
u. fistula
u. jet
u. notching
u. occlusion
u. orifice
u. pelvis
u. perforation
u. perfusion test
u. reflux study
u. renal transplant obstruction
u. seesaw peristalsis
u. spindle
u. stasis
u. stenosis
u. stent
u. stone
u. stricture
ureterectasis
ureteric
u. pelvis
u. rim sign
ureteritis cystica
ureterocele
ectopic u.
orthotopic u.
pyoureter ectopic u.
simple u.
ureterocutaneous fistula
ureterogram
retrograde u.
ureterography
retrograde u.
ureterohydronephrosis

NOTES

U

ureterolysis
ureteroneocystostomy
ureteropelvic
u. junction (UPJ)
u. junction obstruction
ureteroperitoneal fistula
ureteropyelogram
retrograde u.
ureteropyelography
ureteropyelostomy
ureterostomy
ureteroureteral anastomosis
uretero-ureteral reflux
ureterovaginal fistula
ureterovesical
u. junction (UVJ)
u. junction obstruction
urethra
angle of inclination of u.
anterior u.
bulbous u.
cavernous u.
female u.
male u.
membranous u.
pendulous u.
penile u.
posterior u.
prostatic u.
ragged u.
spinning-top u.
urethral
u. atresia
u. crest
u. diverticulum
u. gland
u. groove
u. metallic stent
u. obstruction
u. orifice
u. papilla
u. ridge
u. straddle injury
u. stricture
u. syndrome
u. trauma
u. tumor
u. uterus
u. valve
u. warming
urethritis
urethrocystogram
urethrocystography
u. imaging
retrograde u.
voiding u.
urethrogram
normal fold u.
retrograde u. (RUG)
retrograde u. (RUG)
urethrography
urethroplasty
prostatic u.
retrograde transurethral prostatic u.
urethroscopy
urethrotomy
internal u.
urethrovaginal fistula
urethrovesical angle (UVA)
urgency
sensory u.
uric
u. acid calculus
u. acid nephropathy
urinary
u. bladder
u. bladder adenocarcinoma
u. bladder atony
u. bladder calculus
u. bladder contusion
u. bladder diverticulum
u. bladder exstrophy
u. bladder extrinsic mass
u. bladder fundus
u. bladder hemangioma
u. bladder leiomyoma
u. bladder lymphoma
u. bladder rupture
u. bladder stone
u. bladder trauma
u. bladder tumor
u. bladder wall calcification
u. bladder wall mass
u. bladder wall thickening
u. bladder within a bladder
u. blunt trauma bladder
u. conduit
u. diversion
u. excretion
u. extravasation
u. fistula
u. obstruction
u. stent
u. tract
u. tract anomaly
u. tract calculus
u. tract fibroepithelioma
u. tract gas
u. ulcer
urine
u. ascites
fission track analysis of u.
postvoid residual u.
radiopaque u.
residual u.
retained u.

urinoma
urodynamic study
uroepithelial
u. malignancy
u. tumor
urofollitropin
Urogastrone
urogenital
u. canal
u. diaphragm
u. embryology
u. malignancy
u. sinus
u. tract
u. triangle
Urografin
U. 290 imaging agent
urogram
urographic density
urography
antegrade u.
cystoscopic u.
excretory u. (EU)
u. imaging
intravenous u. (IVU)
magnetic resonance u. (MRU)
retrograde u.
urokinase imaging agent
urolithiasis
Uromiro
Uropac
uropathy
chronic obstructive u.
obstructive u.
uroradiology
Urosellectan
urothelial
u. cancer
u. striation
urothelium
Urovision
Urovist
U. Cysto imaging agent
U. Meglumine imaging agent
U. Sodium imaging agent
ursodeoxycholic acid
US
ultrasonography
ultrasound
USCI
U. PET balloon
U. probe
U. Probe balloon-on-a-wire dilatation system
USO
unilateral salpingo-oophorectomy
USPIO imaging agent
USP XX test
usual
u. interstitial pneumonia (UIP)
u. interstitial pneumonia of Liebow (UIP)
u. interstitial pneumonitis
uteri (*pl. of* uterus)
uteri
cervix u.
corpus u.
fundus u.
uteric fold
uterinae
ostium abdominale tubae u.
uterine
u. adenomyosis
u. agenesis
u. anatomy
u. anomaly
u. aplasia
u. artery
u. artery waveform
u. blood volume flow
u. canal
u. cavity
u. cervical ganglion
u. cervix
u. cervix carcinoma
u. cirsoid aneurysm
u. contraction
u. corpus carcinoma
u. didelphia
u. didelphys
u. fibroid
u. fibroid polyp
u. fundus
u. horn
u. hypoplasia
u. insufficiency
u. isthmus
u. leiomyoma
u. ligament
u. mass
u. myoma
u. papillary serous carcinoma (UPSC)
u. sarcoma metastasis

U

NOTES

uterine *(continued)*
u. size
u. synechia
u. tube
u. wry neck
utero
fetal death in u.
fetal echocardiography in u.
uteroabdominal pregnancy
uterocervical
u. canal
uterogram
uterography
uteropelvic
uteroplacental
u. circulation
u. insufficiency
uterosacral ligament
uterosalpingography
uterotubal pregnancy
uterotubography
uterovaginal
u. canal
u. plexus
uterovesical
u. fossa
u. junction
u. ligament
u. pouch
uterus, pl. **uteri**
adenocarcinoma of u.
anteflexed u.
anteverted u.
aplastic u.
u. arcuatus
bicameral u.
bicornis u.
u. bicornis
bicornuate u.
biforate u.
bilocular u.
bipartite u.
bleeding u.
body of the u.
cervix of u.
cochleate u.
cornu of u.
corpus u.
Couvelaire u.
didelphic u.
double u.
double-mouthed u.
duplex u.
enlargement of u.
fetal u.
fibroid u.
gravid u.
heart-shaped u.
horn of u.
infantile u.
isthmus of u.
large-for-dates u.
pear-shaped u.
pregnant u.
prostatic u.
pubescent u.
retroflexed u.
retroverted u.
ribbon u.
round ligament of u.
saddle-shaped u.
u. subseptus
T-shaped u.
u. unicornis
unicornis unicollis u.
unicornuate u.
urethral u.
utilization
radioiron red cell u.
utricle
large u.
utriculosaccular canal
utriculus
U-tube
U.-t. stent
UVA
urethrovesical angle
uveitis
granulomatous u.
uviofast
uviol
uviometer
uvioresistant
uviosensitive
UVJ
ureterovesical junction
uvula
u. of bladder
cerebellar u.
musculus u.
u. palatina

V
lung volume
ventricular
V pattern
V peak of jugular venous pulse
V phenomenon
V SYNC
μV
microvolt
v
volt
V5M Multiplane transducer
VA
alveolar ventilation
ventriculoatrial
va
volt-ampere
VABES
vasoablative endothelial sarcoma
Vac-Lok patient immobilization system
VACTERL
vertebral, anal, cardiac, tracheal, esophageal, renal limb
VACTERL syndrome
vacuo
hydrocephalus ex v.
vacuole
vacuolization
vacuum
v. arthrography
v. cassette system
v. cleaner sign
v. cleft
v. disk
v. disk phenomenon
v. extraction
facet joint v.
v. joint phenomenon
v. needle biopsy
v. tube
vagale
glomus v.
vagal trunk
vagatomy effect
vagi (*pl. of* vagus)
vagina, pl. **vaginae**
anterior fornix of v.
azygos artery of v.
double v.
fornix of v.
vestibule of v.
vaginae
aditus v.
vaginal
v. agenesis
v. canal
v. carcinoma
v. code irradiation
v. cuff
v. cylinder
v. cyst
v. discharge
v. endosonography
v. fistula
v. fornix
v. fundus
v. hysterectomy
v. intraepithelial neoplasm
v. ligament
v. ligament of hand
v. orifice
v. plexus
v. tampon
v. tumor
v. wall
vaginalis
portio v.
processus v.
tunica v.
vaginectomy
vaginitis emphysematosa
vaginogram
v. imaging
vaginography
barium v.
vaginoperineoplasty
vagus, pl. **vagi**
v. nerve
Valdini method
valence
v. bond
v. electron
electron v.
ionic polar v.
valga
coxa v.
valgum
genu v.
valgus
adolescent hallux v.
v. angulation
bilateral hallux v.
v. carrying angle
congenital convex pes v.
cubitus v.
v. deviation
digitus v.
v. foot
hallux v. (HV)
v. heel

valgus *(continued)*
v. heel deformity
hindfoot v.
v. index
metatarsus v.
pes malleus v.
v. stress
talipes v.
v. tilt
unilateral hallux v.
valgus-external rotation injury
vallecula, pl. **valleculae**
v. cerebelli
vallecular
v. dysphagia
v. narrowing
valley-to-peak dose rate
Valsalva
coronary sinus of V.
V. maneuver
V. muscle
sinus of V.
valsalviana
dysphagia v.
value
attenuation v.
bright pixel v.
comparative v.
CT attenuation v.
dark pixel v.
echo-train v.
v. flip
negative predictive v.
pixel v.
positive predictive v. (PPV)
soft tissue attenuation v.
standard uptake v. (SUV)
tristimulus v.
venous blood gas v.
Valvassori method
valve
absent v.
v. annulus
anterior semilunar v.
aortic v. (AoV)
aortocoronary v.
v. area
artificial cardiac v.
atrioventricular v.
atrioventricular nodal v.
v. attenuation
ball-and-seat v.
ball-occluder v.
ball-type v.
Bauhin v.
bicommissural aortic v.
bicuspid aortic v.
bicuspid atrioventricular v.
bileaflet v.
billowing mitral v.
biological tissue v.
Bjork-Shiley heart v.
blunting of v.
Bunsen-type v.
calcified aortic v.
capillary v.
cardiac v.
caval v.
C-C heart v.
C to E amplitude of mitral v.
v. cinefluoroscopy
cleft mitral v.
v. closure
v. commissure
competent ileocecal v.
composite aortic v.
v. conduit
conduit v.
congenital absence of pulmonary v.
congenital anomaly of mitral v. (CAMV)
convexoconcave heart v.
v. of coronary sinus
coronary sinus v.
v. cusp
v. dehiscence
v. diameter
disk-type v.
doming of v.
dysplastic pulmonary v.
early opening of v.
Ebstein malformation of tricuspid v.
echodense v.
ectatic aortic v.
E-to-F slope of v.
eustachian v.
failed v.
fibroelastoma of heart v.
fishmouth configuration of mitral v.
flail mitral v.
flaplike v.
flexible cardiac v.
floppy aortic v.
floppy mitral v.
foramen ovale v.
frenulum of v.
globular v.
gradient across v.
hammocking of v.
hammock-like posterior bowing of mitral v.
heart v.
v. of Heister

hockey-stick deformity of tricuspid v.
v. of Houston
hypoplastic v.
ileocecal v.
incompetent ileocecal v.
v. leaflet
leaky v.
low-profile mitral v.
v. malformation
mechanical v.
midsystolic buckling of mitral v.
miniaturized mitral v.
mitral v.
monocusp v.
M-shaped pattern of mitral v.
mural leaflet of mitral v.
narrowed v.
native aortic v.
v. of navicular fossa
neoaortic v.
nodules of aortic v.
notching of pulmonic v.
opening of aortic v.
v. opening slope
v. outflow strut
parachute deformity of mitral v.
v. plane
v. pocket
posterior urethral v. (PUV)
premature closure of v.
premature middiastolic closure of mitral v.
preservation of native aortic v.
v. prolapse
prolapse of aortic v.
prolapsed mitral v. (PMV)
prosthetic heart v.
prosthetic mitral v.
pullback across aortic v.
pulmonary v.
pulmonic v. (PV)
pyloric v.
quadricuspid pulmonary v.
rectal v.
regurgitation of v.
v. replacement
retrograde blood flow across v.
rheumatic heart v.
v. ring
sail-like tricuspid v.
semilunar v.
shunt v.
sigmoid v.
spiral v.
spongiosa of mitral v.
Starr-Edwards v.
stenosed aortic v.
stenotic tricuspid v.
stentless porcine aortic v.
stent-mounted allograft v.
stent-mounted heterograft v.
synthetic v.
systolic anterior motion of mitral v.
thebesian v.
thickened aortic v.
v. thickening
tilting-disk v.
v. tip
tissue outflow v.
track v.
tricuspid v. (TV)
tricuspid aortic v.
trileaflet aortic v.
truncal v.
v. tube
unicommissural aortic v.
unicuspid with aortic v.
urethral v.
v. vegetation
venous v.
Vieussens v.
v. of Vieussens
v. wrapping
xenograft v.

valviform

valvoplasty, valvuloplasty

valvotome

spade-shaped v.

valvula, pl. **valvulae**

valvulae conniventes

valvular

v. aortic insufficiency
v. aortic stenosis
v. apparatus
v. atresia
v. cardiac defect
v. damage
v. disease (VD)
v. dysfunction
v. efficiency
v. heart disease
v. incompetence

NOTES

valvular *(continued)*
v. leaflet calcification
v. opening
v. orifice
v. pneumothorax
v. pulmonic stenosis
v. regurgitant lesion
v. regurgitation (VR)
v. scarring
v. sclerosis
valvuloplasty (*var. of* valvoplasty)
VAN
vein, artery, nerve
van
v. Bogaert-Canavan disease
v. Buchem syndrome
V. de Graaf generator
V. der Hoeve syndrome
V. Hoorne canal
v. Neck disease
V. Nuys Prognostic Index for DCIS
V. Rosen view
vanishing
v. bone syndrome
v. lung
v. lung syndrome
v. lung tumor
v. testes syndrome
v. twin
Vanzetti sign
vaporization
plaque v.
Vaquez disease
vara
Blount tibia v.
coxa v.
epiphyseal coxa v.
tibia v.
variability
anatomic v.
beat-to-beat v.
interpretive v.
peak flow v.
variable
v. energy
v. flip-angle excitation
v. intensity
v. projection method (VARPRO)
quantitative exercise thallium-201 v.
v. response rate
v. segment
v. tube current
v. tube potential
variable-angle uniform signal excitation (VUSE)
Varian
V. accelerator
V. Associates 11.7-T, 51-mm bore spectrometer
V. brachytherapy system
V. CT scanner
V. LINAC
V. MLC system
V. NMR spectrometer
variance
v. image
v. imaging
ulnar v.
variant
anatomic bile duct v.
v. angina pectoris
blastic v.
Dandy-Walker v.
electrocardiographic v.
fibrosarcoma v.
labral v.
normal v.
ossification v.
pancreaticobiliary function v.
variation
area/hemidiameter v.
B_O field v.
circadian v.
coefficient of v. (c.v.)
v. in density
exposure v.
field v.
normal anatomic v.
positional v.
pulse width v.
variceal
v. column
v. decompression
v. hemorrhage
v. sclerosis
v. wall
varices (*pl. of* varix)
varicocele
idiopathic v.
Varicocid
varicography
varicoid
v. carcinoma
v. esophageal cancer
varicose
v. aneurysm
v. bronchiectasis
v. vein
varicosity
variocele
v. tumor of breast
varioliform erosion
VARIS radiation oncology system
VariTone

Varivas loop graft
varix, pl. **varices**
v. of aneurysm
arterial v.
arteriovenous v.
Child classification of esophageal varices
colonic v.
Dagradi classification of esophageal varices
downhill v.
duodenal v.
esophageal v.
gastric v.
intraaxial v.
lung v.
Okuda transhepatic obliteration of varices
orbital v.
paraesophageal v.
Pugh Child grading system for bleeding esophageal varices
pulmonary v.
saphenous v.
stomach v.
sublingual v.
umbilical vein v.
uphill v.
VARPRO
variable projection method
varum
genu v.
varus
v. angle
v. angulation
cubitus v.
v. deformity
v. deviation
digitus v.
v. foot
hallux v.
v. heel
v. metatarsophalangeal angle
metatarsus v.
pes v.
rearfoot v.
v. rerotation
v. stress
v. stress laxity
subtalar v.
talipes v.
tibial v.
v. tilt
varus-valgus
v.-v. instability
v.-v. plane
VAS
vestibular aqueduct syndrome
vasa
v. deferentia
v. previa
v. recta
v. vasorum
Vascoray imaging agent
vascular
v. abdominal calcification
v. abnormality
v. access device
v. accident
v. anomaly
v. assessment
v. bed
v. blood
v. blood pool
v. blush
v. bone
v. brain occlusion
v. bud
v. bundle
v. bypass graft
v. catastrophe
v. cell adhesion molecule-1
v. channel
v. cirrhosis
v. colon ectasia
v. compartment
v. compromise
v. congestion
v. cord damage
v. disorder
v. encasement
v. esophageal compression
v. fibrous polyp
v. flask
v. flow imaging
v. goiter
v. hamartoma
v. hemangioma
v. hydraulic conductivity
v. impedance
v. insufficiency
v. insult
v. invasion

NOTES

V

vascular *(continued)*
v. jejunization
v. kidney anatomy
v. leak syndrome
v. leiomyoma
v. lesion
v. lumen
v. malformation
v. markings
v. MR contrast enhancement
v. myxoma
v. necrosis
v. network
v. obstruction
v. occlusive disease
v. origin bone tumor
v. patency
v. pedicle
v. perforation
v. phase
v. placenta space
v. plexus
v. protrusion
v. pterygoid attachment
v. redistribution
v. renal anatomy
v. reserve
v. ring
v. sarcoma
v. sclerosis
v. segmentation
v. segmentation and extraction
v. sheath
v. sling
v. space of the placenta
v. spasm
v. stent
v. structure
v. supply
v. systemic resistance
v. tissue
v. tone
v. tracheal compression
v. transformation
v. trauma
v. tuft
v. tympanic membrane
v. villous atrophy
v. wall
v. xenograft

vascularity
decreased pulmonary v.
femoral head v.
increased pulmonary v.
overcirculation v.
pulmonary v.
sunburst brain v.
tumor v.

vascularization

vasculature
cardiac v.
cerebral v.
depiction of v.
extracranial cerebral v.
increased pulmonary v.
interlobular v.
peripheral v.
pruned appearance of pulmonary v.
pulmonary v.
splanchnic v.

vasculitic
v. lesion
v. rejection

vas deferens

Vasiodone

vasoablative endothelial sarcoma (VABES)

vasoactive
v. intestinal peptide-secreting tumor

vasoactive response

vasoconstriction
hypoxic pulmonary v.
peripheral circulatory v.
peripheral cutaneous v.
pulmonary arteriolar v.
spontaneous transient v.
systemic arterial v.

vasoconstrictor response

vasodepressor
v. response
v. syndrome

vasodilating agent

vasodilation
breakthrough v.

vasodilator administration

vasodilatory
v. capacity
v. effect
v. response

vasogenic
v. edema
v. impotence

vasography

vasomotor
v. change
v. symptom

vasoocclusive angiotherapy (VAT)

vasoreactivity
cerebral v.
pulmonary v.

vasorelaxation of epicardial vessels

vasorum
aortic vasa v.
vasa v.

vasospasm
primary v.

vasospastic vessel
Vasotec
vasovagal
v. phenomenon
v. syndrome
VasoView balloon dissection system
vastus
v. intermedius
v. lateralis
v. lateralis ridge
v. medialis
v. medialis advancement (VMA)
v. medialis muscle
v. medialis obliquus (VMO)
VAT
vasoocclusive angiotherapy
ventricular activation time
video-assisted thoracoscopy
VATER
vertebral, anal, tracheal, esophageal, renal
VATER association
VATER complex
Vater
ampulla of V.
V. diverticulum
V. duct
enterogenous cyst of ampulla of V.
papilla of V.
vaterian segment
vault
cranial v.
plantar v.
rectal v.
VAX 4100 system
VBI
vertebrobasilar insufficiency
VC
vital capacity
VCB
ventricular capture beat
VCF
ventricular contractility function
VCG
vectorcardiogram
VCU, VCUG
voiding cystourethrogram
VCUG
vesicoureterogram
voiding cystourethrogram
VD
valvular disease
VDI
venous distensibility index
VDS
ventral derotating spinal
VDS implant
VDU
video display unit
VE
voluntary effort
VEA
ventricular ectopic activity
VEB
ventricular ectopic beat
vector
bulk magnetization v.
expression v.
v. loop
v. loop vectorcardiography
macroscopic magnetization v.
mean v.
mean cardiac v.
net magnetization v.
QRS v.
spin v.
T v.
vectorcardiogram (VCG)
vectorcardiography
Frank v.
frontal plane v.
v. imaging
sagittal plane v.
spatial v.
transverse plane v.
vector loop v.
vegetation
friable v.
heart valve v.
valve v.
vegetative lesion
veil
tissue v.
veiling glare
vein
absent peripheral v.
accessory cephalic v.
accessory hemiazygos v.
accessory hepatic v.
accessory saphenous v.
accessory vertebral v.
accompanying v.
adrenal v.
anal v.

NOTES

V

vein *(continued)*
anastomotic v.
aneurysmal v.
angular v.
anonymous v.
antebrachial v.
antecubital v.
anterior cardiac v.
anterior internal vertebral v. (AIVV)
anterior jugular v.
anterior terminal v. (ATV)
aplasia of deep v.
appendicular v.
aqueous v.
arciform v.
arcuate v.
arterial v.
v., artery, nerve (VAN)
ascending lumbar v.
auditory v.
auricular v.
autogenous v.
axillary v.
azygos v.
basal placenta v.
basilic v.
basivertebral v.
blind percutaneous puncture of subclavian v.
Boyd perforating v.
brachial v.
brachiocephalic v.
brain bridging v.
branches of v.
bronchial v.
bulb of v.
cannulated central v.
capacious v.
capillary v.
cardiac v.
cardinal v.
carotid v.
caudate v.
cavernous transfer of portal v.
cavernous transformation of portal v.
central v.
cephalic v.
cerebral v.
cervical v.
choroid v.
chronic insufficiency of v.
ciliary v.
circumaortic left renal v.
circumflex v.
Cockett v.
colic v.
common basal v.
common cardinal v.
common facial v.
communicating v.
companion v.
condylar emissary v.
congenital stenosis of pulmonary v.
conjunctival v.
coronary v.
cortical v.
costoaxillary v.
cutaneous v.
cystic v.
deep v.
digital v.
v. dilatation
dilated collateral v.
diploic v.
distended v.
Dodd perforating group of v.'s
dorsal penile v.
dorsispinal v.
duodenal v.
embryonal v.
embryonic umbilical v.
emissary v.
engorged v.
epigastric v.
episcleral v.
esophageal v.
ethmoidal v.
external jugular v. (EJV)
external pudendal v.
extirpation of saphenous v.
extradural vertebral plexus of v.
facial v.
familial varicose v.
feeder v.
femoral v.
fibular v.
flat neck v.
frontal v.
v. of Galen aneurysm
v. of Galen malformation
gastric v.
gastroepiploic v.
v. graft
v. graft occlusion
v. graft stenosis
v. graft thrombosis
great cardiac v.
greater saphenous v.
harvested v.
hemiazygos v.
hemispheric v.
hepatic v.
ileocolic v.
ileofemoral v.

iliac v.
iliofemoral v.
inferior mesenteric v.
inferior ophthalmic v.
inferior pulmonary v.
inferior rectal v.
inferior thyroid v.
v. inflammation
infradiaphragmatic v.
innominate v.
intercostal v.
internal cerebral v. (ICV)
internal jugular v. (IJV)
internal thoracic v.
intraforaminal v.
intussusception of v.
v. intussusception
jugular v.
Labbé v.
labial v.
leaking v.
left hepatic v. (LHV)
left pulmonary v. (LPV)
left retroaortic renal v.
lesser saphenous v.
lobe of azygos v.
marginal v.
Marshall v.
v. of Marshall
median antebrachial v.
mediastinal v.
medullary v.
meningeal v.
mesencephalic v.
mesenteric v.
middle cardiac v.
middle hepatic v. (MHV)
middle rectal v.
v. nodularity
nodularity v.
oblique v.
ophthalmic v.
orbital varix ophthalmic v.
ovarian v.
palmar cutaneous v.
pancreatic v.
parathyroid v.
paraumbilical v.
parent v.
v. patency
patency and valvular reflux of deep v.
penile v.
perforating v.
pericallosal v.
pericardiacophrenic v.
pericardial v.
v.'s of pericardium
perithyroid v.
peroneal v.
petrosal v.
pontomesencephalic v.
popliteal v.
portal v.
posterior auricular v.
posterior cardinal v.
posterior interventricular v.
posterior terminal v. (PTV)
precentral cerebellar v.
prepyloric v.
pudendal v.
pulmonary v.
pulsating v.
quadrigeminal v.
renal v.
retroaortic renal v.
v. of Retzius
Retzius v.
reversed greater saphenous v.
right hepatic v. (RHV)
right pulmonary v. (RPV)
Rosenthal basal v.
saphenous v.
sausaging of v.
v. of Schlesinger
Schlesinger v.
Schwartz test for patency of deep saphenous v.'s
scimitar v.
scrotal v.
septal v.
Servelle v.
v. sign
sludging of retinal v.
small cardiac v.
small saphenous v.
soleal v.
spermatic v.
splenic v.
v. stone
striate v.
subcardinal v.
subclavian v.
subcutaneous v.

NOTES

vein *(continued)*
subependymal v.
superficial femoral v.
superior intercostal v.
superior mesenteric v. (SMV)
superior ophthalmic v.
superior pulmonary v.
superior rectal v.
supracardinal v.
systemic v.
testicular v.
thalamic v.
thalamostriate v.
thebesian v.
thoracoepigastric v.
tibial v.
tortuous v.
transcerebral medullary v.
v. of Trolard
umbilical v.
v. valve wrapping
varicose v.
vermian v.
vertebral v.
velamentous
v. insertion
v. insertion of cord
v. placenta
velocimetry
laser Doppler v.
velocity
acoustic v.
angular v.
blood flow v.
carotid v.
closing v.
coronary blood flow v. (CBFV)
decreased closing v.
diastolic regurgitant v.
v. distribution function (F(v))
v. encoding on brain MR angiography
fiber-shortening v.
flow v.
forward v.
v. gradient
high v.
impact v.
main portal vein peak v. (MPPv)
v. mapping
maximal transaortic jet v.
mean aortic flow v.
mean posterior wall v.
mean pulmonary flow v.
midshunt peak v. (MSPv)
mitral inflow v.
muzzle v.
peak aortic flow v.
peak early diastolic filling v.
peak flow v.
peak late diastolic filling v.
peak pulmonary flow v.
peak regurgitant flow v.
peak systolic v.
peak transmitted v.
portal vein v.
v. profile
regurgitant v.
retrograde blood v.
v. waveform (VWF)
velocity-compensating gradient pulse
velocity-density imaging
velocity-encoded
v.-e. cine MR imaging
v.-e. image
v.-e. sequence
velocity-evaluation phantom
velocity-induced phase shift
velopharyngeal
v. closure
v. insufficiency
velopharynx
Velpeau
V. axillary view
V. deformity
velum
vena, pl. **venae**
v. cava
v. cava anomaly
v. cava syndrome
v. comitans
venae comitantes
venacavagram
venacavography
inferior v.
venacavotony
venae (*pl. of* vena)
venereal lymphogranuloma
venetian blind artifact
venoarterial cannulation
venobiliary fistula
venodilator
venofibrosis
venogram
venography
adrenal v.
antegrade v.
cerebral CT v.
contrast v.
conventional v.
digital free hepatic v.
epidural v.
free hepatic v.
gonadal v.
hepatic v.
iliac v.

v. imaging
intraosseous v.
isotope v.
lower limb v.
magnetic resonance v.
portal v.
radionuclear v.
radionuclide v.
selective v.
spermatic v.
splenic v.
splenic portal v.
technetium Tc99m v.
transjugular v.
transosseous v.
ultrasound v.
vertebral v.
wedged hepatic v.

venolobar syndrome

venospasm

venostasis

venosum

foramen v.

venosus

ductus v.
sinus v.

venotomy

venous

v. access device
v. aneurysm
v. angioma
v. angle
v. anomaly
v. avulsion
v. backflow
v. blood
v. blood gas value
v. brain angiography
v. brain angle
v. calcification
v. cannulation
v. capillary
v. circulation
v. decompression
v. defect
v. distensibility index (VDI)
v. distention
v. Doppler examination
v. drainage
v. edema
v. filling
v. filling time (VFT)
v. fistulogram
v. groove
v. heart
v. heart congestion
v. hemangioma
v. hemorrhage
v. hyperemia
v. hypertension
v. imaging
v. infarct
v. injection
v. insufficiency
v. interposition graft
v. intraplacental lake
v. intravasation
v. intussusception
v. junction
left subclavian central v.
v. ligament
v. motion
v. neck angle
v. network
v. obstruction
v. occlusion
v. oxygen content
v. plethysmography
v. plexus
v. pooling
v. pressure
v. refill time (VRT)
v. return
v. return time (VRT)
right subclavian central v. (RSCVP)
v. scan
v. sclerosis
v. segment
v. sheath
v. sinus
v. sinus thrombosis
v. skull lake
v. spasm
v. stasis
systemic v.
v. thromboembolic disease (VTED)
v. thromboembolization
v. thrombosis embolus
v. ulcer
v. valve
v. vascular malformation
v. ventricle

NOTES

V

venous *(continued)*
v. waveform
v. web
venovenous cannulation
vent
pulmonary arterial v.
thoracic v.
ventilation
airway pressure release v.
alveolar v. (VA)
v. defect
high minute v.
v. image
mask v.
maximal voluntary v. (MVV)
mechanical v.
minute v.
partial liquid v.
v. pneumonitis
pulmonary perfusion and v.
v. radionuclide
reduced alveolar v.
regional v.
v. scintigraphy equilibrium phase
uneven v.
volume-controlled inverse ratio v.
volume-cycled v.
ventilation-perfusion (V/Q)
v.-p. defect
v.-p. imaging
impaired v.-p.
v.-p. inequality
v.-p. lung scan
v.-p. mismatch
v.-p. ratio
v.-p. scan
ventilatory
v. capacity-demand imbalance
v. dysfunction
v. effort
v. failure
venting of heart
ventosa
spina v.
ventral
v. amygdalofugal tract
v. aorta
v. aspect
v. branch
v. bridge
v. cochlear nucleus
v. decubitus position
v. derotating spinal (VDS)
v. derotating spinal implant (VDS implant)
v. duct of Wirsung
v. epidural abscess
v. epidural fat
v. hernia
v. hernia defect
v. horn
v. mesentery
v. muscle
v. pancreas
v. pancreatic anlage
v. pancreatic bud
v. pontine infarct
v. primary ramus
v. root
v. sacrococcygeal ligament
v. sacroiliac ligament
v. spinocerebellar tract
v. spinothalamic tract
v. surface
v. venous pressure line
ventralis
funiculus v.
ventricle
absent v.
akinetic left v.
aortic vestibule of v.
apex of left v.
Arantius v.
atrialized v.
atrium of v.
augmented filling of right v.
auxiliary v.
backrush of blood into left v.
ballooned floor of v.
v. batwing appearance
batwing configuration of v.
bulb of occipital horn of lateral v.
bulb of posterior horn of lateral v.
cephalic v.
cerebral v.
colloid cyst of third v.
compensatory enlargement of v.
dilatation of v.
dilated v.
double-inlet left v.
double-inlet single v.
double-outlet both v.'s (DOBV)
double-outlet left v. (DOLV)
double-outlet right v. (DORV)
dual v.
Duncan v.
dysfunctional v.
v. effacement
effacement of v.
elongation of v.
enlargement of v.
fifth v.
floor of v.
fourth v.
fractional shortening of left v.

frontal horn of lateral v.
Galen v.
high-riding third v.
hourglass v.
hypokinetic left v.
hypoplastic heart v.
hypoplastic left v.
hypoplastic right v.
inflow tract of left v.
ipsilateral lateral v.
laryngeal v.
v. of larynx
lateral v.
left v.
loculated v.
Mary Allen Engle v.
Morgagni v.
morphologic left v.
native v.
outflow of v.
papilloma of the fourth v.
parchment right v.
partial obliteration of lateral v.
pineal v.
primitive v.
right v.
roof of v.
v. root
rudimentary v.
shift of v.
single v.
sixth v.
slit v.
Sylvius v.
temporal horn of lateral v.
terminal v.
thick-walled v.
third v.
thrusting v.
tiny v.
trigone of v.
tubular v.
venous v.
Verga v.

ventricular (V)
v. aberration
v. activation time (VAT)
v. apex
v. aqueduct
v. assist device
v. atresia
v. atrium
v. block
v. branch
v. canal
v. capture beat (VCB)
v. catheter blockage
v. cavity
v. cineangiogram
v. cleft
v. contractility function (VCF)
v. contraction pattern
v. decompensation
v. depression
v. disproportion
v. D-loop
v. drainage
v. dysfunction
v. dysplasia
v. echo
v. ectopic activity (VEA)
v. ectopic beat (VEB)
v. effective refractory period (VERP)
v. ejection fraction
v. electrical instability
v. encasement
v. end-diastolic volume
v. endomyocardial biopsy
v. enlargement
v. escape mechanism
v. failure
v. filling
v. fold
v. free wall
v. free wall rupture
v. free wall thickness
v. function curve
v. function equilibrium image
v. function parameter
v. gradient
v. horn
v. hypertrophy
v. intracerebral hemorrhage
v. inversion
v. irritability
v. isovolumic relaxation time
v. left-handedness
v. ligament
v. loop
v. mass
v. muscle necrosis
v. myocardium
v. myxoma

NOTES

ventricular *(continued)*
v. obstruction
v. outflow tract
v. outlet
v. output
v. paroxysmal tachycardia
v. perforation
v. preexcitation
v. premature beat (VPB)
v. premature complex (VPC)
v. premature contraction (VPC)
v. premature contraction couplet
v. premature depolarization (VPD)
v. pressure
v. pseudoperfusion beat
v. rate
v. repolarization
v. reserve
v. response
v. rhythm
right v.
v. right-handedness
v. segmental contraction
v. septal aneurysm
v. septal defect (VSD)
v. septal rupture
v. septal summit
v. septum (VS)
v. shift
v. size
v. space
v. span
v. standstill
v. status
v. stiffness
v. synchrony
v. system
v. systole
v. transposition
v. tumor
v. underloading
v. view
v. wall dilatation
v. wall motion
v. wall motion echocardiography
ventricularis
sacculus v.
ventricularization of pressure
ventriculoarterial
v. conduit
v. connection
ventriculoatrial (VA)
v. block
v. conduction
v. effective refractory period
v. interval
v. time-out
ventriculocele
ventriculofugal artery
ventriculogmegaly
ventriculogram
axial left anterior oblique v.
bicycle exercise radionuclide v.
biplane v.
bubble v.
cerebral v.
cine left v.
contrast v.
digital subtraction v.
dipyridamole thallium v.
exercise radionuclide v.
first-pass v.
first-pass radionuclide v.
gated blood pool v.
gated nuclear v.
gated radionuclide v.
intraoperative v.
iohexol CT v.
left v. (LVG)
left anterior oblique projection v.
metrizamide v.
radionuclide v. (RNV, RVG, RVN)
retrograde left v.
right anterior oblique position v.
single plane left v.
xenon-133 v.
ventriculography
v. catheter
ventriculoinfundibular fold
ventriculomegaly
fetal v.
teardrop v.
ventriculoradial dysplasia
ventriculotomy
map-guided partial endocardial v.
ventriculus
v. cordis
v. terminalis
ventromedial hypothalamic hamartoma
VentTrak monitoring system
venule
high endothelial v.
postcapillary v.
verae
costae v.
Verga
V. lacrimal groove
V. ventricle
vergae
cavum v.
septum cavum v.
verge
anal v.
vergence
downward v.

vermian
v. agenesis
v. medulloblastoma
v. pseudotumor
v. vein
vermicular
v. appendage
v. appendix
vermiform
v. appendix
v. process
verminous aneurysm
vermis
cerebellar v.
folium v.
hypoplasia v.
v. hypoplasia
vernal edema
Verneuil canal
vernis
vernix membrane
VERP
ventricular effective refractory period
verruciformis
verrucosus
nevus v.
verrucous
v. carcinoma
v. hemangioma
v. nevus
versive motor
vertebra, pl. **vertebrae**
accordion v.
anterior scalloping of v.
arch of v.
articular process of v.
basilar v.
block v.
body of v.
bone-within-bone v.
bony projection from v.
bullet-shaped v.
butterfly v.
caudal v.
cervical v.
coccygeal v.
codfish v.
coin-on-edge v.
coronal cleft v.
cranial v.
displaced v.
dorsal v.
facet surface of v.
false v.
fishmouth v.
fishtail v.
fractured v.
fused vertebrae
ghost v.
hamburger v.
honeycomb v.
hourglass v.
H-shaped v.
ivory v.
last normal v. (LNV)
limbus v.
Lincoln log v.
lumbar v. (L)
midbody of v.
non-rib-bearing v.
olisthetic v.
pear-shaped v.
pedicle of v.
picture frame v.
v. plana
posterior scalloping of v.
rib-bearing v.
rugger jersey v.
sacral v.
sandwich v.
saucerization of v.
scalloping of v.
subluxed v.
thoracic v.
transitional v.
transverse process of v.
true v.
wedge-shaped v.
wedging of olisthetic v.
vertebral
v., anal, cardiac, tracheal, esophageal, renal limb (VACTERL)
v., anal, tracheal, esophageal, renal (VATER)
v. angiography
v. ankylosis
v. arch
v. arch ligament ossification
v. arterial dissection
v. arteriography
v. artery
v. artery of Henry
v. artery occlusion

NOTES

V

vertebral *(continued)*
v. artery stenosis
v. artery syndrome
v. artery system
v. articular sinus
v. body
v. body alignment
v. body bone tumor
v. body collapse
v. body endplate
v. body fracture
v. body line
v. body marrow signal intensity
v. body plate
v. body retrolisthesis
v. body subchondral bone
v. border abnormality
v. canal
v. chordoma
v. collapse
v. column
v. compression fracture
v. cross-section
v. defects, (imperforate) anus, tracheoesophageal (fistula), radial and renal (dysplasia)
v. disk
v. disk interspace
v. endplate abnormality
v. epiphysis ring
v. epiphysitis
v. expansile lesion
v. foramen
v. fusion
v. groove
v. hyperostosis
v. lamina
v. osteochondrosis
v. osteomyelitis
v. plana fracture
v. process
v. rib
v. scalloping
v. segmentation anomaly
v. steal phenomenon
v. stripe
v. vein
v. venography
v. venous plexus
v. wedge compression fracture
vertebrobasilar
v. artery
v. artery syndrome
v. circulation
v. complex
v. disease
v. distribution stroke
v. insufficiency (VBI)
v. ischemia
v. occlusion
v. system
vertebrocostal
v. rib
v. triangle
v. trigone
vertebropelvic ligament
vertebrophrenic angle
vertebrospinous process
vertebrosternal rib
vertex, pl. **vertices**
V. camera
cube v.
v. presentation
vertical
v. axis
v. heart
v. long-axis slice
v. muscle
v. partial laryngectomy
v. plane
v. shear fracture
v. split nondetached tear
v. synchronization pulse (V SYNC)
v. talus
v. talus foot deformity
vertical-long
v.-l. axial image
v.-l. axial imaging
vertices (*pl. of* vertex)
verticosubmental view
VERT software
vesalian bone
vesalianum of vertebral body
Vesalius
V. bone
foramen of V.
vesical
v. distention
v. diverticulum
v. fascia
v. fistula
v. injury
v. neck
v. outlet obstruction
v. stone
v. stone formation
v. venous plexus
vesicancy
vesicant
vesicle
acoustic v.
acrosomal v.
air v.
allantoic v.
auditory v.

brain region v.
cerebral v.
cervical v.
encephalic v.
graafian v.
grape-like v.
malpighian v.
metanephric v.
pulmonary v.
seminal v.
synaptic v.

vesicosacral ligament

vesicoumbilical ligament

vesicoureteral
v. reflux (VUR)
v. scintigraphy

vesicoureterogram (VCUG)

vesicourethral
v. angle
v. canal

vesicouterine
v. ligament
v. pouch

vesicovaginal
v. fistula
v. space

vesicula

vesicular
v. block
v. bronchiolitis
v. emphysema
v. lymph node
v. pattern

vesiculography
v. imaging

vesiculosa appendix

vessel
abdominal great v.
afferent lymph v.
angiographically occult v.
anomalous v.
antegrade filling of v.'s
arcuate v.
atherectomized v.
atraumatic occlusion of v.'s
axillary v.
blood v.
brachiocephalic v.
bronchial v.
caliber of v.
v. caliber
capillary v.
cerebral blood v.
chyle v.
circumflex v.
codominant v.
collateral v.
collecting v.
commencement of v.
complex of v.'s
contralateral v.
corkscrew v.
cranial v.
cross-pelvic collateral v.
culprit v.
curved v.
v. cutoff of contrast material
deep lymph v.
v. diameter
diminutive v.
disease-free v.
displacement of brain v.
v. displacement brain infection
distal runoff v.
dominant v.
eccentric v.
efferent lymph v.
end-on v.
extracranial v.
feeding v.
femoropopliteal v.
v. filling
gastroepiploic v.
great v.'s
hairpin v.
heart and great v.'s
hilar v.
ileocolic v.
iliac v.
increased prominence of pulmonary v.'s
infrapopliteal v.
in-plane v.
intercostal v.
interlobular v.
internal pudendal v.
intimal attachment of diseased v.
intracranial v.
intradural v.
kidney v.
lenticulostriate v.
v. loop
lymphatic v.
mesenteric v.

NOTES

V

vessel *(continued)*
mesocolonic v.
minute v.'s
musculophrenic v.
native v.
nondominant v.
occipital v.
v. occlusion
origin of v.
patency of v.
patent v.
pelvic collateral v.
penile v.
perforator v.
perfusate v.
peripelvic collateral v.
peripheral v.
peroneal v.
pial v.
plump v.
pole of v.
portosystemic collateral v.
posterior lumbar v.
proximal and distal portion of v.
puff-of-smoke v.'s
pulmonary v.
radicular v.'s
reduced prominence of pulmonary v.'s
renal hilar v.
runoff v.
v. runoff
v. rupture
splanchnic v.
splenic v.
subclavian v.
superficial lymph v.
superior gluteal v.
takeoff of v.
telangiectatic v.
v. test
v. topography
tortuous v.
v. tracing
transposition of great v.'s
v. trauma
vasorelaxation of epicardial v.'s
vasospastic v.
vestigial v.
v. wall abnormality
wraparound v.

vest
halo v.

vestibular
v. apparatus
v. aqueduct
v. aqueduct syndrome (VAS)
v. canal
v. division of eighth cranial nerve
v. ganglion
v. labyrinth
v. ligament
v. schwannoma

vestibule
esophageal v.
inner ear v.
large v.
laryngeal v.
v. of larynx
v. of vagina

vestibulocerebellar tract

vestibulocochlear
v. nerve

vestibulospinal tract

vestigial
v. commissure
v. fold
v. left sinoatrial node
v. vessel

VEST system

VFT
venous filling time

VHL
von Hippel-Lindau disease

viability
myocardial tissue v.
tissue v.

viable
v. fetus
v. myocardium

vial
multidose v.
reaction v.

vibration
v. frequency
lattice v.

vibratory motion

vibrio

vicarious
v. contrast excretion
v. excretion of contrast material

Vicq
V. d'Azyr stripe
V. d'Azyr tract

Victoreen dosimeter

Vidar scanner

video
v. digital gastrointestinal radiography
v. display camera
v. display unit (VDU)
v. fluoroscopy
v. proctogram
v. radiography imaging
v. signal generator

videoangiography
  digital v.
video-assisted thoracoscopy (VAT)
videoconferencing
  teleradiology v.
videodensitometry
videodensity curve
videofluoroscopic imaging
videofluoroscopy
  spinal v.
videoradiography
videothoracoscopy
vidian
  v. artery
  v. canal
  v. nerve
vidicon
  V. camera tube
  x-ray sensitive v.
Vieussens
  annulus of V.
  V. annulus
  ansa of V.
  circle of V.
  isthmus of V.
  limbus of V.
  V. loop
  loop of V.
  V. ring
  ring of V.
  valve of V.
  V. valve
view (*See* viewing)
  abdominal v.
  afferent v.
  air-contrast v.
  Alexander v.
  amputated-foot v.
  anterior feet v.
  anteroposterior v.
  apical lordotic v.
  apical and subcostal four-chambered v.
  apical two-chamber v.
  AP inversion stress vagina v.
  AP supine portable v.
  Arcelin v.
  axial v.
  axial sesamoid v.
  axillary tail v.
  ball catcher v.
  base v.
  baseline v.
  beam's eye v. (BEV)
  Beath v.
  biplane orthogonal v.
  bird's eye v.
  Böhler v.
  Böhler calcaneal v.
  v. box
  Breuerton v.
  Broden v.
  brow-down skull v.
  brow-up skull v.
  Bucky v.
  Caldwell v.
  Caldwell occipitofrontal v.
  cardiac long axis v.
  cardiac short axis v.
  carpal tunnel v.
  Carter-Rowe v.
  caudal v.
  caudocranial v.
  cephalic tilt v.
  cerebellar v.
  cervical spine dens v.
  Chamberlain-Towne v.
  Chassard-Lapine v.
  Chausse v.
  Chaussier v.
  chest v.
  cine v.
  cineradiographic v.
  classic carpal tunnel v.
  clenched fist v.
  Cleopatra v.
  closed-mouth v.
  close-up v.
  coalition v.
  comparison v.
  coned-down v.
  contact lateral v.
  coronal v.
  coronal bending v.
  coronal reconstruction v.
  couch v.
  cranial angled v.
  craniocaudal v.
  crosstable lateral v. (CTLV)
  decubitus v.
  dens v.
  dorsiflexion v.
  dorsoplantar v.
  Dunlop-Shands v.

NOTES

V

view *(continued)*
efferent v.
Eklund v.
en face v.
equilibrium v.
erect v.
exaggerated craniocaudal v.
expiration v.
expiratory v.
extended field of v.
extension v.
external rotation v.
fan-shaped v.
FCS v.
full cervical spine view
femoral v.
Ferguson v.
fetal echocardiographic v.
field of v. (FOV)
first-pass v.
Fleckinger v.
flexion v.
flexion and extension v.'s
fluoroscopic v.
followthrough v.
four-chamber apical v.
frogleg lateral v.
frontal v.
Fuchs odontoid v.
full cervical spine v. (FCS view)
full-column v.
full-length v.
Garth v.
gated v.
Granger v.
Grashey shoulder v.
half axial v.
Hampton v.
Harris v.
Harris-Beath axial hindfoot v.
heavily penetrated v.
Heinig v.
hemiaxial v.
hepatoclavicular v.
hip-to-ankle v.
Hobb v.
Hughston v.
ice-pick v.
infrapatellar v.
inspiratory v.
v. insufficiency artifact
internal rotation v.
intraoperative v.
inversion ankle stress v.
Jones v.
Jude pelvic v.
Judet v.
knee v.
KUB v.
large field of v. (LFV)
lateral anterior drawer stress v.
lateral bending v.
lateral decubitus v.
lateral extension v.
lateral flexion v.
lateral oblique v.
lateral tilt stress ankle v.
lateromedial oblique v.
Laurin x-ray v.
Law v.
left anterior oblique (LAO) v.
limited v.
long axial oblique v.
long axis v.
long-axis parasternal v.
lordotic v.
Low-Beers v.
lumbar spine v.
magnification v.
Mayer v.
medial oblique v.
mediolateral oblique v.
Merchant v.
v. microtomography
mortise v.
MPR v.
multiplanar reformatting view
Mukherjee-Sivaya v.
multiplanar reformatting v. (MPR view)
navicular v.
Neer lateral v.
Neer transscapular v.
nonforeshortened angiographic v.
nonstanding lateral oblique v.
nonweightbearing v.
notch v.
oblique v.
occipital v.
odontoid v.
open-mouth odontoid v.
optimally positioned v.
orthogonal v.
outlet v.
overcouch v.
overhead oblique v.
Owen v.
Panorex v.
parallax v.
parasternal long-axis v.
parasternal short-axis v.
patellar skyline v.
pelvic v.
Pillar v.
plain v.
planar v.

plantar axial v.
plantarflexion stress v.
plumbline v.
portable v.
posterior skull v.
posteroanterior v.
posterooblique v.
postevacuation v.
postoperative v.
postreduction v.
postvoid v.
preliminary v.
preoperative v.
prereduction v.
prone lateral v.
push-pull ankle stress v.
push-pull hip v.
ray-sum v.
reconstruction v.
rectangular field of v.
recumbent v.
retroflexed v.
retromammary space v.
Rhese v.
rib v.
right anterior oblique v.
right lateral decubitus v.
right ventricular inflow v.
Rokus v.
rolled v.
room's eye v. (REV)
routine magnification v.
Rumstrom v.
sagittal v.
sagittal and coronal reconstruction v.
Schatzki v.
Schüller v.
scottie dog v.
scout v.
selective coronary arteriography v.
semiupright v.
serendipity v.
v. shadow projection microtomographic system
short-axis parasternal v.
single-breath v.
sitting-up v.
skijump v.
skyline v.
spider x-ray v.
spot compression v.
standing dorsoplantar v.
standing lateral v.
standing postvoid v.
standing weightbearing v.
static v.
steep left anterior oblique v.
Stenvers v.
stereoscopic v.
sternal v.
stress Broden v.
stress eversion v.
stress inversion v.
Stryker notch v.
subcostal four-chamber v.
subcostal long-axis v.
subcostal short-axis v.
submaxillary v.
submental vertex v.
subtalar v.
subxiphoid echocardiography v.
sunrise v.
sunset v.
supine full v.
suprasternal notch v.
swimmer's v.
tangential scapular v.
thoracic v.
tomographic v.
Towne v.
transaxillary lateral v.
transcranial alteral v.
transscapular v.
transverse v.
transverse/neutral v.
true lateral v.
tunnel v.
two-plane v.
ulnar deviation v.
upright postvoid v.
Van Rosen v.
Velpeau axillary v.
ventricular v.
verticosubmental v.
von Rosen v.
washout v.
Waters v.
weeping willow v.
weightbearing dorsoplantar v.
West Point v.
White leg-length v.

NOTES

view *(continued)*
whole-body imaging with magnified v.'s
x-ray v.
Y v.
Zanca v.
viewbox
virtual reality v.
viewing
cine-based v.
film-based v.
fly-through v.
group v.
PVR fly-through v.
v. wand
Viewmax software
Viewnex software
vignetting
cone of v.
vigorous achalasia
VIII nerve complex
Villaret-Mackenzie syndrome
villi (*pl. of* villus)
villoglandular polyp
villotubular adenoma
villous
v. atrophy
v. carcinoma
v. colon adenoma
v. duodenal adenoma
v. esophageal adenoma
v. frond
v. hypertrophy
v. papilloma
v. placenta
v. proliferation
v. stomach polyp
v. tumor
villus, pl. **villi**
anchoring v.
arachnoid v.
duodenal v.
fingerlike v.
floating v.
gallbladder v.
hydropic v.
intestinal v.
leaflike v.
placental v.
ridged-convoluted v.
tongue-shaped v.
vinculum
v. breve
v. longum
Vingmed
V. Sound CFM ultrasound system
V. ultrasound
violation
articular cartilage v.
VIPoma
viral esophagitis
Virchow
V. hydatid
V. law of skull growth
V. metastasis
V. perivascular space
V. plane
V. psammoma
V. sentinel node
V. thrombosis triad
Virchow-Robin
perivascular space of V.-R.
V.-R. space
V.-R. space dilatation
V.-R. space of brain
Virchow-Troisier node
virtual
v. colonoscopy
v. endoscopy
v. reality imaging
v. reality simulator
v. reality viewbox
Virtuoso portable three-dimensional imaging system
virulent atherosclerosis
viscera (*pl. of* viscus)
visceral
v. angiogram
v. angiomatosis
v. arteriography
v. artery
v. brain large migrans
v. cholesterol embolization syndrome
v. edema
v. embolus
v. heterotaxia
v. larva migrans
v. layer
v. lesion
v. lymph node
v. muscle
v. pelvic fascia
v. pericardial calcification
v. pericardium
v. peritoneum
v. pleura
v. pleurisy
v. situs solitus
v. skeleton
v. surface of liver
visceromegaly
visceroptosis
viscerum
situs inversus v.

viscid
viscosity coefficient
Viscous
PMS-Lidocaine V.
viscus, pl. **viscera**
abdominal viscera
abdominopelvic viscera
hollow viscera
hollow v.
intraabdominal viscera
intraperitoneal viscera
mediastinal viscera
pelvic viscera
perforated hollow v.
retroperitoneal viscera
ruptured hollow v.
strangulated v.
visible
v. anterior motion
v. peristalsis
VISI deformity
VISION
V. high-performance gradient system
vision
V. camera
V. MRI scanner
stereoscopic v.
V. Ten V-scan scanner
Visipaque
Vistaril
Vistec x-ray detectable sponge
visual
v. cortex
v. shimmering
visualization
breakthrough v.
delayed v.
direct v.
v. of imaging agent
inadequate v.
intraoperative x-ray v.
needle v.
optimal v.
poor v.
selective v.
suboptimal v.
visualized
suboptimally v.
vita glass
vital
v. capacity (VC)
v. sign
vitamin
v. D-dependent rickets
v. D-resistant rickets
vitelline
v. duct
v. fistula
Viterbi decoding
Vitrea
V. 3D imaging
V. 3D system
vitreitis
vitreous
v. hemorrhage
v. lymphoma
primary v.
vivo
depiction in v.
hydrolysis in v.
in v.
measurement in v.
Vladimiroff-Mikulicz amputation
VMA
vastus medialis advancement
VMO
vastus medialis obliquus
vocal
v. cord
v. cord cancer
v. cord paralysis
v. ligament
v. muscle
vocalis muscle
Vogt
V. bone free projection
V. cephalosyndactyly
VoiceRAD clinical reporting system
void
v. determination
flow v.
signal v.
voiding
v. cystogram
v. cystourethrogram (VCU, VCUG)
v. cystourethrography imaging
v. dysfunction
v. sequence
v. study
v. urethrocystography

NOTES

volar
v. angulation
v. capsule
v. carpal ligament
v. dislocation
v. intercalated segment instability
v. plate
v. rim
v. rim distal radial fracture
v. wrist
volarflexed
v. intercalated segment instability
v. intercalated segment instability deformity (VISI deformity)
volarward
Volkmann
V. canal
V. deformity
V. fracture
V. ischemic contracture
V. subluxation
volt (v)
billion electron v.'s (BEV)
electron v. (eV, ev)
Volta effect
voltage
pulse v.
volt-ampere (va)
volume
v. acquisition
adequate stroke v.
alveolar v.
amnionic fluid v.
aortic flow v.
aqueductal CSF stroke v.
articular cartilage v.
Arvidsson dimension-length method for ventricular v.
atrial emptying v.
augmented stroke v.
v. averaging
back stroke v.
blood v.
capillary blood v.
caudate v.
cavity v.
central blood v.
cerebellar v.
cerebral blood v. (CBV)
cerebrospinal fluid v.
chamber v.
circulating blood v.
circulation v.
clinical target v. (CTV)
closing v.
v. coil
decreased stroke v.
decreased tidal v.
determination of lung v.
diastolic atrial v.
diminished lung v.
Dodge area-length method for ventricular v.
v. element
end-diastolic v.
end-expiratory lung v.
endocardial v.
end-systolic v. (ESV)
end-systolic pressure/end-systolic v. (ESP/ESV)
end-systolic residual v.
epicardial v.
v. estimation
expiratory reserve v. (ERV)
extracellular fluid v.
fetal aortic flow v.
flow v.
fluid v.
forced expiratory v.
forward stroke v. (FSV)
fractional moving blood v.
gas v.
gland v.
gross tumor v. (GTV)
heart stroke v.
hippocampal v.
image v.
v. implant calculation
increased extracellular fluid v.
inspiratory reserve v. (IRV)
interstitial lung disease with increased lung v.
left atrial maximal v.
left ventricular chamber v.
left ventricular end-diastolic v.
left ventricular inflow v. (LVIV)
left ventricular maximal v.
left ventricular outflow v. (LVOV)
left ventricular stroke v.
v. loss
lung v. (V)
mean corpuscular v.
minimal v.
minute v.
v. overload
patient v.
pericardial reserve v.
ping-pong heart v.
planning target v. (PTV)
plasma v.
postvoid residual urine v.
prism method for ventricular v.
pulmonary blood v.
pyramid method for ventricular v.
quantitative amniotic fluid v.
radioactivity per v.

radionuclide stroke v.
reduced plasma v.
reduced stroke v.
regional cerebral blood v. (rCBV)
v. regulation
regurgitant stroke v. (RSV)
v. rendering
residual v. (RV)
respiratory v.
right ventricular end-diastolic v. (RVEDV)
right ventricular end-systolic v. (RVESV)
right ventricular stroke v.
scan v.
sensitive v.
Simpson rule method for ventricular v.
slice v.
stroke v. (SV)
systolic atrial v.
Teichholz equation for left ventricular v.
thermodilution stroke v.
thin cylindrical uniform field v.
thoracic gas v.
three-dimensional v.
tidal inspiratory flow v.
total stroke v. (TSV)
transit v.
tumor v.
ventricular end-diastolic v.
voxel v.

volume-controlled inverse ratio ventilation
volume-cycled ventilation
volume-rendered
v.-r. image
v.-r. imaging
volume-selective excitation
volumetric
v. analysis
v. computed tomography
v. data set
v. function
v. image
v. image data
v. imaging
v. interstitial hyperthermia
v. mapping technique
v. minimally invasive stereotaxis
v. multiplexed transmission holography
v. resampling
v. scan
volumetry
CT-aided v.
hippocampal magnetic resonance v.
tumor v.
voluming artifact
voluntary
v. effort (VE)
v. muscle
volvulus
cecal v.
colonic v.
gastric v.
mesenteroaxial v.
midgut v.
organoaxial v.
sigmoid v.
sigmoid colon v.
small bowel v.
stomach v.
Volz wrist
vomer
v. bone
vomerine canal
vomerorostral canal
vomerovaginal canal
von
v. Gierke disease
v. Hippel-Lindau disease (VHL)
v. Hippel-Lindau syndrome
v. Hippel retina tumor
v. Meyenburg complex
prefrontal bone of v. Bardeleben
v. Recklinghausen syndrome
V. Rokitansky syndrome
v. Rosen view
Voorhoeve disease
vorticity
Voshell sign
Vostal
V. classification of radial fractures
V. radial fracture classification
voxel
adjacent v.'s
v. array
cubic v.
v. element
v. gradient rendering
isotropic v.

NOTES

voxel *(continued)*
seed v.
v. size
v. volume
voxel-gradient rendering image
Voxel-Man software
VoxelView
V. software
V. system
Voxgram multiple-exposure holography
VPB
ventricular premature beat
VPC
ventricular premature complex
ventricular premature contraction
VPD
ventricular premature depolarization
V/Q
ventilation-perfusion
V/Q imaging
V/Q lung segment scan
V/Q mismatch
VR
valvular regurgitation
VRT
venous refill time
venous return time
VS
ventricular septum
VSD
ventricular septal defect
V-shaped
V.-s. fracture
V.-s. ulcer
V-sign of Naclerio
VTED
venous thromboembolic disease
VT multinuclear spectrometer
vulgaris
thermoactinomyces v.
vulva, pl. **vulvae**
epidermoid carcinoma of v.
preinvasive disease of cervix, vagina, and v.
vulvae
synechia v.
vulvar
v. adenoid cystic adenocarcinoma
v. carcinoma
v. intraepithelial neoplasm
v. malignancy
v. melanoma
vulvectomy
radical v.
vulvouterine canal
vulvovaginal carcinoma
VUR
vesicoureteral reflux
VUSE
variable-angle uniform signal excitation
V-wave pressure
VWF
velocity waveform
Doppler VWF

^{188}W
tungsten-188
w
watt
Waardenburg syndrome
Waddell sign
wafer of endocardium
Wagner line
Wagstaffe fracture
waist
w. in balloon
cardiac w.
w. of phalanx
w. of scaphoid bone
waistlike constriction
waiter's tip palsy
Walcher position
Waldenström disease
Waldeyer
W. fascia
fossa of W.
W. fossa
W. ring
W. ring lesion
W. ring lymphoma
W. space
Walker
W. carcinoma
W. carcinosarcoma
W. magnet
walking
w. pneumonia
w. saturation band
walking-stick appearance
wall
w. of aneurysm
aneurysmal w.
anterior abdominal w.
anterolateral abdominal w.
apical w.
arterial w.
axial w.
bladder w.
body w.
bowel w.
bullous edema of bladder w.
w. calcification
capillary w.
carotid w.
cavity w.
chest w.
cystic w.
fetal abdominal w.
w. filter
friable w.
full-thickness button of aortic w.
gallbladder w.
w. hypokinesis
inferior w.
inferoapical w.
intestinal w.
left anterior chest wall w.
left ventricular w. (LVW)
left ventricular free w. (LVFW)
left ventricular posterior w. (LVPW)
luminal w.
midabdominal w.
w. motion
w. motion abnormality (WMA)
w. motion score
w. motion study
multiple bull's eye lesions bowel w.
myocardial w.
nasal cavity w.
orbital w.
pelvic w.
posterior w. (PW)
posterior abdominal w.
posterior free w.
posterolateral w.
septal w.
w. shear stress
w. sign
stomach w.
thickened bladder w.
thickened gallbladder w.
w. thickening
w. thickness
thoracic w.
thoracoabdominal w.
vaginal w.
variceal w.
vascular w.
ventricular free w.
wall-echo
w.-e. shadow (WES)
w.-e. shadow (WES) triad
Wallenberg lateral medullary syndrome
wall-motion
w.-m. imaging
w.-m. score index
Wallstent biliary endoprosthesis
Walt Disney dwarfism
Walter-Murdoch wrist sign
Walther
W. fracture
W. oblique ligament
Waltman loop

wand
programmer w.
viewing w.
wandering
w. gallbladder
w. goiter
w. heart
w. kidney
w. liver
w. pneumonia
w. spleen
Wang applicator
Wang-Binford edge detector
Warburg
W. disease
W. effect
Ward triangle
warming
urethral w.
warm nodule
Wartenberg sign
Warthin
W. tumor
washboard effect
washing
endometrial jet w.'s
peritoneal w.'s
wash-in phase
washout
w. curve
delayed w.
w. gradient
w. kinetics
w. liver sign
lung w.
nitrogen w.
w. phase
w. phase ventilation scan
teboroxime resting w. (TRW)
w. view
wasp-tail deformity
Wassel classification of thumb polydactyly
wastage
pregnancy w.
wasting
cerebral salt w.
muscle fiber w.
Watanabe
W. classification of discoid meniscus
W. discoid meniscus classification
water
w. bolus
w. bottle heart configuration
w. density
w. density area
w. density line
doped w.
heavy w.
w. intoxication
intracellular w.
ion-bound w.
irrotationally bound w.
w. lily lung sign
w. on the brain
oxygen-free w.
w. path
w. perfusable tissue index
polar-bound w.
purified w.
w. range
w. retention
w. selective spin-echo imaging
w. signal on magnetic resonance imaging scan
structured w.
superbound w.
total body w. (TBW)
water-bottle heart
water-contrast
w.-c. computed tomography
w.-c. CT
waterfall
w. appearance
w. hilum
w. right hilum sign
w. stomach
water-infusion esophageal manometry catheter
waterlike signal intensity
Waters
W. position
W. projection
W. view
water-selective SE imaging sequence
watershed
w. area
w. brain infarct
w. mechanism
water-siphon test
water-soluble
w.-s. contrast enema
w.-s. contrast esophageal swallow
w.-s. contrast medium
w.-s. iodinated imaging agent
w.-s. nonionic positive imaging agent
Waterston groove
water-suppression technique
water-trap
duodenum w.-t.
w.-t. duodenum
w.-t. stomach
Watson-Jones
W.-J. classification

W.-J. classification of tibial tubercle avulsion fractures
watt (w)
wave
abdominal fluid w.
acoustic w.
aperiodic w.
circular polarization w.
constant tilt w.
continuous w. (CW)
electromagnetic w.
energy w.
w. of excitation
extracorporeal shock w.
fluid w.
longitudinal acoustic w.
peristaltic w.
pressure w.
primary peristaltic w.
pulsed w.
rapid filling w. (RFW)
reference w.
secondary w.
w. sign
sine w.
slice excitation w. (SEW)
slow filling w.
sound w.
square w.
standing w.
systolic S w.
tertiary w.
transverse acoustic w.
ultrasonic w.
waveform
apiculate w.
arterial w.
dampened w.
Doppler w.
Doppler spectral w.
flow velocity w.
gradient w.
low-resistance spectral w.
pressure w.
pulsed Doppler w.
pulse volume w.
segmental bronchus renal artery w.
sinusoidal w.
spectral w.
tardus-parvus w.
triphasic w.
tube voltage w.
uterine artery w.
velocity w. (VWF)
venous w.
wavelength (Λ)
Compton w.
de Broglie w.
energy w.
psoralen plus ultraviolet light of A w. (PUVA)
readout w.
unit of w.
wavelet
w. compression
w. encoding
w. scalar quantization (WSQ)
w. subband
w. transform
wavelet-encoded
w.-e. magnetic resonance imaging
wax phantom
waxy liver
WBC
white blood cell
indium-111 WBCs
In-111 oxine WBCs
radiolabeled WBCs
technetium-99m-labeled WBC
WBRT
whole-brain radiation therapy
weak
w. carotid upstroke
w. signal
weakened artery
weakness
respiratory muscle w.
structural w.
wear-and-tear degeneration
web
antral w.
w. contracture
duodenal w.
esophageal w.
fibrous w.
finger w.
hepatic w.
intestinal w.
laryngeal w.
lateral w.
postcricoid w.
w. space
terminal w.

W

NOTES

web *(continued)*
thumb w.
venous w.
webbed
w. finger
w. neck
w. penis
Weber
W. C fracture
circle of W.
Weber-Christian
W.-C. breast disease
W.-C. mesentery
weblike appearance
wedge
w. arteriography
w. bond
w. compression fracture
dynamic w.
w. factor
w. filter
w. flexion-compression fracture
w. hepatic venous pressure (WHVP)
w. isodose angle
matchline w.
mediastinal w.
w. pressure
w. resection
step w.
wedged hepatic venography
wedged-pair
w.-p. beam
w.-p. technique
wedge-shaped
w.-s. defect
w.-s. density
w.-s. infarct
w.-s. lesion
w.-s. lobe
w.-s. mass
w.-s. support
w.-s. vertebra
w.-s. zone
wedging
w. deformity
w. of olisthetic vertebra
w. of vertebral interspace
weeping willow view
Wegener granulomatosis
Wegner line
Wehlin method
Weibel-Palade body
weight
estimated fetal w. (EFW)
fetal w.
normal spleen w.
thymus w.
weightbearing
w. acetabular dome
w. axis
w. bone
w. dome of acetabulum
w. dorsoplantar view
w. film
w. joint
w. rotational injury
w. surface
weighted
spin density w.
w. spin-echo column
weighting
human visual sensitivity w.
Weil
W. disease
W. syndrome
Weill
W. sign
W. sign of pneumonia
Weill-Marchesani syndrome
Weinberg-Himelfarb syndrome
Weisenburg syndrome
Weiss-Baker syndrome
Weiss sign
Weitbrecht
W. cord
W. foramen
W. ligament
Welcher basal angle
Welcker method
weld
callus w.
welder's lung
Welin technique
well
w. counter
96-w. scanning fluorometer
well-circumscribed
w.-c. breast mass
w.-c. carcinoma
w.-c. lesion
w.-c. neoplasm
w.-c. tumor
well-defined
w.-d. lesion
w.-d. mass
well-demarcated scar
well-differentiated
w.-d. adenoma
w.-d. astrocytoma
w.-d. carcinoma
w.-d. polycystic Wilms tumor
well-inflated lung
well-preserved ejection fraction
well-type ionization chamber

Wenckebach
W. AV block
W. cardioptosis
W. phenomenon
Werdnig-Hoffmann disease
Werner
W. classification
W. disease
W. syndrome
Wernicke area
Wernicke-Korsakoff syndrome
Wertheim hysterectomy
WES
wall-echo shadow
West
W. Point view
zones 1–4 of W.
Westberg space
Westermark sign
"western boot" in open fracture
Western Neuroradiological Society
Westphal-Strümpell disease
Westphal zone
wet
w. bowel preparation
w. brain
w. laser imaging
w. leather sign
w. lung
w. lung disease
w. pleurisy
w. stomach
w. swallow
w. x-ray reading
wet-lung syndrome
Wetzel test
WFRT
wide-field radiation therapy
Wharton
W. duct
W. gland
W. tumor
Wheatstone bridge
wheelchair artifact
whettle bone
whiplash
w. injury
Whipple
W. operation
W. procedure
W. triad
whirlpool sign
whirl sign
whistling deformity
Whitacre spinal needle
Whitaker test
white
w. blood cell (WBC)
w. blood cell imaging
w. blood cell labeling
w. blood cell with indium-111 scintigraphy
w. cerebellum sign
w. commissure
w. commissure of spinal cord
w. echo writing
w. epidermoid
w. epithelium
W. leg-length view
w. light pattern projector
w. line
w. line of Fränkel
w. line of Simpson
w. lung
w. matter
w. matter abnormality
w. matter demyelination
w. matter disease
w. matter edema
w. matter hypodensity
w. matter infarct
w. matter lesion
w. matter shearing injury
w. matter sign
w. matter signal hyperintensity
w. matter thinning
w. metastasis
w. noise
w. noise artifact
w. pneumonia
w. point
w. star breast lesion
white-appearing blood pool
Whitehead deformity
white-lung syndrome
white-out
Whitfield test
WHO
World Health Organization
WHO classification
whole-body
w.-b. counter
w.-b. ^{29}FDG scanning

NOTES

W

whole-body *(continued)*
w.-b. imaging with magnified views
w.-b. inflammatory response
w.-b. irradiation
w.-b. PET scan
w.-b. scan imaging
w.-b. thallium imaging
w.-b. 3T MRI system scanner
w.-b. 1.5-T Siemens Vision scanner
whole-brain
w.-b. irradiation
w.-b. radiation therapy (WBRT)
w.-b. radiotherapy
whole-breast irradiation
whole-volume coil
Wholey steerable guide wire
whorl
coccygeal w.
whorled appearance
whorling
WHVP
wedge hepatic venous pressure
Wiberg
W. angle
capital epiphysis angle of W.
CE angle of W.
center-edge angle of W.
W. classification of patellar types
W. patellar types classification
Wickham-Miller nephroscope
wide
w. caliber
w. field lesion
w. rib
w. suture
w. tortuous aorta
w. window setting
wide-based, blunt-ended right-sided atrial appendage
wide-beam
w.-b. scan imaging
w.-b. scanning
wide-field radiation therapy (WFRT)
wide-latitude film
widely patent
wide-mouth sac
widened
w. anterior meningeal index
w. cardiac silhouette
w. collecting system
w. duodenal sweep
w. heart shadow
w. joint space
w. mediastinum
w. retrogastric space
w. sacroiliac joint
w. sulcus
w. superior orbital fissure
w. sweep duodenum
w. symphysis pubis
w. teardrop distance
w. thoracic outlet
widening
acute mediastinal w.
ankle mortise w.
w. of aorta
crural cistern w.
growth plate w.
infundibulum w.
interpedicular distance w.
interspinous w.
joint w.
mediastinal w.
sacroiliac joint w.
scapholunate w.
widespread metastasis
width
collimation w.
isodose w.
line w.
prevertebral w.
pulse w. (PW)
spectral w.
window w.
Wiedemann-Beckwith syndrome
Wiener
W. MRI filter
W. spectrum
Wigby-Taylor position
Wigle scale for ventricular hypertrophy
Wilcoxon signed-rank test
Wilkie syndrome
Wilkins
W. classification of radial fractures
W. radial fracture classification
Wilkinson syndrome
Williams
W. elfin facies syndrome
W. sign
W. syndrome
Williams-Beuren syndrome
Williams-Campbell syndrome
Williamson sign
Willis
antrum of W.
W. antrum
arterial circle of W.
artery of W.
circle of W.
W. pancreas
W. pouch
Willisii
chordae W.
willow fracture
Wilmad reference standard

Wilms benign congenital tumor
Wilson
W. block
W. bone disease
W. cloud chamber
W. fracture
W. muscle
W. sign
Wilson-Mikity syndrome
Wiltze angle
Wimberger
W. ring
W. sign
Winchester disk
windblown deformity
winding
Y w.
zero-pitch solenoidal w.
window
acoustic w.
acquisition w.
aortic w.
aortopulmonary w.
apical w.
biologic w.
bone w.
brain w.
w. center
cortical w.
CT bone w.
w. ductus
w. efficiency
energy w.
esophageal w.
gastric w.
w. level
localization w.
lung w.
mediastinal w.
oval w.
parasternal w.
pericardial w.
w. period
pulmonary parenchymal w.
soft tissue w.
spectral w.
subcostal w.
subdural w.
suprasternal w.
w. width
xenon energy w.
windowing
intensity w.
window/level settings
window-period phenomenon
windshield wiper sign
windsock
w. aneurysm
w. appearance
w. appearance of duodenum
w. sign
windswept
w. deformity
w. hand
windup injury
wineglass
w. appearance
w. pelvis
w. shape
wing
absent greater sphenoid w.
absent sphenoid w.
champagne glass iliac w.
greater sphenoid w.
iliac w.
sphenoid w.
w. of sphenoid bone
winged
w. configuration
w. scapula
winging
scapular w.
Winiwarter-Buerger disease
winking owl spinal sign
Winquist-Hansen
W.-H. classification of femoral fractures
W.-H. femoral fracture classification
Winslow
foramen of W.
W. ligament
W. pancreas
Winston-Lutz for LINAC-based radiosurgery
Winter-King-Moe scoliosis
Wintrich sign
Winwarter-Manteuffel-Buerger disease
wire (*See* guide wire)
w. fixation
^{192}Ir w.
iridium w.
w. localization
pacemaker w.

NOTES

W

wire *(continued)*
- sternotomy w.
- temporary atrial pacing w.

wire-fixation buckle
wire-loop lesion
wire-related defect
wiring
- intraosseous w.

Wirsung
- W. dilatation
- W. duct
- duct of W.
- ventral duct of W.

wisdom teeth
Wiseman classification
wispy connection
withdrawal pressure
within-view motion
Wits cephalometric measurement
WMA
wall motion abnormality
Wolfe
- W. breast carcinoma classification
- W. mammographic parenchymal pattern

Wolff-Chaikoff effect
wolffian
- w. cyst
- w. duct
- w. duct carcinoma
- w. ridge

Wolff law
Wolff-Parkinson-White syndrome
Wolf-Hirschhorn syndrome
Wolf Piezolith 2200 lithotripter
Wolin meniscoid lesion
Wolman xanthomatosis
womb
- w. stone

Wood
- W. lamp
- W. light
- W. unit
- W. unit index
- W. units index of resistance

wooden
- w. shoe configuration
- w. shoe sign

woody mass
wool
- w. coil
- w. tail

woolsorter's
- w. inhalation disease
- w. pneumonia

work
- left ventricular stroke w. (LVSW)
- myocardial w.
- right ventricular stroke w. (RVSW)

working
- w. diagnosis
- w. film
- W. Formulation classification
- w. sheath

workstation
- DIMAQ integrated ultrasound w.
- imaging w.
- ISG medical imaging w.
- MacSpect real-time NMR w.
- Pegasys w.
- RADstation radiology w.
- Shebele physician reporting w.
- stacked-metaphor w.
- Sun w.
- Unix/X11 w.

World Federation of Neuroradiological Societies
World Health Organization (WHO)
World Health Organization classification
worm aneurysm
wormian bone
wormy appearance
wound
- exit w.
- gunshot w. (GSW)
- high-velocity gunshot w.
- missile w.
- penetrating w.
- perforating w.
- stag w.
- surgical w.

woven bone
wrap
- aortic w.
- no frequency w.

wraparound
- w. ghosting artifact
- w. vessel

wrapped aneurysmal sac
wrapping
- valve w.
- vein valve w.

Wratten 6B filter
W ray
wrenched knee
wrestler's elbow
wrinkle artifact
wrinkled pleura
wrinkler muscle
Wrisberg
- W. cardiac ganglion
- intermediate nerve of W.
- W. ligament
- ligaments of Henry and W.

wrist
- articular disorders w.
- capholunate arthritic collapse w.
- w. capsule
- w. dislocation
- w. extensor compartment
- gymnast's w.
- w. joint
- palmar w.
- scapholunate arthritic collapse w.
- SLAC w.
- w. triquetrum bone
- volar w.
- Volz w.

wristdrop

writing
- black echo w.
- white echo w.

wryneck

W-shaped ileal pouch

WSQ
- wavelet scalar quantization

Wyburn-Mason
- W.-M. arteriovenous malformation
- W.-M. syndrome

NOTES

W

X
Kienböck unit
magnification
xanthosine
X axis
X gradient
X trough
xanthelasma
xanthoastrocytoma
pleomorphic x. (PXA)
xanthogranuloma
bone x.
juvenile x.
xanthogranulomatous
x. cholecystitis
x. pyelonephritis
xanthoma, pl. **xanthomata**
gastric x.
malignant fibrous x.
x. tuberosum simplex
xanthomatosis
cerebrotendinous x.
x. of long bone
primary familial x.
Wolman x.
xanthomatous
x. granuloma
x. pseudotumor
xanthosarcoma
xanthosine (X)
XCCL
exaggerated craniocaudal lateral
XCT
x-ray computed tomography
Xe
xenon
^{127}Xe
xenon-127
^{133}Xe
xenon-133
XeCl (xenon chloride) excimer
XeCT
xenon computed tomography
xenograft
bovine heart x.
porcine heart x.
x. valve
vascular x.
xenon (Xe)
x. computed tomography (XeCT)
x. CT measurement
x. CT scanning
x. energy window
x. imaging agent
x. trap system
x. washout study
xenon-127 (^{127}Xe)
xenon-133 (^{133}Xe)
x. SPECT imaging
x. ventriculogram
xenon-enhanced
x.-e. computed tomography
x.-e. CT
xenotransplantation
xerography
xeromammogram
chest wall lateral x.
xeromammography
xeroradiograph
xeroradiographic
x. selenium plate
x. technique
xeroradiography
x. imaging
x-height
Xillix
X. LIFE-GI fluorescence endoscopy imaging
X. LIFE-GI fluorescence endoscopy system
Ximatron
X. simulator
XIP
x-ray in plaster
xiphicostal ligament
xiphisternal joint
xiphogus
xiphoid
x. angle
x. appendix
x. bone
x. cartilage
x. ligament
x. process
x. process syndrome
xiphoidalgia
xiphopubic area
x-irradiation
XKnife stereotactic radiosurgery system
XL
inductive reactance
X-linked
XOP
x-ray out of plaster
X-Prep bowel preparation
Xpress/SW helical CT scanner
Xpress/SX helical CT scanner
XRA
x-ray arteriography

x-radiation
x-ray
x.-r. arteriography (XRA)
x.-r. attenuation
baseline chest x.-r.
batch reading of x.-r.'s
x.-r. beam
x.-r. beam size
bitewing x.-r.
characteristic x.-r.
chest x.-r. (CXR)
x.-r. computed tomography (XCT)
x.-r. crystallography
x.-r. detector
x.-r. diffraction
x.-r. diffraction analysis
x.-r. dosimetry
E sign on x.-r.
x.-r. film jacket
five-view chest x.-r.
four-view chest x.-r.
x.-r. generator
Jude pelvic x.-r.
x.-r. mammography
x.-r. out of plaster (XOP)
x.-r. in plaster (XIP)
portable x.-r.
postreduction x.-r.
prereduction x.-r.
scanning-beam digital x.-r. (SBDX)
x.-r. sensitive vidicon
x.-r. shadow projection microtomographic system
x.-r. spectrometer
x.-r. spectrum
x.-r. therapy
x.-r. tomographic microscope (XTM)
x.-r. topography
x.-r. tube
x.-r. tube housing
x.-r. tube rating chart
two-view chest x.-r.
x.-r. view
x-ray-sensitive vidicon imaging
X-terminal
XTM
x-ray tomographic microscope
X′-wave pressure
XXY syndrome
XY
X. plane
xylenol
x. orange
x. orange imaging agent
xylol pulse indicator
Xylo-Pfan
XY syndrome
xyxoid
X, Y, and Z coordinates for target lesion

Y
yttrium
^{50}Y
yttrium-50
^{90}Y
yttrium-90
Y axis
Y bone plate
Y cartilage
Y fracture
Y trough
Y view
Y winding
Yaba tumor
YAG
yttrium-aluminum-garnet
YAG laser
Yakolev
terminal zone of the Y.
Yb
ytterbium
yellow cartilage
yellow-out
Yergason test
yield
y. comparison
low y.
Y-jaws
YLF
yttrium lithium fluoride
yoke bone
yolk
y. sac
y. sac ovary tumor
y. sac (YS) diameter
yo-yo
y.-y. esophageal peristalsis
y.-y. ureteral peristalsis
Y-shaped
Y.-s. acetabulum
Y.-s. distortion
Y.-s. ligament
Y-T fracture
ytterbium (Yb)
ytterbium-169 DTPA
ytterbium-90 microsphere
yttrium (Y)
ferritin-labeled y.
y. lithium fluoride (YLF)
y. radioactive source
yttrium-50 (^{50}Y)
yttrium-90 (^{90}Y)
y. microsphere
yttrium-aluminum-garnet (YAG)
y.-a.-g. laser
yttrium-90-labeled
Yuge
oculosubcutaneous syndrome of Y.
Yunis-Varon syndrome
Y view
Y-wave pressure

Z

Z. axis
Z. band
Z. disk
Z. gradient
Z. line

Zaglas ligament

Zahn

Z. anomaly
pocket of Z.
Z. pocket

Zanca view

Zanelli position

Zang space

Z-axis

Z-dependent

Z.-d. computed tomography
Z.-d. CT

zebra

z. stripe artifact
z. stripe image

Zeek syndrome

Zeeman hamiltonian function

Zellballen

Zellweger syndrome

Zener diode

Zenker

Z. degeneration
Z. diverticulum
Z. necrosis
Z. pouch

zeolite pneumoconiosis

zero

z. filling
z. line
z. net flow
z. phase
z. time of the x-ray apparatus

zero-field splitting

zero-fill artifact

zero-pitch solenoidal winding

zeroth moment

zeugmatography

Fourier transformation z.
rotating-frame z.

Zickel

Z. fracture
Z. fracture classification
Z. fracture classification system

Ziegler syndrome

Zielke derotation level

Zieve syndrome

zig-zag stent

Zimmerman arch

Zimmer method

zinc

irradiated z.

zinc-65 (^{65}Zn)

Zinn

Z. ligament
Z. ring
tendon of Z.
Z. tendon

Zinner syndrome

Z-interpolation algorithm

zipper artifact

zirconium granuloma

ZK44012 contrast medium

Zlatkin grading system

Z-line of esophagus

Zlotsky-Ballard

Z.-B. acromioclavicular injury classification
Z.-B. classification of acromioclavicular injury

Z-Med balloon catheter

^{65}Zn

zinc-65

Zollinger-Ellison

Z.-E. syndrome
Z.-E. tumor

zona, pl. **zonae**

z. fasciculata
z. glomerulosa
z. orbicularis
z. reticularis

zonal

z. gastritis
z. prostate anatomy
z. sampling
z. uterine anatomy

zone

arrhythmogenic border z.
basal z.
bilaminar z.
border z.
clear z.
convergence z.
cross-sectional z.
detection z.
dorsal root entry z. (DREZ)
echo-free central z.
entry z.
epileptogenic z.
esophageal transition z.
focal z. (FZ)
z. focusing
fracture z.
Fraunhofer z.
high-intensity z. (HIZ)

zone *(continued)*
hypoechoic z.
hypovascular z.
z. of ischemia
ischemic z.
junctional z.
lipid z.
Looser z.'s
Looser transformation z.
lung z.
mid-lung z.
no-therapy z.
patchy z.
penumbra z.
z. phenomenon
posterior root entry z. (PREZ)
prostatic transition z.
pyramidal hemorrhagic z.
Rolando z.
root entry z.
root exit z. (REZ)
rough z.
z. of slow conduction (ZSC)
sonolucent z.
therapy z.
transformation z.
transition z.
transradiant z.
Trümmerfeld z.
wedge-shaped z.
z.'s 1–4 of West
Westphal z.
zonography
zonular space
zoster pneumonia
Z-point pressure
ZSC
zone of slow conduction
Zucker catheter
Zuckerguss
Zuckerkandl
Z. bodies
Z. convolution
Z. fascia
Z. organ
organs of Z.
zwitterion
zygapophyseal
z. articulation
z. joint
zygoma
zygomatic
z. arch
z. bone
z. process
zygomaticofacial
z. canal
z. foramen
zygomaticofrontal suture
zygomaticomalar
z. area
z. complex fracture
z. reconstruction
zygomaticomaxillary fracture
zygomaticotemporal
z. canal
z. suture
zygomaxillary
ZY plane

Appendix 1
Anatomical Illustrations

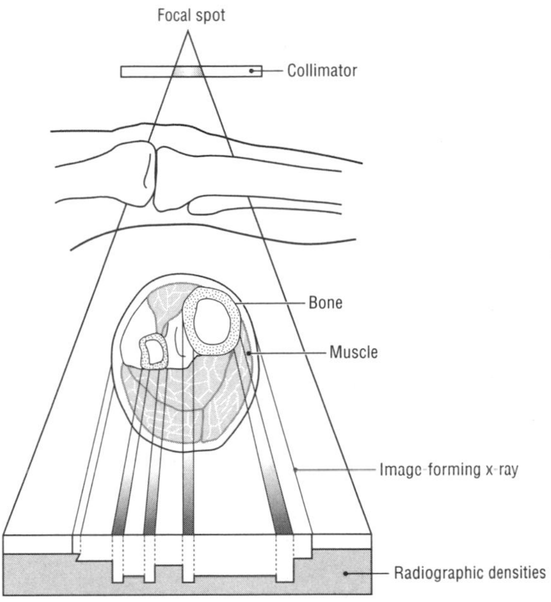

Figure 1. X-Rays pass through body part with the denser structures absorbing more x-rays, resulting in the lighter areas on the radiograph.

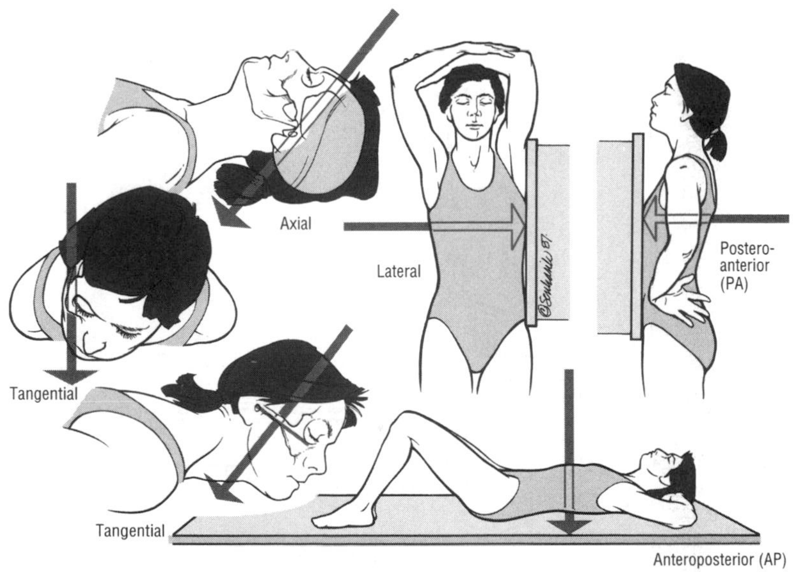

Figure 2. Radiographic projections.

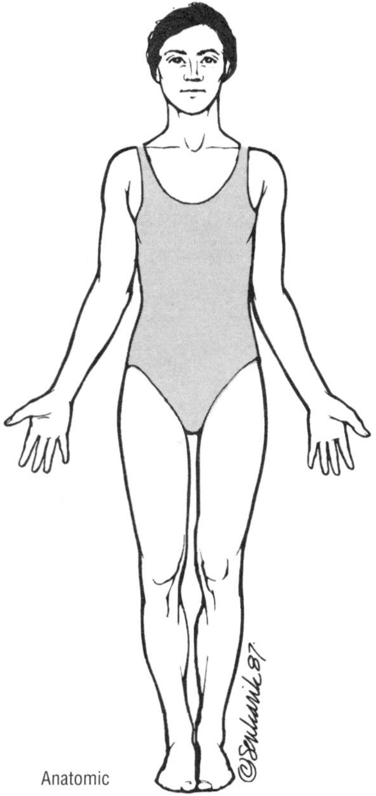

Anatomic

Figure 3. Patient positions.

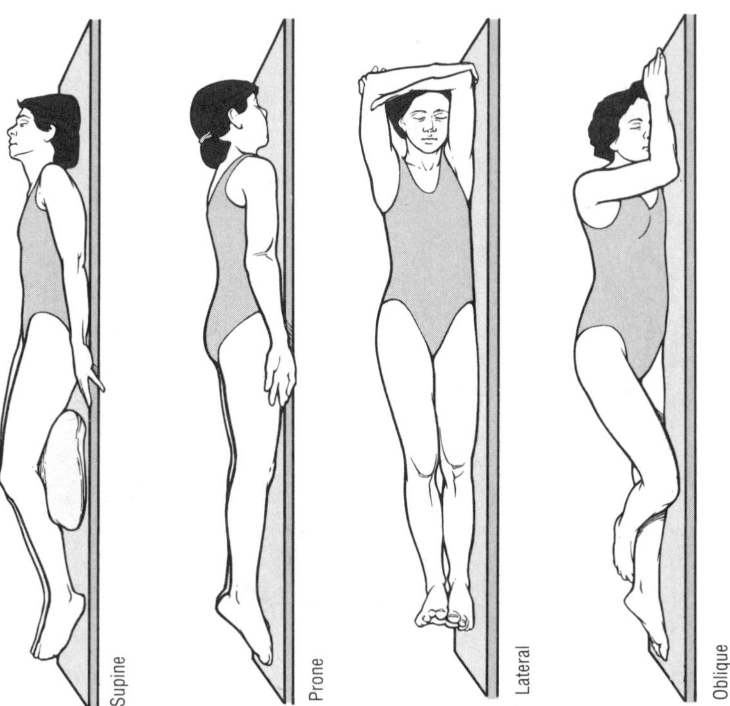

Figure 4. Patient positions.

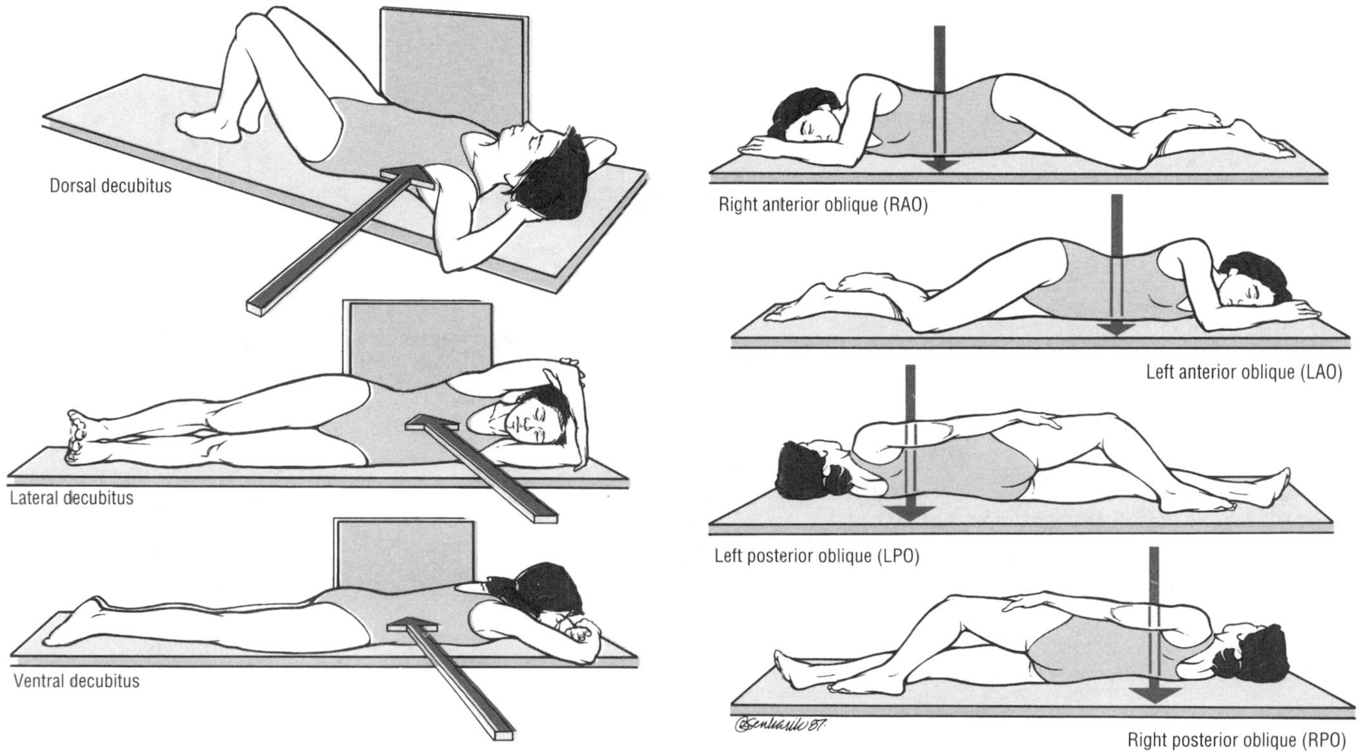

Figure 5. Patient positions.

Figure 6. Patient positions.

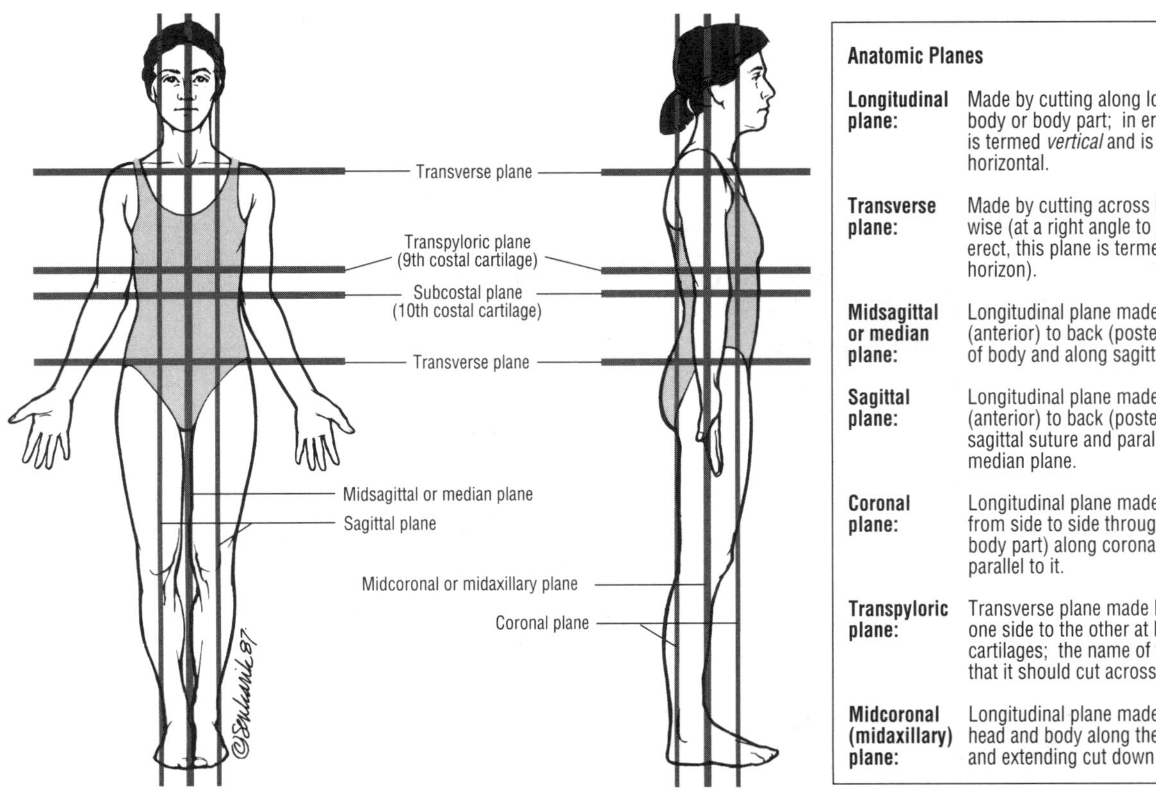

Anatomic Planes

Longitudinal plane:	Made by cutting along long (longitudinal) axis of body or body part; in erect position, this plane is termed *vertical* and is perpendicular to horizontal.
Transverse plane:	Made by cutting across body or body part cross-wise (at a right angle to long axis); if patient is erect, this plane is termed *horizontal* (parallel to horizon).
Midsagittal or median plane:	Longitudinal plane made by cutting from front (anterior) to back (posterior) along median line of body and along sagittal suture of skull.
Sagittal plane:	Longitudinal plane made by cutting from front (anterior) to back (posterior) on either side of sagittal suture and parallel to midsagittal or median plane.
Coronal plane:	Longitudinal plane made by cutting lengthwise from side to side through head and body (or body part) along coronal suture of skull or parallel to it.
Transpyloric plane:	Transverse plane made by cutting across from one side to the other at level of 9th costal cartilages; the name of this plane reflects fact that it should cut across pylorus of stomach.
Midcoronal (midaxillary) plane:	Longitudinal plane made by cutting through head and body along the coronal suture of head and extending cut down the body.

Figure 7. Terms of relationship. Anatomic planes.

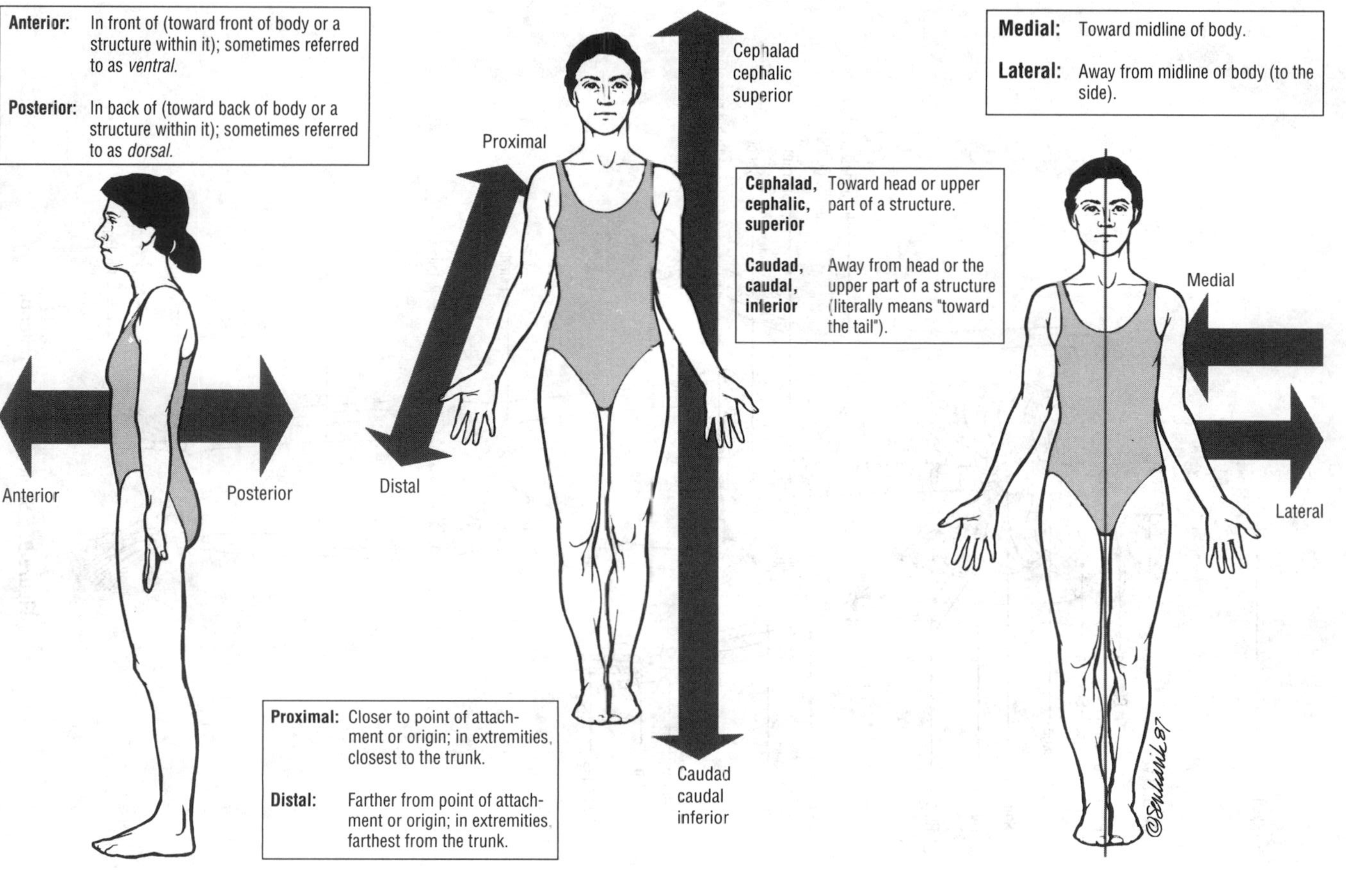

Figure 8. Terms of relationship. Body part terminology.

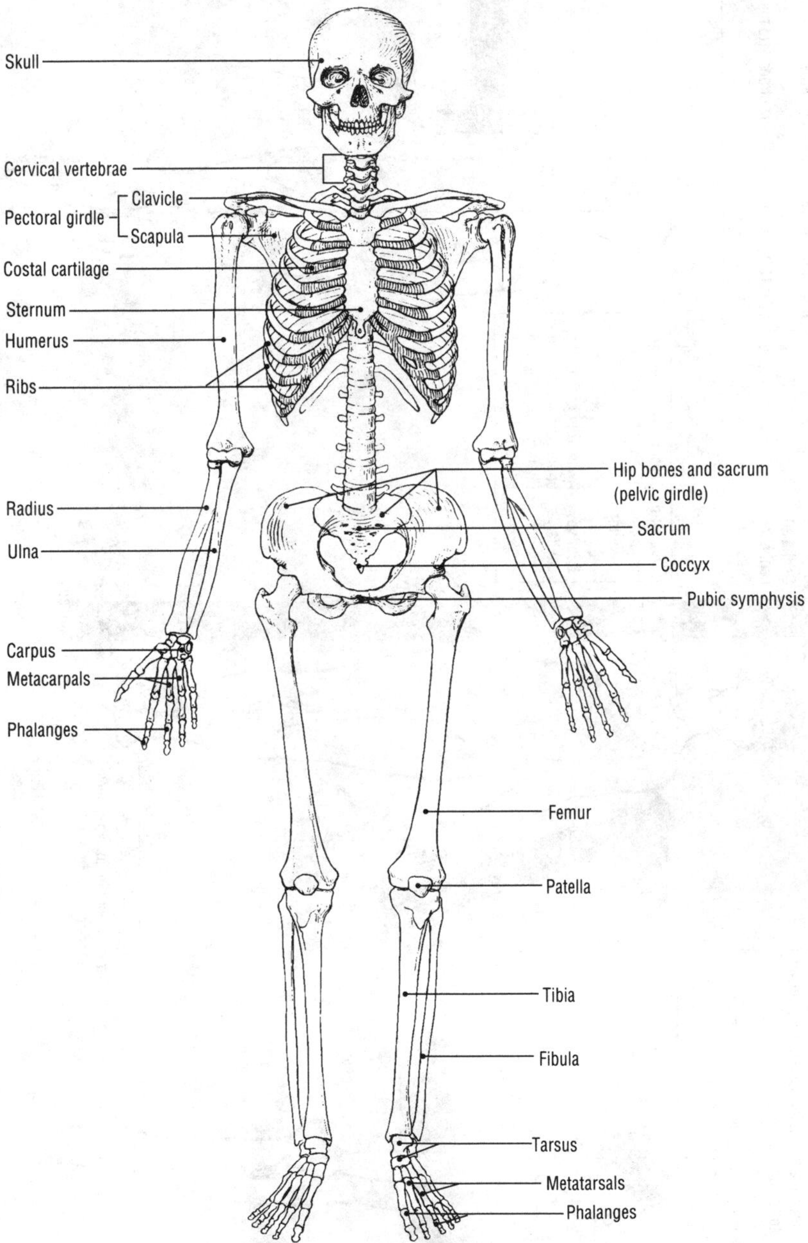

Figure 9. Skeleton, adult, anterior.

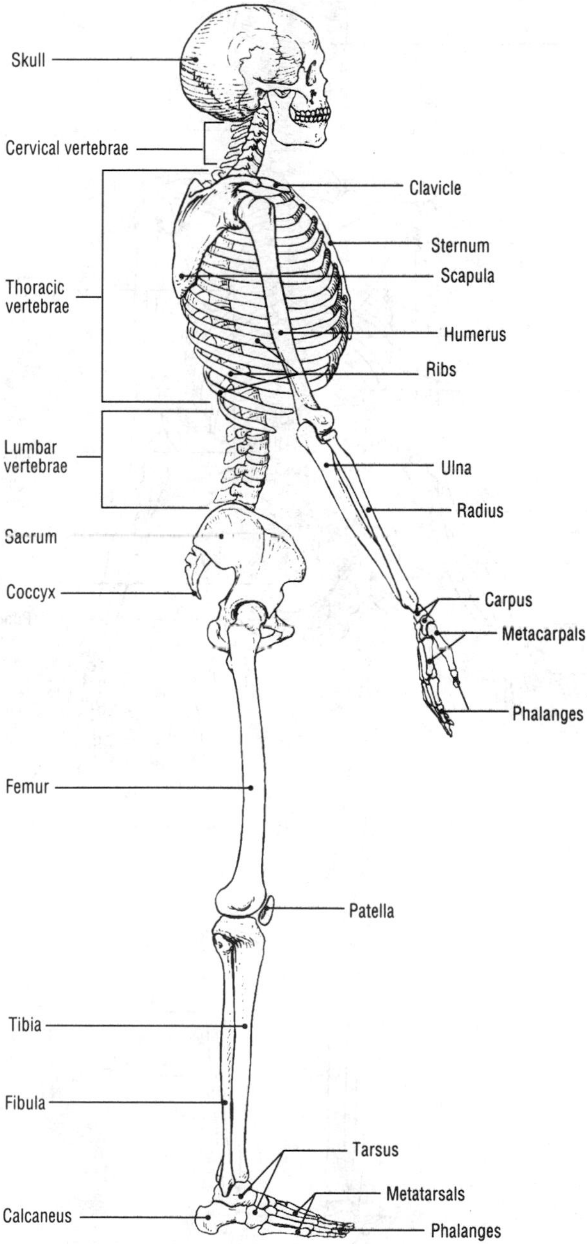

Figure 10. Skeleton, adult, lateral.

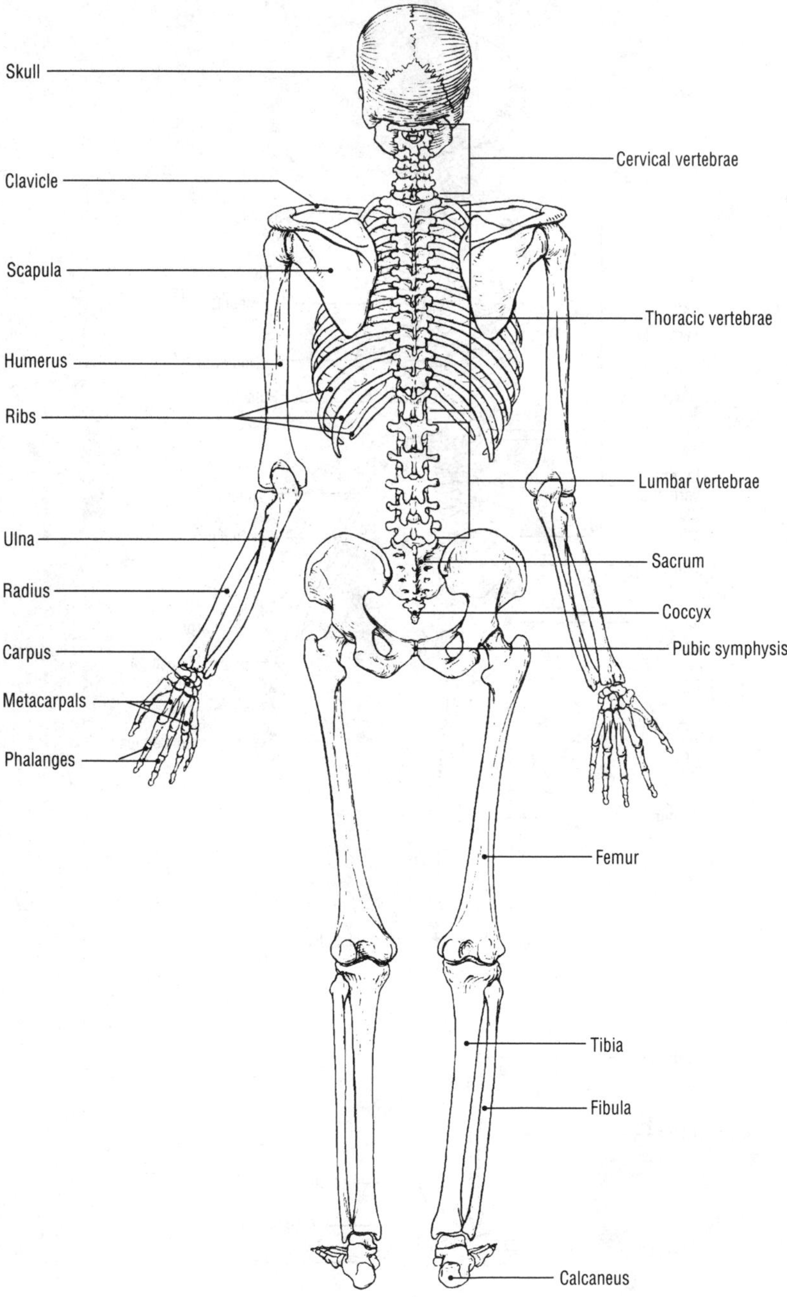

Figure 11. Skeleton, adult, posterior.

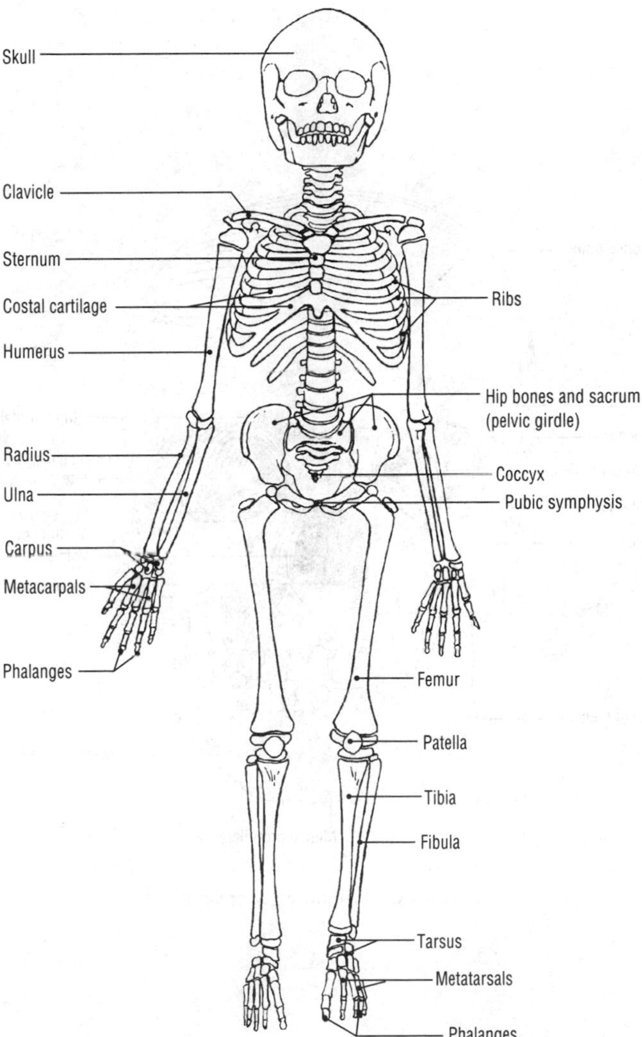

Figure 12. Skeleton, child, anterior.

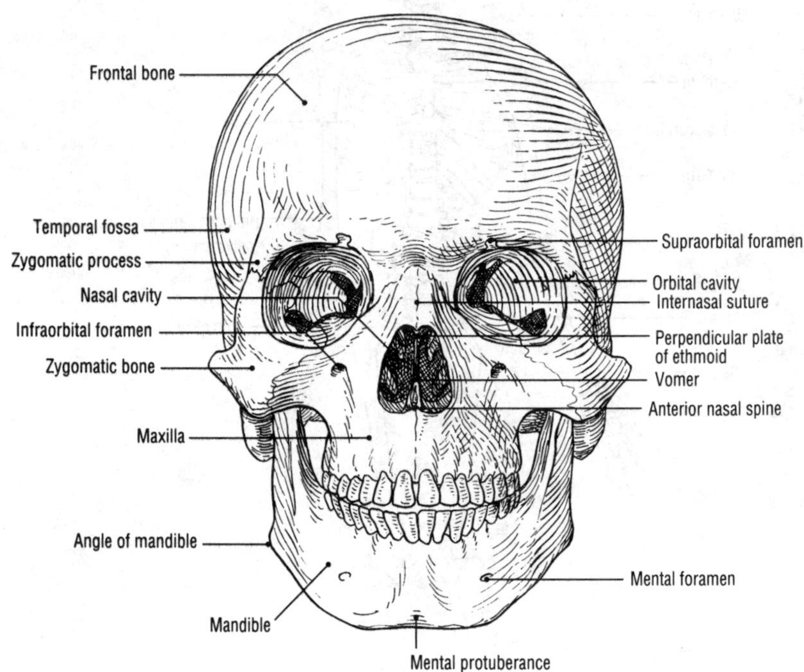

Figure 13. Frontal view of skull.

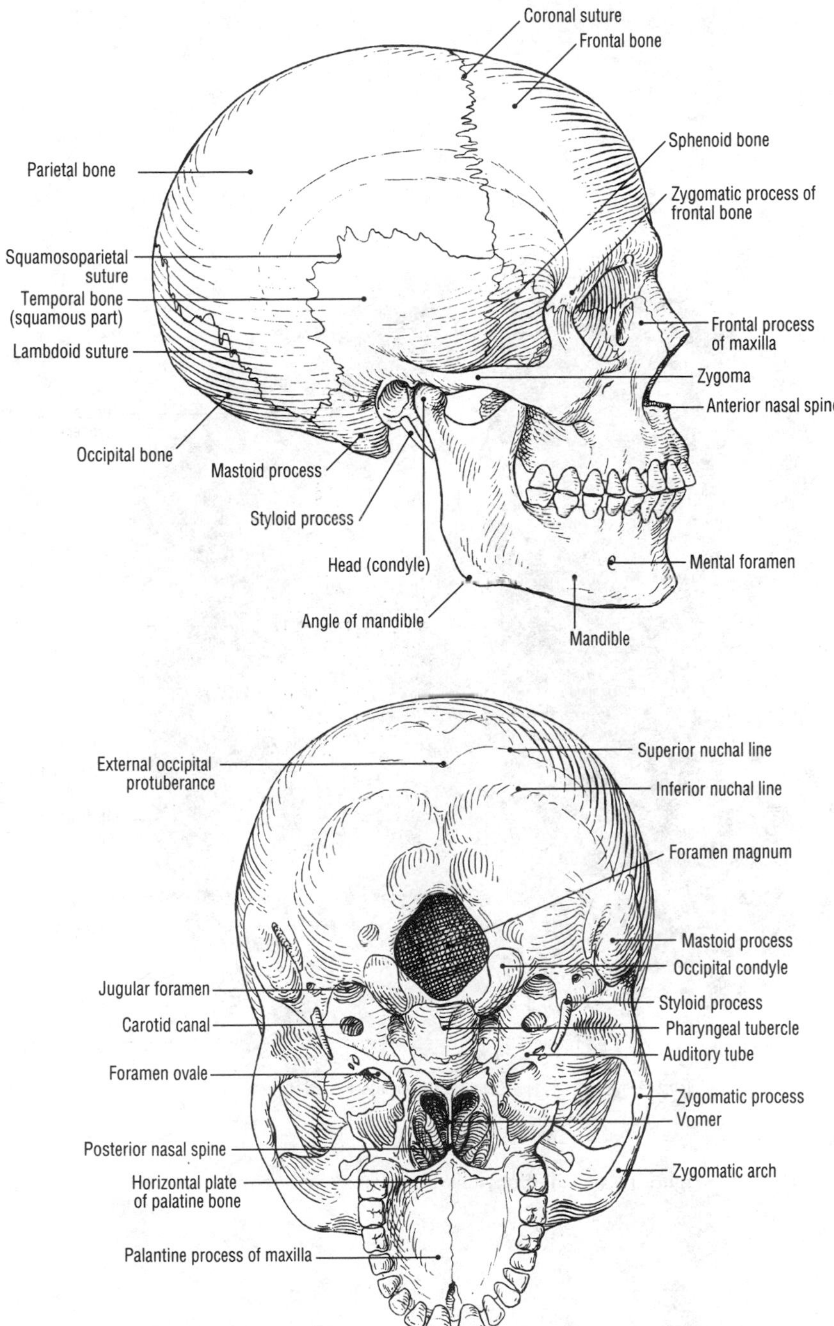

Figure 14. Skull. Top, lateral view. Bottom, inferior view.

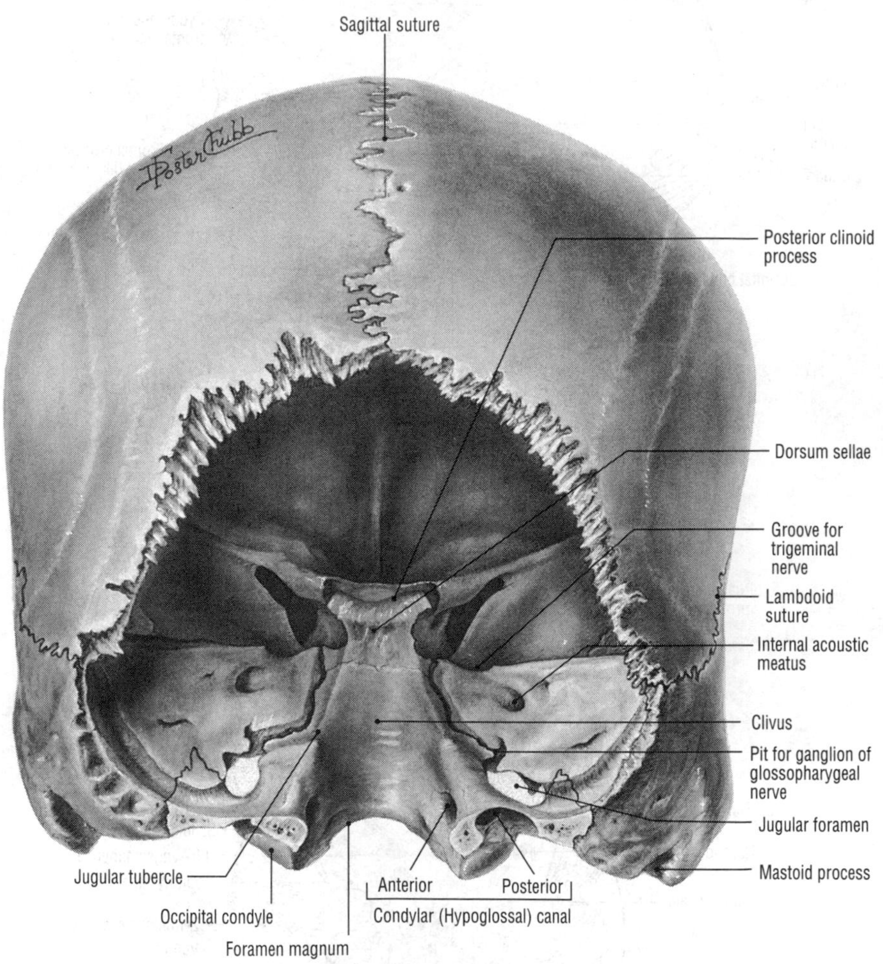

Figure 15. Skull. Bony features of posterior cranial fossa.

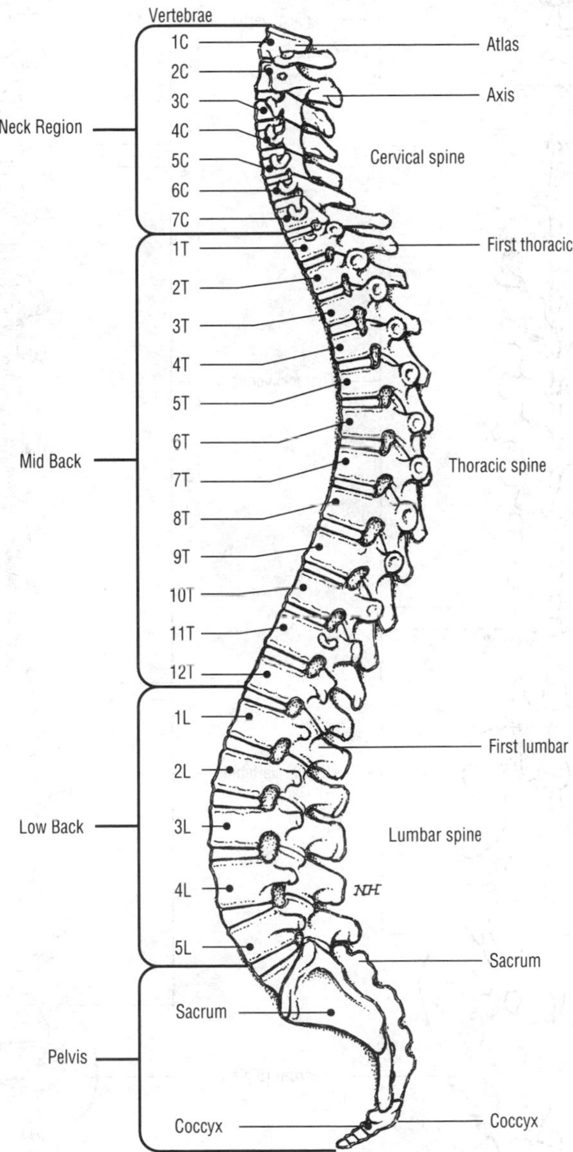

Figure 16. Vertebral column, lateral view.

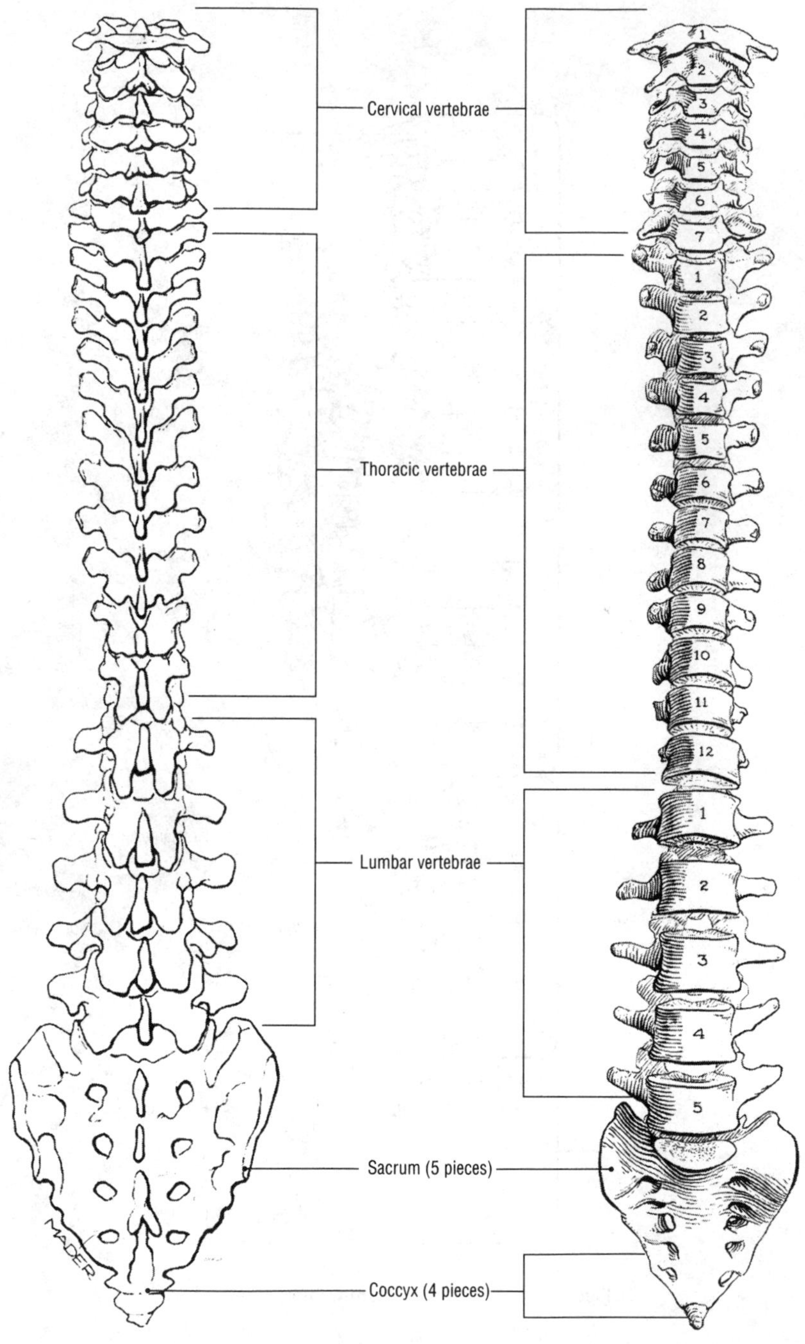

Figure 17. Vertebral column, posterior and anterior views.

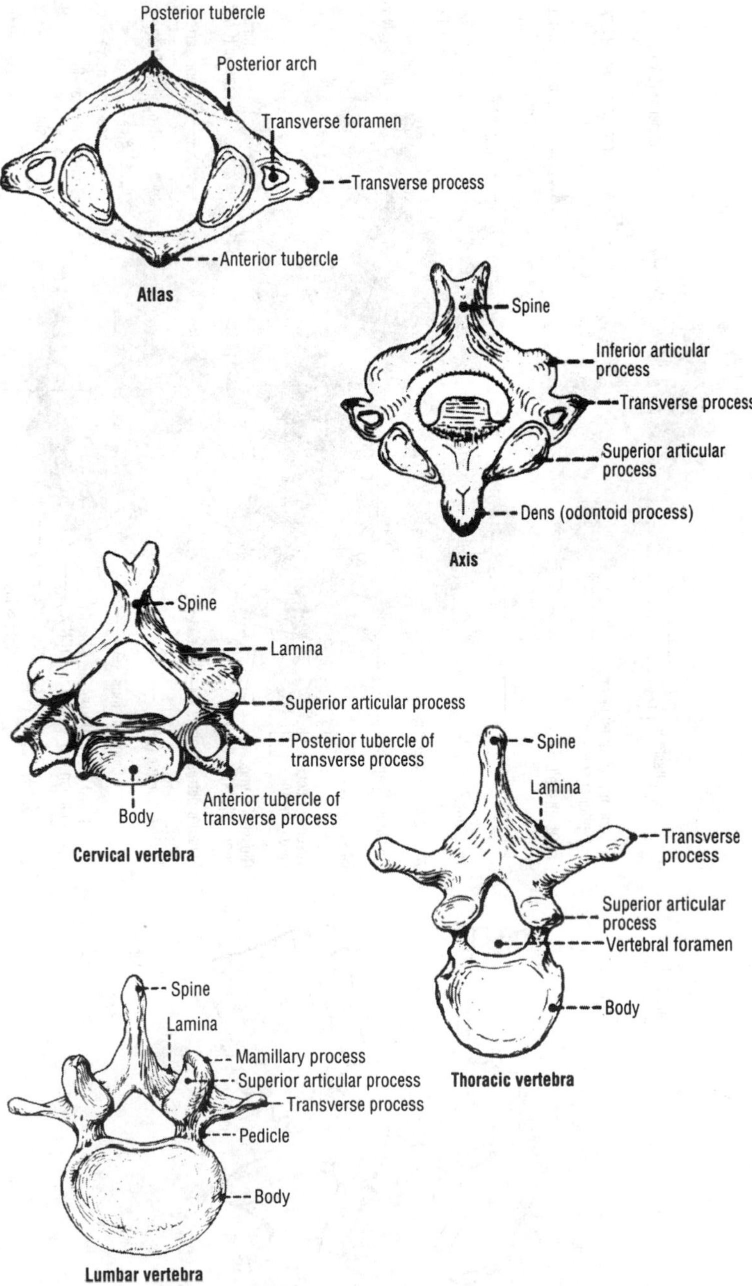

Figure 18. Typical cervical, thoracic, and lumbar vertebrae.

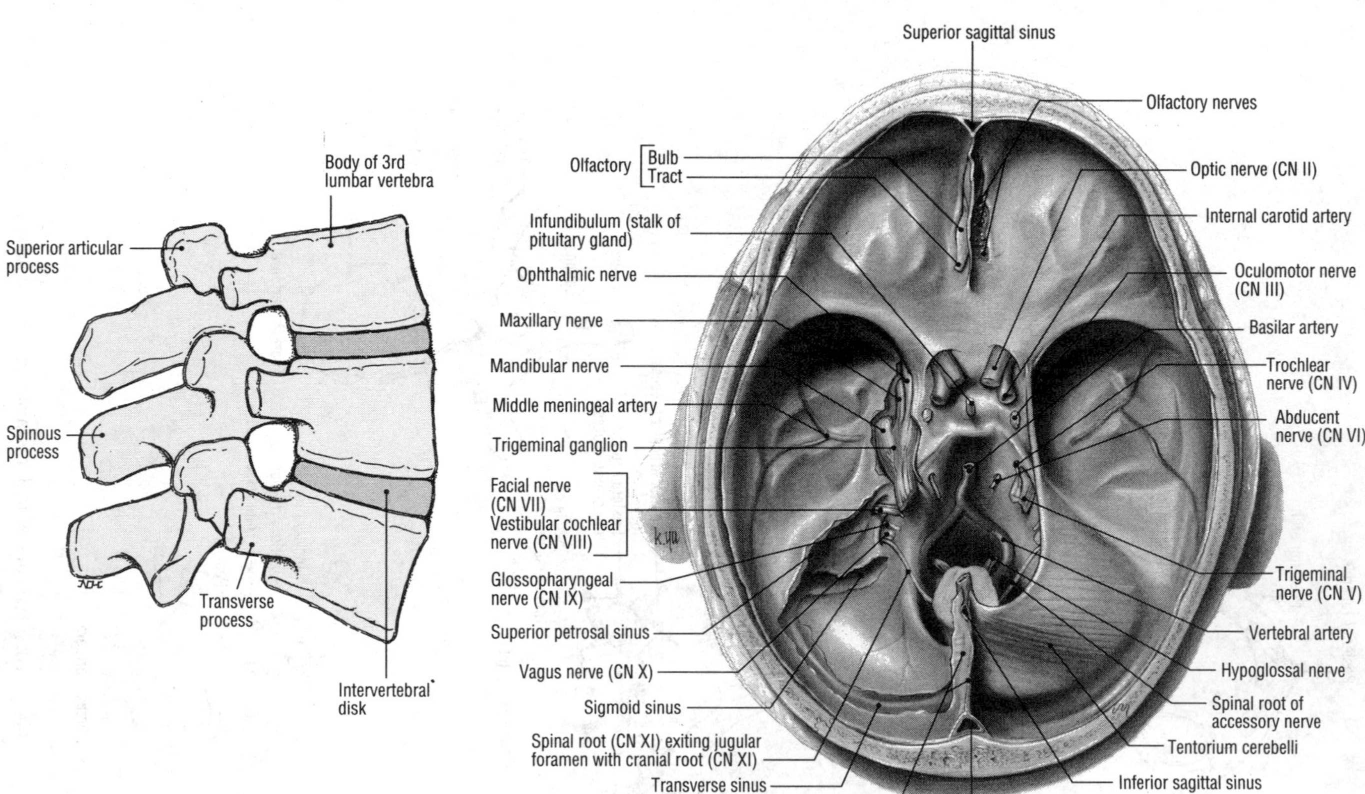

Figure 19. Vertebral processes in three lumbar vertebrae.

Figure 20. Nerves and vessels of the interior of base of skull, superior view.

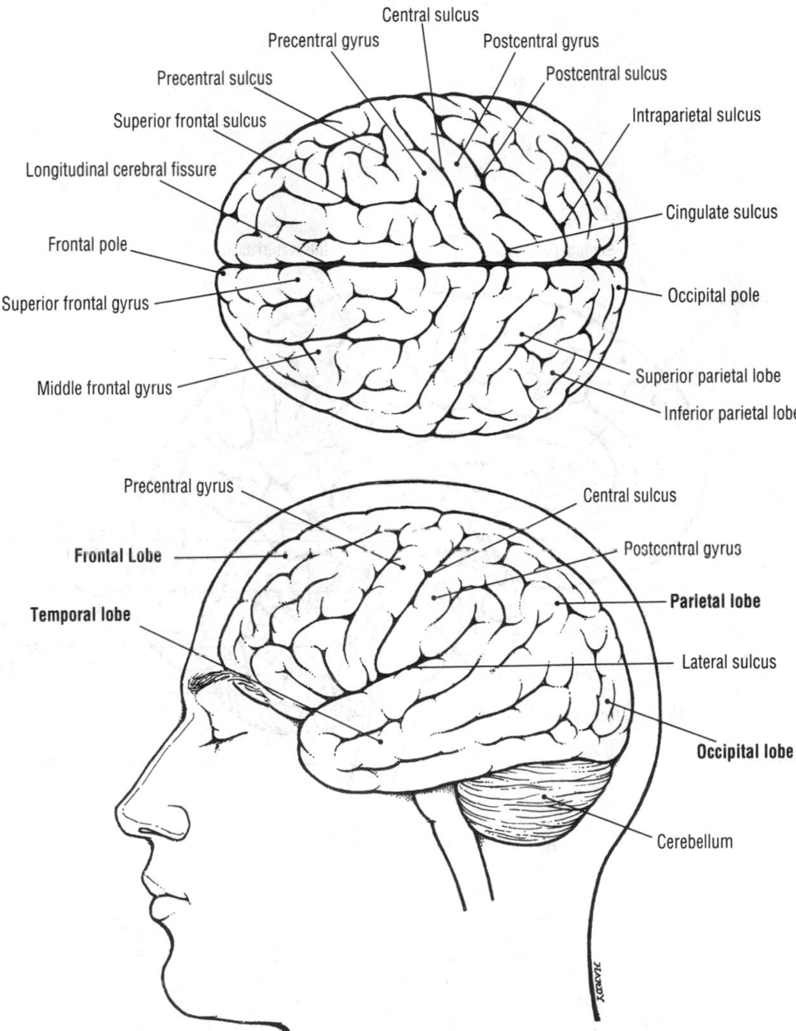

Figure 21. Brain. Top, superior view. Bottom, lateral view.

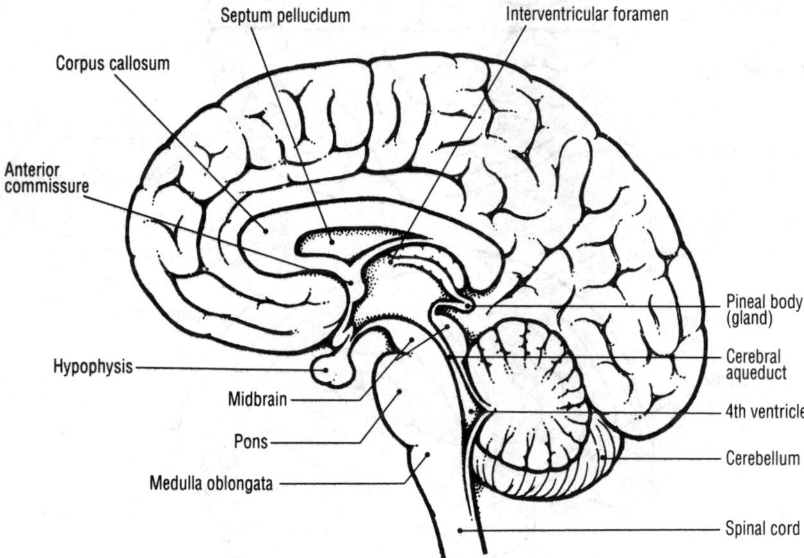

Figure 22. Brain, medial view.

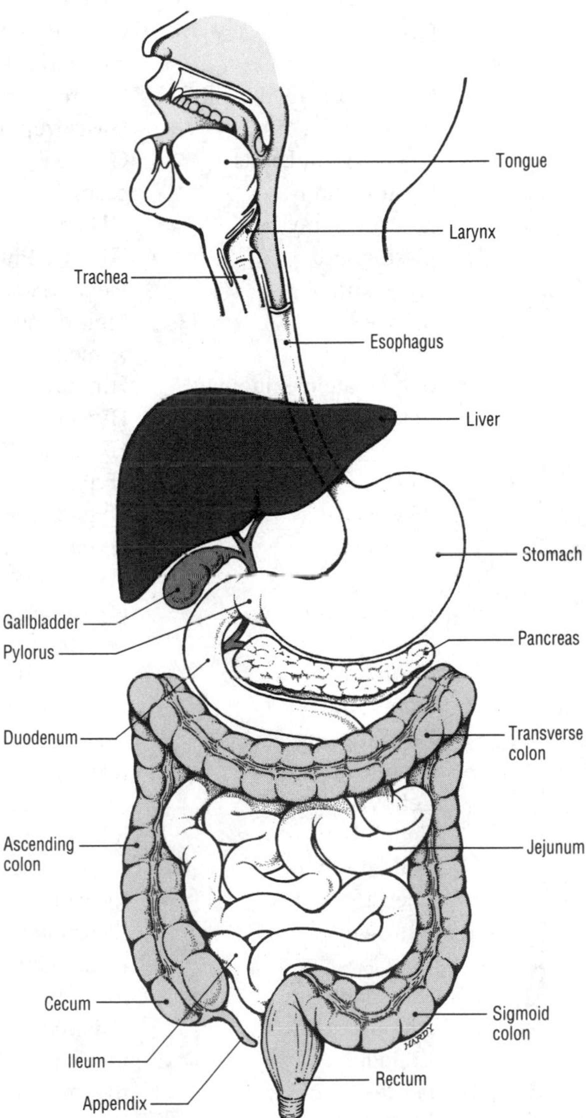

Figure 23. Digestive organs and associated structures.

Appendix 2
Contrast Media

Abrodil
acetrizoate
acetrizoic acid
adipiodone
amidotrizoic acid
Amipaque
Anatrast
Angio Conray
Angiografin
Angiovist 282, 292, 370
Baricon
barium sulfate
Barobag
Baro-CAT
Baroflave
Barosperse
Bar-Test
benzoic acid
Biligrafin
Biligram
Biliodyl
Bilivist
Bilivistan
Bilopaque
Biloptin
bismuth
Bracco
brominized oil
bunamiodyl
calcium
Cardio-Conray
Cardiografin
Cardiolite
CardioTec
CEA-Tc 99m
  (^{99m}Tc CEA)
cerium
Cholebrine
Chografin
Cholografin Meglumine
Cholovue
Clysodrast
Conray
Conray 30, 43, 325, 400
Crystografin
Crystografin Dilute
Cysto-Conray
Cysto-Conray II
Cystografin
Cystokon
diaginol
diatrizoate
diatrizoate meglumine
diatrizoate sodium
diatrizoic acid
diodine
diodone
Diodrast
Dionosil
Dionosil Oily
diprotrizoate
disofenin
Duografin
Duroliopaque
dysprosium
Echovist
Endobile
Endografin
Enecat
Entrobar
Epi-C
Ethiodane
ethiodized oil
Ethiodol
Feridex
Flo-Coat
gadodiamide
gadolinium
  diethylenetriamine-
  penta-acetate
gadopentetate
  dimeglumine
gadoteridol
Gastrografin
Gastrozepine
Gd-DTPA
glucagon
HD 85
HD 200 Plus
Hexabrix
high-osmolar contrast
  medium
Hippuran
Hypaque
Hypaque-76
Hypaque-Cysto
Hypaque-M
Hypaque Meglumine
Hypaque Sodium
Hytrast
Intropaque
Imagent BP
Imagent GI
Imagent LN
Imagent US
indium 111
iobenzamic acid
iobutoic acid
iocarmate meglumine
iocarmic acid
iocetamate
iocetamic acid
iodamic acid
iodamide
iodamide meglumine
iodatol
iodide
iodine 131 MIBG
iodipamide
iodipamide meglumine

iodipamide methylglucamine
iodized oil
iodoalphionic acid
iodohippurate
iodomethamate
iodophendylate
iodophthalein
iodopyracet
iodoxamate
iodoxamic acid
iodoxyl
ioglicate
ioglicic acid
ioglucol
ioglucomide
ioglunide
ioglycamic acid
ioglycamide
iogulamide
iohexol
iopamidol
iopanoate
iopanoic acid
iophendylate
iophenoxic acid
ioprocemic acid
iopromide
iopronic acid
iopydol
iopydone
iosefamate
iosefamic acid
ioseric acid
iosulamide
iosumetic acid
iotasul
ioteric acid
iothalamate
iothalamate meglumine
iothalamate sodium
iothalamic acid
iotrol
iotroxamide
iotroxic acid
ioversol
ioxaglate
ioxaglic acid
ioxithalamate
ioxithalamic acid
iozomic acid
ipodate
ipodate calcium
ipodate sodium
ipodic acid
IR-192
iridium
Iriditope
Isopaque
isosulfan blue
Isovue
Isovue-128, -200, -300, -370
Isovue-M
Isovue-M 200
Isovue-M 300
Kinevac
Kontrast U
Levolist
Lipiodol
Liquid Barosperse
Liquipake
Lymphazurin
Lymphazurin 1%
Macrotec
magnesium
Magnevist
manganese chloride
MD-60
MD-76
MD-Gastroview
meglumine
meglumine diatrizoate
Metastron
methiodal
methylglucamine
metrizamide
metrizoate
metrizoic acid
Micropaque
Microtrast
Monophen
MyoDil
Myoscint
Neo-Iopax
Neurolite
Niopam
Novopaque
Nyegaard
OctreoScan
Omnipaque
Omniscan
OncoRad OV103
OncoScint CR103
OncoScint CR/OV
OncoScint OV103
OncoScint PR
OncoTrac
Optiray
Optiray 160
Optiray 240
Optiray 320
Orabilex
Oragrafin
Oragrafin Calcium
Oragrafin Sodium
Oravue
Osbil
Pantopaque
Perchloracap
Pertscan 99m
phenobutiodil
phentetiothalein
potassium bromide
potassium perchlorate
Praestholm
Prepcat
Prograf
ProHance

propyliodone
radioactive iodide
radiopaque polyvinyl chloride
Raybar 75
Rayvist
Renografin-60
Renografin-76
Reno-M-30
Reno-M-60
Reno-M-Dip
Renotec
Renovist
Renovist II
Renovue
Renovue-65
Renovue-DIP
Retro-Conray
Salpix
satumomab pendetide
sincalide
Sinografin
Sitzmarks
Skiodan
Skiodan Acacia
sodium
Solu-Biloptin
Solutrast
Steripaque-BR
Steripaque-V
tacrolimus
tantalum-178
TcHIDA
teboroxime
Techneplex
Technescan MAG3
technetium Cardiolite
technetium 99m or ^{99m}Tc
technetium-99m albumin
technetium-99m albumin aggregated
technetium-99m albumin colloid
technetium-99m bicisate
technetium-99m colloid
technetium-99m disofenin
technetium-99m etidronate
technetium-99m ferpentetate
technetium-99m furifosmin
technetium-99m glucepate
technetium-99m HIDA
technetium-99m iron-ascorbate-DTPA
technetium-99m lidofenin
technetium-99m macroaggregated albumin
technetium-99m medronate
technetium-99m mertiatide
technetium-99m oxidronate
technetium-99m penetate
technetium-99m pertechnetate sodium
technetium-99m PIPIDA
technetium-99m pyrophosphate
technetium-99m sestamibi
technetium-99m siboroxime
technetium-99m sodium
technetium-99m succimer
technetium-99m sulfur colloid
technetium-99m teboroxime
technetium-99m tetrofosmin
technetium stannous pyrophosphate (TSPP)
technetium-tagged Cardiolite
Telebrix
Telepaque
Teridax
Tesuloid
tetrabromophenolphthalein
tetraiodophenolphthalein
thallium 201
thorium dioxide
thorium tartrate
Thorotrast
Tomocat
Tonopaque
triiodobenzoic acid
Triosil
tyropanoate
tyropanoate sodium
tyropanoic acid
Umbradil
Urografin
Uromiro
Uropac
Urovision
Urovist Cysto
Urovist Meglumine
Urovist Sodium 300
Vascoray
Vasiodone

Appendix 3

Common Radiation Oncology Terms

absolute dose
adjacent field
adjuvant therapy
algorithm
alloy
alpha cradle
American Society of Therapeutic Radiation and Oncology (ASTRO)
angle
annealing
applicator
Aquaplast
arc
asymmetric collimation
backscatter
beam
beam's eye view
beam modifier
belly board
beta radiation
Betatron
bite block
block
block film
bolus
boost
brachytherapy
breast board
buildup region
calculation
calipers
catheter
centigray (cGy)
central axis
Cerrobond
Certified Medical Dosimetrist (CMD)
cesium
cesium-137 (Cs137)
cesium teletherapy unit
chemoradiotherapy
Clinac 2100C
Clinac-6
clinical target volume (CTV)
clinical tumor volume (CTV)
cobalt
cobalt-60 (Co60)
cobalt teletherapy unit
cold spot
collimator
collimator leaf
compensator
composite plan
coned down
conformal radiotherapy
contour
convergence
coplanar beam arrangement
couch angle
couch kick
craniospinal irradiation
CT simulator
curative
curative intent care
Cyclotron
decay
Delclos applicator
depth dose
desquamation
digitally composited radiographs (DCR)
digitally reconstructed radiographs
diode
divergence
divergent beams
dose calculation
dose distribution
dose escalation
dose-volume histograms
dosimetrist
dosimetry
Dwell

Dwell point
Dynamic multileaf collimator
Dynamic wedge
electron
electron beam radiation therapy (EBRT)
electron cones
Ellis filter
equal weighting
extended distance
external beam radiation therapy (XRT)
eye shield
facial mask
field
field arrangement
film digitizer
Fletcher-Suit applicator
fraction
fractionated external beam radiation therapy
gamma knife
gamma radiation
gantry
gap
gap calculation
geometry
gold-198 (Au198)
Gray (Gy)
gross target volume (GTV)
gross tumor volume (GTV)
half beam block
half-life
half valve layer
half valve thickness
hand block
headrest (sizes range from A to F)
Heyman capsule
high dose
high-dose-rate remote afterloading
high dose rate (HDR)
high linear energy transfer (LET) radiation
hot spot
hyperfractionation
hyperthermia
image fusion
immobilization device
implant
independent collimator
informed consent
intensity modulated radiation therapy (IMRT)
interstitial
interstitial brachytherapy
interstitial implant
intracavitary
intracavitary irradiation
intracavitary therapy
intraluminal implant
intraoperative radiation therapy (IRT)
iodine
iodine-125 (I-125)
ionization chamber
irregular fields
iridium
iridium-192 (Ir192)
irradiation
isocenter
isocentric
isodose
isodose curve
isodose plan
isotherm
isotope
Karnofsky Performance Status (KPS)
kilovolt (kV)
laser
laser alignment system
lead
LINAC (*lin*ear *ac*celerator)
local-regional
low dose rate (LDR)
lucite filter
mantle field
megavolts (MV or MeV)
missing tissue compensator
mold

monitor units (MU)
mucositis
multileaf collimator
multiplanar reconstruction
neutron
non-coplanar beam arrangements
oblique
off-axis factor
orthogonal pair
orthovoltage
ovoid
palliation
palliative
palliative intent care
paraaortic field
parallel opposed fields
particle beam
particle beam treatment
penumbra
percentage depth dose (PDD)
permanent implant
photon
photon beam radiation therapy
planning target volume (PTV)
point calculation
port
portal
port film
portal imaging
pre-port
prostate seed implant
proton
radiation therapy planning
radiation therapy technologist (RTT)
radiation biology
radiation field
radiation oncology
radiation physics
radiation portal
radiation protectors
radiation therapy
Radiation Therapy Oncology Group (RTOG)
radiobiology
radioimmunotherapy (RIT)
radiolabeled antibodies
radionuclide
radioprotectors
radiosensitizer
radiotherapy
radioiodine seeds (I-125)
radium
red journal (International Journal of Radiation Oncology/Biology/Physics—IJROBP)
ribbon
rotational therapy
separation
shield
simulation
simulator
source
source axis distance (SAD)
source film distance (SFD)
source surface distance (SSD)
stereotactic head frame
stereotactic radiosurgery (SRS)
stereotactic radiotherapy (SRT)
stereotaxis
strontium 89 (Sr89)
strontium 90 (Sr90)
superficial machine
surface mold
systemic radiation therapy
tandem
target localization
tattoo
teletherapy
testicular shield
thermoluminescent dosimeter (TLD)
thermoplastics
three-dimensional conformal radiation therapy
three-dimensional radiotherapy treatment planning (3DRTP)

two-dimensional radiotherapy treatment planning (2DRTP)
total body irradiation (TBI)
total skin electron (TSE) irradiation
treatment plan
treatment time
tumor volume
tungsten
unequal weighting
vaginal cylinder
verification film
volumetric calculation
wedge
wing board
X-knife

Appendix 4
Sample Radiology Reports

Sample Bone Scan

Reason for Study: A 61-year-old woman with history of esophagus cancer. Has a compression fracture at T8, questionably pathologic. Bone scan to assess for other bony lesions.

Following the administration of 20 mCi of technetium-labeled MDP, a whole-body scan was done. There is marked increased tracer concentration in the eighth thoracic vertebra. The bone scan is otherwise unremarkable.

Conclusion: Solitary bone lesion at T8. Metastatic disease is not excluded, but there are no other bony lesions on this bone scan.

Sample CT Scan of the Abdomen and Pelvis

History: Testicular neoplasm.

Technique: Axial CT images of the abdomen and pelvis were obtained with intravenous and oral contrast.

Findings: Images of the lung bases are normal. Images of abdomen show the liver, spleen, gallbladder, pancreas, and adrenal glands to be normal. No mass is seen. There is no evidence of cholelithiasis. A retroaortic left renal vein is seen. No obvious mass or enlarged lymph nodes are noted in the retroperitoneum. Mesenteric structures appear normal. A prominent inferior vena cava is seen. Gas is identified in the left inguinal structures, likely representing previous left orchidectomy and removal of the inguinal ring. No enlarged lymph node is identified in the pelvis.

Impression: Left retroaortic renal vein. No adenopathy is noted within the abdomen or pelvis. No enlarged lymph node is seen; no mass is identified.

SAMPLE CT SCAN OF THE BRAIN

HISTORY: Left hand numbness.

TECHNIQUE: Multiple sequential axial images were obtained from the skull base up through the vertex without the use of intravenous contrast material.

FINDINGS: The ventricular system, sulci, and cisterns are appropriate in size. There is no evidence of intracranial hemorrhage. No extraaxial fluid collection is seen. Good gray-white differentiation is seen throughout. No mass lesion or midline shift is identified.

Evaluation of the bony structures and soft tissues is unremarkable.

IMPRESSION: No significant abnormality is detected throughout.

SAMPLE CT SCAN OF THE CERVICAL SPINE

HISTORY: A 61-year-old male status post motor vehicle accident. Evaluate C4 through T2.

TECHNIQUE: Axial noncontrast CT images were performed from C3 to T2.

FINDINGS: Bone alignment and mineralization are normal. There is no fracture or subluxation. Bony rings of the C3 through T2 vertebral bodies are intact. Calcification is seen in the nuchal ligament from the C4–5 level to the C6–7 level. Spinous processes appear intact. There is no significant soft tissue swelling.

Large anterior osteophytes are seen at the C5–6, C6–7, and C7-T1 levels. Right eccentric osteophyte mildly indents the thecal sac at C4–5. Concentric osteophyte at C5–6 mildly indents the thecal sac.

IMPRESSION

1. Degenerative disk changes in the lower cervical spine as described.
2. Calcification in the nuchal ligament in the lower cervical region. No spinous process fracture identified.

SAMPLE CT SCAN OF THE CHEST AND ADRENALS WITH CONTRAST

HISTORY: Left pulmonary nodule on chest x-ray.

TECHNIQUE: Helical transaxial images, 7 mm, of the chest were obtained after the administration of oral and intravenous contrast.

FINDINGS: Patient's chest x-rays from February 24 and 25 were reviewed. There is an ill-defined opacity suggested in the left mid-lung zones on those studies, including oblique views.

Within the left lower lobe laterally, there is an approximately 2-cm area of parenchymal density which has the appearance of interstitial changes without findings of significant nodule or mass. This finding can relate to scarring. There is no other nodule, mass, or effusion. Within the mediastinum, there is no evidence of adenopathy seen. The heart and great vessels are normal in appearance. There is a suggestion of minimal pericardial thickening anteriorly which is not specific. Osseous structures show degenerative changes with osteophyte formation at multiple levels in the thoracic spine.

Visualized upper abdominal structures including liver, spleen, kidneys, pancreas, aorta, and paraaortic retroperitoneum, show no specific finding. The adrenal glands are not enlarged.

IMPRESSION: Small focal area of increased parenchymal density which has interstitial pattern. There is no significant nodule or mass. This is suggestive of scarring. There is no nodule, mass, effusion, or adenopathy seen. Consider chest x-ray followup of this lesion to assess stability.

Sample CT Scan of the Paranasal Sinuses

History: A 37-year-old female with sinusitis.

Technique: Coronal noncontrast CT images of the paranasal sinuses were performed.

Findings: Patient is status post bilateral uncinectomies and partial ethmoidectomies and turbinectomies. Mild scattered frontal ethmoid and maxillary mucosal thickening is present. A 15-mm polyp is seen in the left sphenoid sinus. There is filling of a residual right anterior ethmoid air cell. Orbital walls are intact. Mucosal thickening is seen along the nasal septum which is deviated to the left.

Impression

1. Scattered paranasal sinus mucosal disease including a 15-mm polyp in the left sphenoid sinus.
2. Status post bilateral uncinectomies, turbinectomies and partial ethmoidectomies.
3. Mucosal thickening along the nasal septum which is deviated to the left.

Sample Iodine Uptake Test

Reason for Study: A 25-year-old female with symptoms of hyperthyroidism.

Following the oral administration of 106 mCi of iodine-131, the 24-hour iodine uptake is 32% (normal 9% to 29%).

Conclusion: Elevated 24-hour radioiodine uptake.

Sample MRI of the Brain with Gadolinium

History: Hyponatremia due to resetting of her osmostat.

Technique: Axial FLAIR and T2 and coronal T2-weighted images of the brain were performed. Sagittal and coronal T1-weighted pre- and post-gadolinium images were performed through the sella and parasellar regions. The study was terminated prior to obtaining adequate post-contrast images because the patient complained of severe headache and could not tolerate further imaging.

Findings: The exam was limited with post-contrast images severely degraded by motion artifact.

Images through the brain show normal sulci and ventricles. There is no mass lesion, mass effect, hemorrhage or infarction. White matter structures have normal configuration and signal characteristics. The brain stem and cerebellum are normal.

Orbits, visualized paranasal sinuses, and mastoid air cells are normal.

Images through the sella and parasellar regions show no evidence of mass. Pituitary gland has normal size and configuration. Normal high signal of the posterior pituitary is demonstrated. Pituitary infundibulum is midline. Suprasellar cistern and optic chiasm are normal. Floor of the anterior third ventricle and region of the hypothalamus appear within normal limits.

IMPRESSION: Essentially normal MRI of the brain and pituitary. Post-contrast images are significantly degraded by patient motion artifact.

SAMPLE MRI OF THE THORACIC SPINE

HISTORY: Esophageal cancer with compression fractures in the thoracic spine.

TECHNIQUE: Sagittal and axial T1, T2, post gadolinium-enhanced T1 and additional sagittal STIR sequences were performed.

FINDINGS: In comparison to the previous study, there has been further decrease in the amount of enhancement and signal abnormality within the previously noted T8 vertebral body compression fracture. There is no significant change in the tiny focus of enhancement in the anterior posterior T10 vertebral body. No significant loss of height is seen at this level. No soft tissue mass is discerned. A tiny disk bulge is also seen at the T7-T8 intervertebral disk level which is unchanged from the previous study and does not cause significant mass effect upon the spinal canal.

No intrinsic abnormality of the visualized spinal cord is noted.

IMPRESSION: There has been further resolution of abnormal enhancement and abnormal signal intensity within the T8 vertebral body. This is most consistent with healing benign compression fracture. A 2- to 3-mm focus of enhancement in the inferior anterior T10 vertebral body is again noted and unchanged in degree or appearance, and this remains of uncertain clinical significance.

Sample Myocardial Perfusion Scan

Reason for Study: A 69-year-old female with diabetes and coronary artery disease admitted with substernal chest pain.

Adenosine Stress Test: Increased coronary circulation was induced pharmacologically with a 4-minute infusion of 140 mcg/kg per minute of adenosine. At 3 minutes, 30 mCi of technetium Cardiolite was injected. Mild shortness of breath resolved when the infusion was complete.

The baseline ECG revealed nonspecific ST changes and possible anterior scar. There was no change in the ECG during the procedure.

Conclusion: Adenosine stress test without chest pain or diagnostic ischemic ECG changes.

Myocardial Perfusion Scan: A 1-day protocol was followed. Cardiolite 10 mCi was given for the rest study. There is normal distribution of the Cardiolite throughout the myocardium. Variable R-R interval on the ECG prevented a wall motion study.

Conclusion: Normal myocardial perfusion scan.

Sample Thoracic Aortogram with Cerebral Angiography

History: An 82-year-old man with thoracic aneurysm and carotid stenosis.

A 20-minute consultation was utilized explaining risks, benefits and alternatives of angiography. All the patient's questions were answered, and he had given informed consent prior to the procedure. The patient was premedicated with IM Demerol and Phenergan. Buffered lidocaine was used for local anesthesia. Sedation was not required.

A 5-French pigtail catheter was advanced into the aorta via the right femoral artery with standard Seldinger technique. With the tip of the catheter in the ascending aorta, aortogram with digital subtraction technique was obtained in the left anterior projection. AP frontal view of the intracranial circulation was also obtained from an arch injection. Catheter was then exchanged over a guide wire for a 5-French Simmons II catheter. The carotid and left vertebral artery were selectively catheterized and injected with contrast for digital subtraction filming. In the right common carotid, it was initially difficult to get stable catheter position, and various combinations of guide wires and a Simmons III catheter were used to obtain selective catheterization. After all images were reviewed, the catheter was removed, and direct pressure was applied to the puncture site until complete hemostasis was achieved.

Total contrast load was 132 cc of Isovue. Fluoroscopy time was 41.5 minutes.

FINDINGS: The ascending aortic arch is dilated and has a more normal diameter just after the left subclavian catheter, and then the descending thoracic aorta enlarges again. There is no evidence of intimal dissection. The origins from the arch are patent. The right carotid bifurcation is slightly irregular; however, no hemodynamically significant stenosis is observed in the right internal carotid. The right external carotid is open. The left external carotid is completely occluded. The left internal carotid has 75% reduction of its cross-sectional area near its origin. On selective injections, it is interesting to note that the right anterior cerebral artery does not fill from the right carotid injection, but both anterior cerebral arteries fill from the left carotid injection. Vertebral arteries are patent. The left vertebral artery is larger. No obvious intracranial abnormality is observed.

IMPRESSION: There is 75% stenosis of the left internal carotid. Complete occlusion, left external carotid. Very mild irregularity of the right internal carotid. Widely patent right external carotid. Both vertebral arteries are patent.

SAMPLE THREE-PHASE BONE SCAN OF FEET

REASON FOR STUDY: A 52-year-old female with chronic severe pain in the right heel, most likely plantar fasciitis. Rule out calcaneal stress fracture.

Following the IV administration of 20 mCi of Tc-labeled MDP, a three-phase bone scan of the feet was acquired. There is symmetrical appearance time and concentration of the agent during the blood flow phase. Immediate blood pool images are normal except for moderate increased tracer concentration at the inferior anterior surface of the right calcaneus. The 2-hour delayed bony phase shows intense increased uptake at the insertion of the plantar aponeurosis to the right calcaneus, typical of plantar fasciitis. The calcaneal bone itself does not show any increased tracer concentration.

CONCLUSION: Abnormal three-phase bone scan consistent with plantar fasciitis of the right foot.

Sample Thyroid Ultrasound

Clinical Information: Thyroid nodule.

Findings: The right lobe of the thyroid measures 4 cm long × 1.1 cm in AP dimension. The right lobe of the thyroid contains a 1 × 0.75 × 1.1-cm hypoechoic solid mass in the posterior aspect of the right lobe of the thyroid adjacent to the great vessels. A second isoechoic nodule measuring 1.6 × 1.5 cm is seen in the right lobe of the thyroid.

The left lobe measures almost 4 × 1.2 cm. It contains a 0.4 × 0.4 × 0.4-cm hypoechoic nodule laterally located adjacent to the great vessels. A small 0.2 × 0.2 × 0.3-cm simple cyst is seen in the midbody of the thyroid on the left side, more anteriorly placed.

Conclusion

1. At least two solid nodules are seen in the right lobe of the thyroid as discussed above. In light of the patient's history of follicular thyroid carcinoma, correlation with previous ultrasound examination and nuclear medicine scan is recommended.
2. Two very small hypoechoic nodules in the left lobe of the thyroid.

Sample Ventilation/Perfusion Lung Scan

Reason for Study: A 64-year old female admitted with shortness of breath and chest pain. Past history of DVT.

Technique: Xenon-133, 20 mCi, was inhaled for the ventilation study, and 6 mCi of Tc-99m MAA was injected for the perfusion study.

Findings: The ventilation study done in the anterior and posterior projections, including single-breath, equilibrium, and washout phases, shows xenon retention in the lower lung fields bilaterally. There appears to be marked cardiomegaly.

The perfusion scan demonstrates irregular areas of diminished perfusion in the lower lung fields bilaterally, corresponding to the abnormalities noted on the ventilation scan. The heart is enlarged.

Conclusion: Abnormal lung scan demonstrating matched defects in the lower lung fields and an enlarged heart. Low-probability lung scan for pulmonary emboli.

Appendix 5
Common Terms by Procedure

Bone Scan
mCi
technetium-labeled MDP
tracer

CT Scan of the Brain
axial
cisterns
extra-axial
intracranial hemorrhage
sequential
sulci
vertex

CT Scan of the Cervical Spine
axial
mineralization
nuchal ligament
osteophyte
subluxation
thecal sac

CT Scan of the Paranasal Sinuses
air cell
coronal
ethmoidectomies
turbinectomies
uncinectomies

Iodine Uptake Test
hyperthyroidism
iodine-131
iodine uptake
mCi
radioiodine

MRI of the Brain with Gadolinium
axial FLAIR
brain stem
cerebellum
coronal T2-weighted images
gadolinium
hypothalamus
optic chiasm
osmostat
parasellar
pituitary infundibulum
sella
sulci
suprasellar cistern
T2
ventricles

MRI of the Thoracic Spine
focus of enhancement
gadolinium
intervertebral disc
sagittal
sagittal STIR sequences

Myocardial Perfusion Scan
adenosine stress test
infusion
mCi
myocardial perfusion
technetium Cardiolite

Thoracic Aortogram with Cerebral Angiography
aneurysm
angiography
aortogram
arch injection
bifurcation
digital subtraction technique
fluoroscopy
guide wire
hemodynamic
hemostasis

intimal dissection
Isovue
patent
pigtail catheter
Seldinger technique
selective catheterization
Simmons II catheter
Simmons III catheter
stenosis

Three-Phase Bone Scan of Feet

aponeurosis
blood flow phase
blood pool
mCi
plantar fascitis
stress fracture
Tc-labeled MDP
tracer
uptake

Thyroid Ultrasound

follicular thyroid carcinoma
hypoechoic
nodule

Ventilation/Perfusion Lung Scan

cardiomegaly
DVT (deep venous thrombosis)
emboli
equilibrium
mCi
perfusion
retention
Tc-99m MAA
ventilation/perfusion lung scan
washout
xenon-133